This book is for every new graduate or experienced nurse new to oncology. I hope this edition of Cancer Basics *provides you with a source for the knowledge you need to develop your own passion to care for patients with a cancer diagnosis and their families.*

Contributors

Editor

Julia Eggert, PhD, RN, AGN-BC, GNP, AOCN®, FAAN
Professor and Doctoral Coordinator
Clemson University
Clemson, South Carolina
Advanced Genetics Nurse
Cancer Risk Screening Program
St. Francis Bon Secours Cancer Center
Greenville, South Carolina
Chapter 1. Biology of Cancer; Chapter 10. Precision Medicine: Biologics and Targeted Therapies

Authors

Patricia L. Adams, RN, MSN, AOCNS®
Advanced Practice Nurse, Medical Oncology
University of Cincinnati
Cincinnati, Ohio
Chapter 22. Hematologic Issues

Virginia Aguilar, RN, MSN, FNP-BC, AOCNP®
Oncology Solid Tumor Nurse Practitioner
Parkland Hospital
Dallas, Texas
Chapter 11. Hormone Therapy

Lisa Anderson-Shaw, DrPH, MA, MSN
Director, Clinical Ethics Consult Service
Assistant Clinical Professor
University of Illinois Hospital and Health System
Chicago, Illinois
Chapter 30. Ethical Issues

Lanell M. Bellury, PhD, RN, AOCNS®, OCN®
Associate Professor
Georgia Baptist College of Nursing of Mercer University
Atlanta, Georgia
Chapter 19. Fatigue

Jane C. Clark, PhD, RN, AOCN®, OCN®, GNP-BC
Independent Oncology Nursing Consultant
Atlanta, Georgia
Chapter 19. Fatigue

Georgia M. Decker, MS, RN, ANP-BC, FAAN
Founder and Nurse Practitioner
Integrative Care
Albany, New York
Chapter 13. Complementary and Alternative Medicine

Diane Drake, PhD, RN
Nurse Research Scientist
Consultant
San Juan Capistrano, California
Chapter 7. Surgery

Elizabeth Prechtel Dunphy, DNP, CRNP, BC, AOCN®
Gastrointestinal Oncology Nurse Practitioner
Abramson Cancer Center
Penn Presbyterian Medical Center
Senior Lecturer B
Adult Oncology Specialty Minor/Post Master's Certificate, Advanced Practice Oncology Nurse
University of Pennsylvania School of Nursing
Philadelphia, Pennsylvania
Chapter 20. Gastrointestinal Symptoms; Chapter 23. Hepatic Toxicity

Nancy Rankin Ewing, DNP, APRN, ACNS-BC
Senior Lecturer
Clemson University
Clemson, South Carolina
Chapter 34. Caring for the Cancer Survivor

Anecita Fadol, PhD, RN, FNP-BC, FAANP
Assistant Professor, Departments of Nursing and Cardiology
University of Texas MD Anderson Cancer Center
Houston, Texas
Chapter 16. Cardiac Toxicity

Christopher L. Farrell, PhD
Associate Professor
Presbyterian College School of Pharmacy
Clinton, South Carolina
Chapter 6. Pharmacogenomics

Ellen Giarelli, EdD, RN, CRNP
Associate Professor
Drexel University College of Nursing and Health Professions
Philadelphia, Pennsylvania
Chapter 32. Psychosocial Issues

Stephanie Jacobson Gregory, FNP-C, BMTCN®
Nurse Practitioner
Augusta University Medical Center
Augusta, Georgia
Chapter 14. Hematopoietic Stem Cell Transplantation

Janet Harden, PhD, RN
Associate Professor
Wayne State University
Detroit, Michigan
Chapter 29. Developmental Life Stage Issues

Catherine Jansen, PhD, RN, AOCNS®
Oncology Clinical Nurse Specialist
Kaiser Permanente Medical Center, San Francisco
San Francisco, California
Chapter 17. Cognitive Changes

Anne Katz, PhD, RN, FAAN
Clinical Nurse Specialist and Sexuality Counselor
CancerCare Manitoba
Manitoba, Canada
Editor, *Oncology Nursing Forum*
Oncology Nursing Society
Pittsburgh, Pennsylvania
Chapter 33. Sexual and Reproductive Issues

Kristine B. LeFebvre, MSN, RN, AOCN®
Oncology Clinical Specialist
Oncology Nursing Society
Pittsburgh, Pennsylvania
Chapter 2. Staging and Performance Status

Billie Lynes, MSN, RN, FNP-C
Professor of Nursing
Mt. San Antonio College
Walnut, California
Nurse Practitioner, Gynecologic Oncology
City of Hope
Duarte, California
Chapter 7. Surgery

Suzanne M. Mahon, RN, DNSc, AOCN®, AGN-BC
Professor, Internal Medicine/Division of Hematology/Oncology
Professor, Adult Nursing, School of Nursing
Saint Louis University
St. Louis, Missouri
Chapter 3. Cancer Epidemiology and Prevention; Chapter 4. Genetic Risk for Developing Cancer; Chapter 5. Cancer Detection Measures

Diana McMahon, MSN, RN, OCN®
Director of Professional Practice
The Ohio State University Wexner Medical Center
James Cancer Hospital and Solove Research Institute
Columbus, Ohio
Chapter 25. Oncologic Emergencies

Courtney L. Meuth, PharmD, BCPS
Medical Science Liaison
Chiesi USA
Cary, North Carolina
Chapter 16. Cardiac Toxicity

Vickie Connelly Murphy, PA-C
Physician Assistant–Certified
Department of Pulmonology
University of Texas MD Anderson Cancer Center
Houston, Texas
Chapter 28. Pulmonary Toxicities

Colleen M. O'Leary, MSN, RN, AOCNS®
Associate Director, Nursing Education and Evidence-Based Practice
The Ohio State University Wexner Medical Center
James Cancer Hospital and Solove Research Institute
Columbus, Ohio
Chapter 25. Oncologic Emergencies

MiKaela Olsen, APRN-CNS, MS, AOCNS®
Oncology and Hematology Clinical Nurse Specialist
Sidney Kimmel Comprehensive Cancer Center
Johns Hopkins Hospital
Baltimore, Maryland
Chapter 9. Chemotherapy

Denise Portz, MSN, RN, ACNS-BC, AOCNS®
Clinical Nurse Specialist
Froedtert & Medical College of Wisconsin
Milwaukee, Wisconsin
Chapter 15. Alopecia

Rachelle W. Rodriguez, RN, MSN, FNP-BC
Nurse Practitioner
Health in Balance Integrative Medicine
Laguna Beach, California
Chapter 11. Hormone Therapy

Teresa A. Savage, PhD, RN
Clinical Associate Professor
University of Illinois at Chicago, College of Nursing
Chicago, Illinois
Chapter 30. Ethical Issues

Melissa F. Saxon, RN, MSN, FNP, AOCNP®
Nurse Practitioner
GHS Cancer Institute
Seneca, South Carolina
Chapter 27. Peripheral Neuropathy

Anne Marie Shaftic, MSN, RN, AOCNP®
Nurse Practitioner, Oncology
Holy Name Medical Center
Teaneck, New Jersey
Chapter 8. Radiation Therapy

Vickie Shannon, MD
Professor
Department of Pulmonology
University of Texas MD Anderson Cancer Center
Houston, Texas
Chapter 28. Pulmonary Toxicities

Christy R. Smith, MSN, ACNP-BC
Clinical Educator
QuintilesIMS
Parsippany, New Jersey
Chapter 34. Caring for the Cancer Survivor

Matthew Tedder, PhD(c)
Graduate Research Assistant
Healthcare Genetics Doctoral Program
Clemson University
Clemson, South Carolina
Chapter 1. Biology of Cancer

Pamela Hallquist Viale, RN, MS, CS, ANP
Oncology Nurse Practitioner and Consultant
Goleta, California
Associate Clinical Professor (Volunteer)
Department of Physiological Nursing
University of California, San Francisco
San Francisco, California
Chapter 18. Dermatologic Complications; Chapter 24. Hypersensitivity

Suzanne Walker, CRNP, MSN, AOCN®, BC
Nurse Practitioner/Coordinator for Thoracic Malignancies
Penn Presbyterian Medical Center
Senior Lecturer B
Adult Oncology Specialty Minor/Post Master's Certificate, Advanced Practice Oncology Nurse
University of Pennsylvania School of Nursing
Philadelphia, Pennsylvania
Chapter 20. Gastrointestinal Symptoms; Chapter 26. Pain

Joan Westendorp, MSN, OCN®, CCRP
Chief Nursing Officer
West Michigan Cancer Center
Kalamazoo, Michigan
Chapter 12. Clinical Trials

Julia J. Yates, MSN, RN, OCN®
Oncology Nurse Manager, Surgical Oncology
Greenville Health System
Greenville, South Carolina
Chapter 34. Caring for the Cancer Survivor

Ruth R. Zalonis, RN, MSN, OCN®, CHPN, GC-C
Staff Nurse and Member of Palliative and Supportive Care Team
Jefferson Hospital
Jefferson Hills, Pennsylvania
Chapter 31. Palliative Care

Amy Y. Zhang, PhD
Associate Professor of Nursing
Frances Payne Bolton School of Nursing
Case Western Reserve University
Cleveland, Ohio
Chapter 21. Genitourinary Symptoms

Disclosure

Editors and authors of books and guidelines provided by the Oncology Nursing Society are expected to disclose to the readers any significant financial interest or other relationships with the manufacturer(s) of any commercial products.

A vested interest may be considered to exist if a contributor is affiliated with or has a financial interest in commercial organizations that may have a direct or indirect interest in the subject matter. A "financial interest" may include, but is not limited to, being a shareholder in the organization; being an employee of the commercial organization; serving on an organization's speakers bureau; or receiving research funding from the organization. An "affiliation" may be holding a position on an advisory board or some other role of benefit to the commercial organization. Vested interest statements appear in the front matter for each publication.

Contributors are expected to disclose any unlabeled or investigational use of products discussed in their content. This information is acknowledged solely for the information of the readers.

The contributors provided the following disclosure and vested interest information:

Julia Eggert, PhD, RN, AGN-BC, GNP, AOCN®, FAAN: Self Family Foundation, research funding
Lanell M. Bellury, PhD, RN, AOCNS®, OCN®: Emory Saint Joseph's Hospital Atlanta, consultant or advisory role
Elizabeth Prechtel Dunphy, DNP, CRNP, BC, AOCN®: Bayer, Celgene, honoraria; Carevive, consultant or advisory role
Christopher L. Farrell, PhD: eLab Solutions, consultant or advisory role
Stephanie Jacobson Gregory, FNP-C, BMTCN®: Astellas, Midatech Pharma, consultant or advisory role
Kristine B. LeFebvre, MSN, RN, AOCN®: American Nurses Credentialing Center, employment or leadership position
MiKaela Olsen, APRN-CNS, MS, AOCNS®: BD, consultant or advisory role
Anne Marie Shaftic, MSN, RN, AOCNP®: Kyowa Kirin, honoraria
Christy R. Smith, MSN, ACNP-BC: Novartis, employment or leadership position
Pamela Hallquist Viale, RN, MS, CS, ANP: Advanced Practitioner Society for Hematology and Oncology, leadership role, consultant or advisory role
Suzanne Walker, CRNP, MSN, AOCN®, BC: Carevive, consultant or advisory role
Joan Westendorp, MSN, OCN®, CCRP: National Cancer Institute Central Institutional Review Board, consultant or advisory role

Contents

Preface

The first edition of this book was developed to offer basic information about cancer care to nurses who had recently graduated and were starting their first jobs in oncology as well as for experienced nurses looking to develop their knowledge in the specialty. This second edition of *Cancer Basics* continues the focus on the fundamentals of cancer and its treatment but incorporates expanded information as well as updates with the current state of the knowledge to better address the specialized content needs of nurses in all oncology settings. Each chapter now features a list of key points to assist readers in identifying the important topics for nursing practice. At the end of each chapter are study questions that have been added to test your knowledge of the topic. The rationale for the correct answer is provided, as well as an explanation of why the other answers are incorrect. These questions can also be used as tools to supplement preparation for the oncology certified nurse (OCN®) examination.

Chapters on fatigue and palliative care have been added to provide a more comprehensive review. The previously combined Cardiac and Pulmonary Toxicity chapter was divided into separate chapters that incorporate expanded content, including the addition of new images in the Pulmonary Toxicities chapter to demonstrate those found in patients with cancer and receiving treatment. Additional color images are used in some chapters to better show the reality of toxicities seen in patients being treated for a variety of cancers.

The development of the first edition of *Cancer Basics* was led by Barbara Sigler, the Director of Publications for the ONS Publishing Division at the time. The authors hope this second edition continues to exemplify her vision, perseverance, and desire to address the knowledge needs of nurses new to oncology.

Acknowledgments

Thank you to all the authors who have dedicated time to share their knowledge, experience, and expertise on the topics important in the care of patients with a cancer diagnosis and their families.

Thank you to the ONS Publications Department staff, who have expertly guided me through this process for the second time.

Thank you to my husband, who has fixed our meals, run the household, and bought me chocolate. He truly is "the wind beneath my wings."

SECTION I

Foundations

CHAPTER

1 Biology of Cancer

Matthew Tedder, PhD(c), and Julia Eggert, PhD, RN, AGN-BC, GNP, AOCN®, FAAN

Introduction

Many in the lay public describe a diagnosis of "cancer" as if it is one disease. In reality, it encompasses more than 200 diseases that will occur at different ages with different rates of growth, differentiation, abilities to be detected, invasiveness, capacities to spread or metastasize, treatment responses, and prognoses. However, at the cellular and molecular levels, cancer is beginning to be viewed as a few diseases caused by genetic alterations and defective cell function that are actually very similar (Muñoz-Pinedo, El Mjiyad, & Ricci, 2012). These alterations can be associated with "nature," such as inherited cancer syndromes like hereditary breast and ovarian cancer syndrome or immune deficiencies. Or, the genetic alterations can be caused by "nurture," which includes obesity, poor diet, and social habits, such as smoking. A malignant growth is the result of changes in DNA, gene transcription, or translation. The resultant defective protein or proteins lead to transformation of normal cell components into uncontrolled proliferation, spread, or metastasis (Muñoz-Pinedo et al., 2012). This chapter focuses on a description of the malignant changes of a cell that will provide nurses new to oncology with a foundation for understanding the growth of cancer and its treatment, along with the basis to provide education to patients and their families.

Models of Cancer Development

Two models are commonly used to describe how a cancer develops. The first is the Stochastic Model, previously including Knudson's random "two hit" model. This model suggests that each cancer cell has the ability to multiply and form new tumors. The malignant cells have a selective advantage over their normal neighbors and begin to proliferate rapidly, accumulating genetic damage with each generation. As the damage collects, the most aggressive characteristics promote immortalized growth and the formation of a tumor (Beck & Blanpain, 2013; Hanahan & Weinberg, 2011).

The individual cancer stem cell is the focus of the second model. This model states that many different types of cancer cells exist in addition to endothelial, hematopoietic, stromal, and other types of cells to meet the functioning needs of the tumor, demonstrating heterogeneity. With proliferation, cell division occurs. All of these cells have the ability to multiply, but only one cell type—the cancer stem cell—has the ability to become a new tumor (Kreso & Dick, 2014). This is becoming the model most supported by cancer researchers. Once the new tumor is established, the heterogeneous cells begin to proliferate, allowing the tumor to enlarge, and the cancer stem cell moves into the resting phase (G_0) of the cell cycle. Cells in this phase are resistant to treatment and would remain as one surviving cancer cell while treatment destroys the other rapidly dividing noncancer stem cells (Junttila & de Sauvage, 2013). Thus, months or years later, the "resting" cancer stem cell could move into the active phases of the cell cycle, proliferate, and cause exacerbation of the once-dormant cancer believed to be destroyed during the original treatment (Kreso & Dick, 2014). See Figures 1-1 and 1-2 for comparison of these theories of tumor development.

An update of the cancer stem cell model is known as the Plasticity Model of Cancer Stem Cells. This newer model suggests that plasticity (the ability to change throughout the life of the cell) allows cancer stem cells to become heterogeneous with the ability to come out of remission, whereas noncancer stem cells have very low potential to become tumorigenic (Marjanovic, Weinberg, & Chaffer, 2013).

Structure and Function of DNA and Chromosomes

The human genome consists of 23 pairs of chromosomes. Each chromosome is a single double-helix DNA molecule with millions

Figure 1-1. Knudson "Two Hit" Theory of Cancer Development

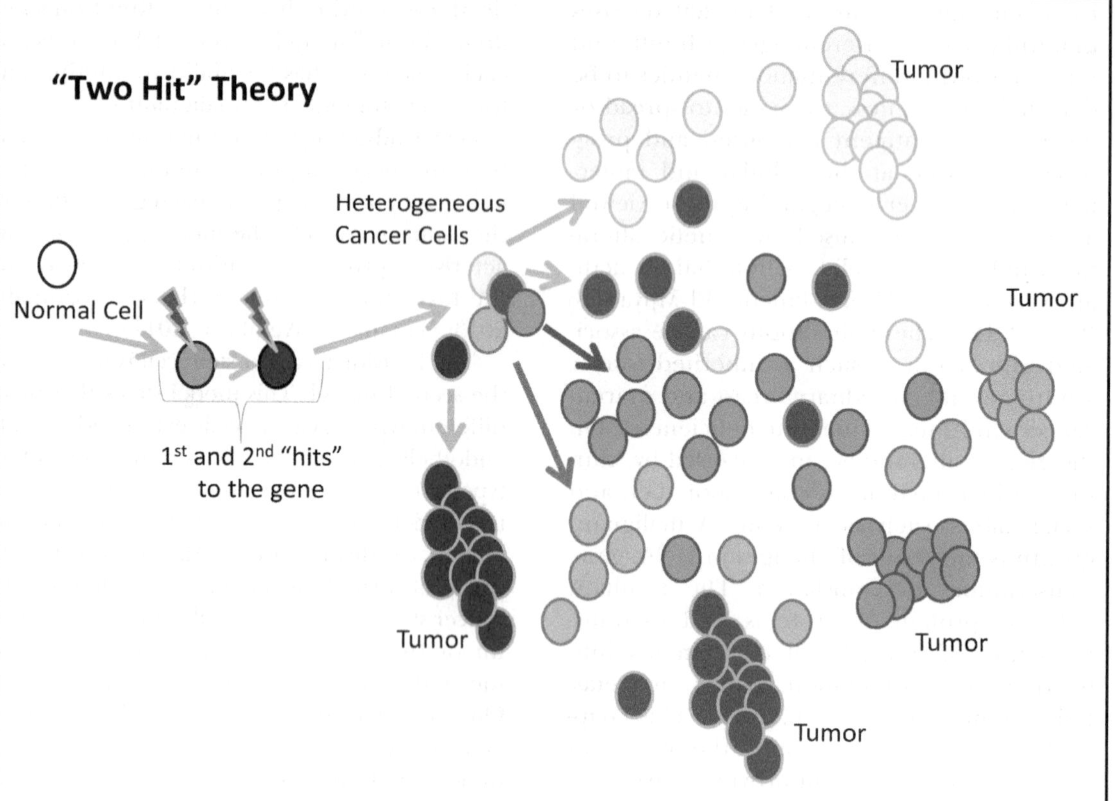

Theory: Two genes within a cell, one on each of a pair of chromosomes, each receive damage-causing hits prior to the development of cancer. The malignant cells are heterogeneous and all have the capability of developing a tumor.

Note. Based on information from Hanahan & Weinberg, 2011; Knudson, 1971; Reya et al., 2001; Wicha et al., 2006.

Figure 1-2. Cancer Stem Cell Theory of Cancer Development

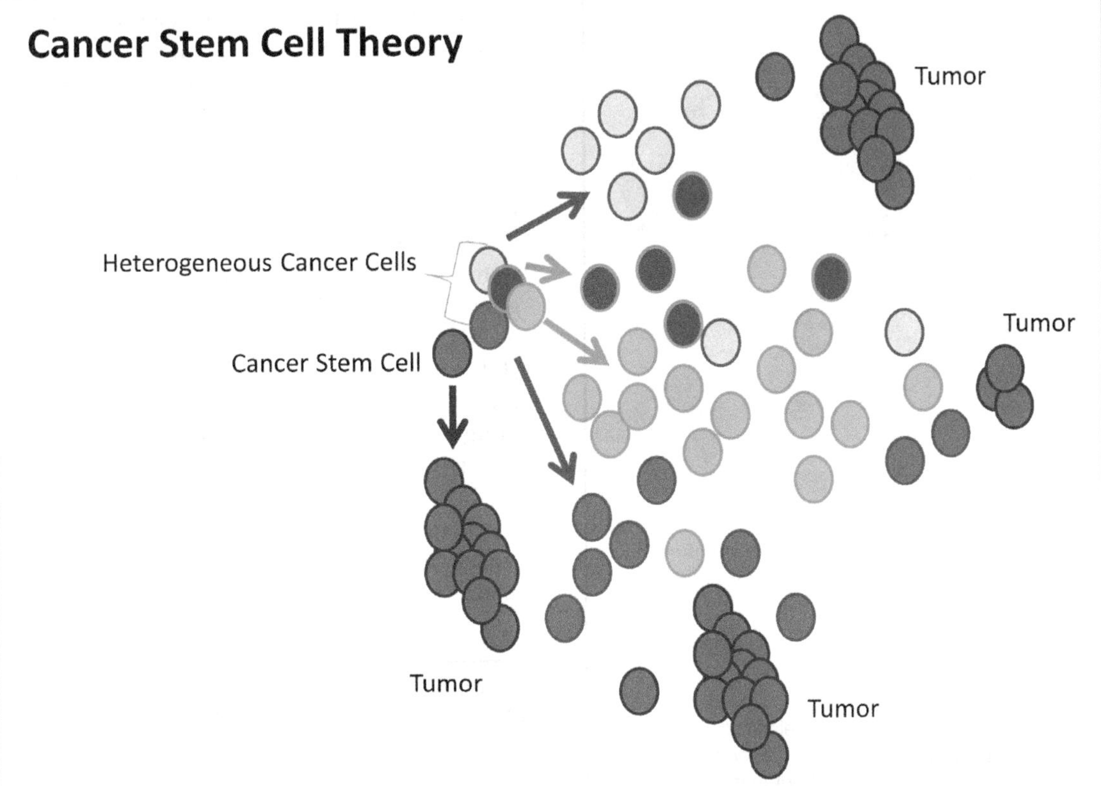

Theory: Cancer stem cells are the only type of heterogeneous cancer cells to develop into tumors.

Note. Based on information from Reya et al., 2001; Wicha et al., 2006.

of base pairs connected in a long, unbroken string that intricately coils back on itself and is scattered with proteins, called *histones* (see Figure 1-3).

Similar to sewing bobbins, histones organize and control the long threads of DNA, wrapping them into a tight coil so that the DNA is able to fit inside the nucleus of a cell. The coiling is necessary because the strands of DNA in a person's body would stretch about five feet but would be only fifty-trillionths of an inch (2 nanometers [nm]) wide. For comparison, the "membrane" of a brightly colored soap bubble is between 100–400 nm wide (UCSB ScienceLine, n.d.). This long but thin physical structure would be extremely fragile, hence the need for tight packaging to keep the DNA message intact. Once it is coiled around the histones, DNA continues twisting back upon itself (much like the continued twisting of a jump rope) until it is tightly wound, forming the chromatid seen in Figure 1-3. These chromatids enable the chromosomes to be visualized for karyotyping during the metaphase of cell division (Klug & Cummings, 2003).

Within the nucleus of each normal human cell, 23 pairs of chromosomes are present. These consist of 22 pairs of nonsex chromo-

Figure 1-3. DNA Packaging

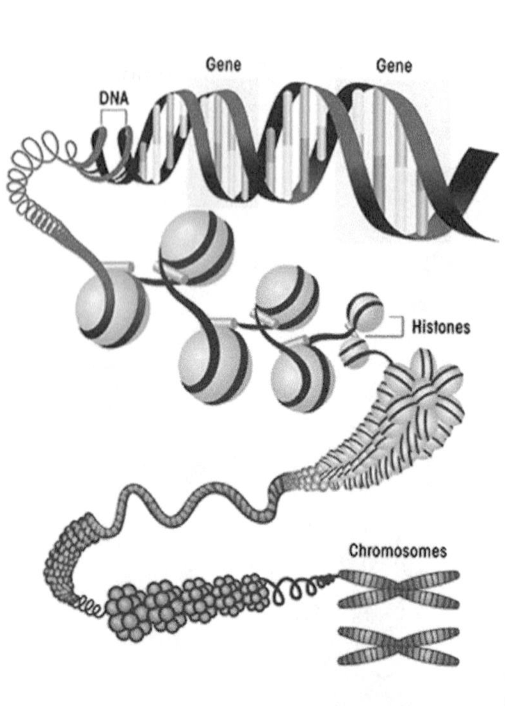

DNA is tightly wound around proteins called histones and packaged into cells' nuclei in the form of chromosomes. Genes are sections of DNA that, under the right circumstances, can be transcribed into proteins. Epigenetics determines which genes each cell transcribes at any given moment.

Note. From "Epigenetics—A New Frontier for Alcohol Research," by National Institute on Alcohol Abuse and Alcoholism, *Alcohol Alert, 86,* p. 2. Retrieved from http://pubs.niaaa.nih.gov/publications/aa86/aa86.htm.

somes (autosomes) and one pair of sex chromosomes (XX for female, XY for male). A person inherits one chromosome of the pair from the father and the other from the mother. A chromosome has a short arm (*p* for "petite") and a long arm (*q* because it follows *p* in the alphabet) with a unique banding pattern that identifies specific regions. These regions are numbered from the centromere to the end of each arm (Genetics Home Reference, 2016c). For example, the breast cancer gene (*BRCA1*) is found on chromosome 17, with a band position of q21 on the long arm (see Figure 1-4). If the position of a gene is uncertain, a range might be noted, such as 17q21–24 (Genetics Home Reference, 2016a). *BRCA2* is located on chromosome 13 at band position 13.2 on the long arm (q) as seen in Figure 1-5 (Genetics Home Reference, 2016b).

The central dogma of molecular biology states that DNA (adenine [A], cytosine [C], guanine [G], and thymine [T]) is transcribed to RNA (adenine [A], cytosine [C], guanine [G], and uracil [U] instead of thymine) and then translated into proteins (Klug & Cummings, 2003) (see Figure 1-6). For example, the DNA (ACTGTC) would be transcribed as RNA (ACUGUC) and then to messenger RNA (mRNA), where it is divided into codons (three nucleotides used to specify an amino acid) (UGA CAG) for translation from amino

Figure 1-4. *BRCA1* Gene Location

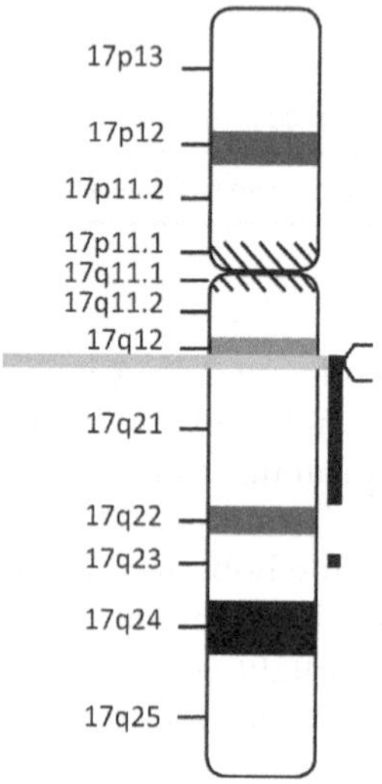

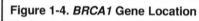

Note. From "Ideogram: Breast Cancer 1 (BRCA1)," by NCBI Map Viewer, n.d. Retrieved from http://www.ncbi.nlm.nih.gov/projects/mapview/maps.cgi?TAXID=9606&CHR=17&MAPS=genes-r%2Cpheno%2Cmorbid%2Cgenec&QUERY=BRCA1&BEG=17q21.1&END=17q21.1&thmb=on.

Figure 1-5. *BRCA2* Gene Location

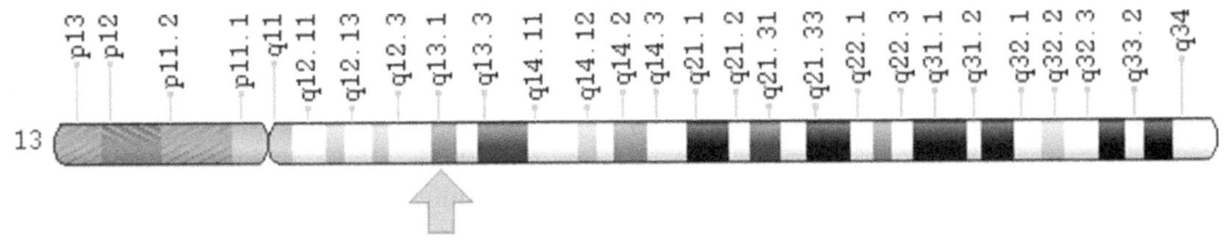

Note. From "Ideogram: Breast Cancer 2 (BRCA2)," by NCBI Map Viewer, n.d. Retrieved from https://ghr.nlm.nih.gov/gene/BRCA2#location.

Figure 1-6. Modified Central Dogma of DNA Model

DNA Transcription →→→ **Messenger RNA Translation** →→ **Protein**

DNA Replication

Protein regulation also occurs with small pieces of RNA, miRNA, and siRNA.

miRNA—microRNA; siRNA—small interfering RNA

Note. Based on information from Crick, 1970; Hayes et al., 2014.

acid to protein. This is important to remember because any changes in the codon "spelling" (mRNA triplet) could change the protein outcome. Some amino acids have multiple codon spellings. One example is leucine, which has six spellings (Algorithmic Arts, n.d.). These would allow several mistakes without creating a problem protein. However, tryptophan has one spelling (Algorithmic Arts, n.d.). Any error in this codon spelling would cause the assembly of a dysfunctional or nonfunctional protein (Adams, 2014).

Changes in DNA nucleotides can be either a mutation or a polymorphism. The distinction depends on the frequency with which the change occurs in the general population: If it occurs in at least 1% of the population, it is called a *polymorphism*. If it occurs in less than 1%, it is labeled as a *mutation* (National Cancer Institute [NCI], n.d.).

To further explain, a normal length of DNA is similar to a recipe for the most common type of cake—for example, a chocolate cake. Although this is the most common, other types of cakes exist, including strawberry, white, spice, pineapple upside-down, and lemon. These would be polymorphisms. They are good-tasting cakes but are not the most common. Sometimes the recipe is misread, and the cake comes out of the oven as a pudding (see Figure 1-7). This is uncommon and not the desired outcome. This is a mutation (NCI, n.d.).

Several types of mutations exist. The most common type is the *point mutation*, in which only one nucleotide base is altered. A *nonsense mutation* occurs when there is a premature termination of the protein. This happens when the stop codon, which signals termination of the length of amino acids, has been "spelled" incorrectly and gives an early or late signal to

Figure 1-7. Polymorphisms Versus Mutations

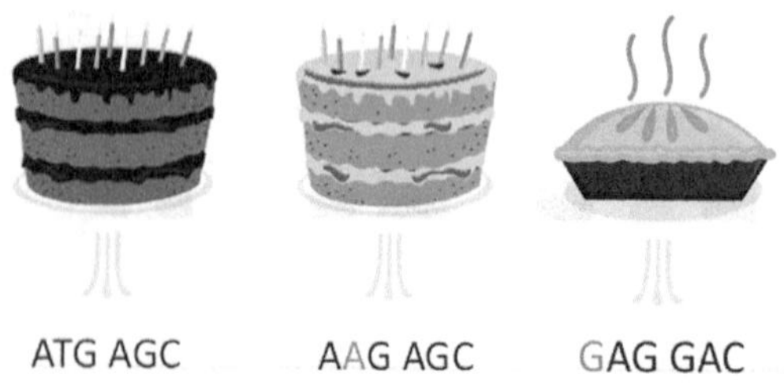

The wild-type genotype is transcribed to a codon that correctly spells a protein (e.g., recipe for a chocolate cake). When there is a polymorphism in the codon spelling, it can still spell a correct amino acid (e.g., a cake, just a different flavor). When the amino acid spelling is rare and uncommon, it is a mutation and creates an undesirable outcome (e.g., cookie, pie, or another undesired result).

end the compilation of amino acids into a protein (NCI, n.d.).

Mutations that occur within any of the cells of the body are labeled as *somatic*. They accumulate over a lifetime and are believed to cause sporadic cancers, which typically occur after an individual has reached 50 years of age. Mutations that are present in the ova or sperm are labeled as *germ line* and are associated with inherited cancers, which typically occur in people younger than 50 years old (see Table 1-1). The results of this genomic instability affect all future generations, depending on the pattern of inheritance (NCI, n.d.).

Most patterns of inheritance follow the dominant or recessive model developed by Gregor Mendel (Klug & Cummings, 2003). Each individual normally has two sets of chromosomes. On each chromosome is a gene, or allele, for a particular characteristic. Although an allele may have a collection of many different traits (such as blue, green, hazel, or brown eyes), each chromosome can exhibit only one of these. So, one chromosome may have the blue-eyes allele, and the second chromosome could have the brown-eyes allele. All of the other eye colors are still allelic options but are not displayed by this set of chromosomes. Each allele is either a dominant type or a recessive type; for example, the brown-eyes allele is dominant over the recessive blue-eyes allele. If the dominant allele is inactivated or lost, then the recessive allele will become active (Klug & Cummings, 2003).

Sometimes an individual will have the dominant allele without it being expressed. This is known as *incomplete penetrance*. The gene is there, but the phenotype (the observable physical trait) is not expressed. An example that illustrates this is a house in a fog; the house is there but is not visible because of the denseness of the low-lying cloud cover. Age, modifier genes, carcinogens, repair enzymes, and hormonal or reproductive factors affect penetrance (Klug & Cummings, 2003).

New descriptions of mutations associated with cancer include "drivers" and "passengers." Driver mutations (such as *TP53*) are commonly

Table 1-1. Somatic Versus Germ-Line Mutations

Somatic Cell	Germ-Line Cell (Egg or Sperm)
No known DNA damage is present at conception.	DNA in egg or sperm already has mutation at conception.
DNA damage may occur in one cell (not an egg or sperm) and accumulate over an extended period of time, after conception.	As cells duplicate, DNA damage is incorporated into every body cell and tissue type of the offspring.
DNA damage is replicated in cell lineage and a tumor develops in one organ or tissue type.	Potential for malignancy exists in multiple tissue types over time.
It is not inheritable.	It is passed to future generations.

Note. Based on information from National Cancer Institute, 2015.

associated with the development of cancer (oncogenesis) and are known to offer clonal advantage in the microenvironment of the evolving cancer cell. Within the same tumor, passenger mutations are found but do not offer growth advantage and at this point have no known contribution to the development of the cancer type. They seem to be "along for the ride" (Merid, Goranskaya, & Alexeyenko, 2014; Stratton, Campbell, & Futreal, 2009). Different cancers may have a varying mixture of driver and passenger mutations but still appear with similar phenotypes. The drivers in this group of mutated gene sets are the ones targeted for treatment either individually or in a staggered approach (Lee et al., 2012; Merid et al., 2014; Stratton et al., 2009).

In healthy cells, driver and passenger mutations can be restored to predamage level by normal DNA repair mechanisms, which are obviously important for cancer-free survival. These systems include (a) the nucleotide excision repair groups with mutations associated with xeroderma pigmentosum, (b) mismatch repair genes accompanying inherited colorectal cancer predisposition, (c) DNA crosslink repair genes (Fanconi anemia), and (d) the well-known DNA repair genes exemplified by the breast cancer genes (*BRCA1* and *BRCA2*). Approximately 130 genes are linked to DNA repair (Goldstein & Kastan, 2015).

Much of the scientific evidence about the development of cancer and its progression suggests that genomic instability is a precursor to changes associated with transformation of a cell into malignancy. Of question in this hypothesis is how the instability circumvents the careful security provided within the cell to monitor and guarantee genomic stability and purity for continued survival of the human cell. These protective teams include DNA monitoring and repair enzymes. Checkpoint gatekeepers function at significant points in the active phases of the cell cycle prior to DNA synthesis (S phase) and mitosis (M phase) to guarantee the accuracy of the genome and cell cycle processes. If an error is present, the P53 or retinoblastoma protein (pRB) tumor suppressor proteins cause cell cycle arrest for repair or apoptosis (programmed cell death) if too much damage has occurred (Feitelson et al., 2015; Hanahan & Weinberg, 2011).

Much research has confirmed that most human cancers have loss of function in the P53 tumor suppressor pathway. Other genes involved in targeting and repairing DNA damage also have been found to have loss of function in multiple cancers (American Cancer Society, 2014; Jeggo, Pearl, & Carr, 2016). Acquiring genomic damage permits evolving populations of precancerous cells to gain functional capabilities associated with malignant transformation. These include (a) self-sufficiency in growth signals, (b) insensitivity to antigrowth signals, (c) evasion of apoptosis, (d) sustained angiogenesis, (e) tissue invasion and metastasis, and (f) limitless replicative potential (Hanahan & Weinberg, 2011).

Epigenetics

Changes that occur to DNA activity beyond the actual sequence of the base pairs are termed *epigenetics* (Hanahan & Weinberg, 2011). These changes occur "above and over" the DNA so there is no effect to the basic sequence and the genotype is not changed, although the phenotypic outcome may be altered. These phenotypic changes occur through loosening or alteration of the tightly wound chromatin by binding of different chemicals in such a way that can determine when and where genes might be expressed, or turned on (Dawson & Kouzarides, 2012).

Chromatin consists of proteins and DNA as part of the chromosomes (Tonna, El-Osta, Cooper, & Tikellis, 2010). The major proteins of chromatin are histones, which are responsible for compacting the primary DNA by twisting it tightly like a jump rope while wrapping it tightly (like thread on a spool) so it fits within the nucleus of the cell. These continuous strands of DNA and histones appear like "beads on a string" (euchromatin) (see Figure 1-3). Multiple histones wrapped tightly together (heterochromatin) prevent transcription and contain inactive genes (Dawson & Kouzarides, 2012; Tonna et al., 2010). The nucleosome is composed of eight separate histone molecules with two loops of DNA wrapped around each group of eight histones (Dawson & Kouzarides, 2012). Figure 1-8 shows some epigenetic modifications of DNA and histones by chemical tags. The changes associated with epigenetics are caused when both the DNA and the histone proteins become modified with addition or removal of chemical groups (tags). Methyl groups can be added to DNA at the cytosine and guanine nucleotides (CpG islands) and cause silencing or stopping of transcription. Acetyl groups loosen the interactions between histones and DNA, allowing easier access to the DNA for transcription (Ho, Turcan, & Chan,

Figure 1-8. Epigenetics

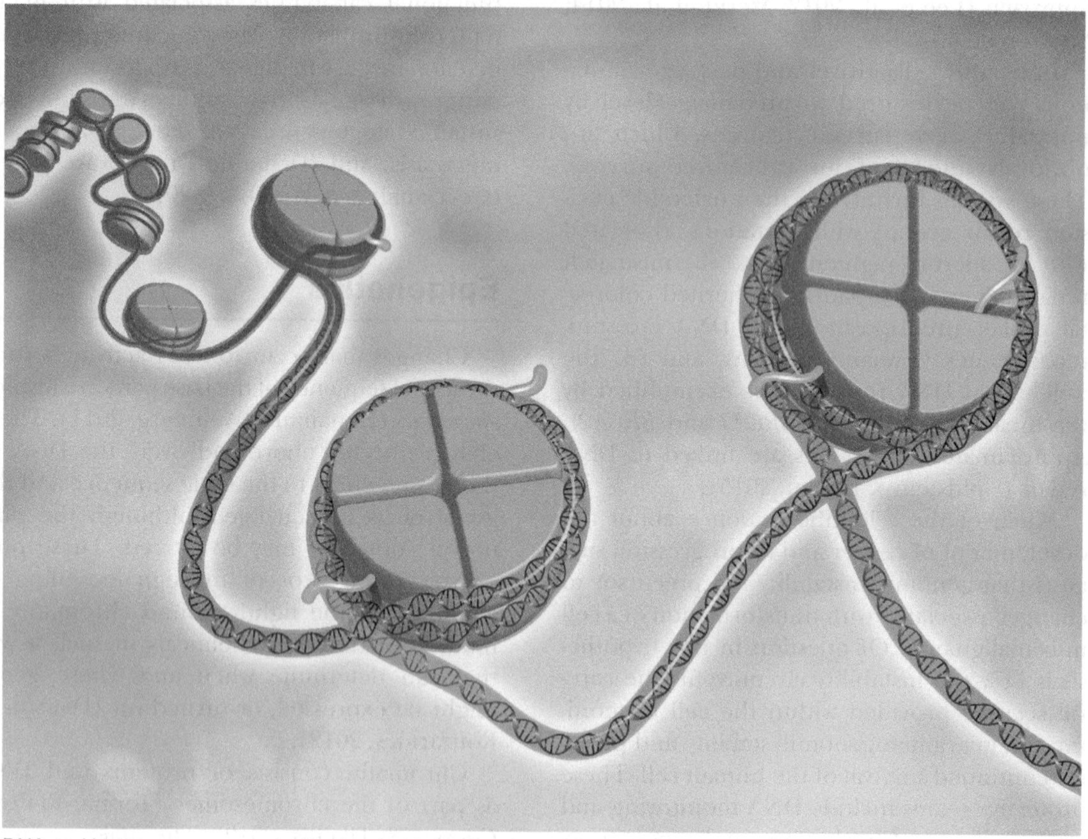

DNA and histones are covered with chemical tags. A variety of tags affect how histones interact with DNA. Some will open a gap between for transcription and others will close a gap to prevent transcription.

Note. Image by Darryl Leja, National Human Genome Research Institute. Retrieved from https://www.genome.gov/dmd/img.cfm?node=Photos/Graphics/Illustrations&id=97352.

2013). Because histones are proteins, they can be modified after translation by attachment of acetyl, phosphate, or ubiquitin groups (Rodríguez-Paredes & Esteller, 2011). The genome tightly wraps genes to make them unreadable, and, when relaxed, the active genes are easily accessible.

Recently, collections of enzymes were identified to have functions as readers, writers, and erasers in the epigenome. Epigenetic "readers" are types of enzymes that look for specific marks on post-translational histones or DNA where they can be modified with chemical groups. Tightly packed histones do not allow changes, so DNA translation is prevented. "Writers" promote attachment of the chemical groups, like acetyl groups, to cause loose packing of the histones for DNA expression (writing) with active protein growth. These chemical groups cause changes that alter the shape of the chromatin in specific places on the genome, making some areas more available to gene expression. "Erasers" are collections of enzymes that remove (erase) histone modifiers (Dawson, Kouzarides, & Huntly, 2012; Gillette & Hill, 2015).

Self-Sufficiency in Growth Signals

Growth Factors

Cell behavior is controlled by circulating proteins known as growth factors (ligands) that have the ability to act as chemical signals. They direct cell growth, differentiation, and survival in addition to determining tissue architecture and morphology. Growth factors must interact with their particular receptor to accomplish signaling (Kolch, Halasz, Granovskaya, & Kholodenko, 2015; Reimand, Wagih, & Bader, 2013).

Growth factors associated with the development of cancer include epidermal growth factor, transforming growth factor, and colony-stimulating factor. Other growth factors exist that are overproduced and are associated with different types of cancer. For example, platelet-derived growth factor is associated with sarcomas and glioblastomas (Kolch et al., 2015).

Growth Factor Receptors

As the first component in signaling pathways, growth factors bind to receptors to initiate signal transduction across the cell membrane. Once a growth factor is bound to a receptor, a signal activates other markers in the cytoplasm, causing transmission of a message to the cell nucleus. The message causes a change in the expression of certain genes that help to usher the cell through its growth cycle (Kolch et al., 2015; Reimand et al., 2013). Overproduction of some growth factors causes altered cellular communication and is associated with cancers. One of these, vascular endothelial growth factor (VEGF), has an important role in tumor neoangiogenesis—that is, the new growth of vessels on a tumor.

Tumor cells induce hypoxia. This lack of oxygen leads to transcription of the VEGF-α protein by binding to its designated cell surface receptors. The binding trips a signal indicating the need for increased blood vessel permeability, resulting in angiogenesis with even more proliferation of cells (Goel & Mercurio, 2013). VEGF is overexpressed in metastases of breast and colorectal cancers.

Tyrosine Kinase Activity

Many cancer-related growth factor receptors are stationed on the surface of the cell. Once they are bound by a ligand that causes activation, proliferative signals are sent into the cytoplasm. Most growth factor receptors possess tyrosine kinase (TK) activity, which leads to reactions that stimulate mitotic cell division, thereby allowing rapid growth of the malignant cell (Kolch et al., 2015; Reimand et al., 2013).

Examples of growth factor receptors that are cancer-causing (oncogenic) when overexpressed are epidermal growth factor receptor (EGFR), human epidermal growth factor receptor 2 (HER2), and transforming growth factor-beta (TGF-β). A variety of cancers express EGFR, including non-small cell lung cancer and breast, ovarian, and colorectal cancers. Approximately 80%–100% of head and neck cancers overexpress EGFR, which also is associated with lower survival. Increased HER2 expression corresponds with more aggressive cancers, including ovarian and breast cancers. When EGFR and TGF-β are both expressed, it is a prognostic marker for tumor relapse and decreased survival (Kolch et al., 2015; Reimand et al., 2013).

Nonreceptor Tyrosine Kinases

Some oncogenes do not require a receptor to initiate TK activity at the cell membrane. One example is the *SRC* gene family. The protein from this gene initiates TK activity at the C-terminus of the DNA where biosynthesis is supposed to end. Because no endpoint exists, the protein function persists, allowing continued signaling to the cell nucleus and persistent cell growth. Such *SRC*-initiated activity is increased in colon cancer and other malignancies such as neuroblastoma, small cell lung cancer, breast adenocarcinomas, and rhabdomyosarcoma (GeneCards, n.d.-b; Wiener & Gallick, 2012).

Intercellular Signaling Enzymes

Oncoproteins with certain enzyme activity are important for sending signals within cells and are called *intracellular signaling enzymes.* A common example is the enzymatic protein produced by the *RAF1* gene (GeneCards, n.d.-a). In the cytoplasm, TK activates the *RAF1* enzyme. Once activated, the enzyme acts as a mediator between the *RAS* (associated with the *RAS* oncogene) receptor on the cell membrane and the processes occurring in the cell nucleus by activating a series of other kinases, including mitogen-activated protein (referred to as MAP) kinases. These kinases are critical for regulating the onset of cell division, apoptosis, differentiation, and migration (GeneCards, n.d.-a; Kolch et al., 2015; Reimand et al., 2013).

Membrane-Associated G Proteins

The guanine nucleotide-binding proteins (G proteins) are products of a family of genes, the *RAS* proto-oncogenes, which normally act as "on-off switches" for cell-surface growth factor receptors. Instead of being transmitted inside the cell membrane, they transform adjacent G protein subunits below the membrane surface, which then begin the signaling cascade inside the cell (O'Hayre et al., 2013; Stephen, Esposito, Bagni, & McCormick, 2014).

When the *RAS* gene mutates into the "on" position, it becomes a cancer-causing gene (oncogene), and the changes interrupt a cascade of normally occurring signals that take place in the cell cytoplasm. Normal *RAS* genes wait for prompting to send stimulatory signals from growth factor receptors to other proteins. Mutant *RAS* genes activate signaling pathways even when unprompted. Mutant *RAS* is found in virtually all types of human cancer and occurs in approximately two-thirds of all malignant tumors (Stephen et al., 2014). G proteins act at the cell membrane to cause malignant transformation (O'Hayre et al., 2013; Stephen et al., 2014).

Transcription Factors

Proteins that bind to DNA and cause changes in gene expression are called *transcription factors.* These proteins have structures that can recognize specific DNA sequences (genes) involved in growth and survival. Mutation of the transcription factors that bind to genes involved in cell growth and survival allows for the malignant transformation found in many tumors. Examples of cancers caused by this mechanism include Ewing sarcoma, clear cell sarcoma, alveolar rhabdomyosarcoma, and many kinds of leukemia. Many of the transcription factor–induced cancers are characterized by translocation of chromosomes (Byrne et al., 2014). One of the tumor suppressor genes, *TP53*, also acts as a transcription factor. In this role, *TP53* "senses" DNA damage and halts cell division by controlling the expression of other genes that directly regulate the cell cycle (Feitelson et al., 2015).

Tumor Suppressor Genes

Tumor suppressor genes (also called antioncogenes) normally suppress or negatively regulate cell proliferation by encoding proteins that block the action of growth-promoting proteins. Using the example of a car, with cell growth caused by the accelerator, the tumor suppressor genes are the brakes, which can prevent cellular proliferation or suppress malignant transformation. At the cellular level, mutations in the cell cause tumor suppressor genes to lose function of both alleles. In other words, the loss of function or mutation of both copies of the gene is required for uncontrolled cell growth, leading to tumorigenesis (National Center for Biotechnology Information [NCBI], n.d.).

Loss of Heterozygosity

Homozygosity refers to the similarity between alleles. If there is an inherited mutation of a tumor suppressor gene, it is termed *heterozygous* because the alleles are different. Because a normal allele is present, the function of the gene and its protein product is maintained. Once the remaining allele is mutated, the gene and its product will lose normal functioning. The heterozygosity has been further altered and is now labeled as *loss of heterozygosity* (LOH). Cells can experience LOH with the loss of an entire chromosome, translocation of a piece of the chromosome, reduplication of a piece of chromosome that already has an abnormal gene, or the development of a point mutation in the second functioning allele. LOH is associated with cancer susceptibility genes, such as oncogenes and tumor suppressor genes (e.g., *TP53*). Basic research is identifying an increasing number of tumor suppressor genes that, when mutated, are closely associated with the development and progression of human cancers (American Cancer Society, 2014; Burrell, McGranahan, Bartek, & Swanton, 2013; NCI, n.d.; NCBI, n.d.).

The tumor suppressor gene *TP53* (located on 17p13) commonly has deletions and mutations associated with a wide variety of cancers, including lung, breast, esophageal, liver, bladder, and ovarian carcinomas; brain tumors; sarcomas; lymphomas; and leukemias. It is believed to contribute to half of all sporadic human cancers, making *TP53* the most common genetic target for mutations leading to cancers (NCBI, n.d.). When *TP53* is inherited in the germ line as a mutation, it is transmitted in an autosomal dominant fashion, a hallmark of Li-Fraumeni syndrome. This is a rare disorder causing multiple types of cancers, including soft tissue sarcomas, osteosarcomas, breast cancers, and different types of leukemias (Genetics Home Reference, 2016d; NCBI, n.d.).

Specific Functions of Tumor Suppressor Genes

Tumor suppressor gene products have specific functions in the cell nucleus and cytoplasm. If deregulation of the cell cycle occurs, which results in excess cell proliferation, the normal *TP53* gene can halt cell division and induce apoptosis (NCBI, n.d.) (see also Apoptosis later in this chapter).

Tumor suppressor genes also can encode for proteins in the cytoplasm. The *NF1* (neurofibromatosis) gene encodes a protein similar to the proteins that modulate the *RAS* oncogene function (Genetics Home Reference, 2016e). Loss of *NF1* may keep *RAS* activated and prolong the signal for cell proliferation (Yap et al., 2014). Loss of other tumor suppressor genes, such as *NF2* and *APC* (adenomatous polyposis coli), may cause cellular disorganization that leads to abnormal cell proliferation.

Insensitivity to Antigrowth Signals

In a normal cell, antigrowth signals move the cell out of the cell cycle growth phases into the resting from proliferation, or G_0, phase. The TGF-β, referred to as both *tumor* or *transforming growth factor*, pathway is the best example of a signaling mechanism that causes inhibition of cell growth and proliferation. This occurs in two ways in the normal pathway. First, TGF-β prevents inactivation of pRB, a tumor suppressor protein, and synthesis of the proteins from the tumor suppressor genes $p15^{INK4\alpha}$ and *p21*. Second, if cyclins are blocked, then cells are not able to move into and through the cell cycle. If the p15 protein is not synthesized, cyclins are not blocked, thereby allowing cells to continuously move into the active cell cycle with growth and proliferation. Finally, pRB tumor suppressor function is lost. Any of these interfering mechanisms, alone or in combination, allow continued cell growth and proliferation (Feitelson et al., 2015; Genetics Home Reference, 2016f).

Much like lights on a Christmas tree, when the circuit works well, all of the lights will come on and blink or not blink based on their function. In a cell, the signal is turned on at the gene/protein level, and as long as the pathway is active, all of the cell functions correctly. If an interruption occurs because of a genetic mutation or protein dysfunction, the pathway is interrupted and the "light" is not turned on, causing poor function or a nonfunctional pathway. As an option, another pathway could be available but lead to a different, potentially cancer-causing outcome. Examples are nonproliferation of cells versus continued proliferation of cells, or apoptosis versus no cell death, both leading to cancer.

If the Hedgehog, Notch, or Wnt pathways overexpress the wild-type (normal) signaling molecules or have activated mutations, malignant conversion of adult stem cells to cancer stem cells occurs (Takebe et al., 2015). Mutation of *BRCA1* can prevent DNA repair. If *PTEN* is mutated or deleted, it can result in increased expression of genes that promote continued movement through the cell cycle (Laukkanen & Castellone, 2016). New therapies are targeting some of these and other signaling pathways, potentially initiating programmed cell death (see also Chapter 10).

Evasion of Programmed Cell Death

Three types of "programmed" cell death are controlled by internal cell mechanisms: autophagy, apoptosis, and necrosis.

Autophagy

During stress, autophagy degrades parts of the cell (e.g., proteins, endoplasmic reticulum) that are dysfunctional or damaged (Glick, Barth, & Macleod, 2010). This begins with the formation of an autophagosome that surrounds the macromolecules and organelles destined for recycling (Liu, Lin, Yu, Liu, & Bao, 2011). Different from apoptosis and programmed necrosis, autophagy regulates starvation, cell differentiation, and cell survival in addition to other physiologic processes in the cell (Ouyang et al., 2012) (see Figures 1-9 through 1-11).

Apoptosis

When DNA damage is not repairable, apoptosis is the major type of cell death to occur. With this process, cell death is a controlled, deliberate, and distinct series of biochemical and cellular changes that allow an organism to remove old, dead, or unwanted cells. No inflammation occurs, and some of the cellular materials are ingested by neighboring cells and reused. Apoptosis is a normal process that occurs in the presence of severe or irreparable damage to the DNA to prevent duplication of inaccurate messages. This process comprises cell shrinkage, nuclear condensation and fragmentation, and blebbing of the cell membrane with loss of adhesion to neighboring cells plus cleavage of the chromosomal DNA into fragments (Ouyang et al., 2012). When a death signal occurs, the proteins of the *BCL2* family of genes (such as Bax, Bak, Bad, Bid, Bik, Bim, and Hrk) are modified, activated, and translocated to the mitochondria, where apoptosis is initiated by the release of these proapoptotic molecules (see Figure 1-10). Increased expression of *BCL2* is associated with resistance to chemotherapy and radiation therapy (Ouyang et al., 2012).

MicroRNAs (miRNAs) have been found to have both oncogenic (e.g., miRNA21) and tumor suppressor capabilities with the ability to promote apoptosis. Some miRNAs (e.g.,

Figure 1-9. Autophagy

Stress signal from the cell

↓

Formation of membrane from the cytoplasm to become phagosome

↓

Fusion of phagosome with lysosome

↓

Autophagy

Note. Based on information from Mizushima, 2014.

Figure 1-10. Apoptosis

Cell shrinkage

↓

Chromatin condensation

↓

Membrane blebbing

↓

Nuclear collapse and DNA fragmentation

↓

Apoptosis

↓

Phagocytosis of apoptotic cells and fragments

Note. Based on information from Ouyang et al., 2012.

Figure 1-11. Programmed Necrosis/Necroptosis

Organelle dysfunction

↓

Formation of necrosome

+

Cell swelling

↓

Packaging of poorly or nonfunctioning organelles

↓

Increased reactive oxygen species production

↓

Permeability of the mitochondrial membrane

↓

Programmed necrosis/necroptosis

Note. Based on information from Su et al., 2015.

miR15a–miR16-1) act as tumor suppressors to target *BCL2,* influence Bax and Bak, and ultimately promote apoptosis (Lin & Gregory, 2015; Ouyang et al., 2012). (See also Chapter 10 for a discussion of miRNAs in targeted therapies.)

Cells that lose their ability to signal apoptosis contribute to early tumorigenesis because they are unable to repair problems in the DNA to eliminate genetically damaged cells. Without repair, damaged cells survive, ultimately leading to tumorigenesis (Venkatanarayanan, Keyes, & Forster, 2013). Inactivation of the *TP53* gene leads to decreased apoptosis and rapid tumor progression. The loss of *TP53* function may indirectly contribute to tumor development by permitting the proliferation of mutated cells (Hanahan & Weinberg, 2011; Venkatanarayanan et al., 2013).

Follicular lymphoma, a type of indolent (slow-growing) non-Hodgkin lymphoma, is an example of the loss of apoptosis. This slow-growing lymphoma accounts for approximately 20% of all non-Hodgkin lymphomas and commonly has a rearrangement of the *BCL2* gene. The overexpression of the BCL-2 protein inhibits apoptosis, allowing continued cellular proliferation and making destruction of this lymphoma difficult (NCI, 2016). It is hypothesized that restoration of apoptosis may provide an approach to cancer therapy.

Programmed Necrosis (Necroptosis)

The third type of programmed cell death associated with cancer is programmed necrosis, or necroptosis. Programmed necrosis is caused by activation of the TNF receptor family, T-cell receptors, interferon receptors, Toll-like receptors, cellular metabolic and genotoxic stress, or multiple types of anticancer agents (Su, Yang, Xu, Chen, & Yu, 2015). The first step in programmed necrosis is formation of the necrosome. This can be blocked or initiated at three checkpoints (Su et al., 2015). Caspases are not part of programmed necrosis. Morphologic features include cell swelling, organelle dysfunction, and cell lysis (Ouyang et al., 2012). This type of cell death is associated with packaging of poorly functioning or nonfunctioning organelles and engages the formation of a cascade of molecules to interact with specialized enzymes that enhance metabolism. Production of reactive oxygen species increases, leading to permeability of the mitochondrial membrane and programmed necrosis. Other molecules, such as PARP1, modulate this complicated process and ultimately programmed necrosis (Ouyang et al., 2012). Impaired programmed necrosis has been associated with chronic lymphocytic leukemia and non-Hodgkin lymphoma (Su et al., 2015).

Sustained Angiogenesis

Tumor cells have limitations in oxygen supply that cause areas of hypoxia. This boosts the need for glucose uptake and glycolysis to generate energy, resulting in lactate production. Although this supports the use of positron-emission tomography in nuclear medicine to identify increased metabolism, it also can result in decreased adenosine triphosphate production and ultimately contribute to the fatigue experienced by patients with a malignancy (Goel & Mercurio, 2013). This lack of oxygen also curtails the proliferation of malignant cells (Hanahan & Folkman, 1996). For tumors to grow to a larger size, they need to develop a microcirculatory system through the process of angiogenesis (Hanahan & Weinberg, 2011).

VEGF causes the growth of new vessels, forming a microcirculatory system in a tumor (i.e., angiogenesis). Tumor cells induce hypoxia, leading to the transcription of VEGF-α, which binds to cell surface receptors and ultimately causes increased blood vessel permeability, angiogenesis, and the proliferation of cells (Goel & Mercurio, 2013). Multiple malignancies, including metastatic breast and colorectal cancers, overexpress VEGF.

Tissue Invasion and Metastasis

Altered Cytoskeletal Control

Cells have a skeleton with interior and exterior functions. The cell's shape and ability to move are included in the external function of the cytoskeleton. The internal function of the cytoskeleton permits substances to move within the cell. On the exterior membrane, microtubules evoke a rigidity to add strength to the membrane surface. Internally, they promote movement of organelles within the cytoplasm. During mitosis, the microtubules are arranged in a centriole as nine bundles of three microtubules each. These form the spindle fibers, which are responsible for separation of the chromosomes prior to the actual splitting of the cell (McCance, 2014). With a malignancy, the cell loses external cytoskeleton control. This causes it to lose rigidity and become more amenable to continued cellular division. In addition, the cytoskeleton is needed for spindle microtubule formation, mitosis, and cellular growth. Multiple protein types participate in these changes associated with malignant transformation (Hanahan & Weinberg, 2011; Liaw, Chang, & Kavallaris, 2007).

Altered Mobility of Membrane Components

Proteins, glycoproteins, and glycolipids are known to have altered mobility on the membrane of a malignant cell. One outcome of this change enables the cancer to avoid immune surveillance. Other outcomes could promote spread and metastasis (Hanahan & Weinberg, 2011; Wallach, 1968).

Modified Contact Adhesion and Inhibition of Movement

After replication, normal cells contact the adjacent cell membrane and are inhibited from growing. Malignant cells lose this characteristic and continue to proliferate even though they are touching the cell next to them. This contributes to the lack of control in malignant cells (Hanahan & Weinberg, 2011; McCance, 2014).

Altered Surface Charge Density

Malignant cell membranes have a lower level of electrical potential than that of normal cells. This is because of the increased amounts of negatively charged phospholipids in the cell membrane (Venkatanarayanan et al., 2013). Positively charged sodium and calcium channels contribute to apoptosis (Williams & Djamgoz, 2005). Changes in the charge of the cell membrane inhibit apoptosis and contribute to the longevity of malignant cells.

Increased Lectin Agglutinability

Alterations in lectin binding enable leukocytes to adhere to and cover malignant cells. This change allows malignant cells to escape surveillance and travel to distant sites in the body as a bolus of normal and abnormal cells (Hanahan & Weinberg, 2011; McCance, 2014).

Limitless Replicative Potential

One factor allowing for limitless replicative potential is the expression of telomerase. This enzyme prevents destruction of the telomere. Because telomeres protect chromosomes, cells with increased telomerase are associated with longer telomeres and longevity of cell life. Short telomeres are associated with a shorter life span. Cancer stem cells have increased levels of telomerase and thus have an extended life enhanced by the protected telomeres at the ends of the chromosome. This also protects the cell from apoptosis (Hanahan & Weinberg, 2011).

Conclusion

The curricula in undergraduate nursing programs do not typically include molecular biology. With completion of the sequencing of the human genome in 2003, many diagnostics and treatments have been developed that require an understanding of certain characteristics of cells, the central dogma, and how cell signaling and communication occur. This knowledge is important for oncology nurses and helps them to anticipate the symptoms of cancer in their patients, to be aware of how the treatments work, and to have a basic foundation when developing teaching plans related to individualized treatment plans for their patients. This chapter has provided a description of how malignancies develop and some of the molecular biology used for diagnostics and treatment in oncology. These include self-sufficiency in growth signals, insensitivity to antigrowth signals, evasion of apoptosis, sustained angiogenesis, tissue invasion and metastasis, and limitless replicative potential (Hanahan & Weinberg, 2011). For people new to oncology or for those who simply want to review and close some gaps in their knowledge, an understanding of the biology of cancer will be useful as they care for patients and their families.

References

Adams, J.U. (2014). The functions of proteins are determined by their three-dimensional structure. In C. O'Connor (Ed.), *Essentials of cell biology*. Retrieved from http://www.nature.com/scitable/ebooks/essentials-of-cell-biology-14749010/122996920

Algorithmic Arts. (n.d.). 20 amino acids, their single-letter data-base codes (SLC), and their corresponding DNA codons. Retrieved from http://algoart.com/aatable.htm

American Cancer Society. (2014). Oncogenes and tumor suppressor genes. Retrieved from http://www.cancer.org/cancer/cancercauses/geneticsandcancer/genesandcancer/genes-and-cancer-oncogenes-tumor-suppressor-genes

Beck, B., & Blanpain, C. (2013). Unravelling cancer stem cell potential. *Nature Reviews Cancer, 13,* 727–738. doi:10.1038/nrc3597

Burrell, R.A., McGranahan, N., Bartek, J., & Swanton, C. (2013). The causes and consequences of genetic heterogeneity in cancer evolution. *Nature, 501,* 338–345. doi:10.1038/nature12625

Byrne, M., Wray, J., Reinert, B., Wu, Y., Nickoloff, J., Lee, S.-H., … Williamson, E. (2014). Mechanisms of oncogenic chromosomal translocations. *Annals of the New*

Key Points

- Cancer is a heterogenic disease because of diverse cell types and genetic and epigenetic differences between cancer cells.
- Several models have been developed to explain the heterogeneity seen in cancer, such as the clonal model, the cancer stem cell model, the plasticity model, and the inflammatory model.
- A genetic change present in at least 1% of the population is termed a *polymorphism* and is likely benign, whereas a genetic change present in less than 1% of the population is termed a *mutation* and is more likely to have negative effects.
- Germ-line mutations occur in the ova or sperm and are present in every cell in the body, whereas somatic mutations are not inherited and can be present in any cell in the body except the sex cells.
- Epigenetic changes are chemical modifications to the DNA molecule that are not inherited and do not alter the sequence of the cellular DNA.
- Driver mutations are those that provide the cell with a selective growth advantage and help to establish the malignancy. Passenger mutations do not contribute to the malignant phenotype and seem to be "along for the ride."
- Cancer cells have many characteristics associated with malignancy, including self-sufficiency in growth signals, insensitivity to antigrowth signals, evasion of apoptosis, sustained angiogenesis, tissue invasion and metastasis, and limitless replicative potential.

York Academy of Sciences, 1310, 89–97. doi:10.1111/nyas.12370

Crick, F. (1970). Central dogma of molecular biology. *Nature, 227,* 561–563.

Dawson, M.A., & Kouzarides, T. (2012). Cancer epigenetics: From mechanism to therapy. *Cell, 150,* 12–27. doi:10.1016/j.cell.2012.06.013

Dawson, M.A., Kouzarides, T., & Huntly, B.J.P. (2012). Targeting epigenetic readers in cancer. *New England Journal of Medicine, 367,* 647–657. doi:10.1056/NEJMra1112635

Feitelson, M.A., Arzumanyan, A., Kulathinal, R.J., Blain, S.W., Holcombe, R.F., Mahajna, J., ... Nowsheen, S. (2015). Sustained proliferation in cancer: Mechanisms and novel therapeutic targets. *Seminars in Cancer Biology, 35*(Suppl.), S25–S54. doi:10.1016/j.semcancer.2015.02.006

GeneCards. (n.d.-a). *RAF1* gene. Retrieved from http://www.genecards.org/cgi-bin/carddisp.pl?gene=Raf1

GeneCards. (n.d.-b). *SRC* gene. Retrieved from http://www.genecards.org/cgi-bin/carddisp.pl?gene=SRC

Genetics Home Reference. (2016a). *BRCA1* gene. Retrieved from https://ghr.nlm.nih.gov/gene/BRCA1

Genetics Home Reference. (2016b). *BRCA2* gene. Retrieved from https://ghr.nlm.nih.gov/gene/BRCA2

Genetics Home Reference. (2016c). Chromosome. Retrieved from https://ghr.nlm.nih.gov/primer/basics/chromosome

Genetics Home Reference. (2016d). Li-Fraumeni syndrome. Retrieved from http://ghr.nlm.nih.gov/condition=lifraumenisyndrome

Genetics Home Reference. (2016e). *NF1* gene. Retrieved from https://ghr.nlm.nih.gov/gene/NF1

Genetics Home Reference. (2016f). *RB1* gene. Retrieved from http://ghr.nlm.nih.gov/gene=rb1

Gillette, T.G., & Hill, J.A. (2015). Readers, writers, and erasers: Chromatin as the whiteboard of heart disease. *Circulation Research, 116,* 1245–1253. doi:10.1161/CIRCRESAHA.116.303630

Glick, D., Barth, S., & Macleod, K.F. (2010). Autophagy: Cellular and molecular mechanisms. *Journal of Pathology, 221,* 3–12. doi:10.1002/path.2697

Goel, H.L., & Mercurio, A.M. (2013). VEGF targets the tumour cell. *Nature Reviews Cancer, 13,* 871–882. doi:10.1038/nrc3627

Goldstein, M., & Kastan, M.B. (2015). The DNA damage response: Implications for tumor responses to radiation and chemotherapy. *Annual Review of Medicine, 66,* 129–143. doi:10.1146/annurev-med-081313-121208

Hanahan, D., & Folkman, J. (1996). Patterns and emerging mechanisms of the angiogenic switch during tumorigenesis. *Cell, 86,* 353–364. doi:10.1016/S0092-8674(00)80108-7

Hanahan, D., & Weinberg, R.A. (2011). Hallmarks of cancer: The next generation. *Cell, 144,* 646–674. doi:10.1016/j.cell.2011.02.013

Hayes, J., Peruzzi, P.P., & Lawler, S. (2014). MicroRNAs in cancer: Biomarkers, functions and therapy. *Trends in Molecular Medicine, 20,* 460–469. doi:10.1016/j.molmed.2014.06.005

Ho, A.S., Turcan, S., & Chan, T.A. (2013). Epigenetic therapy: Use of agents targeting deacetylation and methylation in cancer management. *OncoTargets and Therapy, 6,* 223–232. doi:10.2147/OTT.S34680

Jeggo, P.A., Pearl, L.H., & Carr, A.M. (2016). DNA repair, genome stability and cancer: A historical perspective. *Nature Reviews Cancer, 16,* 35–42. doi:10.1038/nrc.2015.4

Junttila, M.R., & de Sauvage, F.J. (2013). Influence of tumour micro-environment heterogeneity on therapeutic response. *Nature, 501,* 346–354. doi:10.1038/nature12626

Klug, W.S., & Cummings, M.R. (2003). *Genetics: A molecular perspective.* Upper Saddle River, NJ: Prentice Hall.

Knudson, A.G., Jr. (1971). Mutation and cancer: Statistical study of retinoblastoma. *Proceedings of the National Academy of Sciences of the United States of America, 68,* 820–823. doi:10.1073/pnas.68.4.820

Kolch, W., Halasz, M., Granovskaya, M., & Kholodenko, B.N. (2015). The dynamic control of signal transduction networks in cancer cells. *Nature Reviews Cancer, 15,* 515–527. doi:10.1038/nrc3983

Kreso, A., & Dick, J.E. (2014). Evolution of the cancer stem cell model. *Cell Stem Cell, 14,* 275–291. doi:10.1016/j.stem.2014.02.006

Laukkanen, M.O., & Castellone, M.D. (2016). Hijacking the hedgehog pathway in cancer therapy. *Anti-Cancer Agents in Medicinal Chemistry, 16,* 309–317. doi:10.2174/1871520615666151007160439

Lee, M.J., Ye, A.S., Gardino, A.K., Heijink, A.M., Sorger, P.K., MacBeath, G., & Yaffe, M.B. (2012). Sequential application of anticancer drugs enhances cell death by rewiring apoptotic signaling networks. *Cell, 149,* 780–794. doi:10.1016/j.cell.2012.03.031

Liaw, T.Y.E., Chang, M.H.Y., & Kavallaris, M. (2007). The cytoskeleton as a therapeutic target in childhood acute leukemia: Obstacles and opportunities. *Current Drug Targets, 8,* 739–749. doi:10.2174/138945007780830836

Lin, S., & Gregory, R.I. (2015). MicroRNA biogenesis pathways in cancer. *Nature Reviews Cancer, 15,* 321–333. doi:10.1038/nrc3932

Liu, J.-J., Lin, M., Yu, J.-Y., Liu, B., & Bao, J.-K. (2011). Targeting apoptotic and autophagic pathways for cancer therapeutics. *Cancer Letters, 300,* 105–114. doi:10.1016/j.canlet.2010.10.001

Marjanovic, N.D., Weinberg, R.A., & Chaffer, C.L. (2013). Cell plasticity and heterogeneity in cancer. *Clinical Chemistry, 59,* 168–179. doi:10.1373/clinchem.2012.184655

McCance, K.L. (2014). Cellular biology. In K.L. McCance & S.E. Huether (Eds.), *Pathophysiology: The biologic basis for disease in adults and children* (7th ed., pp. 363–395). St. Louis, MO: Elsevier Mosby.

Merid, S.K., Goranskaya, D., & Alexeyenko, A. (2014). Distinguishing between driver and passenger mutations in individual cancer genomes by network enrichment analysis. *BMC Bioinformatics, 15,* 308. doi:10.1186/1471-2105-15-308

Mizushima, N. (2014). Sugar modification inhibits autophagosome-lysosome fusion. *Nature Cell Biology, 16,* 1132–1133. doi:10.1038/ncb3078

Muñoz-Pinedo, C., El Mjiyad, N., & Ricci, J.-E. (2012). Cancer metabolism: Current perspectives and future directions. *Cell Death and Disease, 3,* e248. doi:10.1038/cddis.2011.123

National Cancer Institute. (n.d.). *NCI dictionary of cancer terms.* Retrieved from https://www.cancer.gov/publications/dictionaries/cancer-terms

National Cancer Institute. (2015). The genetics of cancer. Retrieved from http://www.cancer.gov/about-cancer/causes-prevention/genetics#syndromes

National Cancer Institute. (2016). Adult non-Hodgkin lymphoma treatment (PDQ®) [Health professional version]. Retrieved from http://www.cancer.gov/cancertopics/pdq/treatment/adult-non-hodgkins/HealthProfessional/page3

National Center for Biotechnology Information. (n.d.). The p53 tumor suppressor protein. Retrieved from http://www.ncbi.nlm.nih.gov/books/NBK22268

O'Hayre, M., Vázquez-Prado, J., Kufareva, I., Stawiski, E.W., Handel, T.M., Seshagiri, S., & Gutkind, J.S. (2013). The emerging mutational landscape of G proteins and G-protein-coupled receptors in cancer. *Nature Reviews Cancer, 13,* 412–424. doi:10.1038/nrc3521

Ouyang, L., Shi, Z., Zhao, S., Wang, F.-T., Zhou, T.-T., Liu, B., & Bao, J.-K. (2012). Programmed cell death pathways in cancer: A review of apoptosis, autophagy and programmed necrosis. *Cell Proliferation, 45,* 487–498. doi:10.1111/j.1365-2184.2012.00845.x

Reimand, J., Wagih, O., & Bader, G.D. (2013). The mutational landscape of phosphorylation signaling in cancer. *Scientific Reports, 3,* 2651. doi:10.1038/srep02651

Reya, T., Morrison, S.J., Clarke, M.F., & Weissman, I.L. (2001). Stem cells, cancer, and cancer stem cells. *Nature, 414,* 105–111.

Rodríguez-Paredes, M., & Esteller, M. (2011). Cancer epigenetics reaches mainstream oncology. *Nature Medicine, 17,* 330–339. doi:10.1038/nm.2305

Stephen, A.G., Esposito, D., Bagni, R.K., & McCormick, F. (2014). Dragging Ras back in the ring. *Cancer Cell, 25,* 272–281. doi:10.1016/j.ccr.2014.02.017

Stratton, M.R., Campbell, P.J., & Futreal, P.A. (2009). The cancer genome. *Nature, 458,* 719–724. doi:10.1038/nature07943

Su, Z., Yang, Z., Xu, Y., Chen, Y., & Yu, Q. (2015). Apoptosis, autophagy, necroptosis, and cancer metastasis. *Molecular Cancer, 14,* 48. doi:10.1186/s12943-015-0321-5

Takebe, N., Miele, L., Harris, P., Jeong, W., Bando, H., Kahn, M., ... Ivy, S.P. (2015). Targeting Notch, Hedgehog, and Wnt pathways in cancer stem cells: Clinical update. *Nature Reviews Clinical Oncology, 12,* 445–464. doi:10.1038/nrclinonc.2015.61

Tonna, S., El-Osta, A., Cooper, M.E., & Tikellis, C. (2010). Metabolic memory and diabetic nephropathy: Potential role for epigenetic mechanisms. *Nature Reviews Nephrology, 6,* 332–341. doi:10.1038/nrneph.2010.55

UCSB ScienceLine. (n.d.). How long and wide is DNA? Retrieved from http://scienceline.ucsb.edu/getkey.php?key=144

Venkatanarayanan, A., Keyes, T.E., & Forster, R.J. (2013). Label-free impedance detection of cancer cells. *Analytical Chemistry, 85,* 2216–2222. doi:10.1021/ac302943q

Wallach, D.F.H. (1968). Cellular membranes and tumor behavior: A new hypothesis. *Proceedings of the National Academy of Sciences of the United States of America, 61,* 868–874. doi:10.1073/pnas.61.3.868

Wicha, M.S., Liu, S., & Dontu, G. (2006). Cancer stem cells: An old idea—A paradigm shift. *Cancer Research, 66,* 1883–1890. doi:10.1158/0008-5472.CAN-05-3153

Wiener, J.R., & Gallick, G.E. (2012). Nonreceptor tyrosine kinases and their roles in cancer. In D.A. Frank (Ed.), *Signaling pathways in cancer pathogenesis and therapy* (pp. 39–53). doi:10.1007/978-1-4614-1216-8_4

Williams, E.L., & Djamgoz, M.B.A. (2005). Nitric oxide and metastatic cell behaviour. *BioEssays, 27,* 1228–1238. doi:10.1002/bies.20324

Yap, Y.-S., McPherson, J.R., Ong, C.-K., Rozen, S.G., Teh, B.-T., Lee, A.S.G., & Callen, D.F. (2014). The *NF1* gene revisited—From bench to bedside. *Oncotarget, 5,* 5873–5892. doi:10.18632/oncotarget.2194

Chapter 1 Study Questions

1. A patient's tumor has a mutation in a copy of her *p53* gene. The mutation results in a shortened, nonfunctional protein. What type of mutation does the patient most likely have?
   A. Point mutation
   B. Missense mutation
   C. Nonsense mutation
   D. Insertion

2. A new tumor suppressor protein has recently been discovered. What could be a possible function of this new protein?
   A. A transcription factor for epidermal growth factor
   B. A tyrosine kinase in the RAS–RAF pathway
   C. An inhibitor of *NF1* function
   D. An upregulator of *BAX* expression

3. Which of the following procancer traits is associated with increased inflammation?
   A. Upregulation of growth factors
   B. Enzymes that alter the extracellular matrix
   C. Promotion of apoptosis evasion
   D. All of the above

4. The use of positron-emission tomography scans in identifying cancer is based on what characteristic of malignancy?
   A. Cytoskeletal changes
   B. Changes to cellular metabolism
   C. Increased angiogenesis
   D. Evasion of apoptosis

5. Loss of heterozygosity refers to which of the following?
   A. Loss of the second allele (gene)
   B. Wild type of the allele (gene)
   C. Mutation of many zygotes
   D. Shift of the DNA base pair sequences

CHAPTER 2

Staging and Performance Status

Kristine B. LeFebvre, MSN, RN, AOCN®

Introduction

Although often viewed as a single illness, cancer is a collection of more than 100 related diseases involving the abnormal growth of cells that can occur anywhere within the human body (American Cancer Society [ACS], 2015; National Cancer Institute [NCI], 2015c). The word *cancer* is thought to have developed from the Greek reference to the crab, believed to have been adopted because of the finger-like projections sometimes seen with a cancer (ACS, 2014; Kumar, Abbas, & Aster, 2015).

On presentation, a tumor is determined to be benign or malignant. Benign tumors remain localized, grow slowly, and do not spread to other sites within the body. If symptoms occur, they are frequently caused by pressure and obstruction. Benign tumors often are capsulated and can be surgically removed. In contrast, malignant, or cancerous, tumors grow rapidly and in an uncontrolled manner. They are able to invade and destroy tissues and lymph nodes around them and spread to distant sites (Vogel, 2018).

This chapter will review the steps taken to diagnose cancer and determine the type and name. It also will explain staging classification and performance status, as well as the nursing role in this process.

Diagnosis of Cancer

Accurate diagnosis is essential for effective cancer treatment. When cancer is suspected, a diagnostic workup, including relevant tests and studies, is completed to determine the presence or extent of disease. The studies done will vary depending on the type of cancer suspected. National guidelines, such as those from the National Comprehensive Cancer Network® (www.nccn.org) and the American College of Radiology (www.acr.org), can assist in determining the examinations needed.

Workup begins with a comprehensive patient history and physical examination with specific focus on any signs and symptoms of disease and an evaluation of the individual's general health and performance status. Laboratory tests on blood, urine, and other body fluids may be done to determine organ function and any organ malfunctions (Tschanz & Sugarman, 2016; Vogel, 2018). Laboratory tests may include blood chemistries, liver function tests, blood cell counts, and other tests as appropriate.

Depending on the type of cancer suspected, patients may be tested for tumor markers, also called *biomarkers* or *diagnostic markers* (Vogel, 2018). These substances are produced by a tumor or the body in response to a tumor and can be found in the blood, urine, stool, tumor tissue, or other tissues or fluids within the body (NCI, 2015b). Markers include hormones, antigens, proteins, genetic materials, and other substances that help clinicians to diagnose disease, make treatment decisions, or monitor disease progression (Edge et al., 2010; Febbo et al., 2011; Tschanz & Sugarman, 2016; Vogel, 2018; Yamamoto, Viale, Roesser, & Lin, 2005). Table 2-1 lists examples of tumor markers.

Radiologic and nuclear medicine imaging techniques play an important part of the evaluation of the presence or extent of disease. These may include x-rays, ultrasound, or computed tomography scans. For an accurate reading of the disease, however, more detailed tests often are required, which may include magnetic resonance imaging or positron-emission tomography scans (Vogel, 2018).

Surgical procedures are used to obtain tissue for histologic examination. The characteristics and location of the tumor determine the approach. Several surgical approaches to obtain tissue samples exist (Davidson, 2014; Lester, 2018):

- Fine needle aspirate—insertion of a small-gauge needle into a mass under local anesthesia to obtain cells or fluid for examination
- Core-needle biopsy—use of a core-cutting needle to remove tissue
- Incisional biopsy—open procedure to remove all or part of a lesion
- Excisional biopsy—open procedure to remove an entire lesion, mass, or lymph node to obtain clear margins
- Diagnostic endoscopy or laparoscopy—technique performed to visualize structures and obtain fluid or tissue samples

Table 2-1. Sample Listing of Tumor Markers

Marker	Type of Cancer	Source	Uses
Alpha-fetoprotein (AFP)	Germ cell tumors, liver cancer	Blood	Diagnosis, prognosis, monitoring
Beta-human chorionic gonadotropin (β-hCG)	Choriocarcinoma, testicular cancer	Urine or blood	Diagnosis, prognosis, monitoring
Cancer antigen 125 (CA-125)	Ovarian cancer	Blood	Monitoring
Carcinoembryonic antigen (CEA)	Colorectal cancer, breast cancer, lung cancer	Blood	Monitoring, prognosis
CD20	Non-Hodgkin lymphoma	Blood	Determination of therapy
Estrogen receptor (ER)/ progesterone receptor (PR)	Breast cancer	Tumor	Determination of endocrine therapy
HER2	Breast cancer, gastric cancer, esophageal cancer	Tumor	Determination of anthracycline and trastuzumab therapy
Immunoglobulins	Multiple myeloma, Waldenström macroglobulinemia	Urine or blood	Monitoring
Lactate dehydrogenase (LDH)	Germ cell tumors	Blood	Diagnosis, staging, prognosis, monitoring
Prostate-specific antigen (PSA)	Prostate cancer	Blood	Screening, monitoring

Note. Based on information from National Cancer Institute, 2015b; Yamamoto et al., 2005.

A pathologist (a physician who specializes in the examination of cells and tissues) studies the cellular and genetic features to obtain the correct diagnosis (NCI, 2010). The pathologist will evaluate both the overall (gross) appearance of the tissue and the cellular (microscopic) data to determine the presence of cancer cells in the tissue and at the margins of the tissue, as well as the cell type and origin. Cells may come from a biopsy, the tumor itself, or fluid obtained from an aspirate. Examples of fluid studied include bone marrow, cerebrospinal fluid, abdominal fluid (ascites), and other sources. Findings are shared with the oncologist through the pathology report (NCI, 2010).

To accurately diagnose and treat cancer, the healthcare team combines information from these sources to accurately identify the type of cancer. The cell type and characteristics, size, location, and biologic behavior are then used to name and treat the disease.

Types of Cancer

Several factors influence the naming of a tumor. Most often, names are generated from the tissue the cells originated from and the biologic behavior of the cells or tumor (Kumar et al., 2015; Vogel, 2018). Benign tumors often are named according to the tissue of origin, adding the suffix of "-oma." An example would be a benign fatty tumor, called a *lipoma*. Malignant tumors also are named according to the tissue they originated from. For example, cancerous tumors developed from solid tissue, such as bone and muscle, are sarcomas. Hematologic cancers are named by the blood cell at their origin, for example, leukemia, which develops from the leukocytes, or white blood cells (see Table 2-2).

Exceptions to these naming patterns exist (Tschanz & Sugarman, 2016). Some cancers are named for the researcher who discovered the cell type, such as Hodgkin lymphoma or Kaposi sarcoma, or by the appearance of the cells under a microscope, such as hairy cell or oat cell. At the cellular level, hundreds of different types of cancer exist, but they are grouped into six major categories: carcinoma, sarcoma, myeloma, leukemia, lymphoma, and mixed types (NCI, n.d.-b).

The process of metastasis involves a cancer cell breaking away from the original tumor and growing in a new location. These cells retain the histologic characteristics of the primary tumor (Eggert, 2018). Therefore, metastasis is identified as a spread of the original tumor. For example, breast cancer that has spread to the lung would be considered breast

Table 2-2. Classification of Malignant Tumors

Classification	Origin	Prefix or Name
Carcinoma	Epithelial	
	• Glandular epithelium	*Adeno-*
	• Squamous epithelium	*Squamous*
Sarcoma	Connective tissue	
	• Bone	*Osteo-*
	• Cartilage	*Chondro-*
	• Fat	*Lipo-*
	• Skeletal muscle	*Rhabdo-*
	• Smooth muscle	*Leiomyo-*
Hematologic	Blood components	
• Leukemia	Hematopoietic cells	
	• Lymphoid origin	*Lympho-*
	• Myeloid origin	*Myelo-*
• Lymphoma	Lymphocytes	*Hodgkin* *Non-Hodgkin*
• Multiple myeloma	Plasma cells	–

Note. Based on information from Kumar et al., 2015; Vogel, 2018.

cancer metastasis to the lung rather than lung cancer.

Staging

Staging is performed to determine the extent of disease following a diagnosis of cancer and serves several purposes. It enables healthcare providers to effectively communicate disease status, assists with the comparison of treatment options between centers, and assists with research by facilitating evaluation of results of treatment and clinical trials. Staging also helps clinicians to determine the patient's prognosis and the appropriate treatment based on the outcomes of similar cases (Asare, Washington, Gress, Gershenwald, & Greene, 2015; Edge et al., 2010).

Several types of staging exist and are performed at different times in the cancer trajectory (Edge et al., 2010). Clinical staging is most common. It is done before treatment begins and is used to help guide treatment options. Clinical staging uses the physical examination, imaging studies, biopsy findings, laboratory results, and other information obtained before the primary treatment begins. Occasionally, the staging will be adjusted based on findings from surgery, after a pathologist studies the resected tissues to provide precise and objective data. This is called pathologic staging. A patient may also be restaged after therapy or neoadjuvant therapy, with retreatment, on recurrence, or by autopsy. Factors such as gender, age, the length of time symptoms have been present, overall health status, type and grade of the cancer, and any unique biologic traits of the cancer also influence staging (Edge et al., 2010).

Although a tumor may change over time, treatment is based on the clinical staging done at diagnosis to better allow for a common language in treatment and research. Cancer registries, such as NCI's Surveillance, Epidemiology, and End Results Program or the National Cancer Database, which is sponsored jointly by the American College of Surgeons and ACS, collect data on staging, treatment, and outcomes (American College of Surgeons, n.d.; NCI, n.d.-a).

The American Joint Committee on Cancer (AJCC) and the Union for International Cancer Control have collaborated to develop and refine the staging system used most widely around the world, called the TNM classification system (Asare et al., 2015; Edge et al., 2010). It comprises three features: the size of the primary or largest tumor, the presence of disease within the lymph nodes, and whether the disease has spread, or metastasized, outside of the original region to other parts of the body (Edge et al., 2010).

- Tumor (T)—tumor size, as measured either through imaging studies or when removed during surgery. The size will determine whether the tumor is T1, T2, T3, or T4. T1 would be the smallest. Tumor size may have a large prognostic implication in breast cancer but little effect in colon cancer.
- Nodes (N)—the extent to which the tumor has spread to regional lymph nodes. N1 would indicate spread, and N3 would be extensive spread.
- Metastasis (M)—the presence or absence of disease spread outside of the original area. It is noted as M0 (no spread) or M1 (the presence of distant metastasis).

While the TNM classification is considered an anatomic measure of disease, some diagnoses use additional nonanatomic information to determine prognosis. Examples of these include tumor markers, tumor location, and surgical margins that included cancer cells between the edge of the tumor and the excision edge (Edge et al., 2010).

Some cancers use other systems to measure the extent of disease to determine diagnosis and treatment. Staging for brain and spinal cord cancers is done using the cell type and grade (NCI, 2015a). Some hematologic malignancies, such as leukemia, use the World

Health Organization classification, which identifies cell lineage and chromosomal abnormalities (Swerdlow et al., 2008). Lymphoma uses the Ann Arbor Staging System, which factors in the patient's age, sex, and laboratory results (Edge et al., 2010). Gynecologic cancers are staged using the International Federation of Gynecology and Obstetrics (known as FIGO) system (Edge et al., 2010; Kato et al., 2012). Figure 2-1 provides examples of staging systems used for various cancer types.

Grading

Tumor grade reflects how closely a tumor resembles the tissue of origin, also known as *differentiation.* A grade 1 tumor is well differentiated and retains many of the behaviors and functions of the normal cells in the tissue of origin. Tumor cells that are well differentiated usually are less aggressive and more responsive to treatment. A grade 3 or 4 tumor is considered poorly differentiated or undifferentiated. The cells are more abnormal and the prognosis is worse (Edge et al., 2010; NCI, 2013; Vogel, 2018). If a site-specific grading system is not identified, the grading system noted in Figure 2-2 generally is used.

Figure 2-1. Staging Systems Used for Various Cancer Types

Brain and Spinal Cord
- World Health Organization

Leukemia
- French-American-British Classification
- World Health Organization

Lymphoma
- Ann Arbor Staging System
- Kiel classification
- Rappaport system
- World Health Organization

Multiple Myeloma
- International Staging System

Gynecologic Cancers
- International Federation of Gynecology and Obstetrics

Childhood Cancers
- Children's Oncology Group

Note. Based on information from Edge et al., 2010; Greipp et al., 2005; Kato et al., 2012; Louis et al., 2007; National Cancer Institute, 2015a; Olsen & Zitella, 2013; Swerdlow et al., 2008.

As the science advances, more precise grading options are becoming available based on specific characteristics of the cancer type (Asare et al., 2015; Edge et al., 2010). Evaluation of a specific cancer may include the nuclear grade, or the mitotic count. The pathologist counts the number of mitoses in the specimen to determine the growth rate of the cancer. Grade also may be based on histologic differences in the cell, as seen with tubule formation in breast cancer (Edge et al., 2010). Grading systems are continually being studied and reevaluated to provide the best information possible (Asare et al., 2015; Edge et al., 2010; Schymura, Sun, & Percy-Laurry, 2014).

The Gleason scoring system used in the grading of prostate cancer is one of the most widely accepted grading systems worldwide (Shah, 2009). When the pathologist reviews tissue samples from a biopsy, several different types of tissue may be present. The two most prevalent tissue patterns are identified and graded. The two grades are added together to obtain the Gleason score. A lower score indicates a less aggressive cancer, whereas a higher score indicates one that is more likely to spread. This information is combined with the anatomic (TNM) staging and the prostate-specific antigen level to determine the best treatment (Edge et al., 2010; Shah, 2009).

Stage Grouping

Once a tumor has been staged according to its size and characteristics, the TNM and grading systems are grouped to provide

Figure 2-2. Staging and Grading

Staging: TNM Classification
T = Tumor
T0—No evidence of primary tumor
Tis—Carcinoma in situ
T1, T2, T3, T4—Increasing size and/or local extension of the primary tumor
TX—Primary tumor cannot be assessed

N = Regional Lymph Nodes
N0—No regional lymph node metastasis
N1, N2, N3—Increasing number or extent of regional lymph node involvement
NX—Regional lymph nodes cannot be assessed

M = Distant Metastasis
M0—No distant metastases
M1—Distant metastases present
MX—Metastasis cannot be measured

Stage Groupings
Stage 0—Carcinoma in situ, also called CIS. Abnormal cells are present but have not spread to nearby tissue. CIS is not cancer, but it may become cancer.
Stage I, stage II, and stage III—The higher the number, the larger the tumor size and the more it has spread into nearby tissues.
Stage IV—The cancer has spread to other parts of the body.

Grading System
GX—Grade cannot be assessed (undetermined grade)
G1—Well differentiated (low grade)
G2—Moderately differentiated (intermediate grade)
G3—Poorly differentiated (high grade)
G4—Undifferentiated (high grade)

Note. Based on information from Edge et al., 2010; National Cancer Institute, 2013, 2015a.

an overall staging level. Smaller tumors with fewer nodes and no metastasis will be staged at a lower number than larger tumors with local or distant spread. A lower stage confers a better prognosis than a higher one. See Figure 2-3 for the AJCC staging criteria for breast cancer.

Using the appropriate staging algorithm, anatomic (TNM) and nonanatomic (tumor markers, histologic data) are combined to determine the overall disease stage (Edge et al., 2010). Cancers of the same type with similar prognoses are grouped based on their assigned TNM categories. Depending on the type of cancer, a higher-numbered group usually holds a worse prognosis. Tumors that remain at the primary site without spread to regional lymph nodes or other parts of the body will usually be assigned as stage I and have a better prognosis. Larger tumors with spread to regional lymph nodes often are classified as stage II or III. If distant metastasis is present, the stage will be IV. These groupings may be further identified as subsets based on prognostic information, such as stage IIA or IIB. A stage 0 may be assigned if the tumor is considered carcinoma in situ, which is an early-stage cancer that has not spread. Grouping classifications may be used by different diseases. For example, colon and rectal cancer may be grouped following the Dukes criteria or the modified Astler-Coller classification, as noted in Table 2-3 (Edge et al., 2010).

Performance Status

In addition to the extent of disease noted, a person's overall health and performance status can significantly influence treatment outcome and will be considered when determining treatment (Tschanz & Sugarman, 2016). Poor performance status has been shown to be a risk for complications following cancer treatment (O'Leary, 2015).

Performance status information reflects how a disease and its treatment affect the patient's day-to-day activities. Performance status describes the level of functioning in terms of a patient's physical activity and ability to care for oneself (ECOG-ACRIN Cancer Research Group, n.d.). Performance scales are used to determine eligibility for treatment and participation in clinical trials. Perfor-

Figure 2-3. Breast Cancer Staging

BREAST STAGING FORM

CLINICAL *Extent of disease before any treatment*	STAGE CATEGORY DEFINITIONS	PATHOLOGIC *Extent of disease through completion of definitive surgery*
❑ y clinical – staging completed after neoadjuvant therapy but before subsequent surgery	TUMOR SIZE: ________ LATERALITY: ☐ left ☐ right ☐ bilateral	❑ y pathologic – staging completed after neoadjuvant therapy AND subsequent surgery
	PRIMARY TUMOR (T)	
❑ TX	Primary tumor cannot be assessed	❑ TX
❑ T0	No evidence of primary tumor	❑ T0
❑ Tis	Carcinoma *in situ*	❑ Tis
❑ Tis (DCIS)	Ductal carcinoma *in situ*	❑ Tis (DCIS)
❑ Tis (LCIS)	Lobular carcinoma *in situ*	❑ Tis (LCIS)
❑ Tis (Paget's)	Paget's disease of the nipple is NOT associated with invasive carcinoma and/or carcinoma *in situ* (DCIS and/or LCIS) in the underlying breast parenchyma. Carcinomas in the breast parenchyma associated with Paget's disease are categorized based on the size and characteristics of the parenchymal disease, although the presence of Paget's disease should still be noted	❑ Tis (Paget's)
❑ T1	Tumor ≤ 20 mm in greatest dimension	❑ T1
❑ T1mi	Tumor ≤ 1 mm in greatest dimension	❑ T1mi
❑ T1a	Tumor > 1 mm but ≤ 5 mm in greatest dimension	❑ T1a
❑ T1b	Tumor > 5 mm but ≤ 10 mm in greatest dimension	❑ T1b
❑ T1c	Tumor > 10 mm but ≤ 20 mm in greatest dimension	❑ T1c
❑ T2	Tumor > 20 mm but ≤ 50 mm in greatest dimension	❑ T2
❑ T3	Tumor > 50 mm in greatest dimension	❑ T3
❑ T4	Tumor of any size with direct extension to the chest wall and/or to the skin (ulceration or skin nodules)*	❑ T4
❑ T4a	Extension to the chest wall, not including only pectoralis muscle adherence/invasion	❑ T4a
❑ T4b	Ulceration and/or ipsilateral satellite nodules and/or edema (including peau d'orange) of the skin which do not meet the criteria for inflammatory carcinoma	❑ T4b
❑ T4c	Both T4a and T4b	❑ T4c
❑ T4d	Inflammatory carcinoma**	❑ T4d
	**Note*: Invasion of the dermis alone does not qualify as T4. ***Note:* Inflammatory carcinoma is restricted to cases with typical skin changes involving a third or more of the skin of the breast. While the histologic presence of invasive carcinoma invading dermal lymphatics is supportive of the diagnosis, it is not required, nor is dermal lymphatic invasion without typical clinical findings sufficient for a diagnosis of inflammatory breast cancer.	
	REGIONAL LYMPH NODES (N)	
❑ NX	Regional lymph nodes cannot be assessed (e.g., previously removed)	NX
pNX	Regional lymph nodes cannot be assessed (e.g., previously removed, or not removed for pathologic study)	❑ pNX*
❑ N0	No regional lymph node metastases	N0
pN0	No regional lymph node metastasis identified histologically	❑ pN0
pN0(i-)	No regional lymph node metastases histologically, negative IHC	❑ pN0(i-)
pN0(i+)	Malignant cells in regional lymph node(s) no greater than 0.2 mm (detected by H&E or IHC including ITC)	❑ pN0(i+)
pN0(mol-)	No regional lymph node metastases histologically, negative molecular findings (RT-PCR)	❑ pN0(mol-)
pN0(mol+)	Positive molecular findings (RT-PCR), but no regional lymph node metastases detected by histology or IHC	❑ pN0(mol+)

HOSPITAL NAME/ADDRESS	PATIENT NAME/INFORMATION

(Continued on next page)

Figure 2-3. Breast Cancer Staging *(Continued)*

BREAST STAGING FORM

❑	N1	Metastases to movable ipsilateral level I, II axillary lymph node(s)	N1
	pN1	Micrometastases; or metastases in 1 to 3 axillary lymph nodes; and/or in internal mammary nodes with metastases detected by sentinel lymph node biopsy but not clinically detected**	❑ pN1
	pN1mi	Micrometastases (greater than 0.2 mm and/or more than 200 cells, but none greater than 2.0 mm)	❑ pN1mi
	pN1a	Metastases in 1 to 3 axillary lymph nodes, at least one metastasis greater than 2.0 mm	❑ pN1a
	pN1b	Metastases in internal mammary nodes with micrometastases or macrometastases detected by sentinel lymph node biopsy but not clinically detected**	❑ pN1b
	pN1c	Metastases in 1 to 3 axillary lymph nodes and in internal mammary lymph nodes with micrometastases or macrometastases detected by sentinel lymph node biopsy but not clinically detected**	❑ pN1c
❑	N2	Metastases in ipsilateral level I, II axillary lymph nodes that are clinically fixed or matted; or in clinically detected* ipsilateral internal mammary nodes in the *absence* of clinically evident axillary lymph node metastases	
	pN2	Metastases in 4 to 9 axillary lymph nodes; or in clinically detected*** internal mammary lymph nodes in the *absence* of axillary lymph node metastases	❑ pN2
❑	N2a	Metastases in ipsilateral axillary lymph nodes fixed to one another (matted) or to other structures	
	pN2a	Metastases in 4 to 9 axillary lymph nodes (at least one tumor deposit greater than 2.0 mm)	❑ pN2a
❑	N2b	Metastases only in clinically detected*** ipsilateral internal mammary nodes and in the *absence* of clinically evident axillary lymph node metastases	
	pN2b	Metastases in clinically detected*** internal mammary lymph nodes in the *absence* of axillary lymph node metastases	❑ pN2b
❑	N3	Metastases in ipsilateral infraclavicular (level III axillary) lymph node(s) with or without level I, II axillary lymph node involvement; or in clinically detected* ipsilateral internal mammary lymph node(s) with clinically evident level I, II axillary lymph node metastases; or metastases in ipsilateral supraclavicular lymph node(s) with or without axillary or internal mammary lymph node involvement	
	pN3	Metastases in 10 or more axillary lymph nodes; or in infraclavicular (level III axillary) lymph nodes; or in clinically detected*** ipsilateral internal mammary lymph nodes in the *presence* of 1 or more positive level I, II axillary lymph nodes; or in more than 3 axillary lymph nodes and in internal mammary lymph nodes with micrometastases or macrometastases detected by sentinel lymph node biopsy but not clinically detected**; or in ipsilateral supraclavicular lymph nodes	❑ pN3
❑	N3a	Metastases in ipsilateral infraclavicular lymph node(s)	
	pN3a	Metastases in 10 or more axillary lymph nodes (at least one tumor deposit greater than 2.0 mm); or metastases to the infraclavicular (level III axillary lymph) nodes	❑ pN3a
❑	N3b	Metastases in ipsilateral internal mammary lymph node(s) and axillary lymph node(s)	
	pN3b	Metastases in clinically detected*** ipsilateral internal mammary lymph nodes in the *presence* of 1 or more positive axillary lymph nodes; or in more than 3 axillary lymph nodes and in internal mammary lymph nodes with micrometastases or macrometastases detected by sentinel lymph node biopsy but not clinically detected**	❑ pN3b
❑	N3c	Metastases in ipsilateral supraclavicular lymph node(s)	

HOSPITAL NAME/ADDRESS	PATIENT NAME/INFORMATION

(Continued on next page)

Figure 2-3. Breast Cancer Staging *(Continued)*

BREAST STAGING FORM

pN3c	Metastases in ipsilateral supraclavicular lymph nodes *Classification is based on axillary lymph node dissection with or without sentinel lymph node biopsy. Classification based solely on sentinel lymph node biopsy without subsequent axillary lymph node dissection is designated (sn) for "sentinel node," for example, pN0(sn). ***Note: Not clinically detected* is defined as not detected by imaging studies (excluding lymphoscintigraphy) or not detected by clinical examination. ****Note: Clinically detected* is defined as detected by imaging studies (excluding lymphoscintigraphy) or by clinical examination and having characteristics highly suspicious for malignancy or a presumed pathologic macrometastasis based on fine needle aspiration biopsy with cytologic examination. Confirmation of clinically detected metastatic disease by fine needle aspiration without excision biopsy is designated with an (f) suffix, for example, cN3a(f). Excisional biopsy of a lymph node or biopsy of a sentinel node, in the absence of assignment of a pT, is classified as a clinical N, for example, cN1. Information regarding the confirmation of the nodal status will be designated in sitespecific factors as clinical, fine needle aspiration, core biopsy, or sentinel lymph node biopsy. Pathologic classification (pN) is used for excision or sentinel lymph node biopsy only in conjunction with a pathologic T assignment. *Note:* Isolated tumor cell clusters (ITC) are defined as small clusters of cells not greater than 0.2 mm, or single tumor cells, or a cluster of fewer than 200 cells in a single histologic cross-section. ITCs may be detected by routine histology or by immunohistochemical (IHC) methods. Nodes containing only ITCs are excluded from the total positive node count for purposes of N classification but should be included in the total number of nodes evaluated	☐ pN3c
	DISTANT METASTASIS (M)	
☐ M0	No clinical or radiographic evidence of distant metastases (no pathologic M0; use clinical M to complete stage group)	
☐ cM0(i+)	No clinical or radiographic evidence of distant metastases, but deposits of molecularly or microscopically detected tumor cells in circulating blood, bone marrow or other non-regional nodal tissue that are no larger than 0.2 mm in a patient without symptoms or signs of metastases	
☐ M1	Distant detectable metastases as determined by classic clinical and radiographic means and/or histologically proven larger than 0.2 mm	☐ M1

HOSPITAL NAME/ADDRESS	PATIENT NAME/INFORMATION

(Continued on next page)

Figure 2-3. Breast Cancer Staging *(Continued)*

BREAST STAGING FORM

ANATOMIC STAGE • PROGNOSTIC GROUPS

CLINICAL

GROUP	T	N	M
❑ 0	Tis	N0	M0
❑ IA	T1*	N0	M0
❑ IB	T0	N1mi	M0
	T1*	N1mi	M0
❑ IIA	T0	N1**	M0
	T1*	N1**	M0
	T2	N0	M0
❑ IIB	T2	N1	M0
	T3	N0	M0
❑ IIIA	T0	N2	M0
	T1*	N2	M0
	T2	N2	M0
	T3	N1	M0
	T3	N2	M0
❑ IIIB	T4	N0	M0
	T4	N1	M0
	T4	N2	M0
❑ Stage IIIC	Any T	N3	M0
❑ Stage IV	Any T	Any N	M1

* T1 includes T1mi
** T0 and T1 tumors with nodal micrometastases only are excluded from Stage IIA and are classified Stage IB.

❑ Stage unknown

PATHOLOGIC

GROUP	T	N	M
❑ 0	Tis	N0	M0
❑ IA	T1*	N0	M0
❑ IB	T0	N1mi	M0
	T1*	N1mi	M0
❑ IIA	T0	N1**	M0
	T1*	N1**	M0
	T2	N0	M0
❑ IIB	T2	N1	M0
	T3	N0	M0
❑ IIIA	T0	N2	M0
	T1*	N2	M0
	T2	N2	M0
	T3	N1	M0
	T3	N2	M0
❑ IIIB	T4	N0	M0
	T4	N1	M0
	T4	N2	M0
❑ Stage IIIC	Any T	N3	M0
❑ Stage IV	Any T	Any N	M1

* T1 includes T1mi
** T0 and T1 tumors with nodal micrometastases only are excluded from Stage IIA and are classified Stage IB.

❑ Stage unknown

PROGNOSTIC FACTORS (SITE-SPECIFIC FACTORS)

REQUIRED FOR STAGING: None

CLINICALLY SIGNIFICANT:

Paget's disease: ____________________

Tumor grade (Scarff-Bloom-Richardson system): ____________________

Estrogen receptor and test method (IHC, RT-PCR, other): ____________________

Progesterone receptor and test method (IHC, RT-PCR, other): ____________________

HER2 status and test method (IHC, FISH, CISH, RT-PCR, other): ____________________

Method of lymph node assessment (e.g., clinical, fine needle aspiration; core biopsy; sentinel lymph node biopsy): ____________________

IHC of regional lymph nodes: ____________________

Molecular studies of regional lymph nodes: ____________________

Distant metastases method of detection (clinical, radiographic, biopsy): ____________________

Circulating Tumor Cells (CTC) and method of detection (RT-PCR, immunomagnetic separation, other): ____________________

Disseminated Tumor Cells (DTC; bone marrow micrometastases) and method of detection (RT-PCR, immunohistochemical, other): ____________________

Multi-gene signature score: ____________________

Response to neoadjuvant therapy will be collected in the registry but does not affect the post-neoadjuvant stage: ____________________

General Notes:
For identification of special cases of TNM or pTNM classifications, the "m" suffix and "y," "r," and "a" prefixes are used. Although they do not affect the stage grouping, they indicate cases needing separate analysis.

m suffix indicates the presence of multiple primary tumors in a single site and is recorded in parentheses: pT(m)NM.

y prefix indicates those cases in which classification is performed during or following initial multimodality therapy. The cTNM or pTNM category is identified by a "y" prefix. The ycTNM or ypTNM categorizes the extent of tumor actually present at the time of that examination. The "y" categorization is not an estimate of tumor prior to multimodality therapy.

r prefix indicates a recurrent tumor when staged after a disease-free interval, and is identified by the "r" prefix: rTNM.

a prefix designates the stage determined at autopsy: aTNM.

HOSPITAL NAME/ADDRESS	PATIENT NAME/INFORMATION

(Continued on next page)

Figure 2-3. Breast Cancer Staging *(Continued)*

BREAST STAGING FORM

Histologic Grade (G) *(also known as overall grade)*

Grading system	***Grade***
❑ 2 grade system	❑ Grade I or 1
❑ 3 grade system	❑ Grade II or 2
❑ 4 grade system	❑ Grade III or 3
❑ No 2, 3, or 4 grade system is available	❑ Grade IV or 4

ADDITIONAL DESCRIPTORS

Lymphatic Vessel Invasion (L) and Venous Invasion (V) have been combined into Lymph-Vascular Invasion (LVI) for collection by cancer registrars. The College of American Pathologist (CAP) Checklist should be used as the primary source. Other sources may be used in the absence of a Checklist. Priority is given to positive results.

❑ Lymph-Vascular Invasion Not Present (absent)/Not Identified
❑ Lymph-Vascular Invasion Present/Identified
❑ Not Applicable
❑ Unknown/Indeterminate

Residual Tumor (R)

The absence or presence of residual tumor after treatment. In some cases treated with surgery and/or with neoadjuvant therapy there will be residual tumor at the primary site after treatment because of incomplete resection or local and regional disease thatextends beyond the limit of ability of resection.

❑ RX Presence of residual tumor cannot be assessed
❑ R0 No residual tumor
❑ R1 Microscopic residual tumor
❑ R2 Macroscopic residual tumor

General Notes (continued):

surgical margins is data field recorded by registrars describing the surgical margins of the resected primary site specimen as determined only by the pathology report.

neoadjuvant treatment is radiation therapy or systemic therapy (consisting of chemotherapy, hormone therapy, or immunotherapy) administered prior to a definitive surgical procedure. If the surgical procedure is not performed, the administered therapy no longer meets the definition of neoadjuvant therapy.

❑ Clinical stage was used in treatment planning (describe): ______________________

❑ National guidelines were used in treatment planning ❑ NCCN ❑ Other (describe): ______________________

____

Physician signature ______________________ Date/Time ______________________

HOSPITAL NAME/ADDRESS	PATIENT NAME/INFORMATION

(Continued on next page)

Figure 2-3. Breast Cancer Staging *(Continued)*

BREAST STAGING FORM

Illustration

Indicate on diagram primary tumor and regional nodes involved.

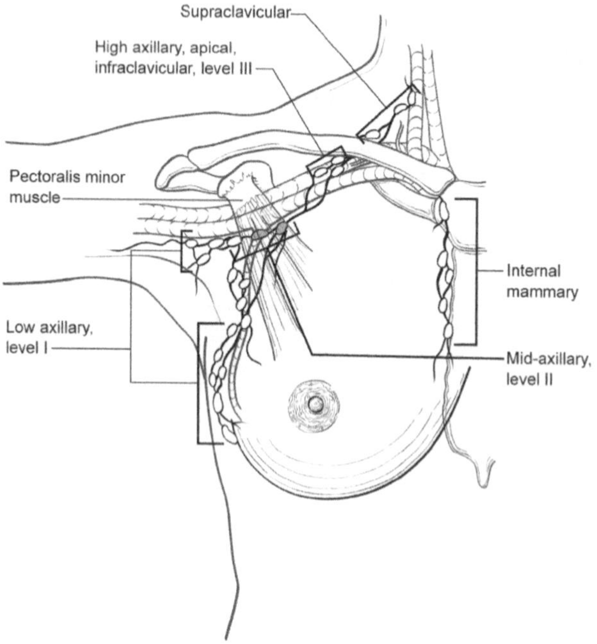

HOSPITAL NAME/ADDRESS	PATIENT NAME/INFORMATION

Note. From *AJCC Cancer Staging Manual* (7th ed., pp. 32-1–32-6), by S.B. Edge, D.R. Byrd, C.C. Compton, A.G. Fritz, F.L. Greene, and A. Trotti III (Eds.), 2010, New York, NY: Springer Science and Business Media, www.springer.com. Copyright 2010 by American Joint Committee on Cancer. Reprinted with permission of the American Joint Committee on Cancer, Chicago, Illinois.

Table 2-3. Comparison of Prognostic Groups in Colon and Rectal Cancer Staging

Stage	T	N	M	Dukes*	MAC*
0	Tis	N0	M0	–	–
I	T1	N0	M0	A	A
	T2	N0	M0	A	B1
IIA	T3	N0	M0	B	B2
IIB	T4a	N0	M0	B	B2
IIC	T4b	N0	M0	B	B3
IIIA	T1–T2	N1/N1c	M0	C	C1
	T1	N2a	M0	C	C1
IIIB	T3–T4a	N1/N1c	M0	C	C2
	T2–T3	N2a	M0	C	C1/C2
	T1–T2	N2b	M0	C	C1
IIIC	T4a	N2a	M0	C	C2
	T3–T4a	N2b	M0	C	C2
	T4b	N1–N2	M0	C	C3
IVA	Any T	Any N	M1a	–	–
IVB	Any T	Any N	M1b	–	–

Note: cTNM is the clinical classification, pTNM is the pathologic classification. The y prefix is used for those cancers that are classified after neoadjuvant pretreatment (e.g., ypTNM). Patients who have a complete pathologic response are ypT0N0cM0 that may be similar to Stage Group 0 or 1. The r prefix is to be used for those cancers that have recurred after a disease-free interval (rTNM).

* Dukes B is a composite of better (T3 N0 M0) and worse (T4 N0 M0) prognostic groups, as is Dukes C (Any T N1 M0 and Any T N2 M0). MAC is the modified Astler-Coller classification.

Note. From *AJCC Cancer Staging Manual* (7th ed., p. 155), by S.B. Edge, D.R. Byrd, C.C. Compton, A.G. Fritz, F.L. Greene, and A. Trotti III (Eds.), 2010, New York, NY: Springer Science and Business Media, www.springer.com. Copyright 2010 by American Joint Committee on Cancer. Reprinted with permission of the American Joint Committee on Cancer, Chicago, Illinois.

mance status also should be checked periodically to monitor response to the disease and treatment (Vogel, 2018). Two common measures of performance status are the Karnofsky Performance Status scale and the Eastern Cooperative Oncology Group performance status scale (see Figure 2-4).

Nursing Implications

Nurses are in an ideal position to support patients during the often confusing and frightening time of cancer diagnosis and staging. Explaining the tests and studies in the diagnostic workup, interpreting the medical terminology used in cancer care, and providing education and support for the steps to come with cancer treatment can have a significant impact on the patient experience.

Nursing assessment and knowledge of the patient's ability to complete daily activities can add objective information to the performance status (Vogel, 2018). Nurses should begin with a baseline assessment of performance status and reassess with each visit to monitor the impact and tolerance of treatment.

Conclusion

Cancer staging is an essential step in the treatment of cancer. Information gathered during the diagnostic workup, including the history and physical, laboratory and imaging tests, and pathologic examination of tissue samples, provides the data needed to accurately diagnose the illness. Ongoing collaboration between AJCC and the Union for International Cancer Control on accurate staging and data collection will continue to serve as a means to communicate disease staging clearly and provide the best opportunity for effective treatment.

Nurses can serve as a resource and guide through the diagnostic and staging experience by providing patient and family education, clarifying confusing information, and documenting assessment of patient status.

Figure 2-4. Comparison of Performance Scales

ECOG Performance Status	Karnofsky Performance Status
0—Fully active, able to carry on all predisease performance without restriction	100—Normal, no complaints; no evidence of disease 90—Able to carry on normal activity; minor signs or symptoms of disease
1—Restricted in physically strenuous activity but ambulatory and able to carry out work of a light or sedentary nature, e.g., light house work, office work	80—Normal activity with effort, some signs or symptoms of disease 70—Cares for self but unable to carry on normal activity or to do active work
2—Ambulatory and capable of all self-care but unable to carry out any work activities; up and about more than 50% of waking hours	60—Requires occasional assistance but is able to care for most of personal needs 50—Requires considerable assistance and frequent medical care
3—Capable of only limited self-care; confined to bed or chair more than 50% of waking hours	40—Disabled; requires special care and assistance 30—Severely disabled; hospitalization is indicated although death not imminent
4—Completely disabled; cannot carry on any self-care; totally confined to bed or chair	20—Very ill; hospitalization and active supportive care necessary 10—Moribund
5—Dead	0—Dead

Karnofsky D, Burchenal J, The clinical evaluation of chemotherapeutic agents in cancer. In: MacLeod C, ed. *Evaluation of Chemotherapeutic Agents.* New York, NY: Columbia University Press; 1949:191–205.
Zubrod C, et al. Appraisal of methods for the study of chemotherapy in man: Comparative therapeutic trial of nitrogen mustard and thiophosphoramide. *Journal of Chronic Diseases*; 1960:11:7-33.

ECOG—Eastern Cooperative Oncology Group

Note. From "ECOG Performance Status," by ECOG-ACRIN Cancer Research Group, n.d. Retrieved from http://ecog-acrin.org/resources/ecog-performance-status.

Key Points

- Diagnosis of a benign tumor usually has a more favorable prognosis than a malignant tumor.
- Accurate diagnosis and staging will help to determine the best treatment for cancer.
- A diagnostic workup for cancer may include physical examination, laboratory tests, radiology studies, and tissue samples.
- Cancer staging is performed at diagnosis to determine the prognosis and best treatment.
- Tumor-node-metastasis, or TNM, classification is based on tumor size, regional lymph node involvement, and the distant spread of cancer cells.
- Grading identifies the similarity of cancer cells to normal cells and helps to determine the aggressiveness of a tumor.
- Performance status is one way to measure how a disease or treatment is affecting an individual.

The author would like to acknowledge Julia Eggert, PhD, RN, AGN-BC, GNP, AOCN®, FAAN, for her contribution to this chapter that remains unchanged from the first edition of this book.

References

American Cancer Society. (2014, June 12). The history of cancer. Retrieved from http://www.cancer.org/acs/groups/cid/documents/webcontent/002048-pdf.pdf

American Cancer Society. (2015, December 8). What is cancer? Retrieved from http://www.cancer.org/cancer/cancerbasics/what-is-cancer

American College of Surgeons. (n.d.). National Cancer Database. Retrieved from https://www.facs.org/quality%20programs/cancer/ncdb

Asare, E.A., Washington, M.K., Gress, D.M., Gershenwald, J.E., & Greene, F.L. (2015). Improving the quality of cancer staging. *CA: A Cancer Journal for Clinicians, 65,* 261–263. doi:10.3322/caac.21284

Davidson, G.W. (2014). Overview. In G.W. Davidson, J.L. Lester, & M. Routt (Eds.), *Surgical oncology nursing* (pp. 1–11). Pittsburgh, PA: Oncology Nursing Society.

ECOG-ACRIN Cancer Research Group. (n.d.). ECOG performance status. Retrieved from http://ecog-acrin.org/resources/ecog-performance-status

Edge, S.B., Byrd, D.R., Compton, C.C., Fritz, A.G., Greene, F.L., & Trotti, A., III. (Eds.). (2010). *AJCC cancer staging manual* (7th ed.). Chicago, IL: Springer.

Eggert, J.A. (2018). Biology of cancer. In C.H. Yarbro, D. Wujcik, & B.H. Gobel (Eds.), *Cancer nursing: Principles and practice* (8th ed., pp. 3–24). Burlington, MA: Jones & Bartlett Learning.

Febbo, P.G., Ladanyi, M., Aldape, K.D., De Marzo, A.M., Hammond, E., Hayes, D.F., ... Birkeland, M.L. (2011). NCCN Task Force report: Evaluating the clinical utility of tumor markers in oncology. *Journal of the National Comprehensive Cancer Network, 9*(Suppl. 5), S1–S32. Retrieved from http://www.jnccn.org/content/9/Suppl_5/S-1.long

Greipp, P.R., San Miguel, J., Durie, B.G.M., Crowley, J.J., Barlogie, B., Bladé, J., ... Westin, J. (2005). International Staging System for multiple myeloma. *Journal of Clinical Oncology, 23,* 3412–3420. doi:10.1200/JCO.2005.04.242

Kato, T., Watari, H., Endo, D., Mitamura, T., Odagiri, T., Konno, Y., ... Sakuragi, N. (2012). New revised FIGO 2008 staging system for endometrial cancer produces better discrimination in survival compared with 1988 staging system. *Journal of Surgical Oncology, 106,* 938–941. doi:10.1002/jso.23203

Kumar, V., Abbas, A.K., & Aster, J.C. (2015). Neoplasia. In V. Kumar, A.K. Abbas, & J.C. Aster (Eds.), *Robbins and Cotran pathologic basis of disease* (9th ed., pp. 265–340). Philadelphia, PA: Elsevier Saunders.

Lester, J. (2018). Surgical oncology. In C.H. Yarbro, D. Wujcik, & B.H. Gobel (Eds.), *Cancer nursing: Principles and practice* (8th ed., pp. 243–266). Burlington, MA: Jones & Bartlett Learning.

Louis, D.N., Ohgaki, H., Wiestler, O.D., Cavenee, W.K., Burger, P.C., Jouvet, A., ... Kleihues, P. (2007). The 2007 WHO classification of tumours of the central nervous system. *Acta Neuropathologica, 114,* 97–109. doi:10.1007/s00401-007-0243-4

National Cancer Institute. (n.d.-a). Overview of the SEER program. Retrieved from http://seer.cancer.gov/about/overview.html

National Cancer Institute. (n.d.-b). SEER training modules: Cancer classification. Retrieved from http://training.seer.cancer.gov/disease/categories/classification.html

National Cancer Institute. (2010, September 23). Pathology reports. Retrieved from https://www.cancer.gov/about-cancer/diagnosis-staging/diagnosis/pathology-reports-fact-sheet

National Cancer Institute. (2013, May 3). Tumor grade. Retrieved from http://www.cancer.gov/about-cancer/diagnosis-staging/prognosis/tumor-grade-fact-sheet

National Cancer Institute. (2015a, March 9). Staging. Retrieved from http://www.cancer.gov/about-cancer/diagnosis-staging/staging

National Cancer Institute. (2015b, November 4). Tumor markers. Retrieved from http://www.cancer.gov/about-cancer/diagnosis-staging/diagnosis/tumor-markers-fact-sheet

National Cancer Institute. (2015c, February 9). What is cancer? Retrieved from http://www.cancer.gov/about-cancer/what-is-cancer

O'Leary, C. (2015). Neutropenia and infection. In C.G. Brown (Ed.), *A guide to oncology symptom management* (2nd ed., pp. 483–504). Pittsburgh, PA: Oncology Nursing Society.

Olsen, M., & Zitella, L.J. (Eds.). (2013). *Hematologic malignancies in adults.* Pittsburgh, PA: Oncology Nursing Society.

Schymura, M.J., Sun, L., & Percy-Laurry, A. (2014). Prostate cancer collaborative stage data items—their definitions, quality, usage, and clinical implications: A review of SEER data for 2004–2010. *Cancer, 120*(Suppl. 23), 3758–3770. doi:10.1002/cncr.29052

Shah, R.B. (2009). Current perspectives on the Gleason grading of prostate cancer. *Archives of Pathology and Laboratory Medicine, 133,* 1810–1816.

Swerdlow, S.H., Campo, E., Harris, N.L., Jaffe, E.S., Pileri, S.A., Stein, H., ... Vardiman, J.W. (Eds.). (2008). *WHO classification of tumours of haematopoietic and lymphoid tissues* (4th ed.). Lyon, France: IARC Press.

Tschanz, J.A., & Sugarman, C. (2016). Carcinogenesis. In J.K. Itano (Ed.), *Core curriculum for oncology nursing* (5th ed., pp. 24–38). St. Louis, MO: Elsevier.

Vogel, W.H. (2018). Diagnostic evaluation, classification, and staging. In C.H. Yarbro, D. Wujcik, & B.H. Gobel (Eds.), *Cancer nursing: Principles and practice* (8th ed., pp. 169–203). Burlington, MA: Jones & Bartlett Learning.

Yamamoto, D.S., Viale, P.H., Roesser, K., & Lin, A. (2005). The clinical use of tumor markers in select cancers: Are you confident enough to discuss them with your patients? *Oncology Nursing Forum, 32,* 1013–1025. doi:10.1188/05.ONF.1013-1025

Chapter 2 Study Questions

1. A woman treated for stage III breast cancer is found to have cancer cells in her liver. Which of the following diagnoses would be correct?
   A. Breast cancer with metastasis to the liver
   B. Liver cancer of breast origin
   C. Metastatic liver cancer
   D. Metastatic cancer of unknown primary

2. Which of the following will determine a cancer diagnosis?
   A. Pathologic examination of biopsy cells
   B. Positron-emission tomography–computed tomography scan
   C. Fine needle aspirate
   D. Measure of CA-125 levels

3. Which of the following cancer types is most likely to be staged using the TNM classification?
   A. Multiple myeloma
   B. Lung cancer
   C. Non-Hodgkin lymphoma
   D. Ovarian cancer

4. Which of the following is consistent with a tumor considered "well differentiated"?
   A. Most often grade 3 or 4
   B. Cells retain behavior of the tissue of origin
   C. Poor prognosis
   D. Grossly abnormal appearance

5. Which of the following is true of performance status?
   A. Reflects the impact of the treatment on the disease
   B. May be used to diagnose cancer
   C. If poor, may lead to metastatic disease
   D. May influence treatment decisions

CHAPTER

3 Cancer Epidemiology and Prevention

Suzanne M. Mahon, RN, DNSc, AOCN®, AGN-BC

Introduction

Although great strides have been made in reducing the morbidity and mortality associated with the diagnosis, cancer remains a significant health problem. More than 1.6 million cancers are diagnosed annually and an estimated 1,600 people die daily from cancer, accounting for one out of every four deaths in the United States (American Cancer Society [ACS], 2016b). Ideally, cancer is prevented or detected early, when treatment is most likely to be effective and less toxic to the patient. This chapter will provide an overview of basic cancer epidemiology, concepts related to risk assessment, and strategies to promote cancer prevention.

Epidemiology is defined as the study of how disease is distributed in a population, factors that influence its distribution in a population, and trends over time. The goals of epidemiology are shown in Figure 3-1. The study of epidemiology encompasses not only the basis of disease but also the impact of treatment, screening, and preventive measures on the natural history of the disease (Gordis, 2014). Instead of focusing on a single patient, epidemiology typically centers on identifying the exposure or source that caused the illness, the number of other individuals who may have been similarly exposed, the potential for further spread in the community, and interventions to prevent additional cases or recurrences (Centers for Disease Control and Prevention, 2012). An understanding of epidemiology is critical to understanding the biology of a disease and possible risk factors and, ultimately, to developing prevention, detection, and treatment strategies.

Figure 3-1. Goals of Epidemiologic Studies

- Study the natural history of disease.
- Determine the extent of disease in a community, region, or defined area.
- Identify potential etiologic sources of a disease and risk factors for the disease.
- Study the prognosis of the disease with and without treatment or intervention.
- Evaluate both existing and new prevention and treatment measures and methods of healthcare delivery.
- Quantify and describe risk factors for a disease.
- Examine the cost-effectiveness of various prevention and treatment strategies.
- Identify disparities in access to care in defined populations.
- Provide accurate data for the basis for public health policy and regulatory decisions regarding healthcare spending and environmental issues.

Note. Based on information from Centers for Disease Control and Prevention, 2012; Gordis, 2014.

Epidemiologic studies have demonstrated that illness, disease, or poor health care are not necessarily random events. Some people have factors that place them at risk for developing disease (ACS, 2014, 2015a, 2015b, 2015c, 2016a, 2016b, 2016c). Thus, risk assessment is a significant component of epidemiology and ultimately directs the science of cancer prevention and early detection.

Epidemiologic Terms and Concepts

Incidence

The *incidence* of cancer is the number of cancers that develop in a population during a defined period, such as a year. *Prevalence* is the number of cancers that exist in a population, including diagnosed and undiagnosed cancers. For example, ACS (2016b) estimated that 246,660 women will be diagnosed with invasive breast cancer and an estimated additional 61,000 women will be diagnosed with in situ breast cancer in the United States in 2016. Incidence numbers can be helpful when trying to understand what overall portion of the general population is at risk for developing a specific cancer. The four most common cancers diagnosed in the United States, excluding basal cell and squamous cell skin cancers, are cancers of the lung, breast, prostate, and colon (ACS, 2016b).

Mortality

The *mortality rate* is the number of people who die of a particular cancer during a defined period. For example, the estimated mortality for breast cancer for women in 2016 is 40,890 deaths, which is 15% of all cancer deaths in women in the United States (ACS, 2016b). For men, the cancers associated with the highest mortality are those of the lung, prostate, and colon. For women, the highest mortality rates are associated with cancers of the lung, breast, and colon. These four cancers account for half of the total cancer deaths in the United States among men and women (ACS, 2016b). Mortality rates provide insight into the strengths of early detection measures for a particular cancer and the effectiveness of current standard therapies. If an incidence rate is high and a mortality rate is low, the implication is that there is a means to detect the malignancy early or there is effective treatment. If the incidence and mortality rates are similar, it might be concluded that there are limited means for early detection or limited options for effective treatment. Current estimates are that one in four Americans dies of cancer or complications related to cancer (ACS, 2016b).

Sources of Epidemiologic Information

ACS publishes projected incidence and mortality rates for common cancers in its annual *Cancer Facts and Figures* publications (ACS, 2014, 2015a, 2015b, 2016a, 2016b). Figure 3-2 shows examples of data that oncology nurses might find useful regarding the major cancer sites. Incidence and mortality figures also are readily available through the Surveillance, Epidemiology, and End Results (SEER) Program, which updates data continually at http://seer.cancer.gov. Data from the SEER geographic areas are used to represent an estimated 28% of the U.S. population (National Cancer Institute, n.d.). The database contains information on more than 86,355,485 cases diagnosed since 1973, and the data can be viewed in multiple ways, including over time as shown in Figure 3-3 through Figure 3-8. The data are viewable in many formats, including by trends and state or geographic areas, which often makes it easier to discuss risk of a specific cancer or cancers with both the public and other healthcare providers. ACS and SEER data can be extremely beneficial when planning programs, conducting educational presentations, providing indi-

Figure 3-2. Selected Epidemiologic Facts About the Major Cancers

Breast Cancer

- 246,660 estimated new cases of invasive cancer and 61,000 new cases of in situ breast cancer occur annually in women.
- 2,600 estimated new cases occur annually in men.
- Breast cancer is the most frequently diagnosed cancer in women.
- 40,450 estimated deaths occur annually (second leading cause of cancer death in women).
- 61% of new cases are diagnosed at a localized stage, for which the 5-year relative survival rate is 99%.
- The 5-year survival rates are 85% for regional-stage cancer and 25% for metastatic disease.
- For all stages combined, the 5-, 10-, and 15-year relative survival rates for breast cancer are 89%, 83%, and 78%, respectively.

Cervical Cancer

- 12,990 estimated new cases occur annually; incidence rates are decreasing gradually in all races.
- 4,120 estimated deaths occur annually.
- Almost half of patients (46%) are diagnosed when the cancer is localized, for which the 5-year survival is 92%.
- Cervical cancer is more often diagnosed at a localized stage in Caucasians (48%) than in African Americans (39%) and in women younger than 50 years old (59%) than in women 50 or older (33%).

Colorectal Cancer

- 95,270 estimated new cases of colon cancer and 39,220 estimated new cases of rectal cancer occur annually.
- It is the third most common cancer in men and women.
- 49,190 estimated deaths occur annually, accounting for 9% of all cancer deaths.
- It is the third most common cause of cancer mortality in men and women.
- More than 1.25 million Americans are alive with a history of colorectal cancer.
- Incidence rates have dropped in the past two decades, which is attributed to increased screening and removal of colorectal polyps.
- The 5-year survival rate for localized cancer is 90%, but only 39% of cancers are diagnosed at this stage.
- The 5-year survival rate for metastatic disease is 13%.

Leukemia

- 60,140 estimated new cases occur annually.
- 91% of cases are diagnosed in adults aged 20 years and older.
- An estimated 24,400 deaths occur annually.
- Overall 5-year survival rate is 26% for acute myeloid leukemia and 84% for chronic lymphocytic leukemia.

Lung Cancer

- 224,390 estimated new cases occur annually.
- Lung cancer is responsible for 14% of all cancer diagnoses.
- Incidence rate is decreasing by 3% per year in men and 2.2% per year in women.
- The probability of developing invasive lung cancer is 7.4 for men (1 in 13 men) and 6.2 for women (1 in 16 women).
- 158,080 estimated deaths occur annually (27% of all cancer deaths).
- With fewer people smoking, the mortality rate from lung cancer is slowly dropping.
- The 1-year survival rate is 44%, and the 5-year survival rate is 17%.
- Only 16% of cases are diagnosed at the localized stage.

Lymphoma

- 81,080 estimated new cases occur annually (72,580 cases of non-Hodgkin lymphoma and 8,500 cases of Hodgkin lymphoma).
- 21,279 estimated deaths occur annually.
- Overall 5-year survival rate is 85% for Hodgkin lymphoma and 70% for non-Hodgkin lymphoma.

(Continued on next page)

Figure 3-2. Selected Epidemiologic Facts About the Major Cancers *(Continued)*

Oral Cancer
- 48,330 estimated new cases occur annually.
- Incidence is two times higher in men.
- 9,570 estimated deaths occur annually.
- The 5- and 10-year relative survival rates for cancer of the oral cavity or pharynx are 63% and 52%, respectively.

Ovarian Cancer
- 22,280 estimated new cases occur annually.
- 14,240 estimated deaths occur annually.
- Overall, the 5- and 10-year relative survival rates for patients with ovarian cancer are 46% and 35%, respectively.
- If detected at a localized stage, overall survival is 92%, but only 15% are detected at this stage.
- 61% of cases are diagnosed at a distant stage, for which the 5-year survival rate is 27%.

Pancreatic Cancer
- 53,070 estimated new cases occur annually.
- 41,780 estimated deaths occur annually.
- For all stages combined, the 1- and 5-year relative survival rates are 26% and 7%, respectively.
- For the 9% of people diagnosed with local disease, the 5-year survival is only 26%.
- 53% of patients are diagnosed at a distant stage, for which 1- and 5-year survival rates are 15% and 2%, respectively.

Prostate Cancer
- 180,890 estimated new cases occur annually.
- Prostate cancer is the most frequently diagnosed cancer in men.
- 26,120 estimated deaths occur annually.
- 93% of cases are diagnosed at the localized or local/regional stage.
- The 5-year survival rate for localized disease is almost 100%.
- Over the past 25 years, the 5-year relative survival rate for all stages combined has increased from 68% to almost 100%.

Skin Cancer
- More than 1 million estimated new cases of basal cell and squamous cell cancers occur annually.
- 76,380 estimated new cases of melanoma occur annually.
- Melanoma is 10 times more common in Caucasians than in other races.
- 10,130 estimated deaths occur annually from melanoma.
- Basal cell and squamous cell cancers are nearly 100% curable if detected at the localized stage.
- The 5- and 10-year relative survival rates for melanoma are 91% and 89%, respectively.
- For localized melanoma (84% of melanoma cases), the 5-year survival rate is 98%.
- Overall survival rates are 63% and 16% for regional and metastatic stage disease, respectively.

Note. Based on information from American Cancer Society, 2014, 2015a, 2016b.

vidual patient risk assessments, or targeting specific populations for outreach efforts.

Levels of Prevention

Three levels of prevention exist: primary, secondary, and tertiary. Although the term *prevention* is used frequently in cancer control, it is important to distinguish the different levels of prevention because of the different focus for each.

Primary cancer prevention encompasses a healthy lifestyle and includes all measures to avoid carcinogen exposure and promote health. Primary prevention is what individuals typically consider when the term *prevention* is

Figure 3-3. Female Breast Cancer Incidence and Mortality

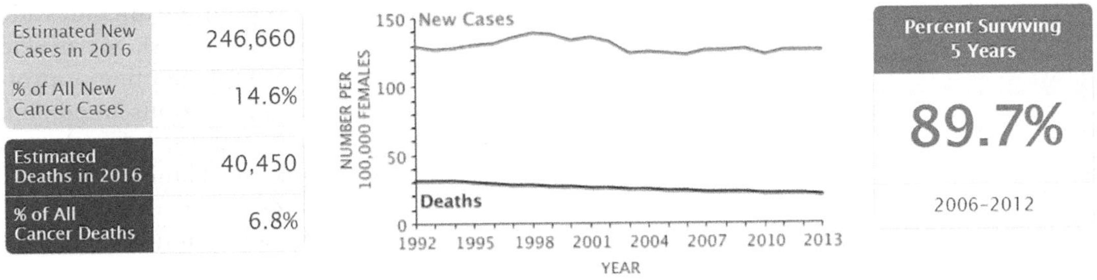

Number of New Cases and Deaths per 100,000: The number of new cases of female breast cancer was 125.0 per 100,000 women per year. The number of deaths was 21.5 per 100,000 women per year. These rates are age-adjusted and based on 2009–2013 cases and deaths.

Lifetime Risk of Developing Cancer: Approximately 12.4 percent of women will be diagnosed with female breast cancer at some point during their lifetime, based on 2011–2013 data.

Prevalence of This Cancer: In 2013, there were an estimated 3,053,450 women living with female breast cancer in the United States.

Note. From "SEER Stat Fact Sheets: Female Breast Cancer," by National Cancer Institute Surveillance, Epidemiology, and End Results Program, n.d. Retrieved from http://seer.cancer.gov/statfacts/html/breast.html.

Figure 3-4. Female Breast Cancer Survival by Stage

Cancer stage at diagnosis, which refers to extent of a cancer in the body, determines treatment options and has a strong influence on the length of survival. In general, if the cancer is found only in the part of the body where it started, it is *localized* (sometimes referred to as stage 1). If it has spread to a different part of the body, the stage is *regional* or *distant*. The earlier female breast cancer is caught, the better chance a person has of surviving five years after being diagnosed. For female breast cancer, 61.4% are diagnosed at the local stage. The 5-year survival for localized female breast cancer is 98.8%.

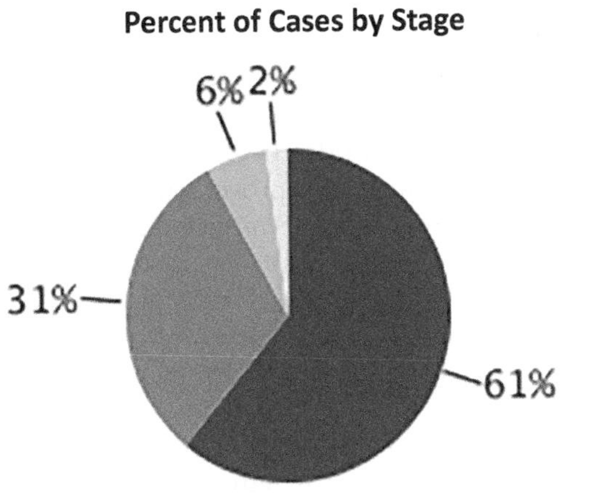

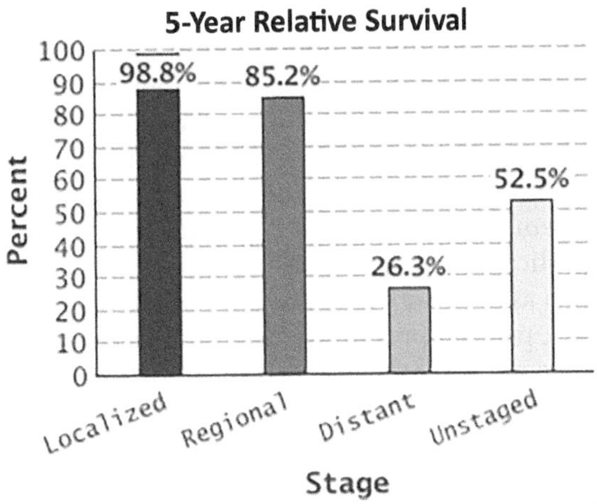

Note. From "SEER Stat Fact Sheets: Female Breast Cancer," by National Cancer Institute Surveillance, Epidemiology, and End Results Program, n.d. Retrieved from http://seer.cancer.gov/statfacts/html/breast.html.

Figure 3-5. Percent of New Breast Cancer Cases by Age

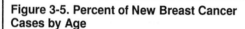

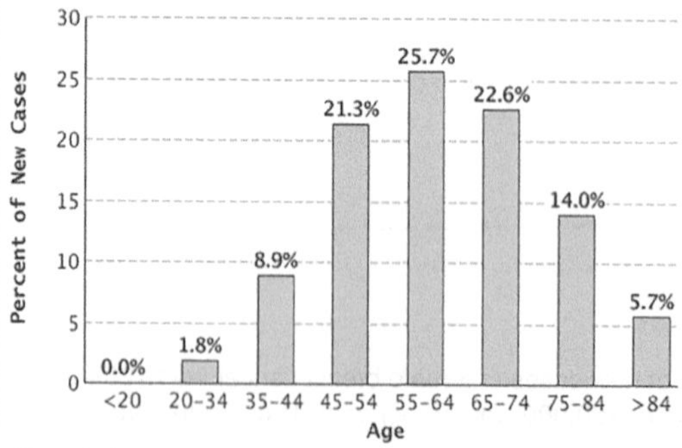

Female breast cancer is most common in middle-aged and older women. Although rare, men can develop breast cancer as well. The number of new cases of female breast cancer was 125.0 per 100,000 women per year based on 2009–2013 cases.

Note. From "SEER Stat Fact Sheets: Female Breast Cancer," by National Cancer Institute Surveillance, Epidemiology, and End Results Program, n.d. Retrieved from http://seer.cancer.gov/statfacts/html/breast.html.

used. It refers to measures for the prevention of disease, such as immunizing against childhood diseases, avoiding tobacco products, eating a healthy diet, exercising regularly, and reducing exposure to ultraviolet rays. Primary prevention measures for malignancy reduce the risk of developing cancer; however, even when such measures are implemented consistently, some individuals will still develop malignancy. The focus of primary prevention is to prevent a cancer from ever developing or to delay the development of a malignancy. For individuals with a particularly high risk of developing a cancer (such as those with a known genetic predisposition), primary prevention may include the use of chemopreventive agents or prophylactic surgery to prevent or significantly reduce the risk of developing a malignancy (ACS, 2014, 2015c; Rodriguez-Bigas & Möeslein, 2013; Zagouri et al., 2013).

Secondary cancer prevention refers to the early detection and treatment of subclinical, asymptomatic, or early disease in people without obvious signs or symptoms of cancer. Secondary cancer prevention includes identifying people who are at risk for developing malignancy and implementing appropriate screening recommendations based on the risk assessment (Craft, 2014; Edwards et al., 2013; Smith, Brooks, Cokkinides, Saslow, & Brawley, 2013). Screening may include physical examinations, self-examinations, radiologic procedures, laboratory tests, or other examinations. Examples of secondary cancer prevention include the use of the Pap test to detect cervical cancer, mammography to detect a nonpalpable breast cancer, or colonoscopy to detect and remove a polyp or early colon cancer (ACS, 2016b).

Screening tests seek to decrease the morbidity and mortality associated with cancer (ACS, 2016b; Plescia, Richardson, & Joseph, 2012; Smith et al., 2014). Following a positive screening test, further diagnostic testing is required to determine if a malignancy exists. More recently, screening for genetic or molecular markers that put one at high risk for developing cancer includes a specialized form of cancer screening that allows for risk clarification in an individual or family (see Chapter 4).

The focus of secondary cancer prevention is to detect a cancer before symptoms are readily evident. The premise of early detection is that treatment will be less complicated, associated with fewer side effects and decreased morbidity, and lead to improvement in both quality and quantity of life (Smith et al., 2014).

Tertiary cancer prevention includes monitoring for and preventing recurrence of the originally diagnosed cancer and screening for second primary cancers and long-term effects of treatment in cancer survivors (Corkum et al., 2013). Examples of tertiary prevention include monitoring for early signs of recurrence using tumor markers or detecting second primary malignancies early in long-term survivors. Because of the ever-growing population of can-

Figure 3-6. Number of New Cases of Breast Cancer by Race/Ethnicity (Per 100,000 Women)

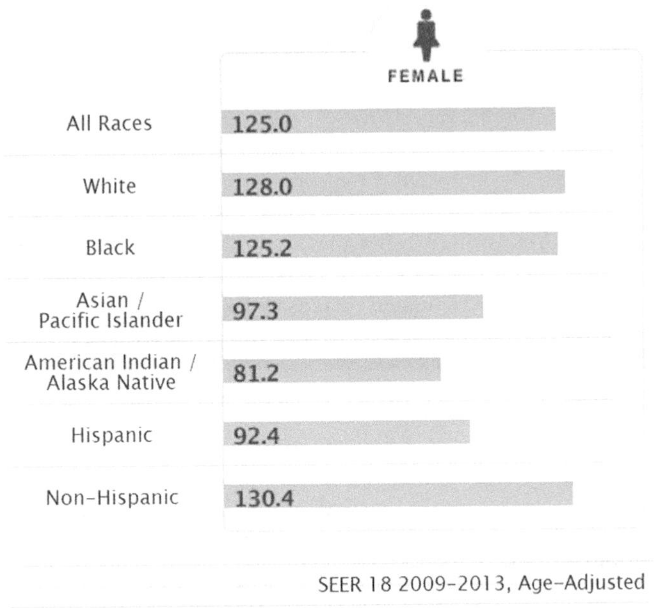

Note. From "SEER Stat Fact Sheets: Female Breast Cancer," by National Cancer Institute Surveillance, Epidemiology, and End Results Program, n.d. Retrieved from http://seer.cancer.gov/statfacts/html/breast.html.

cer survivors, tertiary prevention is becoming more important. The aim of this form of prevention is to detect complications and second cancers in long-term survivors when treatment is most likely to be effective and to ultimately improve their quality of life. More and more efforts are being focused on helping survivors engage in healthier behaviors to prevent additional cancers, especially through weight control, healthier diets, exercise, tobacco cessation, and avoidance of exposure to ultraviolet light (ACS, 2016c). The National Cancer Institute established the Office of Cancer Survivorship in 1996 to help address the needs of this large population. Current estimates suggest that at least 14.5 million Americans with a history of cancer were alive as of January 2014 (ACS, 2016b). See Chapter 34 for more information on cancer survivorship.

Figure 3-7. Percent of Breast Cancer Deaths by Age Group

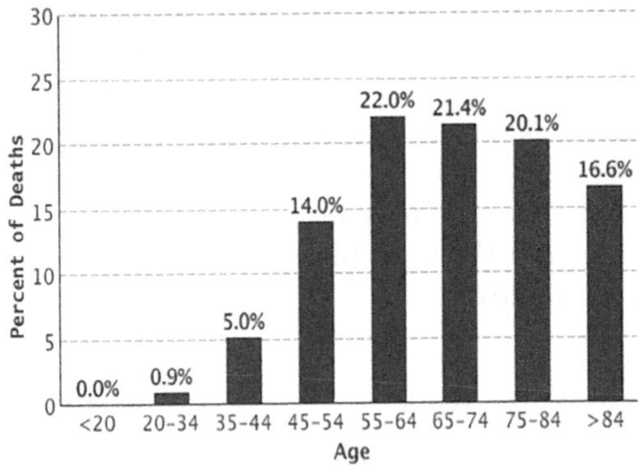

Note. From "SEER Stat Fact Sheets: Female Breast Cancer," by National Cancer Institute Surveillance, Epidemiology, and End Results Program, n.d. Retrieved from http://seer.cancer.gov/statfacts/html/breast.html.

Figure 3-8. Recent Trends in Breast Cancer Incidence, Mortality, and Survival

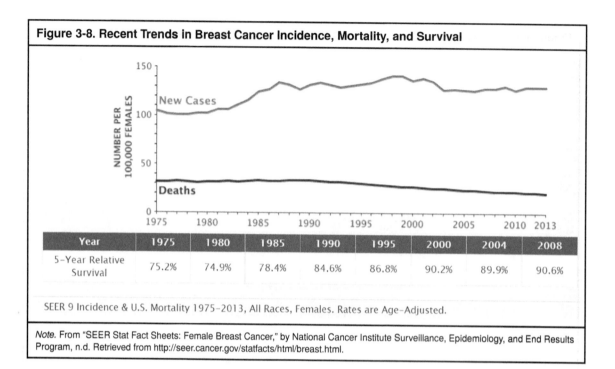

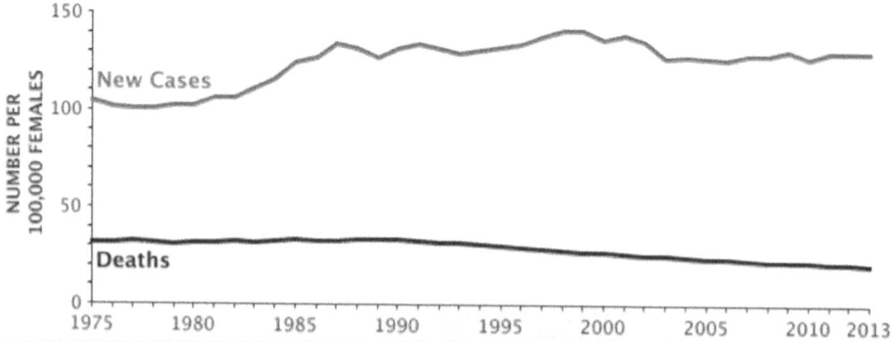

Year	1975	1980	1985	1990	1995	2000	2004	2008
5-Year Relative Survival	75.2%	74.9%	78.4%	84.6%	86.8%	90.2%	89.9%	90.6%

SEER 9 Incidence & U.S. Mortality 1975–2013, All Races, Females. Rates are Age-Adjusted.

Note. From "SEER Stat Fact Sheets: Female Breast Cancer," by National Cancer Institute Surveillance, Epidemiology, and End Results Program, n.d. Retrieved from http://seer.cancer.gov/statfacts/html/breast.html.

Risk Factors and Risk Assessment

A risk factor is a trait or characteristic that is associated with a statistically significant increased likelihood of developing a disease. Risk factors do not predict who will certainly have a cancer, but rather who has an increased chance of developing the disease. Individuals who develop a malignancy may have multiple risk factors or none at all. The risk factor assessment is important because it guides recommendations for cancer prevention and early detection (Weitzel, Blazer, MacDonald, Culver, & Offit, 2011).

Absolute Risk

Absolute risk is a measure of the occurrence of cancer, either incidence (new cases) or mortality (deaths), in the general population. Absolute risk is helpful when a patient needs to understand what the chances are for all people in a population of developing or dying of a particular disease. Absolute risk can be expressed either as the number of cases for a specified denominator (e.g., 131 cases of breast cancer per 100,000 women annually) or as a cumulative risk up to a specified age (e.g., one in eight women will develop breast cancer if they live to age 85) (ACS, 2016b). See Table 3-1 for a list of absolute risk factor figures.

Another way to express absolute risk is to discuss the average risk of developing a cancer at a certain age. This is also referred to as *cumulative risk.* It is a helpful statistic when trying to give an individual a perspective on risk for a specific cancer both in the present and projected over time (see Figure 3-5). For example, a woman's risk of developing breast cancer may be 2% at age 50, but at age 85, it might be approximately 13%. Risk estimates will be much different for a 50-year-old woman than for an 85-year-old woman, as approximately 50% of the cases of breast cancer occur after the age of 65 (ACS, 2015a, 2016b).

Table 3-1. Absolute Risk Figures for Selected Cancers

Cancer	Males	Females
Breast	–	1 in 8
Prostate	1 in 7	–
Colorectal	1 in 21	1 in 23
Lung	1 in 14	1 in 17
Melanoma	1 in 33	1 in 52
Uterus	–	1 in 3
Ovary	–	1 in 66
Cervix	–	1 in 157
Leukemia	1 in 57	1 in 82
Kidney	1 in 49	1 in 83
All sites	1 in 2	1 in 3

Note. Based on information from American Cancer Society, 2016b; Smith et al., 2014.

Individuals need to understand that certain assumptions are made to reach an absolute risk figure for a particular cancer. For example, the one-in-eight figure describes the "average" risk of breast cancer in Caucasian American women, and the calculation takes into consideration other causes of death over the life span (see Table 3-2). This figure will overestimate breast cancer risk for some women with no risk factors and underestimate the risk for women with several risk factors. For those with a genetic predisposition for developing the disease, it will greatly underestimate the risk. What this statistic actually means is that the average woman's breast cancer risk is 0.5% to age 40, 1.4% to age 50, 2.3% to age 60, 3.5% to age 70, and 4.6% from age 70 on. The 12.3% or one-in-eight risk is obtained by adding the risk in each age category (0.5 + 1.4 + 2.3 + 3.5 + 4.6 = 12.3). When a woman who has an average risk reaches age 40 without a diagnosis of breast cancer, she has passed through 0.5% of her risk, so her lifetime risk is 12.3% minus 0.5%, which equals 11.8%. Thus, when she reaches age 70 without a diagnosis of breast cancer, her risk is 4.6% (12.3 – 0.5 – 1.4 – 2.3 – 3.5 = 4.6%). Time must always be considered for the cumulative absolute risk figure to be meaningful (ACS, 2016b; Gordis, 2014).

Relative Risk

The term *relative risk* refers to a comparison of the incidence or deaths among those with a particular risk factor compared to those without the risk factor. By reviewing relative risk factors, individuals can determine their risk factors and thus better understand their personal chances of developing a specific cancer as compared to individuals without such risk factors. If the risk for a person with no known risk factors is 1.0, one can evaluate the risk of those with risk factors in relation to this figure. Relative risk is only helpful if the anchor to which the comparison is being made is clearly identified. In general, it is a comparison to someone who does not have the risk factor. A number greater than 1.0 suggests increased risk; a num-

Table 3-2. Absolute Risk of Women Developing Breast Cancer Over Time

Age (Years)	Risk
Up to 40	0.76% (1 in 169)
41–50	1.9% (1 in 53)
51–59	2.3% (1 in 44)
60–69	3.49% (1 in 29)
70 and older	3.84% (1 in 15)
Over lifetime	12.29% (1 in 8)

Note. Based on information from American Cancer Society, 2015a, 2016b.

ber less than 1.0 suggests a possible protective factor (ACS, 2016b; Gordis, 2014).

Table 3-3 illustrates some of the relative risk factors for developing colorectal cancer. The data show that a smoker is 1.2 times more likely to develop colorectal cancer than a nonsmoker. A person who takes aspirin daily may be less likely to develop colorectal cancer; this relative risk factor implies that aspirin may be protective against colorectal cancer. It is not possible in most cases to mathematically add up risk factors. However, if a person has multiple risk factors, especially those with a higher relative risk, screening guidelines may need to be modified (ACS, 2016b).

Table 3-3. Selected Relative Risk Factors for Colorectal Cancer

Risk Factor	Relative Risk
Smoking	1.2
Obesity (body mass index 30+)	1.2
Physical activity (20+ hours/week)	0.7*
High vegetable consumption (5+ servings/day)	0.9*
Red meat consumption (2+ servings/week as a main dish)	1.2
Alcohol consumption (> 1 drink per day)	1.6
Diabetes	1.2
One first-degree relative with colorectal cancer	2.2
More than one first-degree relative with colorectal cancer	4.0
Relative with colorectal cancer diagnosed before age 45	3.9
Regular daily use of aspirin or nonsteroidal anti-inflammatory drugs	0.6–0.7*
No sigmoidoscopy or colonoscopy in last 10 years in an individual 60 years or older	1.4–3.9

* A number less than 1.0 indicates a protective effect or risk reduction.

Note. Based on information from American Cancer Society, 2014; Aune et al., 2011; Freedman et al., 2009.

For breast cancer, models are available that calculate one's risk based on multiple factors. The most commonly used is the Gail model, which has undergone multiple revisions and is available at www.cancer.gov/bcrisktool (Gail & Mai, 2010). It requires the clinician to ensure that data are collected as accurately as possible. The tool generates and communicates results in both five-year and lifetime risks and provides an explanation as to why the risk is increased. It encourages the woman to discuss the results with her healthcare provider.

However, the Gail model excludes some well-known predictors. The method used by the Breast Cancer Risk Assessment Tool (Gail model) to calculate the risk of invasive breast cancer is not accurate for women with a history of ductal or lobular carcinoma in situ. In addition, the tool cannot accurately predict the risk of another breast cancer developing in women who have a previous history of breast cancer. It does not include family history of ovarian cancer, ages at which relatives were diagnosed with breast cancer, affected second-degree relatives, or paternal family history. Because of these limitations, the model underestimates risk for women who have genetic mutations and overestimates risk for women who have some family history of breast cancer but do not have a genetic mutation. The Gail model is best used for women with a minimal to moderate family history of breast cancer and represents an attempt to combine relative risk factors for a commonly diagnosed cancer (Gail & Mai, 2010; Matsuno et al., 2011).

For most of the major cancers, relative risk data are available. The National Cancer Institute provides fact sheets that explain specific cancer risk factors for the general public, which can be helpful for patient education. This list is continually updated at www.cancer.gov/publications/fact-sheets#Risk+Factors+and+Possible+Causes.

Attributable Risk

Attributable risk is the amount of disease within a population that could be prevented by the alteration of a risk factor. Attributable risk has important implications for public health policy. A risk factor could be associated with a very large relative risk but be restricted to a few individuals, so changing it would only benefit a small group. Conversely, some risk factors that can be altered could potentially decrease the morbidity and mortality associated with malignancy in a large number of people. Smoking is a perfect example. ACS has estimated that one in five (443,000) premature deaths each year in the United States can be attributed to smoking (ACS, 2016b). An additional 8.9 million people are affected by chronic disease related to smoking. Smoking accounts for 30% of all cancer deaths and 87% of lung cancer deaths (U.S. Public Health Service, 2014). Clearly, altering this risk factor could significantly affect cancer-associated morbidity and mortality in the future.

Risk Factor Assessment

Goals of Risk Assessment

The goals of cancer risk assessment and counseling are to (a) provide accurate information about the genetic, biologic, and environmental factors related to an individual's risk of developing cancer, (b) formulate appropriate recommendations for primary and secondary prevention, and (c) offer emotional and psychosocial support to facilitate adjustment to risk information and promote adherence to prevention and early detection recommendations (Fagerlin, Zikmund-Fisher, & Ubel, 2011). Risk quantification also guides public policy for the allocation of funds for screening. Screening is most likely to be recommended for cancer sites for which reasonable screening tests exist, incidence is substantial, risks are understood, and screening directly affects the morbidity and mortality associated with the disease (Smith et al., 2014).

Risk assessment drives the recommendations for screening. It is crucial for patients and healthcare providers alike to understand the importance of an accurate assessment. Patients need to understand that the more complete and accurate the data, the better the risk assessment and the more likely that appropriate screening and prevention strategies will be selected. If risk is underestimated, routine screening maneuvers may not be adequate. If risk is overestimated, expensive and potentially unnecessary screening may be implemented (Croswell, Ransohoff, & Kramer, 2010).

An example of the importance of accurate risk assessment and recommendation of subsequent screening modalities would be the use of breast magnetic resonance imaging (MRI) in women with an increased risk (greater than 20%) or a documented genetic predisposition for developing breast cancer. ACS recommends the use of breast MRI with mammography starting at age 30 in such women (ACS, 2015a). The National Comprehensive Cancer Network® (NCCN®) recommends annual breast MRI starting at age 25 and breast MRI alternating with mammography starting at age 30 (NCCN, 2016). If a woman does not have a genetic predisposition or substantially increased risk for developing breast cancer, such screening is probably unnecessary, exposes the woman to additional radiation, and is very costly. However, in a woman with a high risk for developing breast cancer, the use of mammography and breast MRI starting at age 30 may be a very effective strategy to detect breast cancer early, when it is most likely to be treatable. Thus, the risk assessment demands that the patient provide accurate and complete information. The healthcare professional collecting the data needs to ask questions in such a way that elicits complete information. The healthcare provider also must use the information to select the appropriate screening test so that resources are used wisely and the patient has a reasonable expectation of the early detection of cancer. Finally, the healthcare provider needs to explain what the risk factors mean to the patient in understandable terms and how the risk factors guide decisions for screening recommendations.

Risk factor assessment is challenging to do and is not complete until the patient has an accurate understanding of his or her risk. Risk assessment can be confusing and frightening to patients. Not all risk factors are amenable to change. This is the case with many risk factors for breast cancer. Individuals cannot change their sex, age, family history, or age at menarche. If the risk factors are perceived as great in number, the individual may be too overwhelmed to engage in screening. If the risk factors can be modified or eliminated (such as tobacco and alcohol use or a high-fat diet), it is possible for an individual to decrease the risk of developing cancer. In such cases, it is important for the nurse to provide education and support to modify risk factors whenever possible.

Elements of Risk Assessment

Basic elements of a cancer risk assessment include the patient's medical history, history of exposure to carcinogens in daily living, and detailed family history (see Figure 3-9). Once all information is gathered, it must be communicated to the patient in understandable terms. Often this is accomplished by using various risk calculations, such as absolute risk, relative risk, attributable risk, or specific models for various cancers (such as the Gail model for breast cancer risk). It is important for patients to understand that a general limitation of risk assessment is that no model completely and accurately explains an individual's risk for developing a particular cancer (Fagerlin et al., 2011).

The family history should focus on first- and second-degree relatives and include at least three generations (Bennett, French, Resta, & Doyle, 2008). This includes an assessment of both paternal and maternal families because many autosomal dominant syndromes can be passed through either the father or mother (Riley et al., 2012). This typically is displayed in a pedigree (see Figure 3-10). First-degree relatives include parents, siblings, and children. Because first-degree relatives share 50% of their genes, these relatives are most likely to inherit similar genetic information. Information about second-degree relatives also can be helpful. Second-degree relatives include grandparents, aunts, and uncles. Second-degree relatives have 25% of their genes in common. In particular, older second-degree relatives can provide important information about genetic risk because they would have been expected to manifest an early-onset cancer if a hereditary trait is present in the family. The pedigree also should include nieces and nephews because these younger family members can provide information about childhood cancers, which also has implications for the genetic risk assessment. Third-degree relatives (cousins, great-aunts and great-uncles, and great grandparents) also can be included, but the accuracy of reports on these relatives is not always high. These relatives share 12.5% of the same genes. Once documented, this information should be stored in a standard pedigree format (see Figure 3-10). Pedigrees can be helpful in families with multiple cases of malignancy to teach concepts of genetics, clarify relationships, and provide a quick reference. They can be drawn by hand or by using computer software and should be updated on a regular basis.

The family history provides an organized way to document the risk factors related to family history, such as if a relative is alive or dead, age at death if applicable, significant medical diagnoses, or a diagnosis of cancer. Space can be provided to describe in detail the specific type of cancer, age at diagnosis, and other character-

Figure 3-9. Suggested Elements in a Cancer Screening Form

This includes the information a healthcare provider may want to have accessible in a chart and components to be documented for a cancer risk assessment. The provider needs to document not only risk but also what education and counseling were provided.

Face Sheet
- Name
- Social Security number
- Address
- Occupation
- Telephone number(s)
- Primary physician
- Date of birth
- Sex
- Past surgeries and medical problems

Family History
- Father
- Mother
- Sisters
- Brothers
- Maternal
  - Grandmother
  - Grandfather
  - Aunts
  - Uncles
- Paternal
  - Grandmother
  - Grandfather
  - Aunts
  - Uncles
- Children
- Grandchildren

Male Risk Assessment
- Family history of cancer
  - Prostate
  - Colon/polyps
  - Testicular
  - Skin/melanoma
  - Breast/gynecologic
- Medical history
  - Human papillomavirus (HPV) vaccination
  - Previous cancer screening
  - History of colorectal polyps
- Lifestyle history
  - High-fat diet
  - Chemical exposure
  - Light/fair complexion
  - Previous skin cancer/nevi removal
  - Previous x-ray exposure
  - Sun exposure
  - Tanning bed use
  - Tobacco use
  - Alcohol use

Female Risk Assessment
- Family history of cancer
  - Breast
  - Colon/polyps
  - Ovarian
  - Uterine
  - Skin/melanoma
- Reproductive history
  - Menarche
  - Menopause
  - Hormone history
  - Pregnancy history
  - Early parity
  - Previous breast biopsies
  - Early first coitus; multiple partners
  - History of cervical dysplasia
  - Exposure to diethylstilbestrol
  - Infertility
  - HPV vaccination
- Medical history
  - Previous cancer screening
  - History of colorectal polyps
  - Hypertension
  - Diabetes
  - Obesity
- Lifestyle history
  - High-fat diet
  - Chemical exposure
  - Light/fair complexion
  - Previous skin cancer/nevi removal
  - Previous x-ray exposure
  - Sun exposure
  - Tanning bed use
  - Tobacco use
  - Alcohol use

Risk Assessment Calculations
- Pedigree
- Risk calculations for developing a particular cancer
- Risk calculations for having a mutation

Note. From "Cancer Risk Assessment: Conceptual Considerations for Cancer Genetics," by S.M. Mahon, 1998, *Oncology Nursing Forum, 25,* p. 1544. Copyright 1998 by Oncology Nursing Society. Adapted with permission.

Figure 3-10. Pedigree Demonstrating Potential Hereditary Risk

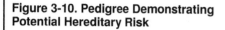

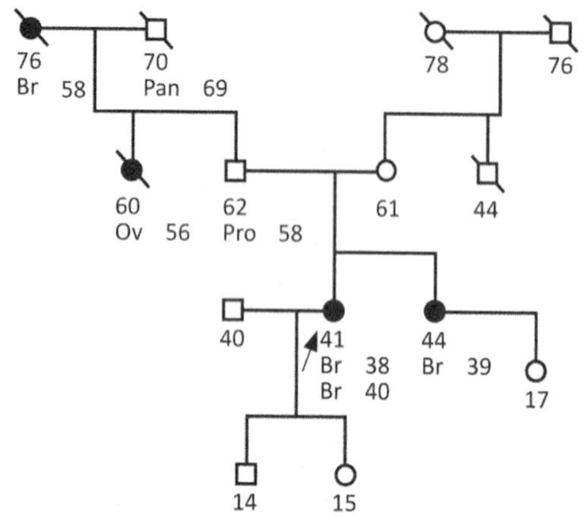

This is a typical pedigree. The arrow points to the proband, which is the spokesperson for the family and the point of reference for calculating risk of developing cancer and hereditary risk. Circles represent females and squares represent males. A slash represents a deceased person. Filled-in circles and squares represent people affected with the cancer(s) of interest. The age at diagnosis and site of cancer is recorded, as well as the current age or the age at death. A pedigree typically includes three generations.

istics, such as if a breast cancer was premenopausal or bilateral. The *proband* is the spokesperson for any family receiving a hereditary risk assessment. The proband may or may not be diagnosed with cancer. Specific knowledge may influence recommendations for screening. Taking a detailed family history is not only useful for cancer risk assessment but also is the first step in identifying families with a possible hereditary predisposition to malignancy and other illnesses. Healthcare providers should ask patients about specific relatives and their health individually rather than asking a more general question such as "Have any of your relatives been diagnosed with cancer?" After gathering the family history, it is important to recheck whether any of the patient's relatives have been diagnosed with these cancers. Patients often forget to provide this information, and reiterating this question provides valuable information. Key indicators of hereditary cancer are shown in Figure 3-11 and are discussed in more detail in Chapter 4 (Weitzel et al., 2011).

Assessment of past medical history and personal history factors that may increase the risk of developing cancer should be documented. This can include information such as menstrual history, hormonal exposures, or exposures to other carcinogens such as ultraviolet light or tobacco. Many of these risk factors (such as age at menarche) are not within an individual's control and are not amenable to primary prevention efforts. However, some lifestyle factors are within the individual's con-

Figure 3-11. Key Indicators of a Hereditary Predisposition for Developing Cancer

The following factors should be considered after gathering the family history. The presence of one or more criteria may suggest a hereditary predisposition and warrant a referral to a genetics professional.

- A cluster of the same cancer in close relatives (breast, colon, uterine, ovarian, melanoma)
- Cancer occurring at a younger age than expected in the general population (breast cancer before age 45; colon cancer before age 50)
- More than one primary cancer in one person (colon and endometrial; breast and ovarian)
- Evidence of autosomal dominant inheritance (two or more generations affected, with both males and females affected)
- Bilateral cancer in any paired organ (bilateral breast cancer)
- Cancers in an organ that are multifocal (multiple, early breast cancers)
- Any pattern of cancer associated with a known cancer syndrome
- Cancers occurring more frequently in a family than are expected by chance in the absence of known environmental and lifestyle risk factors
- Rare cancers such as male breast cancer, ovarian cancer, or pheochromocytomas
- Presence of premalignant conditions (more than 20 lifetime colorectal adenomas, dysplastic nevi)

Note. Based on information from Mahon, 2011; Riley et al., 2012; Weitzel et al., 2011.

trol and serve as a framework for providing education about primary prevention efforts (ACS, 2015c, 2016b).

Risk Communication

After all risk data are collected, the clinician must assimilate the risk factors and provide the patient with information about them for each of the major cancers. For example, early menarche, nulliparity, and late menopause are risk factors for both breast and endometrial cancer. Patient communication should include a discussion of the risk for developing both of these cancers. Risk can be communicated to patients in different formats, including pie charts, graphs, and risk ladders, as well as through highlighting the pedigree, and it often is best to use several means (Edwards et al., 2013; Klein & Stefanek, 2007). This can include absolute, relative, and attributable risk.

Primary Cancer Prevention

Overall, an estimated 25%–30% of cancers are due to tobacco use, 30%–35% are linked to diet and inactivity, and about 15%–20% are due to infections, radiation, stress, and environmental pollutants (ACS, 2015c, 2016b). Many cancers undoubtedly could be prevented by adopting a healthier diet and lifestyle, as well as large-scale use of direct prevention measures such as the human papillomavirus vaccine. A large portion of the Healthy People 2020 guidelines that pertain to cancer could be achieved with implementation of primary cancer practices (see Figure 3-12) (Healthy People 2020, n.d.).

Figure 3-12. Summary of Healthy People 2020 Objectives for Cancer

- Increase the number and quality of population-based cancer registries.
- Reduce the following death rates:
  - Overall cancer death rate from 179.3 to 161.4 per 100,000 population
  - Lung cancer death rate from 50.6 to 45.5 per 100,000 population
  - Breast cancer death rate from 23 to 20.7 per 100,000 females
  - Cervical cancer death rate from 2.4 to 2.2 per 100,000 females
  - Colorectal cancer death rate from 17.1 to 14.5 per 100,000 population
  - Oral cancer death rate from 2.5 to 2.3 per 100,000 population
  - Prostate cancer death rate from 24.2 to 21.8 per 100,000 males
  - Melanoma death rate from 2.7 to 2.4 per 100,000 population
- Increase the following secondary prevention measures:
  - Proportion of women aged 40 and older who have had breast screening based on the current guidelines from 73.7% to 81.1%
  - Number of females who have had cervical cancer screening based on the most current guidelines from 84.5% to 93%
  - Proportion of adults who undergo colorectal cancer screening based on the most current guidelines from 51.2% to 70.5%

Note. Based on information from Healthy People 2020, n.d.

Diet and Exercise

Evidence suggests that one-third of the more than 589,000 cancer deaths in the United States each year can be attributed to diet and physical activity habits, including being overweight or obese (ACS, 2015c). ACS has published recommendations for a healthier lifestyle to reduce cancer risk; these same guidelines are likely to also reduce risk from cardiovascular problems (see Figure 3-13).

A diet rich in fruits and vegetables appears to be important for cancer risk reduction. Research suggests that the body uses certain nutrients in fruits and vegetables to protect the body against the tissue damage that occurs constantly as a result of normal metabolism (oxidation). Because such damage is associated with increased cancer risk, the so-called antioxidant nutrients are thought to protect against cancer (Kushi et al., 2012). Antioxidants include vita-

Figure 3-13. Summary of American Cancer Society Recommendations for Diet and Exercise

Maintain a healthy weight throughout life.
- Balance caloric intake with physical activity.
- Avoid excessive weight gain throughout life.
- Achieve and maintain a healthy weight if currently overweight or obese.

Adopt a physically active lifestyle.
- Adults: Engage in at least 150 minutes of moderate-intensity or 75 minutes of vigorous-intensity activity each week.
- Children and adolescents: Engage in at least 1 hour of moderate- or vigorous-intensity activity each day, with vigorous-intensity activity occurring at least 3 days each week.
- Limit sedentary activity.

Eat a healthy diet, with an emphasis on plant sources.
- Eat 5 or more servings of a variety of vegetables and fruits each day.
- Choose whole grains instead of processed (refined) grains.
- Limit consumption of processed and red meats.
- Drink no more than 1 alcoholic drink per day for women or 2 per day for men.

Note. Based on information from American Cancer Society, 2015c, 2016b; Kushi et al., 2012.

min C, vitamin E, carotenoids, and many phytochemicals.

Being overweight or obese is clearly associated with an increased risk for developing many cancers, including breast cancer in postmenopausal women, colon cancer, endometrial cancer, adenocarcinoma of the esophagus, and kidney cancer (ACS, 2016b). Evidence is highly suggestive that obesity also increases the risk for cancers of the pancreas, gallbladder, thyroid, ovary, and cervix, and for multiple myeloma, Hodgkin lymphoma, and aggressive prostate cancer (ACS, 2015c).

The link between body weight and cancer risk is believed to stem from multiple effects on fat and sugar metabolism, immune function, hormone levels (including insulin and estradiol), and cell growth (Kushi et al., 2012). Recent studies have suggested that losing weight may reduce the risk of breast cancer (ACS, 2015c). Although knowledge about the relationship between weight loss and cancer risk is still limited, individuals who are overweight or obese should be encouraged and supported in their efforts to reduce their weight (Thompson, 2010).

Educating individuals about ways to achieve a healthy body weight is an important nursing responsibility. Many individuals know this is important but need encouragement and support from a healthcare provider to actually implement effective interventions. To achieve this goal, one must balance energy intake (food and beverage consumption) with energy expenditure (physical activity). Excess body fat can be reduced by decreasing caloric intake and increasing physical activity. For most adults, a reduction of 50–100 calories per day may prevent gradual weight gain, whereas a reduction of 500 or more calories per day is a common initial goal in weight loss programs (Kushi et al., 2012). Research suggests that up to 60 minutes per day of physical activity at a moderate to vigorous intensity may be needed to prevent weight gain, but as much as 60–90 minutes per day of moderate-intensity physical activity may be needed to help sustain weight loss for previously overweight people (ACS, 2015c; Kushi et al., 2012). Patients should receive information about the importance of regular physical activity.

Alcohol Use

People who drink alcohol should limit their intake to no more than two drinks per day for men and one drink a day for women (ACS, 2015c; Kushi et al., 2012). The recommended limit is lower for women because of their smaller body size and slower metabolism of alcohol. A drink is defined as 12 ounces of beer, 5 ounces of wine, or 1.5 ounces of 80-proof distilled spirits. Alcohol consumption is a known etiologic factor associated with cancers of the mouth, pharynx, larynx, esophagus, and liver, especially with intake of more than two drinks per day, and also is associated with an increased risk of breast and colorectal cancer (Kushi et al., 2012).

Tobacco Cessation

Tobacco use remains the single largest preventable cause of disease and premature death in the United States (ACS, 2015c). Smoking accounts for $193 billion in healthcare expenditures and productivity losses (ACS, 2015c). A goal of the Healthy People 2020 initiative is to reduce the lung cancer death rate from 50.6 deaths per 100,000 people to 45.5 deaths per 100,000 people (Healthy People 2020, n.d.). Approximately 87% of lung cancer deaths are attributed to smoking (ACS, 2015c). More people die of lung cancer than of colon, breast, and prostate cancers combined. Tobacco use also increases the risk of cancers of the mouth, nasal cavities, larynx, pharynx, esophagus, stomach, pancreas, kidney, bladder, and cervix, as well as leukemia.

The addictive properties of tobacco should not be underestimated (ACS, 2015c; U.S. Public Health Service, 2014). Most smokers become addicted to tobacco before they are old enough to legally buy cigarettes. Addiction develops rapidly in those who experiment with tobacco. Most adolescents who become regular smokers continue to smoke into adulthood. Because the likelihood of developing smoking-related cancers such as lung cancer increases with the duration of smoking, those who start at a younger age and continue to smoke are at highest risk.

People who stop smoking before age 50 cut their risk of dying in the next 15 years in half compared to those who continue to smoke (ACS, 2015c; Wallace, 2011). Individuals who are current smokers also should be informed that the more immediate preventive health priority is the elimination of tobacco use altogether, as smoking cessation offers the most effective means of reducing the risk of premature mortality from lung cancer (Cokkinides et al., 2009).

Secondhand smoke also increases the risk for lung cancer. A nonsmoker who lives with a smoker has about a 20%–30% greater risk of developing lung cancer. Secondhand smoke is the attributed cause for more than 3,000 lung cancer deaths annually (ACS, 2015c).

Comprehensive tobacco control programs aim to reduce tobacco use and the disease, disability, and death associated with it. The goals of comprehensive tobacco control include preventing the initiation of tobacco use, especially in young people; promoting tobacco cessation in current users; and eliminating secondhand smoke. These goals are best accomplished by applying a mix of economic, policy, regulatory, educational, social, and clinical strategies. Effective interventions to reduce tobacco use that currently are mandated by law in many states include increases in excise taxes, restrictions on smoking in public places, and anti-tobacco media campaigns (ACS, 2015c; U.S. Public Health Service, 2014).

Ethnic Differences

Knowledge of the overall trends in cancer incidence and mortality rates, particularly among individuals in certain age groups or racial and ethnic groups, can help oncology nurses to identify populations who are at risk. These data are readily available in ACS's *Cancer Facts and Figures* publications, as well as through the SEER Program (ACS, 2015b, 2016a). These populations may require specialized prevention or early detection programs. If these individuals live within certain communities, efforts can be made to provide targeted prevention and early detection strategies that are culturally acceptable.

Conclusion

Knowledge and integration of epidemiologic concepts is essential in oncology nursing practice. These concepts have implications for risk assessment, prevention recommendations, screening strategies, and monitoring of the effectiveness of various therapies. See the case study for an example of a risk assessment and recommendations.

Epidemiologic data are presented in numerous formats. Nurses can use this information when educating patients, devising screening or prevention programs, conducting clinical research, and monitoring the effectiveness of therapy.

Risk assessment is central to making appropriate recommendations for the prevention and early detection of cancers. Nurses need to provide patients with accurate information about risks and the various risk estimates.

The importance of primary cancer prevention efforts should not be underestimated. Nurses serve as key educators of the importance of these measures, especially primary prevention efforts targeted at improving diet, increasing physical activity, reducing alcohol intake, and eliminating tobacco use.

Case Study

A 39-year-old African American woman presents to the Cancer Screening Center for risk assessment and recommendations for the prevention and early detection of cancer. The clinician gathers her family history, medical history, and lifestyle factors. The clinician then constructs a pedigree and completes the Gail model for breast cancer risk assessment. Risk factors for the major cancers are noted. The patient receives recommendations for cancer screening.

Risk Assessment

- Family history of cancer
  - Breast: paternal grandmother, mother, maternal aunt
  - Colon/polyps: maternal uncle
  - Ovarian: none
  - Uterine: none
  - Skin/melanoma: none
- Reproductive history
  - Age at menarche: 12
  - Age at menopause: not applicable; regular menses
  - Hormone history: no endogenous hormone use
  - Pregnancy history: G0
  - Early parity: not applicable
  - Previous breast biopsies: age 36—atypical hyperplasia
  - Early first coitus/multiple partners: denies
  - History of cervical dysplasia: no history of abnormal Pap tests; done on annual basis without exception
  - Exposure to diethylstilbestrol: denies
  - Infertility: unsure; has not attempted to get pregnant
- Medical/lifestyle history
  - Hypertension: denies, blood pressure = 126/72 mm Hg
  - Diabetes: denies
  - Obesity: height = 58 inches; weight = 166 pounds
  - Exercise: walks an average of 20 minutes per day
  - High-fat diet: states eats meat daily and some fast food two to three times per week

– Light/fair complexion: no
– Previous skin cancer/nevi removal: denies
– Previous x-ray exposure: denies
– Sun exposure: moderate
– Tanning bed use: denies
– Chemical exposure: denies
– Tobacco use: denies
– Alcohol use: less than three beverages per month
– Surgeries: none except breast biopsy
– Current medications: none

Risk Assessment (Increased Risk)
- Uterine: nulliparous
- Ovarian: nulliparous
- Cervix: none identified
- Colon: family history of polyps
- Head and neck: none identified
- Skin/melanoma: none
- Breast: family history, nulliparous, previous breast biopsy, increased risk per Gail model

Gail Model
- 5-year risk of developing breast cancer
  – This woman (age 39): 1.8%
  – Average woman (age 39): 0.5%
  – Explanation: Based on the information provided, the woman's estimated risk for developing invasive breast cancer over the next 5 years is 1.8% compared to a risk of 0.5% for a woman of the same age and race/ethnicity from the general U.S. population. This calculation also means that the woman's risk of NOT getting breast cancer in the next 5 years is 98.2%.
- Lifetime risk of developing breast cancer
  – This woman (to age 90): 27.3%
  – Average woman (to age 90): 10%
  – Explanation: Based on the information provided, the woman's estimated risk of developing invasive breast cancer over her lifetime (to age 90) is 27.3% compared to a risk of 10% for a woman of the same age and race/ethnicity from the general U.S. population.

Recommendations
- Consider referral to a genetics professional because of family history of triple-negative breast cancer.
- Encourage a plan of a low-fat diet high in vegetables and fruits.
- Continue regular exercise and try to increase intensity.
- Decrease ultraviolet light exposure, use sunscreen and protective clothing, and assess skin regularly for changes.
- Consider annual mammography and professional examination and monthly breast self-examination. Begin mammography certainly by age 40, maybe earlier, based on genetics professional's recommendation. Gail model suggests that magnetic resonance imaging might be a consideration depending on breast density and difficulty of clinical examination given the increased lifetime risk of developing breast cancer.
- Obtain annual Pap test and pelvic examination.
- Obtain colonoscopy every 10 years starting at age 50.

Risks for developing the major cancers were discussed. The assessment suggests a potentially increased risk for developing breast cancer. Recommendations for the general population were modified for breast cancer.

Key Points

- The *incidence* of cancer is the number of cancers that develop in a population during a defined period, such as a year. The *mortality rate* is the number of people who die of a particular cancer during a defined period. *Prevalence* of cancer refers to the number of people alive on a specific date with a previous diagnosis of cancer, including newly diagnosed patients and survivors.
- *Primary cancer prevention* encompasses a healthy lifestyle and includes all measures to avoid carcinogen exposure and promote health, such as including at least 150 minutes of intentional exercise per week, eating a diet high in fresh fruits and vegetables, maintaining a proper weight, avoiding ultraviolet light exposure, limiting alcohol use, and avoiding tobacco products.
- *Secondary cancer prevention* refers to the early detection and treatment of subclinical, asymptomatic, or early disease in people without obvious signs or symptoms.
- *Tertiary cancer prevention* includes monitoring for and preventing recurrence of the originally diagnosed cancer and screening for second primary cancers and long-term treatment effects in cancer survivors.
- A *risk factor* is a trait or characteristic that is associated with a statistically significant increased likelihood of developing a disease.
- *Absolute risk* is a measure of the occurrence of cancer, either incidence (new cases) or mortality (deaths), in the general population.
- *Relative risk* refers to a comparison of the incidence or deaths among those with a particular risk factor compared to those without the risk factor.
- *Attributable risk* is the amount of disease within a population that could be prevented by alteration of a risk factor.
- Key elements of a cancer risk assessment include a review of medical history, a history of exposure to carcinogens in daily living, and a detailed family history.
- The goals of cancer risk factor assessment and counseling are to provide information about the biologic basis of risk, provide recommendations for cancer prevention, and promote adherence to prevention and early detection recommendations.

References

American Cancer Society. (2014). *Colorectal cancer facts and figures 2014–2016.* Atlanta, GA: Author.

American Cancer Society. (2015a). *Breast cancer facts and figures 2015–2016.* Atlanta, GA: Author.

American Cancer Society. (2015b). *Cancer facts and figures for Hispanics/Latinos 2015–2017.* Atlanta, GA: Author.

American Cancer Society. (2015c). *Cancer prevention and early detection facts and figures 2015–2016.* Atlanta, GA: Author.

American Cancer Society. (2016a). *Cancer facts and figures for African Americans 2016–2018.* Atlanta, GA: Author.

American Cancer Society. (2016b). *Cancer facts and figures 2016.* Atlanta, GA: Author.

American Cancer Society. (2016c). *Cancer treatment and survivorship facts and figures 2016–2017.* Atlanta, GA: Author.

Aune, D., Chan, D.S.M., Lau, R., Vieira, R., Greenwood, D.C., Kampman, E., & Norat, T. (2011). Dietary fibre, whole grains, and risk of colorectal cancer: Systematic review and dose-response meta-analysis of prospective studies. *BMJ, 343,* d6617. doi:10.1136/bmj.d6617

Bennett, R.L., French, K.S., Resta, R.G., & Doyle, D.L. (2008). Standardized human pedigree nomenclature: Update and assessment of the recommendations of the National Society of Genetic Counselors. *Journal of Genetic Counseling, 17,* 424–433. doi:10.1007/s10897-008-9169-9

Centers for Disease Control and Prevention. (2012). *Principles of epidemiology in public health practice: An introduction to applied epidemiology and biostatistics* (3rd ed.). Atlanta, GA: Author.

Cokkinides, V., Bandi, P., McMahon, C., Jemal, A., Glynn, T., & Ward, E. (2009). Tobacco control in the United States—Recent progress and opportunities. *CA: A Cancer Journal for Clinicians, 59,* 352–365. doi:10.3322/caac.20037

Corkum, M., Hayden, J.A., Kephart, G., Urquhart, R., Schlievert, C., & Porter, G. (2013). Screening for new primary cancers in cancer survivors compared to noncancer controls: A systematic review and meta-analysis. *Journal of Cancer Survivorship, 7,* 455–463. doi:10.1007/s11764-013-0278-6

Craft, M. (2014). Cancer screening in the older adult: Issues and concerns. *Nursing Clinics of North America, 49,* 251–261. doi:10.1016/j.cnur.2014.02.010

Croswell, J.M., Ransohoff, D.F., & Kramer, B.S. (2010). Principles of cancer screening: Lessons from history and study design issues. *Seminars in Oncology, 37,* 202–215. doi:10.1053/j.seminoncol.2010.05.006

Edwards, A.G.K., Naik, G., Ahmed, H., Elwyn, G.J., Pickles, T., Hood, K., & Playle, R. (2013). Personalised risk communication for informed decision making about taking screening tests. *Cochrane Database of Systematic Reviews, 2013*(2). doi:10.1002/14651858.CD001865.pub3

Fagerlin, A., Zikmund-Fisher, B.J., & Ubel, P.A. (2011). Helping patients decide: Ten steps to better risk communication. *Journal of the National Cancer Institute, 103,* 1436–1443. doi:10.1093/jnci/djr318

Freedman, A.N., Slattery, M.L., Ballard-Barbash, R., Willis, G., Cann, B.J., Pee, D., ... Pfeiffer, R.M. (2009). Colorectal cancer risk prediction tool for white men and women without known susceptibility. *Journal of Clinical Oncology, 27,* 686–693. doi:10.1200/JCO.2008.17.4797

Gail, M.H., & Mai, P.L. (2010). Comparing breast cancer risk assessment models. *Journal of the National Cancer Institute, 102,* 665–668. doi:10.1093/jnci/djq141

Gordis, L. (2014). *Epidemiology* (5th ed.). Philadelphia, PA: Elsevier Saunders.

Healthy People 2020. (n.d.). 2020 topics and objectives: Cancer. Retrieved from http://www.healthypeople.gov/2020/topics-objectives/topic/cancer

Klein, W.M.P., & Stefanek, M.E. (2007). Cancer risk elicitation and communication: Lessons from the psychology of risk perception. *CA: A Cancer Journal for Clinicians, 57,* 147–167. doi:10.3322/canjclin.57.3.147

Kushi, L.H., Doyle, C., McCullough, M., Rock, C.L., Demark-Wahnefried, W., Bandera, E.V., ... American Cancer Society 2010 Nutrition and Physical Activity Guidelines Advisory Committee. (2012). American Cancer Society guidelines on nutrition and physical activity for cancer prevention: Reducing the risk of cancer with healthy food choices and physical activity. *CA: A Cancer Journal for Clinicians, 62,* 30–67. doi:10.3322/caac.20140

Mahon, S.M. (2011). Managing families with a hereditary cancer syndrome. *Oncology Nursing Forum, 38,* 641–644. doi:10.1188/11.ONF.641-644

Matsuno, R.K., Costantino, J.P., Ziegler, R.G., Anderson, G.L., Li, H., Pee, D., & Gail, M.H. (2011). Projecting individualized absolute invasive breast cancer risk in Asian and Pacific Islander American women. *Journal of the National Cancer Institute, 103,* 951–961. doi:10.1093/jnci/djr154

National Cancer Institute Surveillance, Epidemiology, and End Results Program. (n.d.). Cancer incidence. Retrieved from http://seer.cancer.gov

National Comprehensive Cancer Network. (2016). *NCCN Clinical Practice Guidelines in Oncology (NCCN Guidelines®): Genetic/familial high-risk assessment: Breast and ovarian* [v.2.2017]. Retrieved from https://www.nccn.org/professionals/physician_gls/pdf/genetics_screening.pdf

Plescia, M., Richardson, L.C., & Joseph, D. (2012). New roles for public health in cancer screening. *CA: A Cancer Journal for Clinicians, 62,* 217–219. doi:10.3322/caac.21147

Riley, B.D., Culver, J.O., Skrzynia, C., Senter, L.A., Peters, J.A., Costalas, J.W., ... Trepanier, A.M. (2012). Essential elements of genetic cancer risk assessment, counseling, and testing: Updated recommendations of the National Society of Genetic Counselors. *Journal of Genetic Counseling, 21,* 151–161. doi:10.1007/s10897-011-9462-x

Rodriguez-Bigas, M.A., & Möeslein, G. (2013). Surgical treatment of hereditary nonpolyposis colorectal cancer (HNPCC, Lynch syndrome). *Familial Cancer, 12,* 295–300. doi:10.1007/s10689-013-9626-y

Smith, R.A., Brooks, D., Cokkinides, V., Saslow, D., & Brawley, O.W. (2013). Cancer screening in the United States, 2013. *CA: A Cancer Journal for Clinicians, 63,* 87–105. doi:10.3322/caac.21174

Smith, R.A., Manassaram-Baptiste, D., Brooks, D., Cokkinides, V., Doroshenk, M., Saslow, D., ... Brawley, O.W. (2014). Cancer screening in the United States, 2014: A review of current American Cancer Society guidelines and current issues in cancer screening. *CA: A Cancer Journal for Clinicians, 64,* 30–51. doi:10.3322/caac.21212

Thompson, R. (2010). Preventing cancer: The role of food, nutrition and physical activity. *Journal of Family Health Care, 20,* 100–102.

U.S. Public Health Service. (2014). *The health consequences of smoking—50 years of progress: A report of the Surgeon General: Executive summary.* Retrieved from http://www.surgeongeneral.gov/library/reports/50-years-of-progress/exec-summary.pdf

Wallace, H.N. (2011). *Guidelines for treating and controlling tobacco use and dependence.* New York, NY: Nova Science Publishers.

Weitzel, J.N., Blazer, K.R., MacDonald, D.J., Culver, J.O., & Offit, K. (2011). Genetics, genomics, and cancer risk assessment: State of the art and future directions in the era of personalized medicine. *CA: A Cancer Journal for Clinicians, 61,* 327–359. doi:10.3322/caac.20128

Zagouri, F., Chrysikos, D.T., Sergentanis, T.N., Giannakopoulou, G., Zografos, C.G., Papadimitriou, C.A., & Zografos, G.C. (2013). Prophylactic mastectomy: An appraisal. *American Surgeon, 79,* 205–212.

Glossary

absolute risk—Measure of the occurrence of cancer, either incidence (new cases) or mortality (deaths), in the general population.

asymptomatic—Both the person being screened and the examiner are unaware of any signs or symptoms of cancer in the individual prior to initiating the screening test.

cumulative risk—Measure of the total risk that a particular event will happen during a given time period or over a lifetime. It often is expressed as the likelihood that a person who is free of a certain type of cancer will develop that cancer by a specific age.

epidemiology—Study of how disease is distributed in a population, factors that influence its distribution in a population, and trends over time.

incidence—Number of cancers that develop in a population during a defined period, such as a year.

mortality—Number of people who die of a particular cancer during a defined period.

prevalence—Number of cancers that exist in a defined population at a given point in time.

primary prevention—Measures to avoid carcinogen exposure, improve health practices, and, in some cases, use chemoprevention agents. Primary prevention also may include the use of prophylactic surgery to prevent or significantly reduce the development of a malignancy in individuals with extremely elevated risk (usually due to known hereditary risk).

relative risk—Comparison of the incidence or deaths among those with a particular risk factor compared to those without the risk factor.

risk factor—Trait or characteristic that is associated with a statistically significant increased likelihood of developing a disease.

secondary prevention—Identification of individuals at risk for developing malignancy and the implementation of appropriate screening recommendations. Terms often used interchangeably with secondary cancer prevention are *early detection* and *cancer screening*.

tertiary prevention—Measures aimed at individuals with a history of malignancy, including monitoring for and preventing recurrence and screening for second primary cancers. In many cases, these individuals have had a diagnosis of cancer or carry a mutation in a cancer susceptibility gene and are known to be at significantly higher risk for developing a second malignancy.

Chapter 3 Study Questions

1. The nurse tells a woman that "one in eight women will be diagnosed with breast cancer if they live to be age 85." What is this an example of?
   A. Relative risk
   B. Attributable risk
   C. Absolute risk
   D. Incidence risk

2. The nurse is counseling a 32-year-old woman about cancer risks and prevention. She recommends 150 minutes of intentional exercise per week. What is this an example of?
   A. Primary prevention
   B. Secondary prevention
   C. Tertiary prevention
   D. Quaternary prevention

3. What level of cancer prevention is applied to cancer survivors?
   A. Primary prevention
   B. Secondary prevention
   C. Tertiary prevention
   D. Quaternary prevention

4. The nurse is conducting a risk factor assessment on a 42-year-old man without a history of cancer. A risk factor assessment is important to:
   A. Determine if he will develop a cancer.
   B. Select appropriate screening recommendations.
   C. Determine when he is most likely to develop a particular cancer.
   D. Select appropriate prevention recommendations.
   E. Determine if he should be referred for genetic testing.
   F. Answers A, B, and D
   G. Answers D and E
   H. Answers B, D, and E

5. A patient is scheduled for a colonoscopy because she just turned 50 years old. What is this an example of?
   A. Primary prevention
   B. Secondary prevention
   C. Tertiary prevention
   D. Quaternary prevention

CHAPTER

4 Genetic Risk for Developing Cancer

Suzanne M. Mahon, RN, DNSc, AOCN®, AGN-BC

Introduction

The Human Genome Project will continue to greatly affect oncology nursing practice. Genetics is an ever-growing field in oncology. An estimated 10% of all cancers have a hereditary component (Weitzel, Blazer, MacDonald, Culver, & Offit, 2011). Cancer genetics includes the identification of at-risk populations, referrals for hereditary cancer evaluation, assistance with the implementation of cancer prevention and detection measures, and management of the psychosocial ramifications of testing (Riley et al., 2012). Genetic testing is now readily and commercially available for hereditary breast and ovarian cancer (HBOC), hereditary nonpolyposis colorectal cancer (HNPCC), familial adenomatous polyposis (FAP) syndromes, and multiple other hereditary cancer syndromes (Ku, Cooper, Ziogas, et al., 2013). Additionally, predisposition genes for many unique or rare syndromes have been identified, and testing is available on a more limited or research basis (Rizzo & Buck, 2012).

Identification of a mutation in a family can be very helpful for risk management and treatment planning for both individuals with cancer and at-risk unaffected family members. Genetic testing is not a tool to be used in routine screening in a population because of the expense of testing and the complex counseling needs of these families. It is best used to help select individuals from high-risk families to make informed decisions about cancer screening and prevention strategies (Greco & Mahon, 2011). A primary nursing responsibility is to identify individuals who are at risk for a genetic predisposition and refer them to a healthcare provider with expertise in genetics (Consensus Panel on Genetic/Genomic Nursing Competencies, 2009; Greco, Tinley, & Seibert, 2012). Figure 4-1 shows the key indicators of a hereditary predisposition for developing cancer.

Genetic Basis of Cancer

Cancer is a disease of abnormal gene function. Genes are segments of DNA that contain instructions on how to make the proteins the body needs to function. They govern hereditary traits, such as hair color, eye color, and height, as well as susceptibility to certain diseases, such as cancer (Gunder & Martin, 2011).

In humans, genes are located on 23 pairs of chromosomes. One of each chromosome pair comes from the mother, and the other is from the father. Each chromosome can contain hun-

Figure 4-1. General Indicators of a Hereditary Predisposition for Developing Cancer

The following factors should be considered after gathering family history, and if one or more criteria are present, it may be prudent to refer the patient to a healthcare provider with expertise in cancer genetics.

- Cancer occurring at a younger age than expected in the general population
- More than one primary cancer in one person
- Evidence of autosomal dominant inheritance (two or more generations affected, with both men and women affected)
- Bilateral cancer in any paired organ
- Any pattern of cancer associated with a known cancer syndrome
- Occurrence of cancers more frequently in a family than expected by chance in the absence of known environmental and lifestyle risk factors
- Multifocal cancers in an organ
- Presence of premalignant conditions such as more than 20 colorectal adenomatous polyps
- A diagnosis of a cancer associated with hereditary risk, such as male breast cancer, ovarian cancer, or a pheochromocytoma
- A cluster of the same cancer in close relatives
- Specific clinical characteristics of a tumor associated with hereditary cancer syndromes, such as microsatellite instability in a colon cancer or triple-negative breast cancer

Note. Based on information from Lindor et al., 2008; Mahon, 2011; Weitzel et al., 2011.

dreds or thousands of genes that are passed from the parents to the child. These genes are in every cell of the body (Wiggs, 2009).

Genes serve two major roles in cancer: some contribute to the development of cancer, and others stop cancer from developing or growing. Genes that can cause cancer are *oncogenes.* Genes that stop or suppress cancer growth are *tumor suppressor genes* (Gunder & Martin, 2011).

A *mutation* is a change in genetic material. Some mutations do not cause disease or problems but are changes in the genetic material; these are referred to as *polymorphisms.* Other mutations can result in disease or other significant changes because of alterations in protein function. These mutations are referred to as *deleterious* because the cell cannot function correctly (Sijmons, Greenblatt, & Genuardi, 2013).

Two types of mutations lead to the development of cancer. Individuals can be born with healthy genes that become changed (mutated) over the course of their life. These mutations are referred to as *somatic* and account for approximately 90% of all cancers. Somatic mutations can occur from exposure to carcinogens, such as chemicals, ultraviolet light, hormones, dietary elements, or radiation. Sporadic cancers occur from multiple somatic mutations in a cell (Gunder & Martin, 2011). If the mutation arises in a body cell, copies of the mutation will exist only in descendants of that particular cell. The older an individual is, the more likely he or she is to have acquired gene mutations. This is why cancer risk increases with age.

The second type of mutation that predisposes humans to developing a disease such as cancer is a *germ-line* mutation and is present at conception in the ova or sperm. When reproductive germ cells containing mutations combine to produce offspring, the mutation will be present in all the offspring's body cells. Because every cell in the body carries the germ-line mutation, cancer typically occurs earlier than expected and often more than once in people with this type of mutation. Because of variable penetrance, having a germ-line mutation does not mean an individual will definitely develop the cancer. *Penetrance* is an indication of the probability that a given mutation will produce disease. For example, the HBOC genes, *BRCA1* and *BRCA2*, confer an 85% risk of developing breast cancer by age 70 (Lindor, McMaster, Lindor, & Greene, 2008). Most inherited cancers are transmitted in an autosomal dominant pattern, so only one parent is responsible for passing the gene that confers the increased risk. The offspring of these individuals have a statistical 50% chance of having the same mutation (Wiggs, 2009).

An accurate family history combined with predisposition genetic testing can help to differentiate somatic and germ-line mutations (Bennett, French, Resta, & Doyle, 2008). Identifying people with germ-line mutations is important because of their increased risk for second primary cancers and the potential risk to other close relatives. These families are routinely identified during cancer risk assessments as described in Chapter 3. The biology of cancer, including a discussion of genetics, is discussed in Chapter 1.

Genetic Risk Assessment

Identifying and managing people who are at risk for hereditary cancer syndromes has become an integral part of oncologic prevention, early detection, and treatment. With proper assessment, testing, and implementation of aggressive screening and prevention measures, healthcare providers can significantly affect the future health of patients and their families with a hereditary risk for cancer development.

As many as 5%–10% of people may have a personal or family health history suggestive of a hereditary cancer syndrome (Weitzel et al., 2011). Some family histories do not suggest a specific syndrome such as HBOC or HNPCC, but the history has a larger number of malignancies than would be expected by chance or explained by environmental exposures. An unusual constellation of cancer types also may be present. It is best to refer to a healthcare provider with expertise in genetics to consider rare syndromes and possible testing strategies or research studies to help these families better define their risk (Mahon, 2013b).

Selection of the appropriate genetic test depends on the risk factor assessment. This includes an assessment of the risk of developing the cancer and, in many cases, calculations of the risk of carrying a mutation. The commercial availability of genetic testing for the cancer susceptibility genes associated with hereditary cancer syndromes has greatly changed oncology practice. Cancer susceptibility genetic testing has the potential to identify whether a person is at increased risk for a particular cancer or cancers associated with a hereditary cancer syndrome. These tests, however, cannot predict when, where, or if a cancer will be diagnosed. One of the challenges in the communication of genetic risk information and genetic test results is that probabilities and uncertainties surround genetic information (Wiseman, Dancyger, & Michie, 2010).

Whether an individual might benefit from predisposition genetic testing will depend on the person's degree of genetic risk, whether testing is likely to address the individual's needs, and the availability of an appropriate test. Because of the high cost of some genetic tests, reimbursement factors also need to be considered. Most insurers cover some or all of the cost of testing for people who meet eligibility criteria set by the insurer. The final testing decision, however, will depend on the patient's understanding of the potential risks and benefits and whether the person wants to proceed (Plutynski, 2012).

Family history and mathematical models can be used to calculate one's risk for developing cancer and carrying a mutation, but ultimately, genetic testing is the only means available to potentially determine who has inherited a germ-line mutation. A number of professional organizations and government agencies have issued position statements regarding genetic testing. Some are more general, but many set forth conditions for offering specific cancer predisposition testing, most often *BRCA1* and *BRCA2* testing. These recommendations are updated frequently, and it is important to consult the individual agency for updates. In general, genetic testing is offered when the family or personal history suggests a hereditary risk, a test is available that can be interpreted, and the results will influence management. The American College of Medical Genetics and Genomics and the National Society of Genetic Counselors have compiled an extensive resource that outlines conditions in which patients and families should be referred for genetic testing (Hampel, Bennett, Buchanan, Pearlman, & Wiesner, 2014). Clinicians should refer to this reference regularly to make appropriate referrals for genetic evaluation.

Provision of Cancer Genetic Education and Counseling

Providing education, counseling, and support is a central nursing responsibility when caring for people with a hereditary predisposition for developing cancer. This education must be tailored to the individual needs and learning capabilities of each family member. It usually is a labor-intensive process, and families should anticipate at least one to three 60–90-minute sessions prior to testing to ensure they have adequate information to make a decision that is congruent with their own individual needs and provide informed consent (Mahon, 2013a). In most cases, families should be referred to a genetic healthcare professional, such as a certified genetic counselor or an advanced practice nurse with additional training in cancer genetics. Such advanced practice nurses are now credentialed through the American Nurses Credentialing Center and have the advanced genetics nursing–board certified (AGN-BC) credential. Figure 4-2 shows a comparison of the roles and responsibilities for oncology nurses caring for people with a hereditary predisposition for developing cancer (Consensus Panel on Genetic/Genomic Nursing Competencies, 2009; Greco & Mahon, 2011; Greco et al., 2012; National Coalition for Health Professional Education in Genetics, 2007).

This credentialing denotes the attainment of additional education and training in managing people with genetic susceptibility. Some of these nurses are also members of the National Society of Genetic Counselors. Some insurance companies require that patients receive genetic counseling from a credentialed genetic healthcare professional prior to reimbursement for genetic testing costs.

When patients do not receive counseling and services from a credentialed genetic healthcare professional, the risk of errors increases substantially (Brierley et al., 2010). These errors include having the wrong or incomplete testing ordered, having results interpreted incorrectly, ordering unnecessary testing, and having inadequate counseling to understand the implications of such testing for both the patient and other family members. Having a comprehensive evaluation by a credentialed genetic healthcare professional has been shown to decrease these errors (Brierley et al., 2012). Genetic professionals also have the training and expertise to identify at-risk family members and provide patients with tools to inform and educate family members. They also can provide referrals to genetic professionals to ensure that all at-risk family members are informed of their risk and offered the option of genetic testing (Bensend, Veach, & Niendorf, 2014; Riley et al., 2012).

Assessment of Hereditary Risk

Cancer genetic education includes a number of steps. During the assessment for hereditary risk, families are asked to provide detailed information about family history and cancer diagnoses. It often is helpful to inform patients of the need for a detailed family history prior to the appointment. Every family who presents for genetic counseling or testing should designate a spokesperson, or *proband*, for the family. The proband may or may not have cancer but serves as a point of reference when discussing risk. Typically, the proband for the family should be instructed to gather information about all cancer diagnoses, ages at diagnoses, and current ages or ages at death for all first- and second-degree relatives. Often this requires that the proband communicate with multiple family members. Obtaining this information before the appointment saves time and allows the advanced practice nurse to make

Figure 4-2. Comparison of Roles for Nurses Caring for Patients With a Hereditary Predisposition for Developing Cancer

General Oncology Nurse
- Perform risk assessments that include personal, medical, occupational, environmental, and family history risk factors.
- Refer families with a potential hereditary predisposition to a genetic healthcare professional.
- Assist with implementation of recommendations for prevention and early detection prescribed by the genetic healthcare professional.
- Provide psychological support and encouragement to patients and families pursuing genetic testing.

Advanced Practice Nurse
- Perform basic risk assessments, and identify risk factors that suggest a hereditary predisposition.
- Initiate collection of data for a three-generation pedigree.
- Answer general questions about genetics.
- Refer at-risk families to a genetic healthcare professional.
- Provide psychological support.
- Assist with evaluating and monitoring the impact of genetic testing, and ensure recommended screening and prevention measures are carried out.

Advanced Practice Nurse With Subspecialty Credentialing in Genetics
- Conduct in-depth assessments of family history.
- Construct pedigrees with cancers verified through medical records and death certificates.
- Assess patients' risk of developing cancer based on personal and family history.
- Assess patients' risk of having a mutation, and evaluate their eligibility and appropriateness for genetic testing.
- Provide genetic counseling, including pre- and post-test counseling as needed.
- Provide information to ensure informed consent regarding the strengths, risks, and limitations of testing.
- Conduct physical assessments from a genetics perspective.
- Identify the best person to initiate testing within the family.
- Select and order the appropriate genetic test or tests.
- Interpret the test results and make recommendations based on personal health history, family history, and genetic testing results.
- Coordinate follow-up care based on genetic testing results.
- Assess and develop strategies to facilitate coping with any adverse psychological consequences of a diagnosis of a hereditary cancer syndrome.
- Identify other family members who might benefit from genetic testing.
- Assist with enrolling families with unusual syndromes in research studies.

Note. Based on information from Consensus Panel on Genetic/Genomic Nursing Competencies, 2009; Greco & Mahon, 2011; Greco et al., 2012; National Coalition for Health Professional Education in Genetics, 2007.

preliminary risk calculations and identify areas where more information is needed. This information should be confirmed by pathology reports or death certificates because families often have incomplete or incorrect information about cancer diagnoses. Without accurate information regarding the diagnoses, it is impossible to accurately assess risk and select the correct genetic test. Taking a detailed family history is the first step in identifying families with a possible hereditary predisposition to malignancy and other illnesses. Healthcare providers should ask patients about specific relatives and their health individually rather than asking a more general question such as "Have any of your relatives been diagnosed with cancer?" The nurse needs to be aware of key indicators of hereditary cancer syndromes, especially when cancers are diagnosed at a younger age than expected, the same cancer or cluster of cancers occurs in multiple family members, or multiple generations are affected. Ethnic background is an additional consideration when deciding if testing may be appropriate. Individuals from an Ashkenazi Jewish background are at higher risk for having several specific mutations associated with HBOC or FAP (Tkatch et al., 2014; Weitzel et al., 2011).

Once the family history information is gathered, it is best organized into a three-generation pedigree, as discussed in Chapter 3. The pedigree is an excellent means to educate a family about autosomal dominant transmission. It also is often required for insurance reimbursement or if the family plans to enroll in a clinical trial. Healthcare providers can use computer programs to construct pedigrees or draw them by hand (Scheuner et al., 2009).

Programs and models are available that help to calculate statistical risks for developing cancer and for carrying a mutation related to hereditary predisposition (see Figure 4-3). These usually are calculated by a genetic professional and included in the risk assessment information. Patients need to understand the risk for developing the disease in the general population (i.e., absolute risk) and also their relative risk compared to people who do not have risk factors. Using relative risk is complicated in people with a family history of cancer. If the individual did not inherit the predisposition gene, the relative risk score will overestimate the person's risk. If the individual did inherit the gene, it will probably underestimate the risk. Patients need to be informed of these potential and significant limitations.

Patients should receive a calculation of their risk for having a genetic mutation as well as their relative risk for developing cancer. If no testing has been done in a family, the calculation of risk usually is based on the number of family members diagnosed with a specific constellation of cancers, ethnicity, and age at diagnosis. Several different models are used (see Figure 4-3), and the patient typically receives the risk estimate in a range. Each method has distinct strengths and limitations. It is especially important to note whether the family is small with few women, as these models usually will underestimate the risk of having a mutation (Riley et al., 2012; Wiseman et al., 2010). Once a mutation is detected in a family, the healthcare provider can offer the statistical risk based on Mendelian patterns of inheritance. In the case of autosomal dominance, first-degree relatives have a statistical 50% chance of having inherited the predisposition gene. If a mutation is not detected in the family, calculation of the risks of developing cancer can be helpful in selecting recommendations for cancer prevention and early detection. Figure 4-4 shows other components of the cancer genetic education and counseling process.

Basic Genetic Information

For families to make informed decisions about testing, they need a basic background in genetics. At minimum, this includes information about autosomal dominant transmission, penetrance, statistical risks, and the difference between germ-line and somatic mutations. Pictures and diagrams are useful when conveying this information. A copy of the pedigree also is useful to share with the family so that they can better understand principles of autosomal dominant transmission. Other materials to share with families include copies of risk calculations, especially if these calculations help the family to understand how their risk compares with that of the general population and estimates of risk over time (Fagerlin, Zikmund-Fisher, & Ubel, 2011).

Prevention Strategies

Before obtaining genetic testing, patients need a clear understanding of the recommendations and guidelines for management of risk if they test positive and if they do not. This anticipatory guidance helps patients to prepare for all the potential ramifications of testing so that they can make an informed choice about whether to pursue genetic testing.

Figure 4-3. Common Risk Model Calculations for Hereditary Cancer Syndromes

Models to Estimate Breast Cancer Risk and Screen for Hereditary Breast or Ovarian Cancer (HBOC)
- Claus Model: Estimates breast cancer risk in 10-year increments in women without a diagnosis of breast cancer who have a family history
- Gail Model: Estimates breast cancer risk over 5-year increments and lifetime in women without a diagnosis of cancer who have a minimal to moderate family history of breast cancer; has known limitation of not considering paternal history or ovarian cancer history
- Pedigree Assessment Tool: Screening tool that uses a simple point-scoring system to identify women who may be at risk for HBOC

Models to Estimate Risk of a *BRCA1* Mutation
- Couch Model: Estimates risk of *BRCA1* mutation; considers the average age at onset of breast cancer and ethnicity
- Shattuck-Eidens Model: Estimates risk of a mutation in women with a strong family history of breast and/or ovarian cancer; does not consider ethnicity

Models to Estimate Risk of a *BRCA1* and/or *BRCA2* Mutation
- Berry Model: Estimates risk of a *BRCA1* or *BRCA2* mutation in women with a family history of breast and/or ovarian cancer
- Frank Model: Estimates risk of a *BRCA1* or *BRCA2* mutation in women diagnosed with breast cancer before age 50
- Manchester Model: Estimates risk of a *BRCA1* or *BRCA2* mutation in non-Jewish women with a family history of breast and/or ovarian cancer
- Penn II Model: Estimates risk of a *BRCA1* or *BRCA2* mutation in women with personal and family history of breast and/or ovarian cancer

Models to Identify Families at Risk for Hereditary Colorectal Cancer
- Amsterdam Criteria: Suggests recommendation to offer genetic testing based on presence of specific family history criteria
- Bethesda Model: Suggests recommendation to offer testing based on presence of a cluster of defined criteria
- MMPro Model: Predicts people who may benefit from genetic testing for *MSH2* or *MLH1* mutations

Models to Estimate Risk of Hereditary Colorectal Cancer
- PREMM Model: Estimates risk of carrying an *MSH2* or *MLH1* mutation in people with a family history of colorectal and gynecologic cancer
- Wijnen Model: Estimates risk of carrying an *MSH2* or *MLH1* mutation in people with a family history of breast and/or endometrial cancer

Note. Based on information from Balmaña et al., 2010; Berry et al., 2002; Claus et al., 1994, 1996; Evans et al., 2004; Gail & Mai, 2010; Kastrinos et al., 2013; Lindor et al., 2010; Matsuno et al., 2011; National Comprehensive Cancer Network, 2016; Parmigiani et al., 2007; Shattuck-Eidens et al., 1997; Ståhlbom et al., 2012; Teller et al., 2010; Umar et al., 2004.

Patients often are interested in prevention, but this area can involve difficult choices. For many cancers with a hereditary predisposition, prevention is best achieved by prophylactic surgery, such as mastectomy, hysterectomy, colectomy, or oophorectomy. Each of these procedures carries not only the risks associated with surgery and anesthesia, but also psychosocial concerns, significant body image changes, and alterations in body function. It is important to explore a patient's feelings, concerns, and openness about these preventive measures prior to testing (Twomey, 2011; Wevers et al., 2011).

Prevention measures also may include chemoprevention if a strategy exists. Patients need to be aware of the risks, side effects, and potential benefits of such agents. This usually requires a discussion of current research. It is important to explore whether the individual is willing to commit to taking the chemopreven-

Figure 4-4. Typical Components of Cancer Genetic Education and Counseling

- Detailed family history and construction of pedigree
- Risks for cancers in the population (absolute risk)
- Individual's risks for a particular cancer (relative risk)
- Potential genetic mutations, calculations of risk of having those mutations, and possibility that the test will be uninformative
- Factors that limit the interpretation and calculation of risk, such as limited family history, adoption, or incomplete information about family members
- Information about and rationale for ordering specific genetic tests, including technical accuracy
- Implications of a positive, negative, or uninformative test result
- Options, risks, benefits, and limitations of prevention and early detection strategies
- Alternatives to testing, including not testing
- Risks to other family members
- Fees for testing and counseling/education
- Privacy and confidentiality issues
- Potential discrimination risks for insurance or employment
- Strategies for disclosing results and information to other at-risk family members
- Potential psychological risks and benefits of testing
- Possibility of enrolling in variant studies or research studies depending on family history

Note. Based on information from Cohen et al., 2012; Greco et al., 2012; Levy et al., 2009; Riley et al., 2012; Twomey, 2011.

tive agent long term, even though the effectiveness may not be immediately evident (Iwuji et al., 2014).

Finally, prevention measures may include lifestyle measures, such as a healthy diet, weight management, exercise, smoking cessation, and sunscreen use and other ultraviolet light–protecting measures. For interventions to be effective, patients need specific information, planning, and detailed approaches and recommendations to implement these behaviors. Lack of provider recommendation is a major barrier to cancer screening (Spruce & Sanford, 2012). Oncology nurses can remove this barrier by conscientiously and consistently recommending cancer prevention measures and role modeling healthy habits (Spruce & Sanford, 2012). Lack of discussion about prevention and early detection often occurs because of the acute and sporadic nature of many visits, the lack of a tracking system to ensure that prevention measures are ordered, and the incorrect assumption by healthcare providers that patients are not interested in being screened. In the case of complicated screening recommendations, such as with colorectal cancer screening, research suggests that the provider needs to streamline decisions and make recommendations for the patient (American Cancer Society [ACS], 2015b; Klabunde et al., 2007; Saslow et al., 2012; Spruce & Sanford, 2012). Detailed information about cancer prevention recommendations is readily available (ACS, 2015b; "A Healthy Diet and Physical Activity Help Reduce Your Cancer Risk," 2012; Kushi et al., 2012).

Early Detection Strategies

Families and individuals with hereditary predisposition need specific information regarding how to detect cancer in the earliest stages, when treatment is most likely to be effective. This includes signs and symptoms to report promptly, as well as screening measures. Each recommended screening measure requires a discussion of the sensitivity and specificity of the test along with the expected benefits and risks. Guidelines for the general population may require modification in high-risk families. It is important that families clearly understand that screening will not prevent a cancer but is hoped to result in sufficiently early detection for the cancer to be treated with limited morbidity and mortality (ACS, 2016; National Comprehensive Cancer Network® [NCCN®], 2016).

Testing Process

Historically, testing for germ-line hereditary predisposition syndromes has involved Sanger DNA sequencing. The introduction of next-generation sequencing (NGS) panels that analyze less common high- and intermediate-penetrance cancer susceptibility genes has led to reduced cost and turnaround time with the simultaneous testing of multiple genes in the genetic testing process (Rizzo & Buck, 2012). NCCN has updated its recommendations to include NGS for HBOC and other cancers. However, because of the complexity and variety of results interpretation, NCCN and other groups strongly recommend that these panels should be ordered only in consultation with a genetic healthcare professional (American College of Medical Genetics and Genomics, 2012; NCCN, 2016).

Many hereditary cancer syndromes have confusing clinical presentations, and it can be challenging to select the correct test. Simultaneous testing for germ-line mutations associated with hereditary cancer syndromes using an NGS-targeted platform may be more efficient, cost-effective, and effective in identifying a mutation and ultimately providing the patient and family with useful information to manage risk. This emerging technology has made the detection of more mutations possible, especially in less common, lower-penetrance genes, but it has greatly increased the complexity of the genetic counseling and testing process, as well as the interpretation of test results. For example, multiple genes are associated with varying degrees of risk for developing breast cancer. Historically, a woman with a personal or family history of breast or ovarian cancer would have been offered genetic testing for *BRCA1* and *BRCA2*, the two genes commonly associated with hereditary breast cancer. Now, instead of testing for just *BRCA1* and *BRCA2*, NGS panels for breast cancer might include testing for the following genes: *ATM, BARD1, BRCA1, BRCA2, BRIP1, CDH1, CHEK2, EPCAM, FANCC, MLH1, MSH2, MSH6, NBN, PALB2, PMS2, PTEN, RAD51C, RAD51D, STK11, TP53,* and *XRCC2* (see Table 4-1). Genetic healthcare professionals must carefully consider the personal and family history to order an NGS panel that is most likely to provide informative information. The clinical implications of a mutation in some of the genes in NGS panels are poorly understood. In addition, recognizing intermediate-penetrance (two- to fivefold increased risk) genes, their contribution to cancer, and the subsequent management of mutation carriers continues to pose a challenge in clinical management because of a lack of published guidelines.

Patients who decide to proceed with genetic testing need information about the test or tests being ordered, potential management strategies, and the potential risks, benefits, and limitations of testing. Patients usually must sign a consent form to document that they understand the ramifications of testing and are not being coerced. A number of agencies have made recommendations about the need for informed consent and consultation with a qualified health professional with expertise in genetics (American College of Medical Genetics and Genomics, 2012; American College of Obstetricians and Gynecologists, 2008; NCCN, 2016; Riley et al., 2012).

Ideally, an affected family member will be the first one to be tested. A person who has been diagnosed with a cancer within the constellation of tumors that have been clearly linked to a particular cancer syndrome or syndromes will be the most informative for the rest of the family. If this relative has been tested and found to carry a deleterious mutation known to be associated with increased cancer risk, then at-risk family members are likely to benefit from testing for the same mutation. This is referred to as *single-site mutation testing* and is considerably less expensive. Sometimes the decision is simple in cases of clear maternal or paternal transmission over several generations with one or two tumor types.

Because testing usually is expensive and insurance reimbursement is variable, preauthorization is desirable so that the patient understands his or her potential financial responsibilities. Preauthorization frequently requires a letter of medical necessity. Typical components

Table 4-1. Common Genetic Syndromes

Gene/Syndrome*	**Associated Cancers†**
APC (familial adenomatous polyposis)	Colon (93%), small bowel (5%), thyroid, pancreatic, brain
ATM	Breast, colon, pancreatic, ataxia telangiectasia
BARD1	Breast, ovarian
BMPR1A	Colon (50%), gastric (20%)
BRCA1	Breast—female (90%), ovarian (50%), pancreatic, prostate, melanoma, breast—male, endometrial
BRCA2	Breast—female (85%), ovarian (35%–40%), pancreatic (8%), prostate (35%), melanoma, breast—male (8%), endometrial
BRIP1	Breast, ovarian
CDH1	Gastric (50%–85%), breast (30%–50%), colon
CDK4	Melanoma, pancreatic, breast, nonmelanoma skin
CDKN2A	Melanoma, pancreatic
CHEK2	Breast—female (30%–50%), prostate, colon, breast—male, ovarian, thyroid
EPCAM (hereditary nonpolyposis colorectal cancer [HNPCC], also known as Lynch syndrome)	Colon (60%–75%), endometrial (40%–55%), ovarian, gastric, pancreatic, biliary tract, urothelium, small bowel, brain, sebaceous neoplasms
FANCC	Breast—female
MEN1 (multiple endocrine neoplasia type 1)	Parathyroid (85%), pancreatic (40%), adrenal (15%–35%), pituitary (30%–80%)
MLH1 (HNPCC)	Colon (80%), endometrial (60%), ovarian (12%–20%), gastric (20%), pancreatic, biliary tract, urothelium, small bowel, brain, sebaceous neoplasms
MSH2 (HNPCC)	Colon (25%–80%), endometrial (55%), ovarian (12%–24%), gastric (10%), pancreatic, biliary tract, urothelium, small bowel, brain, sebaceous neoplasms
MSH6 (HNPCC)	Colon (45%), endometrial (45%), ovarian (11%), gastric, pancreatic, biliary tract, urothelium, small bowel, brain, sebaceous neoplasms
MUTYH (MUTYH-associated polyposis—recessive syndrome)	Colon (50%–80%), small bowel (5%), endometrial, ovarian
NF1 (neurofibromatosis type 1)	Neurofibromas (100%), breast
NF2 (neurofibromatosis type 2)	Vestibular schwannomas
PALB2	Breast—female (60%), pancreatic, colon

(Continued on next page)

Table 4-1. Common Genetic Syndromes *(Continued)*

Gene/Syndrome*	Associated Cancers†
PMS2 (HNPCC)	Colon (20%–30%), endometrial (15%), ovarian, gastric, pancreatic
PTEN (Cowden syndrome)	Breast—female (50%), thyroid (10%), endometrial (10%), colon, gastric, melanoma
RAD51D	Breast, ovarian
RB1	Retinoblastoma, osteosarcoma, melanoma, pineoblastoma
SDHA (paraganglioma-pheochromocytoma [PGL-PCC] syndrome)	Paraganglioma (48%–84%), pheochromocytoma
SDHAF2 (PGL-PCC)	Paraganglioma (40%–65%), pheochromocytoma
SDHB (PGL-PCC)	Paraganglioma (68%), pheochromocytoma
SDHC (PGL-PCC)	Paraganglioma (15%–25%), pheochromocytoma
SDHD (PGL-PCC)	Paraganglioma (15%), pheochromocytoma
SPRED1 (Legius syndrome)	Neurofibromas
RET (multiple endocrine neoplasia type 2)	Medullary thyroid (100%), pheochromocytoma (40%–50%), parathyroid (30%)
STK11 (Peutz-Jeghers syndrome)	Breast—female (55%), colon (40%), pancreatic (40%), gastric (20%), small bowel (13%), endometrial
TP53 (Li Fraumeni syndrome)	Breast, sarcoma, brain, hematologic malignancies, adrenocortical malignancies
VHL (von Hippel-Lindau syndrome)	Renal (70%), pancreatic (17%) neuroendocrine tumors, hemangioblastoma, pheochromocytoma
XRCC2	Breast, pancreatic

*All syndromes are autosomal dominant unless noted otherwise.

†Penetrance rates, when known, are indicated in parentheses.

Note. Based on information from Axilbund & Wiley, 2012; Chan-Smutko, 2012; Chun & Ford, 2012; Daniels, 2012; Eng, 2016; Gabree & Seidel, 2012; Jasperson, 2012; Mahon & Waldman, 2012; Murray & Davies, 2013; Narod, 2010; Pilarski & Nagy, 2012; Senter, 2012; Shannon & Chittenden, 2012; Weissman, Burt, et al., 2012.

of a letter of medical necessity include the test being ordered, why it is appropriate, and how the results will influence the care and management of the patient's risk.

Once preauthorization is obtained, a blood specimen or buccal wash is obtained and sent to the testing laboratory. Some laboratories will hold the specimen until preauthorization is final. Each laboratory has specific rules for collecting and transporting the specimen depending on the test being ordered.

In most cases, results are available in two to five weeks depending on the laboratory and the complexity of the test or tests. Disclosure of results is best done in person. In some cases, telephone disclosure may be acceptable and associated with an equally acceptable outcome, but this needs to be discussed and determined during the pretest phase (Baumanis, Evans, Callanan, & Susswein, 2009; Bradbury et al., 2011). Depending on the outcome, additional sessions may be needed to discuss management strategies and provide coordination of care for other family members.

Genetic testing for a hereditary cancer syndrome has implications for other family members. Therefore, a clear plan must be developed before testing as to how other family members will be informed of risk. Genetic test results are confidential medical information. The proband will need to inform other at-risk relatives, and the genetic healthcare professional assists the proband with this process (Greco et al., 2012; Mahon, 2011).

A related issue that families sometimes confront is the testing of minor children. Something to consider before testing is that knowledge of test results might change prevention and screening behaviors; therefore, this is an important consideration for minor children. In the case of HBOC, HNPCC, and most genetic testing for hereditary cancer syndromes, knowledge of mutation status will not alter behaviors. Minor children would probably not be candidates for mammography or prophylactic surgery. It would not be necessary to know mutation status to recommend following a low-fat, high-fiber diet or reducing ultraviolet light exposure. These recommendations would be appropriate for any member of the population. In most cases, genetic counselors will make these recommendations to both the parents and minor children. When children reach an age to legally consent and are mature enough, following adequate counseling, they can make their own decision regarding testing. One exception to this is families with a known mutation associated with *APC* or *TP53*. For example, in the case of a mutated APC, associated with FAP, these individuals can begin forming polyps prior to their teenage years, and colonoscopy often is initiated before the individual reaches the legal age to provide consent. With careful counseling of both the minor child and parents, families sometimes will decide to test the child. In this case, the parents would consent because knowing the results of mutation status may provide support for regular colonoscopy at a young age or may eliminate the need for this invasive screening procedure (Twomey, 2011).

Potential Risks, Benefits, and Limitations of Testing

The biggest risks of testing involve loss of privacy and psychosocial distress. In most cases, pretest counseling aids in the identification of potential problems so that they can be addressed prior to testing.

Efforts to protect confidentiality are essential. Concerns about confidentiality and potential discrimination often are paramount for patients and in some cases make it difficult for patients to even begin to learn about testing. These fears keep some individuals and families from seeking genetic services or participating in genetic research (Greco et al., 2012).

Federal laws exist that help to protect patients' genetic information. The Health Insurance Portability and Accountability Act of 1996 (referred to as HIPAA) specifically addresses genetic discrimination. Group health insurance plans cannot use genetic information to deny or limit eligibility for coverage or to increase premiums. This information cannot be considered a preexisting condition. The protection has gaps and does not apply to people who have individual or self-insured plans. Employment discrimination was addressed with the passage of the Genetic Information Nondiscrimination Act of 2008. Genetic information could no longer be used to prevent employment or insurance coverage as of November 21, 2009, and May 21, 2010, respectively (U.S. Department of Health and Human Services, 2009). Currently, life, long-term care, and disability insurance coverage is not protected under this legislation. Prior to testing, patients should receive counseling about the risks and potential problems with obtaining life, long-term care, or disability insurance. Failure to disclose a genetic condition may result in cancellation of a policy. Some people may opt to purchase or increase coverage before undergoing testing to avoid possible problems.

The informed consent process for predisposition genetic testing needs to include both educational and decision-making components. The entire education and counseling process that occurs when a patient faces a complicated decision, such as whether to pursue predisposition genetic testing, is integral to informed, shared decision making between the patient and the healthcare provider. Components of informed consent for genetic testing include the risks, benefits, cost, accuracy, and purpose of the specific test being ordered; alternatives to genetic testing; implications of a positive, negative, or uncertain test result; how results will be communicated; psychosocial implications; confidentiality issues; and options for medical surveillance and risk reduction (Twomey, 2011).

Outcomes of Testing

Testing has three possible outcomes: negative, positive, or a variant of indeterminate significance (see Table 4-2). Following disclosure of results, patients need to know the implications of the results. Recommendations for follow-up, prevention, and early detection are based on the results of testing and, in many cases, the personal and family history. For individuals who test positive for a mutation, aggressive screening and prevention measures are recommended and indicated. For those who test negative for a known mutation in a family, recommendations for screening and prevention that would be appropriate for the general population should be given, such as those from ACS (2015b, 2016). For those who test negative and the family does not have a known mutation, recommendations for prevention are based on potential risks after considering the patient's personal and family history, followed by a balanced discussion of the potential risks and benefits of such recommendations. This result is uninformative. It means the patient tested negative for a gene or genes associated with hereditary risk. The family could still have another gene associated with increased risk for which testing was not ordered or is not available, or the family may not have a hereditary predisposition to developing cancer. These families may benefit from enrollment in a hereditary cancer research registry with the hope of identifying a mutation through research.

For those who receive results of a variant of indeterminate significance, individuals may experience confusion and disappointment because risk has not been clarified. It is not immediately clear if the individual may have benign polymorphisms that most likely will not be reported when the variant is reclassified. Alternatively, the individual may not have a germ-line mutation or may have a germ-line mutation for which testing is not currently available, or the cancer is due to another gene or hereditary syndrome.

The risk of a variant of indeterminate significance may be higher in NGS, as less is known about some of the genes (Ku, Cooper, Ziogas, et al., 2013). Rates of variants of indeterminate significance may approach 20% and may be even higher in minority populations because they are not as well represented in databases (Murray, Cerrato, Bennett, & Jarvik, 2011). Patients need to be informed of the increased risk of a variant of indeterminate significance during the pretest process. Often the laboratory will want to test other family members, and if this is an option, it can be offered to families. Some of these families may be able to enroll in a research registry but may not receive useful information in a timely fashion. These families will need recommendations for prevention and early detection based on risks, with a discussion of the

Table 4-2. Implications of Genetic Testing Results

Result	Implications for Individual	Implications for Family	Other Considerations
Positive	At increased risk for developing cancer(s)	In autosomal disorders, first-degree relatives have a statistical 50% chance of having the mutation. Single-site testing would clarify if the family member has the mutation and associated increased risk. Single-site testing is lower in cost.	Does not inform about what type of cancer will develop or when, only that the risk is higher Enables individual to make decisions about prevention and early detection
True negative—no mutation detected in a person with a known mutation in family	Will not need screening greater than that recommended for the general population Will not need to consider prophylactic surgery or chemoprevention	Offspring from this individual are not at risk in autosomal dominant syndromes. No further testing is necessary.	Provides a more accurate cancer risk assessment Provides psychological relief regarding risk for developing cancer and that offspring will not inherit the mutation Creates risk of individuals having a false sense of security that they will not develop cancer, resulting in failure to get screening recommended for those of average risk May cause individuals to feel guilty that they "escaped" the mutation ("survivor guilt")
Negative—no mutation identified in family	No mutation detected in an individual in a family with no known mutations Usually occurs when the first individual in a family is tested The cancer is the result of a different mutation than the one tested, or the cancer seen in the family occurs because of nonhereditary reasons. Results are difficult to interpret and must be considered in conjunction with personal risk factors and family history.	Testing will not be available to other unaffected members in the family, as they will also test negative.	Creates uncertainty about the usefulness of cancer risk reduction strategies Individuals may consider participating in research studies or high-risk registries.

(Continued on next page)

Table 4-2. Implications of Genetic Testing Results *(Continued)*

Result	Implications for Individual	Implications for Family	Other Considerations
Variant of indeterminate significance	Test identifies a mutation; it is not clear if it is a polymorphism or deleterious. Results do not provide meaningful information. May provoke anxiety	Meaningful testing will not be available to other family members.	Creates uncertainty about the usefulness of cancer risk reduction strategies Requires recommendations for cancer prevention and detection needs based on personal risk factors and family history with careful information about potential benefits and risks Individuals may consider participation in a research study or hereditary cancer registry.
Variant—likely benign	Strong evidence suggesting that the genetic change is not associated with increased susceptibility for developing a disease	Meaningful testing will not be available to other family members.	Requires recommendations for cancer prevention and detection needs based on personal risk factors and family history with careful information about potential benefits and risks
Variant—likely pathogenic	Strong evidence that the genetic change is capable of causing increased risk for developing disease but more evidence needed to classify as pathogenic	Changes medical management, especially screening recommendations. Prevention measures may be offered depending on what is known about the variant. At-risk family members can be offered targeted testing to help them clarify risk.	Does not inform about what type of cancer will develop or when, only that the risk is higher Enables individual to make decisions about prevention and early detection

Note. Based on information from Eggington et al., 2014; Mahon, 2015; Selkirk et al., 2014; Sijmons et al., 2013.

potential risks and benefits of these recommendations (Moghadasi et al., 2013; Radice, De Summa, Caleca, & Tommasi, 2011; Richards et al., 2008).

Psychosocial Concerns

When deciding whether to pursue cancer predisposition genetic testing, each patient and family member must weigh the options, risks, and benefits in light of his or her unique situation. The decision is a very personal one, and the issues will be different for each patient. Just because a person has a personal or family history that creates increased risk for carrying a genetic mutation does not mean the individual will wish to know his or her genetic status. For another person, the uncertainty may cause great anxiety or interfere with the individual's ability to make informed choices about his or her health. The physical risks of having a blood sample drawn are minimal. The real risks are associated with the psychological and psychosocial impact of knowing one's genetic status

(Eijzenga, Hahn, Aaronson, Kluijt, & Bleiker, 2014).

Psychosocial issues are associated with cancer genetic counseling and testing and need to be recognized and addressed (Eijzenga et al., 2014; Rew, Kaur, McMillan, Mackert, & Bonevac, 2010). Patients found to carry a cancer susceptibility mutation may experience anxiety, depression, anger, and feelings of vulnerability or guilt about possibly having passed the mutation to children. Those who test negative for a known mutation in a family may experience guilt, known as *survivor guilt*, especially if close family members are found to carry the mutation (Greco & Mahon, 2011). Survivor guilt occurs when people who test negative question why they were fortunate enough to test negative when another sibling or relative tested positive. Individuals also may experience regrets regarding making major life decisions, such as prophylactic surgery, prior to testing (Eijzenga et al., 2014; Metcalfe et al., 2012).

Psychological issues to consider include fear of cancer or medical procedures, past negative experiences with cancer, unresolved loss and sorrow, feelings of guilt about passing on a mutation to children, anxiety about learning test results, and concern about the effect of results on other family members. Family dynamics are important to consider. Although one individual in a family may pursue testing, the results have implications for many (Lapointe et al., 2012).

A primary objective of genetic counseling and education is to help individuals and families weigh the options, risks, and benefits of testing in their unique situations. Identifying potential psychosocial concerns is a substantial component of the counseling process. Testing is not in itself good or bad, right or wrong. For some people, testing is appropriate and will have positive outcomes, whereas for others, testing creates a significant risk for major psychosocial distress (Greco & Mahon, 2011).

Patients may experience increased anxiety and fear while waiting for their test results (Wevers et al., 2011). Individuals may need increased support during this time period. Patients have reported that they find it helpful to have written brochures, a letter summarizing recommendations, and guidance about how to share risk information and testing outcomes with other relatives and healthcare professionals.

Prior experiences with cancer influence perceptions of genetic risk. People who have experienced loss related to cancer often find it particularly difficult to learn about the risks and benefits of genetic testing (Mahon, 2011). People who have lost a relative and then test positive often have difficulty coping, as they fear the same outcome and that their children will lose a parent early. Those who test negative after having lost a parent often have difficulty accepting a negative test result because they assume they will have the same outcome. For these patients, it often takes time to reframe their personal identity (Twomey, 2011).

Some patients who have positive results feel empowered and relieved because they can make appropriate decisions about prevention strategies and feel they exercise some control. Other patients who thought they were prepared for positive results can be overwhelmed by the outcome and require much counseling and support. A major concern for many people who test positive is not as much for their own health conditions and fears but rather feelings of guilt if a child inherits the gene (Eijzenga et al., 2014).

People who receive a result with a variant of indeterminate significance or an inconclusive negative result can experience a wide range of feelings. Many experience frustration because they feel they must make decisions about prevention and early detection without clear information. Others with an inconclusive result feel relief because they believe the malignancy may not be related to a hereditary cause.

Many patients will experience generalized anxiety during the counseling, testing, and short-term follow-up periods even with counseling (Bjorvatn, Eide, Hanestad, Hamang, & Havik, 2009; Vadaparampil, Miree, Wilson, & Jacobsen, 2007). These patients may need psychosocial support during the testing process and in the short term during the follow-up period. Long-term follow-up and support usually are associated with improved knowledge of cancer risks and testing, which in most cases ultimately leads to improved satisfaction with testing decisions and adjustment to risk (Eijzenga et al., 2014). Providing anticipatory guidance prior to the visit is associated with lower feelings of anxiety and an increased sense of control. For those undergoing prophylactic surgical procedures, the need for psychosocial support may be longer. If other individuals in the family are diagnosed with malignancy, additional support may be required. For this reason, many genetic counselors and educators encourage people to contact them again if questions or concerns arise. Families with children may contact the counselor for additional care as teenagers become old enough to consider their own risks and options for testing. Because of these long-term needs, genetic healthcare professionals may follow families intermittently for years with some periods of more intense service (Metcalfe et al., 2012; Rew et al., 2010).

Common Cancer Genetic Predisposition Syndromes

Oncology nurses will encounter some hereditary cancer predisposition syndromes fairly regularly, including HBOC, HNPCC, FAP, and hereditary pancreatic cancer. Oncology nurses must be able to readily identify families who are at risk for these predisposition syndromes, know how to refer them for education services when indicated, and provide support for families as they make complex, difficult decisions about genetic testing and treatment measures.

Hereditary Breast and Ovarian Cancer Syndromes

An estimated 70% of breast cancer is sporadic; 15%–20% is familial, meaning that one or two family members can have breast cancer without an obvious pattern of autosomal dominant transmission being present; and approximately 10% is due to known genetic predisposition (Shannon & Chittenden, 2012). Among women, an estimated 5%–10% of breast cancers and 10%–15% of ovarian cancers are caused by inherited mutations in the *BRCA1* and *BRCA2* genes (Lindor et al., 2008). Mutations in these genes occur in about 1 in every 300–500 individuals (Christinat & Pagani, 2013). Other genes associated with an increased risk of developing breast or ovarian cancer include *ATM*, *BARD1*, *BRIP1*, *CDH1*, *CHEK2*, *EPCAM*, *FANCC*, *MLH1*, *MSH2*, *MSH6*, *NBN*, *PALB2*, *PMS2*, *PTEN*, *RAD51C*, *RAD51D*, *STK11*, *TP53*, and *XRCC2*.

Many studies have estimated the risk of people with *BRCA1* or *BRCA2* mutations developing cancer. The risk for younger women to develop breast cancer is estimated to be 33%–50% by age 50 (Euhus, 2012). The cumulative risk for developing breast cancer by age 70 is estimated to be about 87%, and the risk is as high as 44% for ovarian cancer (Lindor et al., 2010; Shannon & Chittenden, 2012). The risk of developing a second primary cancer (breast or ovarian) also is elevated (Bougie & Weberpals, 2011; Vencken et al., 2013). The degree of risk depends on the first primary malignancy, as well as the current age and other comorbidities of the affected carrier. Figure 4-5 provides teaching points for families who are at risk for HBOC.

Men who have a mutation in *BRCA1* or *BRCA2* have been shown to have an increased risk for developing prostate cancer that might be more aggressive, have nodal involvement, and be associated with a poorer survival when compared with men who do not have a mutation (Euhus, 2012). The risk of prostate cancer in *BRCA1* carriers has been estimated to be approximately double that observed in the general population for men younger than 65 years old and five to seven times as high in *BRCA2* carriers based on results from the international IMPACT (Identification of Men With a Genetic Predisposition to Prostate Cancer) study (Mitra et al., 2011). Lifetime breast cancer risk is estimated at 1.8% for men with *BRCA1* mutations and 8.3% for those with *BRCA2* mutations (Euhus & Robinson, 2013).

Membership in some populations confers increased risk for having a *BRCA1* or *BRCA2* mutation. Founder mutations have been noted in those of Ashkenazi Jewish, Dutch, and Icelandic descent. An estimated 1 in 40 Ashkenazi women carries one of three mutations (185delAG and 5382insC on *BRCA1* and 6174delT on *BRCA2*) (NCCN, 2016).

Women who are at high risk for HBOC typically initiate mammography at age 25. Women need clear instruction on the limitations of mammography in younger age groups because of the density of the breast tissue (Lowry et al., 2012). Mammography, even when combined with ultrasound, may still be ineffective in detecting breast cancer early in HBOC. Breast magnetic resonance imaging (MRI) may result in higher sensitivity, especially when combined with mammography and ultrasound in high-risk women (ACS, 2015a; Morrow, Waters, & Morris, 2011). Breast MRI should be offered to patients with a balanced discussion of the potential risks, including an increased number of false-positive readings necessitating biopsy, and the benefits, including earlier detection of malignancy. Currently, ACS recommends a mammogram and MRI every year for women at high risk (greater than 20% lifetime risk). Women at moderately increased risk (15%–20% lifetime risk) should talk with their doctors about the benefits and limitations of adding MRI screening to their yearly mammogram (ACS, 2015a).

Prophylactic mastectomy can result in a 90%–95% reduction in breast cancer risk (Bougie & Weberpals, 2011; Evans et al.,

Figure 4-5. Summary Points for Hereditary Breast and Ovarian Cancer

Genetic Testing: *BRCA1*, *BRCA2*
Penetrance: 87% breast cancer; 44% ovarian cancer

Key Indicators
- Personal and/or family history of breast cancer diagnosed at age 50 or younger
- Personal and/or family history of ovarian cancer diagnosed at any age
- Women of Ashkenazi Jewish ancestry diagnosed with breast and/or ovarian cancer at any age, regardless of family history
- Personal and/or family history of male breast cancer
- Affected first-degree relatives with a known *BRCA1* or *BRCA2* mutation
- Bilateral breast cancer, especially if the diagnosis was at an early age
- Breast and ovarian cancer in the same woman
- Women with triple-negative breast cancer

Potential Surveillance Recommendations
- Monthly breast self-examination beginning at age 18
- Biannual clinical breast examination beginning at age 20
- Annual mammography beginning at age 25
- Consider other breast imaging strategies, including breast magnetic resonance imaging.
- Biannual pelvic examination beginning at age 25
- Annual or biannual transvaginal ultrasound with color Doppler beginning at age 25
- Consider annual or biannual serum CA-125 testing beginning at age 25.
- Consider pancreatic cancer screening.
- Consider melanoma screening.

Potential Prevention Measures
- Consider prophylactic mastectomy (risk reduction of up to 95%).
- Women with known *BRCA2* mutations can consider tamoxifen for chemoprevention.
- Consider prophylactic oophorectomy between ages 35–40 (risk reduction of up to 85%–96%).

Note. Based on information from Bougie & Weberpals, 2011; Gadducci et al., 2010; National Comprehensive Cancer Network, 2016; Olbrys, 2013; Shannon & Chittenden, 2012; Zagouri et al., 2013.

2013). This may be an appropriate option for many women, especially those who have already been diagnosed with cancer, have undergone multiple breast biopsies, or have breasts that are abnormal or difficult to examine clinically or on mammography. Prophylactic mastectomy may lead to significant overall survival in mutation carriers diagnosed with cancer. However, it is an irreversible procedure that can be emotionally difficult for many women (Gopie et al., 2013). In most cases, a prophylactic mastectomy includes total mastectomy without an axillary node dissection. Skin-sparing and nipple-sparing procedures sometimes are offered with informed consent that documents that the more breast tissue that is left intact, the less effective the procedure (Tokin, Weiss, Wang-Rodriguez, & Blair, 2012). Women who undergo a prophylactic mastectomy can opt for immediate reconstruction with a flap or implant or can use prosthetics.

Prophylactic bilateral salpingo-oophorectomy (BSO) may be a prudent choice for women who are at risk for ovarian cancer, especially considering the limited effectiveness of ovarian cancer screening (Antoniou et al., 2009; Gadducci, Biglia, Cosio, Sismondi, & Genazzani, 2010). A BSO is associated with as much as a 90% reduction in ovarian cancer risk and a 50% reduction in breast cancer risk (Shannon & Chittenden, 2012). The ideal age seems to be between age 35 and 40 if childbearing is complete. Approximately 2%–6% of mutation-positive women in this age group will have occult ovarian cancers at the time of prophylaxis (Finch et al., 2013). This prophylactic surgical decision should be considered after a careful discussion of the potential benefits of reduced risk of breast and ovarian cancers and the consequences of early menopause, which is associated with increased vasomotor symptoms and potential bone loss. Preliminary data suggest that short-term hormone replacement therapy following BSO might be safe and does not negate the protective effect of the surgery while decreasing vasomotor symptoms (NCCN, 2016).

Men who test positive for a *BRCA* mutation should undergo clinical breast examination every six months, perform monthly breast self-examination, and consider mammography (Mohamad & Apffelstaedt, 2008). Mammography sometimes is offered to men with gynecomastia. Men should initiate annual prostate screening, including a digital rectal examination and prostate-specific antigen testing, at age 40 (Castro et al., 2013; Ruddy & Winer, 2013).

Hereditary Nonpolyposis Colorectal Cancer Syndrome

The autosomal dominant syndrome known as HNPCC, or Lynch syndrome, accounts for 3%–5% of all colorectal cancers (Senter, 2012). It also is associated with endometrial, ovarian, gastric, bile duct, small bowel, renal pelvis, and ureter cancers (Barrow, Hill, & Evans, 2013). The majority of mutations responsible for HNPCC occur in four mismatch repair genes: *MSH2*, *MLH1*, *PMS2*, and *MSH6*. The *EPCAM* gene is a recently discovered contributor to Lynch syndrome, accounting for an estimated 1%–3% of all detectable HNPCC mutations because of large deletions in the end of this gene, which is located directly upstream of *MSH2* and can lead to a loss of *MSH2* expression, resulting in HNPCC syndrome (Gala & Chung, 2011; Ligtenberg, Kuiper, Geurts van Kessel, & Hoogerbrugge, 2013).

Patients with an HNPCC-associated mutation have an 80% lifetime risk of developing colorectal cancer compared with a 6% risk in the general population. Women with mutations in these genes have a 60% lifetime risk for developing endometrial cancer (Lindor et al., 2008). Lifetime risk of stomach cancer is 1%–13% compared to 1% in the general population (Chun & Ford, 2012; Patel & Ahnen, 2012). Risk of ovarian cancer is 12%–20%

compared to 1% in the general population (Weissman, Weiss, & Newlin, 2012). Figure 4-6 includes teaching points for HNPCC.

Although HNPCC is not associated with large numbers of polyps, people with HNPCC who do form adenomatous polyps are more likely to do so at an earlier age, are more likely to develop right-sided colon cancer, and exhibit a very rapid progression to malignancy in 1–3 years instead of the pattern of 5–10 years seen in the general population (Patel & Ahnen, 2012; Weissman, Burt, et al., 2012).

Risk assessment for HNPCC is approached in several ways. The Amsterdam and Bethesda criteria assess the number of relatives affected by colorectal cancer or other HNPCC-related cancers with particular emphasis on the age at onset (Weissman, Burt, et al., 2012). The Amsterdam criteria require that one member of the family be diagnosed with colorectal cancer before age 50, two generations are affected, three relatives are affected, with one of them being a first-degree relative of the other two, and FAP is excluded. The Bethesda criteria require that colorectal cancer be diagnosed in an individual younger than age 50. Other criteria include the presence of colorectal cancers and other HNPCC tumors in the same individual or that multiple generations are affected and two or more first-degree relatives are affected.

Microsatellites are another marker used to identify possible cases of HNPCC. Microsatellites are repeated sequences of DNA. Although the length of microsatellites is highly variable from person to person, each individual has microsatellites of a set length. These repeated sequences are common and normal. In cells with mutations in DNA repair genes, however, some of these sequences accumulate errors and become longer or shorter. The appearance of abnormally long or short microsatellites in an individual's DNA is referred to as *microsatellite instability* (MSI). About 90% of tumors from people who have HNPCC show MSI (Buecher et al., 2013). Tests are available

Figure 4-6. Summary Points for Hereditary Nonpolyposis Colorectal Cancer (HNPCC)

Genetic Testing: *MLH1, MSH2, MSH6, PMS2, EPCAM*

Penetrance: 40%–85% colorectal cancer; 40%–60% endometrial cancer; 13% stomach cancer; 12%–20% ovarian cancer

Key Indicators

- Personal history of colorectal and/or endometrial cancer diagnosed before age 50
- First-degree relative with colorectal cancer diagnosed before age 50
- Two or more relatives with colorectal cancer or an HNPCC-associated cancer, which includes endometrial, ovarian, gastric, hepatobiliary, small bowel, renal pelvis, or ureter cancer. At least two of the relatives must be first-degree relatives of each other.
- Colorectal cancer occurring in two or more generations on the same side of the family
- A personal history of colorectal cancer and a first-degree relative with adenomas diagnosed before age 50
- An affected relative with a known HNPCC mutation

Potential Surveillance Recommendations

- Annual colonoscopy with removal of polyps starting between ages 20–25
- Consider gastroscopy and upper endoscopy with colonoscopy.
- Biannual pelvic examination beginning at age 25
- Annual or biannual transvaginal ultrasound with color Doppler beginning at age 25
- Annual or biannual serum CA-125 testing
- Consider urinary screening with urinalysis and/or pelvic ultrasound.

Potential Prevention Measures

- Consider chemoprevention with aspirin or nonsteroidal anti-inflammatory drugs.
- Consider colectomy in patients who cannot or will not undergo regular colonoscopy.
- Consider chemoprevention with oral contraceptives if possible.
- Strongly recommend consideration of a prophylactic hysterectomy including bilateral salpingo-oophorectomy between ages 35–40 or when childbearing is complete.

Note. Based on information from Barton, 2012; de Vos tot Nederveen Cappel et al., 2013; Haanstra et al., 2013; Power et al., 2010; Rodriguez-Bigas & Möeslein, 2013; Shia et al., 2013; Weissman, Burt, et al., 2012.

that detect MSI in tumor cells, and numerous longer or shorter microsatellite regions in these cells suggests the presence of a mutated DNA mismatch repair gene, which is suggestive of HNPCC. Thus, testing a tumor sample for MSI often can help to determine whether genetic testing for HNPCC is appropriate. An MSI-high phenotype is reported in 85%–92% of HNPCC colon cancers and approximately 15% of sporadic cancers (Weissman, Burt, et al., 2012). If a patient's tumor cells show no evidence of MSI, it is unlikely that he or she has a mutated mismatch repair gene. In such cases, genetic tests are unlikely to yield useful information and rarely are worth the time and expense.

Another strategy often employed is immunohistochemistry (IHC) staining, which can be done on tumor tissue from individuals who fulfill the Bethesda criteria to determine the presence or absence of MLH1, MSH2, MSH6, and PMS2 proteins (Kastrinos & Syngal, 2012; Schneider, Schneider, Kloor, Fürst, & Möslein, 2012). If IHC is abnormal, this indicates that one of the proteins is not expressed, and an inherited mutation may be present. If either the IHC or MSI tests are abnormal, then further testing with germ-line DNA analysis would be appropriate.

HNPCC is associated with an accelerated carcinogenesis in which polyps can develop into carcinomas in 2–3 years instead of the typical 8–10 years seen in the general population (Haanstra, Kleibeuker, & Koornstra, 2013). Because of this potentially rapid development of malignancy, annual colonoscopy is recommended beginning at age 20–25 (Levin et al., 2008). Research clearly shows that regular colonoscopy decreases the overall mortality rate by about 65% (de Vos tot Nederveen Cappel et al., 2013).

Because HNPCC also is associated with increased risks to the endometrium and ovaries, women with the mutation need to consider careful surveillance. This usually includes annual or semiannual transvaginal ultrasound of the endometrium and ovaries with concurrent endometrial aspiration for pathologic evaluation and CA-125 testing (Vasen et al., 2013). In particular, women need to be informed of the low sensitivity and specificity of ultrasound and CA-125 testing for ovarian cancer. Ultrasound has limited utility in evaluating endometrial thickness in premenopausal women because of cyclic changes. Although individuals with HNPCC may be at risk for other cancers, no other standard screening recommendations exist at this time (Bernstein & Myrhøj, 2013). Some families with an increased number of urinary tract malignancies consider adding ultrasound and urine cytology (de Vos tot Nederveen Cappel et al., 2013). Similarly, many clinicians will recommend upper endoscopy and gastroscopy, but no formal recommendations currently exist.

Another strategy these families sometimes consider is chemoprevention. The exact efficacy of nonsteroidal anti-inflammatory drugs and aspirin in decreasing gastrointestinal cancers is unknown (Barton, 2012). These measures are based largely on information gained from people with FAP. Because the use of oral contraceptive pills has been associated with decreased risk of developing ovarian and endometrial cancers, some women consider this strategy. Individuals considering chemoprevention strategies for colon or gynecologic cancers need a carefully balanced discussion of the potential benefits and risks associated with the proposed agent. These individuals also may want to consider enrolling in a research study. Patients with an HNPCC-associated mutation may benefit from recommendations on adopting a healthy diet and exercise to reduce the risk of cancer development (see ACS, 2015b) because such behaviors may contribute to overall health and well-being.

Prophylactic colectomy in HNPCC is controversial. It is not associated with a large increase in life expectancy over annual colonoscopy (Rodriguez-Bigas & Möeslein, 2013). It generally is reserved for people in whom colonoscopy is not technically possible or for individuals who refuse to undergo regular screening.

Because the risks for endometrial and ovarian cancers are substantial and screening may be ineffective, many women will consider a total abdominal hysterectomy with BSO at age 35 or older if childbearing is complete (Rodriguez-Bigas & Möeslein, 2013). These women need to be aware of the risks of premature menopause and the need for four to eight weeks of recuperation.

Familial Adenomatous Polyposis Syndromes

FAP, an autosomal dominant trait, is characterized by numerous (usually more than 100) adenomatous colonic polyps and accounts for about 1% of all cases of colorectal cancer (Lindor et al., 2008). The *FAP* gene is nearly 100% penetrant, so if a person is not treated, he or she will develop colorectal cancer because of the sheer number of polyps. The mean age at onset of cancer is 39, but as many as 75% of patients will have developed adenomas by age 20 (Jasperson, 2012). A less severe form of FAP called attenuated familial adenomatous polyposis (AFAP) is characterized by less than 100 polyps (usually about 20) at presentation and later onset of colorectal cancer. More than 800 mutations in the *APC* gene are associated with FAP. Deleterious mutations in this tumor suppressor gene result in the premature truncation of the APC protein (Patel & Ahnen, 2012). Approximately 25% of individuals with FAP have a de novo mutation (Kastrinos & Syngal, 2011). Figure 4-7 lists key indicators of FAP and AFAP and related teaching points.

Figure 4-7. Summary Points for Familial Adenomatous Polyposis (FAP) and Attenuated Familial Adenomatous Polyposis (AFAP)

Genetic Testing: *APC*
Penetrance: 100% for FAP

Key Indicators
- Clinical diagnosis of FAP (100 or more polyps)
- Suspected FAP or AFAP (15–99 polyps)
- First-degree relative with FAP or AFAP
- An affected relative with a known *APC* or *MYH* mutation
- Any number of adenomas in an individual in a family with FAP

Potential Surveillance Recommendation
- Baseline colonoscopy at time of genetic testing or by age 12–15. If no polyps are present, repeat at age 20 and then annually.

Potential Prevention Measures
- Consider chemoprevention with aspirin, nonsteroidal anti-inflammatory drugs, or sulindac to suppress polyp formation.
- Consider prophylactic total proctocolectomy with ileoanal pouch.

Note. Based on information from Dupont et al., 2007; Gala & Chung, 2011; Jasperson, 2012; Patel & Ahnen, 2012.

An autosomal recessive gene on chromosome 1 called *MUYTH* is also associated with polyposis (Lindor et al., 2008). It should be a consideration in anyone with multiple colon polyps. Having mutations in both copies is associated with an 80% lifetime risk of developing colon cancer, 50% risk of developing duodenal cancer, and an increased risk of developing endometrial cancer (Jasperson, 2012). Mutations in *MUYTH* should be a consideration if the patient tests negative for mutations in the *APC* gene. Recommendations for management are similar to those with FAP.

Medical and surgical management of FAP syndromes is complex because the risk of developing colorectal cancer is virtually 100% and the onset can occur before age 20. In general, people with FAP usually receive a recommendation to begin screening with colonoscopy at puberty and to undergo colectomy when symptomatic or when the number of adenomas is considered worrisome. Prophylactic colectomy is an option. Nonsteroidal drugs sometimes are used prophylactically to prevent or delay polyp formation (Dupont, Arguedas, & Wilcox, 2007; Jasperson, 2012).

Pancreatic Cancer

Pancreatic cancer can be seen in different hereditary cancer syndromes. When predominantly pancreatic cancer is seen, the most common mutations are in the *PALB2* and *BRCA2* genes (Axilbund & Wiley, 2012). Other genes associated with hereditary pancreatic cancer include *APC, ATM, BRCA1, CDK4, CDKN2A, EPCAM, MLH1, MSH2, MSH6, PMS2, STK11, TP53, VHL*, and *XRCC2*. These other genes should be considered when selecting a genetic test in a family with suspected hereditary pancreatic cancer.

Pancreatic screening is not typically offered to the general population but has been used in high-risk patients from families with two or more cases of pancreatic cancer and in patients with inherited cancer syndromes associated with hereditary pancreatic cancer. This recommendation comes with a clear discussion of the strengths and limitations of screening so that individuals can make the decision that is best for their situation. Pancreatic cancer surveillance modalities include serum biomarkers, such as CA 19-9 and carcinoembryonic antigen; external imaging, including MRI and computed tomography scan; and internal imaging, such as endoscopic ultrasound, endoscopic retrograde cholangiopancreatography, and magnetic resonance cholangiopancreatography, with or without fine needle aspiration (Shin & Canto, 2012). Data suggest that in high-risk individuals (those with at least 16% lifetime risk for developing pancreatic cancer), endoscopic ultrasound and MRI or magnetic resonance cholangiopancreatography can detect asymptomatic precursor benign and early invasive malignant pancreatic neoplasms that are more likely to be resectable compared to symptomatic tumors (Shin & Canto, 2012; Templeton & Brentnall, 2013).

At this time, no standardized guidelines exist for managing patients at high risk for developing pancreatic cancer, including the age at which screening should be initiated, the modalities used, or how often screening should be conducted (Templeton & Brentnall, 2013). Some experts recommend that high-risk individuals initiate screening at age 35–45 or 10–15 years before the earliest diagnosis of pancreatic cancer in the family (Larghi, Verna, Lecca, & Costamagna, 2009).

Nursing Implications

Oncology nurses implement knowledge and help to manage patients and families with a hereditary predisposition for developing cancer (see Figure 4-2). It is important to remember that all oncology nurses, regardless of practice setting, have a responsibility to refer patients to genetic healthcare professionals and to understand the influence of genetics in health care. Genetics greatly influence the practice of oncology not only in the evaluation and referral of families with a hereditary predisposition but also in pharmacogenetics and tumor characteristics. As the field of genetics is ever-growing, oncology nurses need to continually update their education through journal articles and continuing education courses.

In many cases, oncology nurses will assist in managing the care of people with hereditary risk after they have undergone genetic testing or consultation with a genetic healthcare professional. Oncology nurses are often responsible for ensuring that recommendations for screening are carried out. They also may assist with the care, education, and support of people considering prevention measures, especially prophylactic surgery.

Some patients with hereditary risk may be enrolled in clinical trials and variant reclassification studies. Oncology nurses often assist patients with enrolling in trials and understanding the implications of research findings.

Families with hereditary risk benefit greatly when counseled and encouraged to adopt primary prevention measures, especially those associated with a healthier lifestyle. Incorporation of an appropriate comprehensive prevention and risk reduction plan into the care of a person with a hereditary high risk for cancer can potentially decrease morbidity and mortality associated with cancer (Weitzel et al., 2011). ACS has recommendations for nutrition and physical activity that may be appropriate to share with these families, who are often motivated to engage in such behaviors ("A Healthy Diet and Physical Activity Help Reduce Your Cancer Risk," 2012; Kushi et al., 2012).

Unfortunately, current criteria and risk models do not always correctly categorize those who might be at risk for having a deleterious germline mutation (Wiseman et al., 2010). In addition, family history information changes and evolves over time. A patient may initially present with a history that does not meet the criteria for genetic testing, but if the personal or family history (maternal or paternal) changes, the patient may become eligible for genetic testing or be considered for testing of mutations in other less common genes. Updates in genetic testing technology also necessitate the need to reevaluate whether a patient or family might benefit from additional testing (American College of Medical Genetics and Genomics, 2012; Ku, Cooper, Iacopetta, & Roukos, 2013).

Families with suspected or known hereditary susceptibility to developing malignancy have many psychosocial needs (Cameron & Muller, 2009; Eijzenga et al., 2014). These are ongoing and often change over time. Regular assessment to determine how families are managing their risk and the associated uncertainty, body image changes, and reproductive concerns is important to address issues promptly and appropriately and to help these families to have the best possible outcome (Rew et al., 2010). Oncology nurses have a major role in identifying reputable resources, including written materials, support groups, and websites.

Families who have undergone genetic testing in which a mutation was not detected in one or two of the more common genes should be offered more complete NGS panels for the genes in which they had not previously had testing but might be appropriate given the patient's personal and family history. Such "catch-up" testing might result in the isolation and identification of a less common susceptibility gene and more appropriate, tailored recommendations for prevention and early detection. This testing also may enable other family members to have meaningful single-site genetic testing.

Unfortunately, NGS panels greatly increase the possibility of detecting a variant of indeterminate significance, and it is important for patients and families to understand that the result is uninformative. Indeterminate results can be stressful, confusing, disappointing, and frustrating to families (Mahon, 2015). Recommendations for cancer prevention and surveillance are based on personal risk factors and the family history for both the proband and other family members, as testing of at-risk family members is not recommended when the results are indeterminate.

Conclusion

Genetics is an ever-growing subspecialty in oncology. NGS testing has greatly changed the landscape of genetic testing. When tests are ordered correctly, the possibility that a mutation will be detected is much greater. Unfortunately, the clinical implications of many of these genetic mutations are not always clear. Families will need long-term follow-up as more becomes known about these mutations and management recommendations evolve. NGS testing also has resulted in many more variants of indeterminate significance. Families with a variant of indeterminate significance will need follow-up as more becomes known about the variant, and recommendations for prevention and early detection may need to be modified. As more cancer susceptibility genes are identified, the need will increase for oncology nurses to identify patients who are at risk and refer them to genetic healthcare professionals for further evaluation. Oncology nurses also have important roles in physical assessment, screening, education about prevention strategies, and follow-up care after prophylactic surgery. Families with a known hereditary predisposition need psychosocial support to facilitate adjustment to the diagnosis of a hereditary syndrome. Oncology nurses will continually be challenged to stay current on advances in oncology genetics science.

References

American Cancer Society. (2015a). *Breast cancer facts and figures 2015–2016.* Atlanta, GA: Author.

American Cancer Society. (2015b). *Cancer prevention and early detection facts and figures 2015–2016.* Atlanta, GA: Author.

American Cancer Society. (2016). *Cancer facts and figures 2016.* Atlanta, GA: Author.

American College of Medical Genetics and Genomics. (2012). Policy statement: Points to consider in the clinical application of genomic sequencing. Retrieved from http://www.acmg.net/StaticContent/PPG/Clinical_Application_of_Genomic_Sequencing.pdf

American College of Obstetricians and Gynecologists. (2008). ACOG Committee Opinion No. 410: Ethical issues in genetic testing. *Obstetrics and Gynecology, 111,* 1495–1502. doi:10.1097/AOG.0b013e31817d252f

Antoniou, A.C., Rookus, M., Andrieu, N., Brohet, R., Chang-Claude, J., Peock, S., ... Goldgar, D.E. (2009). Reproductive and hormonal factors, and ovarian cancer risk for *BRCA1* and *BRCA2* mutation carriers: Results from the International *BRCA1/2* Carrier Cohort Study. *Cancer Epidemiology, Biomarkers and Prevention, 18,* 601–610. doi:10.1158/1055-9965.EPI-08-0546

Axilbund, J.E., & Wiley, E.A. (2012). Genetic testing by cancer site: Pancreas. *Cancer Journal, 18,* 350–354. doi:10.1097/ppo.0b013e3182624694

Balmaña, J., Diez, O., Rubio, I., & Castiglione, M. (2010). *BRCA* in breast cancer: ESMO clinical practice guidelines. *Annals of Oncology, 21*(Suppl. 5), v20–v22. doi:10.1093/annonc/mdq161

Barrow, E., Hill, J., & Evans, D.G. (2013). Cancer risk in Lynch syndrome. *Familial Cancer, 12,* 229–240. doi:10.1007/s10689-013-9615-1

Key Points

- Identification of a mutation in a family can be very helpful for risk management and treatment planning for both individuals with cancer and at-risk unaffected family members.
- Genetic testing is not a tool to be used for routine screening in a population because of the expense of testing and the complex counseling needs.
- Somatic mutations occur due to carcinogen exposure and account for approximately 90% of all cancers. Germ-line mutations are in the egg or sperm and can be passed to subsequent generations and account for approximately 10% of all malignancies.
- Taking a detailed family history is the first step to identifying families with a possible hereditary predisposition to malignancy and other illnesses.
- The three-generation pedigree is an excellent means to educate a family about autosomal dominant transmission. It is necessary to calculate the risk of carrying a mutation.
- If patients decide to proceed with genetic testing, they need information about the test or tests being ordered, potential management strategies, and the potential risks, benefits, and limitations of testing.
- Components of informed consent for genetic testing include the risks, benefits, cost, accuracy, and purpose of the specific genetic test being ordered; alternatives to genetic testing; implications of a positive, negative, or uncertain test result; how results will be communicated; psychosocial implications; confidentiality issues; options for medical surveillance; and risk reduction.
- Possible outcomes of testing include a positive test, a variant of indeterminate significance, a true negative for a known family mutation, or an uninformative negative in the first person tested in the family.

Barton, M.K. (2012). Daily aspirin reduces colorectal cancer incidence in patients with Lynch syndrome. *CA: A Cancer Journal for Clinicians, 62,* 143–144. doi:10.3322/caac.21136

Baumanis, L., Evans, J.P., Callanan, N., & Susswein, L.R. (2009). Telephoned *BRCA1/2* genetic test results: Prevalence, practice, and patient satisfaction. *Journal of Genetic Counseling, 18,* 447–463. doi:10.1007/s10897-009-9238-8

Bennett, R.L., French, K.S., Resta, R.G., & Doyle, D.L. (2008). Standardized human pedigree nomenclature: Update and assessment of the recommendations of the National Society of Genetic Counselors. *Journal of Genetic Counseling, 17,* 424–433. doi:10.1007/s10897-008-9169-9

Bensend, T.A., Veach, P.M., & Niendorf, K.B. (2014). What's the harm? Genetic counselor perceptions of adverse effects of genetics service provision by non-genetics professionals. *Journal of Genetic Counseling, 23,* 48–63. doi:10.1007/s10897-013-9605-3

Bernstein, I.T., & Myrhøj, T. (2013). Surveillance for urinary tract cancer in Lynch syndrome. *Familial Cancer, 12,* 279–284. doi:10.1007/s10689-013-9634-y

Berry, D.A., Iversen, E.S., Jr., Gudbjartsson, D.F., Hiller, E.H., Garber, J.E., Peshkin, B.N., ... Parmigiani, G. (2002). BRCAPRO validation, sensitivity of genetic testing of *BRCA1/BRCA2,* and prevalence of other breast cancer susceptibility genes. *Journal of Clinical Oncology, 20,* 2701–2712. doi:10.1200/JCO.2002.05.121

Bjorvatn, C., Eide, G.E., Hanestad, B.R., Hamang, A., & Havik, O.E. (2009). Intrusion and avoidance in subjects undergoing genetic investigation and counseling for hereditary cancer. *Supportive Care in Cancer, 17,* 1371–1381. doi:10.1007/s00520-009-0594-6

Bougie, O., & Weberpals, J.I. (2011). Clinical considerations of *BRCA1*- and *BRCA2*-mutation carriers: A review. *International Journal of Surgical Oncology, 2011,* Article ID 374012. doi:10.1155/2011/374012

Bradbury, A.R., Patrick-Miller, L., Fetzer, D., Egleston, B., Cummings, S.A., Forman, A., ... Daly, M.B. (2011). Genetic counselor opinions of, and experiences with telephone communication of *BRCA1/2* test results. *Clinical Genetics, 79,* 125–131. doi:10.1111/j.1399-0004.2010.01540.x

Brierley, K.L., Blouch, E., Cogswell, W., Homer, J.P., Pencarinha, D., Stanislaw, C.L., & Matloff, E.T. (2012). Adverse events in cancer genetic testing: Medical, ethical, legal, and financial implications. *Cancer Journal, 18,* 303–309. doi:10.1097/ppo.0b013e3182609490

Brierley, K.L., Campfield, D., Ducaine, W., Dohany, L., Donenberg, T., Shannon, K., ... Matloff, E.T. (2010). Errors in delivery of cancer genetics services: Implications for practice. *Connecticut Medicine, 74,* 413–423.

Buecher, B., Cacheux, W., Rouleau, E., Dieumegard, B., Mitry, E., & Lièvre, A. (2013). Role of microsatellite instability in the management of colorectal cancers. *Digestive and Liver Disease, 45,* 441–449. doi:10.1016/j.dld.2012.10.006

Cameron, L.D., & Muller, C. (2009). Psychosocial aspects of genetic testing. *Current Opinion in Psychiatry, 22,* 218–223. doi:10.1097/YCO.0b013e3283252d80

Castro, E., Goh, C., Olmos, D., Saunders, E., Leongamornlert, D., Tymrakiewicz, M., ... Eeles, R. (2013). Germline *BRCA* mutations are associated with higher risk of nodal involvement, distant metastasis, and poor survival outcomes in prostate cancer. *Journal of Clinical Oncology, 31,* 1748–1757. doi:10.1200/JCO.2012.43.1882

Chan-Smutko, G. (2012). Genetic testing by cancer site: Urinary tract. *Cancer Journal, 18,* 343–349. doi:10.1097/ppo.0b013e31826246ac

Christinat, A., & Pagani, O. (2013). Practical aspects of genetic counseling in breast cancer: Lights and shadows. *Breast, 22,* 375–382. doi:10.1016/j.breast.2013.04.006

Chun, N., & Ford, J.M. (2012). Genetic testing by cancer site: Stomach. *Cancer Journal, 18,* 355–363. doi:10.1097/ppo.0b013e31826246dc

Claus, E.B., Risch, N.J., & Thompson, W.D. (1994). Autosomal dominant inheritance of early-onset breast cancer. Implications for risk prediction. *Cancer, 73,* 643–651. doi:10.1002/1097-0142(19940201)73:3<643::AID-CNCR2820730323>3.0.CO;2-5

Claus, E.B., Schildkraut, J.M., Thompson, W.D., & Risch, N.J. (1996). The genetic attributable risk of breast and ovarian cancer. *Cancer, 77,* 2318–2324. doi:10.1002/(SICI)1097-0142(19960601)77:11<2318::AID-CNCR21>3.0.CO;2-Z

Cohen, S.A., Gustafson, S.L., Marvin, M.L., Riley, B.D., Uhlmann, W.R., Liebers, S.B., & Rousseau, J.A. (2012). Report from the National Society of Genetic Counselors Service Delivery Model Task Force: A proposal to define models, components, and modes of referral. *Journal of Genetic Counseling, 21,* 645–651. doi:10.1007/s10897-012-9505-y

Consensus Panel on Genetic/Genomic Nursing Competencies. (2009). *Essentials of genetic and genomic nursing: Competencies, curricula guidelines, and outcome indicators* (2nd ed.). Silver Spring, MD: American Nurses Association.

Daniels, M.S. (2012). Genetic testing by cancer site: Uterus. *Cancer Journal, 18,* 338–342. doi:10.1097/ppo.0b013e3182610cc2

de Vos tot Nederveen Cappel, W.H., Järvinen, H.J., Lynch, P.M., Engel, C., Mecklin, J.-P., & Vasen, H.F.A. (2013). Colorectal surveillance in Lynch syndrome families. *Familial Cancer, 12,* 261–265. doi:10.1007/s10689-013-9631-1

Dupont, A.W., Arguedas, M.R., & Wilcox, C.M. (2007). Aspirin chemoprevention in patients with increased risk for colorectal cancer: A cost-effectiveness analysis. *Alimentary Pharmacology and Therapeutics, 26,* 431–441. doi:10.1111/j.1365-2036.2007.03380.x

Eggington, J.M., Bowles, K.R., Moyes, K., Manley, S., Esterling, L., Sizemore, S., ... Wenstrup, R.J. (2014). A comprehensive laboratory-based program for classification of variants of uncertain significance in hereditary cancer genes. *Clinical Genetics, 86,* 229–237. doi:10.1111/cge.12315

Eijzenga, W., Hahn, D.E.E., Aaronson, N.K., Kluijt, I., & Bleiker, E.M.A. (2014). Specific psychosocial issues of individuals undergoing genetic counseling for cancer—A literature review. *Journal of Genetic Counseling, 23,* 133–146. doi:10.1007/s10897-013-9649-4

Eng, C. (2016). *PTEN* hamartoma tumor syndrome. In R.A. Pagon & M.P. Adam (Eds.), *GeneReviews.* Retrieved from http://www.ncbi.nlm.nih.gov/books/NBK1488

Euhus, D.M. (2012). Managing the breast in patients who test positive for hereditary breast cancer. *Annals of Surgical Oncology, 19,* 1738–1744. doi:10.1245/s10434-012-2258-x

Euhus, D.M., & Robinson, L. (2013). Genetic predisposition syndromes and their management. *Surgical Clinics of North America, 93,* 341–362. doi:10.1016/j.suc.2013.01.005

Evans, D.G.R., Eccles, D.M., Rahman, N., Young, K., Bulman, M., Amir, E., ... Lalloo, F. (2004). A new scoring system for the chances of identifying a *BRCA1/2* mutation outperforms existing models including BRCAPRO. *Journal of Medical Genetics, 41,* 474–480. doi:10.1136/jmg.2003.017996

Evans, D.G.R., Ingham, S.L., Baildam, A., Ross, G.L., Lalloo, F., Buchan, I., & Howell, A. (2013). Contralateral mastectomy improves survival in women with *BRCA1/2*-associated breast cancer. *Breast Cancer Research and Treatment, 140,* 135–142. doi:10.1007/s10549-013-2583-1

Fagerlin, A., Zikmund-Fisher, B.J., & Ubel, P.A. (2011). Helping patients decide: Ten steps to better risk communication. *Journal of the National Cancer Institute, 103,* 1436–1443. doi:10.1093/jnci/djr318

Finch, A., Metcalfe, K.A., Chiang, J., Elit, L., McLaughlin, J., Springate, C., ... Narod, S.A. (2013). The impact of prophylactic salpingo-oophorectomy on quality of life and psychological distress in women with a BRCA mutation. *Psycho-Oncology, 22,* 212–219. doi:10.1002/pon.2041

Gabree, M., & Seidel, M. (2012). Genetic testing by cancer site: Skin. *Cancer Journal, 18,* 372–380. doi:10.1097/PPO.0b013e3182624664

Gadducci, A., Biglia, N., Cosio, S., Sismondi, P., & Genazzani, A.R. (2010). Gynaecologic challenging issues in the management of BRCA mutation carriers: Oral contraceptives, prophylactic salpingo-oophorectomy and hormone replacement therapy. *Gynecological Endocrinology, 26,* 568–577. doi:10.3109/09513590.2010.487609

Gail, M.H., & Mai, P.L. (2010). Comparing breast cancer risk assessment models. *Journal of the National Cancer Institute, 102,* 665–668. doi:10.1093/jnci/djq141

Gala, M., & Chung, D.C. (2011). Hereditary colon cancer syndromes. *Seminars in Oncology, 38,* 490–499. doi:10.1053/j.seminoncol.2011.05.003

Gopie, J.P., Mureau, M.A.M., Seynaeve, C., ter Kuile, M.M., Menke-Pluymers, M.B.E., Timman, R., & Tibben, A. (2013). Body image issues after bilateral prophylactic mastectomy with breast reconstruction in healthy women at risk for hereditary breast cancer. *Familial Cancer, 12,* 479–487. doi:10.1007/s10689-012-9588-5

Greco, K.E., & Mahon, S.M. (2011). The state of genomic health care and cancer: Are we going two steps forward and one step backward? *Annual Review of Nursing Research, 29,* 73–97. doi:10.1891/0739-6686.29.73

Greco, K.E., Tinley, S., & Seibert, D. (2012). *Essential genetic and genomic competencies for nurses with graduate degrees.* Silver Spring, MD: American Nurses Association and International Society of Nurses in Genetics.

Gunder, L.M., & Martin, S.A. (2011). *Essentials of medical genetics for health professionals.* Burlington, MA: Jones & Bartlett Learning.

Haanstra, J.F., Kleibeuker, J.H., & Koornstra, J.J. (2013). Role of new endoscopic techniques in Lynch syndrome. *Familial Cancer, 12,* 267–272. doi:10.1007/s10689-013-9610-6

Hampel, H., Bennett, R.L., Buchanan, A., Pearlman, R., & Wiesner, G.L. (2014). A practice guideline from the American College of Medical Genetics and Genomics and the National Society of Genetic Counselors: Referral indications for cancer predisposition assessment. *Genetics in Medicine, 17,* 70–87. doi:10.1038/gim.2014.147

A healthy diet and physical activity help reduce your cancer risk [Patient page]. (2012). *CA: A Cancer Journal for Clinicians, 62,* 68–69. doi:10.3322/caac.20139

Iwuji, C., Howells, L., Thomasset, S., Brown, K., Steward, W., Barwell, J., & Thomas, A. (2014). Cancer chemoprevention: Factors influencing attitudes towards chemopreventive agents in high-risk populations. *European Journal of Cancer Prevention, 23,* 594–601. doi:10.1097/CEJ.0000000000000061

Jasperson, K.W. (2012). Genetic testing by cancer site: Colon (polyposis syndromes). *Cancer Journal, 18,* 328–333. doi:10.1097/ppo.0b013e3182609300

Kastrinos, F., Balmaña, J., & Syngal, S. (2013). Prediction models in Lynch syndrome. *Familial Cancer, 12,* 217–228. doi:10.1007/s10689-013-9632-0

Kastrinos, F., & Syngal, S. (2011). Inherited colorectal cancer syndromes. *Cancer Journal, 17,* 405–415. doi:10.1097/PPO.0b013e318237e408

Kastrinos, F., & Syngal, S. (2012). Screening patients with colorectal cancer for Lynch syndrome: What are we waiting for? *Journal of Clinical Oncology, 30,* 1024–1027. doi:10.1200/JCO.2011.40.7171

Klabunde, C.N., Lanier, D., Breslau, E.S., Zapka, J.G., Fletcher, R.H., Ransohoff, D.F., & Winawer, S.J. (2007). Improving colorectal cancer screening in primary care practice: Innovative strategies and future directions. *Journal of General Internal Medicine, 22,* 1195–1205. doi:10.1007/s11606-007-0231-3

Ku, C.S., Cooper, D.N., Iacopetta, B., & Roukos, D.H. (2013). Integrating next-generation sequencing into the diagnostic testing of inherited cancer predisposition. *Clinical Genetics, 83,* 2–6. doi:10.1111/cge.12028

Ku, C.S., Cooper, D.N., Ziogas, D.E., Halkia, E., Tzaphlidou, M., & Roukos, D.H. (2013). Research and clinical applications of cancer genome sequencing. *Current Opinion in Obstetrics and Gynecology, 25,* 3–10. doi:10.1097/GCO.0b013e32835af17c

Kushi, L.H., Doyle, C., McCullough, M., Rock, C.L., Demark-Wahnefried, W., Bandera, E.V., ... American Cancer Society 2010 Nutrition and Physical Activity Guidelines Advisory Committee. (2012). American Cancer Society guidelines on nutrition and physical activity for cancer prevention: Reducing the risk of cancer with healthy food choices and physical activity. *CA: A Cancer Journal for Clinicians, 62,* 30–67. doi:10.3322/caac.20140

Lapointe, J., Abdous, B., Camden, S., Bouchard, K., Goldgar, D., Simard, J., & Dorval, M. (2012). Influence of the family cluster effect on psychosocial variables in families undergoing *BRCA1/2* genetic testing for cancer susceptibility. *Psycho-Oncology, 21,* 515–523. doi:10.1002/pon.1936

Larghi, A., Verna, E.C., Lecca, P.G., & Costamagna, G. (2009). Screening for pancreatic cancer in high-risk individuals: A call for endoscopic ultrasound. *Clinical Cancer Research, 15,* 1907–1914. doi:10.1158/1078-0432.CCR-08-1966

Levin, B., Lieberman, D.A., McFarland, B., Smith, R.A., Brooks, D., Andrews, K.S., ... Winawer, S.J. (2008). Screening and surveillance for the early detection of colorectal cancer and adenomatous polyps, 2008: A joint guideline from the American Cancer Society, the US Multi-Society Task Force on Colorectal Cancer, and the American College of Radiology. *CA: A Cancer Journal for Clinicians, 58,* 130–160. doi:10.3322/CA.2007.0018

Levy, D.E., Garber, J.E., & Shields, A.E. (2009). Guidelines for genetic risk assessment of hereditary breast and ovarian cancer: Early disagreements and low utilization. *Journal of General Internal Medicine, 24,* 822–828. doi:10.1007/s11606-009-1009-6

Ligtenberg, M.J.L., Kuiper, R.P., Geurts van Kessel, A., & Hoogerbrugge, N. (2013). *EPCAM* deletion carriers constitute a unique subgroup of Lynch syndrome patients. *Familial Cancer, 12,* 169–174. doi:10.1007/s10689-012-9591-x

Lindor, N.M., Johnson, K.J., Harvey, H., Pankratz, V.S., Domchek, S.M., Hunt, K., ... Couch, F. (2010). Predicting *BRCA1* and *BRCA2* gene mutation carriers: Comparison of PENN II model to previous study. *Familial Cancer, 9,* 495–502. doi:10.1007/s10689-010-9348-3

Lindor, N.M., McMaster, M.L., Lindor, C.J., & Greene, M.H. (2008). Concise handbook of familial cancer susceptibility syndromes—Second edition. *Journal of the National Cancer Institute Monographs, 2008*(38), 3–93. doi:10.1093/jncimonographs/lgn001

Lowry, K.P., Lee, J.M., Kong, C.Y., McMahon, P.M., Gilmore, M.E., Chubiz, J.E.C., ... Gazelle, G.S. (2012). Annual screening strategies in *BRCA1* and *BRCA2* gene mutation carriers: A comparative effectiveness analysis. *Cancer, 118,* 2021–2030. doi:10.1002/cncr.26424

Mahon, S.M. (2011). Managing families with a hereditary cancer syndrome. *Oncology Nursing Forum, 38,* 641–644. doi:10.1188/11.ONF.641-644

Mahon, S.M. (2013a). Allocation of work activities in a comprehensive cancer genetics program. *Clinical Journal of Oncology Nursing, 17,* 397–404. doi:10.1188/13.CJON.397-404

Mahon, S.M. (2013b). Ordering the correct genetic test: Implications for oncology and primary care healthcare professionals. *Clinical Journal of Oncology Nursing, 17,* 128–131. doi:10.1188/13.CJON.128-131

Mahon, S.M. (2015). Management of patients with a genetic variant of unknown significance. *Oncology Nursing Forum, 42,* 316–318. doi:10.1188/15.ONF.316-318

Mahon, S.M., & Waldman, L. (2012). Von Hippel-Lindau syndrome: Implications for nursing care. *Oncology Nursing Forum, 39,* 533–536. doi:10.1188/12.ONF.533-536

Matsuno, R.K., Costantino, J.P., Ziegler, R.G., Anderson, G.L., Li, H., Pee, D., & Gail, M.H. (2011). Projecting individualized absolute invasive breast cancer risk in Asian and Pacific Islander American women. *Journal of the National Cancer Institute, 103,* 951–961. doi:10.1093/jnci/djr154

Metcalfe, K.A., Mian, N., Enmore, M., Poll, A., Llacuachaqui, M., Nanda, S., ... Narod, S.A. (2012). Long-term follow-up of Jewish women with a *BRCA1* and *BRCA2* mutation who underwent population genetic screening. *Breast Cancer Research and Treatment, 133,* 735–740. doi:10.1007/s10549-011-1941-0

Mitra, A.V., Bancroft, E.K., Barbachano, Y., Page, E.C., Foster, C.S., Jameson, C., ... Eeles, R.A. (2011). Targeted prostate cancer screening in men with mutations in *BRCA1* and *BRCA2* detects aggressive prostate cancer: Preliminary analysis of the results of the IMPACT study. *BJU International, 107,* 28–39. doi:10.1111/j.1464-410X.2010.09648.x

Moghadasi, S., Hofland, N., Wouts, J.N., Hogervorst, F.B.L., Wijnen, J.T., Vreeswijk, M.P.G., & van Asperen, C.J. (2013). Variants of uncertain significance in *BRCA1* and *BRCA2* assessment of in silico analysis and a proposal for communication in genetic counseling. *Journal of Medical Genetics, 50,* 74–79. doi:10.1136/jmedgenet-2012-100961

Mohamad, H.B., & Apffelstaedt, J.P. (2008). Counseling for male BRCA mutation carriers—A review. *Breast, 17,* 441–450. doi:10.1016/j.breast.2008.05.001

Morrow, M., Waters, J., & Morris, E. (2011). MRI for breast cancer screening, diagnosis, and treatment. *Lancet, 378,* 1804–1811. doi:10.1016/S0140-6736(11)61350-0

Murray, A.J., & Davies, D.M. (2013). The genetics of breast cancer. *Surgery, 31,* 1–3. doi:10.1016/j.mpsur.2012.10.019

Murray, M.L., Cerrato, F., Bennett, R.L., & Jarvik, G.P. (2011). Follow-up of carriers of *BRCA1* and *BRCA2* variants of unknown significance: Variant reclassification and surgical decisions. *Genetics in Medicine, 13,* 998–1005. doi:10.1097/GIM.0b013e318226fc15

Narod, S.A. (2010). Testing for *CHEK2* in the cancer genetics clinic: Ready for prime time? *Clinical Genetics, 78,* 1–7. doi:10.1111/j.1399-0004.2010.01402.x

National Coalition for Health Professional Education in Genetics. (2007). *Core competencies in genetics for health professionals* (3rd ed.). Retrieved from http://www.nchpeg.org/documents/Core_Comps_English_2007.pdf

National Comprehensive Cancer Network. (2016). *NCCN Clinical Practice Guidelines in Oncology (NCCN Guidelines®): Genetic/familial high-risk assessment: Breast and ovarian* [v.2.2017]. Retrieved from https://www.nccn.org/professionals/physician_gls/pdf/genetics_screening.pdf

Olbrys, K.M. (2013). Identifying patients at risk for hereditary breast cancer. *Journal for Nurse Practitioners, 9,* 66–67. doi:10.1016/j.nurpra.2012.10.001

Parmigiani, G., Chen, S., Iversen, E.S., Jr., Friebel, T.M., Finkelstein, D.M., Anton-Culver, H., ... Euhus, D.M. (2007). Validity of models for predicting *BRCA1* and *BRCA2* mutations. *Annals of Internal Medicine, 147,* 441–450. doi:10.7326/0003-4819-147-7-200710020-00002

Patel, S.G., & Ahnen, D.J. (2012). Familial colon cancer syndromes: An update of a rapidly evolving field. *Current Gastroenterology Reports, 14,* 428–438. doi:10.1007/s11894-012-0280-6

Pilarski, R., & Nagy, R. (2012). Genetic testing by cancer site: Endocrine system. *Cancer Journal, 18,* 364–371. doi:10.1097/ppo.0b013e3182609458

Plutynski, A. (2012). Ethical issues in cancer screening and prevention. *Journal of Medicine and Philosophy, 37,* 310–323. doi:10.1093/jmp/jhs017

Power, D.G., Gloglowski, E., & Lipkin, S.M. (2010). Clinical genetics of hereditary colorectal cancer. *Hematology/Oncology Clinics of North America, 24,* 837–859. doi:10.1016/j.hoc.2010.06.006

Radice, P., De Summa, S., Caleca, L., & Tommasi, S. (2011). Unclassified variants in BRCA genes: Guidelines for interpretation. *Annals of Oncology, 22*(Suppl. 1), i18–i23. doi:10.1093/annonc/mdq661

Rew, L., Kaur, M., McMillan, A., Mackert, M., & Bonevac, D. (2010). Systematic review of psychosocial benefits and harms of genetic testing. *Issues in Mental Health Nursing, 31,* 631–645. doi:10.3109/01612840.2010.510618

Richards, C.S., Bale, S., Bellissimo, D.B., Das, S., Grody, W.W., Hegde, M.R., ... Ward, B.E. (2008). ACMG recommendations for standards for interpretation and reporting of sequence variations: Revisions 2007. *Genetics in Medicine, 10,* 294–300. doi:10.1097/GIM.0b013e31816b5cae

Riley, B.D., Culver, J.O., Skrzynia, C., Senter, L.A., Peters, J.A., Costalas, J.W., ... Trepanier, A.M. (2012). Essential elements of genetic cancer risk assessment, counseling, and testing: Updated recommendations of the National Society of Genetic Counselors. *Journal of Genetic Counseling, 21,* 151–161. doi:10.1007/s10897-011-9462-x

Rizzo, J.M., & Buck, M.J. (2012). Key principles and clinical applications of "next-generation" DNA sequencing. *Cancer Prevention Research, 5,* 887–900. doi:10.1158/1940-6207.CAPR-11-0432

Rodriguez-Bigas, M.A., & Möeslein, G. (2013). Surgical treatment of hereditary nonpolyposis colorectal cancer (HNPCC, Lynch syndrome). *Familial Cancer, 12,* 295–300. doi:10.1007/s10689-013-9626-y

Ruddy, K.J., & Winer, E.P. (2013). Male breast cancer: Risk factors, biology, diagnosis, treatment, and survivorship. *Annals of Oncology, 24,* 1434–1443. doi:10.1093/annonc/mdt025

Saslow, D., Solomon, D., Lawson, H.W., Killackey, M., Kulasingam, S.L., Cain, J., ... ACS-ASCCP-ASCP Cervical Cancer Guideline Committee. (2012). American Cancer Society, American Society for Colposcopy and Cervical Pathology, and American Society for Clinical Pathology screening guidelines for the prevention and early detection of cervical cancer. *CA: A Cancer Journal for Clinicians, 62,* 147–172. doi:10.3322/caac.21139

Scheuner, M.T., de Vries, H., Kim, B., Meili, R.C., Olmstead, S.H., & Teleki, S. (2009). Are electronic health records ready for genomic medicine? *Genetics in Medicine, 11,* 510–517. doi:10.1097/GIM.0b013e3181a53331

Schneider, R., Schneider, C., Kloor, M., Fürst, A., & Möslein, G. (2012). Lynch syndrome: Clinical, pathological, and genetic insights. *Langenbeck's Archives of Surgery, 397,* 513–525. doi:10.1007/s00423-012-0918-8

Selkirk, C.G., Vogel, K.J., Newlin, A.C., Weissman, S.M., Weiss, S.M., Wang, C.-H., & Hulick, P.J. (2014). Cancer genetic testing panels for inherited cancer susceptibility: The clinical experience of a large adult genetics practice. *Familial Cancer, 13,* 527–536. doi:10.1007/s10689-014-9741-4

Senter, L. (2012). Genetic testing by cancer site: Colon (nonpolyposis syndromes). *Cancer Journal, 18,* 334–337. doi:10.1097/ppo.0b013e31826094b2

Shannon, K.M., & Chittenden, A. (2012). Genetic testing by cancer site: Breast. *Cancer Journal, 18,* 310–319. doi:10.1097/PPO.0b013e318260946f

Shattuck-Eidens, D., Oliphant, A., McClure, M., McBride, C., Gupte, J., Rubano, T., ... Thomas, A. (1997). BRCA1 sequence analysis in women at high risk for susceptibility mutations: Risk factor analysis and implications for genetic testing. *JAMA, 278,* 1242–1250. doi:10.1001/jama.1997.03550150046034

Shia, J., Holck, S., DePetris, G., Greenson, J.K., & Klimstra, D.S. (2013). Lynch syndrome-associated neoplasms: A discussion on histopathology and immunohistochemistry. *Familial Cancer, 12,* 241–260. doi:10.1007/s10689-013-9612-4

Shin, E.J., & Canto, M.I. (2012). Pancreatic cancer screening. *Gastroenterology Clinics of North America, 41,* 143–157. doi:10.1016/j.gtc.2011.12.001

Sijmons, R.H., Greenblatt, M.S., & Genuardi, M. (2013). Gene variants of unknown clinical significance in Lynch syndrome. An introduction for clinicians. *Familial Cancer, 12,* 181–187. doi:10.1007/s10689-013-9629-8

Spruce, L.R., & Sanford, J.T. (2012). An intervention to change the approach to colorectal cancer screening in primary care. *Journal of the American Academy of Nurse Practitioners, 24,* 167–174. doi:10.1111/j.1745-7599.2012.00714.x

Ståhlbom, A.K., Johansson, H., Liljegren, A., von Wachenfeldt, A., & Arver, B. (2012). Evaluation of the BOADICEA risk assessment model in women with a family history of breast cancer. *Familial Cancer, 11,* 33–40. doi:10.1007/s10689-011-9495-1

Teller, P., Hoskins, K.F., Zwaagstra, A., Stanislaw, C., Iyengar, R., Green, V.L., & Gabram, S.G.A. (2010). Validation of the Pedigree Assessment Tool (PAT) in families with *BRCA1* and *BRCA2* mutations. *Annals of Surgical Oncology, 17,* 240–246. doi:10.1245/s10434-009-0697-9

Templeton, A.W., & Brentnall, T.A. (2013). Screening and surgical outcomes of familial pancreatic cancer. *Surgical Clinics of North America, 93,* 629–645. doi:10.1016/j.suc.2013.02.002

Tkatch, R., Hudson, J., Katz, A., Berry-Bobovski, L., Vichich, J., Eggly, S., ... Albrecht, T.L. (2014). Barriers to cancer screening among Orthodox Jewish women. *Journal of Community Health, 39,* 1200–1208. doi:10.1007/s10900-014-9879-x

Tokin, C., Weiss, A., Wang-Rodriguez, J., & Blair, S.L. (2012). Oncologic safety of skin-sparing and nipple-sparing mastectomy: A discussion and review of the literature. *International Journal of Surgical Oncology, 2012,* Article ID 921821. doi:10.1155/2012/921821

Twomey, J. (2011). Ethical, legal, psychosocial, and cultural implications of genomics for oncology nurses. *Seminars in Oncology Nursing, 27,* 54–63. doi:10.1016/j.soncn.2010.11.007

Umar, A., Boland, C.R., Terdiman, J.P., Syngal, S., de la Chapelle, A., Rüschoff, J., ... Srivastava, S. (2004). Revised Bethesda guidelines for hereditary nonpolyposis colorectal cancer (Lynch syndrome) and microsatellite instability. *Journal of the National Cancer Institute, 96,* 261–268. doi:10.1093/jnci/djh034

U.S. Department of Health and Human Services. (2009, April 6). *The Genetic Information Nondiscrimination Act of 2008: Information for researchers and health care professionals.* Retrieved from https://www.genome.gov/pages/policyethics/geneticdiscrimination/ginainfodoc.pdf

Vadaparampil, S.T., Miree, C.A., Wilson, C., & Jacobsen, P.B. (2007). Psychosocial and behavioral impact of genetic counseling and testing. *Breast Disease, 27,* 97–108. doi:10.3233/BD-2007-27106

Vasen, H.F.A., Blanco, I., Aktan-Collan, K., Gopie, J.P., Alonso, A., Aretz, S., ... Möslein, G. (2013). Revised guidelines for the clinical management of Lynch syndrome (HNPCC): Recommendations by a group of European experts. *Gut, 62,* 812–823. doi:10.1136/gutjnl-2012-304356

Vencken, P.M.L.H., Kriege, M., Hooning, M., Menke-Pluymers, M.B., Heemskerk-Gerritsen, B.A.M., van Doorn, L.C., ... Seynaeve, C. (2013). The risk of primary and contralateral breast cancer after ovarian cancer in *BRCA1/BRCA2* mutation carriers: Implications for counseling. *Cancer, 119,* 955–962. doi:10.1002/cncr.27839

Weissman, S.M., Burt, R., Church, J., Erdman, S., Hampel, H., Holter, S., ... Senter, L. (2012). Identification of individuals at risk for Lynch syndrome using targeted evaluations and genetic testing: National Society of Genetic Counselors and the Collaborative Group of the Americas on Inherited Colorectal Cancer joint practice guideline. *Journal of Genetic Counseling, 21,* 484–493. doi:10.1007/s10897-011-9465-7

Weissman, S.M., Weiss, S.M., & Newlin, A.C. (2012). Genetic testing by cancer site: Ovary. *Cancer Journal, 18,* 320–327. doi:10.1097/ppo.0b013e31826246c2

Weitzel, J.N., Blazer, K.R., MacDonald, D.J., Culver, J.O., & Offit, K. (2011). Genetics, genomics, and cancer risk assessment: State of the art and future directions in the era of personalized medicine. *CA: A Cancer Journal for Clinicians, 61,* 327–359. doi:10.3322/caac.20128

Wevers, M.R., Ausems, M.G.E.M., Verhoef, S., Bleiker, E.M.A., Hahn, D.E.E., Hogervorst, F.B.L., ... Aaronson, N.K. (2011). Behavioral and psychosocial effects of rapid genetic counseling and testing in newly diagnosed breast cancer patients: Design of a multicenter randomized clinical trial. *BMC Cancer, 11.* doi:10.1186/1471-2407-11-6

Wiggs, J.L. (2009). Fundamentals of human genetics. In M. Yanoff & J.S. Duker (Eds.), *Ophthalmology* (3rd ed., pp. 1–9). St. Louis, MO: Elsevier Mosby.

Wiseman, M., Dancyger, C., & Michie, S. (2010). Communicating genetic risk information within families: A review. *Familial Cancer, 9,* 691–703. doi:10.1007/s10689-010-9380-3

Zagouri, F., Chrysikos, D.T., Sergentanis, T.N., Giannakopoulou, G., Zografos, C.G., Papadimitriou, C.A., & Zografos, G.C. (2013). Prophylactic mastectomy: An appraisal. *American Surgeon, 79,* 205–212.

Chapter 4 Study Questions

1. Which of the following is a characteristic of hereditary breast and ovarian cancer?
   A. Onset of breast cancer at an older age
   B. HER2-positive breast cancer
   C. Bilateral breast cancer
   D. Family member with breast cancer

2. A patient tests negative for a known *MSH6* mutation in his family. The patient has never been diagnosed with cancer. What is his risk for developing colon cancer?
   A. He has no risk of colon cancer.
   B. His risk is greater than that of the general population.
   C. His risk cannot be quantified.
   D. His risk is at least that of the general population.

3. A 35-year-old woman whose mother was diagnosed with breast cancer at age 38 asks her primary nurse about genetics testing for hereditary cancer. How should the nurse reply?
   A. That test can be ordered routinely with your yearly bloodwork.
   B. It would probably be best to see a credentialed genetics nurse or genetics counselor for further evaluation.
   C. It is best to check with your insurance company to see if it is a covered benefit before ordering the test.
   D. The pedigree does not suggest hereditary risk.

4. Which of the following is a potential risk of genetic testing when it is ordered outside of formal counseling by a genetics healthcare professional?
   A. Family members may not learn about the test outcome.
   B. The provider may not be able to correctly interpret the clinical meaning of the test.
   C. The test may be expensive.
   D. Patients will know whether or not they have the disease.

5. A critical component of informed consent for cancer genetic testing is:
   A. Confirmation of the family history for cancer.
   B. Overview of the risks, benefits, and limitations of cancer genetic predisposition testing.
   C. A full history and physical to rule out the possibility of malignancy.
   D. Estimation of the chance of carrying a mutation.

CHAPTER

5

Cancer Detection Measures

Suzanne M. Mahon, RN, DNSc, AOCN®, AGN-BC

Introduction

Improved survival from cancer has been a result of both improved treatment and earlier detection. Oncology nurses are becoming increasingly involved in cancer prevention and detection services. Recommendations for the early detection of cancer are based on the cancer risk assessment (see Chapter 3). This chapter will provide an overview of the fundamental principles involved in the early detection of cancer, which also may be referred to as *cancer screening* or *secondary cancer prevention.*

The premise of secondary cancer prevention is to screen for and detect cancer in its earliest stages. Theoretically, treatment should be the least complicated and least toxic and should provide the greatest chance for long-term disease-free survival (American Cancer Society [ACS], 2015b, 2015c). All nurses need to discuss secondary cancer prevention measures with patients and their family members. Nurses need to be able to discuss and instruct patients and families on the principles of screening, the rationale for recommendations from national agencies, and controversies in screening (Plescia, Richardson, & Joseph, 2012). This chapter begins with a discussion of the theoretical foundations of cancer screening followed by a discussion of the major cancers for which screening tests are available. For each of these cancers, information is provided regarding the epidemiology, risk factors, signs and symptoms, patient education, and potential early detection strategies, including the strengths and limitations of the screening tests.

Principles of Secondary Cancer Prevention

Cancer screening is aimed at asymptomatic people with the goal of finding disease and decreasing the morbidity and mortality associated with cancer in its early stages, when treatment is most likely to be effective. Some also consider testing for genetic or molecular markers that put an individual at high risk for developing cancer to be a form of cancer screening (see Chapter 4).

Accuracy of Cancer Screening Tests

The accuracy of a screening test is the degree to which a measurement represents the true value of the characteristic being measured. In the context of cancer screening, results fall into one of the following categories of accuracy: true positive, true negative, false negative, or false positive. A true-positive result indicates the person tested has cancer, and the person actually does have the disease. A true-negative result indicates the person tested does not have cancer, and that person neither has nor develops cancer within a defined period. A false-negative result occurs if the test indicates the individual does not have cancer, but the individual actually does. A false-positive result occurs when the screening test indicates a person has cancer, but the individual actually does not. Information about accuracy categories is necessary to calculate the sensitivity and specificity of a particular screening test (Gordis, 2014). The *sensitivity* of a screening test is its ability to detect those individuals with cancer. It is calculated by taking the number of true positives and dividing it by the total number of cancer cases (true positives plus false negatives). Most people are unwilling to accept a test with a high false-negative rate because the test will miss many cancers. The *specificity* of a test is its ability to identify individuals who actually do not have cancer. It is calculated by dividing the number of true negatives by the sum of the true-negative and false-positive results. A high false-positive rate can result in unnecessary follow-up testing, costs, and anxiety for people who receive false-positive results (Gordis, 2014).

Understanding the principles of sensitivity and specificity helps individuals to realize the strengths and limitations of the screening test they are considering. Nurses and the public must recognize that a perfect screening test does not exist. Even mammography fails to detect at least 10% of all breast cancers (Sinclair, Littenberg, Geller, & Muss, 2011). Failure rates regarding the detection of breast cancer, especially with mammography, may be even higher in women younger than age 50 (ACS, 2015a). Whenever possible, nurses need to communicate to patients, in understandable terms, information about sensitivity and specificity data.

Variations in Cancer Screening Guidelines

A major source of confusion in cancer screening stems from the variations in screening recommendations among the various professional agencies (Basch, Somerfield, Partridge, Schnipper, & Lyman, 2011; Brawley et al., 2011; Evans, Brouwers, & Bell, 2008; Guirguis-Blake et al., 2007). This is an important area for nurses to consider in patient education. First, nurses need to inform patients of the generally agreed-upon requirements and characteristics of acceptable screening testing regarding sensitivity, specificity, and false-positive and false-negative rates (see Figure 5-1). When presenting screening recommendations to individuals, it is important to include the rationale, as well as the strengths and limitations of the test, and to present this information in light of the individual's risk for developing cancer. Healthcare providers can obtain information about the scientific basis and the review process for a guideline from the agency that generated the guideline or at the National Guideline Clearinghouse website (www.guideline.gov). This information is contin-

Figure 5-1. Considerations for Acceptable Cancer Screening Tests

- The natural history of the disease is adequately understood.
- The condition is an important health problem (high incidence, morbidity, or mortality).
- A test is available that can detect the disease or condition in its early stages or pick up signs that the disease may develop later.
- The screening test has acceptable sensitivity and specificity.
- The disease or condition can be treated, and the treatment is more effective, affordable, safe, or acceptable in the earlier stages.
- Facilities for diagnosis and treatment are available.
- The test is acceptable to the population.
- The test does not have a high probability of other problems or risks.
- An agreed-upon policy exists regarding whom to screen and treat.
- The total cost of finding a case is economically balanced in relation to medical expenditure as a whole.
- Cancer screening is a continuous process, not just a "onetime" project.

Note. Based on information from American Cancer Society, 2016a; Brawley et al., 2011; Evans et al., 2008.

ually updated and facilitates comparison of recommendations across agencies.

A screening protocol or recommendation defines how a cancer screening test should be used. For example, ACS (2016a) recommends an annual mammogram for all women beginning at age 45 with an option to begin at age 40. The specific guidelines change over time, but the focus has changed little (Brawley et al., 2011). The focus is still that healthcare providers should be aware of the latest guidelines to select the best screening tests for an individual of average risk and should modify the guidelines for individuals with a particularly high risk for developing a specific malignancy.

Such recommendations can vary among organizations and practitioners. A recommendation generally describes the target population being served, the screening recommendation to be applied, and the interval at which the test should be applied. Clinicians must remember that screening protocols are guidelines and not practice standards to be implemented with every individual. Clinicians also must consider the goals of the agency's recommendations. The goal of the ACS standards is to detect malignancy. The U.S. Preventive Services Task Force (USPSTF) uses very strict criteria for evidence of effectiveness. Cost-effectiveness also is an important consideration for this group. When providing information on cancer screening recommendations, nurses need to inform individuals why they are selecting a certain recommendation.

Informed Consent for Cancer Screening

Patients must have enough information about screening tests to make an informed decision to either undergo or decline screening. Nurses have a key role in interpreting and explaining information regarding the sensitivity, specificity, strengths, risks, and benefits of a screening test to patients (Fagerlin, Zikmund-Fisher, & Ubel, 2011). Nurses need to explain why a particular set of guidelines is recommended for an individual patient. They need to remind each patient that these are guidelines and that modifications may be made based on risk factor assessment and clinical examination findings. With people who are in failing health, it is appropriate to discuss stopping cancer screening, although few guidelines provide specific direction in this area. Clearly, the benefits, risks, and potential limitations of each screening test need to be discussed and tailored to the risk factor assessment so that patients can make an informed decision about what is best for them.

Many individuals, however, will still choose to undergo a screening examination even if it has a lower sensitivity and specificity, in hopes that it will be effective for them. Screening for ovarian cancer is an excellent example. Highly specific and sensitive screening tests are not yet available for the early detection of this cancer. Ovarian cancer has few, if any, early signs and symptoms (ACS, 2016a). Many women, however, still want an annual pelvic examination to assess for ovarian masses. The test is relatively inexpensive to perform and usually well tolerated. Some clinicians are better at detecting ovarian masses than others, and many ovarian cancers cannot be detected using this examination, even when performed by highly skilled clinicians. As long as a woman realizes that the test may fail to detect ovarian cancer and is willing to accept this limitation, utilizing the pelvic examination may be effective. Thus, being informed about a cancer screening examination includes knowledge that not all cancers may be detected and awareness of the potential risks. If patients decline recommended screening, they need to understand that the symptoms of cancer may not be evident until treatment is no longer likely to be effective (Edwards et al., 2013).

If the intended benefits of screening are to be realized, individuals need to have a clear understanding of the implications of screening tests both before screening and after receiving results. The potential benefits of screening are lost if individuals are never informed of test results or the meaning of these results. Providing patients with information about screening results serves as another opportunity for nurses to reinforce information included in the risk factor assessment. After the screening tests, risk may be more apparent, and the clinician may need to revise screening recommendations. For example, a 50-year-old man may have a baseline screening colonoscopy examination that demonstrates a large polyp, which is subsequently biopsied and shows hyperplasia. His risk for developing colon cancer is higher than initially perceived. He should be informed of the risk and be counseled about the recommendations for screening at a more frequent interval than every 10 years (Levin et al., 2008).

Clearly, cancer risk communication influences patients' decisions to undergo cancer screening examinations. When a healthcare provider recommends a particular screening examination, the patient is more likely to have the recommended screening (Sarfaty, Wender, & Smith, 2011).

Table 5-1. Risk Factors for Lung Cancer

Risk Factor	Possible Etiologic Basis
Asbestos exposure	Asbestos fibers are a known carcinogen to lung tissue.
Genetic predisposition	In some families, more lung cancers develop than can be attributed to chance, especially when they occur in nonsmokers without other risk factors. A mutation appears to exist on chromosome 6 that may place some people at higher risk. Genetic testing is not currently available on a commercial basis.
Radiation exposure to the lungs	Risk is increased in people treated for Hodgkin lymphoma and other diseases that would involve chest radiation, which has a direct carcinogenic effect on lung tissue.
Radon exposure	Radon is a naturally occurring radioactive gas that results from the breakdown of uranium in soil and rocks and has a carcinogenic effect on lung tissue.
Tobacco use (cigarettes, smokeless tobacco, cigars, and pipes)	Nicotine, tar, and other chemicals have a direct carcinogenic effect on lung tissue. Risk increases with the length and intensity of exposure.

Note. Based on information from American Cancer Society, 2015b, 2016a; Lo et al., 2013; Papathomas et al., 2011.

Lung Cancer

Lung cancer is a serious public health problem in the United States. It is more common in older adults; the average age at diagnosis is 70 years (ACS, 2016a). Lung cancer is the second most common cancer diagnosed in men and women and accounts for 14% of new cancers in the United States (ACS, 2016a). Unfortunately, lung cancer is by far the leading cause of cancer death among both men and women. More people die of lung cancer than of colon, breast, and prostate cancers combined (ACS, 2016a).

Risk Factors

Known risk factors for lung cancer are shown in Table 5-1. About 87% of lung cancer deaths are attributed to tobacco use (ACS, 2015b). The longer an individual smokes and the more packs smoked per day, the greater the risk. People who stop smoking before age 50 cut their risk of dying in the next 15 years in half compared with those who continue to smoke (ACS, 2015b). Current smokers should be informed that the immediate preventive health priority is the elimination of tobacco use because smoking cessation offers the most effective means of reducing the risk of premature mortality from lung cancer (Smith et al., 2015).

Secondhand smoke also increases the risk for lung cancer. A nonsmoker who lives with a smoker has about a 20%–30% greater risk of developing lung cancer (Alberg, Brock, Ford, Samet, & Spivack, 2013). Secondhand smoke is the attributed cause for more than 3,000 lung cancer deaths in the United States annually (Alberg et al., 2013).

Signs and Symptoms

Figure 5-2 shows the signs and symptoms of lung cancer. The symptoms are nonspecific, and often the diagnosis is not made until the disease has metastasized to the brain, bone, or liver.

Early Detection

Screening for lung cancer is controversial but becoming more common. Routine screening with a chest x-ray is not effective, as lesions usually are large by the time they are seen on a chest x-ray, and treatment is not always effective because of the presence of metastasis. Recent data from the National Lung Screening Trial showed a sensitivity of 93.8% and specificity of 73.4% for low-dose computed tomography (LDCT) and a sensitivity of 73.5% and specificity of 91.3% for chest radiography (National Lung Screening Trial Research Team, 2011). USPSTF recommends that asymptomatic adults aged 55–80 years who have a 30-pack-year smoking history and currently smoke or have quit smoking within the past 15 years undergo annual lung cancer screening with LDCT (Moyer, 2014).

ACS recommends that when high-volume, high-quality lung cancer screening and treatment centers are available, clinicians can consider LDCT screening in patients aged 55–74 years who appear healthy, have at least a 30-pack-year smoking history, and currently smoke or have quit within the past 15 years (Wender et al., 2013). ACS emphasizes that individuals interested in early detection using LDCT should be educated about the potential risks and unknowns of the test and should be encouraged to participate in a clinical trial to better evaluate this technology (ACS, 2016a).

Figure 5-2. Signs and Symptoms of Lung Cancer

Signs of Lung Cancer
- A cough that does not go away
- Chest pain, often made worse by deep breathing, coughing, or laughing
- Hoarseness
- Weight loss and loss of appetite
- Bloody or rust-colored sputum
- Shortness of breath
- Recurring bronchitis or pneumonia
- New onset of wheezing

Signs Often Seen With Metastasis
- Bone pain
- Weakness or numbness of the arms or legs
- Headache, dizziness, or seizure
- Yellow coloring of the skin and eyes
- Lumps near the surface of the body

Note. Based on information from American Cancer Society, 2016a.

Breast Cancer

Breast cancer is the most common cancer among women in the United States. Women fear breast cancer, and most know someone affected by the diagnosis. Approximately 3.1 million people in the United States are breast cancer survivors (ACS, 2015a). The absolute lifetime risk of developing invasive breast cancer is about 1 in 8. Breast cancer is responsible for 14% of all cancer deaths annually (ACS, 2016a).

Risk Factors

Table 5-2 shows the known risk factors for breast cancer. Risk factor assessment is critical in

Table 5-2. Risk Factors for Breast Cancer

Risk Factor	Epidemiology	Modifiable
Age	Approximately 2 out of 3 women are aged 55 or older at diagnosis. Risk increases with age.	No
Alcohol use	Women who consume 1 drink a day have a slightly increased risk. Those who have 2–5 drinks daily have about 1.5 times the risk of women who drink no alcohol.	Yes
Genetic predisposition	About 10% of breast cancers are linked to mutations in genes (especially *BRCA1* and *BRCA2*) that confer up to an 85% lifetime risk of developing breast cancer. More than 20 genes have been identified that are associated with an increased risk of developing breast cancer for which commercial genetic testing is available.	No
Hormone replacement therapy	Long-term use (several years or more) increases the risk of developing breast cancer and may increase the chances of dying of breast cancer. Five years after use is stopped, breast cancer risk seems to return to normal.	Yes
History of breast biopsy	A history of atypia on biopsy increases risk; fibrocystic changes and fibroadenomas do not increase risk.	No
Increased number of menstrual cycles	Risk is increased in women with menarche before age 12 or menopause after age 55.	No
Late parity or nulliparity	Women who have not had children, or who had their first child after age 30, have a slightly higher risk of developing breast cancer. Being pregnant more than once and at an earlier age reduces breast cancer risk. Delivery of a baby is the final step of breast development.	Possibly
Obesity/ inactivity	Increased body weight is associated with increased risk, especially when the increase in weight occurs later in adulthood. It may relate to the presence of more estrogen receptors in fat cells. Studies show that exercise reduces the risk of developing breast cancer; it is not clear if it is a direct effect or if exercise helps to maintain a healthier weight.	Yes
Oral contraceptives	Women who use birth control pills have a slightly greater risk of developing breast cancer than women who have never used them. Ten years after women have stopped taking oral contraceptives, the risk seems to be gone. Exact risk is unclear.	Yes
Prior history of breast cancer	Once a person is diagnosed with breast cancer, the risk of developing a second primary breast cancer is higher.	No
Prior radiation to the chest	Women who have had radiation treatment to the chest area earlier in life have a greatly increased risk of developing breast cancer.	No
Race	Caucasian women are slightly more likely to develop breast cancer, but African American women are more likely to die of it. African American women may have faster-growing tumors.	No
Sex	Breast cancer is 100 times more common in women than men.	No

Note. Based on information from American Cancer Society, 2015b, 2016a; Green, 2013; Nelson et al., 2012; Tan et al., 2012.

breast cancer because it has a significant impact on recommendations for screening and referral for genetic testing (Shannon & Chittenden, 2012). The proper use of screening and genetic testing can potentially decrease the morbidity and mortality associated with breast cancer. Women with a mutation in a known hereditary predisposition gene, such as *BRCA1* or *BRCA2*, will need more aggressive management strategies that might include breast magnetic resonance imaging (MRI), chemoprevention, and prophylactic surgery (ACS, 2016a; see also Chapter 4).

Signs and Symptoms

Screening is appropriate for asymptomatic women (Smith et al., 2015). All women should be educated about the signs and symptoms of breast cancer and instructed to seek further evaluation if they notice any change in their breasts. Symptomatic women (see Figure 5-3) should be referred directly for a diagnostic evaluation, which might include an ultrasound, additional mammographic views, MRI, and biopsy (ACS, 2015a). Men, especially those at increased risk, should be instructed on the importance of immediate evaluation of any mass behind the nipple.

Figure 5-3. Signs and Symptoms of Breast Cancer

- Lump or mass in the breast
- Lump in the axilla
- Lump or mass behind or in the nipple
- Swelling in all or part of the breast
- Skin irritation or dimpling
- Redness, scaliness, or thickening of the nipple or breast skin
- Breast pain
- Nipple pain or nipple inversion (or eversion if normally inverted)
- Nipple discharge other than breast milk

Note. Based on information from American Cancer Society, 2015a.

Early Detection

Screening for breast cancer has historically involved three modalities: breast self-awareness, also referred to as breast self-examination; clinical breast examination (CBE); and mammography (see Table 5-3). The recommendations for breast self-awareness and CBE vary greatly across professional organizations.

ACS recommends that all women be instructed on the option of breast self-awareness at age 20. Each woman must make a decision about the usefulness of the tool and, if the woman desires, should be provided specific, personalized instruction on how to perform breast self-awareness (ACS, 2015a) (see Figure 5-4). The guidelines from the National Comprehensive Cancer Network® (NCCN®) are similar (NCCN, 2016a).

Historically, CBE has been recommended beginning at age 20 in women of average risk with an interval of every one to three years until age 40 and then annually (NCCN, 2016a). Currently, ACS and USPSTF do not recommend CBE. The steps of breast self-awareness and CBE are similar. If a woman desires to practice breast self-awareness, she should be offered the opportunity to learn during a CBE.

ACS recommends that women of average risk should begin mammography at age 45 with an option to start at age 40 (ACS, 2015a). NCCN recommends annual mammography starting at age 40 (NCCN, 2016a). USPSTF recommends mammography every other year starting at age 50 (Siu, 2016). The routine use of mammography is partially responsible for the reduction in mortality rates for breast cancer. It is estimated to reduce the risk of dying from breast cancer by as much as 38% (ACS, 2015b). Mammography can detect breast cancers long before they are palpable. All mammogram facilities should be certified by the American College of Radiology (ACR) and use dedicated mammogram machines. Mammography usually takes two x-rays of each breast from different angles: top to bottom and side to side. In digital tomosynthesis (three-dimensional mammogaphy), the breast is positioned the same way as in a conven-

Table 5-3. Characteristics of Tools for Early Detection of Breast Cancer

Tool	Strengths	Limitations/Risks
Breast self-awareness	Convenient Inexpensive Can detect interval cancers between professional examinations The woman might be most familiar with her body and subtle changes.	Dependent on the skill of the woman Lesions must be palpable or visible to inspection.
Clinical breast examination	Relatively inexpensive Opportunity to teach self-awareness technique during examination Can detect interval cancers between mammograms	Dependent on the skill of the practitioner Lesion must be palpable or visible to inspection.
Mammography	Sensitivity of 80%–95% Specificity of 95%–98% Will detect 80%–90% of cancers in asymptomatic women Is especially effective in women older than age 50	Less effective in younger women, especially those with dense breasts May be uncomfortable for the woman Exposes the woman to a small dose of radiation Average cost of $50–$150 for a standard mammogram; tomosynthesis may be more expensive with variable reimbursement.
Magnetic resonance imaging	More sensitive than mammography for detecting early cancers in high-risk individuals Useful for evaluating breast implants for leaks or ruptures and for assessing abnormal areas seen on a mammogram or felt after breast surgery or radiation therapy Indicated for screening in women with a greater than 20% lifetime risk of developing breast cancer	Very expensive Requires dedicated machine, capability to perform breast biopsies, and trained radiologist Not widely available High false-positive rate Incomplete algorithms for interpreting small lesions Possibility of reaction to the contrast dye Long-term effects of exposure to dye are not known.

Note. Based on information from American Cancer Society, 2015a; Chiarelli et al., 2009; Morrow et al., 2011; Sinclair et al., 2011.

tional mammogram, but the x-ray tube moves in an arc around the breast while multiple images are taken. The images are assembled to produce highly detailed three-dimensional images of the breast. Early data suggest an increased cancer detection rate, especially in women with dense breasts, as well as a decreased recall rate for false positives (Gilbert, Tucker, & Young, 2016). Digital tomosynthesis is approved by the U.S. Food and Drug Administration (FDA) but is not yet considered the standard of care for breast cancer screening, and insurance reimbursement can be variable. Because it is relatively new, its availability is limited in some areas.

When a woman presents for a mammogram, she should anticipate questioning about previous imaging, breast problems, hormone use, and breast surgeries. If examinations have been done at another facility, the woman will need to sign a release for the films to be sent for comparison. The woman should be instructed to avoid using deodorant or antiperspirant, lotions, and creams on the breast area on the day of the examination because some of these contain sub-

Figure 5-4. Steps for Breast Self-Awareness

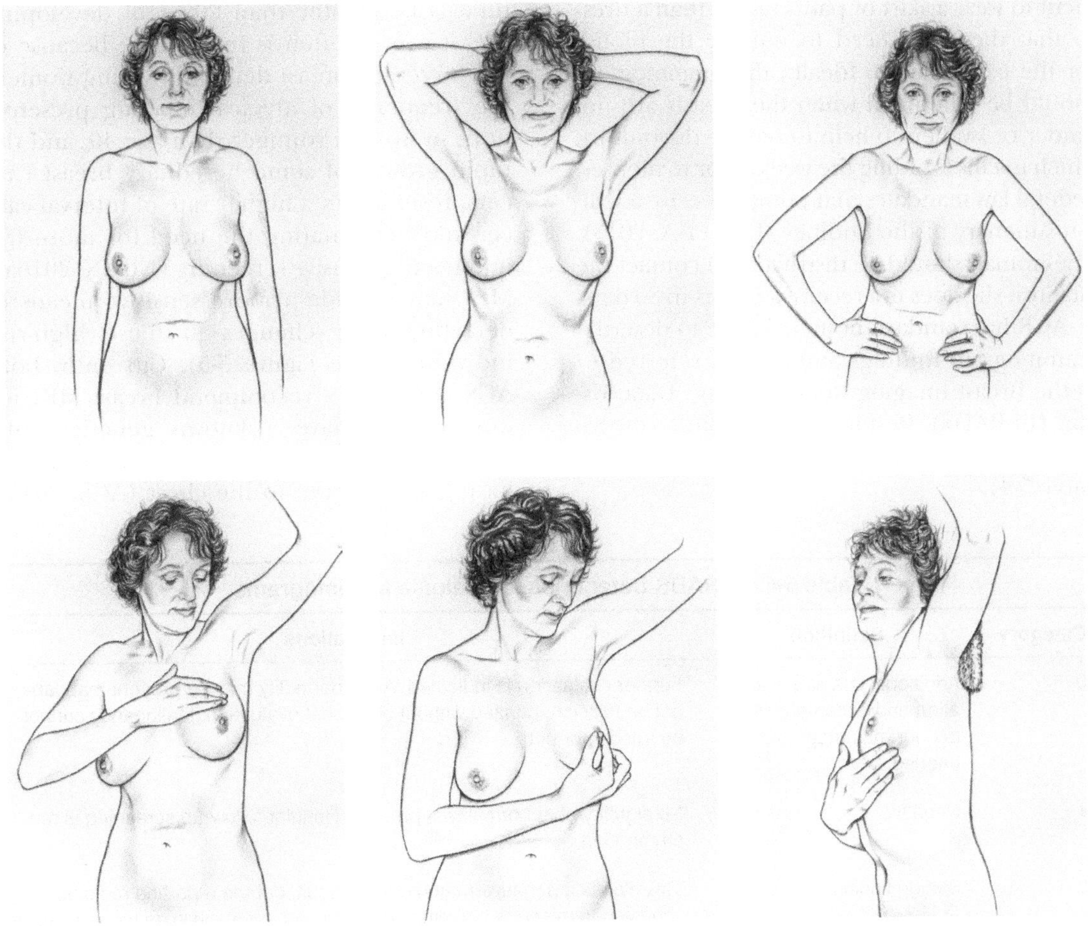

These are the steps for both a professional examination and a breast self-examination. Both examinations are optimally done 7–10 days after the menses start. Begin by examining the breasts with both arms relaxed at sides. One breast is always bigger than the other. The woman should note if this changes. Observe the breast for puckers, dimples, color irregularities, and nipple deviation. Next, the woman should squeeze her arms together at her waist and again observe for changes. The woman should repeat this maneuver with her arms above her head. Next, assess the infraclavicular and supraclavicular areas for palpable lymph nodes. Also assess the axilla for palpable lymph nodes. Palpate the breasts for masses while the woman is sitting up. At this point, assess for nipple discharge. With the woman's arm behind her head and the breast area under a pillow or towel, palpate the entire breast with the pads of the fingers. The palpation should be deep, deeper, and still deeper. The fingers should slide and examine another section of the breast. The entire breast should be assessed from collarbone to midline and inframammary ridge to axilla in a systematic fashion of circles or strips. Finally, palpate the area behind the nipple for lumps and masses.

Note. Figure courtesy of National Cancer Institute. Retrieved from https://visualsonline.cancer.gov/details.cfm?imageid=2146.

stances that can interfere with mammogram interpretation. Some women find it more convenient to wear a skirt or pants rather than a dress so that they only need to remove the blouse for the examination. Ideally, the mammogram should be scheduled when the breasts are not tender or swollen to help to reduce discomfort, which means avoiding the week prior to menses. Federal law mandates that women receive a written summary of the findings (U.S. FDA, 2015). The woman should be instructed to contact the facility if she does not receive a report in 30 days.

ACR has standard nomenclature to describe mammogram findings and results, referred to as the Breast Imaging Reporting and Data System (BI-RADS). Results are sorted into categories numbered 0 through 6 (ACR, 2014) (see Table 5-4).

Conventional screening with mammography for younger women with an increased lifetime risk (greater than 20%) of developing breast cancer often is inadequate because of the increased breast density in young women, the frequency of atypical imaging presentations in women younger than age 40, and the rapid growth of some hereditary breast cancers, resulting in a higher rate of interval cancer and necessitating the need for more frequent and intensive screening (NCCN, 2016a). MRI may provide a more sensitive means of detecting early changes in these high-risk individuals (see Figure 5-5). Currently, both ACS and NCCN recommend breast MRI for women who have a known genetic mutation, have greater than a 20% lifetime risk, or have had radiation to the chest (ACS, 2015a;

Table 5-4. BI-RADS Categories to Evaluate Mammograms

Category	Definition	Implications
0	Additional imaging evaluation and/or comparison to prior mammograms is needed.	Further evaluation is indicated. An abnormality may be present that cannot be fully categorized without additional evaluation. Malignancy cannot be ruled in or out.
1	Negative	No significant abnormality is present. Regular follow-up screening is recommended.
2	Benign finding	This also is a negative mammogram result, but the reporting radiologist is choosing to describe a finding known to be benign, such as benign calcifications, lymph nodes in the breast, or fibroadenomas.
3	Probably benign finding—follow-up in a short time frame is suggested.	The findings in this category have a very high chance (> 98%) of being benign. Because a finding has not been proven by biopsy to be benign, tight, short follow-up is recommended.
4	Suspicious abnormality—biopsy should be considered.	Findings do not definitively appear malignant but could be malignant, and a biopsy is needed to determine the pathology of the lesion. The radiologist is concerned enough to recommend a biopsy.
5	Highly suggestive of malignancy	The findings appear malignant and have an approximate 95% chance of being malignant. Biopsy is necessary and indicated.
6	Known biopsy-proven malignancy	This category is only used for mammogram findings that have already been shown to be cancer by a biopsy. Treatment planning can be initiated based on the radiologic and pathologic findings.

Note. Based on information from Sickles et al., 2013.

Figure 5-5. Comparison of Mammography and Magnetic Resonance Imaging (MRI) in the Evaluation of a Breast Change

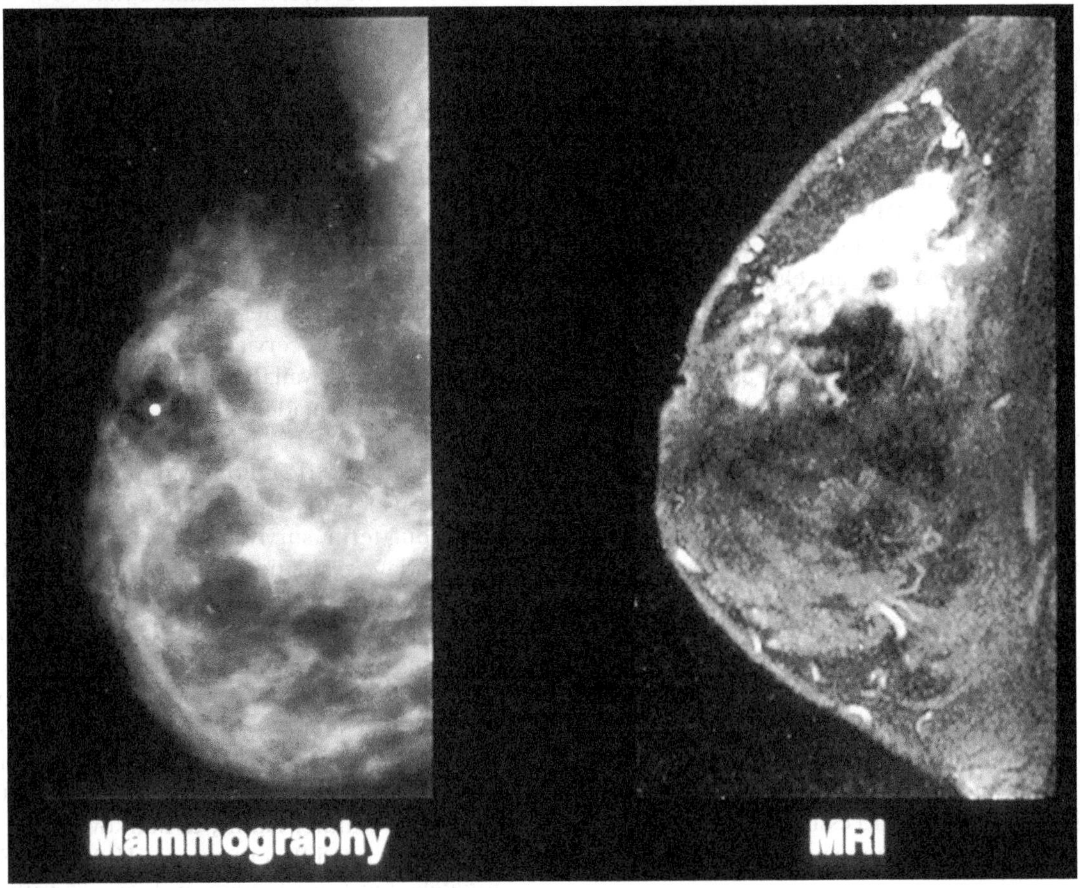

This figure shows mammography on the left and a breast MRI on the right. Note the MRI's enhancement ability to confirm diagnosis.

Note. Figure courtesy of National Cancer Institute, source Mitchell D. Schnall, MD, PhD, University of Pennsylvania. Retrieved from https://visualsonline.cancer.gov/details.cfm?imageid=2705.

NCCN, 2016c). At present, it is not a substitution for mammography, even in high-risk women (Berg et al., 2012). Breast MRI has shown to have utility in the diagnostic workup of women with nonspecific clinical or mammographic abnormalities (ACS, 2015a; Morrow, Waters, & Morris, 2011).

Much of the reduction in breast cancer mortality stems directly from screening efforts (ACS, 2015a). Public awareness of the importance of breast cancer screening is increasing. Government programs exist that promote and fund breast cancer screening, and many private organizations, such as Susan G. Komen and the Avon Breast Cancer Crusade, are dedicated to promoting awareness and screening for breast cancer, especially in underserved populations (Jacobsen & Jacobsen, 2011).

U.S. Congress passed the Breast and Cervical Cancer Mortality Prevention Act of 1990, which resulted in the National Breast and Cervical Cancer Early Detection Program (NBCCEDP). The program provides access to breast and cervical cancer screening and diagnostic services to low-income, uninsured, and underserved women. It is estimated that 8%–11% of U.S. women of screening age are eligible to receive NBCCEDP services (Miller, Hanson, Johnson, Royalty, & Richardson, 2014). Federal guidelines establish an eligibility baseline to direct services to uninsured and underinsured women at or below 250% of the federal poverty level at ages 18–64 for cervical cancer screening and ages 40–64 for breast cancer screening. Services include CBE, mammography, Pap test, diagnostic testing for women whose screening outcome is abnormal, surgical consultation, and referrals for treatment. From 1991 to 2011, the NBCCEDP served more than 4.3 million women, provided more than 710.7 million screening examinations, and diagnosed 54,276 breast cancers (Miller et al., 2014). Oncology nurses should be aware of the many resources in their practice setting and community that serve women with high risk for developing breast cancer, as well as agencies that have programs to increase accessibility through low-cost or free mammography programs.

Cervical Cancer

Screening methods for the early detection of cervical cancer have been available for decades. Despite the widespread use of the Pap test to detect precancerous lesions, women continue to be diagnosed with cervical cancer. Cervical cancer is the second most common cancer among women worldwide, with significantly higher rates seen in developing countries, especially in Africa, the Caribbean, and Latin America (ACS, 2015c).

Cervical cancer is potentially preventable through risk reduction and appropriate screening with the Pap test (ACS, 2016a). The importance of the Pap test should not be underestimated. However, it is estimated that 60%–80% of women with advanced cervical cancer have not had a Pap test during the past five years (ACS, 2015b).

Risk Factors

The natural history of cervical cancer is well known. The most significant risk factor identified is the human papillomavirus (HPV), a sexually transmitted infection present in approximately 99% of cervical cancers. Because of the increasing availability of the Pap test, cervical cancer incidence and mortality rates have decreased 50% in the past three decades (Saslow et al., 2012). For women in whom precancerous lesions are detected through a Pap test, long-term survival is nearly 100% with appropriate evaluation, treatment, and follow-up (ACS, 2015b).

In the United States, HPV is the most common sexually transmitted infection, with an estimated 15% of the population currently infected. The lifetime risk of getting at least one type of HPV infection in sexually active men and women is estimated to be as high as 90% (Chesson, Dunne, Hariri, & Markowitz, 2014). More than 100 different types of HPV exist. Fortunately, most are benign and resolve without treatment. Low-risk HPV types may cause visible benign lesions or warts known as condylomata acuminata. High-risk HPV types tend to persist and are associated with the development of precancerous lesions and cervical cancer. Approximately 15 high-risk HPV types, especially types 16, 18, 33, and 45, are associated with the development of cervical cancer (Saslow et al., 2012). An estimated 70% of cervical cancers are caused by HPV types 16 and 18, and these two types are associated with a more than 200-fold increased risk of developing invasive cervical cancer (Saslow et al., 2012).

Transmission of HPV occurs by genital contact with an infected partner. The virus enters through a break in the squamous epithelium, where infection stimulates the replication of the epithelium. Time from exposure to infection may be one to eight months (Vesco et al., 2011). The risk of acquiring HPV increases with the number of lifetime sexual partners and is not 100% preventable with condom use because the infection can still be transmitted on body surfaces not covered by the condom (Chesson et al., 2014).

Other risk factors associated with the development of cervical cancer include long-term use of oral contraceptives and tobacco exposure (both active and passive) (ACS, 2016a). Women who smoke are about twice as likely as nonsmokers to get cervical cancer. Tobacco by-products have been found in the cervical mucus of women who smoke (ACS, 2015b). Because of the increased risk, it is appropriate to address smoking cessation strategies in all women who smoke. Multiple pregnancies are another risk factor for developing cervical cancer (ACS, 2016a).

Signs and Symptoms

Early cervical cancer generally produces no signs or symptoms. As the cancer progresses, signs might include vaginal bleeding after intercourse, between periods, or after menopause; watery, bloody vaginal discharge that may be heavy and have a foul odor; or pelvic pain or pain during intercourse (ACS, 2016a).

Early Detection

Many organizations have published cervical cancer screening guidelines, but some differences exist among the recommendations. HPV DNA testing is now FDA-approved for adjunct screening with Pap test cytology. ACS recommends HPV screening, but not until women reach age 30 (Saslow et al., 2012). ACS now recommends an initial Pap screening at age 21 (ACS, 2016a). Most organizations recommend annual screening, but ACS and the American College of Obstetricians and Gynecologists (ACOG) make a distinction between women younger than and older than age 30. According to ACS and ACOG, women younger than age 30 may be tested every three years (ACOG, 2016; Saslow et al., 2012). Women aged 30–64 years should have Pap testing every five years with co-HPV testing. If this is not possible, Pap testing should be done every three years. Recommendations for stopping screening are not consistent. ACS recommends that women older than age 70 can stop screening if they have had normal results in the past 10 years, whereas ACOG recommends that testing can stop at age 65 if the woman does not have a history of dysplasia and has had normal tests within the past 10 years (ACS, 2016a; ACOG, 2016). Pap screening after hysterectomy generally is not recommended if the cervix was removed and if the hysterectomy was performed for benign disease.

The HPV test detects HPV infections. The addition of HPV testing to cytology enhances the identification of women with adenocarcinoma of the cervix and its precursors, which often are undetected with traditional Pap test cytology (Saslow et al., 2012). Compared with cytology, HPV testing is more sensitive in identifying women with prevalent CIN3. CIN3 is cervical squamous intraepithelial neoplasia 3, also referred to as stage 0 cervical carcinoma in situ. CIN3 is typically caused by HPV and, if left untreated, progresses to invasive cancer.

The costs of cervical cancer screening cannot be overlooked. These include the provider time to obtain the specimen, laboratory processing fees, and follow-up costs for HPV testing and other diagnostic procedures, such as colposcopy (Saslow et al., 2012). Despite these costs, the Pap test remains an effective means to decrease the morbidity and mortality associated with cervical cancer. Many women do not get regular Pap tests for a variety of reasons, including inability to pay for services, fatalistic attitudes, knowledge deficit, and lack of support. Although many of these factors may not be easily addressed, women should consistently be offered education and support in finding appropriate resources (Warman, 2010). The most significant example of this is the NBCCEDP's program administered by the Centers for Disease Control and Prevention, which provides free or low-cost cervical cancer screening to qualified women. From 1991 to 2011, this program detected 2,554 cervical cancers and 123,563 precancerous cervical lesions, demonstrating the success of this outreach strategy (Miller et al., 2014).

Several points should be considered when scheduling and preparing for a Pap test. These need to be clearly communicated to the woman to be screened. The Pap test should not be collected during a menstrual cycle. Two weeks after the first day of the last period is the optimal time to have the test. Women should be instructed not to douche or use vaginal creams during the three days before the test. Finally, the woman should be instructed to abstain from intercourse within 24 hours before the test because it can cause inaccurate results. Women also should be instructed on how a Pap test is taken. The examiner inserts a speculum to expose the cervix, and an endocervical brush is used to sample the endocervical area in the cervical os.

The most promising tool to reduce the incidence of cervical cancer may be a vaccine against the HPV virus. Three vaccines have been FDA-approved for the prevention of HPV. The most commonly used one provides protection against four HPV types (6, 11, 16, and 18) and is recommended for use in both males and females; another one protects against two HPV types (16 and 18) and is recommended for use in females only (ACS, 2015b). A third vaccine (HPV9) was approved by FDA in December 2014 for both males and females and protects against nine HPV types. Two of the HPV types targeted by all the vaccines (HPV-16 and HPV-18) are responsible for about 70% of the cases of cervical cancer worldwide. The vaccine has been demonstrated to be cost-effective in preventing infections and cervical cancers (ACS, 2015b). The other two HPV types (HPV-6 and HPV-11) cause approximately 90% of the cases of genital warts. The vaccine requires a series of three injections over a six-month period. The second injection is given two months after the first, and the third is given four months after the second. ACS recommends routine HPV vaccination for females aged 11–12 years (Saslow et al., 2012). Females as young as nine years old can receive HPV vaccination. It also is recommended for females aged 13–18 to catch up for missed vaccines or to complete the series.

Endometrial and Ovarian Cancers

ACS estimated 60,050 new diagnoses of endometrial cancer and 22,280 new diagnoses of ovarian cancer in the United States in 2016 (ACS, 2016a). The estimated annual mortality is 10,470 deaths from endometrial cancer and 14,240 from ovarian cancer (ACS, 2016a).

Risk Factors

The risk factors for endometrial and ovarian cancers are similar. Table 5-5 shows a comparison of the risks for developing these two cancers.

Signs and Symptoms

Despite the similarities in risk factors, the signs and symptoms of the two cancers (except in the later stages) are relatively different (see Table 5-6). The hallmark sign of endometrial cancer is unusual spotting, bleeding, or discharge after menopause. Conversely, ovarian cancer typically is a "silent" cancer with few early warning signs (ACS, 2016a). Women need to be educated regarding these signs and symptoms and the importance of reporting them to their healthcare provider.

Table 5-5. Risk Factors for Endometrial and Ovarian Cancers

Risk Factor	Endometrial Cancer	Ovarian Cancer
Age	The risk of developing endometrial cancer increases steadily after age 50.	The risk of developing ovarian cancer increases with age. Ovarian cancer is rare in women younger than age 40. Most ovarian cancers develop after menopause. Half of all ovarian cancers are found in women older than age 63.
Family history of cancer	The risk of endometrial cancer is higher in women with a personal or family history of early-onset endometrial or colorectal cancer, and disease often is associated with hereditary nonpolyposis colorectal cancer (HNPCC) mutations, as well as less common susceptibility genes.	The risk of ovarian cancer is higher in women with a family history of multiple relatives and/or early-onset breast, colon, or endometrial cancer. Women from these families may be at increased risk for *BRCA1* or *BRCA2* mutations or mutations associated with HNPCC, as well as less common susceptibility genes.
Hormone replacement therapy	The use of estrogen alone increases a woman's risk for developing endometrial cancer by as much as five times. Studies now show that giving progesterone-like drugs along with estrogen will avoid this additional risk of endometrial cancer.	Some recent studies have suggested that women using estrogens after menopause have an increased risk of developing ovarian cancer. The risk seems to be higher in women taking estrogen alone (without progesterone) for many years (at least 5 or 10). The increased risk is less certain for women taking both estrogen and progesterone.
Medication history	Tamoxifen is an antiestrogen that acts like an estrogen in the uterus. It can cause the uterine lining to grow, which increases the risk of endometrial cancer (about 1 in 500).	Use of the fertility drug clomiphene citrate for longer than 1 year may increase the risk of developing ovarian tumors. The risk seems to be highest in women who did not get pregnant while on this drug. Women who are infertile may be at higher risk than fertile women, even if they do not use fertility drugs. This may be in part because they have not had children or have not used birth control pills (which are protective).
Obesity	Although most of a woman's estrogen is produced by her ovaries, fat tissue can change some other hormones into estrogens. Having more fat tissue can increase a woman's estrogen levels and therefore increase her endometrial cancer risk. In comparison with women who maintain a healthy weight, endometrial cancer is twice as common in overweight women and more than three times as common in obese women.	Obese women (those with a body mass index of at least 30 kg/m^2) have a higher risk of developing ovarian cancer. The rate of death from ovarian cancer is also higher in obese women. The risk was increased by 50% in the heaviest women.
Prior surgery/radiation therapy	Radiation used to treat some other cancers can damage DNA, sometimes increasing the risk of a second type of cancer, such as endometrial cancer.	The exact risk is not clear but increases with the dose of radiation.

(Continued on next page)

Table 5-5. Risk Factors for Endometrial and Ovarian Cancers *(Continued)*

Risk Factor	Endometrial Cancer	Ovarian Cancer
Reproductive history	Having more menstrual cycles during a woman's lifetime raises her risk of endometrial cancer. Starting menstrual periods (menarche) before age 12 and/or going through menopause later in life raises the risk. During pregnancy, the hormonal balance shifts toward more progesterone. Therefore, having many pregnancies reduces endometrial cancer risk, and women who have not been pregnant have a higher risk.	Women who have had children have a lower risk of ovarian cancer than women who have not had children. The risk gets lower with each pregnancy. Breast-feeding may lower the risk even further. Using oral contraceptives lowers risk.

Note. Based on information from American Cancer Society, 2015a; Cote et al., 2015; Daniels, 2012; Hunn & Rodriguez, 2012; "Oral Contraceptives and Ovarian Cancer Risk," 2008; Weissman et al., 2012.

Early Detection

During a pelvic examination, the healthcare professional feels the ovaries and uterus for size, shape, and consistency. Although a pelvic examination is recommended because it can find some reproductive system cancers at an early stage, most early ovarian tumors are difficult or impossible for even the most skilled examiner to feel (see Figure 5-6) (ACS, 2016a).

Although much research has been done to develop a screening test for ovarian cancer, not much success has occurred to date. Currently, ACS does not have a recommendation for the early detection of ovarian cancer other than an annual pelvic examination, which has low sensitivity and specificity (ACS, 2016a). Transvaginal ultrasonography (TVUS) and CA-125 testing often are offered to women at high risk for developing epithelial ovarian cancer, such as those with a very strong family history.

TVUS is an ultrasound test that can help find a mass in the ovary, but it cannot actually indicate which masses are cancerous. CA-125 is a protein in the blood that is present in higher levels in many women with ovarian cancer. The problem with this test is that other conditions also can cause high levels of CA-125. In addition, someone with ovarian cancer can still have a normal CA-125 level

Figure 5-6. Pelvic Examination

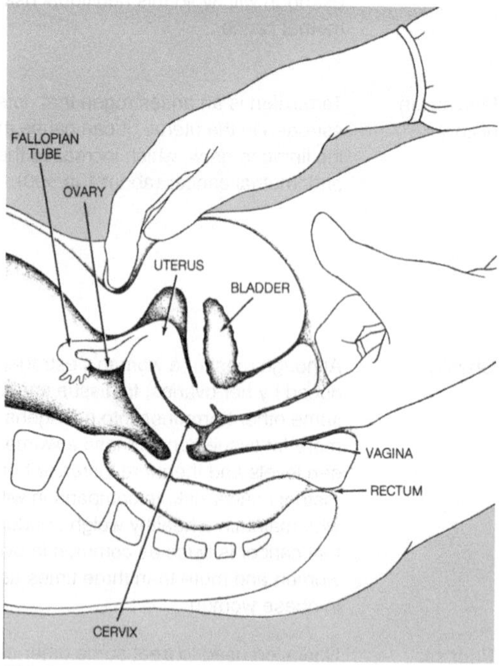

This figure demonstrates pelvic examination of the uterus and ovaries. Note how small and difficult the ovaries are to assess.

Note. Figure courtesy of National Cancer Institute. Retrieved from http://commons.wikimedia.org/wiki/File:Pelvic_exam_nci-vol-1786-300.jpg.

Table 5-6. Signs and Symptoms of Endometrial and Ovarian Cancers

Symptom	Endometrial Cancer	Ovarian Cancer
Back pain	–	Usually a late symptom
Bloating/early satiety	–	Nonspecific relatively early symptom
Constipation	–	Usually a late symptom
Fatigue	Usually a late symptom	Usually a late symptom
Pain during intercourse	–	Usually a late symptom
Pelvic mass	Usually a late symptom	Usually a late symptom
Pelvic pain	Often a late symptom	May be an early or late symptom
Unusual spotting or bleeding	Especially after menopause (90% of cases)	–
Unusual vaginal discharge (not bloody)	May occur in pre- or postmenopausal women (10% of cases)	–
Urinary symptoms	–	Urgency may be an early or late symptom.
Weight loss	A late symptom	Usually a late symptom

Note. Based on information from American Cancer Society, 2016a; Hunn & Rodriguez, 2012.

(Menon et al., 2014). In studies of women who are at average risk for ovarian cancer, these screening tests did not lower the number of deaths caused by the disease. For this reason, TVUS and the CA-125 blood test are not recommended for ovarian cancer screening in women without known strong risk factors (Menon et al., 2014). These tests often are performed in women who are at high risk, but it is not known how helpful they are. For women with a known or suspected *BRCA* mutation, an oophorectomy is recommended at age 35 if childbearing is complete (Gadducci, Biglia, Cosio, Sismondi, & Genazzani, 2010; Menon et al., 2014; NCCN, 2016c).

ACS does not recommend screening for endometrial cancer in most women because no scientific evidence proves that screening methods significantly reduce mortality rates, and the risks and costs of available screening methods outweigh the benefits (ACS, 2016a). Women who are at average risk should be counseled about the risks for and symptoms of endometrial cancer, especially any abnormal or unexpected bleeding or spotting. In addition, no recommended screening measures exist for women considered to be at increased risk, defined as women with a history of unopposed estrogen use, late menopause, tamoxifen use, nulliparity, obesity, diabetes, or hypertension; however, again, healthcare providers are encouraged to discuss risk factors and symptoms with women (ACS, 2016a). For women considered to be at high risk for endometrial cancer—defined as women with or at risk for hereditary nonpolyposis colorectal cancer (HNPCC)—NCCN recommends annual screening with an endometrial biopsy (NCCN, 2016d). Women with a known mutation should be counseled about a prophylactic hysterectomy, including oophorectomy, at age 35 if childbearing is complete (NCCN, 2016d).

Nurses play an important role in educating women about the risk factors and symptoms of endometrial cancer. Education may be the most important tool currently available for early detection. Making women aware of the importance of prompt evaluation of abnormal bleeding could result in early detection of the disease. Nurses need to educate women about the strengths and limitations of the screening tests for ovarian cancer and the importance of persistence if they experience nonspecific gastrointestinal symptoms or unexplained uterine bleeding or discharge.

Colorectal Cancer

In the United States, the cumulative lifetime risk of developing colorectal cancer (CRC) is about 5%. Early detection and removal of adenomatous polyps through regular screening could reduce the CRC mortality rate by 50% (ACS, 2014).

Risk Factors

CRC affects men and women of all races equally, but African Americans have a slightly higher risk of developing CRC. A personal or family history of colorectal polyps, CRC, or inflammatory bowel disease leads to an increased risk compared to that of the general population. The rate of CRC increases significantly in the sixth decade of life in average-risk individuals. For this reason, screening should begin by age 50 (ACS, 2014). This is the basis for various screening protocols for CRC. Risk factors for CRC are stratified and summarized in Table 5-7.

Increasing age is the greatest risk factor for sporadic CRC. Statistics show that 90% of cases occur in people older than 50 years (ACS, 2014). The much higher incidence of CRC in more affluent and industrialized countries compared with less developed countries is associated with lifestyle factors such as obesity and consumption of processed meat and an inverse relationship with physical activity and consumption of fruits and vegetables (Kushi et al., 2012).

In most cases, CRCs arise from dysplastic adenomatous polyps. This occurs during a multistep process that involves the inactivation of multiple genes that suppress tumors and repair DNA and the simultaneous activation of oncogenes. When gene function is altered, normal colonic epithelium can transform to an adenomatous polyp to invasive CRC. This multistep process allows a window of time for screening to detect premalignant lesions and potentially prevent disease. These mutations usually are sporadic and nonhereditary (ACS, 2014).

About 10%–20% of patients describe a family history of CRC but do not show a pattern of inheritance and clinical features consistent with a hereditary cancer syndrome such as familial adenomatous polyposis (FAP) or HNPCC (see Chapter 4). Screening of individuals with this type of medical history should begin at age 40 or 10 years earlier than the age at diagnosis of the youngest affected family member (NCCN, 2016d).

Approximately 10% of the mutations are germ line (inherited) and are associated with HNPCC, FAP, or other unusual syndromes (Kastrinos & Syngal, 2011). HNPCC is characterized by early-onset (before age 50) colorectal, endometrial, ovarian, small intestine, and renal cancers in the family (Senter, 2012). Usually, the number of polyps is not excessive. The interval from polyp to cancer is very short, often 12–18 months. FAP is characterized by the development of hundreds to thousands of adenomatous polyps in the colon and the development of CRC and other cancers in the third and fourth decades of life (Jasperson, 2012). FAP and HNPCC are the most common of the familial cancer syndromes, but together these two syndromes account for fewer than 5% of cases (Patel & Ahnen, 2012). Screening in people with HNPCC usually begins at age 25 with

Table 5-7. Risk Factors for Colorectal Cancer

Risk Factor	Etiology	Stratification
Age	90% occur after age 50.	Average
Alcohol use	Risk is higher in people who drink more than 1 alcoholic beverage per day.	Average
Diabetes	Risk is increased 30%.	Average
Diet	Risk is increased in people who consume a diet high in animal fat, red meat, and processed meats.	Average
Ethnic background	Risk is higher in people of Ashkenazi Jewish background.	Average
Family history of colorectal cancer	Risk is higher if a first-degree relative has a diagnosis of colorectal cancer.	Moderate
Inactivity	Risk is higher in individuals who do not exercise on a regular basis.	Average
Known or suspected familial adenomatous polyposis	Lifetime risk is close to 100%.	High
Known or suspected hereditary nonpolyposis colorectal cancer	Lifetime risk is close to 85%.	High
Personal history of bowel disease	Risk is higher in people with a history of Crohn disease and ulcerative colitis.	Moderate
Personal history of colorectal cancer	Even if the cancer is completely resected, risk of second primary colorectal cancer is increased, especially if the diagnosis is before age 60.	Moderate
Personal history of polyps	Risk is higher in people with large dysplastic or hyperplastic polyps.	Moderate
Race	Incidence and mortality are highest in African Americans.	Average
Tobacco use	Smoking increases risk 30%–40%.	Average
Weight	Risk is increased in overweight and obese people.	Average

Note. Based on information from American Cancer Society, 2014, 2015b, 2016a, 2016b.

annual colonoscopy; for those with FAP, screening often begins at age 10 (NCCN, 2016d).

Signs and Symptoms

The most common symptoms of CRC include abdominal pain, change in bowel habits, rectal bleeding, and anemia (ACS, 2014). Unfortunately, these symptoms also are associated with many more benign gastrointestinal problems, making a diagnostic evaluation necessary. Change in bowel habits is a more common presenting symptom for left-sided cancers caused by a progressive narrowing of the bowel lumen, with diarrhea, a change in stool form, and eventually intestinal obstruction (ACS, 2014). About 10% of patients with iron-deficiency anemia have CRC, most commonly on the right side; thus, iron deficiency in men, and in women who are not menstruating, is an indication for immediate further evaluation (Jellema et al., 2010). The symptom that patients often first recognize is blood in or on the stool. Blood in or on the stool does not absolutely mean CRC is present; bleeding could be related to hemorrhoids, ulcers, a tear, or inflammatory bowel disease. However, when related to CRC, bleeding is seldom associated with early detection of CRC. Ideally, screening should begin before symptoms arise. It may be too late to prevent CRC after symptoms occur (ACS, 2014; Burt et al., 2013).

Early Detection

Screening remains the single most important means to reduce the morbidity and mortality associated with CRC. Extensive research continues to investigate the appropriate interval between screening examinations to obtain the best possible sensitivity and specificity, as well as to reduce the use of costly follow-up procedures (Jeong & Cairns, 2013). ACS makes a distinction between tests that are likely to detect CRC and those likely to detect polyps (ACS, 2014). Tests that primarily find cancer involve testing the stool for signs that cancer may be present. These tests are less invasive and relatively easy to complete but are less likely to detect polyps. Tests that can find both colorectal polyps and cancer examine the structure of the colon to detect any abnormal areas. This is done either with a scope inserted into the rectum or with special imaging (x-ray) tests. Polyps found before they become malignant can be removed, so these tests may prevent CRC. Because of this, these tests are preferred if available and if the patient is willing to complete them. Table 5-8 shows a comparison of the screening tests.

CRC is one of the most preventable cancers. Detection and removal of adenomatous polyps, from which more than 95% of CRCs arise, reduces the risk of being diagnosed with or dying of this disease (Levin et al., 2008). All guidelines for CRC screening require risk assessment as a first step. The approach to screening differs significantly based on risk category (average, increased, or high). The key element of a CRC screening recommendation is to suggest the right test beginning at the correct age for individuals at each risk level (NCCN, 2016b). Screening should be repeated at the proper interval depending on risk level. High-risk patients with hereditary CRC syndromes or inflammatory bowel disease should be referred to specialists early in life (Jasperson, 2012). Those with a suspected hereditary cancer syndrome need to be referred to a genetics expert for genetic testing to clarify risk (Senter, 2012). People who test positive for a deleterious mutation should be managed by a clinician with expertise in these syndromes. Annual screening beginning at a young age will be required (Patel & Ahnen, 2012). Members of these families may consider enrolling in chemoprevention trials.

Regular screening for average-risk individuals should begin by age 50 with guaiac fecal occult blood testing (gFOBT), fecal immunochemical testing (FIT), or stool DNA (sDNA) combined with flexible sigmoidoscopy (FSIG), colonoscopy, double-contrast barium enema (DCBE), or virtual colonoscopy (also called computed tomography colonography [CTC]) (ACS, 2016a).

Stool-Based Tests

Stool blood tests are one of the more common tools used in the detection of CRC. Two types of fecal tests are performed depending on the analysis process: gFOBT or FIT. The premise of fecal testing is that occult blood, although a nonspecific finding, may be the result of bleeding from a larger polyp (greater than 1–2 cm) (Levin et al., 2008). Because small adenomatous polyps do not tend to bleed, and bleeding from cancers or large polyps may be inter-

Table 5-8. Early Detection Strategies for Colorectal Cancer

Test and Frequency	Preparation	Accuracy	Benefits	Risks/Limitations
Flexible sigmoidoscopy; every 5 years	Partial bowel preparation with laxatives and enemas	45%–50% sensitivity	Sedation usually not necessary	Evaluates lower third of colon Potential discomfort Positive screen requires follow-up with colonoscopy. Very small risk of bleeding, infection, or perforation
Colonoscopy; every 1–10 years	Complete bowel preparation	Up to 95% sensitivity	Can usually view entire colon Can biopsy and remove polyps Can diagnose other diseases	Requires patients to miss a day of work Requires conscious sedation Perforation and bleeding; risk increases with polypectomy. Patients need someone to take them to and from the appointment.
Double-contrast barium enema; every 5 years	Complete bowel preparation	48%–73% sensitivity	No sedation needed	Cannot biopsy polyps Positive screen requires follow-up with colonoscopy Rare cases of perforation
Virtual colonoscopy; every 5 years	Complete bowel preparation	55%–59% sensitivity for large polyps	No sedation needed	Positive screen requires follow-up with colonoscopy; if not available the same day, second preparation required. May detect other problems outside of the colon that need evaluation Rare cases of perforation Costly; may not be covered by insurance
Guaiac fecal occult blood testing; annually	Requires collection of at least 2–3 samples	37%–79% sensitivity	No risk of bowel injury Inexpensive Done in privacy of home	Requires avoidance of certain foods and medications 48 hours prior to and during collection, including aspirin, nonsteroidal anti-inflammatory drugs, vitamin C, red meat, poultry, fish, and raw vegetables Positive screen requires further evaluation with colonoscopy.
Fecal immunochemical testing; annually	None	29%–94% sensitivity	No risk of bowel injury Done in privacy of home Relatively inexpensive	Onetime testing is likely to be ineffective. Positive screen requires follow-up with colonoscopy. Requires specific instructions on transport to laboratory
Stool DNA; no recommended interval	None	52%–91% sensitivity; 93%–97% specificity	No risk of bowel injury Done in privacy of home No dietary restrictions	Positive screen requires follow-up with colonoscopy. Requires collection of an adequate sample and proper preservation and shipping to laboratory

Note. Based on information from American Cancer Society, 2016a, 2016b; Jasperson, 2012; Senter, 2012; U.S. Preventive Services Task Force, 2008a.

mittent or is not always detectable in a single sample of stool, the proper use of stool blood tests requires annual testing that consists of collecting multiple specimens from consecutive bowel movements while following a specific dietary regimen (ACS, 2014).

The goal of fecal testing is to examine the stool for hidden blood that occasionally sheds from adenomatous polyps and cancer. One disadvantage of this screening method is that often polyps do not bleed. This test should be done every year by obtaining a three-sample card from a primary care provider; the patient takes the card home to obtain the stool samples for testing. Patients must follow dietary guidelines both before and during this test because if not done properly, the test can produce a false-positive outcome. Additionally, negative results do not necessarily indicate absence of polyps or cancer, just that no blood was detected in the stool. Conversely, positive results do not indicate cancer, only that further screening should be administered to locate the source of bleeding. Any fecal test administered by a doctor using a small stool sample on a single card is inadequate and not recommended as a CRC screening method (Levin et al., 2008). Studies with gFOBT or FIT completed correctly and regularly showed a 30% decrease in mortality between the annually screened group and the control group (NCCN, 2016b). Guaiac-based tests detect blood in the stool through the pseudoperoxidase activity of hemoglobin. A significant advantage of FIT is that it detects human globin, a protein that, along with heme, constitutes human hemoglobin. Thus, FIT is more specific for human blood than guaiac-based tests, which rely on detection of peroxidase in human blood and react to the peroxidase present in dietary constituents such as rare red meat, cruciferous vegetables, and some fruits. A significant difference in the fecal testing is in the processing. FITs usually are processed in a clinical laboratory, whereas gFOBTs can be processed either in the physician's office or a clinical laboratory (Burt et al., 2013).

Adenoma and carcinoma cells that contain altered DNA are continuously shed into the colon and passed out of the body through feces. Because DNA is stable in stool, it can be isolated from bacterial DNA found in the feces (ACS, 2014). A limitation of sDNA testing is that no single gene mutation is present in cells shed by every adenoma or cancer. Thus, a multitarget DNA stool assay is required to achieve adequate sensitivity, and the commercial availability of this test is limited. This is an active area of current research. The exact interval needed for testing remains unclear (Burt et al., 2013; Levin et al., 2008).

Structural Examinations

FSIG is an endoscopic procedure that directly examines the lumen of the lower half of the colon. The scope typically is passed to the transverse colon (approximately 60 cm). FSIG usually is performed without sedation and with a limited bowel preparation. It is an attractive screening tool because it can be performed in the office setting by a variety of healthcare professionals, including nurses with specialized training (Levin et al., 2008). It is documented to have a 60%–80% reduction in CRC mortality for the area of the colon that can be examined. For people who are at higher risk, it is not a sufficient examination because a significant portion of the colon is not evaluated. ACS and NCCN recommend that if sigmoidoscopy is performed for CRC screening, insertion to 40 cm or beyond is required (Burt et al., 2013; Levin et al., 2008; NCCN, 2016b).

In the United States, FSIG has decreased in popularity in the past 15 years, and the use of colonoscopy has increased (ACS, 2014). Much of this shift is attributed to Medicare coverage for colonoscopy, which began in 1998. Colonoscopy has increased in popularity because it not only detects polyps but also makes it possible to remove polyps in one procedure. Adenomatous polyps (a known precursor lesion to CRC) are common in adults older than age 50, accounting for more than one-half of all colorectal polyps. The majority of polyps will not develop into adenocarcinoma, but the removal of such polyps is considered to be a true form of primary cancer prevention, and this is an important teaching point for nurses (Levin et al., 2008).

DCBE is a radiographic technique that evaluates the entire colon by coating the mucosal lumen with barium and distending it with air through a flexible catheter placed in the rectum. Multiple radiographs are obtained. The test usually is completed in 15–20 minutes without sedation. Any positive finding must be evaluated with colonoscopy, which will require an additional bowel preparation. A benefit of DCBE is that it evaluates the entire colon in almost all cases and can detect most cancers and the majority of significant polyps. DCBE also provides an opportunity for a full structural examination for individuals for whom colonoscopy has either failed or cannot be performed for other medical reasons (Levin et al., 2008).

Virtual colonoscopy, or CTC, is a relatively new screening option to detect CRC (Levin et al., 2008). It produces a two- or three-dimensional colorectal image generated using data from a spiral computed tomography scan. This screening method is appealing to many people because it is noninvasive and requires no sedation, and a view of the entire colon and rectum is obtained. The preparation for this procedure requires the same dietary restrictions and bowel cleansing as the colonoscopy, and air insufflation also is needed for a clear view of the colon (NCCN, 2016b).

If an abnormality or polyp is detected, access to immediate colonoscopy is desirable so that the patient does not have to repeat the bowel preparation. Institutions that offer this technology need to have radiologists who are trained in the procedure; thus, access is limited in many geographic areas. CTC is a minimally invasive test, and the risk for colonic perforation during screening is extremely low (less than 0.05%) (USPSTF, 2008a). Another potential benefit that needs to be further evaluated is the possibility of finding extracolonic pathology because CTC produces an image of the upper and lower abdomen as well as the colon. Preliminary research demonstrates that significant extracolonic pathology or findings may occur in 4.5%–11% of all CTCs performed (Levin et al., 2008). The management of CTC findings is controversial, and more defined guidelines are needed. At this time, the recommendation is that all patients with one or more polyps 10 mm or larger or three or more polyps 6 mm or larger should be referred for colonoscopy (NCCN, 2016b). The best management of patients with three or fewer polyps in which the largest polyp is 6–9 mm is unclear.

Implementation of Screening Guidelines

Educating the public about the epidemiology, risk factors, symptoms, and screening options for CRC enables individuals to become advocates for their own health. Typically, individuals in the community setting have many misconceptions about CRC. For instance, many people do not know the difference between a sigmoidoscopy and a colonoscopy, or that fecal testing should be done every year to increase the efficiency of sigmoidoscopy and to help decrease the risk of developing CRC (ACS, 2014). Many individuals believe that CRC inevitably ends in a colostomy. Many do not realize that polypectomy can prevent CRC from developing. Correction of these misconceptions is critical to motivate individuals to engage in CRC screening. As health educators, nurses need to work to alter these perceptions and arm individuals with the correct information. The goal of health education is to promote healthy living and encourage individuals to engage in practices and behaviors that are beneficial to long-term health.

All bowel preparations carry risk. Adequate hydration is critical before and during the bowel purgative process and after colonoscopy, regardless of the preparation. Adequate patient screening and increased patient education, along with reinforcement of the importance of adequate hydration throughout the preparation and postprocedure periods, may reduce the risk of complications. Improved patient acceptance of and compliance with bowel preparation instructions will increase the likelihood of a safe and successful colonoscopy.

Oral Cancers

Oral cancers include cancers of the oral cavity and oropharynx (see Figure 5-7). The oral cavity includes the lips, the inside lining of the lips and cheeks (buccal mucosa), the teeth, the gums, the front two-thirds of the tongue, the floor of the mouth below the tongue, the bony roof of the mouth (hard palate), and the area behind the wisdom teeth (retromolar trigone). The oropharynx begins where the oral cavity stops. It includes the base of the tongue (the back one-third of the tongue), the soft palate (the back part of the roof of the mouth), the tonsils, and the side and back walls of the throat. Although they rarely occur in children, about one-third of oral cancers occur in patients younger than 55 years old (ACS, 2016a).

Figure 5-7. Oral Cavity and Oropharynx

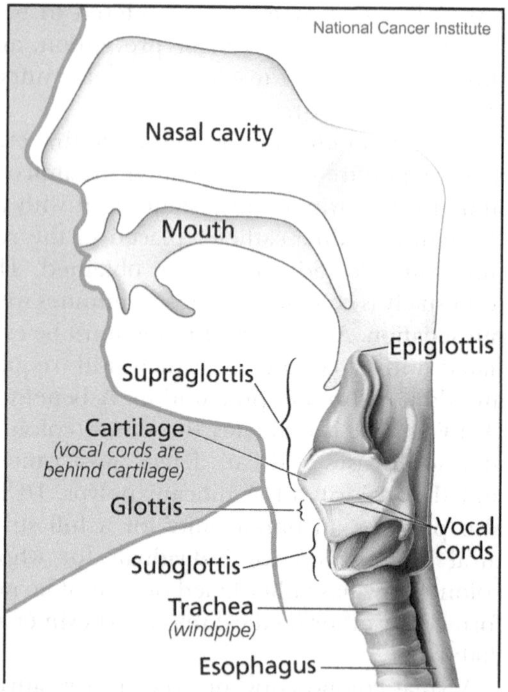

This figure shows areas of oral anatomy that are at risk for cancer. With the exception of the nasal cavity and pharynx, most are accessible for visual inspection by a dentist or other healthcare provider.

Note. Figure courtesy of National Cancer Institute, Alan Hoofring, illustrator. Retrieved from https://visualsonline.cancer.gov/details.cfm?imageid=4357.

Risk Factors

Tobacco and alcohol use are the biggest risk factors for these two cancers (ACS, 2015b). High-risk oral HPV infections are associated with oral cancer and may be responsible for as many as 8,400 oral cancers annually, although these can be prevented with routine HPV vaccination (ACS, 2015b). Ultraviolet (UV) radiation is an important and avoidable risk factor for cancer of the lips, as well as for skin cancer. Avoiding sources of oral irritation (such as ill-fitting dentures) may lower the risk for oral cancer. Poor diet has been related to oral cavity and oropharyngeal cancers, but it is not exactly clear what substances in healthy foods might be responsible for reducing the risk of these cancers. In general, eating a healthy diet is much better than adding vitamin supplements to an otherwise unhealthy diet. ACS recommends eating a healthy diet with an emphasis on at least five daily servings from plant sources (ACS, 2015b).

Signs and Symptoms

Leukoplakia and *erythroplasia* are terms used to describe an abnormal area in the mouth or throat. Leukoplakia is a white area. Erythroplasia is a slightly raised, red area that bleeds easily if scraped. Leukoplakia or erythroplasia may be a cancer, a precancerous condition called *dysplasia* (mild, moderate, or severe), or a completely benign condition. The higher the degree of dysplasia, the more likely it is to progress to cancer and the less likely it is to go away on its own or after treatment. The most frequent causes of leukoplakia and erythroplasia are cigarettes and chewing tobacco. Poorly fitting dentures rubbing against the tongue or the inside of the cheeks also can cause them. Approximately one out of four leukoplakias is either cancerous when first found or has precancerous changes that eventually progress to cancer if not properly treated (ACS, 2016a). As many as 7 out of 10 of these erythroplasia lesions are malignant when biopsied or will develop into cancer later (NCCN, 2016e).

Early Detection

Screening for oral cancers is frequently done by dental providers and primary care providers and includes inspection and palpation of the oral cavity (see Figure 5-7). Any patient with an abnormality should be referred to an otolaryngologist for further evaluation.

Testicular Cancer

ACS estimated about 8,720 new cases of testicular cancer would be diagnosed and 380 men would die of the disease in the United States in 2016 (ACS, 2016a). A man's lifetime chance of developing testicular cancer is about 1 in 300 (ACS, 2016a). The rate of testicular cancer has been increasing in many countries, including the United States. The increase is mostly in seminomas, although the etiologic basis is unclear. If the cancer has not spread outside the testicle, the five-year relative survival rate is 99%. Even if the cancer has spread to nearby lymph nodes, the five-year relative survival rate is 96%. If the cancer has spread beyond the lymph nodes, the five-year survival rate is around 74% (ACS, 2016a).

Risk Factors

One of the main risk factors for testicular cancer is cryptorchidism, or an undescended testicle or testicles. About 10% of cases of testicular cancer occur in men with a history of cryptorchidism. Normally, the testicles develop inside the abdomen of the fetus and descend into the scrotum before birth. In about 3% of boys, however, the testicles do not make it all the way down before the child is born (Lim et al., 2015). Sometimes the testicles remain in the abdomen or groin area. If the testicles have not descended by the time a child turns one year old, they probably will not go down on their own. Sometimes a surgical procedure known as orchiopexy is necessary to bring the testicles down into the scrotum. Some evidence has shown that performing orchiopexy when a child is younger can reduce the risk of developing certain types of germ-cell tumors (Oldenburg et al., 2013). The best time to do this surgery to reduce the risk of testicular cancer is not clear. Experts in the United States recommend that orchiopexy be done soon after the child's first birthday for reasons not related to cancer, such as fertility (Feng et al., 2016).

A family history of testicular cancer increases a person's risk (Chan-Smutko, 2012). If a man has the disease, the likelihood is increased that one or more of his brothers or sons also will develop it. However, only about 3% of testicular cancer cases are actually found to occur in families, so most men are unlikely to pass this disorder to their children (Oldenburg et al., 2013). Testicular cancer may be increased in men with known mutations in the *STK11* and *TP53* genes (Weitzel, Blazer, MacDonald, Culver, & Offit, 2011).

A personal history of testicular cancer is another risk factor. About 3%–4% of men who have been cured of cancer in one testicle will eventually develop it in the other testicle (Curreri, Fung, & Beard, 2015). This may be due to genetic factors or exposure to chemotherapy and radiation. Ninety percent of testicular cancers occur in men aged 20–54 (Sui, Morrow, Bermejo, & Hellenthal, 2015). However, this cancer can affect men of any age, including infants and older adult men. The risk of testicular cancer among Caucasian men is about five and a half times that of African American men and more than three times that of Asian American and American Indian men (Sui et al., 2015). The reason for these differences is not completely clear but may be attributable to cancer biology, access to health care, socioeconomic factors, baseline comorbidities, and healthcare literacy (NCCN, 2016h; Sui et al., 2015).

Signs and Symptoms

Most testicular cancers can be found at an early stage. Commonly, the first sign is a lump on the testicle. Unfortunately, however, some testicular cancers may not cause symptoms until after they have reached an advanced stage (Oldenburg et al., 2013).

Early Detection

ACS recommends testicular examination as part of routine cancer-related checkups (ACS, 2016a). Men need to be aware of testicular cancer and to immediately seek health care if they find a lump (ACS, 2016a). Because regular testicular self-examinations have not been studied enough to show whether they reduce the death rate from this cancer, ACS does not recommend regular testicular self-examinations for men unless they have specific testicular cancer risk factors.

Some healthcare providers believe that finding a lump is an important factor in making a man seek early treatment, and they recommend that all men perform monthly testicular self-examinations after puberty. However, no evidence-based recommendations support this. Each man has to decide whether to perform a monthly self-examination. Figure 5-8 shows the anatomy and describes the basic technique for a professional and self-examination.

Figure 5-8. Basic Testicular Examination

Cross Section of Testicle

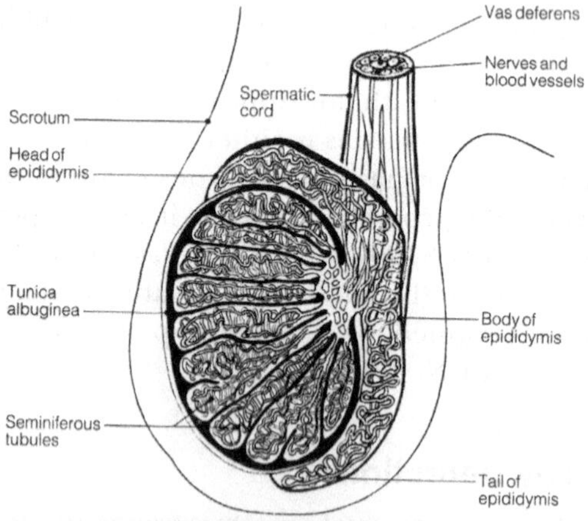

This figure shows the basic anatomy of the testicle. The steps of a self or professional testicular examination are similar. Examine one testicle at a time. Gently roll each testicle (with slight pressure) between the fingers. Place the thumbs over the top of the testicle, with the index and middle fingers of the hand behind the testicle, and then roll it between the fingers. The epididymis feels soft, rope-like, and slightly tender to pressure and is located at the top of the back part of each testicle. This is a normal lump. Remember that one testicle (usually the right one) is slightly larger than the other for most men, and this is normal. Any mass, lump, or asymmetry should be evaluated. It is recommended that self-examination be completed in the shower because the warm water relaxes the skin of the scrotum.

Note. Figure courtesy of National Cancer Institute. Retrieved from https://visualsonline.cancer.gov/details.cfm?imageid=1769.

Prostate Cancer

ACS (2016a) estimated about 180,890 new cases of prostate cancer and 26,120 deaths in the United States in 2016. This means that about 1 in 7 men will be diagnosed with prostate cancer during his lifetime, but only 1 in 35 will die of it. More than two million men in the United States who have been diagnosed with prostate cancer are still alive today. Prostate cancer is the second leading cause of cancer death in American men, behind only lung cancer. An estimated 92% of prostate cancers are found in the local and regional anatomic area. When compared to men the same age and race who do not have cancer, the five-year relative survival rate for these men is nearly 100%. The five-year relative survival rate for men whose prostate cancer has already spread to distant parts of the body at the time of diagnosis is about 28% (ACS, 2016a).

Risk Factors

Older men fear a diagnosis of prostate cancer, and with good reason. Prostate cancer is a significant problem in older men; most cases are diagnosed after age 65 (ACS, 2016a). Table 5-9 shows other risk factors for prostate cancer.

Signs and Symptoms

Early prostate cancer usually causes no symptoms and most often is found by a prostate-specific antigen (PSA) test or digital rectal examination (DRE) (ACS, 2016a). Some advanced prostate cancers can slow or weaken the urinary stream or result in frequent urination. But noncancerous diseases of the prostate, such as benign prostatic hyperplasia, cause these symptoms more often. In advanced prostate cancer, hematuria or pain in the hips, spine, ribs, or other areas may be present. Cancer that has spread to the spine can press on the spinal nerves, which can result in weakness or numbness in the legs or feet, or even loss of bladder or bowel control (NCCN, 2016g).

Early Detection

Prostate cancer often can be found early by testing the amount of PSA in the blood and performing DRE (NCCN, 2016g) (see Figure 5-9). Since the use of early detection tests for prostate cancer became common (circa 1990), the prostate cancer death rate has dropped (ACS, 2016a).

Table 5-9. Risk Factors for Prostate Cancer

Risk Factor	Etiology
Age	Prostate cancer is very rare before age 40, but the chance of having prostate cancer rises rapidly after age 50. About 2 out of 3 prostate cancers are found in men older than age 65.
Diet	A diet high in red meat or high-fat dairy products appears to increase risk.
Family history	Etiology may be associated with hereditary risk. Having a father or brother with prostate cancer more than doubles a man's risk of developing this disease. The risk increases for men with several affected relatives, particularly if their relatives were young at diagnosis.
Obesity	Obese men are more likely to be diagnosed with more advanced disease.
Race/ethnicity	The disease occurs more often in African American men than in men of other races; they also are likely to be diagnosed at an advanced stage and more than twice as likely to die of prostate cancer than Caucasian men. The disease occurs less often in Asian American, American Indian, and Hispanic/Latino men than in non-Hispanic Whites.

Note. Based on information from American Cancer Society, 2016a; Smith et al., 2015.

Figure 5-9. Digital Rectal Examination

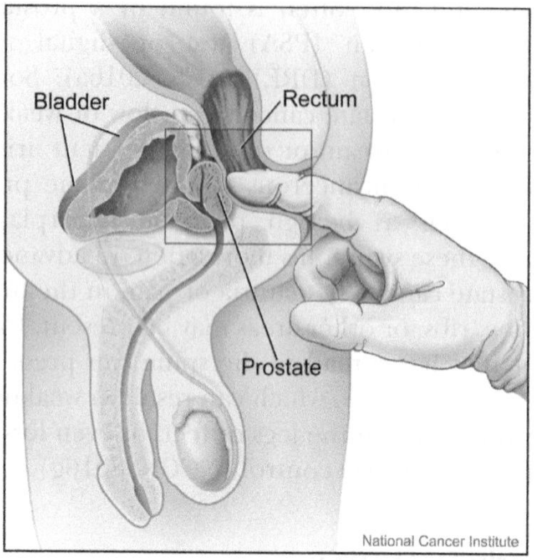

This figure demonstrates the examination of the prostate using the digital rectal examination. The examiner palpates the prostate for size, shape, and the presence of nodularity. A doctor performs a digital rectal examination by inserting a lubricated, gloved finger into the rectum to feel for abnormalities.

Note. Figure courtesy of National Cancer Institute, Alan Hoofring, illustrator. Retrieved from https://visualsonline.cancer.gov/details.cfm?imageid=4351.

The current screening methods have limitations. Neither the PSA test nor the DRE are 100% accurate. Uncertain or false-positive results lead to unnecessary prostate biopsies, which carry some risks and discomfort (see Table 5-10) (ACS, 2016a; NCCN, 2016g; USPSTF, 2008b).

The biggest controversy in prostate cancer screening is that some prostate cancers grow so slowly that they would likely never cause problems (NCCN, 2016g). Because of an elevated PSA level, some men may be diagnosed with a prostate cancer that would never have caused any symptoms or led to their death. But they may still be treated with surgery or radiation, either because the doctor cannot be sure of how aggressive the cancer might be or because the men are uncomfortable with not having any treatment. These treatments can have side effects that seriously affect quality of life. For this reason, before implementing screening recommendations, it is important to consider the individual's age and overall health and to have a discussion that promotes shared decision making (NCCN, 2016g).

No major scientific or medical organizations, including ACS, USPSTF, National Cancer Institute, and NCCN, support routine testing for prostate cancer at this time (ACS, 2016a; NCCN, 2016g; USPSTF, 2008b). USPSTF (2008b) has concluded that studies completed so far do not provide enough evidence to know whether the benefits of testing for early prostate cancer outweigh the possible risks. These groups recommend that healthcare professionals discuss the possible benefits, side effects, and questions about early prostate cancer detection and treatment so that men can make informed decisions, taking into account their own situation and risk. ACS and NCCN recommend that healthcare professionals should offer the option of testing for early detection of prostate cancer to all men who are at least 50 years old, or younger if at higher risk (ACS, 2016a; NCCN, 2016g). In general, testing is not recommended after age 70 (ACS, 2016a).

Skin Cancer

Skin cancer is a major public health problem in the United States and throughout the world (ACS, 2015c). Skin cancers that are not melanoma are sometimes grouped together as nonmelanoma skin cancers because they start from skin cells other than melanocytes. Nonmelanoma skin cancers include basal cell and squamous cell cancers (by far the most common cancers of the skin). Because they rarely spread elsewhere in the body, the annual estimated one million cases of basal cell and squamous cell skin

Table 5-10. Screening Tests for Prostate Cancer

Test	Characteristics
Digital rectal examination	This is a physical examination in which the provider inserts a gloved, lubricated finger into the rectum to feel for any lumps or hard areas that might be a cancer. Sensitivity is 59%.
Prostate-specific antigen (PSA) blood test	PSA is a substance made by cells in the prostate gland (whether they are normal or cancerous). Although PSA is mostly found in semen, a small amount is also found in the blood. Normal level is 4 ng/ml. Levels of 4–10 ng/ml are associated with a 25% risk of having prostate cancer. Levels > 10 ng are associated with a 50% risk of having the disease. Overall sensitivity is 73%.
Percent free PSA (fPSA)	The fPSA is the ratio of how much PSA circulates free compared to the total PSA level. Biopsies are not recommended for men whose fPSA is 10% or less and are recommended if it is 10%–25%.
PSA velocity	PSA velocity is not a separate test. It is a measure of how fast the PSA rises over time. For men whose initial PSA value is < 4 ng/ml, a PSA velocity of 0.35 ng/ml/year or greater may warrant a biopsy. For men whose PSA value is 4–10 ng/ml, a biopsy should be more strongly considered if the level rises faster than 0.75 ng/ml/year.

Note. Based on information from American Cancer Society, 2016a; Kim et al., 2010; Lee & Amling, 2010; National Comprehensive Cancer Network, 2016g; U.S. Preventive Services Task Force, 2008b.

cancers are less threatening and are treated differently than melanoma (ACS, 2016a). An estimated 76,380 new cases and 10,130 deaths from melanoma occurred in the United States in 2016 (ACS, 2016a). Overall, the lifetime risk of developing melanoma is about 2% (1 in 50 people) for Caucasians (NCCN, 2016f).

Risk Factors

Everyone has some risk for developing skin cancer and melanoma. The risk is higher in individuals with a lighter or fair complexion. Table 5-11 shows risk factors for melanoma and nonmelanoma cancers. Those with a significant family history of melanoma should be referred to a genetics professional for additional testing and education. Individuals who come from high-risk families with genetic syndromes require more extensive and frequent monitoring (Narayanan, Saladi, & Fox, 2010).

Signs and Symptoms

Because the prognosis can be favorable when melanoma is detected early, it is important for individuals and healthcare providers to be aware of the early signs and symptoms of melanoma and nonmelanoma skin cancer (see Figure 5-10). Many use the ABCDE rule to teach patients about the early detection of melanoma. With this approach, A stands for asymmetry in a lesion; B stands for border irregularity or jagged borders; C stands for color irregularity or multiple colors; D stands for a diameter greater than 5 mm, which is about the size of a pencil eraser; and E stands for evolving or growing.

Early Detection

Clearly, preventing skin cancer is best. Figure 5-11 outlines skin cancer prevention measures that all individuals should routinely imple-

Table 5-11. Risk Factors for Skin Cancers and Melanomas

Risk Factor	Melanoma	Squamous and Basal Cell Skin Cancers
Age	Risk increases with age, but it is found in all age groups.	Risk is highest in older people, but they can occur in younger age groups.
Family history of cancer	A family history of melanoma increases risk, especially if multiple first-degree relatives are affected. Those with a known *p16* mutation have an 85% lifetime risk of developing melanoma.	People with xeroderma pigmentosum (XP) have a high risk of skin cancer. XP is a rare, inherited condition resulting from a defect in an enzyme that repairs damage to DNA. Because people with XP are less able to repair DNA damage caused by sunlight, they develop huge numbers of cancers on sun-exposed areas of their skin.
History of skin conditions	Lifetime melanoma risk is estimated to be 6%–10% for those with many dysplastic nevi.	Risk is higher in those with a history of many sunburns as a child.
Medications	Individuals taking medicines that suppress the immune system, such as organ transplant recipients, have an increased risk of developing melanoma.	Risk is increased in people taking photosensitizing medications.
Personal history of cancer	A previous history of melanoma increases risk; 5%–10% of people with one melanoma develop a second one.	A previous history of skin cancer increases risk.
Sex	Risk is higher in males.	Risk is higher in males.
Skin tone/hair color	Risk is highest in red- or light-haired people with fair skin.	Risk is higher in red- and light-haired people and those with fair skin.
Ultraviolet radiation (UVR) exposure	UVR exposure is a major risk factor for most melanomas. Sunlight is the main source of UVR, which can damage the genes in skin cells. Tanning lamps and booths also are sources of UVR.	Most skin cancers are caused by unprotected UVR exposure to the area of skin that develops the cancer. Most of this radiation comes from sunlight, but some may come from man-made sources such as tanning booths.

Note. Based on information from American Cancer Society, 2015b, 2016a; Colantonio et al., 2014; Dubas & Ingraffea, 2013; Gandini et al., 2011; Lucas, 2011.

ment. The effectiveness of regular use of a broad-spectrum sunscreen with SPF 30, reduction of UV exposure, and wearing of protective clothing should not be underestimated (ACS, 2015b). Regular sunscreen use can reduce the incidence of solar keratoses, which are precursors of squamous cell carcinoma (Sambandan & Ratner, 2011). The relationship between UV radiation exposure and cutaneous melanoma is less clear (Narayanan et al., 2010; Park et al., 2012). In melanoma, intermittent acute sun exposure leading to sunburn seems to be more damaging; such exposures in childhood or adolescence may be particularly important (Lim et al., 2011).

One way to gauge the intensity of and risk for UV exposure is to know the UV index for the geographic locale. The UV index is a num-

Figure 5-10. Signs and Symptoms of Skin Cancer

- A mole that changes in size, shape, or color
- A mole that has irregular edges or borders
- A mole that is more than one color
- A mole that is asymmetric (if the mole is divided in half, the two halves are different in size or shape)
- A mole that itches
- A mole that oozes, bleeds, or is ulcerated (a hole forms in the skin when the top layer of cells breaks down and the underlying tissue shows through)
- A sore that does not heal
- Areas of the skin that are small, raised, smooth, shiny, and waxy
- Areas of the skin that are small, raised, and red or reddish-brown
- Areas of the skin that are scaly, bleeding, or crusty

Note. Based on information from American Cancer Society, 2016a; U.S. Preventive Services Task Force, 2009; Walton et al., 2014.

Figure 5-11. Skin Cancer Prevention Measures

- Wear protective clothing, including hats and long-sleeved shirts. Dark colors and tightly woven fabrics provide more protection. Clothes are available with special coatings to help absorb UVR.
- Use a sunscreen with SPF 15 or higher that provides protection against UVA and UVB radiation. Most sunscreen products expire within 2–3 years, so it is important to ascertain whether the product is expired. Apply sunscreen generously to dry skin 20–30 minutes before going outside so that the skin has time to absorb the chemicals. When applying it, pay close attention to the face, ears, hands, and arms, and generously coat the skin that is not covered by clothing (about 1 oz for an adult). For best results, most sunscreens must be reapplied at least every 2 hours and more often when swimming or perspiring.
- Wear a hat with at least a 2–3-inch brim all around because it protects areas often exposed to the sun, such as the neck, ears, eyes, forehead, nose, and scalp.
- Wear sunglasses that block UVR. The sunglasses should block 99%–100% of UVA and UVB radiation.
- Limit direct sun exposure between 10 am and 2 pm. UVR reaches the ground even on cloudy days and can pass through water. Seek shade whenever possible.
- Avoid using tanning beds and sunlamps, which can cause serious long-term skin damage and contribute to skin cancer.

UVA—ultraviolet A; UVB—ultraviolet B; UVR—ultraviolet radiation

Note. Based on information from American Cancer Society, 2015b, 2016a; National Comprehensive Cancer Network, 2016f.

ber from 0 to 10+ that indicates the amount of UV radiation reaching the Earth's surface during the hour around noon. The higher the number, the greater the exposure to UV radiation outdoors (U.S. Environmental Protection Agency, 2016). The National Weather Service forecasts the UV index daily in 58 U.S. cities based on local predicted conditions (U.S. Environmental Protection Agency, 2016). The index covers about a 30-mile radius from each city. The information can be accessed through the local newspaper, television and radio news broadcasts, or at www.cpc.noaa.gov/products/stratosphere/uv_index/uv_current.shtml.

USPSTF (2009) has concluded that insufficient evidence exists to recommend for or against routine screening (total body examination by a clinician) to detect skin cancers early. However, USPSTF recommends that clinicians be aware that fair-skinned men and women aged 65 and older and people with atypical moles or more than 50 moles are at greater risk for developing melanoma and that clinicians should remain alert for skin abnormalities when conducting physical examinations for other purposes (USPSTF, 2009). ACS recommends routine inspection of the skin as part of an annual cancer-related checkup (ACS, 2016a). High-risk individuals may be encouraged to perform skin self-examinations to monitor for early changes.

Nursing Implications

To increase the number of cancer survivors, it is necessary to increase the practice of a healthy diet, exercise, the elimination of tobacco use, and protection against UV light exposure. Beyond these measures to prevent cancer, it is necessary to detect cancer in its earliest stages when it is most treatable. The implementation of effective screening programs that provide education that influences health behaviors and improves health outcomes is an important nursing role, in addition to providing case management to ensure follow-up of abnormalities and continuity throughout the process (Benito et al., 2014).

Nurses in inpatient and other healthcare settings should conduct health histories that accurately and adequately assess patients so that appropriate cancer screening recommendations can be made. Additionally, providing appropriate education to patients and families concerning cancer screening is an important nursing role. Family, friends, and other healthcare professionals often rely on information from nurses to assist them in understanding screening options and early cancer detection guidelines.

For each of the cancers discussed, nurses have a vital role in cancer prevention and detection education. First, nurses need to assess individuals for the risk of each cancer and communicate the magnitude of that risk to patients in understandable terms. For families with a significant history of a cancer, referral to a genetics professional can better clarify risk. Individuals need to know the signs and symptoms of each cancer and the importance of reporting these symptoms promptly to a healthcare provider. Depending on the risk, patients need to be instructed on cancer prevention strategies and appropriate screening maneuvers. Nurses who role model these healthy practices and take the time to explain the importance of these behaviors to patients will contribute to decreasing the morbidity and mortality associated with cancer.

Oncology nurses have a large responsibility to teach the public about cancer detection and screening. Individuals need to realize that cancer screening is different from diagnostic examinations for cancer. Individuals also need to understand that cancer screening is not perfect and, even when conducted properly, will fail to detect some malignancies because of the strengths and limitations associated with different screening tests. An understanding of epidemiologic principles, the sensitivity and specificity of various tests, and the rationale for various screening recommendations is necessary to give individuals the information they need to make informed choices about cancer screening.

Research continues to suggest that the single most important factor in whether an individual has ever had a screening test, or has recently had a screening test, is a recommendation from the healthcare provider. When nurses recommend screening to an individual, a far greater chance exists that the individual will go on to have appropriate screening. This recommendation can easily come in the form of patient education about cancer prevention and early detection. In a hectic practice setting, dedicated nurse navigators and advanced practice nurses can play a critical role in improving discussion about options and ultimately improving utilization of cancer screening services, especially in at-risk populations.

Some populations are at increased risk for developing cancer and have difficulty accessing primary and secondary prevention services. The implementation of effective strategies that can potentially influence health behaviors and improve health outcomes in at-risk populations requires sincerely caring about the specific needs of the population and working directly to implement culturally sensitive strategies (Abbott, 2015).

Nurses need to look for teachable moments. Research suggests that when a celebrity is diagnosed with a cancer, increased media coverage heightens awareness about prevention and early detection (Ayers, Althouse, Noar, & Cohen, 2014). Nurses should try to use this media attention to promote prevention programs. More research needs to be done to learn how to sustain the enthusiasm and interest in cancer screening (Noar, Willoughby, Myrick, & Brown, 2014).

Nurses need to recognize barriers to implementing cancer screening programs (Spruce & Sanford, 2012). Difficulties with implementing shared decision making and effective screening programs include lack of time, competing health priorities, lack of patient interest, complexity of screening decisions, poor reimbursement for counseling and education, malpractice concerns, and lack of provider knowledge about screening strengths and limitations. Lack of health insurance and lack of prior screening have been consistently associated with late stage at diagnosis for breast, cervical, and colorectal cancers (ACS, 2016a).

When nurses are providing patients with information on cancer control, it is important to use educational materials that focus on wellness. More and more resources are becoming available both in print and social media formats. Selecting appropriate references that augment education and are cost-effective is a challenge for nurses and merits more research to better understand the best approaches (Lairson, Chung, Smith, Springston, & Champion, 2015). It is inappropriate to provide materials that focus on disease and treatment; some people actually find this distressing (Edwards et al., 2013; Fagerlin et al., 2011). The focus of education and materials should be that early detection is associated with decreased morbidity and mortality and improved quality of life compared to when cancer is detected at later stages. Written materials with a focus on prevention, including nutrition, self-examination technique, Pap tests, and prostate, breast, skin, and CRC screening, are available through ACS and the National Cancer Institute.

Nurses and other healthcare providers need to role model healthy practices and regularly engage in cancer screening behaviors and can positively influence patients to adopt such practices (Oberg & Frank, 2009).

Conclusion

Cancer control requires a large amount of public education to empower individuals to take more responsibility for their health and well-being. This ever-growing subspecialty in oncology has the potential to decrease the morbidity and mortality associated with cancer and ultimately improve the quality of life for many individuals. Oncology nurses have important roles in assessing and interpreting risks; explaining the strengths, limitations, and risks associated with various screening tests; and reinforcing information about possible symptoms of cancer and when to seek evaluation. These education activities should be directed to cancer survivors as well as the general public.

References

Abbott, L.S. (2015). Evaluation of nursing interventions designed to impact knowledge, behaviors, and health outcomes for rural African-Americans: An integrative review. *Public Health Nursing, 32,* 408–420. doi:10.1111/phn.12174

Alberg, A.J., Brock, M.V., Ford, J.G., Samet, J.M., & Spivack, S.D. (2013). Epidemiology of lung cancer: Diagnosis and management of lung cancer, 3rd ed: Ameri-

Key Points

- The accuracy of a cancer screening test can be described in terms of sensitivity and specificity.
- Screening protocols or recommendations define how a cancer screening test should be used and can vary across organizations and professional groups.
- Asymptomatic adults aged 55 years and older who have a 30-pack-year smoking history and currently smoke or have quit smoking within the past 15 years may undergo annual screening for lung cancer with LDCT.
- Mammography can detect breast cancers long before they are palpable. Recommendations for mammography vary across organizations.
- Breast MRI is recommended for women with a greater than 20% lifetime risk of developing breast cancer.
- The most significant risk factor identified for cervical cancer is HPV, a sexually transmitted infection that is present in approximately 99% of cervical cancers. Most cervical cancers could be prevented with better uptake of the HPV vaccine and regular use of the Pap test.
- During a pelvic examination, the healthcare professional feels the ovaries and uterus for size, shape, and consistency. Although a pelvic examination is recommended because it can find some reproductive system cancers at an early stage, most early ovarian tumors are difficult or impossible for even the most skilled examiner to feel.
- Tests that primarily find CRC involve testing the stool for signs that cancer may be present. Tests that can find both colorectal polyps and cancer examine the structure of the colon to detect any abnormal areas, most often with colonoscopy. Polyps found before they become malignant can be removed, so these tests may prevent CRC and are preferred.
- Prostate cancer screening is controversial because some prostate cancers grow so slowly that they would likely never cause problems. Because of an elevated PSA level, some men may be diagnosed and treated for a prostate cancer that would never have caused any symptoms or led to their death.
- Oral cancers are largely preventable by avoiding tobacco use and limiting alcohol intake.
- Skin cancers are largely due to UV light exposure. Effective prevention measures include limiting exposure to UV light, not using artificial tanning devices, and regularly using sunscreen, protective clothing, large-brimmed hats, and ocular protection. The skin is readily accessible to inspection, and prompt evaluation of suspicious lesions, including removal, reduces the morbidity and mortality associated with skin cancer.

can College of Chest Physicians evidence-based clinical practice guidelines. *Chest, 143*(Suppl. 5), e1S–e29S. doi:10.1378/chest.12-2345

American Cancer Society. (2014). *Colorectal cancer facts and figures 2014–2016.* Atlanta, GA: Author.

American Cancer Society. (2015a). *Breast cancer facts and figures 2015–2016.* Atlanta, GA: Author.

American Cancer Society. (2015b). *Cancer prevention and early detection facts and figures 2015–2016.* Atlanta, GA: Author.

American Cancer Society. (2015c). *Global cancer facts and figures* (3rd ed.). Atlanta, GA: Author.

American Cancer Society. (2016a). *Cancer facts and figures 2016.* Atlanta, GA: Author.

American Cancer Society. (2016b). *Cancer treatment and survivorship facts and figures 2016–2017.* Atlanta, GA: Author.

American College of Obstetricians and Gynecologists. (2016). Practice bulletin No. 157: Cervical cancer screening and prevention. *Obstetrics and Gynecology, 127,* e1–e20. doi:10.1097/AOG.0000000000001263

American College of Radiology. (2014). Mammography—Frequently asked questions. In *ACR BI-RADS atlas.* Retrieved from http://www.acr.org/~/media/ACR/Documents/PDF/QualitySafety/Resources/BIRADS/01%20Mammography/03%20%20BIRADS%20Mammography%20FAQs.pdf

Ayers, J.W., Althouse, B.M., Noar, S.M., & Cohen, J.E. (2014). Do celebrity cancer diagnoses promote primary cancer prevention? *Preventive Medicine, 58,* 81–84. doi:10.1016/j.ypmed.2013.11.007

Basch, E., Somerfield, M.R., Partridge, A., Schnipper, L., & Lyman, G.H. (2011). Commentary: Should cost and comparative value of treatments be considered in clinical practice guidelines? *Journal of Oncology Practice, 7,* 398–401. doi:10.1200/JOP.2011.000414

Benito, L., Binefa, G., Lluch, T., Vidal, C., Milà, N., Puig, M., ... Garcia, M. (2014). Defining the role of the nurse in population-based cancer screening programs: A literature review [Online exclusive]. *Clinical Journal of Oncology Nursing, 18,* E77–E83. doi:10.1188/14.CJON.E77-E83

Berg, W.A., Zhang, Z., Lehrer, D., Jong, R.A., Pisano, E.D., Barr, R.G., ... Gabrielli, G. (2012). Detection of breast cancer with addition of annual screening ultrasound or a single screening MRI to mammography in women with elevated breast cancer risk. *JAMA, 307,* 1394–1404. doi:10.1001/jama.2012.388

Brawley, O., Byers, T., Chen, A., Pignone, M., Ransohoff, D., Schenk, M., ... Wender, R. (2011). New American Cancer Society process for creating trustworthy cancer screening guidelines. *JAMA, 306,* 2495–2499. doi:10.1001/jama.2011.1800

Burt, R.W., Cannon, J.A., David, D.S., Early, D.S., Ford, J.M., Giardiello, F.M., ... Freedman-Cass, D. (2013). Colorectal cancer screening. *Journal of the National Comprehensive Cancer Network, 11,* 1538–1575. Retrieved from http://www.jnccn.org/content/11/12/1538.long

Chan-Smutko, G. (2012). Genetic testing by cancer site: Urinary tract. *Cancer Journal, 18,* 343–349. doi:10.1097/PPO.0b013e31826246ac

Chesson, H.W., Dunne, E.F., Hariri, S., & Markowitz, L.E. (2014). The estimated lifetime probability of acquiring human papillomavirus in the United States. *Sexually Transmitted Diseases, 41,* 660–664. doi:10.1097/olq.0000000000000193

Chiarelli, A.M., Majpruz, V., Brown, P., Thériault, M., Shumak, R., & Mai, V. (2009). The contribution of clinical breast examination to the accuracy of breast screening. *Journal of the National Cancer Institute, 101,* 1236–1243. doi:10.1093/jnci/djp241

Colantonio, S., Bracken, M.B., & Beecker, J. (2014). The association of indoor tanning and melanoma in adults: Systematic review and meta-analysis. *Journal of the American Academy of Dermatology, 70,* 847–857. doi:10.1016/j.jaad.2013.11.050

Cote, M.L., Alhajj, T., Ruterbusch, J.J., Bernstein, L., Brinton, L.A., Blot, W.J., ... Olson, S.H. (2015). Risk factors for endometrial cancer in black and white women: A pooled analysis from the Epidemiology of Endometrial Cancer Consortium (E2C2). *Cancer Causes and Control, 26,* 287–296. doi:10.1007/s10552-014-0510-3

Curreri, S.A., Fung, C., & Beard, C.J. (2015). Secondary malignant neoplasms in testicular cancer survivors. *Urologic Oncology: Seminars and Original Investigations, 33,* 392–398. doi;10.1016/j.urolonc.2015.05.002

Daniels, M.S. (2012). Genetic testing by cancer site: Uterus. *Cancer Journal, 18,* 338–342. doi:10.1097/PPO.0b013e3182610cc2

Dubas, L.E., & Ingraffea, A. (2013). Nonmelanoma skin cancer. *Facial Plastic Surgery Clinics of North America, 21,* 43–53. doi:10.1016/j.fsc.2012.10.003

Edwards, A.G.K., Naik, G., Ahmed, H., Elwyn, G.J., Pickles, T., Hood, K., & Playle, R. (2013). Personalised risk communication for informed decision making about taking screening tests. *Cochrane Database of Systematic Reviews, 2013*(2). doi:10.1002/14651858.CD001865.pub3

Evans, W.K., Brouwers, M.C., & Bell, C.M. (2008). Should cost of care be considered in a clinical practice guideline? [Commentary]. *Journal of the National Comprehensive Cancer Network, 6,* 224–226. Retrieved from http://www.jnccn.org/content/6/3/224.long

Fagerlin, A., Zikmund-Fisher, B.J., & Ubel, P.A. (2011). Helping patients decide: Ten steps to better risk communication. *Journal of the National Cancer Institute, 103,* 1436–1443. doi:10.1093/jnci/djr318

Feng, S., Yang, H., Li, X., Yang, J., Zhang, J., Wang, A., ... Qiu, Y. (2016). Single scrotal incision orchiopexy versus the inguinal approach in children with palpable undescended testis: A systematic review and meta-analysis. *Pediatric Surgery International, 32,* 989–995. doi:10.1007/s00383-016-3956-4

Gadducci, A., Biglia, N., Cosio, S., Sismondi, P., & Genazzani, A.R. (2010). Gynaecologic challenging issues in the management of BRCA mutation carriers: Oral contraceptives, prophylactic salpingo-oophorectomy and hormone replacement therapy. *Gynecological Endocrinology, 26,* 568–577. doi:10.3109/09513590.2010.487609

Gandini, S., Autier, P., & Boniol, M. (2011). Reviews on sun exposure and artificial light and melanoma. *Progress in Biophysics and Molecular Biology, 107,* 362–366. doi:10.1016/j.pbiomolbio.2011.09.011

Gilbert, F.J., Tucker, L., & Young, K.C. (2016). Digital breast tomosynthesis (DBT): A review of the evidence for use as a screening tool. *Clinical Radiology, 71,* 141–150. doi:10.1016/j.crad.2015.11.008

Gordis, L. (2014). *Epidemiology* (5th ed.). Philadelphia, PA: Elsevier Saunders.

Green, V.L. (2013). Breast cancer risk assessment, prevention, and the future. *Obstetrics and Gynecology Clinics of North America, 40,* 525–549. doi:10.1016/j.ogc.2013.05.003

Guirguis-Blake, J., Calonge, N., Miller, T., Siu, A., Teutsch, S., & Whitlock, E. (2007). Current processes of the U.S. Preventive Services Task Force: Refining evidence-based recommendation development. *Annals of Internal Medicine, 147,* 117–122. doi:10.7326/0003-4819-147-2-200707170-00170

Hunn, J., & Rodriguez, G.C. (2012). Ovarian cancer: Etiology, risk factors, and epidemiology. *Clinical Obstetrics and Gynecology, 55,* 3–23. doi:10.1097/GRF.0b013e31824b4611

Jacobsen, G.D., & Jacobsen, K.H. (2011). Health awareness campaigns and diagnosis rates: Evidence from National Breast Cancer Awareness Month. *Journal of Health Economics, 30,* 55–61. doi:10.1016/j.jhealeco.2010.11.005

Jasperson, K.W. (2012). Genetic testing by cancer site: Colon (polyposis syndromes). *Cancer Journal, 18,* 328–333. doi:10.1097/PPO.0b013e3182609300

Jellema, P., van der Windt, D.A.W.M., Bruinvels, D.J., Mallen, C.D., van Weyenberg, S.J.B., Mulder, C.J., & de Vet, H.C.W. (2010). Value of symptoms and additional diagnostic tests for colorectal cancer in primary care: Systematic review and meta-analysis. *BMJ, 340,* c1269. doi:10.1136/bmj.c1269

Jeong, K.E., & Cairns, J.A. (2013). Review of economic evidence in the prevention and early detection of colorectal cancer. *Health Economics Review, 3,* 20. doi:10.1186/2191-1991-3-20

Kastrinos, F., & Syngal, S. (2011). Inherited colorectal cancer syndromes. *Cancer Journal, 17,* 405–415. doi:10.1097/PPO.0b013e318237e408

Kim, H.L., Puymon, M.R., Qin, M., Guru, K., & Mohler, J.L. (2010). A method for using life tables to estimate lifetime risk for prostate cancer death. *Journal of the National Comprehensive Cancer Network, 8,* 148–154. Retrieved from http://www.jnccn.org/content/8/2/148.long

Kushi, L.H., Doyle, C., McCullough, M., Rock, C.L., Demark-Wahnefried, W., Bandera, E.V., … American Cancer Society 2010 Nutrition and Physical Activity Guidelines Advisory Committee. (2012). American Cancer Society guidelines on nutrition and physical activity for cancer prevention: Reducing the risk of cancer with healthy food choices and physical activity. *CA: A Cancer Journal for Clinicians, 62,* 30–67. doi:10.3322/caac.20140

Lairson, D.R., Chung, T.H., Smith, L.G., Springston, J.K., & Champion, V.L. (2015). Estimating development cost of an interactive website based cancer screening promotion program. *Evaluation and Program Planning, 50,* 56–62. doi:10.1016/j.evalprogplan.2015.01.009

Lee, A.K., & Amling, C.L. (2010). Appropriate use of nomograms to guide prostate cancer treatment selection. *Journal of the National Comprehensive Cancer Network, 8,* 201–209. Retrieved from http://www.jnccn.org/content/8/2/201.long

Levin, B., Lieberman, D.A., McFarland, B., Smith, R.A., Brooks, D., Andrews, K.S., … Winawer, S.J. (2008). Screening and surveillance for the early detection of colorectal cancer and adenomatous polyps, 2008: A joint guideline from the American Cancer Society, the US Multi-Society Task Force on Colorectal Cancer, and the American College of Radiology. *CA: A Cancer Journal for Clinicians, 58,* 130–160. doi:10.3322/CA.2007.0018

Lim, H.W., James, W.D., Rigel, D.S., Maloney, M.E., Spencer, J.M., & Bhushan, R. (2011). Adverse effects of ultraviolet radiation from the use of indoor tanning equipment: Time to ban the tan. *Journal of the American Academy of Dermatology, 64,* e51–e60. doi:10.1016/j.jaad.2010.11.032

Lim, L.Y., Nah, S.A., Lakshmi, N.K., Yap, T.-L., Jacobsen, A.S., Low, Y., & Ong, C.C.P. (2015). Undescended testis: Level of knowledge among potential referring healthcare providers. *Journal of Paediatrics and Child Health, 51,* 1109–1114. doi:10.1111/jpc.12911

Lo, Y.-L., Hsiao, C.-F., Chang, G.-C., Tsai, Y.-H., Huang, M.-S., Su, W.-C., … Hsiung, C.A. (2013). Risk factors for primary lung cancer among never smokers by gender in a matched case-control study. *Cancer Causes and Control, 24,* 567–576. doi:10.1007/s10552-012-9994-x

Lucas, R.M. (2011). An epidemiological perspective of ultraviolet exposure—Public health concerns. *Eye and Contact Lens Science and Clinical Practice, 37,* 168–175. doi:10.1097/ICL.0b013e31821cb0cf

Menon, U., Talaat, A., Rosenthal, A.N., Macdonald, N.D., Jeyerajah, A.R., Skates, S.J., … Jacobs, I.J. (2014). Performance of ultrasound as a second line test to serum CA125 in ovarian cancer screening. *BJOG: An International Journal of Obstetrics and Gynaecology, 121*(Suppl. 7), 35–39. doi:10.1111/1471-0528.13211

Miller, J.W., Hanson, V., Johnson, G.D., Royalty, J.E., & Richardson, L.C. (2014). From cancer screening to treatment: Service delivery and referral in the National Breast and Cervical Cancer Early Detection Program. *Cancer, 120*(Suppl. S16), 2549–2556. doi:10.1002/cncr.28823

Morrow, M., Waters, J., & Morris, E. (2011). MRI for breast cancer screening, diagnosis, and treatment. *Lancet, 378,* 1804–1811. doi:10.1016/S0140-6736(11)61350-0

Moyer, V.A. (2014). Screening for lung cancer: U.S. Preventive Services Task Force recommendation statement. *Annals of Internal Medicine, 160,* 330–338. doi:10.7326/M13-2771

Narayanan, D.L., Saladi, R.N., & Fox, J.L. (2010). Review: Ultraviolet radiation and skin cancer. *International Journal of Dermatology, 49,* 978–986. doi:10.1111/j.1365-4632.2010.04474.x

National Comprehensive Cancer Network. (2016a). *NCCN Clinical Practice Guidelines in Oncology (NCCN Guidelines®): Breast cancer screening and diagnosis* [v.1.2016]. Retrieved from https://www.nccn.org/professionals/physician_gls/pdf/breast-screening.pdf

National Comprehensive Cancer Network. (2016b). *NCCN Clinical Practice Guidelines in Oncology (NCCN Guidelines®): Colorectal cancer screening* [v.2.2016]. Retrieved from https://www.nccn.org/professionals/physician_gls/pdf/colorectal_screening.pdf

National Comprehensive Cancer Network. (2016c). *NCCN Clinical Practice Guidelines in Oncology (NCCN*

Guidelines®): Genetic/familial high-risk assessment: Breast and ovarian [v.2.2017]. Retrieved from https://www.nccn.org/professionals/physician_gls/pdf/genetics_screening.pdf

National Comprehensive Cancer Network. (2016d). *NCCN Clinical Practice Guidelines in Oncology (NCCN Guidelines®): Genetic/familial high-risk assessment: Colorectal* [v.2.2016]. Retrieved from https://www.nccn.org/professionals/physician_gls/pdf/genetics_colon.pdf

National Comprehensive Cancer Network. (2016e). *NCCN Clinical Practice Guidelines in Oncology (NCCN Guidelines®): Head and neck cancers* [v.2.2016]. Retrieved from https://www.nccn.org/professionals/physician_gls/pdf/head-and-neck.pdf

National Comprehensive Cancer Network. (2016f). *NCCN Clinical Practice Guidelines in Oncology (NCCN Guidelines®): Melanoma* [v.1.2017]. Retrieved from https://www.nccn.org/professionals/physician_gls/pdf/melanoma.pdf

National Comprehensive Cancer Network. (2016g). *NCCN Clinical Practice Guidelines in Oncology (NCCN Guidelines®): Prostate cancer early detection* [v.2.2016]. Retrieved from https://www.nccn.org/professionals/physician_gls/pdf/prostate_detection.pdf

National Comprehensive Cancer Network. (2016h). *NCCN Clinical Practice Guidelines in Oncology (NCCN Guidelines®): Testicular cancer* [v.2.2017]. Retrieved from https://www.nccn.org/professionals/physician_gls/pdf/testicular.pdf

National Lung Screening Trial Research Team. (2011). Reduced lung-cancer mortality with low-dose computed tomographic screening. *New England Journal of Medicine, 365,* 395–409. doi:10.1056/NEJMoa1102873

Nelson, H.D., Zakher, B., Cantor, A., Fu, R., Griffin, J., O'Meara, E.S., ... Miglioretti, D.L. (2012). Risk factors for breast cancer for women aged 40 to 49 years: A systematic review and meta-analysis. *Annals of Internal Medicine, 156,* 635–648. doi:10.7326/0003-4819-156-9-201205010-00006

Noar, S.M., Willoughby, J.F., Myrick, J.G., & Brown, J. (2014). Public figure announcements about cancer and opportunities for cancer communication: A review and research agenda [Editorial]. *Health Communication, 29,* 445–461. doi:10.1080/10410236.2013.764781

Oberg, E.B., & Frank, E. (2009). Physicians' health practices strongly influence patient health practices. *Journal of the Royal College of Physicians of Edinburgh, 39,* 290–291. doi:10.4997/JRCPE.2009.422

Oldenburg, J., Fosså, S.D., Nuver, J., Heidenreich, A., Schmoll, H.-J., Bokemeyer, C., ... Kataja, V. (2013). Testicular seminoma and non-seminoma: ESMO clinical practice guidelines for diagnosis, treatment and follow-up. *Annals of Oncology, 24*(Suppl. 6), vi125–vi132. doi:10.1093/annonc/mdt304

Oral contraceptives and ovarian cancer risk. (2008). *CA: A Cancer Journal for Clinicians, 58,* 127–128. doi:10.3322/CA.2008.0004

Papathomas, M., Molitor, J., Richardson, S., Riboli, E., & Vineis, P. (2011). Examining the joint effect of multiple risk factors using exposure risk profiles: Lung cancer in nonsmokers. *Environmental Health Perspectives, 119,* 84–91. doi:10.1289/ehp.1002118

Park, S.L., Le Marchand, L., Wilkens, L.R., Kolonel, L.N., Henderson, B.E., Zhang, Z.-F., & Setiawan, V.W. (2012). Risk factors for malignant melanoma in White and Non-White/Non–African American populations: The multiethnic cohort. *Cancer Prevention Research, 5,* 423–434. doi:10.1158/1940-6207.CAPR-11-0460

Patel, S.G., & Ahnen, D.J. (2012). Familial colon cancer syndromes: An update of a rapidly evolving field. *Current Gastroenterology Reports, 14,* 428–438. doi:10.1007/s11894-012-0280-6

Plescia, M., Richardson, L.C., & Joseph, D. (2012). New roles for public health in cancer screening. *CA: A Cancer Journal for Clinicians, 62,* 217–219. doi:10.3322/caac.21147

Sambandan, D.R., & Ratner, D. (2011). Sunscreens: An overview and update. *Journal of the American Academy of Dermatology, 64,* 748–758. doi:10.1016/j.jaad.2010.01.005

Sarfaty, M., Wender, R., & Smith, R. (2011). Promoting cancer screening within the patient centered medical home. *CA: A Cancer Journal for Clinicians, 61,* 397–408. doi:10.3322/caac.20125

Saslow, D., Solomon, D., Lawson, H.W., Killackey, M., Kulasingam, S.L., Cain, J., ... ACS-ASCCP-ASCP Cervical Cancer Guideline Committee. (2012). American Cancer Society, American Society for Colposcopy and Cervical Pathology, and American Society for Clinical Pathology screening guidelines for the prevention and early detection of cervical cancer. *CA: A Cancer Journal for Clinicians, 62,* 147–172. doi:10.3322/caac.21139

Senter, L. (2012). Genetic testing by cancer site: Colon (nonpolyposis syndromes). *Cancer Journal, 18,* 334–337. doi:10.1097/PPO.0b013e31826094b2

Shannon, K.M., & Chittenden, A. (2012). Genetic testing by cancer site: Breast. *Cancer Journal, 18,* 310–319. doi:10.1097/PPO.0b013e318260946f

Sickles, E.A., D'Orsi, C.J., Bassett, L.W., & American College of Radiology BI-RADS Committee. (2013). ACR BI-RADS® mammography. In *ACR BI-RADS® Atlas: Breast Imaging Reporting and Data System* (5th ed.). Reston, VA: American College of Radiology.

Sinclair, N., Littenberg, B., Geller, B., & Muss, H. (2011). Accuracy of screening mammography in older women. *American Journal of Roentgenology, 197,* 1268–1273. doi:10.2214/AJR.10.5442

Siu, A.L. (2016). Screening for breast cancer: U.S. Preventive Services Task Force recommendation statement.

Annals of Internal Medicine, 164, 279–296. doi:10.7326/M15-2886

Smith, R.A., Manassaram-Baptiste, D., Brooks, D., Doroshenk, M., Fedewa, S., Saslow, D., ... Wender, R. (2015). Cancer screening in the United States, 2015: A review of current American Cancer Society guidelines and current issues in cancer screening. *CA: A Cancer Journal for Clinicians, 65,* 30–54. doi:10.3322/caac.21261

Spruce, L.R., & Sanford, J.T. (2012). An intervention to change the approach to colorectal cancer screening in primary care. *Journal of the American Academy of Nurse Practitioners, 24,* 167–174. doi:10.1111/j.1745-7599.2012.00714.x

Sui, W., Morrow, D.C., Bermejo, C.E., & Hellenthal, N.J. (2015). Trends in testicular cancer survival: A large population-based analysis. *Urology, 85,* 1394–1398. doi:10.1016/j.urology.2015.03.022

Tan, M.-H., Mester, J.L., Ngeow, J., Rybicki, L.A., Orloff, M.S., & Eng, C. (2012). Lifetime cancer risks in individuals with germline *PTEN* mutations. *Clinical Cancer Research, 18,* 400–407. doi:10.1158/1078-0432.CCR-11-2283

U.S. Environmental Protection Agency. (2016, March 21). Sun safety. Retrieved from https://www.epa.gov/sunsafety

U.S. Food and Drug Administration. (2015, July 22). Frequently asked questions about MQSA. Retrieved from http://www.fda.gov/Radiation-EmittingProducts/MammographyQualityStandardsActandProgram/ConsumerInformation/ucm113968.htm

U.S. Preventive Services Task Force. (2008a). Screening for colorectal cancer: U.S. Preventive Services Task Force recommendation statement. *Annals of Internal Medicine, 149,* 627–637. doi:10.7326/0003-4819-149-9-200811040-00243

U.S. Preventive Services Task Force. (2008b). Screening for prostate cancer: U.S. Preventive Services Task Force recommendation statement. *Annals of Internal Medicine, 149,* 185–191. doi:10.7326/0003-4819-149-3-200808050-00008

U.S. Preventive Services Task Force. (2009). Screening for skin cancer: U.S. Preventive Services Task Force recommendation statement. *Annals of Internal Medicine, 150,* 188–193. doi:10.7326/0003-4819-150-3-200902030-00008

Vesco, K.K., Whitlock, E.P., Eder, M., Burda, B.U., Senger, C.A., & Lutz, K. (2011). Risk factors and other epidemiologic considerations for cervical cancer screening: A narrative review for the U.S. Preventive Services Task Force. *Annals of Internal Medicine, 155,* 698–705. doi:10.7326/0003-4819-155-10-201111150-00377

Walton, A.E., Janda, M., Youl, P.H., Baade, P., Aitken, J.F., Whiteman, D.C., ... Neale, R.E. (2014). Uptake of skin self-examination and clinical examination behavior by outdoor workers. *Archives of Environmental and Occupational Health, 69,* 214–222. doi:10.1080/19338244.2013.771247

Warman, J. (2010). Cervical cancer screening in young women: Saving lives with prevention and detection. *Oncology Nursing Forum, 37,* 33–38. doi:10.1188/10.ONF.33-38

Weissman, S.M., Weiss, S.M., & Newlin, A.C. (2012). Genetic testing by cancer site: Ovary. *Cancer Journal, 18,* 320–327. doi:10.1097/PPO.0b013e31826246c2

Weitzel, J.N., Blazer, K.R., MacDonald, D.J., Culver, J.O., & Offit, K. (2011). Genetics, genomics and cancer risk assessment: State of the art and future directions in the era of personalized medicine. *CA: A Cancer Journal for Clinicians, 61,* 327–359. doi:10.3322/caac.20128

Wender, R., Fontham, E.T.H., Barrera, E., Jr., Colditz, G.A., Church, T.R., Ettinger, D.S., ... Smith, R.A. (2013). American Cancer Society lung cancer screening guidelines. *CA: A Cancer Journal for Clinicians, 63,* 106–117. doi:10.3322/caac.21172

Chapter 5 Study Questions

1. What would be the primary purpose of gathering data on a patient's personal colorectal cancer risk?
   A. To determine appropriate colon cancer screening and primary prevention guidelines
   B. To convince the patient he needs a colonoscopy
   C. To convince the patient to have his siblings undergo a colonoscopy
   D. To determine if the patient can obtain more life insurance

2. The nurse reviews the risk assessment for a 41-year-old woman. The patient's sister and mother have been diagnosed with breast cancer, but a mutation cannot be identified in the family. The patient's lifetime risk of developing breast cancer is estimated to be 32% by the Gail model. Which of the following would be appropriate to consider?
   A. Mammography every six months
   B. Adding breast magnetic resonance imaging (MRI) alternating with mammography every other year
   C. MRI instead of mammography every year
   D. Mammography alternating with breast MRI every six months

3. The nurse considers whether a 57-year-old man should be offered lung cancer screening. He has a 40-pack-year smoking history. Based on the risk factor assessment, it should be anticipated that the patient should have which of the following?
   A. Annual chest x-ray
   B. Annual low-dose computed tomography
   C. Annual chest MRI
   D. Annual sputum cytology

4. Which one of the following people would have the highest risk for developing skin cancer?
   A. A 15-year-old African American student
   B. A 30-year-old Asian teacher
   C. A 70-year-old Hispanic factory worker
   D. A 75-year-old Caucasian wheat farmer from the Midwest

5. Which of the following is a major risk factor for cervical cancer?
   A. Obesity
   B. History of breast cancer
   C. History of a human papillomavirus infection
   D. Skipping a pelvic examination for three years

CHAPTER

6 Pharmacogenomics

Christopher L. Farrell, PhD

Introduction

Many of the traditional chemotherapy agents used in the treatment of cancer are nonspecific and have narrow therapeutic windows with frequent side effects and toxicities. Doses of these agents needed to eradicate malignant cells also can damage normal cells. In addition, patients respond differently to the same drugs and dosages because of genetic variability in both tumor and normal cells. In an effort to develop more effective treatment with improved outcomes, healthcare providers are increasingly using personalized cancer therapy so that chemotherapy agents can better target tumor cells. This emphasizes the need for oncology nurses to understand how drugs work, why they need to assess for unusual responses found in patients receiving the same medications, and the role of an individual gene or multiple genes in cancer therapy (Petros & Evans, 2004). This chapter will review terminology relevant to pharmacogenomics, categories of drug responses attributable to genetic variances, and implications for nurses in the oncology setting.

History

Pythagoras first noted the variable responses that individuals have to medication, and even food, in 510 BC. Fava beans were a dietary staple for people in his region of Egypt. Although most individuals had no reaction to the beans, a few developed hematuria. The problem was not understood at the time, but it is now known that the blood in the urine was caused by a deficiency of the glucose-6-phosphate dehydrogenase (known as G6PD) enzyme (Deye & Magill, 2014; Sweeney, 2005). This deficiency affects approximately 14% of African Americans, causing African American soldiers serving in World War II to develop hemolysis and hematuria when receiving primaquine to prevent malaria, a common disease in many areas where combat had occurred (Deye & Magill, 2014; Sweeney, 2005).

In 1902, using Mendelian genetics (basic concepts describing transmission of inheritance from parent to child), Archibald Garrod was the first to hypothesize that a human gene could determine if an individual would respond positively or negatively to the ingestion of chemical substances. In the 1940s, researchers discovered the link between isoniazid and peripheral neuropathy (Mancinelli, Cronin, & Sadée, 2000). In 1957, researchers identified the link between administration of the anesthetic agent succinylcholine and acetyl cholinesterase deficiency, causing prolonged paralysis after administration. Two years later, "slow acetylators" (slow metabolizers) were identified in patient populations. Also in 1959, Friedrich Vogel coined the term *pharmacogenetics*. In 1962, an article was published that linked pharmacology and genetics with research describing the difference between phenylthiocarbamide "non-tasters" and "tasters" (Sweeney, 2005). For cancer treatment, the first polymorphism associated with chemotherapy treatment occurred in the early 1980s, when it was discovered that variants of the *TPMT* gene in patients with leukemia caused toxicity when they were treated with thiopurine drugs (Weinshilboum & Sladek, 1980). In the same decade, researchers identified that the activation of certain proteins in the tumor cells through somatic alterations caused an increase in the promotion of cancer growth. Discovery of these activating proteins led to the development of two drugs that were able to target the activating or oncogenic proteins in tumor cells. Trastuzumab, a DNA-derived, humanized monoclonal antibody, was the first biologic drug to target an activating protein in breast cancer cells. This drug was identified in clinical trials to increase the survival for many patients with breast cancer and received U.S. Food and Drug Administration approval in 1998 (Kumar & Badve, 2008). Imatinib, a tyrosine kinase inhibitor, was another targeted therapy found to inhibit the activity of an abnormal fusion protein, *BCR-ABL*, in the tumor cells of patients with leukemia (Wong & Witte, 2004). This tyrosine kinase inhibitor treatment received U.S. Food and Drug Administration approval in 2001. Since then, the study of pharmacogenetics has led to pharmacogenomics in cancer therapy, where researchers and clinicians are discovering countless polymorphisms and somatic variants associated with interindividual variability (Mancinelli et al., 2000; Motulsky & Qi, 2006; Sweeney, 2005).

Pharmacogenetics and Pharmacogenomics

Pharmacogenetics and *pharmacogenomics* are terms often used when describing the variation of a drug response based on a patient's DNA. The term *pharmacogenetics* describes a study for a specific gene or set of genes involved in a drug response. With advancing technology in detecting genetic markers, pharmacogenomics has become an emerging field of genomic medicine in which healthcare professionals can use the patient's whole genome to identify the appropriate drug therapy. Because a single gene rarely causes most drug responses, a comprehensive approach of scanning the entire genome in combination with environmental influences is a better method to personalize the treatment. To better understand the role of pharmacogenomics in oncology nursing, it is important to review key terminology and concepts (Howington, Riddlesperger, & Cheek, 2011).

With the completion of the human genome sequencing project in 2003, researchers and clinicians now understand that more than 99.9% of all genetic material is identical. Differences among individuals are caused by less than 0.1% of a person's DNA (Collins, Guyer, & Chakravarti, 1997). The basic components of the DNA sequence are a phosphate group, sugars, and four nucleotides—adenine, cytosine, guanine, and thymine (also referred to as the letters A, C, G, and T). Phosphate groups and sugars make up the backbone of the DNA. The nucleotides are bound to these sugars through bonds to form a single strand. For DNA to form a double-strand helix, two opposite strands have to bind together through the attachment of nucleotides, which is referred to as *base pairing*. This base pairing occurs with the joining of adenine and thymine, as well as the binding of the cytosine and guanine (Watson & Crick, 1954).

The sequences of the DNA are broken into genes, which hold the information for the protein sequences. The structure of a gene sequence consists of exons, introns, and promoter regions. The exons, or coding regions, contain the genetic information needed for the protein sequence. The introns are the spaces found between the exons of a gene. The promoter region plays an important role in initiating the process for sending the message of protein translation (Smale & Kadonaga, 2003). The process of translating the DNA to a protein starts with the unwinding of the DNA helix. The DNA is then separated into single strands, and an enzyme, called an RNA polymerase, attaches to the promoter region (see Figure 6-1). The nucleotides are transcribed into messenger RNA (mRNA), and thymine in the mRNA is replaced by uracil (U). Once the message is complete, the mRNA is released (expressed) from the DNA as a single-stranded sequence with the exon and intron segments. The intron segments are then removed through a splicing process. Once the splicing process is complete, the mRNA containing only the exon sequences is ready for translation (Clancy & Brown, 2008).

The strand of mRNA is read in triplets (called codons); for example, "AUCCGTATA" is read as "AUC CGT ATA," translated by ribosome complex into strings of amino acids, which are cut by enzymes once the protein sequence is complete (National Institutes of Health National Institute of General Medical Sciences, 2012). The "codon spelling" of amino acids can have several or only one triplet spelling (Algorithmic Arts, 2006) (see Table 6-1).

Polymorphisms are the genetic changes that make the population diverse and also cause every individual to have a unique genomic sequence. Several different types of polymorphisms exist, such as single nucleotide polymorphisms (SNPs, pronounced "snips"), copy number variants, and repeated sequences (Gonzaga-Jauregui, Lupski, & Gibbs, 2012). A SNP is a single nucleotide change that occurs in a particular position of the DNA sequence. This could be the difference of adenine replaced by thymine, or cytosine replaced by guanine, on the genomic sequence. These simple changes could have great or limited effect based on where the nucleotide substitution occurs in the triplet codon or the type of nucleotide change (Hicks, Wheeler, Plon, & Kimmel, 2011). For example, if the following sentence "THE BIG FAT CAT ATE THE RAT" is used as the triplet codon spelling for a protein, a SNP change could lead to "THE BIG F*I*T CAT ATE THE RAT." A small change in the meaning occurred, but the end result is still the same; the amino acid and thus the pro-

Figure 6-1. Central Dogma of Biology

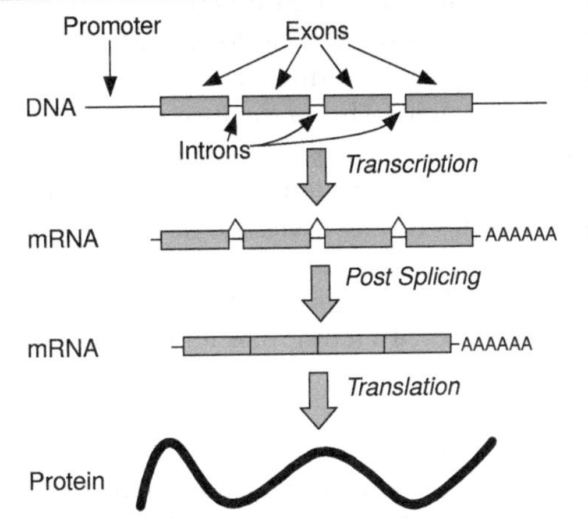

DNA—deoxyribonucleic acid; mRNA—messenger ribonucleic acid

Note. Based on information from Crick, 1970.

Table 6-1. Examples of Codon Spelling for Some Amino Acids

Amino Acid	Codon Spelling
Leucine	CTT, CTC, CTA, CTG, TTA, TTG
"Start amino acid assembly" message and methionine	ATG
Tyrosine	TAT, TAC
Tryptophan	TGG
Threonine	ACT, ACC, ACA, ACG
"Stop or termination" message for amino acid assembly	TAA, TAG, TGA

Note. Based on information from Algorithmic Arts, 2006.

tein do not change. (Remember, amino acids may have several codon spellings.) When the protein sequence is unaffected by the change, this is referred to as a *silent* or *nonsynonymous* variant (see Table 6-2). When a SNP leads to an amino acid substitution, this is referred to as a *missense variant.* Based on the type of amino acid change, a missense variant may have a major impact on protein function or no effect at all. A SNP also may lead to an early termination in the protein sequence, which results in a smaller protein. The premature stop, or nonsense variant, has the potential of causing a devastating effect on protein activity. For example, the protein with the nonsense variant could be so small that it is nonfunctional. SNPs can also be observed as a single deletion in the nucleotide sequence. Deleting one letter could alter the message to "THE BIG FTC ATA TET HER AT." Everything shifts, and that sentence (protein) does not make sense. The addition of a SNP creates a similar problem. The protein goes from "THE BIG FAT CAT ATE THE RAT" to "TBH EBI GFA TCA TAT ETH ERA T," again creating an abnormal protein. Abnormal proteins do not function appropriately, and a variety of outcomes are problematic to the human biologic system, such as a variable response or idiosyncratic reaction (Pepper, 2005). All reference SNPs are cataloged by the Short Genetic Variations database, known as dbSNP (Sherry, Ward, & Sirotkin, 1999). The SNPs in this database are given a reference ID number or rs number. For example, the CYP 450s are a group of heme-conforming enzymes responsible for phase I metabolic reactions. The *CYP2D6* gene has a SNP in the coding region referenced as rs28371703.

Table 6-2. Examples of Variants

Type of Variant	Example of Changes
Missense	TPMT*3B (alanine 154 → threonine)
Nonsense	CYP2D6—rs147960066 (arginine 293 → STOP)
Silent	CYP2C19—rs17885098 (arginine 227 → arginine)
Insertion	CYP2D6—rs4244285 (tryptophan 152 → X)
Deletion	CYP2D6—rs35742686 (arginine 237 → X)

Note. Based on information from PharmGKB, n.d.

Copy number variants are larger deletions or insertions in the genomic sequence. Deletion of a gene causes the individual to only have one gene copy and can result in decreased protein activity. Having more than two gene copies, also referred to as *gene duplication,* causes an increase in the activity of the encoded protein (Gonzaga-Jauregui et al., 2012).

Repeated sequences, or *microsatellites,* consist of one to six nucleotides observed in a repetitive pattern along the DNA sequence. These repeated sequences are informative as a DNA fingerprint in forensic science, but in medicine the repeats may affect protein activity in two ways. When a change is observed in the promoter region, or intron, of the gene, the length of the repeats could potentially reduce the expression of the gene, causing lower protein activity in the cell. Repeated sequences also can affect the coding sequence, which could lead to devastating results, such as a deletion or insertion in the sequence, as seen in certain inherited diseases (Gonzaga-Jauregui et al., 2012).

Pharmacokinetics and Pharmacodynamics

The sequencing of the human genome in 2003 has affected two processes common to pharmacology. *Pharmacokinetics* (PK) focuses on the movement of drugs in the body from entrance to exit by studying the absorption, distribution, metabolism, and excretion of the drug. Absorption describes how much drug is available in the vascular system for distribution and use by the cells. Enzymes participate in the metabolic transformation of the drug structure by changing it into an active or inactive form. The drug and its metabolites are removed from the body via excretion. Thus, PK determines the concentration of drug available for attachment to the targeted proteins and the uptake of the drug by the cells. Any genetic variation to the PK process can affect how an individual will respond to medication; this could lead to a decrease in efficacy or an increase in side effects (Evans & McCleod, 2003; Farinde, 2016; Lee, Lockhart, Kim, & Rothenberg, 2005).

Pharmacodynamics (PD) is the study of what a drug does to the body through the binding of direct and indirect targets. These targets include receptors, enzymes, signal proteins, and other interactions. Physiologic changes influenced by disorders, aging, and other drugs can affect the PD. Genetic variation in cancer also can change the PD through receptor binding (such as *BCR-ABL* translocation), increased levels of binding proteins (such as HER2/neu overexpression), and decreased receptor sensitivity (Farinde, 2016) (see Figure 6-2).

Drug metabolism converts foreign substances, known as *xenobiotics*, into active drug or water-soluble metabolites that are more easily excreted (Sweeney, 2005). Typically, the pathways of metabolism are classified as either phase I or phase II. Phase II reactions are typically responsible for detoxification (or inactivation) of drugs and other ingested molecules, whereas the phase I pathway consists of oxidation, reduction, and hydrolysis and includes the P450 enzymes. In most cases, these reactions lead to the active metabolism of drugs (Sarlis & Gourgiotis, 2005).

Figure 6-2. Factors Contributing to Response of a Drug

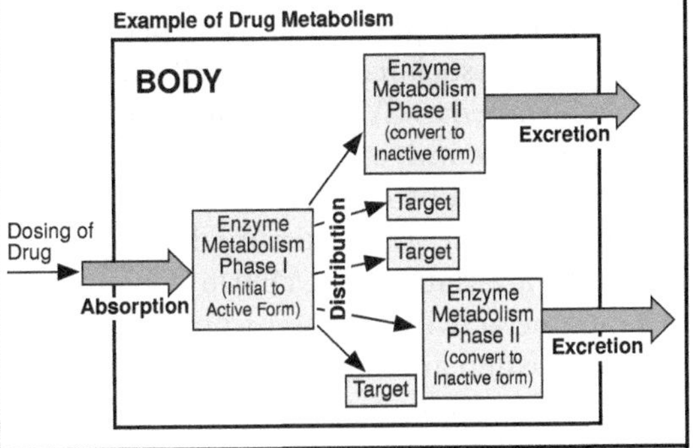

Note. Based on information from Undevia et al., 2005.

Cytochrome P450 Metabolizers

A cytochrome is a class of hemoprotein involved in electron transport that enables drug metabolism. The cytochrome P450 (CYP) system is a superfamily of enzymes and the most important enzymes that catalyze phase I reactions (Sweeney, 2005). Enzymes are types of proteins primarily located in the membranes of the smooth endoplasmic reticulum in the liver, small intestine, lungs, and kidneys. As noted earlier, these enzymes can be changed as a result of genetic variation. In the oncology setting, the P450 cytochromes (a) include key enzymes involved in cancer formation because of their ability to mediate metabolic activation of precarcinogens, (b) participate in the metabolism of different cancer treatments, and (c) have the ability to both inhibit and induce anticancer drugs (Rodriguez-Antona & Ingelman-Sundberg, 2006). This group of metabolic enzymes has a classification system to help identify which family of cytochromes is involved in the response of a specific drug.

Fifty-seven of the CYP genes are designated as individual families based on their similarity in the positions of amino acids (Sweeney, 2005). The CYP label indicates a human cytochrome. This designation is followed by the family number (CYP1, CYP2), a capital letter for the subfamily (CYP2A), and a second number to identify the gene coding the enzyme (CYP2A3). The most common type is designated as *1 (e.g., CYP2A3*1). Any other variation is assigned *2, *3, and so on, depending on the number of SNPs that have been identified in the gene. If an unexpected drug response is associated with a SNP variation, it would be noted as CYP2A3*2, or for a different drug response with another SNP variation, the notation would be CYP2A3*3. For example, a recent research study identified that individuals with a variation in CYP2D6*4 had low or no enzyme activity. Women who were treated with tamoxifen and possessed this variant were found to be at a higher risk for a relapse (Wegman et al., 2007).

The CYP enzymes have the ability to activate or inactivate drugs. A CYP enzyme with the ability to "inhibit" will prevent or decrease the activity of the drug. This means if the drug is not degraded or inactivated, more drug is available, which may cause increased toxicities for the patient. Other CYP enzymes "induce," or increase the enzyme activity. If more of the drug is deactivated, then less of the drug is available for therapeutic effect. If it is a chemotherapy agent, the patient may receive a lesser amount of the drug than needed to combat the cancer (Pepper, 2005; Roden et al., 2006) (see Table 6-3).

Non-Cytochrome P450 Metabolizers

The SNPs in genes can code for other metabolizing drug enzymes besides the CYP enzymes. Two non-CYP drug-metabolizing proteins include a phase I metabolizer, dihydropyrimidine dehydrogenase (DPD), and a phase II metabolizer, thiopurine methyltransferase (TPMT). Like the CYP enzymes, these can affect the toxicities and efficacy of anticancer drugs and their side effects (Diasio, Beavers, & Carpenter, 1988; Salonga et al., 2000; Tai, Krynetski, Schuetz, Yanishevski, & Evans, 1997).

A commonly used chemotherapy agent, 5-fluorouracil (5-FU), is inactivated to a metabolite by the DPD enzyme coded from *DYPD.* The activity of this gene product (enzyme) has been associated with up to 20-fold differences in drug metabolism among humans. The DYPD*2A is found over the exon–intron junction (referred to as a *splice site modification*) and is associated with low (heterozygous—one allele has *2A) or no (homozygous—both alleles have *2A) enzyme activity. Patients with low or no enzyme activity who are treated with 5-FU will accumulate active metabolites, causing a significantly greater risk of hematopoietic, neurologic, and gastrointestinal toxicities, which can be fatal. Genetic testing for the gene causing the enzyme deficiency prior to receiving 5-FU treatment is commercially available (Sadée & Dai, 2005).

As a phase II metabolizing drug, 6-mercaptopurine (6-MP) is catalyzed by TPMT to form inactive metabolites so that antimetabolites do not incorporate into the DNA or RNA of healthy cells. Three main variants (*3A, *3B, and *3C) are associated with low levels of TPMT enzymatic activity. If a patient possesses one of these variants (heterozygous), less drug degradation and increased toxicities will occur and the patient would need some reduction in dosage. If the patient has two of the same variants (homozygosity), he or she may require significant dose reductions or alternative treatment options (Relling et al., 2011). In the United States, 10% of Caucasians and African Americans have intermediate (heterozygous) TPMT activity. One in 300 individuals has low or undetectable (homozygous) TPMT activity (Weinshilboum & Wang, 2004). Applying this information to a patient situation, a young child being treated for acute lymphoblastic leukemia could receive 6-MP. If this child has low TPMT enzyme activity, life-threatening neutropenia and thrombocytopenia could occur (Maitland, Vasisht, & Ratain, 2006). Prospective genetic testing is available to identify members of this at-risk population. Children who experience myelosuppression after their initial dose of

Table 6-3. Changes in Oncology Drug Response Based on Cytochromes and Single Nucleotide Polymorphisms

Metabolic Activity	Enzymes and/or Gene Symbols	Single Nucleotide Polymorphisms (SNPs)	Effect on Drug Response
Phase I	*CYP 2D6*† *CYP 2C9*† *CYP 2C19* *CYP 3A5* *CYP 2B6*† *CYP 2E1*	Numerous and frequent functional polymorphisms (e.g., CYP2D6*3, CYP2D6*4, and CYP2D6*10 or CYP3A5*1 and CYP3A5*5)	Metabolism of CYP substrates varies with enzyme specificity. Ethnic groups have varying allele frequencies. Decreased sensitivity to tamoxifen dosing occurs if CYP2D6 activity is poor.
	Dihydropyrimidine dehydrogenase (*DYPD*)	Multiple polymorphisms including DYPD*2A	*2A increases 5-FU toxicity.
Phase II	Thiopurine methyltransferase (*TPMT*)†	Multiple polymorphisms including TPMT*3A, *3B, and *3C	Hematopoietic 6-MP toxicity in homozygous individuals (found in 1 of 300 individuals)
	UDP-glycosyltransferase 1A1 (*UGT1A1*)†	Multiple polymorphisms including UGT1A1*28	Increased irinotecan toxicity Dose-limiting diarrhea and leukopenia Increased unconjugated serum bilirubin
Drug transport	Multidrug resistant gene 1 (*ABCB1*)†	Multiple polymorphisms	Higher altered drug transport activity Poor patient outcomes
	Breast cancer–related protein (*BCRP*) (also known as *ABCG2*)	Polymorphisms such as rs2622604 and a deletion	Enhanced drug sensitivity (e.g., irinotecan and gefitinib)
Drug targets/ pathway	Methylenetetrahydrofolate reductase (*MTHFR*)	rs1801131 and rs1801133	Increased toxicity to methotrexate
	BCR-ABL translocation (t[9;22])†	Translocation of chromosome 9 to 22 (Philadelphia chromosome)	In chronic myeloid leukemia, Philadelphia chromosome responds to imatinib mesylate.
	HER2/neu (*ERBB2*)†	Overexpression of protein	Breast cancers with overexpression of *ERBB2* respond to trastuzumab.
	Epidermal growth factor receptor (*EGFR*)†	Mutations	Lung cancers with mutations respond to gefitinib.

* Genetic variant, SNP

† Genotyping tests for genes or protein are used in clinical practice or under consideration.

Note. Based on information from Higgins et al., 2009; Nakagawa et al., 2006; Petros & Evans, 2004; Sadée & Dai, 2005.

6-MP should be considered for genetic testing (Sadée & Dai, 2005).

Another phase II metabolizer, UDP-glycosyltransferase 1A1 (UGT1A1), is associated with devastating toxicities for patients who are either homozygous or heterozygous for the UGT1A1*28 allele. This variant is a sequence of seven TA nucleotide repeats in the promoter region of the *UGT1A1* gene versus the six repeats in the wild-type sequence. Individuals with the variant can have 1,000-fold greater inhibition of topoisomerase, causing diarrhea and leukopenia when dosed with irinotecan. In addition, unconjugated serum bilirubin levels are increased. Genetic testing is available, but it has not been confirmed that dose reduction based on test results will not affect the efficacy of treatment (Gold, Hall, Blinder, & Schackman, 2009; Petros & Evans, 2004) (see Table 6-4).

Drug Transport and Other Metabolic Protein Genes

Polymorphisms in drug transporter genes also can affect outcomes of intracellular transport. Membrane proteins facilitate passage of many naturally derived toxins, including anticancer drugs. One of these transporters is the multidrug resistance gene *ABCB1*, which encodes the P-glycoprotein found on the membrane of the cell. This protein pumps lipophilic compounds such as anthracycline, taxane, and vinca alkaloid anticancer drugs out of the cell. P-glycoprotein, also referred to as MDR1 (multidrug resistant 1), is responsible for reducing intestinal absorption and brain uptake while increasing drug excretion via the biliary, intestinal, and renal routes. Several SNPs in P-glycoprotein have been associated with variations in drug response, but the results have been conflicting (Hoffmeyer et al., 2000; Morita, Yasumori, & Nakayama, 2003).

Breast cancer resistant protein (BCRP) is another transporter that may affect the drug response of cancer agents, such as methotrexate, gefitinib, and irinotecan metabolite (SN-38) (Cusatis & Sparreboom, 2008; Han, Lim, Park, Lee, & Lee, 2009). BCRP is encoded by the

Table 6-4. Necessity of Pharmacogenetic Testing for Some Approved Oncology Agents

Pharmacogenetic Biomarker	Cancer Target	Oncology Agent
Tests Required Prior to Treatment		
EGFR expression	Metastatic colon cancer, head and neck cancer	Cetuximab
HER2 overexpression	Breast cancer	Trastuzumab
Presence of Philadelphia chromosome	Chronic myeloid leukemia	Dasatinib
Tests Recommended for Treatment Decision		
TPMT variants	Acute lymphoblastic leukemia, acute myeloid leukemia	Mercaptopurine, thioguanine
UGT1A1 variants	Colorectal cancer	Irinotecan
Tests for Information Only		
c-Kit expression	Kit+ gastrointestinal stromal tumors	Imatinib
CYP2D6 variants	Breast cancer	Tamoxifen
DPD deficiency	Colorectal or breast cancers	Capecitabine, 5-fluorouracil
Philadelphia chromosome deficiency	Chronic myeloid leukemia	Busulfan
PML/RAR gene expression	Promyelocytic leukemia	Tretinoin

Note. Based on information from U.S. Food and Drug Administration, 2016.

ABCG2 gene and expressed in many of the same areas as P-glycoprotein. This transporter protein is also expressed in the placenta as a protective mechanism for the fetus that removes toxins and foreign agents. The SNP rs2622604 has been associated with adverse reactions to gefitinib and irinotecan metabolite (SN-38). Patients receiving either of these cancer agents have reactions, such as diarrhea. These genes can be identified using routine laboratory assays, but the application in clinical practice is still under consideration (Petros & Evans, 2004; Sadée & Dai, 2005). Finally, drug transport and its effect on signaling pathways is another important mechanism that can affect patient outcomes. One example is the enzymatic target of methotrexate, methylenetetrahydrofolate reductase, the gene product of the *MTHFR* gene. The SNPs rs1801131 and rs1801133 are associated with methotrexate toxicity (Song, Bae, & Lee, 2014). About 10% of the Caucasian population can have a *MTHFR* variant genotype that causes reduced enzyme function and increased toxicity when receiving methotrexate. These toxicities may include cardiovascular, neurologic, dermatologic, hematologic, hepatic, and gastrointestinal symptoms. Depending on the genotype identified in genetic testing, dose reductions may be recommended for children with acute lymphoblastic leukemia (Donnelly, 2004; Krajinovic et al., 2004) (see Table 6-4).

Nursing Implications

Pharmacogenomics is an emerging field with important implications for oncology nurses. Because nurses have the most contact with their patients, they play an important role as educators in explaining how genetic variants may influence the efficacy or side effects of a drug therapy. Education on pharmacogenomics will be a challenge for nurses. They will need to be able to explain the complex concepts to individuals who are unfamiliar or uneducated in the area of genetic medicine.

Assessment information about the patient should include questions about previous problems with a poor or unusual response to any drugs or a family history of similar responses to these drugs. Individuals with no response to treatment, nonresponders, will require additional support and may be treated differently for their cancer or medication side effects. Nurses will need to be aware of these potential nonresponders so that these patients do not die or have serious adverse reactions to the drug therapy.

Another concern is patient insurability. The Genetic Information Nondiscrimination Act of 2008 prevents employers and insurance companies from discriminating based on genetic information, but this has focused on diseases and disorders. How will it affect insurability when nonresponders require a more expensive drug because of a genetic variation? Questions will arise for nurses regarding how to advocate and explain the sometimes-confusing governmental policy statements (U.S. Department of Health and Human Services, 2009). Monitoring changing policies, both state and federal, will become increasingly important for nurses to provide answers for patients who test positive for a genetic variation.

Education regarding prevention through genetic testing will become a component of parenting. Children may begin to be tested for allelic variations that will affect their responses to drugs. Policies will need to be developed to identify the ethical implications for testing adolescents and children aged 18 and younger. Informed consent and confidentiality issues will be paramount to protecting patients' rights.

Finally, what are the implications for SNPs with uncertain significance (i.e., not enough data are available to know whether they are associated with a condition or just an individual trait) that are later identified to be associated with risk for a disease? Who is responsible for contacting these individuals, who may not have been seen for 30 years since the initial testing? Who is responsible for their counseling and follow-up care? These issues will need to be addressed by the healthcare providers who are caring for patients and families, even outside the oncology setting.

Conclusion

This chapter provided a simple introduction to a complex subject that is becoming important in the day-to-day pharmacologic care of patients with cancer. The history and basic concepts of pharmacogenomics and pharmacogenetics were presented, the principles of PK and PD were discussed, and a brief explanation of the cytochrome nomenclature was provided with a short review of the phases of drug metabolism as applicable to drugs used in the oncology setting. Drugs were identified for which genetic testing is currently available or under development, with rationale for directing the care of the patient. Finally, a discussion of the need for nurses to be advocates for patients, as pharmacogenomics and pharmacogenetics become more predominant in oncology, was emphasized. Genetics is an increasingly complex field of medicine. Nurses need to understand basic pharmacogenomics in order to educate patients about the importance of family history of typical and unexpected drug responses, the rationale for differences in drugs and drug doses between patients with the same cancer diagnosis, and the need to report unexpected side effects.

The author would like to acknowledge Julia Eggert, PhD, RN, AGN-BC, GNP, AOCN®, FAAN, for her contribution to this chapter that remains unchanged from the first edition of this book.

Key Points

- *Pharmacogenomics* is a term used to describe the tailoring of medication based on the patient's whole genome.
- Oncology nurses need to be familiar with the key genetic terminology such as polymorphisms/variants and the concepts of transcription and translation.
- Pharmacokinetics describe the absorption, distribution, metabolism, and excretion of drugs through the individual's body, and pharmacodynamics explain how the patient responds to the treatment when a drug binds to direct and indirect targets.
- The CYP enzymes are able to catalyze the phase I drug reactions for different treatments, including cancer treatment, and also have the ability to both inhibit and induce anticancer drugs.
- DPD, a phase I non-CYP enzyme, normally inactivates 5-FU, causing lower adverse effects to patients, but patients with DYPD*2A have lower enzyme activity, which leads to higher toxicity of the drug therapy.
- TPMT, a phase II drug metabolizing enzyme, inactivates 6-MP into an inactive metabolite, but patients with TPMT*3A, TPMT*3B, or TPMT*3C have low levels of TPMT enzymatic activity, which is associated with higher toxicity of 6-MP.
- UDP-glycosyltransferase 1A1 (UGT1A1) is associated with devastating toxicities for patients who are either homozygous or heterozygous for the UGT1A1*28 allele when dosed with irinotecan.
- Protein transporter genes such as *ABCB1* and *ABCG2* also can affect the efficacy of chemotherapy agents through variants in these genes.
- The *MTHFR* gene, which encodes for methylenetetrahydrofolate reductase, has two SNPs, rs1801131 and rs1801133, which are associated with methotrexate toxicity.
- Nurses need a basic understanding of pharmacogenomics in order to educate patients about the associated genetic variations and drug responses.

References

Algorithmic Arts. (2006). 20 amino acids, their single-letter data-base codes (SLC), and their corresponding DNA codons. Retrieved from http://algoart.com/aatable.htm

Clancy, S., & Brown, W. (2008). Translation: DNA to mRNA to protein. *Nature Education, 1,* 101.

Collins, F.S., Guyer, M.S., & Chakravarti, A. (1997). Variations on a theme: Cataloging human DNA sequence variation. *Science, 278,* 1580–1581. doi:10.1126/science.278.5343.1580

Crick, F. (1970). Central dogma of molecular biology. *Nature, 227,* 561–563. doi:10.1038/227561a0

Cusatis, G., & Sparreboom, A. (2008). Pharmacogenomic importance of *ABCG2. Pharmacogenomics, 9,* 1005–1009. doi:10.2217/14622416.9.8.1005

Deye, G.A., & Magill, A.J. (2014). Primaquine for prophylaxis of malaria: Has the CYP sailed? *Journal of Travel Medicine, 21,* 67–69. doi:10.1111/jtm.12080

Diasio, R.B., Beavers, T.L., & Carpenter, J.T. (1988). Familial deficiency of dihydropyrimidine dehydrogenase. Biochemical basis for familial pyrimidinemia and severe 5-fluorouracil-induced toxicity. *Journal of Clinical Investigation, 81,* 47–51. doi:10.1172/JCI113308

Donnelly, J.G. (2004). Pharmacogenetics in cancer chemotherapy: Balancing toxicity and response. *Therapeutic Drug Monitoring, 26,* 231–235. doi:10.1097/00007691-200404000-00026

Evans, W.E., & McCleod, H.L. (2003). Pharmacogenomics—Drug disposition, drug targets, and side effects. *New England Journal of Medicine, 348,* 538–549. doi:10.1056/NEJMra020526

Farinde, A. (2016). Overview of pharmacodynamics. In *The Merck manual of diagnosis and therapy.* Retrieved from http://www.merck.com/mmpe/sec20/ch304/ch304a.html

Gold, H.T., Hall, M.J., Blinder, V., & Schackman, B.R. (2009). Cost effectiveness of pharmacogenetic testing for uridine diphosphate glucuronosyltransferase 1A1 before irinotecan administration for metastatic colorectal cancer. *Cancer, 115,* 3858–3867. doi:10.1002/cncr.24428

Gonzaga-Jauregui, C., Lupski, J.R., & Gibbs, R.A. (2012). Human genome sequencing in health and disease. *Annual Review of Medicine, 63,* 35–61. doi:10.1146/annurev-med-051010-162644

Han, J.-Y., Lim, H.S., Park, Y.H., Lee, S.Y., & Lee, J. (2009). Integrated pharmacogenetic prediction of irinotecan pharmacokinetics and toxicity in patients with advanced non-small cell lung cancer. *Lung Cancer, 63,* 115–120. doi:10.1016/j.lungcan.2007.12.003

Hicks, S., Wheeler, D.A., Plon, S.E., & Kimmel, M. (2011). Prediction of missense mutation functionality depends on both the algorithm and sequence alignment employed. *Human Mutation, 32,* 661–668. doi:10.1002/humu.21490

Higgins, M.J., Rae, J.M., Flockhart, D.A., Hayes, D.F., & Stearns, V. (2009). Pharmacogenetics of tamoxifen: Who should undergo CYPD6 genetic testing? *Journal of the National Comprehensive Cancer Network, 7,* 203–213. Retrieved from http://www.jnccn.org/content/7/2/203.long

Hoffmeyer, S., Burk, O., Von Richter, O., Arnold, H.P., Brockmöller, J., Johne, A., ... Brinkmann, U. (2000). Functional polymorphisms of the human multidrug-resistance gene: Multiple sequence variations and correlation of one allele with P-glycoprotein expression and activity *invivo. Proceedings of the National Academy of Sciences of the United States of America, 7,* 3473–3478. doi:10.1073/pnas.050585397

Howington, L., Riddlesperger, K., & Cheek, D.J. (2011). Essential nursing competencies for genetics and genomics: Implications for critical care. *Critical Care Nurse, 31,* e1–e7. doi:10.4037/ccn2011867

Krajinovic, M., Lemieux-Blanchard, E., Chiasson, S., Primeau, M., Costea, I., & Moghrabi, A. (2004). Role of polymorphisms in MTHFR and MTHFD1 genes in the outcome of childhood acute lymphoblastic leukemia. *Pharmacogenomics Journal, 4,* 66–72. doi:10.1038/sj.tpj.6500224

Kumar, G.L., & Badve, S.S. (2008). Milestones in the discovery of HER2 proto-oncogene and trastuzumab (Herceptin™). *Connection, 13,* 9–14.

Lee, W., Lockhart, A.C., Kim, R.B., & Rothenberg, M.L. (2005). Cancer pharmacogenomics: Powerful tools in cancer chemotherapy and drug development. *Oncologist, 10,* 104–111. doi:10.1634/theoncologist.10-2-104

Maitland, M.L., Vasisht, K., & Ratain, M.J. (2006). *TPMT, UGT1A1* and *DPYD*: Genotyping to ensure safer cancer therapy? *Trends in Pharmacological Sciences, 27,* 432–437. doi:10.1016/j.tips.2006.06.007

Mancinelli, L., Cronin, M., & Sadée, W. (2000). Pharmacogenomics: The promise of personalized medicine. *AAPS Journal, 2,* 29–41. doi:10.1208/ps020104

Morita, N., Yasumori, T., & Nakayama, K. (2003). Human MDR1 polymorphism: G2677T/A and C3435T have no effect on MDR1 transport activities. *Biochemical Pharmacology, 65,* 1843–1852. doi:10.1016/S0006-2952(03)00178-3

Motulsky, A.G., & Qi, M. (2006). Pharmacogenetics, pharmacogenomics and ecogenetics. *Journal of Zhejiang University—Science B, 7,* 169–170. doi:10.1631/jzus.2006.B0169

Nakagawa, H., Saito, H., Ikegami, Y., Aida-Hyugaji, S., Sawada, S., & Ishikawa, T. (2006). Molecular modeling of new camptothecin analogues to circumvent ABCG2-mediated drug resistance in cancer. *Cancer Letters, 234,* 31–39. doi:10.1016/j.canlet.2005.05.052

National Institutes of Health National Institute of General Medical Sciences. (2012). Studying genes. Retrieved from https://www.nigms.nih.gov/education/pages/factsheet_studyinggenes.aspx

Pepper, G.A. (2005). Pharmacokinetics and pharmacodynamics. In E.Q. Youngkin, K.J. Sawin, J.F. Kissinger, & D.S. Israel (Eds.), *Pharmacotherapeutics: A primary care clinical guide* (2nd ed., pp. 7–42). Upper Saddle River, NJ: Pearson Prentice Hall.

Petros, W.P., & Evans, W.E. (2004). Pharmacogenomics in cancer therapy: Is host genome variability important? *Trends in Pharmacological Sciences, 25,* 457–464. doi:10.1016/j.tips.2004.07.007

PharmGKB. (n.d.). The Pharmacogenetics Knowledge Base. Retrieved from http://www.pharmgkb.org

Relling, M.V., Gardner, E.E., Sandborn, W.J., Schmiegelow, K., Pui, C.-H., Yee, S.W., ... Klein, T.E. (2011). Clinical Pharmacogenetics Implementation Consortium guidelines for thiopurine methyltransferase genotype and thiopurine dosing. *Clinical Pharmacology and Therapeutics, 89,* 387–391. doi:10.1038/clpt.2010.320

Roden, D.M., Altman, R.B., Benowitz, N.L., Flockhart, D.A., Giacomini, K.M., Johnson, J.A., ... Weiss, S.T. (2006). Pharmacogenomics: Challenges and opportunities. *Annals of Internal Medicine, 145,* 749–757. doi:10.7326/0003-4819-145-10-200611210-00007

Rodriguez-Antona, C., & Ingelman-Sundberg, M. (2006). Cytochrome *P*450 pharmacogenetics and cancer. *Oncogene, 25,* 1679–1691. doi:10.1038/sj.onc.1209377

Sadée, W., & Dai, Z. (2005). Pharmacogenetics/genomics and personalized medicine. *Human Molecular Genetics, 14*(Suppl. 2), R207–R214. doi:10.1093/hmg/ddi261

Salonga, D., Danenberg, K.D., Johnson, M., Metzger, R., Groshen, S., Tsao-Wei, D.D., ... Danenberg, P.V. (2000). Colorectal tumors responding to 5-fluorouracil have low gene expression levels of dihydropyrimidine dehydrogenase, thymidylate synthase, and thymidine phosphorylase. *Clinical Cancer Research, 6,* 1322–1327. Retrieved from http://clincancerres.aacrjournals.org/content/6/4/1322.long

Sarlis, N.J., & Gourgiotis, L. (2005). Hormonal effects on drug metabolism through the CYP system: Perspectives on their potential significance in the era of pharmacogenomics. *Current Drug Targets—Immune, Endocrine and Metabolic Disorders, 5,* 439–448. doi:10.2174/1568008054774912971

Sherry, S.T., Ward, M., & Sirotkin, K. (1999). dbSNP—Database for single nucleotide polymorphisms and other classes of minor genetic variation. *Genome Research, 9,* 677–679. Retrieved from http://genome.cshlp.org/content/9/8/677.long

Smale, S.T., & Kadonaga., J.T. (2003). The RNA polymerase II core promoter. *Annual Review of Biochemistry, 72,* 449–479. doi:10.1146/annurev.biochem.72.121801.161520

Song, G.G., Bae, S.-C., & Lee, Y.H. (2014). Association of the MTHFR C677T and A1298C polymorphisms with methotrexate toxicity in rheumatoid arthritis: A meta-analysis. *Clinical Rheumatology, 33,* 1715–1724. doi:10.1007/s10067-014-2645-8

Sweeney, B.P. (2005). Pharmacogenomics: The genetic basis for variability in drug response. In J.N. Cashman & R.M. Grounds (Eds.), *Recent advances in anaesthesia and intensive care* (Vol. 23, pp. 1–34). London, England: Cambridge University Press.

Tai, H.-L., Krynetski, E.Y., Schuetz, E.G., Yanishevski, Y., & Evans, W.E. (1997). Enhanced proteolysis of thiopurine *S*-methyltransferase (TPMT) encoded by mutant alleles in humans (*TPMT*3A, TPMT*2*): Mechanisms for the genetic polymorphism of TPMT activity. *Proceedings of the National Academy of Sciences of the United States of America, 94,* 6444–6449. doi:10.1073/pnas.94.12.6444

Undevia, S.D., Gomez-Abuin, G., & Ratain, M.J. (2005). Pharmacokinetic variability of anticancer agents. *Nature Reviews Cancer, 5,* 447–458. doi:10.1038/nrc1629

U.S. Department of Health and Human Services. (2009, April 6). "GINA": The Genetic Information Nondiscrimination Act of 2008: Information for researchers and health care professionals. Retrieved from http://www.genome.gov/Pages/PolicyEthics/GeneticDiscrimination/GINAInfoDoc.pdf

U.S. Food and Drug Administration. (November 7). Table of pharmacogenomic biomarkers in drug labeling. Retrieved from http://www.fda.gov/Drugs/ScienceResearch/ResearchAreas/Pharmacogenetics/ucm083378.htm

Watson, J.D., & Crick, F.H.C. (1953). The structure of DNA. *Cold Spring Harbor Symposia on Quantitative Biology, 18,* 123–131. doi:10.1101/SQB.1953.018.01.020

Wegman, P., Elingarami, S., Carstensen, J., Stål, O., Nordenskjöld, B., & Wingren, S. (2007). Genetic variants of *CYP3A5, CYP2D6, SULT1A1, UGT2B15* and tamoxifen response in postmenopausal patients with breast cancer. *Breast Cancer Research, 9,* R7. doi:10.1186/bcr1640

Weinshilboum, R.M., & Sladek, S.L. (1980). Mercaptopurine pharmacogenetics: Monogenic inheritance of erythrocyte thiopurine methyltransferase activity. *American Journal of Human Genetics, 32,* 651–662. Retrieved from https://www.ncbi.nlm.nih.gov/pmc/articles/PMC1686086/pdf/ajhg00191-0015.pdf

Weinshilboum, R.M., & Wang, L. (2004). Pharmacogenomics: Bench to bedside. *Nature Reviews Drug Discovery, 3,* 739–748. doi:10.1038/nrd1497

Wong, S., & Witte, O.N. (2004). The BCR-ABL story: Bench to bedside and back. *Annual Review of Immunology, 22,* 247–306. doi:10.1146/annurev.immunol.22.012703.104753

Chapter 6 Study Questions

1. Which of the following genes encodes for a metabolic enzyme involved in the inactivation of irinotecan and has a polymorphism of seven TA repeats (instead of six) in the promoter region?
   A. *CYP2D6*
   B. *TPMT*
   C. *DYPD*
   D. *UGT1A1*

2. What kind of polymorphism causes the substitution of one nucleotide base for another nucleotide base and leads to a change in the protein sequence of one amino acid to another amino acid?
   A. Splice site alteration
   B. Nonsense
   C. Silent
   D. Missense

3. What important role will the oncology nurse play in tailoring treatment with genetic variants?
   A. Performing the genetic test in the laboratory
   B. Translating the genetic results to the pharmacist
   C. Educating patients about their genetic variants
   D. Identifying the panel of genetic variants for pharmacogenomic testing

4. What transporter may affect the drug response of cancer agents such as methotrexate, gefitinib, and irinotecan metabolite and possesses the polymorphism rs2622604?
   A. Breast cancer resistant protein
   B. Methylenetetrahydrofolate reductase
   C. Butyrylcholinesterase
   D. Dihydropyrimidine dehydrogenase

5. What drug is degraded by dihydropyrimidine dehydrogenase and becomes toxic in patients who possess a variant in the splice site (exon–intron modification) of the *DYPD* gene?
   A. Capecitabine
   B. 5-Fluorouracil
   C. Irinotecan
   D. Thiopurine

SECTION II

Treatment Options

CHAPTER

7 Surgery

Diane Drake, PhD, RN, and Billie Lynes, MSN, RN, FNP-C

Introduction

Surgery is the oldest and most consistently effective method to treat and cure various types of cancer. Surgical procedures are ubiquitous in cancer diagnoses, treatments, rehabilitation, and palliation. Cancer surgery is most commonly combined with nonsurgical modalities to increase survival, improve quality of life, and improve treatment outcomes for all patients.

Multidisciplinary healthcare teams specializing in surgical oncology have advanced the treatment of many cancer types, such as lung, sarcoma, breast, and colorectal. Oncology nurses are important members of patient-centered and multidisciplinary surgical oncology care teams, which often include radiologists, pathologists, surgical oncologists, general and reconstructive surgeons, medical oncologists, radiation oncologists, anesthesiologists, psycho-oncologists, rehabilitation specialists, and oncology pharmacists (Pollock, Choti, & Morton, 2010).

Advances in collaborative clinical research with surgical oncology fellowship training programs in the United States and Canada with molecular science investigations and individualized cancer treatments have introduced a new era for surgical oncology (Society of Surgical Oncology, n.d.). A look at these advances, including cancer surgery rationale, types of cancer operations, perioperative nursing considerations, and selected cancers in surgical oncology, will be explored in this chapter.

Cancer Surgery Rationale

Patients often are informed of a solid tumor cancer diagnosis by a surgeon following the results of pathologic analysis of a lesion or tumor biopsy. Confirmation of the initial pathology is recommended before new treatment. Commonly used biopsy methods include needle biopsy (fine needle aspiration [FNA] or core) with or without radiologic guidance, open incisional biopsy, and excisional biopsy (Pollock et al., 2010) (see Table 7-1). FNA is a cytologic technique using a syringe and needle to aspirate cells from a tumor. It can be performed using image-directed guidance for relatively inaccessible lesions, such as deep visceral tumors. Tissue obtained by FNA is disaggregated cells (separated without damage) rather than intact tissue; therefore, other biopsy techniques may be more appropriate (Pollock et al., 2010). Cutting-core biopsy retrieves a small piece of intact tumor tissue and is the simplest method of histologic diagnosis (not cytologic diagnosis). Cutting-core biopsy is used for subcutaneous and muscular masses, as well as for internal biopsy of the liver, kidney, and pancreas (Pollock et al., 2010). Incisional biopsy is the removal of a small portion of the tumor via surgical resection. Incisional biopsy is used for deep subcutaneous or intramuscular tumor masses when initial needle biopsy fails to establish a diagnosis. Excisional biopsy completely removes the local tumor mass with adequate margins and is used when incisional biopsy tissue was inadequate for diagnosis. The accuracy of the initial diagnosis, adequacy of evidence-based practice, and decisions made during surgical consultation initiate a cascade of events that determine cancer treatment, referrals, survival, and patient outcomes (Pollock et al., 2010). The amount of tissue received from the various types of biopsies is another consideration when sending tumors for diagnostics in external laboratories. Some smaller malignancies, such as ductal carcinoma in situ (DCIS), may not have enough physical cancer tissue for biomarkers or genetic testing.

Table 7-1. Biopsy Techniques

Technique	Description
Needle biopsy	
• Radiologic guidance	Use of live computed tomography to view nonpalpable mass and guide needle to site (e.g., lung nodule, breast nodule, adrenal nodule)
• Ultrasound guidance	Use of ultrasound to view area of palpable tumor and guide needle to desired biopsy site (e.g., muscle tumor, breast mass)
• Fine needle aspiration	Use of a needle and syringe to aspirate cells from palpable cyst or mass (e.g., subcutaneous nodule, fluid-filled cysts, palpable nodule underneath skin suspicious for metastasis)
• Cutting-core needle biopsy	Use of a large, open-bore needle to retrieve a small piece of intact tumor tissue (e.g., muscle mass, liver nodule)
Incisional biopsy	Surgical removal of a portion of a tumor for pathologic diagnosis; usually used on larger masses (e.g., subcutaneous mass, muscle mass, abdominal tumor) and may be achieved by surgical incision or through bronchoscopy, colonoscopy, laparoscopy, or thoracoscopy procedures
Excisional biopsy	Surgical removal of an entire mass or lesion with adequate margins for diagnosis (e.g., skin lesions [basal or squamous cell carcinomas, melanoma], breast mass [may be done with radiologic needle localization of mass], metastasis of primary tumor to lung [wedge resection], polypoid lesions of the colon); usually used on discrete masses 2–3 cm in diameter and may be used to control metastatic tumor

Note. Based on information from Cochran et al., 2003; Gipponi et al., 2004; Sabel, 2007.

Tumor staging is specific to the type of cancer and is essential in developing an appropriate therapeutic program (Pollock et al., 2010). Two staging systems are currently in use, the Union for International Cancer Control and the American Joint Committee on Cancer. Both systems use a tumor-node-metastasis (TNM) classification to define a cancer (Pollock et al., 2010) (see Figure 2-2 in Chapter 2). The American Joint Committee on Cancer system categorizes cancers into stages 0 to IV. See Chapter 2 for further discussion of cancer staging.

Types of Cancer Operations

Many types of surgical operations are used in the treatment of cancer. Depending on the specific diagnosis, tumor stage, and tumor location, surgical operations may be recommended for cure, prevention, or palliation. Minimally invasive techniques using robotics and laparoscopy have introduced new surgical options and advances in treatment.

Curative

Resection of the primary tumor, or removing the entire tumor with adequate margins of normal tissue, so that cancer does not recur is the goal of curative surgery (see Figure 7-1). Adequate tumor margins vary according to cancer

Figure 7-1. Rationales for Cancer Surgery

Curative
- Resection of primary tumor to provide curative results; may need neoadjuvant or adjuvant therapies for optimum results
- Localized tumors resected with adequate margins (i.e., lobectomy, mastectomy, hysterectomy)
- May include resection of regional lymph nodes to check for microscopic spread

Preventive
- Prophylactic surgery to reduce risk of cancer in high-risk patients
- Ulcerative colitis: Colon cancer—colectomy
- *BRCA* mutations
  - Breast cancer—bilateral mastectomies
  - Ovarian cancer—bilateral salpingo-oophorectomy
- *MEN2A* and *MEN2B* mutations
  - Multiple endocrine neoplasia and thyroid carcinoma—thyroidectomy

Palliative
- Surgery intended for relief of symptoms, not cure; may be a surgical emergency
- Surgeries for alleviation of pain or bleeding, circumvention or removal of bowel obstruction, decompression, and nutritional support
- Examples
  - Tumor debulking*
  - Removal of primary tumor
  - Gastrostomy or jejunostomy tube placement
  - Vascular access device placement
  - Esophageal stent placement

*Tumor debulking to remove all visible tumor has proved to be curative in some instances (e.g., intraperitoneal metastasis in ovarian carcinomas).

Note. Based on information from Pollock et al., 2010.

type and have evolved following clinical trial implications. A classic example is the evolution of breast cancer surgery. The Halsted mastectomy removed the breast with the pectoralis muscle, regional lymph nodes, and overlying skin in order to improve the local control rate of breast cancer and was often curative (Sabel, 2011). This radical surgery remained the standard of care for decades; however, over time, it became apparent that patient survival did not improve (Sabel, 2011). Clinical trial findings supported more limited resection and provided a model to include other treatment modalities. In some cases, chemotherapy and radiation therapy have replaced surgery as the primary treatment. For example, squamous cell carcinoma and head and neck cancers often are first treated with nonsurgical methods. In other cases, surgical resection is the primary therapy and is enhanced by neoadjuvant or adjuvant chemotherapy or radiation therapy (Sabel, 2011).

Resection of regional lymph nodes is an accepted part of surgical treatment for many solid tumors and is important in cancer staging (Miyoshi, 2013). Regional lymph node dissection often is considered beneficial in local disease control and prophylactic for distant microscopic disease. Some tumors may be indolent, or patients may have impaired quality of life because of symptoms and may benefit from tumor debulking for palliative reasons or prior to treatment. Ultimately, complete debulking of an abdominal tumor would leave no visible or palpable disease (Schorge, McCann, & Del Carmen, 2010). Ovarian carcinomas with intraperitoneal metastasis may benefit from a comprehensive debulking surgery to reduce tumor cells in preparation for postoperative chemotherapy (Schorge et al., 2010). Although this is not a curative procedure, tumor debulking in combination with treatment can improve survival time and quality of life (Berek, Friedlander, & Hacker, 2010; Schorge et al., 2010).

Preventive

Advances in cancer risk analysis and genetic screening have resulted in opportunities for surgical prevention of cancer. Patients with ulcerative colitis may benefit from prophylactic colectomy, and women with increased breast and ovarian cancer risk may benefit from prophylactic bilateral mastectomies or bilateral salpingo-oophorectomy. At-risk family members of patients with multiple endocrine neoplasia syndrome type 2a or 2b with *RET* mutations should have a prophylactic thyroidectomy at an early age (Rosenberg, 2011).

Palliative

Following assessment of the relative risk-benefit ratio, surgical palliation may be used for patients with cancer who are not candidates for surgical cure. For example, resection of a primary tumor to alleviate pain or bleeding, bowel resection for bleeding or obstruction, placement of a gastrostomy tube for decompression, placement of a jejunostomy tube for enteral feedings, or vascular access for hyperalimentation in malnutrition may improve quality of life. Emergency surgical intervention may be indicated to alleviate obstruction, perforation, bleeding, and pain. However, it also may result in unwanted side effects and increased patient risk (Pollock et al., 2010).

Minimally Invasive

Laparoscopic and robotic-assisted procedures offer surgeons significant advantages with improved visualization of disease, reduction in blood loss, lower incidence of wound infection, decreased postoperative pain, and decreased length of hospital stay (Tse & Ngan, 2015). The use of robotics during laparoscopic procedures offers surgeons increased dexterity and improved precision, as well as the avoidance of muscle fatigue and tremor (Tse & Ngan, 2015). Robotics in cancer surgery allows the surgeon to visualize and dissect a tumor that previously could not be adequately removed with laparoscopy. Minimally invasive cancer surgery, whether performed with robotic assistance or conventional laparoscopy, compared to laparotomy, has been shown to have fewer long-term complications with improved body image and better short-term quality of life (Tse & Ngan, 2015) (see Figures 7-2 and 7-3).

Minimally invasive treatments using cryoablation or radiofrequency ablation are reported to be effective treatments in early-stage colorectal cancers (Qian, 2011). Investigations of localized ablation therapy for hepatocellular carcinoma include radiofrequency ablation, microwave coagulation therapy, laser therapy, cryotherapy, and percutaneous injections (Qian, 2011). Advances in surgical technique and minimally invasive treatments have improved treatment outcomes and minimized surgical side effects.

Figure 7-2. Da Vinci® Robot

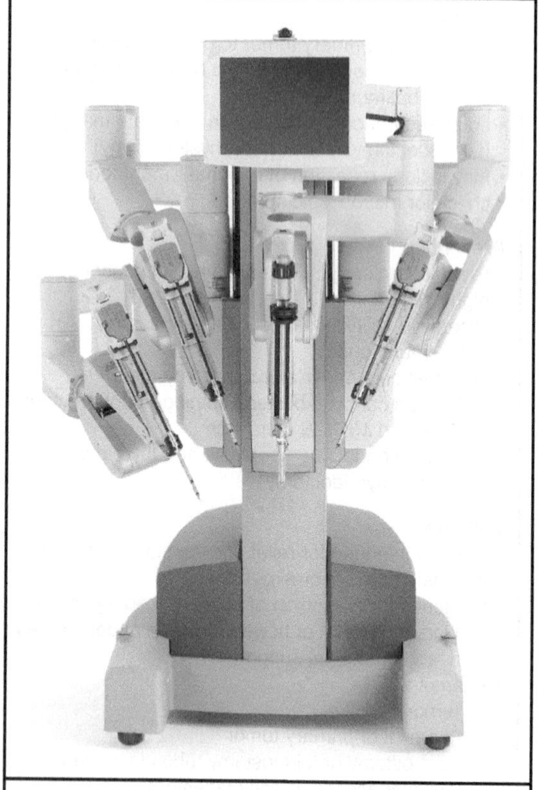

Note. Copyright 2014 by Intuitive Surgical, Inc. Used with permission.

Perioperative Nursing Considerations

Prior to cancer surgery, the healthcare team must compare the realistic benefits of surgery with treatment risks. Factors to be considered include the patient's health status, expected long-term survival, likelihood of cure or pallia-

Figure 7-3. Robotic Instrumentation

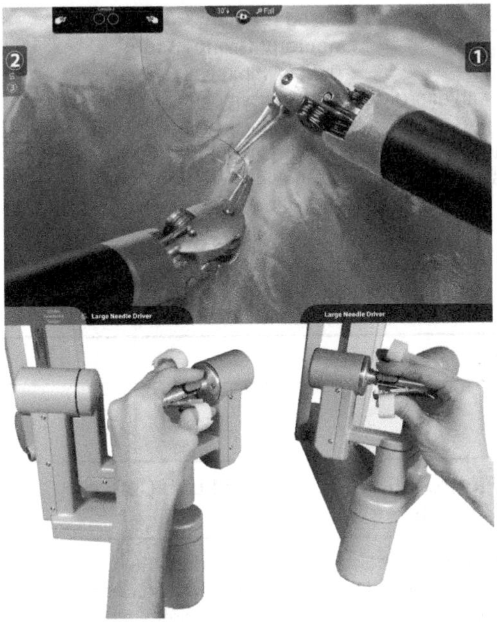

Note. Copyright 2009 by Intuitive Surgical, Inc. Used with permission.

tion, potential risks of intervention, and overall quality-of-life expectations. Performance status represents an assessment of the patient's level of function and can be calculated using either the Karnofsky Performance Scale or the Eastern Cooperative Oncology Group scale (Jang et al., 2014) (see Figure 7-4). The Palliative Performance Scale often is used in palliative care settings (Jang et al., 2014).

Patients with advanced disease may have an increased risk for postoperative surgical complications. Preoperative evaluation and prophylaxis are integral to surgical outcomes. To minimize perioperative complications and avoid delays for postoperative treatment, every effort should be made to correct physiologic and biochemical deficiencies preoperatively (Pollock et al., 2010). Determining the benefits compared to the inherent risks of surgery is a complicated and extensive assessment, especially in patients with poor health status. Complications as a result of neoadjuvant chemotherapy or radiation therapy also must be considered when preparing patients for cancer surgery (Pollock et al., 2010). Morbidity and mortality have decreased in complex cancer operations because of advances in surgical technique, anesthesia, supportive care, and limited cancer resection (Pollock et al., 2010).

Postoperative nursing care considerations may include patient comorbidities, type of disease and surgical procedure, symptoms, education, and quality of life. Common surgical side effects, such as constipation and infection, or symptoms, such as pain and fatigue, are not unique to cancer surgery but may require special interventions. Early referral for rehabilitation services is essential to achieve optimal function in patients who may have residual effects from surgical intervention (Thomas & Ragnarsson, 2010). Specialized concerns and related treatment resources for cancer surgery include an exercise prescription for cancer-related fatigue, therapy for breast cancer–related lymphedema, cryopreservation of sperm cells for testicular cancer, and colostomy care by enterostomal therapists (Thomas & Ragnarsson, 2010).

Perioperative nursing care requires attention to emotional and psychological concerns. Curative surgery may offer years of disease-free survival; however, fear of recurrence and frequent clinical follow-up may be related to depression and anxiety (Reece, Chan, Herbert, Gralow, & Fann, 2013). Palliative surgery intended to ameliorate symptoms and improve quality of life may not result in prolonged survival and may result in added care of physical needs, such as surgical wounds, healing, and rehabilitation.

Cancer surgery and the subsequent pathology are the primary sources of data for cancer statistics (American Cancer Society [ACS], 2016c). The majority of patients with cancer will have a surgical biopsy and undergo surgical treatment. Most surgeons performing cancer-related surgeries are not surgical oncologists,

Figure 7-4. Surgical Oncology Performance Status

Performance Status	Karnofsky Score (%)	Zubrod (Eastern Cooperative Oncology Group) Score
• Normal activity; no specific care • Unable to work • Unable to care for self • Very sick • Moribund • None	• 100 (no symptoms) • 90 (some symptoms) • 80 (some symptoms, activity with effort) • 70 (cares for self) • 60 (needs occasional assistance) • 50 (needs considerable assistance) • 40 (requires medical care) • 30 (disabled) • 20 (requires hospitalization) • 10 (rapid fatal progression) • 0 (death)	• 0 (no symptoms) • 1 (some symptoms) • 2 (in bed less than 50% of the day) • 3 (in bed more than 50% of the day) • 4 (unable to get out of bed)

Note. Based on information from Sabel, 2007; Thomas & Ragnarsson, 2010.

which may contribute to the low enrollment (less than 5%) of patients with cancer in clinical trials (Fouad et al., 2013). Continued support of participation in clinical trials, training of multidisciplinary cancer surgical specialists, and translation of research findings into practice will likely optimize cancer surgery and improve patient outcomes.

Selected Cancers in Surgical Oncology

Lung Cancer

Epidemiology and Etiology

Lung cancer is the most common cause of cancer-related deaths in men and women in the United States, exceeding that of breast, colon, and prostate cancers (ACS, 2016c). Although technology and treatments have improved, changes in survival rates continue to be disappointing, with only 12%–15% of patients being cured of the disease (Prokhorov & Hudmon, 2014). Only 16% of lung cancer cases are diagnosed when the disease is still localized and at an early stage (see Figure 7-5 for definitions of procedures); however, if detected early, when the disease is resectable, the five-year survival is approximately 55% (ACS, 2016c).

Figure 7-5. Definitions of Lung Cancer Procedures

flexible bronchoscopy—Procedure that uses a flexible fiber-optic scope inserted into the trachea to view the supraglottic and glottic areas as well as the tracheal bronchial tree and possibly obtain samples of tissue or body fluids for diagnostic purposes.

mediastinoscopy—Procedure that uses a rigid scope to view the area in front of the lungs directly beneath the sternum and obtain samples of tissue as indicated. Often used prior to lung cancer surgery for mediastinal nodal assessment.

positron-emission tomography (PET) scan—Nuclear three-dimensional imaging that detects areas of increased metabolism through uptake of a radioactive biologic tracer, fluorodeoxyglucose, that has been introduced into the body. Results of a PET-computed tomography scan indicate areas of metastasis in patients with cancer.

sleeve lobectomy—Removal of a lobe of the lung including a portion of the involved main bronchus and reattachment of the bronchial portions and remaining lobes with an anastomosis.

thoracoscopy—Minimally invasive procedure using a small incision to insert a thoracoscope into the thoracic cavity.

thoracotomy—Incision in the thoracic cavity, usually on one side of the chest between the ribs.

wedge resection of the lung—Removal of a portion (in a pie shape) of a lobe of the lung using staples.

Note. Based on information from Blackmon & Vaporciyan, 2012; Lu et al., 2010.

Cigarette smoking is the cause of a majority (80%–90%) of lung cancers (Alberg, Brock, Ford, Samet, & Spivack, 2013). Other exposures, such as secondhand smoke, asbestos, certain metals or chemicals, radiation, and air pollution, also pose a risk (ACS, 2016c; Alberg et al., 2013). See Figure 7-6 for additional risk factors for cancer. A history of prior respiratory disease, such as tuberculosis, asthma, emphysema, or lung cancer, in a first-degree relative increases the risk of lung cancer (Prokhorov & Hudmon, 2014). Examination of the National Institutes of Health–AARP Diet and Health Study cohort found that an increased body mass index in men and women is associated with a decreased lung cancer risk (inverse correlation) among current and former smokers (Smith et al., 2012). In the United States, approximately 16,000–24,000 deaths occur each year from lung cancer in people who have never smoked (ACS, 2016i). The risk of developing lung cancer in a smoker increases with the length of time the individual has smoked. The risk decreases if the person quits smoking. Former and current smokers continue to be at risk; however, the risk decreases depending on the duration of abstinence (Prokhorov & Hudmon, 2014). The importance of screening for the early detection of lung cancer to improve survival rates cannot be overstated. Early trials using sputum cytology and chest x-ray in high-risk, asymptomatic patients indicated that mortality rates did not improve (Tanner, Mehta, & Silvestri, 2012). Consequently, chest x-rays are not recommended for lung cancer screening (Tanner et al., 2012). Two studies, the National Lung Screening Trial and the International Early Lung Cancer Action Program, have had a major impact on lung cancer screening. Both studies identified the ability to use computed tomography (CT) scanning as a screening tool to diagnose lung cancers when the lesion is smaller and at an earlier stage, which allows for early surgery and a chance for cure (Yip, Henschke, Yankelevitz, Boffetta, & Smith, 2015). Based on these results, in 2013, ACS issued guidelines for the screening of lung cancer using low-dose CT scanning (ACS, 2016c).

Typically, people with undiagnosed lung cancer do not have symptoms that can be identified early. The most common symptoms of lung cancer are a long-term or worsening cough; blood or rust-colored sputum (spit or phlegm); deep breathing, coughing, or laughing associated with worsening chest pain; hoarseness; weight loss (not always associated with loss of appetite); loss of appetite; shortness of breath; feeling of extreme fatigue or weakness; lung infections that do not go away or keep coming back; and recently diagnosed wheezing (ACS, 2016f) (see Figure 7-7).

Figure 7-6. Lung Cancer Risk Factors

- Cigarette smoking
- Exposure to carcinogens
  - Secondhand smoke
  - Asbestos
  - Certain metals or chemicals
  - Radiation
  - Air pollution
- Prior respiratory disease
- Lung cancer in a first-degree relative
- Increased body mass index and waist size in women

Note. Based on information from Alberg et al., 2013; American Cancer Society, 2016c.

Staging and Treatment

Pathologic diagnosis and staging prior to treatment may be achieved through several methods, such as bronchoscopy, mediastinoscopy, CT-guided needle biopsy (for a solitary lesion), thoracotomy, thoracoscopy with wedge resection, and immediate frozen section. Mediastinal lymph node disease has been reported in 12%–77% of patients with non-small cell lung cancer (NSCLC) (Cuellar, Marom, & Erasmus, 2014). Lung cancer histology usually is divided into two groups: small cell lung cancer (13%) or NSCLC (85.3%), which includes adenocarcinoma, squamous

Figure 7-7. Lung Cancer Symptoms

- Bone pain
- Chest discomfort
- Cough
- Dysphagia
- Dyspnea
- Fatigue
- Fever
- Hemoptysis
- Hoarseness
- Neurologic symptoms
- Shoulder pain

Note. Based on information from American Cancer Society, 2016f; Lu et al., 2010.

cell carcinoma, and large cell carcinoma (Carr, Finigan, & Kern, 2011). Small cell lung cancer generally is treated with chemotherapy, radiation therapy, or both; however, early-stage single peripheral tumors with negative mediastinal nodes may be treated with surgery and adjuvant chemotherapy (National Comprehensive Cancer Network® [NCCN®], 2016d). NSCLC may be managed surgically when the tumor is localized (Carr et al., 2011). Surgery alone in patients with stage IA/IB NSCLC may achieve five-year survival rates of 73%/58%, respectively (Carr et al., 2011). Resection of tumor in stage I, stage II, and selected stage III cases is the treatment of choice for potential cure (Carr et al., 2011).

Surgical Interventions

Flexible bronchoscopy often is used to diagnose and stage lung cancer and may be used by the thoracic surgeon immediately before surgery to visualize possible lesions in the bronchus. Bronchoscopy is recommended for both central and peripheral lesions (Carr et al., 2011). Samples may be obtained for diagnosis by bronchial washings, cytology brushings, and transbronchial or endobronchial biopsies. Biopsy of mediastinal or hilar nodes may be obtained using endobronchial ultrasound–guided transbronchial needle aspiration (Carr et al., 2011). At the time of bronchoscopy, tumors are stage T3 if there is infiltration within 1 cm of the carina or stage T4 if there is invasion into the trachea (Carr et al., 2011).

Video mediastinoscopy is an outpatient procedure using a suprasternal incision to obtain large samples of lymph nodes for staging in order to determine treatment for lung cancer (Pipkin & Keshavjee, 2014). Enlarged nodes on a chest CT scan or uptake in the mediastinum on a PET scan are indications for mediastinoscopy. However, even with negative scans, positive nodes may be detected during surgery (Pipkin & Keshavjee, 2014). In cases of left upper lobe tumors, the patient may be recommended to undergo a Chamberlain procedure, or anterior mediastinotomy, with an incision at the left second intercostal space in order to sample subaortic, periaortic, and anterior mediastinal nodes (Pipkin & Keshavjee, 2014).

Video-assisted thoracic surgery (VATS) with or without robotic assistance in the surgical treatment of early-stage NSCLC continues to be an alternative to thoracotomy (Blackmon, 2014). When indicated, minimally invasive surgeries can be performed safely in place of a thoracotomy, and patients experience reduced blood loss and pain, a shorter hospital stay, improved independence, preserved pulmonary function, improved inflammatory response, and shorter chest tube duration (Blackmon, 2014). Contraindications to VATS, in which case a thoracotomy may be performed, include an inability to tolerate single-lung ventilation, involvement of the chest wall by tumor, or, in some centers, induction therapy (Hanna, Berry, & D'Amico, 2013).

Colorectal Cancer

Epidemiology and Etiology

Colorectal cancer (CRC) (see Figure 7-8 for definitions) is the third most common cancer in the United States and the third leading cause of cancer deaths among men and

Figure 7-8. Colorectal Cancer Definitions

brachytherapy—A type of radiation therapy delivered inside the body via radioactive seeds that are temporarily (as in colorectal and gynecologic cancers) or permanently (as in prostate cancer) placed strategically into the cancerous tumor.

carcinoembryonic antigen (CEA)—An antigen produced by some cancers that can be detected in the blood. Most commonly, it is elevated in patients with cancers of the gastrointestinal tract; however, it can be elevated in other cancers and certain benign disease processes. CEA also is produced by developing fetuses.

colonoscopy—Insertion of a long, flexible scope into the anus to evaluate the rectum and colon to the cecum.

familial adenomatous polyposis—Familial disease of the colon in which patients develop multiple polyps in the large intestines at an early age. If not treated, the polyps will become malignant.

hereditary nonpolyposis colorectal cancer—Inherited disease in which genetic mutations have occurred that prevent the correction of abnormal DNA synthesis. Abnormal cell growth occurs and develops into colorectal cancer or other types of cancers, such as endometrial cancer in women.

sigmoidoscopy—Insertion of a flexible scope into the anus to examine the lower portion of the colon from the rectum to the sigmoid colon.

Note. Based on information from Church & Mandel, 2011.

women (ACS, 2016c). The number of deaths from CRC has declined over the years, which can be attributed to early detection and prevention through screening and removal of polyps that have the potential to develop into an adenocarcinoma (ACS, 2016c). Risk factors include diets high in red meats and processed foods; foods that have been broiled, fried, or grilled; and heavy use of alcohol. As with lung cancer, heavy smoking for long periods of time has been determined to be a risk factor for colon cancer. Some risk factors are not modifiable, such as age and family or personal history of large adenomatous polyps (see Figure 7-9). Hereditable mutations have also been identified to cause colon cancer (ACS, 2016e) (see also Chapter 4).

Signs and symptoms of colorectal cancer are discussed in detail in Chapter 5. A succinct list is offered in Figure 7-10.

Recommended colonoscopy screening begins at age 50, yet because of low screening rates, only 39% of CRCs are diagnosed at an early stage (ACS, 2016d). If CRC is diagnosed and treated when the disease is localized, the five-year survival rate is 90% (ACS, 2016d). The survival rate is 71% for patients who are diagnosed with regional spread, and 13% for those with metastasis to distant organs (ACS, 2016d).

Figure 7-9. Colorectal Cancer Risk Factors

- Age greater than 50 years
- Hereditary factors
  - Familial adenomatous polyposis
  - Hereditary nonpolyposis colorectal cancer
  - Genetics
- Disease-specific factors
  - Ulcerative colitis
  - Crohn disease
  - History of polyps
  - Chronic inflammatory bowel disease
  - Diabetes
- Family history of colorectal cancer
- High-fat, low-fiber diet
- Cigarette smoking
- Alcohol abuse

Note. Based on information from Padussis et al., 2010.

Figure 7-10. Colorectal Cancer Symptoms

- Abdominal pain
- Anemia
- Anorexia
- Change in bowel habits
- Fatigue
- Fever
- Hematochezia
- Melena
- Nausea and vomiting
- Rectal bleeding
- Right upper quadrant pain
- Weight loss

Note. Based on information from Padussis et al., 2010.

Staging and Treatment

CRCs, most of which are adenocarcinomas, are treated based on tumor location and stage of the disease (Van Schaeybroeck et al., 2014). Pathologic histology grades the tumor to determine the aggressiveness and, consequently, high-grade tumors have been shown to have a poor prognosis (Van Schaeybroeck et al., 2014). Once pathologic diagnosis and staging have been determined, further workup is needed to determine disease progression and preoperative performance status. Imaging studies to be considered to determine potential metastasis include CT of the chest, abdomen, and pelvis; magnetic resonance imaging of the liver; and PET scan (Van Schaeybroeck et al., 2014).

At initial presentation with CRC, 20% of patients will have metastasis at the time of diagnosis (Van Schaeybroeck et al., 2014). The liver is the most common site for metastasis. If this is isolated, 10%–20% of these patients may be candidates for surgically curable disease (Van Schaeybroeck et al., 2014).

Fifty percent of patients diagnosed with CRC have potentially curable disease (Chan, Chong, Lieske, & Tan, 2014). Surgical procedures may be performed laparoscopically with or without robotic assistance or use of laparotomy with comparable long-term results (Chan et al., 2014; Halabi et al., 2013). Procedures performed laparoscopically offer less discomfort, a decrease in length of hospital stay, earlier return of bowel function, and improved quality of life (Chan et al., 2014; Halabi et al., 2013). Laparoscopic resections yield a similar number of resected nodes and distal resection margins as do open procedures (Chan et al., 2014).

Surgical Interventions

Colon cancer: More than 80% of colon cancers may be treated with surgical resection (Van Schaeybroeck et al., 2014). Depending on the location of the tumor, indications for surgery might include a right or right-extended hemicolectomy, transverse colectomy, left hemicolectomy, or low anterior resection. En bloc excisions with adequate lengths of bowel proximal and distal to the cancer, a minimum of 12 lymph nodes, and the vascular structure supplying the segment provide the best evaluation of prognosis (Van Schaeybroeck et al., 2014).

During surgery, it is important to carefully explore the peritoneal cavity and examine the entire length of the colon. If the tumor is attached to adjacent structures, 50% of the cases will have tumor invasion and should have en bloc excision (Van Schaeybroeck et al., 2014). Adjuvant chemotherapy is advised for patients with both high-risk stage II and stage III disease to reduce the risk of recurrence and cancer-related mortality (Van Schaeybroeck et al., 2014).

Rectal cancer: When planning surgery, the healthcare team should consider sexual, urinary, and sphincter preservation to maintain the patient's quality of life. Neoadjuvant radiation and chemotherapy treatment of low rectal carcinomas allows for preservation of the sphincter in 70% of patients (Tarchi, Moretti, & de Manzini, 2013). Low anterior resections with end-to-end anastomosis less than 10 cm from the tumor, regardless of neoadjuvant radiation, may cause impairment in the activity of the sphincter, resulting in incontinence, soiling, or constipation (Tarchi et al., 2013). Neoadjuvant radiation also may result in sphincter changes. Reconstruction with a colonic pouch to improve outcome seems to provide good functional results in 75% of cases, thus preventing colostomy (Tarchi et al., 2013). Postoperatively, adjuvant therapy with chemotherapy with or without radiation therapy may be considered to improve survival.

Prostate Cancer

Epidemiology and Etiology

In the United States, an estimated 3.3 million men were living with a history of prostate cancer as of January 1, 2016 (see Figure 7-11 for definitions) (ACS, 2016d). In the United States, prostate cancer is the most prevalent malignancy in men and the second most common solid cancer mortality (ACS, 2016d). Prostate cancer usually occurs in men older than age 50, and men have a 42% lifetime risk of developing microscopic disease (Turner & Drudge-Coates, 2010). African American men have an increased incidence of prostate cancer as well as increased mortality and recurrence rates compared to Caucasian men (Knipe et al., 2014). If a man has been identified to have a *BRCA* mutation, especially *BRCA2*, he has a higher risk for prostate cancer. Although diet, smoking, obesity, inflammation of the prostate, and exposure to chemicals such as Agent Orange have been identified as potential risks for prostate cancer, the research evidence is not strong and shows both positive and negative correlations (ACS, 2016g) (see Figure 7-12). Detection through prostate-specific antigen (PSA) testing or possibly incidental finding with transurethral resection of the prostate continues to contribute to the number of prostate cancer cases (Turner & Drudge-Coates, 2010). Figure 7-13 presents a succinct list of symptoms. Screening of prostate cancer may be improved with further genotype testing (Knipe et al., 2014).

Figure 7-11. Prostate Cancer Definitions

priapism—Painful prolonged erection not related to sexual function. May be caused by invasion of the penis with solid tumor, such as in prostate cancer.

prostate-specific antigen—A protein produced by the prostate gland that may become elevated in benign as well as cancerous conditions of the prostate gland.

Note. Based on information from Reid & Hamdy, 2008.

Figure 7-12. Prostate Cancer Risk Factors

- Aging
- Diet (high in fat, low in vitamin D)
- Testosterone increase or decrease
- Environmental factors affecting testosterone
- Familial history of prostate cancer

Note. Based on information from National Comprehensive Cancer Network, 2016c.

Figure 7-13. Prostate Cancer Symptoms

- Bone pain
- Fatigue
- Hematuria
- Priapism
- Weight loss

Note. Based on information from Reid & Hamdy, 2008.

Staging and Treatment

Prostate cancer is usually diagnosed when symptoms are absent through digital rectal examination, PSA testing, and finally with transrectal ultrasound core biopsy (Nelson, Carter, DeWeese, Antonarakis, & Eisenberger, 2014). Multiple biopsies are obtained during transrectal ultrasound to minimize the chance of missing cancer (Nelson et al., 2014).

Prostate cancer staging typically uses the TNM staging system and most often occurs after radical prostatectomy (Turner & Drudge-Coates, 2010). Further staging studies, such as bone scan, CT scan, or magnetic resonance imaging for determination of lymph node metastasis, depend on the level of PSA elevation (greater than 20 ng/ml) and histology grading and should be reserved for men with high-risk prostate cancer (Nelson et al., 2014) (see also Chapter 5).

Surgical Interventions

Prostate cancer is treated with radical prostatectomy, radiation therapy, or watchful waiting (NCCN, 2016c). Surgeries may be performed via an open or a minimally invasive approach. Robotic-assisted laparoscopic radical prostatectomy is the most common approach to removal of the prostate and includes a staging pelvic lymphadenectomy, resection of the seminal vesicles, and identification and preservation of the neurovascular bundles necessary for penile erection if indicated (Nelson et al., 2014). Maintenance of urinary continence and sexual potency are of great concern to patients when making a decision for treatment (see also Chapter 33). Robotic-assisted laparoscopic prostatectomy may help to decrease these complications. Men with organ-confined cancer and more than 10 years of life expectancy might be good candidates for radical prostatectomy (Gillitzer & Thüroff, 2013).

Surgical intervention or radiation therapy may not be the first choice of treatment in men with prostate cancer. In men with small volumes of low-grade prostate cancer, the risk is low that the disease will progress within the first 10 years following diagnosis, and a decision to observe may be indicated (Smith, 2013). Watchful waiting, sometimes called active surveillance, occurs with a slow-growing prostate cancer that is being closely monitored (ACS, 2016h). Typically, the cancer would have a low Gleason score (a lower score means the cancer is similar to the tissue of origin and has a low likelihood of spreading) (National Cancer Institute, n.d.).

Breast Cancer

Epidemiology and Etiology

Based on current surveillance research, breast cancer (see Figure 7-14 for definitions) continues to be the most frequent cancer in women, with one in eight women diagnosed in their lifetime (Ban & Godellas, 2014). It is the second leading cause of death in women, and approximately 1.4 million women are diagnosed annually worldwide. The lifetime risk for men to develop breast cancer is 1 in 1,000 (ACS, 2016a). The majority (92%) of women who are diagnosed with breast cancer now survive five years beyond diagnosis because of early detection and treatment (Ban & Godellas, 2014).

Figure 7-14. Breast Cancer Definitions

***BRCA1* and *BRCA2* genes**—Tumor suppressor genes. Individuals with mutations in these genes have an increased risk of breast and ovarian cancers as well as other cancers and disorders. *BRCA1* and *BRCA2* gene mutation is hereditary.

hormone receptor status—Estrogen receptor (ER) and progesterone receptor (PR) status is determined at the time of pathologic diagnosis. Hormone receptor status is important for treatment planning.

stereotactic biopsy—Breast biopsy that is performed with computer-guided imaging.

tamoxifen—A selective ER modulator used in patients with ER-positive breast cancer or, in some cases, as a preventive measure. Blocks estrogen at receptor sites, inhibiting tumor growth.

Note. Based on information from National Comprehensive Cancer Network, 2016a.

Risk factors for breast cancer include age, with only one in eight invasive cancers occurring in women younger than age 45 and one third of cases occurring in women older than age 55. If atypical ductal hyperplasia or atypical lobular hyperplasia are diagnosed after a breast biopsy, breast cancer risk increases by 3.5–5 times. Lobular carcinoma in situ (LCIS) is another type of cellular change and is associated with 7–11 times increase in breast cancer risk. Longer hormone exposure, such as starting menses prior to age 12 or ending menses after age 55, may cause a slightly higher risk for some women. Hormonal exposure such as diethylstilbestrol use to prevent loss of a pregnancy or medroxyprogesterone injections or birth control pills have shown a slight increase of risk over time, but risk typically decreases once the medication is stopped. Recent studies have shown that use of combined hormone therapy (progesterone and estrogen) after menopause increases the risk of breast cancer, but estrogen alone does not. If a woman is overweight after menopause, her risk for developing breast cancer is also increased, perhaps because estrogen is produced by fat cells. Another risk factor is an increased intake of alcohol, such as two to five drinks per day. There is growing evidence from research studies that physical activity, even as little as 2.5 hours per week, decreases risk. Another factor associated with decreased risk of breast cancer is breast-feeding, although the length of time has been difficult to associate with changes in risk (ACS, 2016b) (see Figure 7-15).

Early detection of breast cancers using mammography has advanced the practice of pathologic diagnosis of both nonpalpable and palpable masses. Treatment is more effective when breast cancer is diagnosed at an early stage. Mammographic evaluation will determine if there are masses bilaterally, as well as a suspicion of malignancy based on appearance. NCCN (2016a) guidelines recommend a bilateral diagnostic mammogram and possibly an ultrasound following a diagnosis of early-stage breast cancer. Well-defined, solitary masses found on a mammogram usually are classified as "probably benign"; however, all masses should be further evaluated with ultrasound (Wilson, 2013). For suspicious lesions, an invasive procedure such as FNA, core needle biopsy, or excisional biopsy will be performed.

Some options for diagnosis include needle localization with mammography followed by excision, FNA, ultrasound-guided biopsy, or stereotactic biopsy. A minimally invasive approach is the first choice for diagnosis if possible. In cases of noninvasive breast cancer, DCIS, or invasive breast cancer, it is recommended that women who are at high risk for hereditary breast cancer undergo genetic testing as part of their workup (NCCN, 2016a).

Figure 7-15. Breast Cancer Risk Factors

- Modest risk: Aging women, nulliparity, obesity, alcohol intake, early menarche
- Moderate risk: Atypia, lobular carcinoma in situ, previous breast cancer, ductal carcinoma in situ, family history, long-term hormone replacement therapy use
- High risk: Hereditary syndrome, breast radiation exposure

Note. Based on information from National Comprehensive Cancer Network, 2016a.

Noninvasive Breast Cancer

Ductal carcinoma in situ: DCIS is a proliferation of malignant epithelial cells that are confined to the mammary ducts and accounts for 20%–25% of newly detected breast cancers found with screening examinations, with an estimate of 1 case per 1,300 mammograms (Morrow, 2012). DCIS typically is not palpable and was rarely diagnosed prior to the use of mammograms (Morrow, 2012). Mortality rates are low for women diagnosed with DCIS regardless of treatment, with 1%–2.6% dying of invasive cancer within 8–10 years (Morrow, 2012). According to NCCN (2016a) guidelines, options for the primary treatment of stage 0 DCIS include lumpectomy without lymph node surgery plus whole breast radiation therapy; mastectomy with or without sentinel node biopsy with or without reconstruction; or just lumpectomy. Depending on the pathologic diagnosis, tamoxifen may be recommended postoperatively for five years, and the patient should be followed according to NCCN risk reduction guidelines (NCCN, 2016a). Recommended ongoing follow-up includes annual mammograms and a history and physical every 6–12 months for the first five years and then every 12 months thereafter (NCCN, 2016a).

Lobular carcinoma in situ: LCIS is an intraepithelial proliferation confined to the lobules and usually is found in 0.5%–1.5% of screen-detected lesions (Wells & Arkoumani, 2013). Normally, LCIS is not visible on mammography or detectable on palpation but is found incidentally via biopsy for other breast-related problems (McAuliffe, Andtbacka, Robinson, & Hunt, 2012). Clinical presentation is similar to that of patients with fibroadenomas, benign ductal disease, or DCIS (McAuliffe et al., 2012). Diagnosis with core needle biopsy is recommended based on studies indicating a risk of synchronous invasive breast cancer or DCIS. In cases of aggressive variants of LCIS, risk reduction with bilateral mastectomy and reconstruction is suggested, as 40% of women will have LCIS in the contralateral breast (NCCN, 2016a; Wells & Arkoumani, 2013). Follow-up recommendations are similar to those for DCIS.

Invasive Breast Cancer

The majority of invasive breast cancers are adenocarcinomas arising from the terminal ducts, with the remaining rare histologic types comprising papillary, apocrine, secretory, squamous cell, and spindle cell carcinomas and carcinosarcoma (Kwon, Kelly, & Ching, 2012). The five common variants of mammary adenocarcinoma include infiltrating ductal carcinoma, which accounts for 75% of all breast cancers; infiltrating lobular carcinoma; tubular carcinoma; medullary carcinoma; and mucinous or colloid carcinoma (Kwon et al., 2012).

Once malignancy has been pathologically confirmed, the extent of the disease must be evaluated and the staging determined. This may be achieved through radiographic imaging, such as chest x-ray and bone scans, and laboratory testing, including liver function tests and alkaline phosphatase. A history and physical examination with a review of the bone, liver, lungs, and brain is performed to determine symptomatic indications of metastasis. Palpation and imaging of the tumor will determine the approximate size. Treatment for stage I, IIA, IIB, or T3 N1 M0 disease includes lumpectomy followed by radiation therapy or total mastectomy with axillary staging with or without reconstruction (NCCN, 2016a).

The pathologic diagnosis of the axillary nodes will determine the need for chemotherapy plus radiation, radiation therapy alone, or no further therapy (NCCN, 2016a). Systemic adjuvant hormone or chemotherapy treatment will be determined by pathology, hormone receptor status, and HER2 status (NCCN, 2016a). Neoadjuvant chemotherapy may be used prior to surgical intervention in patients with stage IIIA N2, IIIB, or IIIC disease (NCCN, 2016a).

Surgical Interventions

Breast conservation (lumpectomy): Women with stage I or II breast cancer are excellent candidates for breast-conserving surgery. However, trial results from the National Surgical Adjuvant Breast and Bowel Project (NSABP B-06 trial) revealed that breast-conserving surgery in combination with radiation therapy markedly reduced the recurrence rate from 39% to 10% (Kwon et al., 2012).

Careful consideration of breast size and tumor dimensions is necessary when evaluating a patient for breast-conserving surgery. Patients with small or pendulous breasts might have poor cosmetic results after excision or radiation and may benefit from mastectomy with reconstruction (Kwon et al., 2012). Sentinel lymph node biopsy should be performed prior to lumpectomy in early breast cancers so that the node can be analyzed during the breast resection (Zurrida & Veronesi, 2015). In all patients with invasive breast cancer, axillary staging should be performed to identify metastasis (Kwon et al., 2012).

The sentinel lymph node or group of nodes receive lymphatic drainage from the affected breast and would be the first likely area of metastasis; therefore, lymphatic mapping and sentinel lymph node biopsy may determine whether axillary node dissection should be limited (Kwon et al., 2012). Lumpectomy should be performed with adequate margins (tissue with tumor cell–free space between the tumor and the edge of excision) in order to minimize the need for reexcision (Baker, 2014). Marking of the specimen using a two-point system to maintain orientation is important to evaluate margins (Baker, 2014). If the surgical pathology results determine that the margins cannot be adequately resected, further surgery with mastectomy will be necessary (NCCN, 2016a).

Oncoplastic surgical techniques: Patients with breast cancer are increasingly being cured of their disease, and the postoperative appearance of the breast correlates with improved psychosocial outcomes (Chakravorty et al., 2012). Oncoplastic breast-conserving surgery (oBCS) enhances standard breast-conserving surgery and provides women who meet inclusion criteria the opportunity for positive aesthetic outcomes without mastectomy, even in the case of larger tumors, (Chakravorty et al., 2012). This type of breast conservation removes the breast cancer tissue and reshapes, replaces, or rearranges the noncancerous breast tissue (Tenofsky, Dowell, Topalovski, & Helmer, 2014). The decision to perform oBCS depends on the tumor location, characteristics of the breast, and clinical evaluation (Urban et al., 2011). Women with large breasts who would benefit from bilateral breast reduction or women requiring a breast lift are often good candidates for oBCS, as this allows for a wider excision to encompass a larger tumor as well as wider margins (Urban et al., 2011). The surgeries are performed by a team that may include a breast surgeon with training in all techniques of oBCS or in conjunction with a plastic surgeon (Urban et al., 2011).

Mastectomy and breast reconstruction: After discussing the risks, benefits, and alternatives with the surgeon, the patient may decide a mastectomy with possible breast reconstruction is her first choice for surgical intervention. Genetic testing and early detection of breast disease have given high-risk patients options for the treatment and prevention of breast cancer. Women who test positive for *BRCA1* or *BRCA2* mutations or those with breast cancer who wish to remove the contralateral breast may choose to undergo prophylactic bilateral mastectomies with immediate breast reconstruction. Results of clinical studies indicate that prophylactic mastectomy may reduce the risk of developing breast cancer by 90% or more (Burke, Portschy, & Tuttle, 2015). Immediate breast reconstruction is best if the patient will not be treated with radiation therapy after surgery. If postmastectomy radiation is recommended, it is best to wait until after treatment to proceed with reconstruction because of possible fibrosis, radiation burns, or fat necrosis. In some cases, when the patient understands the possible complications, the psychological benefits of immediate reconstruction may outweigh the risks.

If reconstruction is performed, it is expected that the reconstruction will match the contralateral breast in size, shape, and degree of ptosis (Serletti, Fosnot, Nelson, Disa, & Bucky, 2011). If the tumor is not close to the skin, mastectomy often is performed using a skin-sparing technique to plan for reconstruction by either implantation or an autologous flap (Serletti et al., 2011). The skin-sparing mastectomy also may spare the nipple or include a complete circumareolar incision with or without a lateral extension depending on the need for axillary node dissection (Laronga & Smith, 2014). Autologous reconstruction uses excess skin and subcutaneous fat to shape the breast using either a latissimus dorsi flap, a transverse rectus abdominis myocutaneous (TRAM) flap, or a free flap from a distant site, such as a gluteal flap (Serletti et al., 2011). The pedicled or free flap is used for autologous reconstruction using excess skin and subcutaneous fat from areas routinely used in cosmetic abdominoplasty. The rectus abdominis muscle contains a dual blood supply that allows the TRAM flap to be used as a pedicled flap, creating a tunnel subcutaneously along the chest wall. The tunnel connects the abdominal region with the mastectomy site. The flap, still attached to its blood supply, is pulled through the tunnel to the mastectomy site and is trimmed, shaped into the breast, and sutured into place (Serletti et al., 2011).

Patients are screened for contraindications prior to proceeding with surgery. Patients must have sufficient lower abdominal tissue and no previous surgery that would interrupt the blood supply, and any comorbidities must be evaluated before surgery. Risk factors associated with TRAM flap complications are obesity, a history of smoking, and previous invasive or noninvasive breast cancer with radiation therapy to the surgical site (Laronga & Smith, 2014). The procedure in which the deep inferior epigastric artery is ligated usually is performed during sentinel lymph node biopsy approximately two weeks before mastectomy and reconstruction to increase the superior epigastric vessel diameter (Serletti et al., 2011).

Prophylactic mastectomy: Bilateral prophylactic mastectomy is an option considered for breast cancer risk reduction for individuals with moderate to high risk and may reduce mortality in those with *BRCA* mutations. NCCN guidelines do not recommend prophylactic mastectomy in women with LCIS without additional risk factors (NCCN, 2016b). Bilateral prophylactic mastectomy also is considered for women who have been treated with mantle radiation for Hodgkin lymphoma and for patients with non-*BRCA* hereditary breast cancer syndromes (Burke et al., 2015).

Breast ductal lavage: Ductoscopy is an endoscopic technique that enables direct visualization of the mammary ductal epithelium using fiber-optic microendoscopes inserted through the ductal openings of the nipple and is an important tool to characterize intraductal lesions (Lian et al., 2015). Ductal lavage is a minimally invasive surgical procedure used to identify cellular abnormalities in the epithelial lining of the breast duct (Green, 2015). Following an initial aspiration to identify fluid-yielding breast ducts, a small catheter is placed into the duct and is used to infuse several milliliters of normal saline. The resultant ductal effluent is collected and examined using cytopathology. Researchers offer ductal lavage and ductoscopy to women with a prior history of breast cancer and those at high risk for breast cancer. However, data are insufficient to recommend this as an independent screening tool to determine treatment (Green, 2015).

Conclusion

Because cancer surgery is ubiquitous in the cancer continuum, most oncology nurses are involved in surgical patient care. Through participation in specialized surgical oncology teams, surgical oncology clinical trials, and pal-

Key Points

- Surgery is the most consistently effective method to treat and cure cancer.
- Confirmation of the initial pathology is recommended before beginning a new treatment.
- Tumor staging is specific to the type of cancer and is essential in developing an appropriate therapeutic program.
- Resection of the primary tumor or removal of the entire tumor with adequate margins of normal tissue is the goal of curative surgical treatment.
- Advances in cancer risk analysis and genetic screening have resulted in opportunities for surgical prevention of cancer.
- Laparoscopic and robotic-assisted procedures offer significant surgical advantages.
- CT screening is a significant method to improve the early detection of lung cancer.
- Surgical resection is a common treatment for colorectal cancer.
- Transrectal ultrasound core biopsy is used to obtain multiple biopsies to diagnose prostate cancer.
- Breast-conserving surgery is considered for women with early-stage breast cancer.

liative and end-of-life surgical interventions for symptom management, oncology nurses provide critical and compassionate care to patients with cancer. Nurses are contributors to the advances in multidisciplinary care, clinical trials, laboratory and genetic sciences, and surgical technologies to improve cancer diagnosis, treatment, prevention, rehabilitation, and palliation.

References

Alberg, A.J., Brock, M.V., Ford, J.G., Samet, J.M., & Spivack, S.D. (2013). Epidemiology of lung cancer: Diagnosis and management of lung cancer, 3rd ed: American College of Chest Physicians evidence-based clinical practice guidelines. *Chest, 143*(Suppl. 5), e1S–e29S. doi:10.1378/chest.12-2345

American Cancer Society. (2016a). Breast cancer: Causes, risk factors, and prevention. Retrieved from http://www.cancer.org/cancer/breastcancer/detailedguide/breast-cancer-risk-factors

American Cancer Society. (2016b). Breast cancer in men. Retrieved from http://www.cancer.org/cancer/breastcancerinmen/detailedguide/index

American Cancer Society. (2016c). *Cancer facts and figures 2016.* Atlanta, GA: Author.

American Cancer Society. (2016d). *Cancer treatment and survivorship facts and figures 2016–2017.* Atlanta, GA: Author.

American Cancer Society. (2016e). Colon cancer: Causes, risk factors and prevention. Retrieved from http://www.cancer.org/cancer/colonandrectumcancer/moreinformation/colonandrectumcancerearlydetection/colorectal-cancer-early-detection-risk-factors-for-crc

American Cancer Society. (2016f). Lung cancer: Signs and symptoms of lung cancer. Retrieved from http://www.cancer.org/cancer/lungcancer-non-smallcell/moreinformation/lungcancerpreventionandearlydetection/lung-cancer-prevention-and-early-detection-signs-and-symptoms

American Cancer Society. (2016g). Prostate cancer: Causes, risk factors and prevention. Retrieved from http://www.cancer.org/cancer/prostatecancer/detailedguide/prostate-cancer-risk-factors

American Cancer Society. (2016h). Prostate cancer treatment: Watchful waiting or active surveillance for prostate cancer. Retrieved from http://www.cancer.org/cancer/prostatecancer/detailedguide/prostate-cancer-treating-watchful-waiting

American Cancer Society. (2016i). Why non-smokers sometimes get lung cancer. Retrieved from http://www.cancer.org/cancer/news/features/why-lung-cancer-strikes-nonsmokers

Baker, M.K. (2014). Breast cancer: Surgical management. In J.L. Cameron & A.M. Cameron (Eds.), *Current surgical therapy* (11th ed., pp. 584–586). Philadelphia, PA: Elsevier Saunders.

Ban, K.A., & Godellas, C.V. (2014). Epidemiology of breast cancer. *Surgical Oncology Clinics of North America, 23,* 409–422. doi:10.1016/j.soc.2014.03.011

Berek, J.S., Friedlander, M., & Hacker, N.F. (2010). Epithelial ovarian, fallopian tube, and peritoneal cancer. In J.S. Berek & N.F. Hacker (Eds.), *Berek and Hacker's gynecologic oncology* (5th ed., pp. 443–508). Philadelphia, PA: Wolters Kluwer Health/Lippincott Williams & Wilkins.

Blackmon, S.H. (2014). Minimally invasive resections for lung cancer. In J.A. Roth, W.K. Hong, R.U. Komaki, F. Fastro, A.S. Tsao, J.Y. Chang, & S.H. Blackmon (Eds.), *Lung cancer* (4th ed., pp. 224–235). Hoboken, NJ: John Wiley & Sons. doi:10.1002/9781118468791.ch14

Blackmon, S.H., & Vaporciyan, A.A. (2012). Thoracic malignancies. In B.W. Feig & D.C. Ching (Eds.), *The MD Anderson surgical oncology handbook* (5th ed.). Philadelphia, PA: Wolters Kluwer Health/Lippincott Williams & Wilkins.

Burke, E.E., Portschy, P.R., & Tuttle, T.M. (2015). Prophylactic mastectomy: Who needs it, when and why. *Journal of Surgical Oncology, 111,* 91–95. doi:10.1002/jso.23695

Carr, L.L., Finigan, J.H., & Kern, J.A. (2011). Evaluation and treatment of patients with non–small cell lung cancer. *Medical Clinics of North America, 95,* 1041–1054. doi:10.1016/j.mcna.2011.08.001

Chakravorty, A., Shrestha, A.K., Sanmugalingam, N., Rapisarda, F., Roche, N., Querci della Rovere, G., & MacNeill, F.A. (2012). How safe is oncoplastic breast conservation?: Comparative analysis with standard breast conserving surgery. *European Journal of Surgical Oncology, 38,* 395–398. doi:10.1016/j.ejso.2012.02.186

Chan, D.K.-H., Chong, C.-S., Lieske, B., & Tan, K.-K. (2014). Laparoscopic resection for rectal cancer: What is the evidence? *BioMed Research International, 2014,* Article ID 347810. doi:10.1155/2014/347810

Church, T.R., & Mandel, J.S. (2011). Screening for gastrointestinal cancers. In V.T. DeVita Jr., T.S. Lawrence, & S.A. Rosenberg (Eds.), *Cancer: Principles and practice of oncology* (9th ed., pp. 596–609). Philadelphia, PA: Wolters Kluwer Health/Lippincott Williams & Wilkins.

Cochran, A.J., Roberts, A.A., & Saida, T. (2003). The place of lymphatic mapping and sentinel node biopsy in oncology. *International Journal of Clinical Oncology, 8,* 139–150. doi:10.1007/s10147-003-0333-9

Cuellar, S.L.B., Marom, E.M., & Erasmus, J.J. (2014). Imaging lung cancer. In J.A. Roth, W.K. Hong, R.U. Komaki, F. Fastro, A.S. Tsao, J.Y. Chang, & S.H. Blackmon (Eds.), *Lung cancer* (4th ed., pp. 191–201). Hoboken,

NJ: John Wiley & Sons. doi:10.1002/9781118468791.ch11

Fouad, M.N., Lee, J.Y., Catalano, P.J., Vogt, T.M., Zafar, S.Y., West, D.W., … Kiefe, C.I. (2013). Enrollment of patients with lung and colorectal cancers onto clinical trials. *Journal of Oncology Practice, 9,* e40–e47. doi:10.1200/JOP.2012.000598

Gillitzer, R., & Thüroff, J.W. (2013). Radical perineal prostatectomy. In A. Tewari (Ed.), *Prostate cancer: A comprehensive perspective* (pp. 663–678). London, England: Springer-Verlag. doi:10.1007/978-1-4471-2864-9_55

Gipponi, M., Solari, N., Di Somma, F.C., Bertoglio, S., & Cafiero, F. (2004). New fields of application of the sentinel lymph node biopsy in the pathologic staging of solid neoplasms: Review of literature and surgical perspectives. *Journal of Surgical Oncology, 85,* 171–179. doi:10.1002/jso.20031

Green, V.L. (2015). Breast cancer screening. In E.J. Bieber, J.S. Sanfilippo, I.R. Horowitz, & M.I. Shafi (Eds.), *Clinical gynecology* (2nd ed., pp. 691–722). Cambridge, United Kingdom: Cambridge University Press. doi:10.1017/cbo9781139628938.046

Halabi, W.J., Kang, C.Y., Jafari, M.D., Nguyen, V.Q., Carmichael, J.C., Mills, S., … Pigazzi, A. (2013). Robotic-assisted colorectal surgery in the United States: A nationwide analysis of trends and outcomes. *World Journal of Surgery, 37,* 2782–2790. doi:10.1007/s00268-013-2024-7

Hanna, J.M., Berry, M.F., & D'Amico, T.A. (2013). Contraindications of video-assisted thoracoscopic surgical lobectomy and determinants of conversion to open. *Journal of Thoracic Disease, 5*(Suppl. 3), S182–S189. doi:10.3978/j.issn.2072-1439.2013.07.08

Jang, R.W., Caraiscos, V.B., Swami, N., Banerjee, S., Mak, E., Kaya, E., … Zimmermann, C. (2014). Simple prognostic model for patients with advanced cancer based on performance status. *Journal of Oncology Practice, 10,* e335–e341. doi:10.1200/JOP.2014.001457

Knipe, D.W., Evans, D.M., Kemp, J.P., Eeles, R., Easton, D.F., Kote-Jarai, Z., … Martin, R.M. (2014). Genetic variation in protein specific antigen detected prostate cancer and the effect of control selection on genetic association studies. *Cancer Epidemiology, Biomarkers and Prevention, 23,* 1356–1365. doi:10.1158/1055-9965.EPI-13-0889

Kwon, D.S., Kelly, C.M., & Ching, C.D. (2012). Invasive breast cancer. In B.W. Feig & C.D. Ching (Eds.), *The MD Anderson surgical oncology handbook* (5th ed.). Philadelphia, PA: Wolters Kluwer Health/Lippincott Williams & Wilkins.

Laronga, C., & Smith, P. (2014). Nipple-sparing mastectomy: An oncologic and cosmetic perspective. *Surgical Oncology Clinics of North America, 23,* 549–566. doi:10.1016/j.soc.2014.03.013

Lian, Z.-Q., Wang, Q., Zhang, A.-Q., Zhang, J.-Y., Han, X.-R., Yu, H.-Y., & Xie, S.-M. (2015). A nomogram based on mammary ductoscopic indicators for evaluating the risk of breast cancer in intraductal neoplasms with nipple discharge. *Breast Cancer Research and Treatment, 150,* 373–380. doi:10.1007/s10549-015-3320-8

Lu, D., Onn, A., Vaporciyan, A., Chang, J., Glisson, B., Komaki, R., … Herbst, R. (2010). Cancer of the lung. In W.K. Hong, R.C. Bast Jr., W.N. Hait, D.W. Kufe, R.E. Pollock, R.R. Weichselbaum, … E. Frei III (Eds.), *Holland-Frei cancer medicine* (8th ed., pp. 999–1043). Shelton, CT: People's Medical Publishing House–USA.

McAuliffe, P.F., Andtbacka, R.H.I., Robinson, E.K., & Hunt, K.K. (2012). Noninvasive breast cancer. In B.W. Feig & C.D. Ching (Eds.), *The MD Anderson surgical oncology handbook* (5th ed.). Philadelphia, PA: Wolters Kluwer Health/Lippincott Williams & Wilkins.

Miyoshi, S. (2013). Intraoperative nodal staging: Role of sentinel node technology. *Thoracic Surgery Clinics, 23,* 357–368. doi:10.1016/j.thorsurg.2013.04.002

Morrow, M. (2012). Refining the use of endocrine therapy for ductal carcinoma in situ. *Journal of Clinical Oncology, 30,* 1249–1251. doi:10.1200/jco.2011.40.5514

National Cancer Institute. (n.d.). Gleason score. In *NCI dictionary of cancer terms.* Retrieved from http://www.cancer.gov/publications/dictionaries/cancer-terms?cdrid=45696

National Comprehensive Cancer Network. (2016a). *NCCN Clinical Practice Guidelines in Oncology (NCCN Guidelines®): Breast cancer* [v.2.2016]. Retrieved from http://www.nccn.org/professionals/physician_gls/PDF/breast.pdf

National Comprehensive Cancer Network. (2016b). *NCCN Clinical Practice Guidelines in Oncology (NCCN Guidelines®): Breast cancer risk reduction* [v.1.2016]. Retrieved from https://www.nccn.org/professionals/physician_gls/pdf/breast_risk.pdf

National Comprehensive Cancer Network. (2016c). *NCCN Clinical Practice Guidelines in Oncology (NCCN Guidelines®): Prostate cancer* [v.1.2017]. Retrieved from http://www.nccn.org/professionals/physician_gls/PDF/prostate.pdf

National Comprehensive Cancer Network. (2016d). *NCCN Clinical Practice Guidelines in Oncology (NCCN Guidelines®): Small cell lung cancer* [v.2.2017]. Retrieved from http://www.nccn.org/professionals/physician_gls/PDF/sclc.pdf

Nelson, W.G., Carter, H.B., DeWeese, T.L., Antonarakis, E.S., & Eisenberger, M.A. (2014). Prostate cancer. In J.E. Niederhuber, J.O. Armitage, J.H. Doroshow, M.B. Kastan, & J.E. Tepper (Eds.), *Abeloff's clinical oncology* (5th ed., pp. 1463–1496). Philadelphia, PA: Elsevier Saunders.

Padussis, J.C., Beasley, G.M., McMahon, N.S., Tyler, D.S., & Ludwig, K.A. (2010). Neoplasms of the small intestine, vermiform appendix, and peritoneum, and carcinoma of the colon and rectum. In W.K. Hong, R.C. Bast Jr., W.N. Hait, D.W. Kufe, R.E. Pollock, R.R. Weichselbaum, ... E. Frei III (Eds.), *Holland-Frei cancer medicine* (8th ed., pp. 1172–1193). Shelton, CT: People's Medical Publishing House–USA.

Pipkin, M., & Keshavjee, S. (2014). Staging of the mediastinum. In J.A. Roth, W.K. Hong, R.U. Komaki, F. Fastro, A.S. Tsao, J.Y. Chang, & S.H. Blackmon (Eds.), *Lung cancer* (4th ed., pp. 202–213). Hoboken, NJ: John Wiley & Sons. doi:10.1002/9781118468791.ch12

Pollock, R.E., Choti, M.A., & Morton, D.L. (2010). Principles of surgical oncology. In W.K. Hong, R.C. Bast Jr., W.N. Hait, D.W. Kufe, R.E. Pollock, R.R. Weichselbaum, ... E. Frei III (Eds.), *Holland-Frei cancer medicine* (8th ed., pp. 499–509). Shelton, CT: People's Medical Publishing House–USA.

Prokhorov, A.V., & Hudmon, K.S. (2014). Smoking prevention and cessation. In J.A. Roth, W.K. Hong, R.U. Komaki, F. Fastro, A.S. Tsao, J.Y. Chang, & S.H. Blackmon (Eds.), *Lung cancer* (4th ed., pp. 1–24). Hoboken, NJ: John Wiley & Sons. doi:10.1002/9781118468791.ch1

Qian, J. (2011). Interventional therapies of unresectable liver metastases. *Journal of Cancer Research and Clinical Oncology, 137,* 1763–1772. doi:10.1007/s00432-011-1026-9

Reece, J.C., Chan, Y.-F., Herbert, J., Gralow, J., & Fann, J.R. (2013). Course of depression, mental health service utilization and treatment preferences in women receiving chemotherapy for breast cancer. *General Hospital Psychiatry, 35,* 376–381. doi:10.1016/j.genhosppsych.2013.03.017

Reid, S.V., & Hamdy, F.C. (2008). Epidemiology, pathology, and pathogenesis. In V.H. Nargund, D. Raghavan, & H.M. Sandler (Eds.), *Urological oncology* (pp. 451–469). London, United Kingdom: Springer.

Rosenberg, S.A. (2011). Surgical oncology: General issues. In V.T. DeVita Jr., T.S. Lawrence, & S.A. Rosenberg (Eds.), *Cancer: Principles and practice of oncology* (9th ed., pp. 268–276). Philadelphia, PA: Wolters Kluwer Health/Lippincott Williams & Wilkins.

Sabel, M.S. (2007). Principles of surgical therapy. In M.S. Sabel, V.K. Sondak, & J.J. Sussman (Eds.), *Surgical foundations: Essentials of surgical oncology* (pp. 39–52). Philadelphia: Elsevier Mosby.

Sabel, M.S. (2011). Surgical considerations in early-stage breast cancer: Lessons learned and future directions. *Seminars in Radiation Oncology, 21,* 10–19. doi:10.1016/j.semradonc.2010.08.002

Schorge, J.O., McCann, C., & Del Carmen, M.G. (2010). Surgical debulking of ovarian cancer: What difference does it make? *Reviews in Obstetrics and Gynecology, 3,* 111–117. Retrieved from http://www.ncbi.nlm.nih.gov/pmc/articles/PMC3046749

Serletti, J.M., Fosnot, J., Nelson, J.A., Disa, J.J., & Bucky, L.P. (2011). Breast reconstruction after breast cancer. *Plastic and Reconstructive Surgery, 127,* 124e–135e. doi:10.1097/PRS.0b013e318213a2e6

Smith, J.A., Jr. (2013). Radical treatment for localized disease: An overview of options and strategies for decision making. In A. Tewari (Ed.), *Prostate cancer: A comprehensive perspective* (pp. 609–614). London, UK: Springer-Verlag. doi:10.1007/978-1-4471-2864-9_49

Smith, L., Brinton, L.A., Spitz, M.R., Lam, T.K., Park, Y., Hollenbeck, A.R., ... Gierach, G.L. (2012). Body mass index and risk of lung cancer among never, former, and current smokers. *Journal of the National Cancer Institute, 104,* 778–789. doi:10.1093/jnci/djs179

Society of Surgical Oncology. (n.d.). Program list. Retrieved from http://www.surgonc.org/training-fellows/fellows-education/breast-oncology/program-list

Tanner, N.T., Mehta, H., & Silvestri, G.A. (2012). New testing for lung cancer screening. *Oncology.* Retrieved from http://www.cancernetwork.com/oncology-journal/new-testing-lung-cancer-screening

Tarchi, P., Moretti, E., & de Manzini, N. (2013). Reconstruction. In N. de Manzini (Ed.), *Rectal cancer: Strategy and surgical techniques* (pp. 117–130). Milan, Italy: Springer-Verlag Italia. doi:10.1007/978-88-470-2670-4_9

Tenofsky, P.L., Dowell, P., Topalovski, T., & Helmer, S.D. (2014). Surgical, oncologic, and cosmetic differences between oncoplastic and nononcoplastic breast conserving surgery in breast cancer patients. *American Journal of Surgery, 207,* 398–402. doi:10.1016/j.amjsurg.2013.09.017

Thomas, D.C., & Ragnarsson, K.T. (2010). Principles of cancer rehabilitation medicine. In W.K. Hong, R.C. Bast Jr., W.N. Hait, D.W. Kufe, R.E. Pollock, R.R. Weichselbaum, ... E. Frei III (Eds.), *Holland-Frei cancer medicine* (8th ed., pp. 810–822). Shelton, CT: People's Medical Publishing House–USA.

Tse, K.Y., & Ngan, H.Y.S. (2015). The role of laparoscopy in staging of different gynaecological cancers. *Best Practice and Research: Clinical Obstetrics and Gynaecology, 29,* 884–895. doi:10.1016/j.bpobgyn.2015.01.007

Turner, B., & Drudge-Coates, L. (2010). Prostate cancer: Risk factors, diagnosis and management. *Cancer Nursing Practice, 9*(10), 29–35. doi:10.7748/cnp2010.12.9.10.29.c8126

Urban, C., Lima, R., Schunemann, E., Spautz, C., Rabinovich, I., & Anselmi, K. (2011). Oncoplastic principles in breast conserving surgery. *Breast, 20,* S92–S95. doi:10.1016/s0960-9776(11)70302-2

Van Schaeybroeck, S., Lawler, M., Johnston, B., Salto-Tellez, M., Lee, J., Loughlin, P., ... Johnston, P. (2014). Colorectal cancer. In J.E. Niederhuber, J.O. Armitage, J.H. Doroshow, M.B. Kastan, & J.E. Tepper (Eds.), *Abel-*

off's clinical oncology (5th ed., pp. 1278–1335). Philadelphia, PA: Elsevier Saunders.

Wells, C.A., & Arkoumani, E. (2013). Premalignant and borderline lesions: Ductal and lobular carcinoma in situ. In J.R. Benson, G. Gui, & T.M. Tuttle (Eds.), *Early breast cancer: From screening to multidisciplinary management* (3rd ed., pp. 250–265). Boca Raton, FL: CRC Press. doi:10.1201/b13937-28

Wilson, A.R.M. (2013). Breast masses. In J.R. Benson, G. Gui, & T.M. Tuttle (Eds.), *Early breast cancer: From screening to multidisciplinary management* (3rd ed., pp. 148–155). Boca Raton, FL: CRC Press. doi:10.1201/b13937-17

Yip, R., Henschke, C.I., Yankelevitz, D.F., Boffetta, P., & Smith, J.P. (2015). The impact of the regimen of screening on lung cancer cure: A comparison of I-ELCAP and NLST. *European Journal of Cancer Prevention, 24,* 201–208. doi:10.1097/CEJ.0000000000000065

Zurrida, S., & Veronesi, U. (2015). Milestones in breast cancer treatment. *Breast Journal, 21,* 3–12. doi:10.1111/tbj.12361

Chapter 7 Study Questions

1. Oncology nurses are members of a patient-centered, multidisciplinary surgical oncology cancer care team that often includes which of the following?
   A. Pathologists
   B. Radiologists
   C. Pharmacists
   D. Psychologists
   E. All of the above

2. Preventive surgical practices include all of the following EXCEPT:
   A. Colectomy.
   B. Bilateral mastectomy.
   C. Thyroidectomy.
   D. Medullectomy.

3. Important considerations for discussion with patients prior to cancer surgery include all of the following EXCEPT:
   A. Expected long-term survival.
   B. Likelihood of curative treatment.
   C. Quality of life.
   D. Age at diagnosis.
   E. Surgical risks.

4. Surgical techniques used for lung cancer pathologic diagnosis and staging include all of the following EXCEPT:
   A. Bronchoscopy.
   B. Mediastinoscopy.
   C. Computed tomography–guided needle biopsy.
   D. Colonoscopy.
   E. Thoracotomy.

5. Ductal carcinoma in situ accounts for approximately how many newly detected breast cancers found with screening examinations?
   A. 5%–10%
   B. 20%–25%
   C. 50%
   D. 100%

CHAPTER

8 Radiation Therapy

Anne Marie Shaftic, MSN, RN, AOCNP®

Introduction

More than 60% of patients with cancer will undergo radiation therapy (Ruppert, 2011). For some, it will be the only cancer treatment they need. Radiation can be combined with chemotherapy or used before, during, or after surgery. When combining radiation therapy with other treatments, such as chemotherapy or surgery, it can shrink the tumor, making surgery or chemotherapy more effective. When used after surgery in particular, it destroys any cancer cells that might remain (Moding, Kastan, & Kirsch, 2013). For many patients and family members, the idea of treatment with radiation is frightening. Nuclear accidents, terrorist threats, and the distressing experiences of some patients treated with radiation many years ago all make it difficult for people to think of radiation as safe. Having a basic understanding of the science behind this treatment modality will help nurses to educate patients effectively and dispel the myths and misconceptions.

The Science Behind Radiation Therapy

Radiation Physics

All matter is composed of atoms bound together to form molecules. Each atom has a central nucleus of neutrons and positively charged protons, around which negatively charged electrons orbit (see Figure 8-1). In the normal state, an equal number of protons and electrons are present. If an atom loses or gains an electron, this balance is altered and the atom becomes ionized, with a positive or negative charge. This, in turn, may damage or destroy the molecule (Khan & Gibbons, 2014).

Figure 8-1. Structure of an Atom

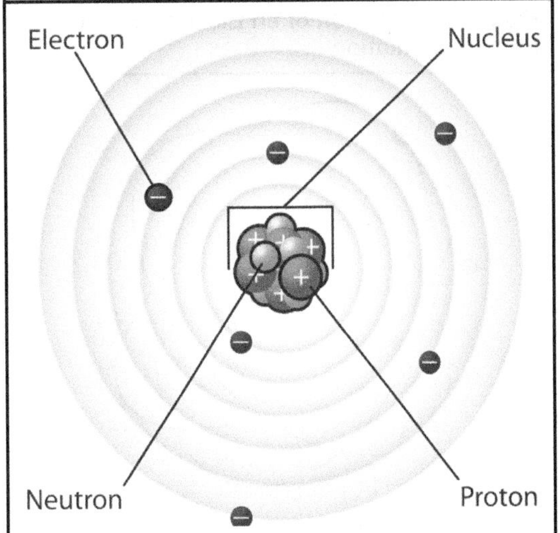

Note. Image copyright 2008 by Memorial Sloan Kettering Cancer Center. Used with permission.

Ionizing radiation is a form of energy radiation with enough energy that during an interaction with an atom, it can remove tightly bound electrons from the orbit of an atom, causing the atom to become charged, or ionized (see Figure 8-2). When patients are treated with radiation therapy, this ionizing energy is used in a controlled way to destroy cancer cells. Ionizing radiation can be in the form of electromagnetic waves or particles (World Health Organization, n.d.).

The electromagnetic energy spectrum includes all types of energy emitted in the form of waves. These waves vary in their lengths and frequencies. Electromagnetic energy includes radio waves, visible light, and ultraviolet light. Waves with the shortest length and highest frequency have the greatest amount of energy and are called *photons*. These include x-rays and gamma rays, both of which cause ionization and are used in treating cancer. X-rays are generated electrically, and gamma rays are emitted from a radioactive source; both are capable of penetrating deeply into the body (Khan & Gibbons, 2014).

Figure 8-2. Ejection of an Electron From Ionizing Radiation

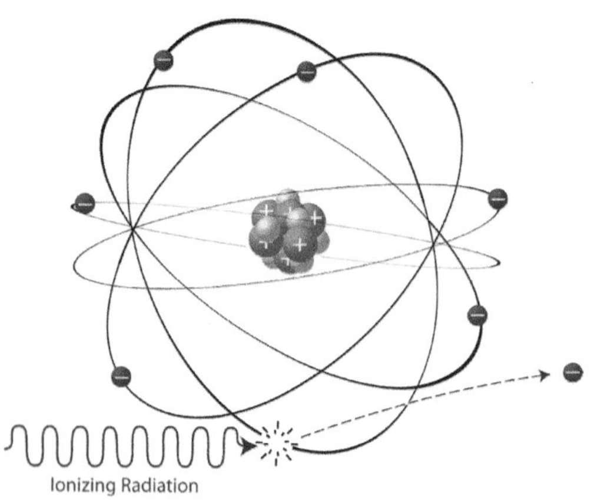

Note. Image copyright 2008 by Memorial Sloan Kettering Cancer Center. Used with permission.

In radiation treatment planning, energy is selected based on the part of the body that will be treated with radiation therapy. Two different radiation delivery methods exist. External beam radiation therapy (EBRT) uses specialized machines (such as the linear accelerator) to deliver a dose of radiation directly to the cancer site from outside of the body. Internal radiation, or brachytherapy, involves radioactive implants placed in the body at the tumor site. Radiation implants can be small tubes, seeds, or capsules filled with different types of sealed radioactive material. Brachytherapy allows for the delivery of higher doses of radiation to a more specific area of the body, such as the cervical canal. Brachytherapy may have fewer side effects than EBRT, plus the overall treatment time is usually shorter. Common sites for use of brachytherapy are cancers of the cervix, prostate, breast, and bronchus (Iwamoto, Haas, & Gosselin, 2012).

A radiation oncologist prescribes radiation, specifying the delivery method and dose of radiation. The dose is calculated in gray (Gy) or centigray (cGy) (1 Gy = 100 cGy) units (American Cancer Society, 2014a). The total dose generally is divided into multiple small doses given daily, Monday through Friday, over a number of weeks. Dividing the total dose is referred to as *fractionation*. Alternative schedules also are used, such as *hyperfractionation*, with smaller doses given two to three times a day, or *hypofractionation*, with larger doses over a shorter total treatment time (Wang et al., 2014). In select situations, such as bone marrow transplantation, the entire treatment can be given as a single high dose.

Radiobiology

Radiobiology describes the physical, chemical, and biologic changes that occur when the body is exposed to ionizing radiation. Irradiated atoms become ionized, damaging the molecules built from those atoms. The DNA molecule is particularly vulnerable (see Figure 8-3).

Figure 8-3. Indirect and Direct Effects of Ionizing Radiation on the DNA Molecule

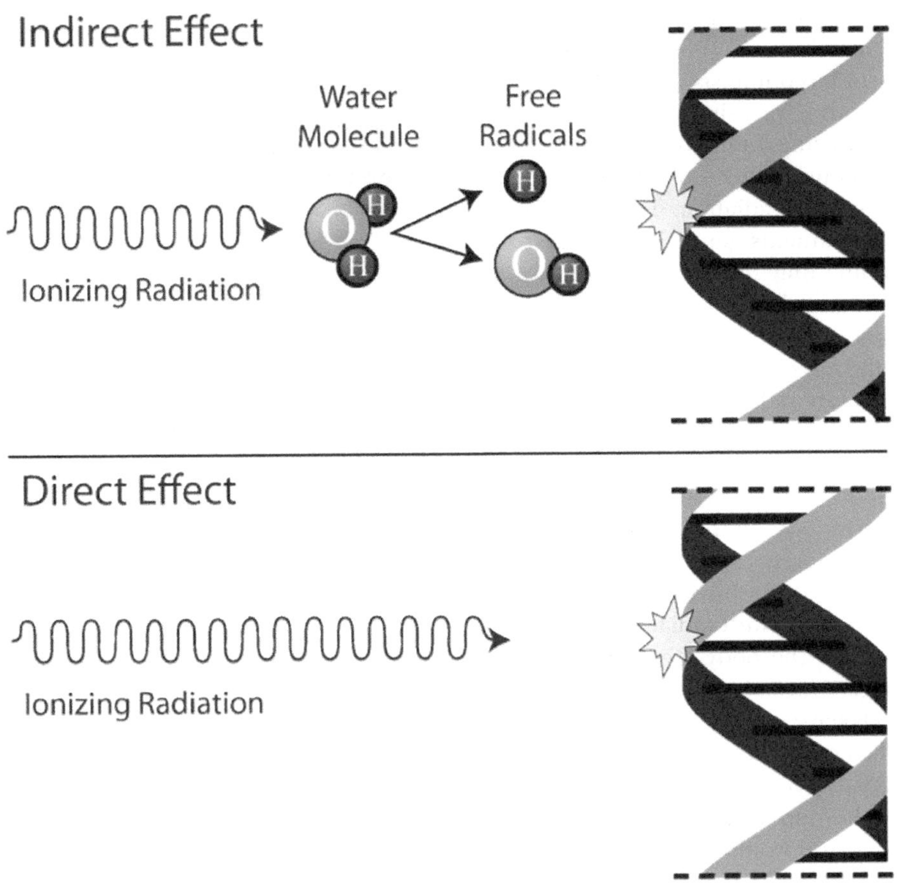

Note. Image copyright 2008 by Memorial Sloan Kettering Cancer Center. Used with permission.

The primary effect is indirect, due to ionization of water molecules in the cells. These water molecules undergo a series of reactions resulting in the formation of free radicals (such as the hydroxyl anion, OH*) with a number of high-energy, unpaired electrons that cause breaks in the DNA strands. Ionizing radiation can have four different effects on the cell, including (a) damage causing the inability of the cell to function, resulting in cell death, (b) loss of the ability to reproduce, (c) DNA damage resulting in the alteration of future copies of chromosomes, or (d) no effect on the cell (Morgan & Sowa, 2013). Some cells are more sensitive to radiation than others; those that multiply rapidly are the most susceptible. Some examples of rapidly multiplying cells are gastrointestinal mucosa, fetal tissue, and cancer cells (Ruppert, 2011). Cells can repair radiation damage, but if the damaged cell splits into two new identical cells before they are able to repair radiation damage, the new cells might not be accurate copies of the healthy one. All cells will attempt to repair the damage and, if effective, will continue to function and divide. However, if the cell is not able to repair itself, it will die, either immediately or at a subsequent time as it attempts to undergo mitosis. Normal cells and cancer cells both have a similar response when exposed to ionizing radiation. Normal cells, however, are better able to repair themselves, ultimately surviving radiation. The time interval between treatments generally is at least six hours, providing time for the repair of normal tissues (Moding et al., 2013).

Some cancer cells and normal cells are more sensitive to the effects of radiation than others. Cells that are more radiosensitive are those that are rapidly dividing, moving through the G_2 or M phase (right before or during mitosis) of the cell cycle, poorly differentiated, and well oxygenated (McBride & Withers, 2008). Understanding the differences in tissue radiosensitivity helps to predict which cancers will best respond to treatment with radiation and which normal tissues in the body are most susceptible to damage. Normal tissues and organs of the body each have unique tolerance to radiation regardless of the tissue volume irradiated (Passmore, 2016). If tissue is exposed to doses of radiation beyond this tolerance, the side effects or toxicities would be too severe to be acceptable. These issues pose major challenges in the use of radiation to treat cancer. One of the goals of radiation therapy is to administer the highest possible dose to the tumor to ensure destruction but to avoid excessive toxicity based on the tolerance of the surrounding normal tissues (Moding et al., 2013).

Clinical Uses of Radiation Therapy

Radiation therapy is used for many patients with cancer, whether the goal is cure, control, or palliation. Table 8-1 lists examples of the clinical uses of radiation therapy.

Table 8-1. Clinical Uses of Radiation Therapy

Goal of Treatment	Clinical Examples
Cure: to eradicate the disease	
• Definitive treatment: Radiation therapy (RT) as the primary treatment, with or without chemotherapy	Early-stage prostate cancer Laryngeal cancer
• Neoadjuvant treatment: RT before surgery to shrink a tumor, increase resectability, and enable less extensive organ-sparing surgery	Locally advanced rectal cancer
• Adjuvant treatment: RT after surgery to destroy gross or microscopic residual disease and prevent tumor recurrence	Early-stage breast cancer
Control: to prolong life and extend the time that patients are without symptoms	Locally advanced pancreatic cancer
Palliation: to relieve symptoms of advanced disease (e.g., pain, obstruction, neurologic symptoms)	Bone metastasis Brain metastasis Lung cancer Spinal cord compression

Note. Based on information from American Cancer Society, 2014a.

In some patients, chemotherapy is given concurrently with radiation to increase the response of the tumor to radiation. This generally is used in patients with locally advanced disease or to allow for organ-sparing treatment (Lawrence, Haffty, & Harris, 2014). Examples of tumors for which chemotherapy is given with radiation include locally advanced cancers of the head and neck, lung, esophagus, pancreas, rectum, anus, bladder, and cervix. Examples of chemotherapy agents used are 5-fluorouracil, cisplatin, paclitaxel, gemcitabine, and irinotecan. Concurrent chemotherapy and radiation therapy is an evolving field, and increasing numbers of agents are being given in a variety of schedules in clinical practice and as investigational protocols (Lawrence et al., 2014).

External Beam Radiation Therapy

Before beginning treatment, patients will have a consultation with the radiation oncologist. During this visit, the clinician will take a history, perform a physical examination, review diagnostic tests, and determine whether radiation therapy is an appropriate treatment. If the patient is to receive radiation therapy with EBRT, the next step would be to schedule an appointment to begin the simulation process.

Simulation

A licensed radiation therapist, working in coordination with the radiation oncologist, will ensure that the radiation beams are directed to the correct part of the body through careful patient positioning that is reproducible for each treatment. Approximately three to seven tattoos are applied to guide direction of the external beam. For some patients, immobilization devices also are used (see Figure 8-4). The position for radiation treatment is corrected by aligning the tattoos and markings on the immobilization device to laser lights coming from the walls and ceiling in the simulation and treatment room (see Figure 8-5).

Once correct positioning is achieved, radiologic images are then obtained to localize the area to be treated. Computed tomography (CT) scans are most commonly used, but for some areas of the body, magnetic resonance imaging or positron-emission tomography scans also are obtained. The images are fused to better demarcate the structures in the area and differentiate malignant from nonmalignant tissue (Leaver, Keller, & Uricchio, 2010).

Treatment Planning

After simulation, the radiation oncologist uses the radiologic images to contour the volumes of the tumor to be treated and to avoid the normal surrounding structures. These images are then used to create virtual three-dimensional reconstructions of the treatment area. Based on these, physicists, in collaboration with the radiation oncologist, develop the treatment plan. They determine the number, angles, and shapes of the multiple overlapping beams (or fields) of radiation to direct to the tumor (Iwamoto et al., 2012).

Based on the treatment plan, physicists calculate the exact dose to be delivered to the tumor and to the normal surrounding structures. As noted previously, the goal of therapy is to deliver the maximal dose to the target area while minimizing the dose to normal surrounding tissue to prevent excessive toxicities (Iwamoto et al., 2012).

The treatment plan is based on the position of the patient during simulation. However, even with immobilization devices and tattoos, a position cannot be reproduced in exactly the same way each day the patient comes in for treatment. In addition, the position of the tumor itself within the body can vary from moment to moment because of organ movement related to respiration (lung or liver), peristalsis (abdominal and pelvic structures), or bladder and rectal fullness (prostate). Furthermore, the volume of the tumor itself can change over time because of shrinkage from treatment (Iwamoto et al., 2012). To accommodate these variations, the targeted area for treatment includes margins of up to 1 cm of normal tissue (Iwamoto et al., 2012).

Setup

Before the first treatment, the patient will come for a "setup" appointment. Radiation therapists position the patient on the treatment couch, using immobilization devices as appropriate, and the couch is moved to align

Figure 8-4. Immobilization Devices

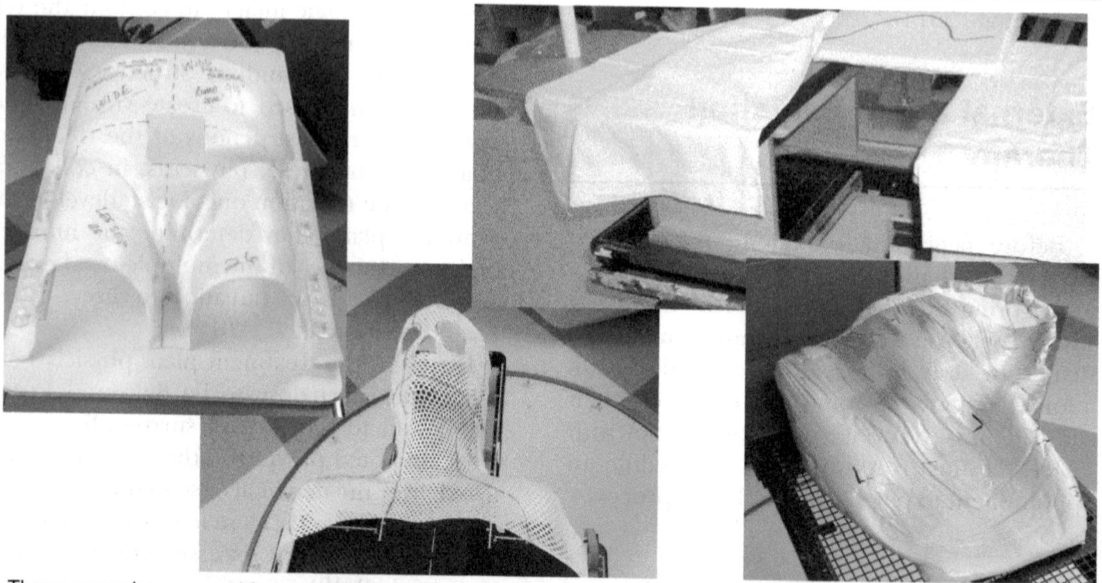

These examples are used for patients being treated for prostate cancer (supine position with mold placed over the abdomen, pelvis, and upper thighs), head and neck cancer (supine position with mold placed over the head, neck, and shoulders), and breast cancer (supine position on top of mold with left arm elevated or prone with breast hanging dependently through the aperture).

Note. Images copyright 2008 by Memorial Sloan Kettering Cancer Center. Used with permission.

the skin tattoos and device markings with the lasers. X-ray or CT images are taken from each beam or field of treatment to ensure that the patient has been set up correctly and that the beams are being directed to the targeted areas as planned. These images are repeated regularly throughout the treatment to ensure that no significant shifts have occurred (Iwamoto et al., 2012).

Treatment Delivery

Licensed radiation therapists administer the EBRT treatment. Each day of treatment, the patient is positioned on the treatment couch in the exact way as during the simulation and setup. The external treatment is most commonly delivered with a linear accelerator that produces x-rays and/or electrons (see Figure 8-6). The gantry is a part of the EBRT machine that can rotate 360°. With movement of the treatment couch and rotation of the gantry, the beam of energy can be directed at any desired angle. The beam exits through the collimator and generally is shaped using a multileaf collimator (MLC). This is composed of a set of tungsten leaves, each of which can move independently to shape the beam for each field of treatment (see Figure 8-7) (Coleman, 2016).

Once the patient and gantry are set up, the radiation therapists leave the room and select the correct beam shape for the MLC. The total beam-on time for most treatments is 3–15 minutes. Patients may hear the machine as it turns on and off between fields, and they can see the gantry move to the different angles defined in their plan. The radiation beam does not create any sensation of heat, burning, or pain. Patients are monitored throughout each treatment with the use of an audiovisual system (Iwamoto et al., 2012).

Patients generally come to the radiation center daily, Monday through Friday, for a predetermined number of treatments based on the prescription written by the radiation oncologist. An example of a prescription for definitive (curative) treatment is a total dose of 5,040 cGy, at 180 cGy per fraction. This patient would receive 28 treatments over five and a half weeks.

Technologic Advances

Technologic advances allow more precise planning and delivery of EBRT. Intensity-modulated radiation therapy (IMRT) uses dynamic MLCs, which break up the radiation beam into small "beamlets" that vary in intensity and enable the beam shape to change during the beam-on time (Coleman, 2016). This allows the dose to be more precisely sculpted to the target. Image-guided radiation therapy (IGRT) incorporates new imaging technology to visualize the target area immediately before every treatment with x-rays or CT scans. If there are no anatomic landmarks to use, small imaging fiducial markers, such as gold seeds, are placed on the body or surgically implanted into the tumor to visualize the target. This makes it possible to adjust the patient's position as needed to minimize variations in treatment setup. With this increased precision, margins are reduced to as little as 2–3 mm, minimizing the dose administered to healthy tissue, thus enabling delivery of very high doses to the tumor without the risk

Figure 8-5. Positioning by Alignment With Laser Lights

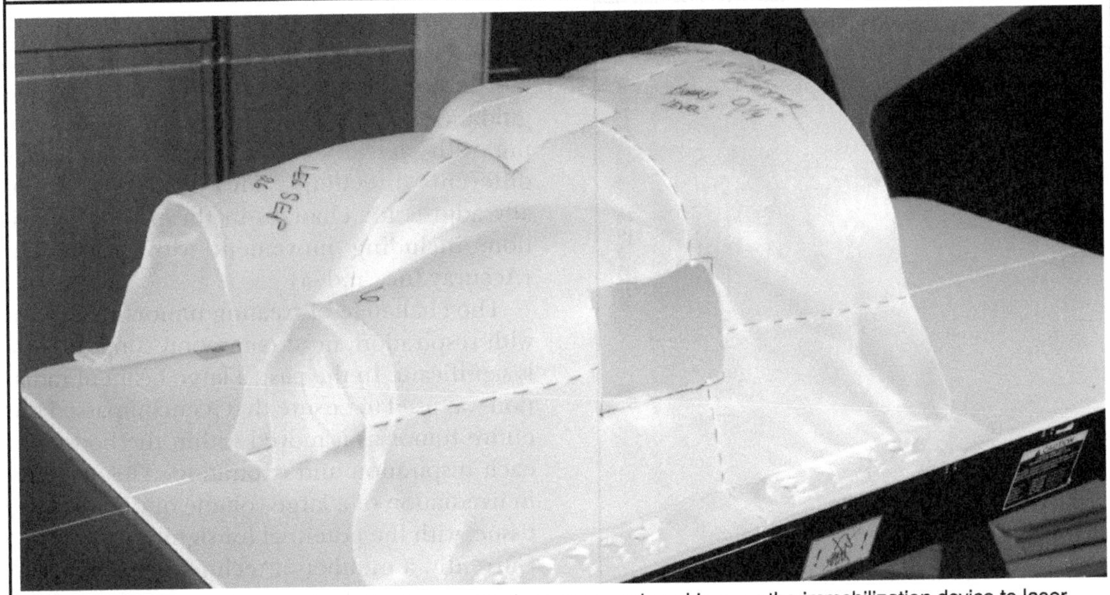

Patients are set up in the correct position by aligning the tattoos and markings on the immobilization device to laser lights coming from the walls and ceiling of the simulation and treatment rooms.

Note. Image copyright 2008 by Memorial Sloan Kettering Cancer Center. Used with permission.

Figure 8-6. Linear Accelerator

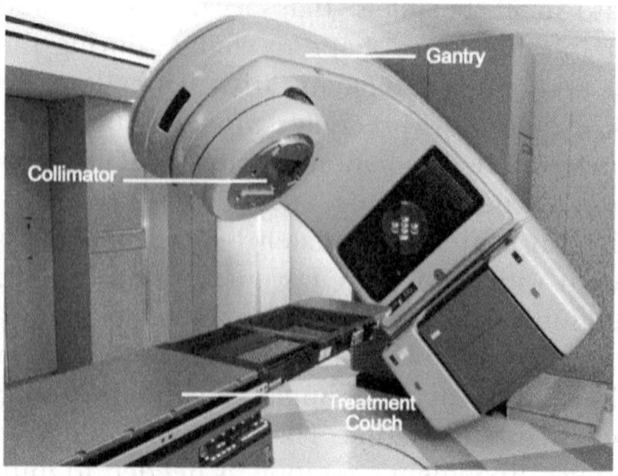

The gantry rotates 360° around the treatment couch. The beam of radiation comes out through the collimator.

Note. Image copyright 2008 by Memorial Sloan Kettering Cancer Center. Used with permission.

Figure 8-7. Multileaf Collimator

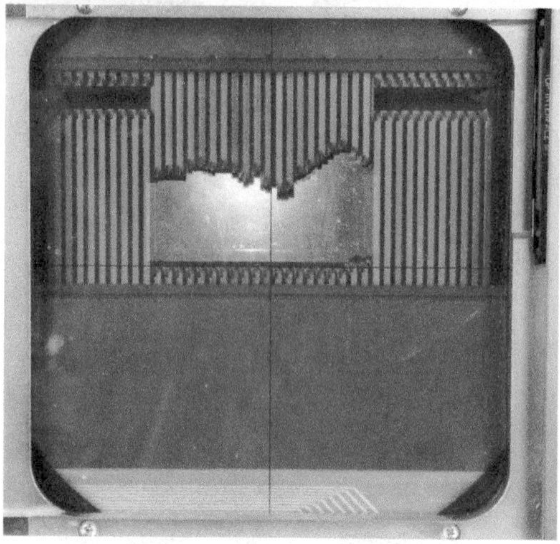

The leaves move independently to shape the beams of radiation emitted from the linear accelerator.

Note. Image copyright 2008 by Memorial Sloan Kettering Cancer Center. Used with permission.

of excessive toxicity (Ahmad, Duke, Jena, Williams, & Burnett, 2012).

By combining IGRT with IMRT, tumors that were once difficult to treat, such as tumors wrapped around the spinal cord, can now be treated. Previously, these tumors could only be treated with relatively low doses and required a course of several weeks. Now, in select cases, they can be more accurately treated with tumoricidal doses in a course lasting only one to five treatments. Other patients who may benefit from these advances include those with primary tumors in the lung and prostate, as well as those with metastatic tumors in the liver or lung (Ahmad et al., 2012).

IGRT and IMRT are most commonly delivered using a linear accelerator, but a number of other systems also are used. The TomoTherapy® system resembles a CT scan. It requires daily pretreatment scans, allowing for adjustment of patient positioning as needed, and has a linear accelerator mounted within the 360° ring gantry of the machine, allowing for continuous delivery of treatment as it moves around the patient (Accuray Inc., n.d.-b). The CyberKnife® system has a small linear accelerator mounted on a robotic arm and an image guidance system, allowing for fast repositioning with delivery of treatment from many different directions. This system continually adjusts for changes in the patient's position, including movement with respiration (Accuray Inc., n.d.-a).

The challenge of treating tumors that move with respiration, most commonly lung tumors, is significant. In the past, a large beam of radiation was used to ensure that it encompassed the entire tumor as it moved within the body with each inspiration and expiration. This resulted in irradiation of a large volume of normal lung tissue, with the potential for significant toxicity. Currently, a number of techniques are used to decrease this volume: (a) compression of the abdomen to minimize diaphragmatic movement, (b) respiratory gating to activate the beam only when the tumor is in a predefined position during the respiratory cycle, and (c) tracking systems that move the collimator or treatment couch with respiratory movement to ensure the beam is focused correctly on the targeted tissue as it moves (Baskar, Lee, Yeo, & Yeoh, 2012).

Another technology is the use of proton therapy. Protons are particles generated by a cyclotron. Because of their high mass, it is possible to control where the protons will deposit their energy as the beam passes through the body. As a result, the normal tissue entrance and exit doses (in front of and behind the target) are reduced or eliminated. This allows for administration of high doses of radiation to the tumor while sparing the surrounding normal tissues, especially tissue in the entrance and exit areas (Baskar et al., 2012). Currently, 23 working proton centers exist in the United States, with an additional 11 under construction (National Association for Proton Therapy, 2016).

Special Uses of External Beam Radiation Therapy

Examples of special uses of EBRT are described in Table 8-2. Several of these build on recent technologic advances in the planning and delivery of radiation therapy treatment.

Internal Radiation Therapy: Radioactive Source Therapy

Each chemical element on earth has a unique atomic structure with a defined number of neutrons, protons, and electrons. Some elements have structural variations with differing numbers of neutrons, which are called *isotopes.* Some isotopes are stable; the nucleus holds together well despite the varying numbers of neutrons. However, some isotopes are unstable or excited and release energy as they decay. This energy is ionizing radiation in the form of beta particles or gamma rays. These unstable isotopes are called *radioactive isotopes* or *radionuclides.* Radioactive source therapy involves placing radioactive isotopes inside the body. Brachytherapy uses sealed sources, whereas radiopharmaceutical therapy uses unsealed sources (Ruppert, 2011).

Brachytherapy

Sealed sources are generally in the form of seeds, ribbons, plaques, or rods. They are placed within or close to the tumor (see Table 8-3). The rate at which the radiation dose is emitted is categorized as a low dose rate (LDR) or high dose rate (HDR). LDR treatment takes days, weeks, or months to deliver the dose; HDR treatment delivers the dose in minutes. Regardless of the type of brachytherapy used, the dose emitted from the source falls off rapidly with increasing distance. In addition, brachytherapy eliminates the need for a beam of radiation to pass through normal tissue to penetrate to a tumor deep inside the body. Thus, brachytherapy can effectively deliver a high dose of radiation to the tumor while sparing the surrounding normal tissue (Ruppert, 2011).

To deliver treatment with brachytherapy, catheters or applicators are first positioned in the body, into which radioactive sources are subsequently placed. Historically, the radioactive sources were placed manually and left for two to five days (i.e., temporary LDR brachytherapy). This required that patients be hospitalized and isolated to minimize staff and visitor exposure to radiation (Smeltzer, Bare, Hinkle, & Cheever, 2010). The radiation sources are stored in a shielded compartment of the computer-driven afterloader when not in use. To deliver treatment, the afterloader, a motorized system, transports the source through cables into the applicator or catheters positioned in the area to be treated, and then retracts the source after the

Table 8-2. Special Uses of External Beam Radiation Therapy

Treatment	Definition	Clinical Use	Key Points
Total body irradiation	Radiation therapy (RT) to the entire body; combined with high-dose chemotherapy prior to bone marrow or stem cell transplant (to destroy residual cancer cells, eradicate the bone marrow, and suppress the immune system to prevent rejection of the donor marrow)	Hematologic malignancies	Patient may be lying down or standing on a special stand. Treatment is given 1–3 times daily over 3–6 days. Treatment takes 20–30 minutes.
Stereotactic radiosurgery	RT given as a onetime treatment to a small, well-defined target volume within the brain	Brain metastasis	Treatment requires placement of a head ring with localizer to define the target and immobilize the head. Treatment can be delivered with a linear accelerator, CyberKnife®, or Gamma Knife®.
Stereotactic body RT	RT given as a high-dose treatment to a small, well-defined target volume outside the brain (extracranial), delivered in 1–5 fractions	Liver metastasis Lung tumor or metastasis Paraspinal tumor	Treatment requires use of a body frame to immobilize the patient, an internal or external marker to localize the target, and an image-guidance system to confirm setup position prior to each treatment. Treatment takes about 20 minutes.
Intraoperative RT	RT given as a single high dose using electrons to an exposed tumor bed at the time of surgery (to improve local control when there is residual gross or microscopic disease)	Neuroblastoma Lung cancer Rectal cancer Retroperitoneal sarcoma	Treatment can be delivered with a dedicated linear accelerator in the operating room or with a mobile linear accelerator. Treatment can be combined with external beam RT.

Note. Based on information from Calvo et al., 2008; Gillin, 2010; Iwamoto et al., 2012; Kavanagh et al., 2008.

Table 8-3. Brachytherapy Treatment Techniques

Technique	Definition	Radionuclide
Interstitial	Placement of seeds into the tumor or tumor bed using thin needles and catheters	Permanent: iodine-125, palladium-103 Temporary: iridium-192
Intracavitary	Placement of a rigid applicator in a body cavity next to the tumor	Cesium-137
Intraluminal	Placement of seeds in a lumen	Iridium-192
Superficial	Placement of a plaque or mold on a body surface	Iodine-125, ruthenium-106

Note. Based on information from Cohen, 2016.

dose is delivered. Patients need to be isolated during the time that the radiation source is in the body. This controls the amount of radiation exposure to nurses and doctors while patients are undergoing brachytherapy as an inpatient. The clinical uses of brachytherapy include cure to eradicate the disease, adjuvant treatment after surgery to destroy any residual disease, salvage therapy to a previously irradiated site, or palliation to relieve symptoms caused by advanced disease (Smeltzer et al., 2010). Examples of clinical uses of brachytherapy are illustrated in Figures 8-8 and 8-9.

Radiopharmaceutical Therapy

Radiopharmaceutical therapy includes two different types of therapy. The first is radiolabeled antibodies. This type of radiation therapy is a combination of a radioactive isotope and a monoclonal antibody. Two radiolabeled antibodies are tositumomab (Bexxar®) and ibritumomab tiuxetan (Zevalin®). Both of these agents are indicated for the treatment of lymphoma given via the IV route. Ibritumomab tiuxetan is given in combination with rituximab, whereas tositumomab is given as a single course of treatment. The safety of multiple courses of the tositumomab therapeutic regimen, or combination of this regimen with other forms of irradiation or chemotherapy, has not been evaluated.

The second type of radiopharmaceutical therapy is often used in the treatment of bone metastases. The three agents are strontium-89 (Metastron®), samarium-153 (Quadramet®), and radium-223 (Xofigo®). These are given via the IV route so they can travel through the body and build up in the areas of the bones affected by the cancer. The radiation treatment kills the cancer cells, helping to ease the pain caused by these bone metastases (American Cancer Society, 2014b). If more than one area of bone is involved, these IV agents are a better option

Figure 8-8. Permanent Interstitial Seed Implant for Treatment of Prostate Cancer

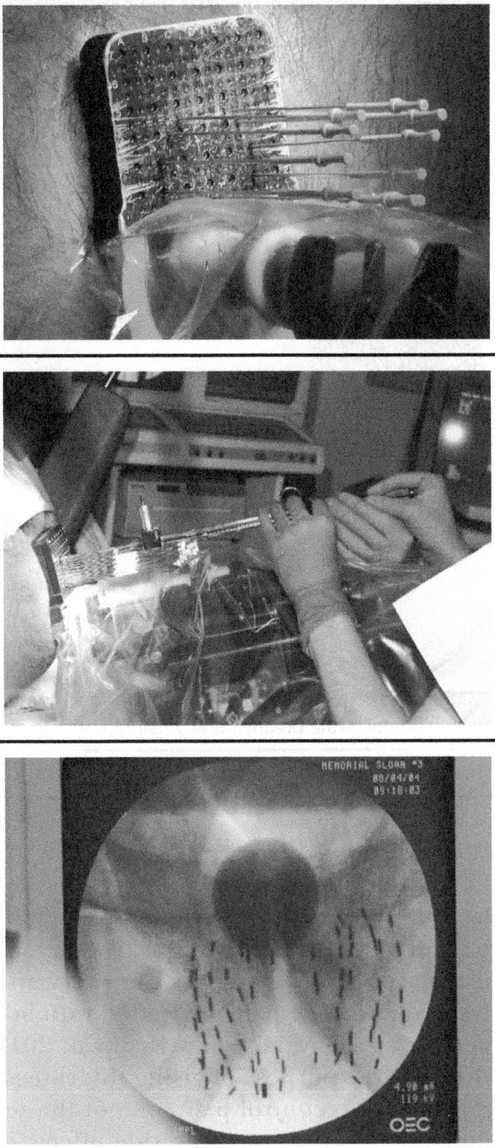

A template is used to guide placement of needles transperineally into the prostate. These are then loaded with iodine-131 seeds. Ultrasound image shows seeds distributed throughout the prostate after needles are removed.

Note. Images copyright 2008 by Memorial Sloan Kettering Cancer Center. Used with permission.

Figure 8-9. High-Dose-Rate Brachytherapy for Treatment of Sarcoma

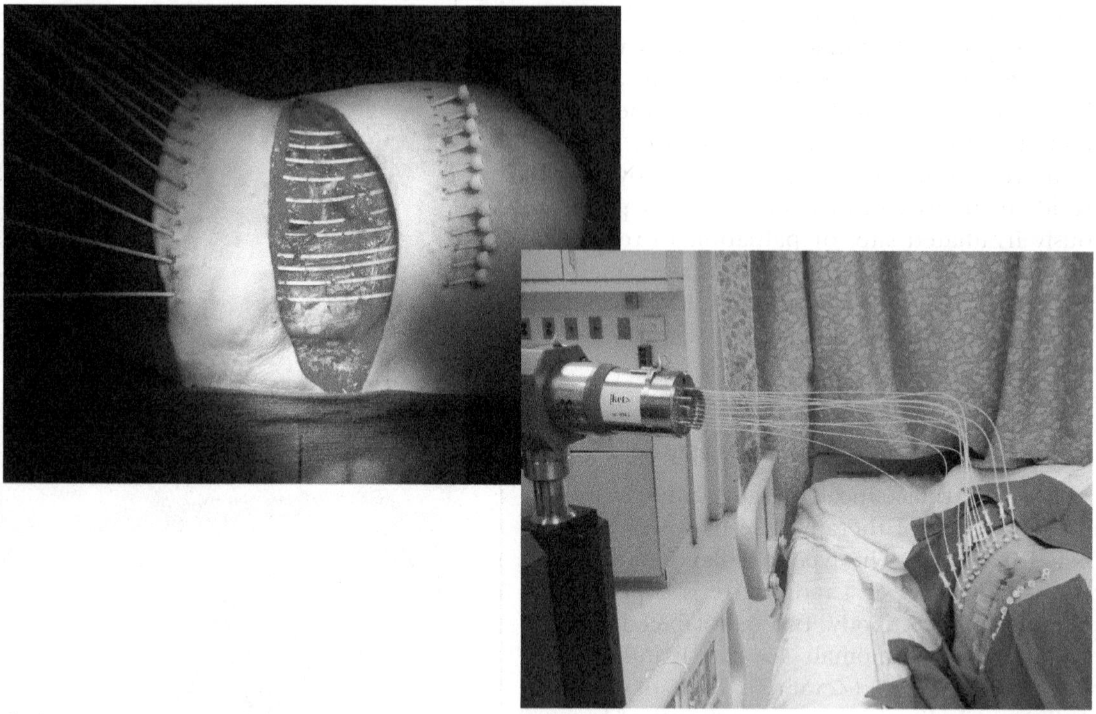

Catheters are positioned at the time of surgery for tumor resection through the tumor bed. The patient is later treated with high-dose-rate brachytherapy using a remote afterloader with iridium-192 sources.

Note. Images copyright 2008 by Memorial Sloan Kettering Cancer Center. Used with permission.

than administering EBRT to multiple areas. Prostate cancer is one type of cancer that can spread to the bone, so this type of radiopharmaceutical therapy has been very effective in controlling pain associated with bone metastases (University of Wisconsin, 2013). Although the purpose of giving this category of agents is to control pain, one of the temporary, though uncommon, side effects can be an increase in bone pain for the first couple of days after treatment. Another possible side effect is lowering of the white blood cell count and platelet count. Patients usually are followed closely for the first weeks to monitor effects of treatment (Abuhanoğlu & Özer, 2012).

Radiation Safety

People are exposed every day to background radiation from the sun, the stars, and the environment, such as minerals in the earth. Healthcare workers are also at risk for occupational exposure to radiation. No risk exists when caring for patients receiving EBRT; however, radioactive source therapy poses a potential risk. Rigorous standards and laws regulate healthcare facilities that use radiation to ensure that staff exposure is limited. Although each organization will have its own policies and procedures, key principles must be followed (American College of Radiology, 2014).

The goal is to keep exposure of caregivers "as low as reasonably achievable," commonly abbreviated as ALARA (Health Physics Society, n.d.). This goal is accomplished by reducing the amount of *time* spent near a radioactive source, by increasing *distance* from the source, and by using *shielding* when directed. To reduce time, caregivers should plan care beforehand and ensure that all needed supplies are available. To reduce distance, caregivers should stand away from the source as much as possible when teaching and assessing the patient (e.g., at the doorway or at the opposite end of the bed). Based on the *inverse square law*, as the person moves from the source, the amount of radiation received is diminished by the inverse of the square of the distance moved (Curtis, 1999). For example, a distance of 5 feet would result in 1/25 of the radiation. If a person moves 2 feet from a source of 120 Gy, they would receive 1/4 of 120 Gy, or 30 Gy. Shielding is not always needed. The institution's radiation safety service will determine the necessity of shielding based on the energy of the source. Lead aprons or standing rolling shields may be used (Iwamoto et al., 2012).

The radiation safety service also will post door signs and chart labels for patients who require special precautions because of potential radiation exposure. These advisories are focused on the type of radioactive material used for the therapy and include a list of staff and patient cautionary instructions. Staff members who are working with potential radiation exposure are given a personal dosimetry monitor to be worn at all times while in the workplace. The badge should be placed on the front of the clothing between the waist and collar (Iwamoto et al., 2012). These badges detect radiation exposure and are replaced each month so that the interval and cumulative doses of exposure can be monitored over time. Pregnant staff members should consult with the radiation safety service to identify additional measures to take to protect the fetus based on potential exposure in the particular work setting.

Side Effects

Normal cells and cancer cells respond similarly when exposed to radiation. Although normal cells are better able to repair themselves, patients may experience side effects from the damaging effects of radiation in the treatment area. Radiation can cause early (acute) effects that occur during treatment, subacute effects that occur several months after completion of treatment, and late effects that occur six months or longer after completion of treatment (McBride & Withers, 2008).

Early effects result from inflammation of the tissues in the treatment field and from depletion of cells in tissues with rapidly proliferating cells (McBride & Withers, 2008). Examples of tissues with rapidly proliferating cells are mucous membranes, skin, and bone marrow. Early effects are common, and the severity ranges from mild to severe. Early effects generally begin about two weeks after the start of treatment and resolve within six months of treatment completion. They are reversible and generally have no long-term sequelae (Poirier, 2013).

Subacute effects may occur in certain tissues in which recovery of the normal tissues from the early effects of radiation takes longer. Examples include the spinal cord, brain, and lung. Subacute effects generally begin several months after treatment is completed. They generally are reversible but can cause serious damage (Poirier, 2013).

Late effects result from permanent damage to normal tissues in the treatment field: the parenchymal cells (affecting organ function), the vasculature (affecting blood supply and delivery of oxygen and nutrients to the organ), and the connective tissues (affecting elasticity of the tissues). This damage may result in dysfunction of affected organs or fibrosis, atrophy, ulceration, fistula formation, or necrosis of the affected tissues (DeSantis et al., 2014). A key component of treatment planning is to ensure that normal tissue exposure during treatment is kept below the tissue tolerance dose to minimize the risk of these problems. The clinical impact will depend on what tissues and organs are affected and the volume of normal tissue irradiated. Late effects generally are quite rare but are irreversible and, in some cases, can cause chronic health problems (DeSantis et al., 2014).

Side effects are differentiated between general side effects that can occur to any patient regardless of the site treated and site-specific side effects that are based on the area being treated. Although variation exists from patient to patient, the type and severity of side effects are based on a number of factors, including type and dose of radiation, fraction size and intervals, duration of treatment course, organs in the treatment field, volume of organ irradiation, use of concurrent chemotherapy, and any comorbid conditions (DeSantis et al., 2014). General and site-specific early side effects and some interventions used to help patients in managing these are described in Tables 8-4 and 8-5. Examples of site-specific late side effects are described in Table 8-6. Among the most challenging of side effects experienced by patients are skin reactions (see Figure 8-10) and oral mucositis (see Figure 8-11).

During treatment, the radiation oncologist and nurse assess patients weekly for the presence of side effects. These assessments continue during follow-up visits after treatment is completed. A standardized scale may be used to grade the severity of each side effect. One widely used example is the Common Terminology Criteria for Adverse Events (National Cancer Institute Cancer Therapy Evaluation Program, 2010). Side effects are graded in severity from 1 to 5 based on specific descriptors for each adverse event.

Nursing Implications

Nurses play a significant role in supporting patients throughout their treatment with radiation therapy. Components of the radiation oncology nursing role include assessment, education, symptom management, emotional support and counseling, physical care, and coordination of care. Nursing involvement begins at the time of consultation, continues through simulation and treatment, and extends through the follow-up period after treatment is completed. Radiation oncology nurses have specific responsibilities at each phase of the continuum. Figure 8-12 lists selected Internet resources that may be used when educating patients.

Throughout treatment, close collaboration occurs with the radiation oncologists, radiation therapists, and physicists to ensure that care is implemented safely and effectively on a day-to-day basis. Nurses collaborate with colleagues from other disciplines to ensure that all patient needs are addressed.

Nurses also participate in clinical and administrative leadership activities within the department. These may include collaborating with physicians and administrators on the implementation of new clinical programs; developing patient education materials, policies, and procedures; leading patient and family support groups; ordering and managing equipment and supplies; and taking part in or leading quality assessment and performance improvement initiatives. In addition, nurses may be involved in clinical research within the department. Specific research responsibilities may include implementation of medical protocols (e.g., participating in informed consent, coordinating care to ensure correct implementation of the protocol, administering investigational agents, assessing for toxicity), developing and implementing independent research protocols, and applying research evidence in practice. The role of the radiation oncology nurse is

Table 8-4. General Early (Acute) Side Effects

Side Effect	Presentation	Prevention and Treatment
Anorexia	Loss of appetite Early satiety	Monitor weight, fluid, and nutritional status. Encourage small, frequent meals and high-calorie, high-protein foods. Encourage oral liquid supplements if patients are not taking in adequate amounts of nutrients. Refer for dietary counseling.
Bone marrow suppression	Thrombocytopenia Neutropenia Anemia	Monitor blood counts. Hold treatment based on physician's parameters. Institute infection and bleeding precautions as needed.
Fatigue	Severity varies; increased with concurrent chemotherapy	Encourage patients to find a balance between maintaining usual activities as much as possible and resting to conserve energy. Encourage patients to exercise within tolerance; a regular walking regimen may lessen fatigue. Treat sleep disorders (e.g., medication, relaxation techniques, maintenance of a regular sleep-wake regimen).
Skin reaction	Erythema Dry desquamation: dry, flaky, itchy skin Moist desquamation: loss of epidermal layer with exposed dermis; erythema with serous exudate and associated with pain	Instruct patients on skin care in the treatment area (entrance and exit sites). In other areas, patients may continue their usual practices. Cleanse skin daily using a mild soap, and pat dry. Apply a water-soluble moisturizer (e.g., Aquaphor®, Eucerin®, products with aloe vera gel, Biafine® RE) 2 times daily but not in the 4 hours preceding treatment. Avoid physical irritants (e.g., shaving; tape; tight, constricting clothing); chemical irritants (e.g., perfumes, deodorants, cosmetics); and thermal irritants (e.g., ice packs, heating pads). Avoid sun exposure to the area for life. Consider medication if indicated: topical steroids for itching and/or topical antibiotics if indicated. For moist desquamation, select product based on presentation: • Minimal exudate: hydrogel gel or dressing (nonadherent; provides moist environment for wound healing) • Moderate or severe exudate: foam dressing (nonadherent, absorbs exudate) • High risk of infection: silver-based products (gels, dressings, or creams such as silver sulfadiazine cream)

Note. Based on information from Bolderston et al., 2006; Kangas et al., 2008; McQuestion, 2006; Mitchell et al., 2014; Wickline, 2004.

Table 8-5. Site-Specific Early (Acute) Side Effects

Side Effect	Presentation	Prevention and Treatment
Brain		
Alopecia	Hair loss begins about 6 weeks after treatment starts. Unless whole brain radiation therapy (RT) is being used, hair loss will only be in areas where beam enters and exits the body.	Instruct patients on care of the scalp: • Wash hair gently with mild shampoo. • Apply moisturizers to the scalp for itching. Manage skin reactions of the scalp in the same way as in other areas of the body. Encourage patients to consider use of hairpieces and scarves after hair loss and to select these before hair loss occurs.
Cerebral edema	Headache Nausea and vomiting Change in mental status Recurrence or increase in presenting neurologic symptoms (e.g., seizure, focal weakness, aphasia)	Monitor for increased intracranial pressure, and consult with physician about use of steroids (e.g., dexamethasone) if indicated, possibly with prophylaxis for secondary gastritis or fungal infection.
Head and Neck		
Oral mucositis	Erythema Pseudomembranes (white patches) Ulcers (isolated or contiguous) Dysphagia (difficulty swallowing) Odynophagia (pain with swallowing)	Instruct patients on mouth care: • Brush teeth four times a day with a soft toothbrush. • Floss daily, if flossed previously. • Rinse mouth four times a day with a bland rinse (e.g., normal saline solution, sodium bicarbonate solution, nonalcoholic unsweetened mouthwash); increase as needed for comfort. • Remove and clean dental appliances each time mouth is cleaned. • Avoid irritants (e.g., tobacco; alcohol; rough, spicy, acidic, or hot foods or fluids). Encourage soft, pureed, or liquid diet, including oral liquid supplements. Refer for dietary counseling. Monitor for pain, and consult with physician about use of topical and/or systemic analgesics if indicated. Monitor for signs of thrush, and consult with physician about use of antibiotics if indicated. Monitor weight, fluid, and nutritional status, and consult with physician about placement of a feeding tube or use of IV hydration if indicated. Instruct patients on swallowing and jaw exercises to maintain swallowing function and prevent jaw tightening.

(Continued on next page)

Table 8-5. Site-Specific Early (Acute) Side Effects *(Continued)*

Side Effect	Presentation	Prevention and Treatment
Xerostomia (may be a permanent long-term effect) (Note: Use of intensity-modulated RT reduces the RT dose to the parotid gland)	Dry mouth Thick, tenacious saliva	Have patients obtain a dental evaluation prior to RT for treatment of preexisting dental caries and prescribing of fluoride treatments to reduce the risk of dental caries. Encourage patients to take frequent sips of water throughout the day and use humidification at night. Advise patients that commercial mouth moisturizers and artificial saliva may be helpful (e.g., Bioténe® and OralBalance® products).
Breast		
Inflammation	Swelling and heaviness of the breast from edema	Instruct patients to wear a surgical compression bra. Instruct patients to take acetaminophen as needed for discomfort. Manage skin reactions of the breast in the same way as in other areas of the body.
Chest		
Esophagitis	Dysphagia (difficulty swallowing) Odynophagia (pain with swallowing)	Encourage soft, pureed, or liquid diet, including oral liquid supplements. Refer for dietary counseling. Monitor weight, fluid, and nutritional status, and consult with physician about IV hydration if indicated. Monitor pain, and consult with physician about use of topical and systemic analgesics or proton pump inhibitors (for symptoms of reflux).
Pneumonitis	Nonproductive cough Dyspnea Low-grade fever Hemoptysis	Instruct patient on strategies to ease dyspnea: • Upright positioning • Breathing exercises • Supplemental oxygen Monitor for dyspnea, and consult with physician about use of medication (e.g., steroids, bronchodilators) if indicated.
Abdomen		
Enteritis: diarrhea	Frequent watery stools: varying frequency and severity depending on amount of small bowel in the field	Instruct patients to alter diet to be low in insoluble fiber (avoid raw fruits and vegetables, whole grains, and nuts; eat rice and noodles), high in soluble fiber (eat bananas and applesauce), low in lactose, and low in fat. Monitor frequency and consistency of bowel movements. Monitor weight, fluid, and nutritional status, and consult with physician about use of IV hydration if indicated. For diarrhea, consult with physician about use of antidiarrheal medication, probiotic oral supplementation, or psyllium fiber supplementation.

(Continued on next page)

Table 8-5. Site-Specific Early (Acute) Side Effects *(Continued)*

Side Effect	Presentation	Prevention and Treatment
Nausea and vomiting	Varying frequency and severity (Note: Patients receiving total body irradiation are at highest risk; patients receiving upper and whole abdomen RT are at moderately high risk.) May occur after first treatment	Instruct patients to avoid spicy, fatty, and salty foods. Refer for dietary counseling if indicated. Monitor frequency and severity of nausea and vomiting. Monitor fluid and nutritional status, and consult with physician about use of IV hydration if indicated. For persistent nausea or vomiting, consult with physician about use of antiemetics (prophylaxis for high-risk patients and as needed for lower-risk patients).
Pelvis		
Cystitis	Frequent urination Urgency Dysuria	Instruct patients to increase fluids. Instruct patients to avoid irritants (e.g., caffeine, spicy foods). Rule out urinary tract infection, and consult with physician about use of antibiotics if indicated. For persistent symptoms, consult with physician about use of medications to reduce bladder spasm (e.g., oxybutynin) and provide topical analgesia (e.g., phenazopyridine).
Enteritis: diarrhea	See previous.	See previous.
Vaginitis	Pain Discharge	Instruct patients on use of sitz baths for comfort and perineal pads to absorb discharge. Rule out vaginal infection, and treat with antibiotics if indicated.
Prostate		
Bladder outlet obstruction	Frequent urination Urgency Nocturia Decrease in force or caliber of urinary stream Dribbling	Differentiate from irritative symptoms using bladder scan to measure postvoid residual urine. Rule out urinary tract infection, and treat with antibiotics if indicated. Consult with physician about use of medication to relax smooth muscle and improve bladder emptying (e.g., tamsulosin, terazosin).
Proctitis	Rectal mucous discharge Inflamed hemorrhoids	Instruct patients on use of sitz baths for comfort. For persistent discomfort, consult with physician about use of topical steroids.

Note. Based on information from Bradley & Movsas, 2004; Clarkson et al., 2010; DiSalvo et al., 2008; Eilers et al., 2014; Feyer et al., 2005; Muehlbauer et al., 2009; Rubenstein et al., 2004; Sonis et al., 2004; Worthington et al., 2011.

Table 8-6. Examples of Site-Specific Late Effects

Site	Late Effects	Presentation
Brain and spinal cord	Necrosis of brain tissue from injury to blood vessels	Increased intracranial pressure
	Cerebral atrophy	Cognitive change
	Myelopathy from injury to myelin sheath	Paresthesias and sensory changes
Head and neck	Xerostomia from injury to parotid gland	Dry mouth, with increased risk of dental caries
	Trismus: injury to muscles and connective tissue around temporomandibular joint resulting in contractions and fibrosis	Reduced mouth opening
Breast	Vascular and fibrotic effects on skin and underlying tissues	Telangiectasia or hypo- or hyperpigmentation Change in breast consistency
Chest	Esophageal stricture from fibrosis of esophageal tissues	Dysphagia
	Pulmonary fibrosis from thickening of alveolar septa and vascular damage; symptoms unlikely unless more than 50% of one lung is irradiated	Dyspnea, with deterioration in pulmonary function studies
Abdomen	Nephritis from glomerular sclerosis and vascular damage	Impaired renal function
Pelvis	Enteritis from fibrosis and damage to villi of small bowel	Chronic diarrhea, with malabsorption and hypermotility
	Vaginal stenosis from fibrosis	Shortening and narrowing of the vagina, with dyspareunia (pain with intercourse)
Prostate	Erectile dysfunction from damage to blood vessels and nerves	Impotence

Note. Based on information from Constine et al., 2008.

rich and varied, offering multiple opportunities to significantly affect the quality of life of patients receiving radiation therapy.

Conclusion

Many nurses will encounter patients receiving radiation therapy during the course of their career. Expertise as a radiation oncology nurse is not required to initiate a discussion about what radiation therapy is, how it is given, and what patients may experience during treatment. Figure 8-12 lists selected Internet resources that nurses and patients may find helpful to learn more about radiation therapy. By dispelling myths and misconceptions and guiding patients in gathering the information they need to make decisions and cope with treatment, nurses can provide a service of great value to patients and their families.

Figure 8-10. Skin Reactions From Radiation Therapy

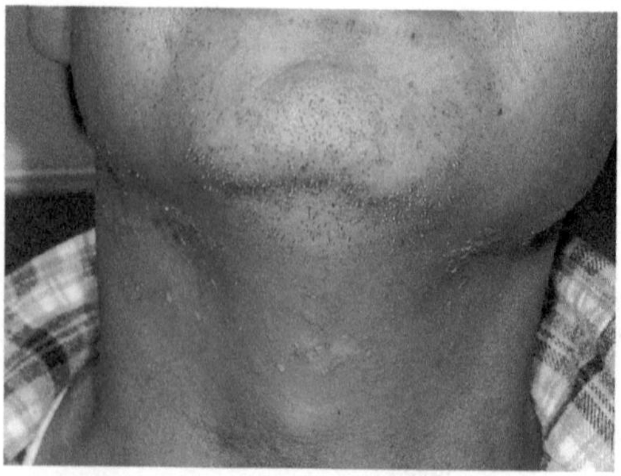

Patient treated to the head and neck developed erythema and small area of moist desquamation

Note. Image copyright 2008 by Memorial Sloan Kettering Cancer Center. Used with permission.

Figure 8-11. Oral Mucositis From Radiation Therapy

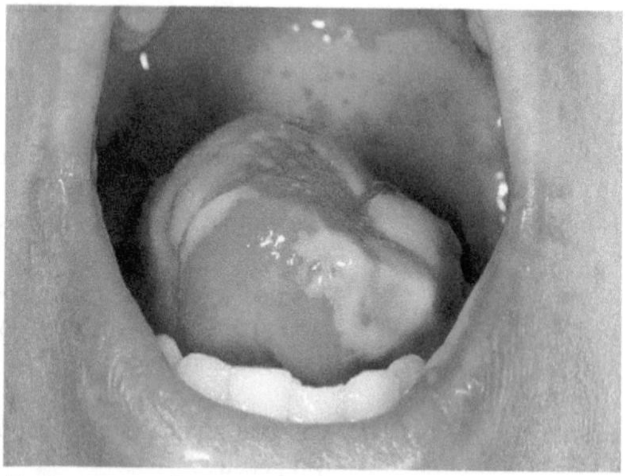

Erythema, confluent pseudomembranes, and ulceration

Note. Image copyright 2008 by Memorial Sloan Kettering Cancer Center. Used with permission.

Figure 8-12. Selected Internet Resources for Educating Patients About Radiation Therapy

- American Cancer Society: www.cancer.org
- American College of Radiology and Radiological Society of North America: www.radiologyinfo.org
- American Society for Radiation Oncology: www.rtanswers.org
- National Cancer Institute: www.cancer.gov
- National Comprehensive Cancer Network: www.nccn.org

Key Points

- The different types of radiation treatments are external beam and internal radiation therapy.
- Different side effects are associated with radiation therapy to different sites of the body. Effects of radiation therapy can be early or acute, subacute, or late and include but are not limited to myelosuppression, fatigue, local skin reactions, oral mucositis, pneumonitis, xerostomia, and pulmonary fibrosis.
- Certain chemotherapy agents act as radiosensitizers. Potential side effects associated with combining treatments include myelosuppression, fatigue, nausea and vomiting, oral mucositis, and local skin reactions.
- Radiation oncology team members include radiation oncologists, radiation nurse practitioners or nurses, dosimetrists, physicists, and radiation oncology technicians.
- The radiation therapy process starts with a consultation with the radiation oncologist and nurse. The simulation is completed at the next visit. During this time, the exact area to be treated is mapped out with small dots or tattoos placed on the patient's body to ensure the exact area is treated every day. This takes about 1–1.5 hours.
- The nursing role in caring for patients undergoing radiation therapy includes managing potential side effects.

The author would like to acknowledge Joanne Frankel Kelvin, MSN, AOCN®, for her contribution to this chapter that remains unchanged from the first edition of this book.

References

Abuhanoğlu, G., & Özer, A.Y. (2012). Adverse reactions to radiopharmaceuticals. *FABAD Journal of Pharmaceutical Sciences, 37,* 43–59. Retrieved from http://dergi.fabad.org.tr/pdf/volum37/issue1/43-59.pdf

Accuray Inc. (n.d.-a). How is the CyberKnife System unique? Retrieved from http://www.cyberknife.com/cyberknife-overview/how-unique.aspx

Accuray Inc. (n.d.-b). The Tomo® process. Retrieved from http://www.tomotherapy.com/process

Ahmad, S.S., Duke, S., Jena, R., Williams, M.V., & Burnett, N.G. (2012). Advances in radiotherapy. *BMJ, 345,* e7765. doi:10.1136/bmj.e7765

American Cancer Society. (2014a). Radiation therapy principles. Retrieved from http://www.cancer.org/treatment/treatmentsandsideeffects/treatmenttypes/radiation/radiationtherapyprinciples/index

American Cancer Society. (2014b). Radiopharmaceuticals. Retrieved from http://www.cancer.org/treatment/treatmentsandsideeffects/treatmenttypes/radiation/radiationtherapyprinciples/radiation-therapy-principles-how-is-radiation-given-radiopharmaceuticals

American College of Radiology. (2014). *ACR–ASTRO practice parameter for radiation oncology.* Retrieved from http://www.acr.org/~/media/7B19A9CEF68F4D6D8F0CF25F21155D73.pdf

Baskar, R., Lee, K.A., Yeo, R., & Yeoh, K.-W. (2012). Cancer and radiation therapy: Current advances and future directions. *International Journal of Medical Sciences, 9,* 193–199. doi:10.7150/ijms.3635

Bolderston, A., Lloyd, N.S., Wong, R.K.S., Holden, L., Robb-Blenderman, L., & Supportive Care Guidelines Group of Cancer Care Ontario Program in Evidence-based Care. (2006). The prevention and management of acute skin reactions related to radiation therapy: A systematic review and practice guideline. *Supportive Care in Cancer, 14,* 802–817. doi:10.1007/s00520-006-0063-4

Bradley, J., & Movsas, B. (2004). Radiation esophagitis: Predictive factors and preventive strategies. *Seminars in Radiation Oncology, 14,* 280–286. doi:10.1016/j.semradonc.2004.06.003

Calvo, F.A., Meirino, R.M., de la Mata, M.D., Serrano, F.J., & Galvez, M. (2008). Intraoperative radiotherapy. In E.C. Halperin, C.A. Perez, & L.W. Brady (Eds.), *Perez and Brady's principles and practice of radiation oncology* (5th ed., pp. 397–406). Philadelphia, PA: Wolters Kluwer Health/Lippincott Williams & Wilkins.

Clarkson, J.E., Worthington, H.V., Furness, S., McCabe, M., Khalid, T., & Meyer, S. (2010). Interventions for treating oral mucositis for patients with cancer receiving treatment. *Cochrane Database of Systematic Reviews, 2010*(8). doi:10.1002/14651858.CD001973.pub4

Cohen, G.N. (2016). Overview of radiobiology. In C.M. Washington & D. Leaver (Eds.), *Principles and practice of radiation therapy* (4th ed., pp. 293–310). St. Louis, MO: Elsevier Mosby.

Coleman, A.M. (2016). Treatment procedures. In C.M. Washington & D. Leaver (Eds.), *Principles and practice of radiation therapy* (4th ed., pp. 156–177). St. Louis, MO: Elsevier Mosby.

Constine, L.S., Milano, M.T., Friedman, D., Morris, M., Williams, J.P., Rubin, P., & Okunieff, P. (2008). Late effects of cancer treatment on normal tissues. In E.C. Halperin, C.A. Perez, & L.W. Brady (Eds.), *Perez and Brady's principles and practice of radiation oncology* (5th ed., pp. 320–355). Philadelphia, PA: Lippincott Williams & Wilkins.

Curtis, R.A. (1999, January). Introduction to ionizing radiation. Retrieved from https://www.osha.gov/SLTC/radiationionizing/introtoionizing/ionizinghandout.html

DeSantis, C.E., Lin, C.C., Mariotto, A.B., Siegel, R.L., Stein, K.D., Kramer, J.L., ... Jemal, A. (2014). Cancer treatment and survivorship statistics, 2014. *CA: A Cancer Journal for Clinicians, 64,* 252–271. doi:10.3322/caac.21235

DiSalvo, W.M., Joyce, M.M., Tyson, L.B., Culkin, A.E., & Mackay, K. (2008). Putting evidence into practice®: Evidence-based interventions for cancer-related dyspnea. *Clinical Journal of Oncology Nursing, 12,* 341–352. doi:10.1188/08.CJON.341-352

Eilers, E., Harris, D., Henry, K., & Johnson, L.A. (2014). Evidence-based interventions for cancer treatment-related mucositis: Putting evidence into practice. *Clinical Journal of Oncology Nursing, 18*(Suppl. 6), 80–96. doi:10.1188/14.CJON.S3.80-96

Feyer, P.C., Maranzano, E., Molassiotis, A., Clark-Snow, R.A., Roila, F., Warr, D., & Olver, I. (2005). Radiotherapy-induced nausea and vomiting (RINV): Antiemetic guidelines. *Supportive Care in Cancer, 13,* 122–128. doi:10.1007/s00520-004-0705-3

Gillin, M.T. (2016). Special procedures. In C.M. Washington & D. Leaver (Eds.), *Principles and practice of radiation therapy* (4th ed., pp. 310–323). St. Louis, MO: Elsevier Mosby.

Health Physics Society. (n.d.). ALARA. Retrieved from http://hps.org/publicinformation/radterms/radfact1.html

Iwamoto, R.R., Haas, M.L., & Gosselin, T. (Eds.). (2012). *Manual for radiation oncology nursing practice and education* (4th ed.). Pittsburgh PA: Oncology Nursing Society.

Kangas, M., Bovbjerg, D.H., & Montgomery, G.H. (2008). Cancer-related fatigue: A systematic and meta-analytic review of non-pharmacological therapies for cancer patients. *Psychological Bulletin, 134,* 700–741. doi:10.1037/a0012825

Kavanagh, B.D., Bradley, J.D., & Timmerman, R.D. (2008). Stereotactic irradiation of tumors outside the central nervous system. In E.C. Halperin, C.A. Perez, & L.W. Brady (Eds.), *Perez and Brady's principles and practice of radiation oncology* (5th ed., pp. 389–396). Philadelphia, PA: Wolters Kluwer Health/Lippincott Williams & Wilkins.

Khan, F.M., & Gibbons, J.P. (2014). *Khan's the physics of radiation therapy* (5th ed.). Philadelphia, PA: Wolters Kluwer Health/Lippincott Williams & Wilkins.

Lawrence, T.S., Haffty, B.G., & Harris, J.R. (2014). Milestones in the use of combined-modality radiation therapy and chemotherapy. *Journal of Clinical Oncology, 32,* 1173–1179. doi:10.1200/JCO.2014.55.2281

Leaver, D., Keller, R., & Uricchio, N. (2010). Conventional (fluoroscopy-based) simulation procedures. In C.M. Washington & D. Leaver (Eds.), *Principles and practice of radiation therapy* (3rd ed., pp. 442–466). St. Louis, MO: Elsevier Mosby.

McBride, W.H., & Withers, H.R. (2008). Biologic basis of radiation therapy. In E.C. Halperin, C.A. Perez, & L.W. Brady (Eds.), *Perez and Brady's principles and practice of radiation oncology* (5th ed., pp. 76–108). Philadelphia, PA: Lippincott Williams & Wilkins.

McQuestion, M. (2006). Evidence-based skin care management in radiation therapy. *Seminars in Oncology Nursing, 22,* 163–173. doi:10.1016/j.soncn.2006.04.004

Mitchell, S.A., Hoffman, A.J., Clark, J.C., DeGennaro, R.M., Poirier, P., Robinson, C.B., & Weisbrod, B.L. (2014). Putting evidence into practice: An update of evidence-based interventions for cancer-related fatigue during and following treatment. *Clinical Journal of Oncology Nursing, 18*(Suppl. 6), 38–58. doi:10.1188/14.CJON.S3.38-58

Moding, E.J., Kastan, M.B., & Kirsch, D.G. (2013). Strategies for optimizing the response of cancer and normal tissues to radiation. *Nature Reviews Drug Discovery, 12,* 526–542. doi:10.1038/nrd4003

Morgan, W.F., & Sowa, M.B. (2013). Non-targeted effects induced by ionizing radiation: Mechanisms and potential impact on radiation induced health effects. *Cancer Letters, 356,* 17–21. doi:10.1016/j.canlet.2013.09.009

Muehlbauer, P.M., Thorpe, D., Davis, A., Drabot, R., Rawlings, B.L., & Kiker, E.S. (2009). Putting evidence into practice: Evidence-based interventions to prevent, manage, and treat chemotherapy- and radiotherapy-induced diarrhea. *Clinical Journal of Oncology Nursing, 13,* 336–341. doi:10.1188/09.CJON.336-341

National Association for Proton Therapy. (2016). Welcome: The voice of the proton community. Retrieved from http://www.proton-therapy.org

National Cancer Institute Cancer Therapy Evaluation Program. (2010). *Common terminology criteria for adverse events* [v.4.03]. Retrieved from https://evs.nci.nih.gov/ftp1/CTCAE/CTCAE_4.03_2010-06-14_QuickReference_5x7.pdf

Passmore, G.C. (2016). Overview of radiobiology. In C.M. Washington & D. Leaver (Eds.), *Principles and practice of radiation therapy* (4th ed., pp. 58–87). St. Louis, MO: Elsevier Mosby.

Poirier, P. (2013). Nursing-led management of side effects of radiation: Evidence-based recommendations for practice. *Nursing: Research and Reviews, 2013*(3), 47–57. doi:10.2147/nrr.s34112

Rubenstein, E.B., Peterson, D.E., Schubert, M., Keefe, D., McGuire, D., Epstein, J., ... Sonis, S.T. (2004). Clinical practice guidelines for the prevention and treatment of cancer therapy–induced oral and gastrointestinal mucositis. *Cancer, 100*(Suppl. 9), 2026–2046. doi:10.1002/cncr.20163

Ruppert, R. (2011). Radiation therapy 101. *American Nurse Today, 6*(1). Retrieved from https://www.americannursetoday.com/radiation-therapy-101

Smeltzer, S.C., Bare, B.G., Hinkle, J.L., & Cheever, K.H. (2010). *Brunner & Suddarth's textbook of medical-surgical nursing* (12th ed.). Philadelphia, PA: Wolters Kluwer Health/Lippincott Williams & Wilkins.

Sonis, S.T., Elting, L.S., Keefe, D., Peterson, D.E., Schubert, M., Hauer-Jensen, M., ... Rubenstein, E.B. (2004). Perspectives on cancer therapy-induced mucosal injury: Pathogenesis, measurement, epidemiology, and consequences for patients. *Cancer, 100*(Suppl. 9), 1995–2025. doi:10.1002/cncr.20162

University of Wisconsin. (2013). Radiation oncology: Targeted radionuclide therapy. Retrieved from http://www.uwhealth.org/radiation-oncology/targeted-radionuclide-therapy/41503

Wang, D., Ho, A., Hamilton, A.S., Wu, X.-C., Lo, M., Fleming, S., ... Owen, J. (2014). Type and dose of radiotherapy used for initial treatment of non-metastatic prostate cancer. *Radiation Oncology, 9,* 47. doi:10.1186/1748-717X-9-47

Wickline, M.M. (2004). Prevention and treatment of acute radiation dermatitis: A literature review. *Oncology Nursing Forum, 31,* 237–247. doi:10.1188/04.ONF.237-247

World Health Organization. (n.d.). What is ionizing radiation? Retrieved from http://www.who.int/ionizing_radiation/about/what_is_ir/en

Worthington, H.V., Clarkson, J.E., Bryan, G., Furness, S., Glenny, A.-M., Littlewood, A., ... Khalid, T. (2011). Interventions for preventing oral mucositis for patients with cancer receiving treatment. *Cochrane Database of Systematic Reviews, 2011*(4). doi:10.1002/14651858.CD000978.pub5

Chapter 8 Study Questions

1. Skin reactions are common in radiation therapy. Nursing recommendations for promoting skin integrity should include all of the following EXCEPT:
   A. Avoid the use of sunscreens when going into direct sunshine.
   B. Use soft cotton fabrics for clothing.
   C. Wash the area with a mild soap and lukewarm water and pat (not rub) dry.
   D. Avoid the application of ointments, powders, and lotions to the area.

2. Which of the following is NOT a teaching guideline regarding radiation therapy?
   A. The therapy is painless.
   B. To promote safety, patients are assisted by therapy personnel while the machine is in operation.
   C. Patients may communicate all their concerns, needs, or discomforts while the machine is operating.
   D. Safety precautions are necessary only during the time of actual irradiation.

3. When caring for a patient on radiation isolation, which of the following policies is NOT important for nurses and doctors?
   A. Provide care in a timely manner, limiting exposure to the patient.
   B. Spend an hour providing education on radiation precautions to the isolated patient.
   C. Spend less than five minutes when caring for patients receiving brachytherapy in isolation.
   D. Limit young children and pregnant women from visiting a patient who is receiving brachytherapy.

4. A patient is scheduled for external beam radiation therapy to the chest wall. The nurse discusses which treatment side effect with the patient?
   A. Xerostomia
   B. Ulceration
   C. Suppuration
   D. Desquamation

5. In discussing the management of dry desquamation with a patient, what treatment is most recommended?
   A. Take hot showers daily and apply baby powder to the area.
   B. Apply an unscented, hydrophilic, lanolin-free cream to the area.
   C. Shave the area to decrease the amount of hair in the radiation field.
   D. Use a soft loofah sponge to gently exfoliate the area and then apply petroleum jelly.

CHAPTER

9 Chemotherapy

MiKaela Olsen, APRN-CNS, MS, AOCNS®

Introduction

When caring for patients who are undergoing chemotherapy, nurses need to understand the mechanism of action and side effects of each drug administered. Oncology nurses should provide patients with evidence-based side effect management strategies for self-care. Many patients with cancer will receive chemotherapy in their disease course. Therefore, nurses need to be knowledgeable in administration, patient teaching, and symptom management to minimize toxicities and increase quality of life to achieve the optimal response.

Chemotherapy is the use of various chemical agents that interfere with replication and other normal functions of cancer cells, causing cell death. The goals of chemotherapy are cure, control, and palliation. Chemotherapy was first discovered early in the 20th century. During World War II, soldiers exposed to nitrogen mustard (a form of chemical warfare) experienced symptoms of myelosuppression (low white blood cell, red blood cell, and platelet counts). These soldiers presented with profound toxicities associated with the low blood counts, including infections, anemia, and bleeding. This led scientists to investigate whether this agent and similar agents could be used to kill rapidly growing cancer cells. The continued development of chemotherapy agents led to major improvements in survival for patients with various cancer types, including childhood leukemia, lymphomas, testicular cancer, and others. See Table 9-1 for a timeline of important chemotherapy developments (Polovich, Olsen, & LeFebvre, 2014).

In the 21st century, cancer care has focused on the combination of treatment modalities (e.g., chemotherapy, radiation therapy, surgery, targeted therapy) to cure or improve the survival of patients with cancer. The discovery and use of combination chemotherapy, using drugs with varying mechanisms of action, led to improvements in patient survival and decreased cancer death rates. As chemotherapy and other molecular-targeted agents continue to be developed and used in combination, it will be necessary to optimize their use to minimize toxicities and improve outcomes for patients with cancer. This chapter will provide an overview of the role of chemotherapy in cancer treatment, describe the mechanism of action of various classifications of agents, and review administration principles.

Chemotherapy and the Cell Cycle

Chemotherapy agents target different phases of the cell cycle, halting growth and division of cells and leading to cell death, or apoptosis. Both normal and cancerous cells enter the cell cycle to reproduce. Cell division can be

Table 9-1. Historical Perspective on Chemotherapy Development

Period	Events
World War I	Mustard gas was first used as chemical warfare in World War I. Soldiers exposed to this chemical developed reversible bone marrow suppression, which led investigators to develop nitrogen mustard (a derivative of mustard gas) as an antineoplastic drug to treat cancer.
1937	The National Cancer Institute was established after Congress passed the National Cancer Act.
1950s	Antitumor antibiotics were discovered.
1960s–1970s	Platinum compounds were developed. Combination chemotherapy was used and led to improved survival; MOPP (nitrogen mustard, vincristine, procarbazine, and prednisone) cured patients with Hodgkin lymphoma.
1980–1990s	Focus during this time was on drug development for supportive care and dose-limiting toxicities, such as myelosuppression and nausea and vomiting. Biologic response modifiers were discovered.
1991	First serotonin receptor antagonist received U.S. Food and Drug Administration (FDA) approval.
1992	Granulocyte–colony-stimulating factor received FDA approval for use after chemotherapy that causes neutropenia.
21st century	New classes of chemotherapy drugs are being identified. Chemotherapy is used in combination with immunotherapy.

Note. Based on information from Polovich et al., 2014; Tortorice, 2018.

separated into two main phases that take place sequentially: interphase (which consists of G_0, G_1, and S [synthesis] phases) and mitosis (M). Prior to division, a cell must duplicate all of its contents and double in mass; most of this growth occurs in interphase.

During interphase, many important processes take place intracellularly, including the production of DNA, RNA, proteins, lipids, and other cellular substances. Interphase is where copies of chromosomes are made. Each of these processes is important to the development of the cell.

Mitosis is nuclear division and cytokinesis, where the cytoplasm and DNA copies divide into two daughter cells. The amount of time to complete cellular division and the amount of time the cell spends in each phase are variable.

Normal cells are highly controlled and divide for only two possible reasons: to replace injured or lost tissue and to develop normal tissue. Functioning "social control genes" and conditions such as nutrients, blood supply, appropriate space, and growth factors must be present for normal cell division. The five phases of reproduction that occur in both normal and malignant cells are the G_0, G_1, S, G_2, and M phases (Temple, 2016).

- The G_0 phase (G = gap) is the resting phase where the cell is not dividing but cellular activity continues, including normal cell function. Substances such as growth factors interact with cell surface receptors to facilitate entry into and out of this phase. The duration of time that cells spend in this phase is variable.
- The G_1 phase is the beginning of growth, when necessary enzymes are produced in preparation for DNA synthesis and transcription of RNA. Once a cell enters the division process, it cannot return to the resting phase, but cell division can be halted at any moment. The G_1 phase can last from hours to days.

- The S phase of the cell cycle is where DNA is synthesized inside the nucleus. Cells can be in the S phase for 10–20 hours.
- The G_2 phase (premitotic) includes RNA and protein synthesis. Cells spend 2–10 hours in this phase.
- The M phase (mitosis) is division of the cell. The nuclear membrane disappears and microtubules, known as spindle fibers, are formed in the cytoplasm to pull chromosomes to opposite sides of the cell. As the normal cell divides, equal numbers of chromosomes go to each daughter cell. Division of the cell occurs in four phases: prophase, metaphase, anaphase, and telophase. The M phase has a short duration of 30–60 minutes.

Chemotherapy agents can be grouped depending on where they exert their effect during the cell cycle and are referred to as cell cycle specific or cell cycle nonspecific (see Figure 9-1).

Cell cycle–specific chemotherapy agents exert their cytotoxic effect in certain phases of the active cell cycle, such as mitosis and DNA synthesis. These agents usually are not effective when the cell is in the resting phase (G_0) and have the greatest cell kill when administered as frequent divided doses or as a continuous infusion to increase the amount of time the cancer cell is exposed to the chemotherapy in the specific phase of division. For example, the antimetabolite cytarabine is used routinely for induction in acute myeloid leukemia because it kills the rapidly dividing leukemic cells in the S phase. Classifications of agents that are cell cycle specific include antimetabolites and plant alkaloids (Polovich et al., 2014).

Cell cycle–nonspecific agents are effective in any cell cycle, including the G_0 resting phase, and can destroy slowly dividing cells, such as those found in larger tumors. With these agents, cell kill may not happen right away, but the drug is taken into the cell, and when the cancer cell attempts to divide, apoptosis (cell death) occurs. These drugs often are administered intermittently to allow the normal cells to repair. The amount of drug given directly affects the number of cells killed; therefore, increased doses cause enhanced toxicities. Drugs in this class include alkylating agents, antitumor antibiotics, and nitrosoureas (Polovich et al., 2014).

Unfortunately, chemotherapy drugs cannot differentiate between a rapidly growing malignant cell and a rapidly growing normal cell. The result is that normal cells and cancer cells are both damaged. Consequently, patients who are undergoing chemotherapy experience acute side effects, such as bone marrow suppression, gastrointestinal mucosal injury, and damage to hair follicles and gonads. After administration of standard doses of chemotherapy, the body will regenerate new cells; thus, the majority of the side effects are transient (Wilkes & Barton-Burke, 2016).

Chemotherapy Classifications

Chemotherapy agents are classified based on their mechanism of action or where they exert their cytotoxic effect on the cancer cell. Each class of agents has unique properties related to their mechanism of action and side effects. Within each of the classifications, agents are further subclassified, usually related to the origin of the drug, such as a plant or metal. The major classifications of chemotherapy agents are alkylating agents, antimetabolites, antitumor antibiotics, topoisomerase inhibitors, mitotic inhibitors, and miscellaneous agents (Tortorice, 2018).

Alkylating Agents

Alkylating agents impair cell function by forming covalent bonds with DNA, RNA, and protein molecules (Gaddis & Gullatte, 2014). These bonds produce a number of cellular and biochemical consequences that cause DNA mutations, strand breakage, and DNA cross-linking, which all interfere with DNA replication, RNA transcription, and messenger RNA translation into protein products. These actions prevent normal cell function, thus leading to

Figure 9-1. Mechanism of Action of Major Chemotherapy Drugs

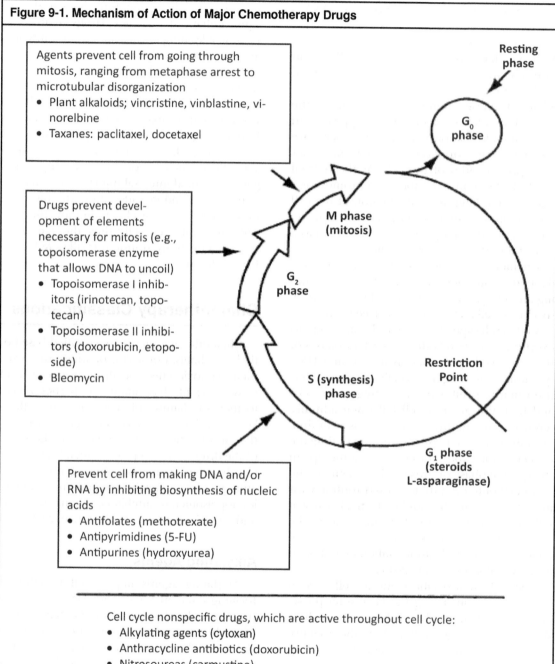

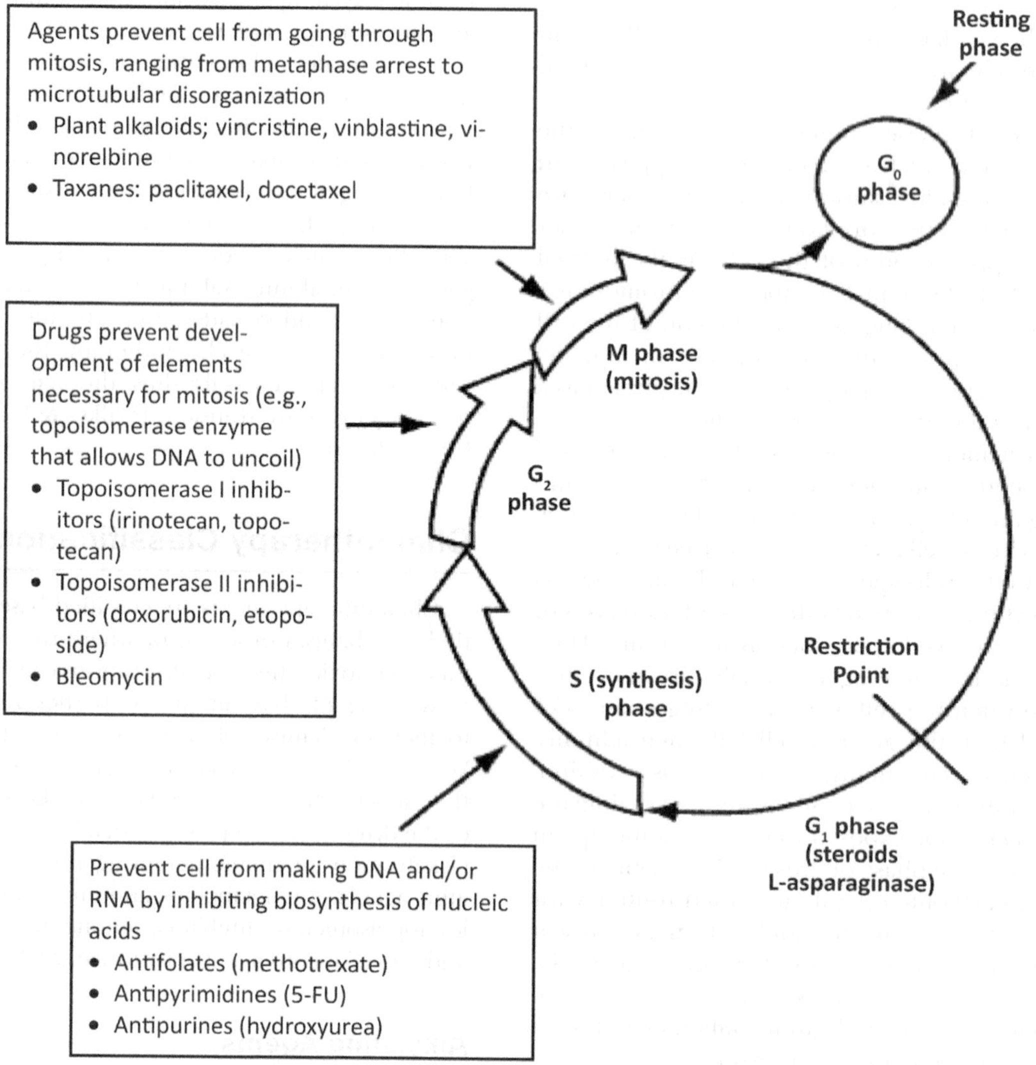
Agents prevent cell from going through mitosis, ranging from metaphase arrest to microtubular disorganization
• Plant alkaloids; vincristine, vinblastine, vinorelbine
• Taxanes: paclitaxel, docetaxel
Resting phase
G_0 phase
M phase (mitosis)
Drugs prevent development of elements necessary for mitosis (e.g., topoisomerase enzyme that allows DNA to uncoil)
• Topoisomerase I inhibitors (irinotecan, topotecan)
• Topoisomerase II inhibitors (doxorubicin, etoposide)
• Bleomycin
G_2 phase
Restriction Point
S (synthesis) phase
G_1 phase (steroids L-asparaginase)
Prevent cell from making DNA and/or RNA by inhibiting biosynthesis of nucleic acids
• Antifolates (methotrexate)
• Antipyrimidines (5-FU)
• Antipurines (hydroxyurea)

Cell cycle nonspecific drugs, which are active throughout cell cycle:

- Alkylating agents (cytoxan)
- Anthracycline antibiotics (doxorubicin)
- Nitrosoureas (carmustine)
- Miscellaneous (cytoxan, dacarbazine, mitomycin-C)

Note. From *2016 Oncology Nursing Drug Handbook* (20th ed., p. 3), by G.M. Wilkes and M. Barton-Burke, 2016, Burlington, MA: Jones & Bartlett Learning. Copyright 2016 by Jones & Bartlett Learning. Reprinted with permission.

cell death (Gaddis & Gullatte, 2014). This class of drugs demonstrates activity in all phases of the cell cycle and therefore is used for a wide variety of cancer types, both slow and rapidly proliferating. The first alkylating agent developed was nitrogen mustard. Alkylating agents also include platinum compounds, cyclophosphamide, melphalan, ifosfamide, and other agents. All of these agents share the same dose-limiting toxicity of myelosuppression. Alkylating agents are associated with an increased risk of second malignancy, most commonly occurring 5–10 years after treatment. Higher cumulative doses and longer length of therapy affect the level of risk (Gaddis & Gullatte, 2014). See Table 9-2 for individual alkylating agents.

Antimetabolites

Antimetabolites have a similar structure as the naturally occurring metabolites that are necessary for DNA and RNA synthesis and exert their effect during the S phase of the cell cycle. Antimetabolites are substituted for metabolites during the synthesis of nucleic acids, inhibiting the replication and repair of DNA. Tumors with a high growth rate, or a high percentage of cells in the S phase, are the most susceptible to antimetabolites. Additionally, normal cells with high division rates, such as gastrointestinal mucosal and bone marrow cells, are sensitive to antimetabolites, which results in side effects such as mucositis, diarrhea, and myelosuppression (Gaddis & Gullatte, 2014; Polovich et al., 2014; Wilkes & Barton-Burke, 2016).

Chemotherapy drugs included in this classification are folate antagonists (e.g., methotrexate), purine antagonists (e.g., 6-mercaptopurine), and pyrimidine antagonists (e.g., 5-fluorouracil). Folate antagonists, such as methotrexate, halt folate metabolism, which is necessary for new cell development and maintenance. Decreased DNA synthesis and interference in cell function lead to cell death. Purine analogs inhibit purine nucleotide synthesis and metabolism, whereas pyrimidine analogs inhibit thymidylate synthase; both subclasses alter the synthesis and function of DNA and RNA. Some antimetabolite agents are most effective when given as a prolonged infusion to target more of

Table 9-2. Alkylating Agents*

Drug	Specific Side Effects/ Toxicities
General class side effects	Myelosuppression, nausea and vomiting, gonadal dysfunction, second malignancies
Bendamustine	Fever, skin reactions, anaphylaxis (second and subsequent cycles)
Carboplatin	Thrombocytopenia, hypersensitivity (sixth dose and higher)
Chlorambucil	Pulmonary fibrosis, skin rash
Cisplatin	Nephrotoxicity, ototoxicity, nausea and vomiting (highly emetogenic), peripheral neuropathy, electrolyte wasting
Cyclophosphamide	Hemorrhagic cystitis
Dacarbazine	Flu-like symptoms, delayed neutropenia nadir Irritant—phlebitis
Ifosfamide	Hemorrhagic cystitis, neurologic toxicity
Mechlorethamine (nitrogen mustard)	Vesicant—potential for necrosis if infiltrated Irritant—phlebitis Fever, chills
Melphalan	Mucositis, pulmonary fibrosis, delayed neutropenia nadir
Oxaliplatin	Neurotoxicity, pharyngolaryngeal dysesthesia, hepatotoxicity, extreme cold sensitivity, pulmonary toxicity

* Table includes only select agents. This is not a comprehensive list of all side effects of each agent.

Note. Based on information from Gaddis & Gullatte, 2014; Polovich et al., 2014.

the cells in the synthesis phase. Table 9-3 lists specific agents in this group (Polovich et al., 2014; Wilkes & Barton-Burke, 2016).

Table 9-3. Antimetabolites*

Drug	Specific Side Effects/Toxicities
General class side effects	Myelosuppression, mucositis, diarrhea, nausea and vomiting, darkening of the veins, photosensitivity
Capecitabine	Palmar-plantar erythrodysesthesia
Cladribine	Hypersensitivity reaction, fever, nephrotoxicity, neurotoxicity
Cytarabine	Cerebellar toxicity when bolus dosing is used Pulmonary toxicity when continuous infusion dosing is used
Fludarabine	Interstitial pneumonitis, neurotoxicity, rash
Fluorouracil	Mucositis, diarrhea, photosensitivity, ocular toxicity, cardiotoxicity (rare), hepatotoxicity
Gemcitabine	Fever, flu-like symptoms, rash, pulmonary toxicity, radiation recall, edema
Mercaptopurine	Mucositis, nausea and vomiting
Methotrexate	Neurotoxicity associated with higher doses, nephrotoxicity
Pemetrexed	Mucositis, nausea and vomiting, rash, nephrotoxicity, hepatotoxicity Vitamin B_{12} and folic administration prior and concurrently can decrease side effects.
Pentostatin	Fever, chills, lymphocytopenia, increased infection risk, hepatotoxicity, nephrotoxicity
Thioguanine	Hepatotoxicity, mucositis

* Table includes only select agents. This is not a comprehensive list of all side effects of each agent.

Note. Based on information from Gaddis & Gullatte, 2014; Polovich et al., 2014.

Antitumor Antibiotics

Antitumor antibiotics interfere with DNA synthesis by binding with DNA at various points and preventing RNA synthesis. These agents also can alter the cell membrane and inhibit specific enzymes. This class of chemotherapy drugs is considered cell cycle nonspecific. Common side effects of this class of drugs include myelosuppression, gastrointestinal toxicity, and alopecia. A number of these agents have lifetime dose limits for individual patients to minimize the risk of long-lasting cardiac or pulmonary toxicity. Examples include doxorubicin, daunorubicin, and bleomycin. A list of antitumor antibiotics appears in Table 9-4.

Topoisomerase Inhibitors

Topoisomerase is a nuclear enzyme essential for maintaining DNA structure during replication, transcription, and translation of genetic materials. Inhibition of this enzyme results in DNA breaks with subsequent cell death. This class is further divided into topoisomerase I and II, depending on whether one or two DNA strands are damaged. These enzymes, found in the nucleus of the cell, are responsible for maintaining the structure and function of DNA. Chemotherapy agents that target the topoisomerase enzyme are classified as topoisomerase inhibitors. Agents in this class include camptothecins, which inhibit topoisomerase I, and epipodophyllotoxins, which inhibit topoisomerase II. See Table 9-5 for examples of topoisomerase inhibitors (Polovich et al., 2014; Wilkes & Barton-Burke, 2016).

Mitotic Inhibitors

Mitotic inhibitors, also known as plant alkaloids, are compounds found in nature. These agents primarily work in the M phase but can cause damage in any cell phase. This class consists of vinca alkaloids, taxanes, and epothilones. Vinca alkaloids (extracts of the

Table 9-4. Antitumor Antibiotics*

Drug	Specific Side Effects/Toxicities
General class side effects	Myelosuppression, stomatitis, diarrhea, nausea and vomiting, alopecia, cardiotoxicity, hepatotoxicity
Bleomycin	Pneumonitis, pulmonary fibrosis, fever, chills, hypersensitivity reactions
Dactinomycin	Radiation recall, hepatotoxicity Vesicant—potential for necrosis if infiltrated
Daunorubicin	Cardiotoxicity, radiation recall, red urine Vesicant—potential for necrosis if infiltrated
Daunorubicin liposomal	Cardiotoxicity, radiation recall, red urine Irritant—phlebitis
Doxorubicin	Cardiotoxicity, radiation recall, red urine Vesicant—potential for necrosis if infiltrated Local hypersensitivity—flare reaction
Doxorubicin liposomal	Palmar-plantar erythrodysesthesia Irritant—phlebitis Hypersensitivity reactions
Epirubicin	Cardiotoxicity, radiation recall, red urine Vesicant—potential for necrosis if infiltrated
Idarubicin	Cardiotoxicity, radiation recall, red urine Vesicant—potential for necrosis if infiltrated
Mitomycin C	Pulmonary fibrosis Vesicant—potential for necrosis if infiltrated Delayed neutropenic nadir
Mitoxantrone	Cardiotoxicity Irritant—phlebitis Blue-green urine

*Table includes only select agents. This is not a comprehensive list of all side effects of each agent.

Note. Based on information from Gaddis & Gullatte, 2014; Polovich et al., 2014.

Madagascar periwinkle plant, *vinca rosea*) bind to microtubular proteins, causing arrest of mitosis and eventual cell death. Taxanes are semisynthetic derivatives of European yew, *Taxus baccata*, and unlike vinca alkaloids, they promote microtubular stability and assembly, which blocks the cell cycle in mitosis. Epothilones act similar to taxanes by stabilizing the microtubules (Goodin, Kane, & Rubin, 2004). Because the liver metabolizes these agents, dose reduction may be necessary to avoid hepatic dysfunction (Gaddis & Gullatte, 2014).

A dose-limiting toxicity common to this class of drugs is damage to peripheral nerves. This is caused by a disruption of the microtubule function of the axons. The damage to the distal axons leads to impaired transport of nerve signals (Krukowski, Nijboer, Huo, Kavelaars, & Heijnen, 2015). See Table 9-6 for examples of mitotic inhibitor agents.

Table 9-5. Topoisomerase Inhibitors*

Drug	Specific Side Effects/ Toxicities
General class side effects	Myelosuppression, diarrhea, nausea and vomiting, alopecia
Etoposide	Hypersensitivity reactions, malaise, fever, hypertension with rapid infusion of higher doses
Irinotecan	Early diarrhea—cholinergic response Late diarrhea—secretory Nausea and vomiting, phlebitis
Teniposide	Hypersensitivity reactions, hepatotoxicity
Topotecan	Neutropenic enterocolitis, interstitial lung disease

*Table includes only select agents. This is not a comprehensive list of all side effects of each agent.

Note. Based on information from Gaddis & Gullatte, 2014; Polovich et al., 2014.

Miscellaneous Agents

Miscellaneous agents include asparaginase and arsenic trioxide (see Table 9-7). Asparaginase is a miscellaneous agent because of its unique mechanism of action. Asparagine is a nonessential amino acid in the human body; however, it is essential for the growth of leukemia cells, specifically lymphoblastic cells (Salzer, Asselin, Plourde, Corn, & Hunger, 2014). Asparaginase is an enzyme derived from bacteria (*Escherichia coli* or *Erwinia chrysanthemi*) that depletes circulating levels of asparagine, resulting in leukemia cell death (Keating, 2013). This unique agent is a key component of acute lymphoblastic leukemia therapy used for the achievement of remission and intensification. Another miscellaneous agent, arsenic trioxide, is used for patients with acute promyelocytic leukemia and has shown activity in myelodysplastic syndrome and multiple myeloma. Arsenic trioxide is a differentiating agent and causes fragmented changes in the DNA, leading to apoptosis. Arsenic trioxide is thought to inhibit the self-renewal of leukemia cells due to free radical formation (Kritharis, Bradley, & Budman, 2013).

Table 9-6. Mitotic Inhibitors*

Drug	Specific Side Effects/Toxicities
General class side effects	Neurotoxicity, hepatotoxicity
Taxanes	
• Cabazitaxel	Hypersensitivity reactions, peripheral neuropathy, nausea and vomiting
• Docetaxel	Fluid retention, rash, nail disorders, hypersensitivity reactions, hyperpigmentation of the vein, phlebitis
• Paclitaxel	Hypersensitivity reactions, peripheral neuropathy, arthralgia, myalgia, alopecia, nausea and vomiting Vesicant-like properties—potential for necrosis if infiltrated
• Paclitaxel-albumin bound	Peripheral neuropathy, arthralgia, myalgia, alopecia, nausea and vomiting
Vinca alkaloids	For IV use; fatal if given via any other route
• Vinblastine	Myelosuppression, peripheral neuropathy Vesicant—potential for necrosis if infiltrated
• Vincristine	Peripheral neuropathy, ileus Vesicant—potential for necrosis if infiltrated
• Vinorelbine	Myelosuppression Irritant—phlebitis Vesicant—potential for necrosis if infiltrated

* Table includes only select agents. This is not a comprehensive list of all side effects of each agent.

Note. Based on information from Gaddis & Gullatte, 2014; Polovich et al., 2014.

Table 9-7. Miscellaneous Agents*

Drug	Specific Side Effects/Toxicities
General class side effects	Myelosuppression, diarrhea, nausea and vomiting, alopecia
Arsenic trioxide	QTc prolongation, fever, nausea and vomiting, headache
Asparaginase	Hypersensitivity reactions, hepatotoxicity, pancreatitis, hyperglycemia

* Table includes only select agents. This is not a comprehensive list of all side effects of each agent.

Note. Based on information from Gaddis & Gullatte, 2014; Polovich et al., 2014.

Factors Affecting Responses to Chemotherapy

Many factors can affect patients' responses to chemotherapy, such as tumor-specific characteristics, patient-specific factors, and resistance.

Tumor-Specific Factors

Tumor-specific factors that affect responses to chemotherapy include the tumor burden and rate of tumor growth. Tumor burden and chemotherapy response have an inverse relationship. The larger the tumor, the lower the response rate, and the smaller the tumor, the greater the response rate (Temple, 2016). With an increasing tumor burden, the growth rate slows, thus decreasing the number of cells actively dividing. Two cellular properties—doubling time and growth fraction—affect growth rate. *Doubling time* is the amount of time it takes for one cancer cell to double (length of the cell cycle). *Growth fraction* refers to the proportion of actively dividing cells (Polovich et al., 2014).

Cell cycle time is the amount of time it takes for a cell to move from G_1 through mitosis. Malignant cells with short cycles are most sensitive to cell cycle–specific agents administered as continuous infusions because a large proportion of these cells are actively dividing (Polovich et al., 2014). The tumor cells will continue to reproduce and even become resistant if they do not pass through the S phase while exposed to chemotherapy. If a tumor has small growth fractions (not many cells actively dividing), it may become resistant to chemotherapy agents. This resistance to chemotherapy cellular kinetics can be overcome by decreasing the tumor load with surgery or radiation and using scheduled, cycled, combination chemotherapy. Chemotherapy drugs are most effective when tumor cells are continually growing, have a high growth fraction, and have a short cell cycle time (Brown, 2014).

Structural characteristics that affect tumor response include the location of the tumor and the blood supply, which affects adequate drug uptake. Locations of malignant cells with poor systemic response to chemotherapy include the peritoneum; the pleural space, because of diffusion; and the brain, because of the blood-brain barrier. The vasculature in a tumor bed tends to be disorganized and leaky, and as solid tumors grow larger, the inside of the mass has a poor blood supply and may become necrotic. These factors affect chemotherapy delivery to the tumor bed, causing cell kill on the outside of the tumor but not the inside, where the cells have a decreased growth fraction resulting from lack of nutrients and oxygen (Brown, 2014).

Patient Factors

Patient factors that affect chemotherapy response include physical status, age, performance status (see Chapter 2), comorbidities, psychological status, and the number of previous therapies. Performance status should be assessed prior to and during chemotherapy. A poor performance status will affect the patient's tolerance of the chemotherapy, leading to increased toxicities (Polovich et al., 2014). The two main ways of measuring performance status are the Eastern Cooperative Oncology Group (ECOG) scale and the Karnofsky Performance Status scale. The ECOG scale rates performance from 0 to 5, with 0 being fully active, 4 being in need of total care and unable to perform any self-care, and 5 being dead (Oken et al., 1982). Karnofsky status is rated on a percentage score, with 100% being able to perform all self-care, 50% being in need of frequent assistance and medical care, and 10% being imminently near death and with a progressing fatal process (Karnofsky & Burchenal, 1949). Before initiating chemotherapy, healthcare providers must assess patients' functional status. If patients have physiologic limitations due to the cancer and the disease is responsive to chemotherapy, they should see an improvement in functional status (e.g., acute leukemia). If patients are experiencing dose-limiting toxicities or symptoms unbearable and their functional status continues to decline despite interventions, the patients and providers will need to discuss the risks and benefits of therapy to decide whether to continue.

Chemotherapy Drug Resistance

Chemotherapy drug resistance results when tumors become inherently resistant to antineoplastic agents (natural resistance) or develop resistance after exposure (acquired resistance) (Brown, 2014). Control of a tumor may be ineffective without extreme toxicity to the host; therefore, resistance is a chief limitation for achieving cure in people with cancer. Chemotherapy resistance is similar to the antimicrobial resistance that develops in microorganisms. Once a cell has been exposed to a chemotherapy agent, the agent is transported across the cell membrane and usually causes cell death. However, in drug resistance, the cell can adapt and develop further tumor cell genetic mutations that make the drug ineffective. Mechanisms of drug resistance are multifaceted and can influence cell membrane transport, intracellular activity, drug concentration, detoxification, and repair of DNA after exposure to chemotherapy and multidrug-resistant phenotypes (Brown, 2014).

Chemotherapy agents enter the cell through a facilitated transport mechanism in which a protein on the cell surface binds with the chemotherapy agent and is transported through the cell membrane, where the agent applies its cytotoxic effects. Tumor cells become resistant by changing the protein transports on the cell surface by either disabling them to prevent transport of chemotherapy into the cell or by decreasing the number of protein receptors on the cell surface such that less chemotherapy is allowed inside the cell (Gottesman, 2002).

Tumor cells can increase the number of intracellular targets for the chemotherapy agent so that concentrations will always be ineffective and cell growth will not be inhibited. Methotrexate exhibits this type of resistance because its action depends on binding to dihydrofolate reductase inside the cell to cause disruption in DNA synthesis; cells that are resistant show an increase in dihydrofolate reductase (Gottesman, 2002). Glutathione S-transferase, an enzyme that is responsible for multiple cellular functions, causes drug resistance by binding with the chemotherapy agent and stopping its mechanism of action.

One cause of resistance involves highly evolved and effective mechanisms for repairing damaged DNA and preventing future damage. When alkylating agents cause alterations in the DNA that would result in apoptosis, the section of damaged DNA is cleaved, and newly synthesized DNA is replaced. Chemotherapy agents such as pyrimidine and purine analogs need to be converted with an enzyme inside the cell to exert their cytotoxic effect. Resistance can occur when a loss of these conversion enzymes occurs, leading to decreased intracellular activation of chemotherapy such as cytarabine, fluorouracil, mercaptopurine, and thioguanine (Gottesman, 2002).

After drug resistance develops, the cell may develop cross-resistance to various unrelated chemotherapy agents; this is called *multidrug resistance.* Molecules that have been identified include P-glycoprotein, an extracellular pump used to transport toxins out of the cell (Gottesman, 2002). P-glycoprotein affects drugs derived from natural substances such as antibiotics and plant alkaloids. Malignant cells that have been exposed to one class of chemotherapy can develop cellular functions that expel other classes of chemotherapy from the inside of the cell or do not allow the agent to enter the cell at all. This is usually caused by naturally occurring compounds such as vinca alkaloids, anthracyclines, and taxanes and is the result of biologic and genetic mutations in the cell, including gene amplification or point mutations (Gottesman, 2002). Cells also may become less responsive because of changes in the environment, such as prior exposure to a toxin. P53 is a tumor suppressor protein that, in a normal cell, stops cellular growth and division and is responsible for cell death if the DNA is damaged. In cancer, loss of P53 protein function has been associated with decreased chemotherapy effectiveness. Single-agent chemotherapy can increase the likelihood of drug-resistant clones (Chu & De Vita, 2017).

Overcoming Drug Resistance

One strategy used to overcome tumor resistance is combination chemotherapy, which is the use of agents in combination to target the cell in different phases of the cell cycle to maximize cell kill and decrease resistance. Agents to select for combination therapy are those that demonstrate efficacy as a single agent to treat a specific cancer and work in different areas of the cell cycle. Using a combination of chemotherapy drugs can provide a broad range of cell kill in order to overcome resistance and prevent or slow the development of new resistant clones. Toxicities of the drugs used in combination therapy should not overlap in order to prevent lethal toxicities and balance safety with efficacy. Combination chemotherapy is effective in patients with large tumor burdens and slow growth fractions because as one agent kills tumor cells, more cells are recruited to proliferate and are injured or destroyed (Temple, 2016).

Administration of combination therapy should be done at constant intervals with the shortest rest time possible to allow for recovery of sensitive normal cells, such as hematopoietic cells in the bone marrow. The drugs should be used at the optimal schedule and dose, which is called *dose intensity* (Polovich et al., 2014). Response to chemotherapy is defined as complete response, partial response, minimal response or stable disease, progression, and relapse (Polovich et al., 2014).

Chemotherapy Treatment Approaches

The goals of cancer therapy need to be identified prior to administration so that both the patient and the healthcare team are in agreement. Three goals of treatment exist: cure, control, and palliation. Cure is the preferred outcome, but is not always possible, and refers to a prolonged absence of disease. *Adjuvant* refers to the use of chemotherapy in conjunction with a primary treatment in patients with minimal or unmeasurable tumor volume in an attempt to eliminate cancer cells and increase the chance of a cure. Cancer control prevents cell growth but does not totally eliminate malignant cells; therefore, a cure is not possible. The aim of cancer control is to extend the length of survival and improve the quality of life. Palliation focuses on comfort when cure or disease control is not possible. Palliative chemotherapy may be used to shrink an obstructing tumor causing significant symptoms (Polovich et al., 2014). Figure 9-2 lists terms used to describe chemotherapy treatment.

Prior to treatment, the nurse must perform a thorough nursing assessment and patient history. The patient history should include a review of previous or recent treatments, including surgery, radiation therapy, and chemotherapy, and a thorough medication history (over the counter, herbal, and prescription). The healthcare team needs to be aware of any complementary therapies the patient is using for symptom management. The nurse also should review the patient's medical and psychiatric history and list all of the patient's allergies, including those to food, drugs, and environmental stimuli. This process includes screening the patient for symptoms experienced during previous treatments, such as fatigue, pain, and nausea and vomiting, so that the nurse can tailor any teaching and interventions (Polovich et al., 2014). See Figure 9-3 for a patient history checklist.

Prior to the administration of chemotherapy, the nurse must obtain vital information to ensure the orders are accurate and the patient is ready to receive the therapy. These include the patient's actual, not stated, height and weight, which must be compared with previous weights. Recent laboratory values, including electrolytes, renal function, and complete blood count with differential, should be thoroughly reviewed before administering chemotherapy, as the dose may need to be

Figure 9-2. Definitions of Chemotherapy Treatment Terms

adjuvant therapy—Therapy administered after the primary treatment modality such as surgery. The goal is to eliminate small sites or microscopic disease for patients who have a high risk of recurrence.

chemoprevention—Selected use of pharmaceutical agents to prevent cancer in high-risk patients.

combination chemotherapy—Use of two or more active agents that increase tumor cell kill, decrease resistance to chemotherapy drugs, and do not increase toxicity.

dose delay—Doses of chemotherapy can be delayed because of toxicities.

dose dense—The dose of chemotherapy is delivered over a shorter period of time. Supportive care, such as growth factors, is necessary.

dose intensity—Smaller doses are given more frequently.

dose reduce—Doses can be reduced by a certain percentage depending on toxicities, such as a low platelet count or impaired renal function.

myeloablation (high-dose chemotherapy)—Obliteration of the bone marrow in preparation for bone marrow or peripheral blood stem cell transplantation.

neoadjuvant therapy—Chemotherapy administered prior to another treatment, such as surgery. The goal is to decrease tumor size for surgical removal.

regional chemotherapy—Delivery of higher doses of chemotherapy to specific tumor sites, such as the peritoneal cavity, pleural space, or liver. Systemic toxicity tends to be reduced.

Note. Based on information from American Cancer Society, n.d.

altered or held if the values are not within acceptable limits (Polovich et al., 2014).

Age is also an important factor to consider. Chemotherapy toxicity in older adults can be higher than in younger adults. Hurria et al. (2011) developed and implemented a self-administered geriatric assessment tool to predict morbidity and mortality risk in older adults. This assessment measures functional status, cognitive function, comorbidity, psychological state, social support, and nutrition status. Similarly valid and reliable tools can be helpful in predicting risk for older patients receiving cancer treatment. Older adults at risk for toxicities should not be denied chemotherapy, but they should be monitored closely.

In addition to a thorough physical assessment, assessment of any spiritual or cultural preferences and coping mechanisms is important. Patient and family views of chemotherapy and previous treatment experience can influence adherence and nursing care and should be explored. Referrals can be made to a social worker; a physical, occupational, or speech ther-

Figure 9-3. Pretreatment Chemotherapy Checklist

Assess for previous and recent treatments.

Medical history
- History of motion sickness or morning sickness with pregnancy (predisposed to increased nausea with chemotherapy)
- Complete physical examination and history
- Comorbid conditions
- Surgeries

Chemotherapy, radiation therapy, hormone therapy, immunotherapy
- Previous treatments
- Tolerance—side effects/toxicities

Medications
- Prescriptions
- Over-the-counter agents
- Herbal substances
- Vitamins

Psychiatric and social history
- History of mental illness, depression, or anxiety
- History of drug or alcohol use
- Support systems

Allergies
- Food
- Drug
- Environmental

Complementary therapies
- Acupuncture, acupressure, aromatherapy, healing touch

Note. Based on information from Polovich et al., 2014.

apist; spiritual care provider; dietitian; and other interprofessional team members (Polovich et al., 2014). It is helpful to assess the patient's understanding of the disease stage and treatment with a question such as, "What has the doctor told you about your disease and treatment?" This open-ended question facilitates further discussion.

Nurses may face many ethical dilemmas when caring for patients undergoing chemotherapy that arise from the patient or the healthcare environment. Informed consent is necessary prior to chemotherapy administration; the patient and family need to be aware of the side effects, toxicities, and possible adverse outcomes of the chemotherapy treatment. Important topics to discuss include infertility, sexuality, short- and long-term effects, and the risk of extravasation or phlebitis if administering a vesicant or irritant. Autonomy also is important to decision making. The patient may not want chemotherapy, or they may want the chemotherapy but not the teaching. The patient may refuse treatment based on many different factors, such as cultural reasons, health beliefs, or lack of education. These scenarios can be difficult for the healthcare team, and it is important to use a team-based approach to find solutions (Polovich et al., 2014).

Ethical dilemmas from the healthcare team can include nurse–physician conflicts when the nurse is advocating for patient wishes that conflict with the current goals of care. A lack of access to health care, inability to afford cancer treatment, patient nonadherence, and reimbursement issues can make the administration of chemotherapy challenging. Patients should be made aware of assistance programs, which may remove financial barriers to treatment. See Chapter 30 for further discussion of ethical issues.

Routes of Chemotherapy

Chemotherapy can be administered via many different routes depending on the drug being administered and the tumor type and location (see Table 9-8). The most frequently used routes

Table 9-8. Routes of Chemotherapy Administration

Route	Considerations
Oral	Route requires attention to patient adherence and drug–drug and food–drug interactions.
Intravenous	Administration requires time for patient and nurse. It is the most common route used. Venous access must be reliable and monitored frequently during infusion.
Subcutaneous or intramuscular	Maximum volumes sometimes require multiple injections. Injection site discomfort can occur.
Intrathecal/intraventricular	Intrathecal route consists of administration into the thecal space and requires a lumbar puncture. Some draws are fatal if mistakenly given intrathecally. Intraventricular administration requires an implanted intraventricular access device, such as an Ommaya reservoir.
Intra-arterial	Route is used for the instillation of chemotherapy into the arterial system of the liver.
Intraperitoneal	Chemotherapy is delivered to the abdominal cavity by a catheter or a port. It also may be delivered in the operating room, where the chemotherapy is heated and perfused in the abdomen.
Intrapleural	Chemotherapy is delivered into the pleural space to prevent recurrent pleural effusions.
Intravesicular	Chemotherapy is administered into the bladder via a Foley catheter.
Topical	Chemotherapy is administered on the skin.

Note. Based on information from Polovich et al., 2014.

are intravenous (IV) and oral (PO). Chemotherapy can be delivered more directly to a specific site of the tumor in higher doses than would be tolerated systemically; this is known as *regional chemotherapy* (Temple, 2016). Each route has its own risks and benefits. Although nurses may not administer chemotherapy via all routes, such as intrathecal, it is necessary to know the risks and benefits to educate patients and families and anticipate their needs.

IV chemotherapy is considered systemic and therefore has the most consistent absorption and dose accuracy. It requires time and resources to administer an IV treatment, which can be taxing on patients and the healthcare system. Administering irritant or vesicant agents intravenously may cause sclerosing of the veins, possible extravasation leading to tissue necrosis, and the need for a central vascular access device. Complications of the IV route include phlebitis, infection, infiltration, local discomfort, extravasation, hypersensitivity, and anaphylaxis (Polovich et al., 2014).

Administration of vesicants can lead to extravasation if they infiltrate the local tissue. Vesicant extravasation is an immediate complication of chemotherapy that can cause severe tissue damage, necrosis, and loss of function. Infiltration of some vesicants can cause binding to DNA, leading to cell death, and these injuries increase in depth and size over time. When administering IV chemotherapy, nurses must know the risk of extravasation and take precautions. Risk factors for extravasation include poor vascular integrity; multiple IV chemotherapy agents; small, fragile veins; failure to accurately cannulate the vein with a vascular access device; patient movement, which dislodges the device; and limited vein selection sites. Signs of extravasation of a vesicant include swelling, lack of blood return, IV fluid that stops or slows, or leaking around the injection site. If vesicant extravasation occurs, the nurse should immediately stop the infusion, aspirate the vesicant, and initiate institutional policies for the management of vesicant extravasation (Polovich et al., 2014).

Oral chemotherapy agents are rapidly emerging and allow for greater patient independence, although drawbacks, including inconsistent absorption and nonadherence, are frequent problems (Polovich et al., 2014). Medication and food interactions can affect the therapeutic level of these oral agents. Patient education coupled with medication reconciliation to assess for interactions is paramount (Polovich et al., 2014). The cost of oral agents and insurance coverage can vary widely, which can lead to significant challenges for patients. Drug assistance programs are available, and patients should be provided access if needed.

Subcutaneous or intramuscular routes of chemotherapy administration can be convenient for patients and are easy to administer. It is important to use the smallest gauge needle and to document and observe the administration sites for signs of infection, pain, hematoma, bleeding, or irritation. Nurses are required to wear personal protective equipment (PPE) during administration of chemotherapy by this and all other routes. The nurse should rotate the sites and use proper technique to facilitate maximal absorption of chemotherapy (Polovich et al., 2014).

Intra-arterial (into an artery) chemotherapy is delivered directly to a tumor or organ by targeting the arterial blood supply to that area. The most common approach is use of the hepatic artery. Chemotherapy is administered into the liver for patients with colorectal liver metastases or nonresectable hepatocellular carcinoma. Chemotherapy via this route can provide targeted treatment to the liver while minimizing whole body side effects; however, it is most effective when combined with IV chemotherapy to treat systemic disease (Karanicolas et al., 2014). Intra-arterial infusion pump placement and chemotherapy administration via this route requires a group of interprofessional healthcare members with specialized expertise to ensure success. Possible complications include pain, hepatic artery injury, bleeding, fatigue, embolism, pump malfunction, and catheter migration (Cahill, 2005).

Floxuridine and oxaliplatin are the most common drugs administered by this route (Karanicolas et al., 2014).

Intrathecal (into the cerebrospinal fluid) chemotherapy is administered via a lumbar puncture procedure or an intraventricular implanted reservoir for either prevention or treatment of central nervous system involvement in select cancers, such as testicular cancer, leukemia, or aggressive lymphomas, or as treatment for leptomeningeal carcinomatosis. For patients with leptomeningeal carcinomatosis, an intraventricular reservoir (Ommaya) is placed to allow long-term access to the cerebrospinal fluid. If chemotherapy is administered via a lumbar puncture, patients should lie flat for 30 minutes after the procedure, and all patients should be monitored for dizziness, headache, blurred vision, nausea, vomiting, bleeding, or signs of infection. Some chemotherapy agents that are administered into the cerebrospinal fluid include methotrexate, cytarabine, liposomal cytarabine, and corticosteroids (Del Principe et al., 2014). Inadvertently administering intrathecal chemotherapy can be fatal; strict caution is advised (Gilbar & Seger, 2012; Goldspiel et al., 2015).

Intraperitoneal chemotherapy is administered when a patient has peritoneal surface malignancy caused by ovarian cancer, peritoneal mesothelioma, appendiceal carcinoma, or peritoneal dissemination from pancreatic, duodenal, or gastric cancer (Al-Quteimat & Al-Badaineh, 2014). The goal of intraperitoneal chemotherapy is to administer chemotherapy through a catheter to destroy cancerous cells in the peritoneum, where other routes of administration have inadequate delivery, while sparing normal healthy cells and decreasing systemic toxicity. For peritoneal cavity cancers, higher chemotherapy drug concentrations are needed to effectively kill the tumor cells than those via the IV route. Intraperitoneal chemotherapy often is used in combination with IV chemotherapy to provide maximum systemic tumor kill. The most common drugs given via this route are cisplatin and paclitaxel, although other agents are used. The slower clearance of chemotherapy via this route allows for better drug exposure in the peritoneum (Al-Quteimat & Al-Badaineh, 2014).

Intrapleural chemotherapy is used for pleurodesis with malignant pleural effusions that are likely to reoccur. Chemotherapy is administered via a chest tube. The chemotherapy aggravates the normal tissues, causing them to adhere to each other and form scar tissue with the goal of preventing recurrent pleural effusions. At the same time, the chemotherapy may kill remaining cancer cells in the area. Talc powder remains the choice agent for pleurodesis; however, bleomycin is also used (Clive, Jones, Bhatnagar, Preston, & Maskell, 2016). Bleomycin given as a sclerotherapy agent can cause pain, fever, and dyspnea (Rafiei et al., 2014).

Intravesicular chemotherapy is instilled into patients with bladder cancer either postoperatively or in cycles via a bladder catheterization. The most common chemotherapy agent administered via this method is mitomycin C. Chemical cystitis can occur, leading to patient complaints of frequency, dysuria, or hematuria. The nurse must use caution to prevent exposure to hazardous drugs while administering chemotherapy via this route. The bladder system should be maintained as a closed system, and drainage should be done into a closed catheter drainage system that can be labeled as cytotoxic waste (Polovich, 2011).

As described, chemotherapy agents can be administered via a variety of routes, and with new combination therapies and clinical trials, treatment may incorporate more than one route of administration. Nurses should have knowledge related to these routes to support patients' understanding.

Administration of Chemotherapy

The administration of chemotherapy is a high-risk procedure because of the narrow therapeutic index and varying dosing regimens and routes of administration (Polovich et al., 2014). If patients receive more than the intended dose of chemotherapy (overdose), they can have toxic effects; if underdosed, they may not achieve maximum response. This is referred to as a narrow therapeutic index. Doses can be reduced or modified for patients based on individual toxicities. A systematic approach to chemotherapy dose determination and administration should be used to decrease variances in practice. It is critical to validate the chemotherapy regimen and dose by cross-referencing with published guidelines (e.g., National Comprehensive Cancer Network® guidelines), institutionally approved protocols, or peer-reviewed journal articles. Safe doses, usually given as ranges in a chemotherapy reference book, can still be wrong in the context of a protocol. Every line of the orders should be critically reviewed for patient identifiers, frequency, date, drug, dose, method of dose determination, route, rate of administration, fluid volume and diluent, and the need for premedications and hydration, if applicable. It is important to determine the vesicant and irritant potential of the agent and check the label, appearance, and expiration times for each drug. Emergency drugs, a spill kit, and extravasation supplies should be readily available during chemotherapy administration (Polovich et al., 2014).

Doses of agents can be calculated by the body surface area (BSA), milligrams per kilogram (mg/kg), or area under the curve (AUC), or measured as units, milligrams, or grams (Polovich et al., 2014). BSA can be calculated using various methods, with the simplest being a calculator with a square root function. Computer programs and BSA calculators can be used. Note that the BSA obtained can vary with different formulas used for calculation; therefore, institutions should use the same dose determination method each time and establish a policy to promote compliance and consistency. The patient should be weighed and measured in kilograms and centimeters to avoid mistakes with calculations. If a significant change (5%–10%) occurs in the BSA, this may lead to a chemotherapy dose change (depending on institutional policy). The prescriber should be notified, and the chemotherapy dose should be recalculated to avoid over- or underdosing (Schulmeister, 2005). Other considerations include the patient's current weight; obese patients may be dosed based on actual, ideal, or adjusted body weight depending on the protocol and institutional guidelines.

Carboplatin, a commonly used chemotherapy agent, is dosed by AUC, which is based on the patient's renal function and excretion of the drug. Calculation of the dose requires the patient's current serum creatinine, age, weight, and sex. To prescribe carboplatin and verify the dose, the creatinine clearance needs to be determined; this is also known as the glomerular filtration rate (Polovich et al., 2014).

Chemotherapy orders should be verified and safety checks completed by two nurses who are trained and competent in the administration of chemotherapy. It is vital to find a quiet area to complete these safety checks. Many different factors can lead to errors with chemotherapy dosing, including stress, lack of staffing, inexperience, lack of resources and experts, unclear or illegible chemotherapy orders, fatigue, and difficulty comprehending drug packaging. Some chemotherapy agents have similar sounding or looking names; for example, vincristine and vinblastine can be confused by illegible handwritten orders or transcriptions. Tall man lettering—writing part of a drug name in upper case letters—should be used with chemotherapy prescribing to help prevent errors with sound-alike, look-alike drugs (e.g., vinCRIStine and vinBLAStine). The use of preprinted chemotherapy orders is critical and can help avoid transcription errors. A small error in the calculation process could have major, if not lethal, consequences for a patient. Double checks throughout the chemotherapy administration process will reduce variance and promote safe administration (Polovich et al., 2014). See Figure 9-4 for an example of a nursing chemother-

Figure 9-4. Chemotherapy Administration Checklist

JOHNS HOPKINS
MEDICINE

THE JOHNS HOPKINS HOSPITAL
600 NORTH WOLFE STREET
BALTIMORE, MD 21287

Chemotherapy
Administration
CHECKLIST

SIGNATURE/TITLE	INITIALS

for addressograph plate

Allergies: ☐ Yes ☐ No List: ____________

Date / Time	Regimen	Order#

Central line present for continuous IV vesicant chemotherapy
☐ Yes ☐ Blood return present ☐ N/A

Weight	Height	BSA	IBW
kg	cm/inches		

CHECKLIST	INITIALS	Comments:
BEFORE ADMINISTRATION OF THE <u>FIRST</u> DOSE OF EACH CHEMOTHERAPY AGENT ORDERED:		
1. Order includes any supportive care medications (eg. Premeds, antiemetics, hydration, growth factors, emergency meds, etc.).		☐ None required per regimen
2. Pediatric oncology patient: order received to proceed with chemotherapy administration.		☐ N/A
3. Confirm presence of consent (if applicable).		☐ N/A
4. Patient, parent and/or caregiver have received written and verbal education.		
5. Patient, parent and/or caregiver understands the treatment plan, toxicities, side effects and wishes to proceed.		
BEFORE <u>EVERY</u> DOSE OF A CHEMOTHERAPY AGENT: (Practitioner administering chemo)		* Document on page 2 of chemo checklist
1. Doses are acceptable based on: ☐ Standard regimen dose ☐ JHMIRB Research protocol ☐ Individual therapy *Web address for Oncology Center research protocols: **JHMCIC.JHMI.edu/oncres**		☐ Reference for dosing of individual chemothe is placed in chart. ☐ If reference doesn't exist for individual chem 2 *attending physicians* have signed treatmen
2. Treatment note/plan includes: Patient name, history #, date, indication for chemo, chemo agents used, doses, schedule, dose modification and rationale for modifications (if applicable). **For standard regimens, e.g. VAD, CHOP, JHH Oncology preprinted chemo orders, <u>doses</u> do not need to be rewritten in note, unless modified.*		Upon initiation of any new therapy or with any ch in treatment plan, a separate physician note must present and co-signed by an attending.
3. Treatment note/plan is written or co-signed by attending physician.		
4. If on research protocol: Treatment note/plan includes protocol name, #, arm and point in therapy (arm, cycle, phase, week, etc.).		☐ N/A
5. Lab values that would modify administration of chemo are WNL (labs should be within 7 days unless otherwise specified). *acceptable values are based on protocol requirements or dept standards.		If laboratory values are not WNL ☐ order received to hold chemo ☐ order received to proceed
6. Assess patient's prior tolerance to chemo and note any existing side effects or toxicities, notify physician if indicated.		
7. Correct drug, dose, route, patient name, history #, birthdate, and patient ID band (JHH Medical ID card in adult outpatient areas) verified with patient and chemo orders at bedside/chair.		
VALIDATION BEFORE <u>EVERY</u> DOSE OF A CHEMOTHERAPY AGENT: (2 practitioners independently check)		*Document the 2 practitioner validation on pg 2 of chemo checklist
1. Chemo orders are written or co-signed by attending physician.		* Do not proceed without physician signature(s) p protocol.
2. Orders contain drug, dose, eg. units/m^2 or units/kg, dosing interval, duration of therapy, diluent type and volume, and rate (if applicable), and Ht, Wt, & BSA (if applicable).		**Pediatric oncology patients:** ☐ dose is written per day eg. units/m^2/day or units/kg ☐ intra-thecal orders contain patient's date of birth
3. Multi-day continuous infusion chemo includes total daily dose and total multi-day hours of infusion. Pediatric oncology: Multi-day infusions include cumulative dose.		☐ N/A
4. Doses based on renal function, ideal or adjusted Wt., or other formulas include calculations.		☐ N/A
5. Chemo dose(s) recalculated independently by two practitioners based on *current* Ht, Wt, BSA (if applicable).		☐ N/A Dose does not require calculation
6. Dosage recalculations are within 10% of the ordered dose (based on dose and current Ht and Wt). *Calculations for BSA are done in OCIS in Oncology and using nomogram elsewhere.		If dosage recalculations are not within 10% of the ordered dose, Attending notified and ☐ Chemo held ☐ Orders re-written
7. Label on chemo matches order, includes; patient name, history #, date, drug, dose, rate, route, volume in bag (ensure volume in bag appears to match stated amount), color of fluid (appears appropriate) # of pills (count each pill).		

JHH 24-957-0011 (Rev 08/10)

(Continued on next page)

Figure 9-4. Chemotherapy Administration Checklist *(Continued)*

PRACTITIONER VALIDATION DOCUMENTATION: ***This section must be used for the 2 practitioner validation of each chemo dose administered. The administering practitioner on Day 1 of chemo completes page 1 of checklist and also signs below. On subsequent days administering practitioner signs below to validate that the required checks have been validated on page 1. Refer to chemo policy MDU001.***

Date/Time	Drug	Practitioner Administering drug	Practitioner validation

JHH 24-957-0011 (Rev 08/10)

Note. Figure courtesy of Sidney Kimmel Comprehensive Cancer Center at Johns Hopkins Hospital, 2011. Used with permission.

apy administration checklist that can be used prior to administration to standardize safety checks and reduce errors.

Documentation of chemotherapy administration and patient care is a fundamental nursing responsibility. Documentation regarding chemotherapy should note the patient and family education provided, including mechanism of action, side effect management, follow-up instructions, and possible adverse events. Anytime a nurse has a conversation with a patient that involves advice, either in person or via telephone, documentation needs to be completed. When administering chemotherapy, the nurse documents the patient's name; the date and time of drug administration, including premedication administration; and chemotherapy details, including drug name, dose, route, length of infusion (start and stop times), and the volume and type of fluids administered. If an IV site is used, documentation needs to include the site, type (e.g., peripheral IV, implanted port), and size (gauge and length of needle) of infusion device. Blood return needs to be verified and documented before, during, and at the conclusion of therapy (Polovich et al., 2014).

Although chemotherapy is therapeutic to the patient, these drugs are hazardous and pose a risk to healthcare providers who handle the drugs or the excreta from patients who have received the drugs. Hazardous drugs have the potential to cause acute and long-term toxicities in individuals who handle them (American Society of Health-System Pharmacists [ASHP], 2006; National Institute for Occupational Safety and Health [NIOSH], 2014). It is essential that healthcare providers follow the guidelines for safe handling of these agents. Agents are defined as hazardous if they have any of the following characteristics: genotoxicity, carcinogenicity, teratogenicity, reproductive toxicity, organ toxicity, or a structure and profile similar to an existing hazardous drug. Genotoxicity is the ability to cause mutagenicity, a mutation in genetic material. Carcinogenicity is the ability of an agent to cause cancer in an animal or human (e.g., cigarettes). Teratogenicity is the ability to cause fetal malformations or defects (ASHP, 2006; NIOSH, 2014).

Healthcare workers should always implement safe handling precautions to decrease their risk of exposure to hazardous drugs. Studies have looked at cohorts of nurses exposed to hazardous agents and various endpoints, such as mutagenic substances in the urine and acute health effects such as headaches, hair loss, and reproductive outcomes (fetal loss, infertility, low birth weight, and congenital malformations) (Polovich, 2011). A meta-analysis of 14 studies from Europe and the United States showed an association between adverse reproductive outcomes and hazardous drug exposure. A significant association existed between spontaneous abortion and exposure, and although incidences of other endpoints were elevated, none were statistically significant (Dranitsaris et al., 2005).

The highest risk for exposure is during drug manufacturing and preparation, whereas the lowest risk for exposure is during handling of patient excreta when drug metabolites are at their lowest concentration (ASHP, 2006). Nurses should take precautions throughout drug preparation and administration and in handling patient excreta to minimize their exposure to hazardous agents. The duration of chemotherapy precautions varies and depends on the agent administered.

Possible short-term effects (hours to days) of occupational exposure include local skin or mucous membrane irritation, contact dermatitis or rash, blurred vision, dizziness, and allergic responses. Long-term effects (months to years) include chromosomal abnormalities, increased risk of cancer, liver damage, and reproductive risks. Direct contact occurs when skin or mucous membranes come in contact directly with a hazardous drug, possibly by contaminated food, inhalation, or touching of contaminated surfaces. Indirect contact can occur when handling excreta of a patient who had chemotherapy within the past 48 hours (Polovich et al., 2014).

Precautions include preparing the drug in a biologic safety cabinet or crushing oral hazardous agents in the biologic safety cabinet. Oral hazardous drugs should not be crushed, mixed, or manipulated outside of a biologic safety cabinet (Polovich et al., 2014). Healthcare providers need to don PPE when coming into contact with hazardous agents or their metabolites, as this is the best way to avoid accidental exposure (NIOSH, 2004). PPE includes gloves that have been tested for use with hazardous agents. Healthcare providers should wear two pairs of powder-free gloves, with the inner glove cuff under the gown and the cuff of the outer glove over the gown to protect the skin of the wrist. If the wrist area cannot be covered, extended-length gloves should be used. Gowns should be made of low-permeability, lint-free material and disposable. Gowns should never be reused. A mask with a face shield should be used to protect the eyes and mouth whenever there is a possibility of spillage or splashing (NIOSH, 2004; Polovich et al., 2014). PPE should be worn during drug preparation, administration, and disposal, and when handling excreta while the patient is on chemotherapy precautions (NIOSH, 2004; Polovich et al., 2014). When the nurse is administering IV chemotherapy, needles should be avoided and locking connections used to prevent accidental exposure. Closed-system devices should also be integrated into the current delivery system for IV and intravesicular chemotherapy administration to decrease aerosolization and droplet exposure (NIOSH, 2004; Polovich et al., 2014). Using PPE and following guidelines while handling hazardous agents will minimize risk and occupational exposure, providing a safe work environment.

Conclusion

Chemotherapy continues to be a standard of care for the treatment of most types of cancer. As new agents are developed and research continues, treatment paradigms will take place. The use of chemotherapy in combination with immunotherapy or other molecular-targeted oral agents is emerging as a viable option in many types of cancer (see Chapter 10). Nurses

Key Points

- At the completion of mitosis, newly developed cells can continue through the cell cycle or enter a resting phase.
- Chemotherapy is most active against actively growing tumor cells.
- Cancer cells may be resistant before treatment or become resistant during or after treatment.
- Chemotherapy drugs that can damage cells in any phase of the cell cycle are referred to as cell cycle–nonspecific drugs.
- The goals of combination chemotherapy are to increase cancer cell kill without increasing toxicities and to decrease resistance.
- Chemotherapy drugs that affect cells in one or more phases of the cell cycle are referred to as cell cycle–specific drugs.
- Doubling time is the amount of time it takes for one cancer cell to double (length of the cell cycle).
- Three goals of treatment exist: cure, control, and palliation.
- The highest risk for exposure is during drug manufacturing and preparation, whereas the lowest risk for exposure is during handling of patient excreta when drug metabolites are at their lowest concentration.
- PPE should be worn during drug preparation, administration, and disposal, and when handling excreta while the patient is on chemotherapy precautions.

must understand the unique side effects and interactions of these different types of cancer therapies used in combination in order to teach and care for patients with cancer.

References

Al-Quteimat, O.M., & Al-Badaineh, M.A. (2014). Intraperitoneal chemotherapy: Rational, applications, and limitations. *Journal of Oncology Pharmacy Practice, 20,* 369–380. doi:10.1177/1078155213506244

American Cancer Society. (n.d.). Glossary: Definitions on phonic pronunciations. Retrieved from http://www.cancer.org/cancer/glossary.html

American Society of Health-System Pharmacists. (2006). ASHP guidelines on handling hazardous drugs. *American Journal of Health-System Pharmacy, 63,* 1172–1191. doi:10.2146/ajhp050529

Brown, D.L. (2014). Cellular mechanisms of chemotherapy. In M.M. Gullatte (Ed.), *Clinical guide to antineoplastic therapy: A chemotherapy handbook* (3rd ed., pp. 1–23). Pittsburgh, PA: Oncology Nursing Society.

Cahill, B.A. (2005). Management of patients who have undergone hepatic artery chemoembolization. *Clinical Journal of Oncology Nursing, 9,* 69–75. doi:10.1188/05.CJON.69-75

Chu, E., & De Vita, V.T. (2017). *Physicians' cancer chemotherapy drug manual 2017* (17th ed). Burlington, MA: Jones & Bartlett Learning.

Clive, A.O., Jones, H.E., Bhatnagar, R., Preston, N.J., & Maskell, N. (2016). Interventions for the management of malignant pleural effusions: A network meta-analysis. *Cochrane Database of Systematic Reviews, 2016*(5). doi:10.1002/14651858.CD010529.pub2

Del Principe, M.I., Maurillo, L., Buccisano, F., Sconocchia, G., Cefalo, M., De Santis, G., ... Venditti, A. (2014). Central nervous system involvement in adult acute lymphoblastic leukemia: Diagnostic tools, prophylaxis and therapy. *Mediterranean Journal of Hematology and Infectious Diseases, 6.* doi:10.4084/mjhid.2014.075

Dranitsaris, G., Johnston, M., Poirier, S., Schueller, T., Milliken, D., Green, E., & Zanke, B. (2005). Are health care providers who work with cancer drugs at an increased risk for toxic events? A systematic review and meta-analysis of the literature. *Journal of Oncology Pharmacy Practice, 11,* 69–78. doi:10.1191/1078155205jp155oa

Gaddis, J.S., & Gullatte, M.M. (2014). Pharmacologic principles of chemotherapy. In M.M. Gullatte (Ed.), *Clinical guide to antineoplastic therapy: A chemotherapy handbook* (3rd ed., pp. 25–46). Pittsburgh, PA: Oncology Nursing Society.

Gilbar, P., & Seger, A.C. (2012). Deaths reported from the accidental intrathecal administration of bortezomib. *Journal of Oncology Pharmacy Practice, 18,* 377–378. doi:10.1177/1078155212453752

Goldspiel, B., Hoffman, J.M., Griffith, N.L., Goodin, S., DeChristoforo, R., Montello, C.M., ... Patel, J.T. (2015). ASHP guidelines on preventing medication errors with chemotherapy and biotherapy. *American Journal of Health-System Pharmacy, 72,* e6–e35. doi:10.2146/sp150001

Goodin, S., Kane, M.P., & Rubin, E.H. (2004). Epothilones: Mechanism of action and biologic activity. *Journal of Clinical Oncology, 22,* 2015–2025. doi:10.1200/JCO.2004.12.001

Gottesman, M.M. (2002). Mechanisms of cancer drug resistance. *Annual Review of Medicine, 53,* 615–627. doi:10.1146/annurev.med.53.082901.103929

Hurria, A., Cirrincione, C.T., Muss, H.B., Kornblith, A.B., Barry, W., Artz, A.S., ... Cohen, H.J. (2011). Implementing a geriatric assessment in cooperative group clinical cancer trials: CALGB 360401. *Journal of Clinical Oncology, 29,* 1290–1296. doi:10.1200/JCO.2010.30.6985

Karanicolas, P.J., Metrakos, P., Chan, K., Asmis, T., Chen, E., Kingham, T.P., ... Ko, Y.J. (2014). Hepatic arterial infusion pump chemotherapy in the management of colorectal liver metastases: Expert consensus statement. *Current Oncology, 21,* e129–e136. doi:10.3747/co.21.1577

Karnofsky, D.A., & Burchenal, J.H. (1949). The clinical evaluation of chemotherapeutic agents in cancer. In C. MacLeod (Ed.), *Evaluation of chemotherapeutic agents* (pp. 191–205). New York, NY: Columbia University Press.

Keating, G.M. (2013). Asparaginase *Erwinia chrysanthemi* (Erwinaze®): A guide to its use in acute lymphoblastic leukemia in the USA. *BioDrugs, 27,* 413–418. doi:10.1007/s40259-013-0051-4

Kritharis, A., Bradley, T.P., & Budman, D.R. (2013). The evolving use of arsenic in pharmacotherapy of malignant disease. *Annals of Hematology, 92,* 719–730. doi:10.1007/s00277-013-1707-3

Krukowski, K., Nijboer, C.H., Huo, X., Kavelaars, A., & Heijnen, C.J. (2015). Prevention of chemotherapy-induced peripheral neuropathy by the small-molecule inhibitor pifithrin-μ. *Pain, 156,* 2184–2192. doi:10.1097/j.pain.0000000000000290

National Institute for Occupational Safety and Health. (2004). *NIOSH Alert: Preventing occupational exposures to antineoplastic and other hazardous drugs in health care settings* (DHHS [NIOSH] Publication No. 2004-165). Cincinnati, OH: Author.

National Institute for Occupational Safety and Health. (2014). *NIOSH list of antineoplastic and other hazardous drugs in healthcare settings, 2014* (DHHS [NIOSH] Publication No. 2014-138). Retrieved from http://www.cdc.gov/niosh/docs/2014-138

Oken, M.M., Creech, R.H., Tormey, D.C., Horton, J., Davis, T.E., McFadden, E.T., & Carbone, P.P. (1982). Toxicity and response criteria of the Eastern Cooperative Oncology Group. *American Journal of Clinical Oncology, 5,* 649–655. doi:10.1097/00000421-198212000-00014

Polovich, M. (2011). *Safe handling of hazardous drugs* (2nd ed.). Pittsburgh, PA: Oncology Nursing Society.

Polovich, M., Olsen, M., & LeFebvre, K.B. (Eds.). (2014). *Chemotherapy and biotherapy guidelines and recommendations for practice* (4th ed.). Pittsburgh, PA: Oncology Nursing Society.

Rafiei, R., Yazdani, B., Ranjbar, S.M., Torabi, Z., Asgary, S., Najafi, S., & Keshvari, M. (2014). Long-term results of pleurodesis in malignant pleural effusions: Doxycycline vs bleomycin. *Advanced Biomedical Research, 3,* 149. doi:10.4103/2277-9175.137831

Salzer, W.L., Asselin, B.L., Plourde, P.V., Corn, T., & Hunger, S.P. (2014). Development of asparaginase *Erwinia chrysanthemi* for the treatment of acute lymphoblastic leukemia. *Annals of the New York Academy of Sciences, 1329,* 81–92. doi:10.1111/nyas.12496

Schulmeister, L. (2005). Ten simple strategies to prevent chemotherapy errors. *Clinical Journal of Oncology Nursing, 9,* 201–205. doi:10.1188/05.CJON.201-205

Temple, S.V. (2016). Nursing implications of chemotherapy. In J.K. Itano (Ed.), *Core curriculum for oncology nursing* (5th ed., pp. 237–250). St. Louis, MO: Elsevier.

Tortorice, P.V. (2018). Cytotoxic chemotherapy: Principles of therapy. In C.H. Yarbro, D. Wujcik, & B.H. Gobel (Eds.), *Cancer nursing: Principles and practice* (8th ed., pp. 375–416). Burlington, MA: Jones & Bartlett Learning.

Wilkes, G.M., & Barton-Burke, M. (2016). *2016 oncology nursing drug handbook* (20th ed.). Burlington, MA: Jones & Bartlett Learning.

Chapter 9 Study Questions

1. Which personal protective equipment should be worn during drug preparation, administration, and disposal and when handling excreta while the patient is on chemotherapy precautions?
   A. Gown and gloves
   B. Gloves and mask with face shield
   C. Gown, double gloves, and mask with face shield
   D. Gown and mask with face shield

2. Cell cycle–specific drugs include which of the following?
   A. Antimetabolites
   B. Alkylating agents
   C. Antitumor antibiotics
   D. Miscellaneous agents

3. Which side effect of vincristine requires an immediate call to the doctor?
   A. Myelosuppression
   B. Mucositis
   C. Petechiae
   D. Constipation

4. Possible acute toxicities from chemotherapy exposure include which of the following?
   A. Nausea
   B. Hair loss
   C. Rash
   D. All of the above

5. Oral chemotherapy can be crushed and mixed in food in the patient's room.
   A. True
   B. False

CHAPTER

10 Precision Medicine: Biologics and Targeted Therapies

Julia Eggert, PhD, RN, AGN-BC, GNP, AOCN®, FAAN

Introduction

The idea that individual differences can be considered to guide prevention and treatment of disease is not new, but a unique perspective recently promoted by President Obama is to use these differences to promote "creative approaches to precision medicine, test them rigorously, and ultimately use them to build the evidence base needed to guide clinical practice" (Collins & Varmus, 2015, p. 793). Oncology has been identified as having a "near-term" impact for precision medicine because cancers are common diseases globally and the incidence increases in accordance with the aging population (Collins & Varmus, 2015). In addition, cancer carries concerns about disfigurement due to surgery, symptoms due to radiation and chemotherapy, and the fear of death. It is also known that all cancer is genetic and that an accumulation of genetic damage over a lifetime contributes to cancer risk (Marjanovic, Weinberg, & Chaffer, 2013). As the mechanisms that contribute to the development of cancer become understood, this new knowledge begins to influence the therapeutic strategies with increasing use of drugs and immune therapies designed to counter the influence of specific molecular drivers of cancer (Collins & Varmus, 2015). Some of these drugs are now designated as targeted therapies and others as immune therapies, but both have been designed to confer benefits as precision medicine. Genetics is beginning to profile tumors to identify the best therapy with the best outcome and least amount of side effects (Ewing, 2014).

Biologic therapy is an important treatment in the fight against cancer, yet is different from chemotherapy. Biologic therapy helps the immune system fight cancer or targets certain biologic areas of the cancer growth process interruption or inhibition, whereas chemotherapy attacks the cancer cells directly. The goal of biotherapy is to enhance the body's natural defense and its ability to fight cancer. It is not completely understood how these therapies destroy cancer, but the treatments are thought to stop or slow the growth of cancer cells, make it easier for the immune system to destroy these cells, and prevent cancer from spreading to other parts of the body (American Society of Clinical Oncology, 2016a, 2016b; Polovich, Olsen, & LeFebvre, 2014).

Molecular-targeted therapies are some of the latest advances in modern cancer care, providing patients the opportunity to receive treatment of greater specificity than with traditional methods alone. These new agents hold great promise for oncology professionals and their patients. Many of these present complications and side effects that differ from those typically observed with traditional cytotoxic chemotherapy.

In this chapter, the basic scientific foundation of biologic therapies will be reviewed, with directions on how to anticipate and manage side effects, thereby empowering oncology nurses with the confidence to provide education to patients. This chapter is not, however, all-inclusive of every targeted therapy. It is hoped that, subsequent to the publication of this book, several other targeted therapies will have been approved.

Historical Perspective

Biologic therapy began with the discovery of immunization more than 200 years ago. Edward Jenner discovered the benefits of injecting humans with fluid taken from sores on a milkmaid's hand infected with cowpox, a disease also known as vaccinia. This fluid contained the viral organisms that produce the disease. The inoculation worked because the cells of the human immune system developed antibodies against the cowpox organism (Baxby, 1999; Bickels, Kollender, Merinsky, & Meller, 2002). About a century later, William Coley, a New York surgeon, started using biologic therapy to treat patients with cancer (Coley, 1893). He noticed a connection between infection and the spontaneous regression of tumors in patients he treated. He concluded that the body's response to the infection must have been exerting some effect on the cancer. He injected patients with cancer with live bacteria, then later with filtered toxins. This induced an infectious response that sometimes led to a remission of their cancer. This method of treatment became known as Coley's toxins and over the past 20 years has become recognized as the basis of cancer immunology. Today it is known that molecules, such as the Toll-like receptors (TLRs), activate the two signaling pathways (TLR4 and TLR9) to produce and trigger production of two types of immune cells, natural killer (NK) cells and cytotoxic T lymphocytes, explaining the mechanism of Coley's toxins (Hennessy, Parker, & O'Neill, 2010; Jin & Yeo, 2014).

Paul Ehrlich, a German Nobel Prize winner, is considered the "father of chemotherapy." In the early 1900s, he theorized that the surfaces of cells carried receptor molecules, or "side chains," which could be bound to drugs (Strebhardt & Ullrich, 2008). Over time, his work evolved to suggest that a variety of receptor types with different chemical structures and binding groups exist on the exterior of cells in order to bind to drugs (Strebhardt & Ullrich, 2008).

In the mid-1980s, the use of interferon (IFN) to treat a rare blood disorder called hairy cell leukemia, named for its appearance under a microscope, produced encouraging results. The U.S. Food and Drug Administration (FDA) approved IFN for the treatment of this disease, as well as for chronic myeloid leukemia (CML), AIDS-related Kaposi sarcoma, and genital warts. This was followed by the approval of granulocyte–colony-stimulating factor (G-CSF) and granulocyte macrophage–colony-stimulating factor (GM-CSF) (National Cancer Institute [NCI], 2013; Polovich et al., 2014).

In 1985, genetically engineered interleukin (IL)-2 received FDA approval for treating advanced kidney cancer (NCI, 2013; Polovich et al., 2014). An extensive number of ILs (IL-1–IL-18) are being studied for their clinical potential in the treatment of cancer. The majority of work is being done with IL-2 because of its ability to mediate antitumor responses (Polovich et al., 2014).

By 1998, a number of monoclonal antibodies (mAbs) were approved for various oncology indications. One of these, rituximab, binds to a specific antigen on B cells and is useful in treating lymphoproliferative disorders. Another mAb, trastuzumab, binds to the human epidermal receptor-2 (HER2) receptor and is effective in treating breast cancer (Polovich et al., 2014; Shuptrine, Surana, & Weiner, 2012).

With the turn of the century, epigenetics was being targeted as a new option for cancer treatment. Normal mechanisms are altered for the malignant process, including transcription for cell maturation and differentiation, cell cycle control, DNA repair, angiogenesis, migration, and promotion of host immunosurveillance (Dawson & Kouzarides, 2012; Falkenberg & Johnstone, 2014). Because tightly wound chromatin prevents transcription of DNA, a variety of epigenetic mechanisms are used to unwind the DNA and enhance these normal functions. These epigenetic mechanisms include histone acetylation, DNA methylation, histone modification, nucleosome remodeling, and RNA-mediated targeting (Dawson & Kouzarides, 2012). All are current and potential targets for precision medicine. In 2011, a team of NCI researchers proved that cell transfer therapy of lymphocytes from patients with metastatic melanoma can facilitate durable complete responses regardless of prior treatment (Rosenberg et al., 2011). To understand biologic and epigenetic therapies, it helps to have basic knowledge about the human immune system and the epigenetics associated with cancer progression and treatment.

Epigenetics

Epigenetics refers to changes that occur to DNA activity beyond the actual sequence of the base pairs (Weinhold, 2006). These changes occur "above and over" the DNA so the basic sequence is not affected; the genotype is not changed, although the phenotypic outcome may be altered. These phenotypic changes occur through loosening or alteration of the tightly wound chromatin by binding of different chemicals in such a way that can determine when and where genes might be expressed, or turned on (Dawson & Kouzarides, 2012). Review Chapter 1 for a description of DNA, including chromatin, histones, and epigenetic mechanisms.

Epigenetic "readers" are types of enzymes that look for specific marks on post-translational histones or DNA where it can be modified. Tightly packed histones do not allow changes, so DNA translation is prevented. "Writers" promote attachment of the chemical groups, such as methyl, acetyl, and lysine-methyl groups, to cause loose packing of the histones for DNA expression with protein growth. The chemical groups cause changes that alter the shape of the chromatin in specific places on the genome, making some areas more available to gene expression. "Erasers" are collections of enzymes that remove histone modifiers (Gillette & Hill, 2015). These types of epigenetic modifications are now the targets of cancer therapy for malignancies such as CML, gastrointestinal (GI) stromal tumors (GISTs), and breast cancer (Ahuja, Sharma, & Baylin, 2016; Dawson, Kouzarides, & Huntly, 2012; Falkenberg & Johnstone, 2014). Epigenetic changes can be reversed, but they also may be transmitted to daughter cells.

Histone Deacetylase Inhibitors

Over the past decade, researchers have gained a better understanding of the mechanisms that govern gene transcription and its relationship with cancer. Histone deacetylase (HDAC) plays an important role in gene expression, and aberrant expression or function of HDAC can be found in many types of cancers. HDAC inhibitors are a class of compounds that interfere with the function of HDAC and are emerging as an exciting new class of potential agents for the treatment of solid and hematologic malignancies (Glass &

Viale, 2013). They impede cell proliferation by inhibiting cell cycle checkpoints and induce differentiation or apoptosis of tumor cells in culture studies and animal models (Khan & La Thangue, 2012; Slingerland, Guchelaar, & Gelderblom, 2014; West & Johnstone, 2014).

HDAC inhibitors have the ability to hyperacetylate both histone and nonhistone targets, resulting in a variety of effects on cancer cells, their microenvironment, and immune responses. To date, responses with single-agent HDAC inhibitors have been predominantly observed in advanced hematologic malignancies, including T-cell lymphoma, Hodgkin lymphoma, and myeloid malignancies. Generally, HDAC inhibitors are well tolerated, with the most common acute toxicities being fatigue, GI toxicities (diarrhea, nausea, vomiting, anorexia, weight loss, constipation), and transient cytopenias (Khan & La Thangue, 2012; Rubin, 2015; Slingerland et al., 2014).

The optimal use of HDAC inhibitors will most likely be in combination with other anticancer therapies. Several studies have shown that HDAC inhibitors can synergize with a large set of other chemotherapy drugs, such as cisplatin, etoposide, bortezomib, and gemcitabine (Khan & La Thangue, 2012). Other therapeutics that exhibit an additive or synergistic effect when used with HDAC inhibitors include differentiation agents such as retinoic acid and all-trans-retinoic acid for the treatment of leukemic cells; imatinib for the treatment of Philadelphia chromosome–positive (Ph+) CML; and trastuzumab for the treatment of breast cancer (Dokmanovic, Clarke, & Marks, 2007).

Small RNAs

MicroRNA (miRNA) was originally discovered in 1993. Since then, more small RNAs have been identified to include three main classes: miRNAs, small interfering RNAs (siRNAs), and Piwi-interacting RNAs (piRNAs). Now, there are even newer classes of these small RNAs involved in cell differentiation, proliferation, and death; chromatin organization; and genome integrity (Rovira, Güida, & Cayota, 2010). The three main classes will be discussed here.

MicroRNA

More than 2,000 pieces of miRNA have been identified (Friedländer et al., 2014). Although these are transcribed from DNA, they are not referred to as proteins but as RNA genes. These miRNA are short pieces, approximately 17–25 nucleotides in length, and are believed to regulate more than 30% of protein coding genes affecting cytokines, transcription, growth and other factors, influencing regulation of the cell cycle, cell proliferation, differentiation, and apoptosis. As the miRNA begins translation of the complementary nucleotide sequences, it is bound with a protein complex called Dicer that chops the already short pieces of miRNA into smaller pieces. A duplex of miRNA is formed with the more abundant and mature form identified as the "star" strand (Hayes, Peruzzi, & Lawler, 2014). This strand is bound to a protein and unwound in order to form the RNA-induced silencing complex (RISC) with degradation of the second strand. As RISC attaches to complementary nucleotide sequences targeted for messenger RNA (mRNA), there is interference, causing rapid degradation of the mRNA and repression of protein translation. Ultimately, this decrease in protein production, which is necessary for homeostasis of the cell, can cause tumorigenesis and the development of malignancies (Hayes et al., 2014; Wang et al., 2017).

Acting as *tumor suppressors*, miRNAs cause loss of function by genomic deletion, mutation, epigenetic silencing, or alteration of processes that lead to malignant change in the cell. For example, the miR-15a/16-1 cluster is associated with a 13q14 deletion common to chronic lymphocytic leukemia (CLL). When associated with *BCL2*, the miRNAs are deleted or downregulated to cause increased cell survival, which can promote leukemogenesis and lymphomagenesis in hematopoietic cells (Hayes et al., 2014; Rovira et al., 2010). If the miRNAs are overexpressed or amplified, they can act as *oncogenes* in the cancer-causing pathway (Lin & Gregory, 2015).

Currently, tumor miRNA profiles can be used to identify differences between tumor subtypes, define patient survival, and monitor response to treatment (Hayes et al., 2014). This has implications as future biomarkers to differentiate treatments and monitor miRNA expression levels to anticipate relapse or predict likelihood of metastasis (Hayes et al., 2014; Pencheva & Tavazoie, 2013). Because miRNA biomarkers are detectable in body fluids and are stable within their clinical samples, they have better utility than other potential markers (Hayes et al., 2014). A clinical trial using miRNA profiling for patient prognosis and clinical response is currently underway (Bouchie, 2013).

Small Interfering RNA

Also known as short interfering RNA or silencing RNA, siRNA is a negatively charged, double-stranded RNA about 20–25 base pairs in length. Succinctly, siRNA gets in the way of the protein product of specific genes by degrading mRNA after transcription, resulting in an absence of protein translation (Wang et al., 2017). Because of its negative charge and small size, siRNA is either unable to cross the cell membrane like other small molecules or is removed by the kidney. Endocytosis is the only mechanism available to transport the siRNA pieces into the cell. Because siRNAs have difficulty exiting from the endosome, they continue to be delivered inside the cell within 5–10 minutes and then eventually are degraded (Wang et al., 2017). To be an effective treatment for cancer, siRNAs need to accumulate and silence the gene within the tumor via targeting or transported to the RISC machinery (Wang et al., 2017).

Currently, 17 clinical trials including siRNAs are either completed or actively recruiting for patients. All but one are phase I studies. A variety of cancers are targeted, all for people with advanced disease (ClinicalTrials.gov, 2016c).

Piwi-Interacting RNA

Like the miRNAs and siRNAs, the piRNAs are a group of small, noncoding RNAs approximately 24–32 nucleotides in length. These small RNAs specifically interact with the Piwi protein subfamily to regulate piRNA biogenesis and regulatory function. Although they were originally identified as germ-line associated, evidence now shows they may also have responsibilities in the somatic tissues, including epigenetic regulation, specifically histone modification and DNA methylation (Ku & Lin, 2014). Some laboratory studies have identified an overexpression of piRNAs in a variety of germ-line and somatic tumors, including testicular, ovarian, endometrial, prostate, breast, and GI cancers in humans (Hashim et al., 2014). Specifically in ovarian cancer, the overexpression of *PiwiL2* is linked to chemotherapy resistance to cisplatin through increased chromatin coiling preventing access by DNA repair machinery (Hashim et al., 2014). This example suggests future profiling use in the clinical setting to prevent usage of agents that cause resistance to chemotherapy in certain cancers. Although much literature suggests the promise of piRNA in future cancer care, only 10 clinical trials have incorporated piRNA technology for screening, profiling, or treatment of cancer (ClinicalTrials.gov, 2016b).

Immune System

Two basic types of defense mechanisms protect the body from foreign invaders such as bacteria, viruses, and cancer cells. The first line of defense is a physical barrier involving the skin, mucous membranes, and the lining of the respiratory tract. This line of defense produces a nonspecific response, identified as *nonspecific* or *natural immunity* because it works regardless of the invader (Kannan, Madden, & Andrews, 2015; McCance & Huether, 2014; Polovich et al., 2014).

The second line of defense, unlike the physical barrier, recognizes invaders and develops *specific* weapons to fight them. It is even able to remember what the invader looks like so that its response will be even swifter the next time it is approached. This precise response is made by immune system cells and is known as *adaptive immunity*. The immune system cells circulate throughout the body and defend it against attacks by foreign invaders. This immune network is one of the body's main defenses against disease and works in a variety of ways. For example, the immune system may recognize the difference between healthy cells and cancer cells in the body and work to eliminate those that become cancerous (McCance & Huether, 2014).

Immune system cells include lymphocytes (one type of white blood cells) and other immune cells (see Figure 14-1 in Chapter 14). Lymphocytes can be categorized into T cells, B cells, and NK cells. At least three types of T cells regulate the immune response by signaling other immune system defenders. When an antigen-presenting cell (APC) encounters a foreign antigen (cancer in this situation), the foreign tissue is processed internally, and the identifying peptides (major histocompatibility complex) are revealed on the APC surface. Dendritic cells can function as APCs to foster the response of the T cells (CD4+ and CD8+). The CD4+ cell includes the T helper type 1 (Th1), which interacts with other T cells (cytotoxic and regulators) plus other mononuclear phagocytes (including dendritic cells in the tissue) to assist with cellular identification and destruction. Using cytokines, CD4+ cells orchestrate the entire immune response. CD8+ cytotoxic cells directly attack infected, foreign, or cancerous cells, while the T suppressor cells (Treg) calm the immune response. The type 2 (Th2) helper cells interact with the B cells, which mature into plasma cells and produce immunoglobulins (IgM, IgG, IgA, IgD, IgE) specific to the foreign tissue antigen. These proteins recognize and attach to foreign antigens to cause cell death (McCance & Huether, 2014).

NK cells are believed to be a type of T cell that produce powerful chemical substances that bind to and destroy any foreign invader. They attack without the need to first recognize a specific antigen. Monocytes are another type of white blood cell that circulate in the bloodstream. When activated, the macrophages (mature monocytes) engulf the invaders and digest them. Another type of phagocytic cell in the tissue is the dendritic cell, which supports the roles of the T and B cells by enhancing their destructive functions (McCance & Huether, 2014; Polovich et al., 2014). Functions of all the immune cells are mediated by cytokines that include a variety of ILs, IFNs, and hormones. Specifically, IL-1 and IL-2 aid in communication among the leukocytes to direct the immune response, whereas IL-12 and IFN gamma target the function of NK cells (McCance & Huether, 2014).

Understanding how immune system cells exchange messages and finding ways to make these messages clearer and stronger are the goals of immunologic research. Each of these components, and each step in the immune response, represents a potential targeted avenue for the development of a cancer therapy.

Definition and Classification of Biotherapy

Biotherapies enhance the work of the immune system by using substances that occur naturally or mimic the signals that normally control cell function in the body. The therapy may stimulate the body to make more of the substance, or the therapy may be a man-made version of a natural substance itself. Other types of therapies use cells from the patient's body, which are then altered in a laboratory and given back to the patient. Alternative names for biologic therapies include biologic agents, biologics, biotherapies, biologic response modifiers, or immunotherapy (American Cancer Society, 2014). In summary, biotherapies use the body's immune system, either directly or indirectly, to fight cancer or to reduce the side effects that may be caused by some cancer treatments.

Biologic Response Modifiers

Biologic response modifiers is a general term used to identify a group of factors that include IFNs, ILs, colony-stimulating factors (CSFs), mAbs, vaccines, and gene therapy, plus nonspecific immunomodulating agents. *Active immunity* occurs when a person is exposed to foreign antigen and an immune response is initiated. *Passive immunity* is obtained when a portion of the immune response is provided to a patient without any participation by the individual's immune system (e.g., maternal antibodies passed to an infant in breast milk or injection of gamma globulin [horse serum]). An example of passive immunity is mAbs.

Cytokines

Cytokines are a class of proteins that are secreted by immune cells and have been called the messengers of the immune system. They can either upregulate (increase a response to a stimulus) or downregulate (reduce or suppress a response to a stimulus) other molecules of the immune system in response to physiologic or pathologic events in the body. Cytokines also have a role in regulating cells involved in innate immunity (e.g., NK cells, macrophages, neutrophils) and acquired immunity (McCance & Huether, 2014; Polovich et al., 2014). Hematopoietic growth factors, IFNs, tumor necrosis factor, and CSFs are all classified as cytokines.

Hematopoietic Growth Factors

Hematopoietic growth factors are naturally occurring proteins in the body that regulate the proliferation and differentiation of the hematopoietic stem cells. These specialized cytokines stimulate the growth of groups of cells (colonies) and are also known as *colony-stimulating factors*, or CSFs. They have the ability to enhance the production and function of their target cells and mediate the inflammatory process (Polovich et al., 2014). Through the use of DNA technology, several growth factors are commercially available as therapies for the prevention and treatment of cytopenias due to cytotoxic treatment such as chemotherapy or radiation therapy. Recombinant technology generally employs the insertion or alteration of a gene to produce a specific biologically active protein (Polovich et al., 2014).

Granulocyte–Colony-Stimulating Factor

G-CSF is a single-lineage growth factor that regulates the proliferation and maturation of colony-forming unit (CFU)–granulocyte (CFU-G) progenitor cells. It has been shown to reduce the incidence, magnitude, and duration of neutropenia following a variety of myelosuppressive chemotherapy regimens. G-CSF enhances the mobilization of mature neutrophils from the bone marrow while providing constant stimulation of stem cell progenitors. It also enhances the migration of neutrophils into the tissues.

Recombinant G-CSF is commercially available and is indicated to decrease the incidence of infection, as manifested by febrile neutropenia, in patients with nonmyeloid malignancies receiving myelosuppressive anticancer drugs associated with a significant incidence of severe neutropenia with fever (Amgen Inc., 2015a; Polovich et al., 2014). G-CSF also is indicated for the following:

- Reducing the time to neutrophil recovery and the duration of fever following induction or consolidation chemotherapy treatment of adults with acute myeloid leukemia
- Reducing the duration of neutropenia and neutropenia-related clinical sequelae in patients with nonmyeloid malignancies undergoing myeloablative chemotherapy followed by bone marrow transplantation
- Mobilizing hematopoietic progenitor cells into the peripheral blood for collection by leukapheresis
- Reducing the incidence and duration of sequelae of neutropenia in symptomatic patients who require long-term therapy for congenital neutropenia, cyclic neutropenia, or idiopathic neutropenia

The most frequent side effect of G-CSF is bone pain, which typically is relieved by administration of acetaminophen (Amgen Inc., 2015a; Polovich et al., 2014). The most common sites of bone pain are those with large marrow reserve (i.e., the sternum, back, pelvis, and limbs).

Filgrastim is a covalent conjugate of recombinant methionyl human G-CSF. Both filgrastim and pegfilgrastim have the same mechanism of action. Pegfilgrastim has reduced renal clearance and prolonged persistence in vivo, which allows a single dose per chemotherapy cycle, compared to daily subcutaneous dosing for up to 14 days with filgrastim. These agents have comparable biologic activity with respect to stimulating neutrophil proliferation and function, as well as with safety and efficacy (Amgen Inc., 2015a, 2016c; Polovich et al., 2014). Both G-CSF products are indicated to decrease the incidence of infection, as manifested by febrile neutropenia, in patients with nonmyeloid malignancies receiving myelosuppressive anticancer drugs associated with a clinically significant incidence of febrile neutropenia (Amgen Inc., 2016c; Polovich et al., 2014).

Pegfilgrastim should be administered 24 hours after and no sooner than 14 days before administration of cytotoxic chemotherapy. Bone pain is the most common side effect, generally reported to be mild to moderate in severity and controlled with non-narcotic analgesics. Splenic rupture, acute respiratory distress syndrome, allergic reactions, sickle-cell crisis, injection site reactions, generalized erythema, and flushing have been observed during the post-approval period (Amgen Inc., 2016c; Polovich et al., 2014).

Granulocyte Macrophage–Colony-Stimulating Factor

GM-CSF, like G-CSF, is a multilineage growth factor that stimulates the growth of CFU-G, erythrocyte, macrophage, megakaryocyte cells (also referred to as CFU-GEMM cells), and CFU-G/macrophage progenitor cells. It works by enhancing the mobilization of mature cells from the bone marrow while providing constant stimulation of the stem cell progenitors. GM-CSF stimulates the production of neutrophils, monocytes, macrophages, basophils, and eosinophils, all of which play a role in the body's inflammatory response system. It is commercially available as sargramostim (Leukine®, Sanofi-Aventis U.S., LLC, 2013). Sargramostim is a recombinant human GM-CSF for use in older adults with acute myeloid leukemia following induction chemotherapy in order to shorten the time to neutrophil recovery and reduce the incidence of severe and life-threatening infections. Sargramostim is used in multiple stem cell transplantation settings, including mobilization and following the transplant of autologous peripheral blood progenitor cells; myeloid reconstitution after autologous bone marrow transplantation; myeloid reconstitution after allogeneic bone marrow transplantation; and bone marrow transplant failure or engraftment delay (Sanofi-Aventis U.S., LLC, 2013).

The side effects of sargramostim administration include fever, lethargy, myalgia, bone pain, anorexia, injection site redness, and rash. A syndrome characterized by respiratory distress, hypoxia, flushing, hypotension, syncope, and tachycardia has been reported following the first administration of sargramostim, which usually resolves with symptomatic treatment and typically does not recur with subsequent doses in the same cycle of treatment (Polovich et al., 2014; Sanofi-Aventis U.S., LLC, 2013).

Erythropoietin

Erythropoietin is a single-lineage growth factor. It is the primary regulator of erythropoiesis, the formation and development of erythrocytes in the bone marrow. Its principal activity is the stimulation of terminal maturation of CFUs. Recombinant erythropoietin (epoetin alfa) was the first recombinant hematopoietic growth factor to receive FDA approval. It has shown effectiveness in the treatment of anemia in cancer, myelosuppressive chemotherapy-induced anemia, and anemia of chronic renal failure. Recombinant human erythropoietin is commercially available as epoetin alfa (Epogen®, Amgen Inc., 2016b; Procrit®, Janssen Products, L.P., 2016) and darbepoetin alfa (Aranesp®, Amgen Inc., 2016a). Erythropoiesis-stimulating agents (ESAs) generally are well tolerated in patients with cancer, as they reduce the need for blood transfusions and alleviate fatigue. Current guidelines recommend initiating therapy when the hemoglobin level is less than 11 g/dl or 2 g/dl or greater below baseline, with the goal of avoiding transfusion with gradual improvement in anemia-related symptoms (National Comprehensive Cancer Network® [NCCN®], 2016; Polovich et al., 2014).

Recently, much discussion has taken place regarding the safety of ESAs. As a result of these safety concerns, the labeling of these agents now includes a black box warning (Amgen Inc., 2016a, 2016b; Janssen Products, L.P., 2016; NCCN, 2016). Therapy should be individualized to achieve and maintain hemoglobin levels of 10–12 g/dl. In patients with cancer, ESAs were shown to shorten overall survival or increase the risk of tumor progression or recurrence in some clinical studies in patients with breast, non-small cell lung, head and neck, lymphoid, and cervical cancers (NCCN, 2016; Polovich et al., 2014). To decrease these risks, as well as the risk of serious cardiovascular and thrombovascular events, the lowest dose needed should be administered to avoid red blood cell transfusion. ESAs should only be used for the treatment of anemia caused by concomitant myelosuppressive chemotherapy. ESAs are not indicated for patients receiving myelosuppressive therapy when the anticipated outcome is cure, and therapy should be discontinued following the completion of a chemotherapy course (Amgen Inc., 2016a, 2016b; Janssen Products, L.P., 2016; NCCN, 2016; Polovich et al., 2014).

Thrombopoietin

Oprelvekin (IL-11, Neumega®) is another type of CSF that stimulates the proliferation of hematopoietic stem cells and megakaryocyte progenitor cells and induces megakaryocyte maturation, resulting in increased platelet production (Pfizer Inc., 2015a). It is given after chemotherapy to prevent severe thrombocytopenia and discontinued when platelet nadir is greater than 50,000/mm^3 or two days before the next chemotherapy cycle (Pfizer Inc., 2015a; Polovich et al., 2014).

Agencies and organizations, including the American Society of Clinical Oncology, the American Society of Hematology, and NCCN, have developed guidelines to help clinicians to continue prescribing these important agents in the care of patients with cancer (NCCN, 2016; Polovich et al., 2014).

Proteins

Romiplostim for subcutaneous injection (Nplate®, Amgen Inc., 2016d), the first FDA-approved peptibody protein, works by raising and sustaining platelet counts, representing a novel approach for the long-term treatment of thrombocytopenia in splenectomized and non-splenectomized adults with chronic immune thrombocytopenic purpura. Romiplostim works similarly to thrombopoietin, a natural protein in the body. It stimulates the thrombopoietin receptor, which is necessary for the growth and maturation of the bone marrow cells that produce platelets (Amgen Inc., 2016d). Romiplostim is given to maintain platelet counts at about 50,000/mm^3 to lower the risk for bleeding. It is not used to make platelet counts normal. Romiplostim is not for use in patients with blood cancers or myelodysplastic syndrome (Amgen Inc., 2016d).

Serious adverse reactions have been associated with romiplostim. Long-term use may lead to bone marrow reticulin deposition. Reticulin is a protein that is normally absent or present at low levels in bone marrow. Elevated reticulin levels could potentially be useful in assessing for the presence of immune thrombocytopenic purpura. The mild form of these bone marrow changes (increased reticulin) may progress to a more severe form (fibrosis). Increased reticulin may not cause problems; however, fibrosis may lead to life-threatening blood problems. Signs of bone marrow changes may appear as abnormalities in blood tests. Worsening thrombocytopenia may occur after romiplostim discontinuation. These effects are most likely to happen shortly after stopping romiplostim and may last about two weeks. The lower platelet counts during this time period may increase the risk of bleeding. Administration of romiplostim may lead to an increased risk of venous thromboembolism if the platelet count increases too much. Healthcare providers should assess patients' complete blood count including platelet count and peripheral blood smear prior to initiation, throughout administration, and following the discontinuation of romiplostim therapy (Amgen Inc., 2016d).

Most adverse events were of mild severity and were related to the underlying thrombocytopenia. Headache was the most commonly reported adverse drug reaction. Others included arthralgia, dizziness, insomnia, myalgia, extremity pain, abdominal pain, shoulder pain, dyspepsia, and paresthesia. As with all therapeutic proteins, patients may develop antibodies to romiplostim (Amgen Inc., 2016d; Hassan & Waller, 2015).

Cytokines

Interferons

IFNs are proteins produced by diverse cells throughout the human body in response to pathologic or physiologic events. Isaacs and Lindenmann (1957) were the first researchers to describe the phenomenon of IFN in the laboratory when they noticed that cells infected by a virus secreted a substance. That substance protected other cells in close proximity from being infected by the virus. The substance was given the name *interferon* because of its ability to "interfere" with viral replication. Over the past six decades, many IFN species have been discovered and described (Polovich et al., 2014).

Five different types of IFNs exist, classified by the receptors they target: alpha (α), beta (β), gamma (γ), omega (ω), and tau (τ). IFN-α has the most applications in cancer therapy. IFN-α and IFN-β have similar biologic activities and bind to type I cell surface receptors. Type I IFNs (alpha and beta) have antiproliferative, antiviral, and immunomodulatory effects by modifying or altering the immune system through inhibition or stimulation. Type II IFNs include gamma, omega, and tau. They bind to different receptors than type I IFNs and have stronger immunomodulatory properties, including macrophage activation (Polovich et al., 2014). With the use of recombinant DNA technology, IFNs have been mass produced and incorporated in cancer therapy since 1986 (Polovich et al., 2014).

IFN alfa-2b (Intron® A) is a commercially approved IFN for cancer therapy (Merck & Co., Inc., 2016b). Specific approved uses for IFN alfa-2b in cancer are treatment of hairy cell leukemia, AIDS-related Kaposi sarcoma, and CML. Approved uses of IFN alfa-2b in cancer therapy include high-risk melanoma, follicular lymphoma, hairy cell leukemia, and AIDS-related Kaposi sarcoma. IFNs have a complex mechanism of action. As discussed earlier, some of these processes are immunomodulatory, antiproliferative, and antiangiogenic. IFNs modulate NK cells and macrophages. They also may activate pathways involved with other cytokines, such as IL-1, IL-2, IL-6, IL-8, and tumor necrosis factor (Polovich et al., 2014). In the presence of IFN-α, NK activity increases and becomes more effective in destroying cancer cells. Toxicities seen with IFNs vary and are based on the route of administration, dose, and frequency of treatment (Polovich et al., 2014).

Side effects less likely to occur, yet cause more concern, include depression, confusion, and slowing of mental function (Polovich et al., 2014). Retinal changes and elevated enzymes are less frequent. Healthcare providers should institute appropriate measures to monitor patients for these more chronic yet uncommon toxicities. Because this agent is intimately linked with multiple cells in the immune system, the side effects experienced are related to the activation of many immune cells. For example, macrophages are activated with transcription of IFN-α (Polovich et al., 2014). These cells are key contributors to the acute inflammatory process. Antidepressants and nonsteroidal anti-inflammatory drugs have been used to combat these side effects (Polovich et al., 2014).

Interleukins

IL-2 is an endogenous protein and cytokine that stimulates and interacts with multiple immune system molecules. Activated helper T cells produce IL-2; therefore, an immune response must already be mounted by T cells via the recognition of an antigen or foreign substance for IL-2 to respond. IL-2 stimulates the production of cytotoxic T cells, NK cells, and monocytes (Polovich et al., 2014). In addition, it also has a role in B-cell growth, antibody production, activation of lymphokine-activated killer cells, and the secretion of additional ILs, including IL-4, IL-5, and IL-6 (Polovich et al., 2014). Many other cells in the human immune system interact with IL-2.

Research on IL-2 began in the 1970s, and since FDA approval of a recombinant IL-2 in 1992, it has been used for the treatment of metastatic renal cell carcinoma and metastatic melanoma (Polovich et al., 2014). Unlike the actions of cytotoxic chemotherapy agents, the mechanism of action of IL-2 is not a direct effect of the drug itself. The benefit of IL-2 is achieved by the effect it has on stimulating the multitude of immune responses in the body, thus causing damage to cancer cells. Aldesleukin (Proleukin®) has been given alone (every eight hours for a maximum of 14 doses) and in combination with other agents in an attempt to establish a maximum benefit (Prometheus Laboratories Inc., 2012).

Cardiovascular side effects that can occur with IL-2 therapy are hypotension (mimicking septic shock), tachycardia, arrhythmias, cardiomyopathy, and capillary leak syndrome. IL-1, tumor necrosis factor, and IFN-γ are hypothesized to cause increased permeability of the vascular walls, leading to vascular leak syndrome and fluid imbalances (Dutcher et al., 2014). Interstitial pulmonary edema and acute respiratory distress syndrome are potential toxicities, and nurses should monitor patients for dyspnea and changes in respiratory status (Dutcher et al., 2014). Additionally, monitoring of electrolytes, urine output, heart rate (tachycardia), blood pressure (hypotension), crackles or rales in lungs, cough, and wheezing also is necessary (Dutcher et al., 2014).

Immunomodulatory Agents

Immunomodulatory drugs (IMiDs) are structural and functional analogs of thalidomide that have shown promise for the treatment of a variety of indications in the hematology, oncology, inflammatory, and autoimmune settings. IMiDs have both immunomodulatory and antiangiogenic properties, which could lead to antitumor and antimetastatic effects. They have been demonstrated to possess antiangiogenic activity through inhibition of basic fibroblast growth factor, vascular endothelial growth factor (VEGF), and tumor necrosis factor-alpha–induced endothelial cell migration because, at least in part, of inhibition of the Akt phosphorylation response to basic fibroblast growth factor (Zhu, Kortuem, & Stewart, 2013). IMiDs also have a variety of immunomodulatory effects, including stimulation of T-cell proliferation; production of IL-2, IL-10, and IFN-γ; inhibition of IL-1 beta and IL-6; and modulation of IL-12 production (Zhu et al., 2013).

Thalidomide

Thalidomide (Thalomid®) is an immunomodulatory agent that possesses immunomodulatory, anti-inflammatory, and antiangiogenic properties (Celgene Corp., 2010). It is approved for acute treatment of the cutaneous manifestations of moderate to severe erythema nodosum leprosum and in combination with dexamethasone for newly diagnosed multiple myeloma (Celgene Corp., 2010; Waters, 1971).

Thalidomide has been used experimentally for many years to treat a variety of autoimmune and inflammatory diseases. In the early 1960s, thalidomide was associated with severe birth defects and was largely responsible for legislation in the United States and other countries to regulate the pharmaceutical industry. The history of this lifesaving drug that was once feared for its teratogenic (capable of causing birth defects) effects is closely tied to the evolution of drug testing and marketing and played a central role in the creation of modern regulations (Stephens & Brynner, 2001).

The label for thalidomide contains two black box warnings. The first addresses severe, life-threatening human birth defects if thalidomide is taken during pregnancy. Because of the potential for severe birth defects, FDA approved the marketing of thalidomide under a restricted distribution program, the Thalomid REMS® program (formerly known as the S.T.E.P.S.® program). This program requires prescribers, patients, and distributing pharmacists to be registered and to agree to comply with the program. Separate warnings exist for prescribers, female patients, and male patients, with detailed pregnancy testing, contraceptive use, and education outlined (Celgene Corp., 2010).

The second black box warning concerns thromboembolic events. The use of thalidomide in multiple myeloma, especially in combination with dexamethasone and other chemotherapy agents, has been associated with an increased risk of venous thromboembolic events (Celgene Corp., 2010). Anticoagulation agents (low-molecular-weight heparin, low-dose warfarin, full-dose warfarin with target international normalized ratio of 2:3) or aspirin may be given to prevent the development of blood clots (Polovich et al., 2014). The American Society of Clinical Oncology (Lyman et al., 2013) and the Mayo Clinic (Dispenzieri et al., 2007) have published recommendations for venous thromboembolic event prophylaxis for patients with cancer based on patient risk factors.

Lenalidomide

Lenalidomide (Revlimid®), a thalidomide analog, is an immunomodulatory agent with antiangiogenic and antineoplastic properties (Celgene Corp., 2015). It is indicated for the treatment of patients with transfusion-dependent anemia caused by low- or intermediate-1–risk myelodysplastic syndrome (based on the International Prognostic Scoring System [IPSS]) associated with a deletion 5q cytogenetic abnormality with or without additional cytogenetic abnormalities (Celgene Corp., 2015; List et al., 2006). The IPSS score provides an indication of the risk of developing leukemia. It is based on three risk factors: the number of bone marrow blasts, the presence of one or more cytopenias, and the presence of specific chromosomal abnormalities (cytogenetics). Each factor is assigned a point score, and the sum total is the patient's risk score. Risk scores can range from 0 to 2.5 or greater and are associated with risk categories of low (0), intermediate-1 (0.5–1), intermediate-2 (1.5–2), and high (2.5 or greater). Healthcare providers may use this score to decide when and how aggressively to treat a patient with myelodysplastic syndrome (Greenberg et al., 1997).

Lenalidomide also is approved in combination with dexamethasone for the treatment of patients with multiple myeloma who have received at least one prior therapy (Celgene Corp., 2015; Dimopoulos et al., 2007; Weber et al., 2007).

Black box warnings for lenalidomide include the potential for human birth defects, hematologic toxicity (neutropenia and thrombocytopenia), and deep vein thrombosis and pulmonary embolism. Lenalidomide is an analog of thalidomide and thus is a known teratogen that causes severe life-threatening birth defects. Therefore, women should be advised to avoid pregnancy while taking lenalidomide. To avoid fetal exposure, lenalidomide is only available under a special restricted distribution program, the Revlimid REMS® program (formerly known as RevAssist®). Under this program, only registered prescribers and pharmacists can prescribe and dispense lenalidomide, and only registered patients who meet all conditions of the program will be able to receive the drug (Celgene Corp., 2015).

Patients with deletion 5q myelodysplastic syndrome treated with lenalidomide have experienced significant neutropenia and thrombocytopenia. Most patients require a dose reduction or treatment delay. Patients should have a complete blood count monitored weekly for the first eight weeks of therapy and at least monthly thereafter. Blood product support or growth factors can be used to prevent the development of hematologic toxicities (Celgene Corp., 2015; Polovich et al., 2014).

Patients with multiple myeloma treated with lenalidomide in combination with high-dose dexamethasone experienced a significant increase in deep vein thrombosis and pulmonary embolism that required immediate medical attention (Polovich et al., 2014; Weber et al., 2007). As with thalidomide, guidelines for anticoagulation prophylaxis are available (Elice, Jacoub, Rickles, Falanga, & Rodeghiero, 2008; Lyman et al., 2013; Wiley, 2007).

Monoclonal Antibodies

The use of antibodies began with Ehrlich, dating back to the early 1900s (Strebhardt & Ullrich, 2008). He envisioned studying and designing a drug that could be directed to a specific cell structure. His aim was to find chemical substances that have special affinities for pathogenic organisms and would be "magic bullets." The therapeutic goal was to identify agents that would directly harm the pathologic organism without causing injury to normal cells (Strebhardt & Ullrich, 2008). In 1975, Georges Köhler and César Milstein described the hybridoma technique for the production of mAbs. *Hybridomas* are cells that have been engineered to produce a desired antibody in large amounts. To produce mAbs, B cells are removed from the spleen of an animal that has been challenged with the relevant antigen. These B cells are fused with myeloma tumor cells by making the cell membranes more permeable. The myeloma cells provide the immortalization for indefinite growth in culture. The fused hybrid cells (hybridomas), being cancer cells, multiply rapidly and indefinitely and produce large amounts of the desired antibodies (Dyer, 2001; Senter & Sievers, 2012). The techniques for the production of mAbs represent some of the most important advances in biomedicine, and for this, Köhler and Milstein received the Nobel Prize in Physiology and Medicine in 1984 (Dyer, 2001). Antibodies were developed in an attempt to replicate the endogenous antibodies our bodies produce to destroy viruses, bacteria, cancer cells, and any substance recognized as abnormal. As of 2015, more than 2,500 tumor antigens had been identified via the analysis of tumor antibodies and other methods (Gubin, Artyomov, Mardis, & Schreiber, 2015).

Murine (mouse) antibodies were the first to be developed and studied. These antibodies are completely foreign to the human body. Therefore, complications of murine antibodies include the development of hypersensitivity and anaphylactic reactions. This limited the application of murine antibodies and led to the use of other methods to manufacture antibodies. From this initial scientific research, several additional types of mAbs were developed. *Chimeric antibodies* are approximately 70% human and 30% foreign, such as murine. *Humanized antibodies* are approximately 90% human, and *fully humanized antibodies* are 100% human. The exact percentage depends on the specific manufactured antibody (Genentech, Inc., n.d.). The type of antibody can be determined by looking at the ending of the generic name (see Table 10-1). If the name of the antibody ends in -momab, it is murine; -ximab is chimeric; -zumab is humanized; and -umab indicates a fully human antibody (Polovich et al., 2014; Shuptrine et al., 2012).

When considering a receptor or antigen on a cell surface for a therapeutic mAb target, four principles determine whether the antigen is an ideal target: the antigen is abundant; it has a role in cell survival; it is not shed or cleaved from the cell; and it is only present on the abnormal cells (Scott, Wolchok, & Old, 2012). Vaccines and mAbs are developed against tumor-associated antigens that have one or more of these characteristics.

Antibodies target a specific receptor, ligand, or growth factor (substance attaching to a receptor that causes a cell response). If the receptor is the target and is present on normal cells, it will be affected by the biologic effect of the antibody. The degree of harm depends on the number of cancer cells and normal cells and the amount of receptors present on these cells (Polovich et al., 2014; Scott et al., 2012; Shuptrine et al., 2012). Manufactured antibodies can be either conjugated or unconjugated (also referred to as *naked*). Conjugated antibodies have a toxic substance attached to them. This toxic substance is intended to cause cell damage and can be a chemotherapy agent, radioisotope, or toxin. Naked antibodies have no additional substance attached to them. Unconjugated antibodies attach themselves to specific receptors or antigens on the cancer cells, marking them for destruction by the immune system (Polovich et al., 2014; Shuptrine et al., 2012).

The therapeutic activity of unconjugated mAbs can include antibody-dependent cell-mediated cytotoxicity, complement-dependent cytotoxicity, apoptosis (cell death), direct antiproliferative effects induced by a mAb binding to the tumor cell, and prevention of ligand–receptor binding. These antibodies prevent rapid growth of cancer cells by blocking other molecules from attaching to the cell. Many of the targeted therapy agents, mAbs, and small tyrosine kinase inhibitors are administered until cancer progresses.

Most cancer therapies, including cytotoxic agents and biologics, carry a risk for infusion reactions, which vary in symptom severity from mild flushing to potentially life-threatening events (Polovich et al., 2014). Infusion reactions typically are mild to moderate in intensity, develop during the infusion or several hours thereafter, and are most commonly associated with a complex of chills, fever, nausea, asthenia, headache, skin rash, and pruritus. Infusion reactions are more common in chimeric mAbs. Severe hypersensitivity reactions may occur in patients receiving mAbs and are characterized by acute onset of bronchospasm, hypotension,

Table 10-1. Nomenclature of Monoclonal Antibodies

Suffix/Name	Type of Antibody	Example
-mab	Monoclonal antibody	
-mo-mab	Mouse mab	
-**xi**-mab	Chimeric mab	Cetu-**xi**-mab
-**zu**-mab	Humanized mab	Bevaci-**zu**-mab
-**mu**-mab	Human mab	Panitu-**mu**-mab
-**tu**-xx-mab	Tumor-directed xx mab	Pani-**tu**-mu-mab
-**li**-xx-mab	Immune-directed xx mab	Inf-**li**-xi-mab
-**ci**-xx-mab	Cardiovascular-directed xx mab	Beva-**ci**-zu-mab
-vi-xx-mab	Virus-directed xx mab	

Note. Table courtesy of Dr. Axel Grothey. Adapted with permission.

urticaria, or cardiac arrest. Because such events can be fatal without appropriate interventions, nurses must recognize the symptoms, understand the pathology, and provide supportive care and patient teaching (Breslin, 2007; Polovich et al., 2014).

Monoclonal Antibodies for Hematologic Malignancies

Rituximab

In 1997, FDA approved the chimeric mAb rituximab for the treatment of patients with indolent lymphoma who had failed previous therapy, making rituximab the first therapeutic antibody to receive approval. The clinical utility of rituximab has outreached its initial indication. Its wide-ranging application in lymphoproliferative disorders is based on laboratory studies and clinical trials, resulting in its acceptance by medical oncologists for the treatment of B-cell malignancies. This section of the chapter will focus on the hematologic indications.

Rituximab (Rituxan®) is a chimeric human mAb directed against the CD20 antigen found on the surface of B lymphocytes (Biogen Idec Inc. & Genentech, Inc., 2012). CD20 is a B-cell–specific surface protein. It is expressed in the pre-B stage and later stages of development, but not on lymphoid stem cells. The expression of CD20 continues through B-cell maturation until the plasmacytoid immunoblast phase, while it is only weakly expressed on plasma cells. CD20 is an ideal antibody target for several reasons (Maloney, 2012; Weiner, Surana, & Wang, 2010): it is integral in the initiation of the cell cycle and in differentiation of the cell, it does not internalize into the cell after antibody binding, and it does not shed into the circulation.

CD20 is expressed on most malignant B cells, with nearly 90% of B-cell lymphomas expressing the CD20 antigen. B-cell acute lymphoblastic leukemia (ALL) is CD20 positive in about 50% of cases. Approximately 20% of multiple myelomas express the CD20 antigen, generally in a weak pattern (Maloney, 2012; Weiner et al., 2010). Most cases of Waldenström macroglobulinemia appear to be CD20 positive. B-cell CLL is usually CD20 positive, but CD20 is less densely expressed in small lymphocytic lymphoma and CLL than in many other B-cell malignancies (Maloney, 2012; Weiner et al., 2010).

Rituximab is indicated for the treatment of patients with relapsed or refractory, low-grade or follicular, CD20-positive, B-cell non-Hodgkin lymphoma (NHL) as a single agent; for previously untreated diffuse large B-cell, CD20-positive NHL in combination with CHOP (cyclophosphamide, doxorubicin, vincristine, and prednisone) or other anthracycline-based chemotherapy regimens; for previously untreated follicular, CD20-positive, B-cell NHL in combination with CVP (cyclophosphamide, vincristine, and prednisone) chemotherapy; and for the treatment of non-progressing (including stable disease), low-grade, CD20-positive, B-cell NHL as a single agent after first-line CVP chemotherapy (Biogen Idec Inc. & Genentech, Inc., 2012; Maloney, 2012).

Rituximab is given as a single agent or combined with chemotherapy. The rationale for combining chemotherapy with rituximab stems from the independent clinical activity and mode of action of each modality, the lack of overlapping toxicity profiles, and the in vitro evidence that rituximab may potentially sensitize lymphoma cells to chemotherapy (Maloney, 2012; Polovich et al., 2014).

Rituximab is well tolerated. Common side effects include fever, headache, rigors, nausea, itching, hives, cough, sneezing, arthralgia, upper respiratory tract infection, and cytopenias. Other possible side effects of rituximab administration include hepatitis B virus reactivation, angina, and irregular heartbeat. Rituximab can increase the rate of infections in patients with cancer (Biogen Idec Inc. & Genentech, Inc., 2012; Polovich et al., 2014).

Rituximab can cause serious side effects, including infusion reactions, such as hives, swelling, dizziness, blurred vision, drowsiness, headache, cough, wheezing, or trouble breathing. Tumor lysis syndrome, caused by the fast breakdown of certain types of cancer cells, can cause kidney failure and result in the need for dialysis treatment. Severe cutaneous reactions, such as painful sores on the skin or in the mouth, ulcers, blisters, or peeling skin, have been observed (Biogen Idec Inc. & Genentech, Inc., 2012; Polovich et al., 2014).

Progressive multifocal leukoencephalopathy, a rare brain infection that usually causes death or severe disability, has been observed on rare occasions in patients treated with rituximab plus combination chemotherapy or as part of a hematopoietic stem cell transplantation. The pathophysiology of rituximab-associated progressive multifocal leukoencephalopathy is unclear, particularly with respect to the role of rituximab. The mechanism underlying viral reactivation following rituximab treatment is likely to be more complex than B-cell depletion (Paolo et al., 2014).

Alemtuzumab

Alemtuzumab (Campath®) is a humanized mAb directed against CD52, an antigen expressed by B and T cells, as well as monocytes and granulocytes (Genzyme Corp., 2014). The cell surface of this mAb is relatively specific for lymphocytes and is neither shed nor internalized, making it an attractive target for antibody-directed immunotherapy. The mechanism of action is not completely understood but involves a number of effects, including complement-mediated cell lysis, antibody-dependent cellular toxicity, and induction of apoptosis. Alemtuzumab has shown efficacy in CLL, with an approved indication as a single agent in the treatment of B-cell CLL (Genzyme Corp., 2014).

Alemtuzumab is given intravenously at an escalated dose. Most infusion-related side effects are mild to moderate and generally occur during the first week of treatment. Rigors, fever, nausea, vomiting, and low blood pressure are common during alemtuzumab treatment and may occur during infusion. These effects can be lessened with premedication of diphenhydramine and acetaminophen, as well as gradual dose escalation (Genzyme Corp., 2014; Pazdur, 2013).

Nurses should instruct patients to immediately report symptoms such as bleeding, easy bruising, occurrence of small reddish or purple blood spots on the body (*petechiae* or *purpura*), paleness, weakness, or fatigue. They also should report any symptoms of infection to the doctor immediately. Other reported side effects include rash, shortness of breath, coughing, diarrhea, hives, headache, loss of appetite, itching, sweating, dizziness, and abdominal pain (Genzyme Corp., 2014; Pazdur, 2013).

Allopurinol should be given with the first treatment for prevention of tumor lysis syndrome. Trimethoprim-sulfamethoxazole (or the therapeutic equivalent) for *Pneumocystis jiroveci* pneumonia (formerly named *Pneumocystis carinii* pneumonia) prophylaxis and famciclovir (or the therapeutic equivalent) for herpes virus prophylaxis also should be administered with alemtuzumab (Genzyme Corp., 2014; Pazdur, 2013).

Radiolabeled Anti-CD20 Monoclonal Antibodies

Radiolabeled mAbs have gone through a long developmental process but have emerged as effective therapeutics, most notably in hematologic malignancies, especially lymphoma. Although solid tumor therapy holds some promise, this area has shown much slower progress than lymphomas, in part because these tumors are less radiosensitive. The concept of radioimmunotherapy (RIT) is that tumor-specific radioactively labeled mAbs will specifically target tumors, allowing IV delivery. Consequently, specific targeted delivery of radiation energy to the tumor will occur. The concept is quite similar to that of external beam radiation, which is to maximize tumor radiation dose while keeping the normal tissue dose below toxic levels (Jacene & Wahl, 2014; Maloney, 2012; Polovich et al., 2014).

The most commonly used radionuclides that have been linked to murine mAbs for administration of RIT are iodine-131 (^{131}I), yttrium-90 (^{90}Y), and copper-67. The mAb is primarily used to focus the radiation on the target cell population while sparing the nearby normal tissue. RIT is a conjugated mAb that is connected or joined with a radioisotope. It destroys the antibody present on B cells but also delivers radiation, which causes a cross-fire effect, killing neighboring cells that may not express the CD20 antigen. The use of RIT has demonstrated tumor regression in patients with NHL with very few side effects in normal organs, except for myelosuppression caused by irradiation of the bone marrow (Jacene & Wahl, 2014; Maloney, 2012).

Proper patient selection criteria for RIT are crucial and include bone marrow involvement of less than 25% with a reasonably healthy bone marrow reserve and overall cellularity greater than 15%. In addition, a circulating platelet count greater than 100,000/mm^3 and an absolute neutrophil count greater than 1,500/mm^3 are required to safely administer RIT (GlaxoSmithKline, 2013).

Two radioimmunoconjugates are available commercially: ^{90}Y ibritumomab tiuxetan (Zevalin®) and ^{131}I tositumomab (Bexxar®) (GlaxoSmithKline, 2013; Spectrum Pharmaceuticals, Inc., 2013). Both are FDA-approved for use in relapsed follicular lymphoma and transformed lymphoma. ^{90}Y ibritumomab tiuxetan is also approved for previously untreated follicular lymphoma in patients who achieved a complete or partial response after frontline chemotherapy (Spectrum Pharmaceuticals, Inc., 2013). Both agents are administered on an outpatient basis in which the patient receives two doses approximately one week apart. The unconjugated (or cold) antibody dose is always administered first, followed by the radioactive dose, called the conjugated (or hot) dose, one week later (GlaxoSmithKline, 2013; Spectrum Pharmaceuticals, Inc., 2013).

Ibritumomab tiuxetan is a murine antibody and, when attached to yttrium, is a beta emitter. Rituximab (the cold or unconjugated antibody) is given on day 1 followed by an indium-111 dose of ibritumomab for imaging. Scans are performed 48–72 hours after the ibritumomab infusion to ensure biodistribution. On day 7 or 8, unlabeled rituximab is given again, followed by the therapeutic (conjugated or hot) dose of ibritumomab (Spectrum Pharmaceuticals, Inc., 2013). Tositumomab is attached to ^{131}I, which emits beta and gamma radiation. The treatment plan is similar to that of ibritumomab with a few exceptions. RIT using ^{131}I tositumomab is administered over seven to eight days. On day 1, tositumomab (the cold or unconjugated antibody) is given followed by a radiolabeled dose of tositumomab, which is used for scanning. Scans are performed on days 0, 2–3, and 6–7 to ensure proper dosing. The therapeutic dose of tositumomab is administered within 7–14 days of the dosimetric dose and consists of 450 mg of tositumomab followed by a 20-minute infusion of the patient-specific dose of ^{131}I tositumomab (GlaxoSmithKline, 2013; Goldsmith, 2010; Polovich et al., 2014; Spectrum Pharmaceuticals, Inc., 2013).

Specific patient teaching is important for ibritumomab tiuxetan, including contact precautions regarding body fluids for the first three days after treatment. Good hand washing should be maintained at all times, particularly during the first week after treatment completion. Barrier precautions should be maintained during sexual intercourse for as long as one year after treatment. Because tositumomab is a beta and a gamma emitter, patients receive potassium iodide before and after treatment to protect against the development of thyroid abnormalities (GlaxoSmithKline, 2013; Goldsmith, 2010; Spectrum Pharmaceuticals, Inc., 2013).

Patients treated with RIT should sleep alone in a separate bed for four to seven days after treatment, maintain a distance of at least six feet from children and pregnant women, and limit exposure to others when traveling in a car. Laundry must be washed separately, and patients should avoid having sexual contact for at least four to seven days after tositumomab administration. RIT-induced myelosuppression requires hematologic supportive care for as long as three months after treatment (Goldsmith, 2010).

Monoclonal Antibodies for Solid Tumors

Epidermal Growth Factor Receptor Family

The epidermal growth factor receptors (EGFRs) are some of the most studied receptors. Several biotherapy agents exist that target either the receptors or their internal pathways. A basic review of EGFRs is helpful in understanding the application of the biotherapy agents that target these receptors or pathways.

Members of the human epidermal growth factor receptor (EGFR, HER, ErbB) family include HER1 (EGFR1 and ErbB1), HER2 (ErbB2, neu), HER3 (ErbB3), and HER4 (ErbB4) (Eccles, 2011). Molecules may be identified by more than one name, often resulting in confusion.

In general, HER family receptors have three functional units. The extracellular portion is the part that sticks out of the cell membrane and is on the surface of the cell. The transmembrane surface is the portion that holds the receptor in place within the cell membrane. The intracellular surface is the portion on the receptor that is inside the cell (Eccles, 2011). They become activated after a ligand molecule attaches to one of the receptors. Specific ligands attach to particular receptors. Epidermal growth factor, transforming growth factor-alpha, and neuregulins are ligands that can bind to HER family receptors (Eccles, 2011). One exception is the

HER2 receptor, as it does not have any known ligands. Regarding the other HER family receptors, attachment of the ligand to the receptor causes the receptor to dimerize, or bind with another member of the HER family. Although HER2 does not have any ligands, it can adopt conformational changes, leading the receptor to dimerization (Eccles, 2011). Dimerization causes activation of the receptor, leading to signaling within internal cell pathways, and in some cases, allows for the receptor to be drawn into the cell.

Homodimerization occurs when one type of receptor dimerizes with another identical receptor (e.g., HER1 and HER1). Heterodimerization arises when the receptor dimerizes with a different HER partner, such as HER1 and HER2. Typically, heterodimerization causes more pronounced cellular activity (Eccles, 2011).

In cancer, overexpression and dysregulation of EGFR have been found in many tumor types, including head and neck, lung, breast, pancreatic, prostate, colorectal, ovarian, and glioblastoma (Mitsudomi & Yatabe, 2010). Increased expression of the extracellular receptor, ligands, amplification of the intracellular gene, and mutations of receptors and genes can direct the aberrant cell activity (Kreamer & Riordan, 2015; Mitsudomi & Yatabe, 2010). See Figure 10-1 for patient resources.

Cetuximab

Cetuximab (Erbitux®) is a chimeric antibody that targets EGFR1 (ImClone LLC, 2016; Polovich et al., 2014). It is approved for use in treating locally advanced oral squamous cell carcinoma of the head and neck in combination with radiation therapy or in patients who have progressed after a platinum therapy; as a single agent in patients with EGFR-expressing metastatic colorectal cancer after failure of both irinotecan and oxaliplatin-based therapies or in those intolerant to irinotecan-based treatments; and in patients with metastatic colorectal cancer who are refractory to irinotecan-based therapy in combination with irinotecan.

Of interest, patients in the middle-southern part of the United States have an increased incidence of severe reactions to cetuximab (Berg, Platts-Mills, & Commins, 2014). Recent studies revealed that a new IgE antibody response to α-gal, a carbohydrate found in meats, is associated with an immediate-onset anaphylaxis during first exposure to IV cetuximab. The study results suggest that a bite from a certain variety of ticks causes IgE antibody responses to α-gal in the United States (Berg et al., 2014).

Patients receiving cetuximab can experience serious infusion reactions such as bronchospasm, angioedema, hypotension, and urticaria (ImClone LLC, 2016; Polovich et al., 2014). Ninety percent of the severe reactions occurred with the first infusion (ImClone LLC, 2016). Hypomagnesemia can occur in patients with low baseline serum magnesium, seven or more cetuximab administrations, and concurrent administration of platinum, such as cisplatin or carboplatin (Enokida, Suzuki, Wakasugi, Yamazaki, & Tahara, 2014; ImClone LLC, 2016; Polovich et al., 2014). Monitoring for electro-

Figure 10-1. Patient Resources for Epidermal Growth Factor Receptor Inhibitor Toxicities

- CancerConnect.com: Relief for Side Effects to Skin For Patients Taking EGFR Inhibitors: http://news.cancerconnect.com/relief-side-effects-skin-patients-egfr-inhibitors
- Cancer.Net: Navigating Cancer Care: Side Effects: www.cancer.net/navigating-cancer-care/side-effects
- National Cancer Institute: About Cancer: www.cancer.gov/about-cancer
- National Cancer Institute: Biological Therapies for Cancer: www.cancer.gov/about-cancer/treatment/types/immunotherapy/bio-therapies-fact-sheet

lyte imbalances, including hypomagnesemia, hypocalcemia, and hypokalemia, is encouraged. Patients with a history of myocardial infarction, congestive heart failure, or arrhythmia should be evaluated for the risk versus benefit of therapy, as hypomagnesemia is associated with increased cardiac events (Polovich et al., 2014).

Panitumumab

Panitumumab (Vectibix®) is a humanized antibody that also binds to EGFR (Amgen Inc., 2015b). This molecule, an IgG2 antibody, is structurally different from cetuximab, an IgG1 antibody. It is indicated as a single agent in the treatment of progressive metastatic colorectal cancer or after failure of fluoropyrimidine, oxaliplatin, and irinotecan regimens. The mechanism of action for panitumumab works by preventing the activation of the EGFR and intracellular signaling pathways. If a *KRAS* mutation exists, the signaling will occur and the benefit of panitumumab is minimized (U.S. FDA Center for Drug Evaluation and Research, 2016). In one retrospective review, the results of three treatment regimens suggested that patients with mutant *KRAS* codon 12 or 13 in metastatic colorectal cancer are unlikely to benefit from panitumumab treatment. Panitumumab therapy should target patients with the wild-type (normal) *KRAS* gene in metastatic colorectal cancer (Peeters et al., 2013; U.S. FDA Center for Drug Evaluation and Research, 2016).

Hypomagnesemia requiring oral or IV replacement can occur in up to 2% of treated patients (Amgen Inc., 2015b; Polovich et al., 2014). Monitoring of magnesium levels is required with panitumumab. Potential severe reactions include infusion reactions and severe skin toxicities with fissures and abscesses (Polovich et al., 2014).

Trastuzumab

Trastuzumab (Herceptin®) is a humanized mAb that targets HER2 (Genentech, Inc., 2016). It is estimated that HER2 is overexpressed in 20%–25% of all breast cancers (Untch et al., 2010). Overexpression is associated with a poorer prognosis, more aggressive disease, and less response to traditional chemotherapies (Untch et al., 2010). Trastuzumab was approved in the United States in 2006 for the adjuvant treatment of high-risk, early-stage, HER2-positive breast cancer as a single agent after multimodality anthracycline-based therapy, or as part of a treatment regimen consisting of doxorubicin, cyclophosphamide, and either paclitaxel or docetaxel or in combination with docetaxel and carboplatin. In the metastatic setting, the indication is as a single agent for the treatment of patients with HER2-overexpressing breast cancer after receiving one or more chemotherapy regimens for metastatic disease, or as first-line treatment with paclitaxel (Genentech, Inc., 2016).

The most commonly reported side effects include fever, nausea, vomiting, infusion reactions, diarrhea, infections, increased cough, headache, fatigue, dyspnea, rash, neutropenia, anemia, and myalgia. Serious toxicities can occur with trastuzumab therapy, including subclinical and clinical heart failure manifested by cardiac heart failure or decreased left ventricular ejection fraction (LVEF) (Bourdeanu & Luu, 2013; Genentech, Inc., 2016; Polovich et al., 2014). Risk for increased cardiac dysfunction occurs when trastuzumab is given concurrently with anthracyclines. LVEF should be evaluated before the initiation of treatment, every three months during therapy, and every six months after completion of therapy. The frequency of monitoring should be increased if the patient's LVEF status changes. A four- to sixfold increase in symptomatic myocardial dysfunction occurs in patients on trastuzumab (Ewer & Ewer, 2010). Trastuzumab also has been shown to induce cardiotoxicity in patients with HER2-positive metastatic esogastric cancers with a higher asymptomatic risk than in those with breast cancer (Martin-Babau et al., 2016).

Specific recommendations about temporarily or permanently holding treatment based on LVEF measurements are found in the package insert. Serious infusion reactions, such as pulmonary toxicities, have been documented. In the majority of cases, these occur within the first 24 hours of administration. Interruption of therapy is required for patients who experience dyspnea or significant hypotension. Discontinuation is appropriate in the occurrence of anaphylaxis, angioedema, interstitial pneumonitis, or acute respiratory distress syndrome (Genentech, Inc., 2016; Polovich et al., 2014).

Bevacizumab

Bevacizumab (Avastin®) is a humanized mAb that differs from the early antibodies that were approved in that it targets a growth factor (or ligand), VEGF, rather than a receptor (or antigen) on the outside surface of a cell (Genentech, Inc., 2015). VEGF is essential in stimulating the production of new blood vessels for the tumor from the established vascular system. Many cancers produce VEGF. Bevacizumab binds to VEGF, thus stopping it from attaching to endothelial cells, and is hypothesized to prevent the formation of new blood vessels and regress existing abnormal vascularity (Hanahan & Weinberg, 2011). Increased permeability of the blood vessels occurs as a result of the activated VEGF signaling the and the immature vascular system. This increased permeability allows fluid, plasma proteins, and other molecules to escape from the blood vessel, thereby creating an abnormal increase in pressure (Hanahan & Weinberg, 2011).

Bevacizumab was the first drug approved that is considered an antiangiogenic agent. It has been approved for the treatment of the following (Genentech, Inc., 2015):

- First- and second-line metastatic colorectal cancer with IV 5-fluorouracil-based therapy
- First-line metastatic, locally advanced, or recurrent lung cancer (non-small cell nonsquamous type) with carboplatin and paclitaxel
- First-line metastatic HER2-negative breast cancer with paclitaxel in patients who have not previously had chemotherapy for metastatic disease
- Metastatic renal cell carcinoma in combination with IFN-α
- Glioblastoma in patients who have progressed after prior therapy

The incidence and severity of toxicities seen with bevacizumab vary based on the chemotherapy regimen and the cancer that is being treated. Women considering treatment with an antiangiogenic agent should be instructed to avoid pregnancy because of the potential harm to fetal development (Azim, Azim, & Peccatori, 2010). Arterial thromboembolic events, including cerebral infarction, transient ischemic attacks, myocardial infarction, and angina, are among the more serious potential side effects. In a pooled analysis, the incidence of arterial thromboembolic events was 4.4% for bevacizumab plus chemotherapy versus 1.9% for chemotherapy alone. The risk (8.5%) is greater for those older than age 65 (Genentech, Inc., 2015). GI perforation also has occurred and is more common in trials with colorectal cancer. In one breast cancer study (Miller et al., 2007), the incidence of GI perforation was 0.5% versus 0%–3.7% across all studies. Severe and fatal hemorrhage has been observed with bevacizumab. This may include hemoptysis, GI bleeding, hematemesis, epistaxis, central nervous system hemorrhage, and vaginal bleeding. The range for hemorrhage of grade 3 or greater listed in the package insert for all indications is 1.2%–4.6% (Genentech, Inc., 2015). Reversible posterior leukoencephalopathy syndrome has been reported (less than 0.1% in clinical studies), and symptoms can include visual and neurologic changes, headache, seizure, lethargy, blindness, confusion, and mild to severe hypertension (Genentech, Inc., 2015). It is diagnosed by magnetic resonance imaging, and its development necessitates discontinuation of bevacizumab. Since the approval of bevacizumab for the treatment of metastatic colorectal cancer in

October 2003, other agents, such as sorafenib and sunitinib, that target multiple pathways, including antiangiogenic pathways, have been developed and approved (Bayer HealthCare Pharmaceuticals Inc., 2014; Pfizer Inc., 2015c).

Recent study results indicate bevacizumab also may be able to profile certain side effects. These include hypertension, vascular imaging, and polymorphisms affecting components of the VEGF pathway in patients receiving bevacizumab (Jubb & Harris, 2010).

Vaccines

The concept of using vaccines to target cancer has been of medical interest for decades. Therapeutic cancer vaccines attempt to destroy the malignancy via the restoration and upregulation of the immune system. Developing vaccines against pathogens is more likely than developing a therapeutic cancer vaccine because antigens on pathogens are found only on a particular pathogen and not on normal cells. Antigens on normal cells that remain a component of the tumor cell may not be recognized as foreign by the immune system, thus providing some cancer cells with protection because the immune system has previously identified these antigens as normal (Gajewski, Schreiber, & Fu, 2013).

Developing a vaccine that is lethal to tumors, spares normal cells, and does not elicit an autoimmune response is a complex issue. The goal of cancer vaccines is to stimulate the patient's immune system to fight or destroy the tumor (Hammerstrom, Cauley, Atkinson, & Sharma, 2011; Liu, 2011). This can be achieved by (a) protecting the body against the pathogens that can cause cancer, (b) enhancing or stimulating the body's immune system, and (c) heightening immunosurveillance by the body's immune system.

Currently, two therapeutic cancer vaccines are approved in the United States. In 2010, sipuleucel-T (Provenge®) was the first to be approved for use in some men with metastatic prostate cancer. In October 2015, talimogene laherparepvec (T-VEC, or Imlygic®), an oncolytic virus therapy, was approved by FDA for the treatment of some patients with metastatic melanoma that cannot be surgically removed. This vaccine is injected directly into melanoma tumors to both infect and lyse cancer cells. Of note, T-VEC also causes responses in noninjected lesions, suggesting, much like other anticancer vaccines, it triggers an antitumor immune response (NCI, 2015).

Three human papillomavirus vaccines have received FDA approval: Gardasil® (strains 6, 11, 16, and 18), Gardasil 9® (strains 6, 11, 16, 18, 31, 33, 45, 52, and 58), and Cervarix® (strains 16 and 18) (GlaxoSmithKline, 2011; Merck & Co., Inc., 2011, 2016a). These human papillomavirus strains are associated with future development of cervical, anal, penile, and head and neck cancer. Hepatitis B vaccines are available for infants, young children, and adults (Centers for Disease Control and Prevention, 2016). Hepatitis B is associated with liver cancer.

Cancer vaccine studies can be found for virtually every tumor type: dendritic vaccines for non-small lung cancer, lymphoma, and prostate cancer; multipeptide vaccines for melanoma and metastatic breast cancer; and allogeneic vaccines for prostate cancer. At least 15 new vaccines are in phase III clinical trials (see NCI, 2015, for additional information about these agents).

Intracellular Targeted Therapies

As the biology of cancer becomes better understood, other therapies in addition to biotherapies are being developed to target the various elements of the molecular biology of the cancer. Targets include cell signaling pathways to the nucleus, cascades of events within the cell, and mutations in specific proteins causing altered cell function with overexpression of membrane-bound tyrosine kinase receptors or overactivation of the cell signal in the absence of growth factors. These targeted treatments are part of precision medicine and work to control the specific causes of cancer cell growth, division, and spread.

Some therapies are both immunotherapies and small molecule targeted therapies. For instance, the growth signal inhibitors include trastuzumab (mAb) for breast cancer and imatinib (small molecule) for chronic myeloid leukemia (American Cancer Society, 2014). In patients with cancer, certain growth factors, such as VEGF, promote growth of the malignant tumor. One type of growth factor inhibitor, bevacizumab, blocks the ability to promote this blood vessel growth (angiogenesis) and causes tumor lysis. This targeted therapy is used to treat colorectal, kidney, and lung cancers (American Cancer Society, 2014).

Another group of targeted therapies is the apoptosis-inducing drugs. When normal cells have accumulated too much damage in their DNA, they induce programmed cell death, or apoptosis. Cancer cells have been reprogrammed to avoid this normal pathway for cell death and become immortalized, thus allowing them to continue to replicate and divide, accumulating further DNA damage.

Small Molecules—Tyrosine Kinase Inhibitors

The receptor tyrosine kinases are primary regulators of cellular processes that are critical to homeostasis and the prevention of cancer. Proliferation and differentiation, cell survival and metabolism, cell migration, and cell cycle control processes are all included and easily identifiable as the mechanisms of escape for malignant transformation (Lemmon & Schlessinger, 2010). The receptor tyrosine kinase family comprises 20 subtypes. All receptor tyrosine kinases bind on the extracellular surface and have at least one transmembrane molecule and a cytoplasmic tyrosine kinase that comes together (dimerization) to activate the intracellular signaling pathway. Once activated, the signaling pathway carries the cellular information and instruction for specific cellular activity to occur (Lemmon & Schlessinger, 2010).

Protein kinase inhibitors are small molecules that work by blocking the binding site on the intracellular portion of a receptor. Adenosine triphosphate (ATP) attaches to a binding site on the intracellular portion of the cell, continuing the cellular instruction to various pathways into the nucleus of the cell. In the treatment of cancer, small tyrosine kinase inhibitors are agents designed to enter the cell membrane and bind at the ATP binding site. This binding prevents cellular instructions to specific pathways such as proliferation, apoptosis, metabolism, differentiation, or cell survival. As mentioned earlier, overexpression of ligands, receptors, genes, and mutations can cause aberrant cell signaling. Ultimately, this can result in uncontrolled proliferation, the prevention of apoptosis, inhibition of tumor suppressor genes, increased cell motility, and irregular metabolism (Lemmon & Schlessinger, 2010). Several intracellular signaling pathways exist. Specific pathways are dysfunctional in certain cancers; some of the receptors have redundant pathways or more than one pathway. Many of these pathways interact with each other. Some of the small tyrosine kinase agents block one pathway, whereas other agents interrupt more than one pathway. Because of the multiple pathways and complexities, it is not possible to explain all the pathways in detail. A sampling of these agents is reviewed in this chapter. A common aspect of these agents is that they are administered orally. This presents some unique toxicities and nursing considerations. Many of these agents are metabolized by cytochrome P450 (CYP) isoenzymes, primarily CYP3A4 in the liver. Specific criteria exist for medications to avoid overdosage or underdosage of small molecule biotherapy agents (Polovich et al., 2014). One unique complication of tyrosine kinase inhibitors recently identified is posterior reversible encephalopathy syndrome, which is manageable if identified early (Przybylyski & Esper, 2016). A thorough review of prescription medications, over-the-counter products, and herbal agents is necessary to prevent any potential drug–drug interactions. Teaching patients about the unique side effects and providing detailed instructions for taking these oral agents are essential. Many of the products have teaching tools and programs, and resources are available from the Oncology Nursing Society and other organizations (Polovich et al., 2014) (see Figures 10-2 and 10-3).

Figure 10-3. Teaching Considerations for Oral Agents

- Complexity of medication regimen
- Oral medication calendar
- Electronic medication reminders
- Alarm reminders, vibrating watches, audio and visual alarms
- What to do when a dose is missed
- Pill boxes (glowing, vibrating, and alarming pill boxes are now available)
- Drug–drug interactions
- Updated list of patient-assistance websites
- List of common side effects with related symptom management sheet
- Handling of oral medications in the home
- Patient diary
- Pill count during patient's office visits
- Tear sheets with information on when and how to take medications
- Oncology Nursing Society's Oral Adherence Toolkit: www.ons.org/practice-resources/toolkits/oral-adherence
- Some websites to consider:
  - American Cancer Society, *Oral Chemotherapy: What You Need to Know*: www.cancer.org/treatment/treatmentsandsideeffects/treatmenttypes/chemotherapy/oral-chemotherapy.html
  - Multinational Association for Supportive Care in Cancer Oral Agent Teaching Tool (MOATT): www.mascc.org/mc/page.do?sitePageId=89760

Note. Based on information from Burhenn & Smudde, 2015; Schneider et al., 2011; Spoelstra & Sansoucie, 2015.

Tyrosine Kinase Inhibitors for Hematologic Malignancies

Imatinib Mesylate

Imatinib mesylate (Gleevec®) has changed the treatment of CML with improvement in survival in all three phases—chronic, accelerated, and blast (Novartis Pharmaceuticals Corp., 2015). Unlike traditional chemotherapy, which is usually nonspecifically cytotoxic, imatinib specifically targets the underlying molecular cause of certain types of cancer (Cilloni & Saglio, 2012). Imatinib is a potent and selective inhibitor of tyrosine kinase–signaling enzymes, including a fusion protein of *abl* with breakpoint cluster region (Bcr-Abl), stem cell or steel factor receptor (c-Kit), and platelet-derived growth factor (PDGF) receptors (Cilloni & Saglio, 2012). Imatinib inhibits the activity of protein tyrosine kinase by binding to the kinase domain, thereby inhibiting signaling activity within malignant cells and promoting cell death. The translocation of genetic material between chromosomes 9 and 22 results in the formation of the Philadelphia chromosome, characterized by the creation of the *BCR-*

Figure 10-2. Implications for Practice for Oral Cancer Agent Adherence

- Promote adherence to oral agents for cancer by enacting patient feedback and monitoring, as well as multicomponent interventions.
- Use automated voice recordings and text messages and treat depression to promote adherence to oral agents.
- Implement evidence-based interventions in the clinical practice within the context of the institution to promote adherence to oral agents.

Note. From "Putting Evidence Into Practice: Evidence-Based Interventions for Oral Agents for Cancer," by S.L. Spoelstra and H. Sansoucie, 2015, *Clinical Journal of Oncology Nursing, 19*(Suppl. 3), p. 66. Copyright 2015 by Oncology Nursing Society. Reprinted with permission.

ABL gene. This gene is transcribed into a protein with tyrosine kinase activity and causes abnormal cellular reproduction. Imatinib mesylate interferes with cellular proliferation and induces apoptosis of *BCR-ABL* cells (Cilloni & Saglio, 2012).

Identification of the molecular cause of CML, the activation of an intracellular protein tyrosine kinase, (Bcr-Abl), provided the conceptual underpinnings for this therapeutic approach (Cilloni & Saglio, 2012). Inhibition of Bcr-Abl tyrosine kinase activity by imatinib in the treatment of CML has been shown to be effective and well tolerated and to lead to an improved quality of life. Imatinib currently is approved for several oncology indications, including all phases of Ph+ CML in adults, Ph+ CML in chronic phase in children, Ph+ ALL, myelodysplastic syndrome associated with *PDGFR* gene rearrangements, myeloproliferative neoplasms, and Kit+ GISTs (Cilloni & Saglio, 2012; Novartis Pharmaceuticals Corp., 2015).

As with most treatments for cancer, the benefits of imatinib come with occasional adverse effects that must be managed in order to improve patients' quality of life and promote adherence to therapy. Adverse effects in patients receiving imatinib typically are mild to moderate in severity, are dose related, and often diminish over time with continued use (Cilloni & Saglio, 2012; Novartis Pharmaceuticals Corp., 2015).

Side effects usually are manageable without dosage reduction or permanent discontinuation. Minimal side effects have been reported with imatinib use and include edema, nausea, vomiting, myelosuppression, rash, muscle cramping, and bone pain. Serious side effects such as severe edema, pleural effusion, ascites, pulmonary edema, and rapid weight gain, have been reported and can be managed by holding imatinib, giving diuretics, and providing supportive measures (Barnes & Reinke, 2011; Novartis Pharmaceuticals Corp., 2015; Polovich et al., 2014).

Symptom management includes antiemetics for nausea, diuretics for edema in lower extremities and the periorbital area, and hemorrhoid preparation wipes or ice packs for periorbital edema (Polovich et al., 2014). Most patients experience intermittent diarrhea that is well controlled with antidiarrheal agents. Bone pain, as well as hand and foot cramps, can be relieved by drinking tonic water and using nonsteroidal anti-inflammatory drugs (Polovich et al., 2014). Skin rashes are well managed with topical and systemic steroids (Polovich et al., 2014). If myelosuppression or liver dysfunction occurs, imatinib should be discontinued until symptoms resolve; the drug can then be resumed at a decreased dosage (Novartis Pharmaceuticals Corp., 2015).

Patients should take imatinib with food and a large glass of water and should remain upright for 30 minutes to prevent reflux and vomiting. Patients should avoid grapefruit products and alcohol because of possible liver toxicity and CYP interaction (Novartis Pharmaceuticals Corp., 2015). Some commonly used drugs may interact with imatinib, including acetaminophen and acetaminophen-containing products, warfarin, erythromycin, and phenytoin (Novartis Pharmaceuticals Corp., 2015).

Dasatinib

Dasatinib (Sprycel®) is indicated for the treatment of adults with chronic, accelerated, myeloid, or lymphoid blast phase CML with resistance or intolerance to prior therapy including imatinib (Bristol-Myers Squibb Co., 2015). The effectiveness of dasatinib is based on hematologic and cytogenetic response rates. Dasatinib also is indicated for the treatment of adults with Ph+ ALL with resistance or intolerance to prior therapy (Bristol-Myers Squibb Co., 2015). Primary care providers need to follow patients receiving first- or second-generation tyrosine kinase inhibitors because unforeseen toxicities may surface, requiring accurate assessment, evaluation, and management (Cilloni & Saglio, 2012).

Myelosuppression is common in all patient populations taking dasatinib. The frequency of grade 3 or 4 neutropenia, thrombocytopenia, and anemia is higher in patients with advanced phase CML or Ph+ ALL. In patients who experience severe myelosuppression, recovery generally occurs following dose interruption or reduction (Bristol-Myers Squibb Co., 2015; Cilloni & Saglio, 2012; Polovich et al., 2014).

Elevations of transaminase or bilirubin, hypocalcemia, and hypophosphatemia have been reported in patients with all phases of CML but occurred with greater frequency in patients with myeloid or lymphoid blast phase CML and Ph+ ALL. Elevations in transaminase or bilirubin usually were managed with dose reduction or interruption. Patients developing grade 3 or 4 hypocalcemia often had recovery with oral calcium supplementation (Bristol-Myers Squibb Co., 2015; Cilloni & Saglio, 2012; Polovich et al., 2014). Certain drugs may increase dasatinib plasma concentrations, including CYP3A4 inhibitors. In patients receiving treatment with dasatinib, close monitoring for toxicity and dose reduction should be considered if systemic administration of a potent CYP3A4 inhibitor cannot be avoided (Bristol-Myers Squibb Co., 2015; Polovich et al., 2014). Drugs that may decrease dasatinib plasma concentrations include CYP3A4 inducers, such as antacids. Simultaneous administration of dasatinib with antacids should be avoided. If antacid therapy is needed, the antacid dose should be administered at least two hours before or two hours after administration of the dose of dasatinib. The administration of H_2 antagonists or proton pump inhibitors (e.g., famotidine and omeprazole) is likely to reduce dasatinib exposure; therefore, concomitant use of H_2 antagonists or proton pump inhibitors with dasatinib is not recommended. The use of antacids should be considered in place of H_2 antagonists or proton pump inhibitors in patients receiving dasatinib therapy (Bristol-Myers Squibb Co., 2015; Polovich et al., 2014).

Drugs that may have their plasma concentration altered by dasatinib include CYP3A4 substrates such as alfentanil, cisapride, cyclosporine, fentanyl, pimozide, quinidine, sirolimus, tacrolimus, or ergot alkaloids (ergotamine, dihydroergotamine) and should be administered with caution in patients receiving dasatinib (Bristol-Myers Squibb Co., 2015; Polovich et al., 2014).

Tyrosine Kinase Inhibitors for Solid Tumors

Erlotinib

Erlotinib (Tarceva®) is a tyrosine kinase inhibitor blocking the kinase binding site for the intracellular domain of the HER1 receptor (OSI Pharmaceuticals, Inc., Astellas Oncology, & Genentech, Inc., 2016). This agent is approved in the treatment of advanced or metastatic non-small cell lung cancer after the failure of at least one prior chemotherapy agent. It also is approved for the treatment of locally advanced, unresectable, or metastatic pancreatic cancer in combination with gemcitabine.

The most common side effects of this agent in the non-small cell lung cancer studies (greater than 50%) were rash, diarrhea, anorexia, and fatigue. In the pancreatic cancer studies, fatigue, rash, nausea, and anorexia were the most common (greater than 50%). Pulmonary interstitial lung disease (ILD) has been reported with this agent, with an overall incidence of 1.1% (OSI Pharmaceuticals, Inc., et al., 2016). Any new or progressive pulmonary symptoms, such as dyspnea, cough, or fever, warrant a diagnostic evaluation for ILD.

Patients with impaired liver function or dehydration prior to starting therapy may be at risk for developing hepatorenal syndromes and should be monitored for dehydration, renal, and liver status changes (e.g., electrolytes, liver enzymes). GI perforation was reported in patients who were also taking antiangiogenic agents, corticosteroids, and nonsteroidal anti-inflammatory agents (OSI Pharmaceuticals, Inc., et al., 2016). Rash is one of the most common toxicities, occurring on the face, upper chest, and back. A 60%–75% incidence is reported, with severe rash accounting for approximately 5%–9% (OSI Pharmaceuticals, Inc., et al., 2016). Myocardial infarction and cerebrovascular accident were reported to occur in 2.3% of patients in the pancreatic cancer trials when erlotinib was combined with gemcitabine. A small incidence (0.8%) of microangiopathic hemolytic anemia with thrombocytopenia also was reported (Eli Lilly & Co., 2014; OSI Pharmaceuticals, Inc., et al., 2016). Other warnings and precautions listed in the package insert include corneal perforation, ulcerations, abnormal eyelash growth, keratitis, and bullous and exfoliative skin disorders. Nurses should monitor for an increase in bleeding events in patients taking concomitant warfarin.

This drug is metabolized by CYP3A4 and to a lesser extent CYP1A2 (OSI Pharmaceuticals, Inc., et al., 2016). Taking other drugs that induce CYP3A4 or CYP1A2 can result in the patient being underdosed, reducing the plasma concentration. Conversely, concurrent use of erlotinib with CYP3A4 inhibitors can cause an increased concentration of the drug (OSI Pharmaceuticals, Inc., et al., 2016). Additionally, patients should be advised to stop smoking; erlotinib levels are reduced with cigarette smoking (OSI Pharmaceuticals, Inc., et al., 2016).

Dual Inhibitors of Kinase Binding Sites

Lapatinib ditosylate (Tykerb®) is a small molecule that inhibits the HER1 (ErbB1) and HER2/neu (ErbB2) receptors by blocking the intracellular kinase binding sites (GlaxoSmithKline, 2015). This drug is approved in combination with capecitabine for use in patients with advanced or metastatic HER2-positive breast cancer who have received a prior anthracycline, taxane, and trastuzumab. Lapatinib has also been approved for use in combination with letrozole in postmenopausal women with hormone receptor–positive breast cancer that overexpresses HER2 (GlaxoSmithKline, 2015). Decreases in LVEF have been reported, and normal LVEF should be established before starting therapy with lapatinib. More than 60% of the LVEF abnormalities occurred within the first nine weeks of therapy (Frankel & Palmieri, 2010; GlaxoSmithKline, 2015).

A prolonged QT interval has been noted, and monitoring of electrocardiogram and electrolytes should be considered (GlaxoSmithKline, 2015). Hepatotoxicity can occur days to months after the initiation of therapy (GlaxoSmithKline, 2015). This agent could cause fetal harm, so patients should be educated on the risk and the appropriate measures to take to avoid pregnancy. ILD and pneumonitis also have occurred in patients taking lapatinib (GlaxoSmithKline, 2015). Dose adjustment recommendations are listed in the package insert in reference to drug–drug interactions in patients taking other inhibitors or inducers of CYP3A4 or CYP2C8 (GlaxoSmithKline, 2015). The package insert for lapatinib ditosylate includes a patient education sheet that can be used to teach patients about the side effects of the drug.

Inhibitors of Multiple Signaling Pathways

Sorafenib

Sorafenib (Nexavar®) blocks the signaling of the Ras-Raf/MEK/ERK pathway, which has a role in proliferation, angiogenesis, and tumor apoptosis (Bayer HealthCare Pharmaceuticals

Inc., 2014; Polovich et al., 2014). Sorafenib inhibits several tyrosine kinases, including VEGF receptor and PDGF-β, FMS-like tyrosine kinase-3 (Flt3), and c-Kit (Bayer HealthCare Pharmaceuticals Inc., 2014; Polovich et al., 2014). Inhibiting these pathways interferes with cellular proliferation, survival, and angiogenesis. Sorafenib is approved for the treatment of advanced renal cell carcinoma and inoperable hepatocellular carcinoma (Bayer HealthCare Pharmaceuticals Inc., 2014).

Cardiac ischemia or infarction, hemorrhage, hypertension, hand-foot syndrome, and GI perforation are potential side effects reported with sorafenib. The risk of these toxicities varies based on the study and the type of cancer. For cardiac events, the incidence was 2.7% in the hepatocellular cancer study and 2.9% in the renal cancer study (Bayer HealthCare Pharmaceuticals Inc., 2014; Polovich et al., 2014). Bleeding from esophageal varices with hepatocellular carcinoma was reported to occur in 2.4% of patients, which was lower than what was reported for the placebo group (Bayer HealthCare Pharmaceuticals Inc., 2014). In the phase III renal cancer study, adverse events included reversible skin rashes, hand-foot skin reaction, and diarrhea (40%, 30%, and 43%, respectively) (Bayer HealthCare Pharmaceuticals Inc., 2014; Polovich et al., 2014).

Several drug–drug interactions occur with this agent and include irinotecan, docetaxel, doxorubicin, 5-fluorouracil, warfarin, and dexamethasone; this is not a complete list of agents (Bayer HealthCare Pharmaceuticals Inc., 2014).

Sunitinib Malate

Sunitinib malate (Sutent®) is indicated for the treatment of GISTs after disease progression or intolerance to imatinib mesylate (Pfizer Inc., 2015c). It also is indicated for the treatment of advanced renal cell carcinoma. This agent inhibits multiple kinases: PDGF-Rα, PDGF-β, VEGF receptor, c-Kit, Flt3, CSF receptor type 1, and glial cell-line–derived neurotrophic factor receptor (Pfizer Inc., 2015c; Polovich et al., 2014).

LVEF declines below normal have occurred. Baseline LVEF measurement and monitoring for signs and symptoms of congestive heart failure are encouraged (Polovich et al., 2014). Prolonged QT intervals, hypertension, hemorrhagic events, and hypothyroidism have occurred with sunitinib therapy (Pfizer Inc., 2015c; Polovich et al., 2014). Clinical assessments should include monitoring for signs and symptoms of hypothyroidism such as dry skin, brittle nails, hair thinning, constipation, weight gain, fatigue, hoarseness, and depression. Hemorrhagic events vary depending on the study population; the incidence was 30% in the metastatic renal cancer study and 18% in the GIST study (Pfizer Inc., 2015c). Epistaxis is the most common bleeding event reported, but upper GI and wound bleeding and rectal, gingival, and tumor-related hemorrhage also can occur (Pfizer Inc., 2015c; Polovich et al., 2014). Monitoring for signs and symptoms of these potential toxicities should be considered standard care with patients on sunitinib.

Signaling Pathway Inhibitors

Mammalian Target of Rapamycin Inhibitors

In the field of oncology, mammalian target of rapamycin (mTOR) inhibition as a therapeutic approach has entered the clinical practice setting in renal cell carcinoma, with approximately 1,096 clinical trials underway to evaluate the efficacy and safety profiles of several mTOR inhibitors in a variety of solid tumors and hematologic cancers (ClinicalTrials.gov, 2016a). Cell survival, growth, and proliferation are regulated through the phosphatidylinositol 3-kinase (PI3K)/Akt (protein kinase B) signaling pathway, of which mTOR is a downstream target (Faivre, Neuzillet, &

Raymond, 2016). It plays a pleiotropic role, including regulation of essential signal-transduction pathways, involvement in cell cycle progression, initiation of mRNA translation, and other aspects of cell growth (Faivre et al., 2016). Studies have indicated that because of its connection to the PI3K/Akt pathway, mTOR may play a pivotal role in tumor growth. Certain tumors, such as those whose growth patterns stimulate the PI3K/Akt/mTOR signal transduction pathway or that harbor mutations that activate the PI3K/Akt pathway, may be especially susceptible to mTOR inhibitors (Faivre et al., 2016).

Sirolimus

Rapamycin (sirolimus) is the archetypical mTOR inhibitor (Pfizer Inc., 2015b). This antifungal agent, produced by the bacteria *Streptomyces hygroscopicus* and originally found in the soil of Easter Island, was studied in the laboratory for other uses before the mTOR kinase had been identified and its association with cancer recognized (Easton & Houghton, 2006; Faivre et al., 2016). Multiple analogs of rapamycin have been developed and are being studied for the treatment of a wide variety of hematologic and solid malignancies (Pfizer Inc., 2015b).

Temsirolimus

Temsirolimus (Torisel®) is one of the newest targeted agents approved in the intracellular kinase pathway (Wyeth Pharmaceuticals Inc., 2015). Activation of this pathway targets translation of cell cycle regulatory proteins and prevents overexpression of angiogenic growth factors (Schulze, Stock, Zaccagnini, Teber, & Rassweiler, 2014). Subsequent to the activation of the pathway, synthesis of cyclin D and hypoxia-inducible factor-1 occurs to regulate the G_1 cell cycle pathway, leading to VEGF production (Hudson et al., 2002). Temsirolimus causes cell cycle arrest in the G_1 phase of the cell cycle and disrupts the proteins directing cell proliferation, growth, and survival (Feitelson et al., 2015; Schulz et al., 2014; Wyeth Pharmaceuticals Inc., 2015). Temsirolimus is indicated for the treatment of advanced renal cell carcinoma (Wyeth Pharmaceuticals Inc., 2015).

Pretreatment with antihistamines is recommended to prevent hypersensitivity reactions (Polovich et al., 2014). Monitoring glucose and lipids for indications of hyperglycemia and hyperlipidemia is recommended (Wyeth Pharmaceuticals Inc., 2015). The most common serious side effects reported are anemia, fatigue, dyspnea, infection, and hyperglycemia, and 9% of patients experienced hypersensitivity reactions (Polovich et al., 2014). ILD, bowel perforation, renal failure, and intracerebral bleeding also are possible but are less commonly seen in patients receiving temsirolimus (Creel, 2014; Wyeth Pharmaceuticals Inc., 2015). Stomatitis can also occur and should be carefully managed (Divers & O'Shaughnessy, 2015; Pilotte, Hohos, Polson, Huftalen, & Treister, 2011). Preventing pregnancy during and up to three months after therapy is recommended because of potential fetal harm (Wyeth Pharmaceuticals Inc., 2015). Patients also should avoid exposure to live vaccines, such as those for measles, mumps, polio, rubella, and intranasal influenza (Polovich et al., 2014; Wyeth Pharmaceuticals Inc., 2015).

Everolimus

Everolimus (Afinitor®) has recently been approved for advanced renal cell carcinoma after sunitinib or sorafenib failure (Novartis Pharmaceuticals Corp., 2012). Everolimus binds to an intracellular protein to cause inhibition of mTOR kinase and reduction of cell proliferation, angiogenesis, and glucose uptake (Dienstmann, Rodon, Serra, & Tabernero, 2014; Novartis Pharmaceuticals Corp., 2012).

Common side effects of oral administration of everolimus include stomatitis, infections, asthenia, fatigue, cough, and diarrhea. Hypophosphatemia, hyperglycemia, hypertriglyceridemia, hypercholesterolemia, anemia, and lymphopenia have been noted; therefore, laboratory values, including complete metabolic profile (including lipid profile) and complete blood counts, should be monitored while on everolimus (Novartis Pharmaceuticals Corp., 2012; Polovich et al., 2014).

Noninfectious pneumonitis, characterized by nonspecific respiratory signs and symptoms (hypoxia, pleural effusion, cough, or dyspnea), is a class effect of rapamycin derivatives and has been noted in patients treated with everolimus (Novartis Pharmaceuticals Corp., 2012). Localized and systemic infections, including pneumonia, other bacterial infections, and invasive fungal infections, have occurred in patients taking everolimus. Some of these infections have been severe and led to respiratory failure and death (Polovich et al., 2014). Patient teaching must include signs and symptoms of infections and instruction to patients to contact their healthcare provider immediately. As with temsirolimus, the use of live vaccines and close contact with those who have received live vaccines should be avoided during treatment (Novartis Pharmaceuticals Corp., 2012).

Patients taking everolimus should avoid the use of concomitant CYP3A4 inducers (i.e., dexamethasone, phenytoin, carbamazepine, rifampin, rifabutin, phenobarbital) as well as CYP3A4 inhibitors (i.e., amprenavir, aprepitant, atazanavir, clarithromycin, delavirdine, diltiazem, erythromycin, fluconazole, fosamprenavir, grapefruit juice, indinavir, itraconazole, ketoconazole, nefazodone, nelfinavir, ritonavir, saquinavir, telithromycin, verapamil, voriconazole) (Novartis Pharmaceuticals Corp., 2012).

Proteasome Inhibitors

Proteasomes are part of an enzyme complex that acts as housekeeping enzymes to degrade (break down) proteins in the cell nucleus when they are no longer needed. These proteins are recycled and used again. Proteasomes are found in every cell of the body and degrade proteins that have a ubiquitin tag. This small protein is active in the ubiquitin–proteasome pathway to regulate protein homeostasis through quality control within the cell (Kisselev, van der Linden, & Overkleeft, 2012). Proteasome inhibitors block this process from occurring, causing the cells to receive conflicting signals for cell regulation. The conflicting messages the cell nucleus receives cause apoptosis of malignant cells, whereas normal cells are less sensitive to the overload and are able to recover. One example is its work in the cell cycle to prevent progression if the proteins are dysfunctional. The proteasome inhibitors are also believed to affect angiogenesis (Kisselev et al., 2012; Kubiczkova, Pour, Sedlarikova, Hajek, & Sevcikova, 2014). Without proteasome activity, it is believed that cells self-induce apoptosis, thereby inhibiting tumor growth.

Bortezomib (Velcade®) was the first approved drug in the inhibitor class of anticancer drugs (Millennium Pharmaceuticals, Inc., 2014). Carfilzomib (Kyprolis®) is a new agent of selective, irreversible proteasome inhibitors used for the treatment of hematologic malignancies and solid tumors. Compared with bortezomib, carfilzomib is longer acting because of the irreversible inhibition of proteasome activity. It has shown activity in relapsed and refractory multiple myeloma, with one study showing longer survival compared to bortezomib (Moreau et al., 2012). At least four other proteasome inhibitors, with other unique structures, are in clinical trials to determine their effectiveness against multiple myeloma solid tumors and during transplant (Kisselev et al., 2012). Neuropathy is a common problem with the proteasome inhibitors. Other side effects include cytopenias (primarily leukopenia and thrombocytopenia), peripheral neuropathy, and potentially nausea and vomiting with dehydration (Polovich et al., 2014).

Telomerase Inhibitors

Telomerase plays an active role in the embryonic development and continued growth of the body over time. Normally, cells in the body only divide 50–70 times over a lifetime. Research has identified that this enzyme prevents chromosome ends from shortening, thereby allowing the cell to live forever. It is well known that this enzyme is active in cancer cells, which enables them to continue to grow and become immortalized. Two oncogenes induce telomerase activity, myc and the Ras-MAPK signaling pathway. Targeting this growth enzyme for inhibition through vaccines and a lipid delivery system has moved into clinical trials for a variety of cancer types (ClinicalTrials.gov, 2016d; Puri & Girard, 2013).

Conclusion

Newer therapies include agents that inhibit the proteasome complex, HDAC, mTOR pathway, the eicosanoid (a signaling molecule made of essential fatty acids) pathway, Raf kinase, protein kinase pathway, matrix metalloproteinase, and telomerase, to name a few. As molecular science evolves and changes the approach to cancer therapy, the demand for understanding the complexity of these agents is increasing. Complex internal cellular pathways, mTOR, Ras, Raf, crosstalk among receptors, constitutively active receptors, redundant pathways, cancer stem cells, ligand binding, and blocking costimulatory receptors are just a few of the terms describing the pathophysiologic targets of newer and experimental cancer agents.

The demand to accelerate understanding of this complex science is one of the challenges nurses face, along with being able to explain the action of these agents in an understandable yet detailed way to patients. With these advancements come the unique toxicities of targeted agents. These side effects are unlike those that nurses have become experts in managing with chemotherapy—in some ways making the nurse educator feel vulnerable and like a neophyte. Maculopapular rash with an etiology different than acneform rash, hand-foot syndrome, and CYP34A inducers and inhibitors—some of these terms were foreign to the oncology profession just a few decades ago. More recently, oncology nurses have become familiar not only with the terminology but also with educating, monitoring, and managing the toxicities from these cutting-edge therapies. Of particular concern are the oral agents for cancer treatment. While these agents are believed to have less toxicity, there remains a lack of knowledge and a need for safe handling of these medications (Lester, 2012; Rudnitzki & McMahon, 2015). Sharing experience and knowledge is necessary to be able to provide excellence in oncology nursing care to patients. It is impossible to cover all of the nuances of biotherapy agents in one chapter. Multiple resources are available via the Internet and professional organizations such as the Oncology Nursing Society to fill gaps in knowledge and lend support and encouragement. (See Polovich et al., 2014, for more information about recommendations for practice for patients receiving any of the medications described in this chapter.) Perhaps as precision medicine evolves at accelerated paces, the use of chemotherapy, at least as a single therapy, will be a distant memory.

The author would like to acknowledge Denise Vranicar Lapka, RN, MS, AOCN®, CNS, and Paula J. Franson, RN, MS, AOCN®, for their contributions to this chapter that remain unchanged from the first edition of this book.

Key Points

- Biologic therapy helps the immune system fight cancer or targets certain biologic areas of the cancer growth process, whereas chemotherapy attacks the cancer cells directly.
- Epigenetic changes occur "above and over" the DNA so that the basic sequence is not affected and the genotype is not changed; however, the phenotypic outcome may be altered.
- Lymphocytes can be categorized into T cells, B cells, and NK cells.
- The type of antibody can be determined by looking at the ending of the generic name. If the name of the antibody ends in -momab, it is murine; -ximab is chimeric; -zumab is humanized; and -umab indicates a fully human antibody.
- MicroRNAs (miRNAs) can function as tumor suppressors or oncogenes.
- Many targeted therapies regulate cell survival, growth, and proliferation.
- The immediate-onset anaphylaxis during first exposure to IV cetuximab is believed to be due to an IgE reaction associated with a previous tick bite.
- Tyrosine kinase inhibitors have changed the treatment of CML with improvement in survival in all three phases—chronic, accelerated, and blast.
- Although oral cancer treatment agents are convenient, patients, caregivers, and healthcare providers face exposure risks similar to those posed by IV chemotherapy.

References

Ahuja, N., Sharma, A.R., & Baylin, S.B. (2016). Epigenetic therapeutics: A new weapon in the war against cancer. *Annual Review of Medicine, 67,* 73–89. doi:10.1146/annurev-med-111314-035900

American Cancer Society. (2014). Evolution of cancer treatments: Immunotherapy. Retrieved from http://www.cancer.org/cancer/cancerbasics/thehistoryofcancer/the-history-of-cancer-cancer-treatment-immunotherapy

American Society of Clinical Oncology. (2016a). Understanding immunotherapy. Retrieved from http://www.cancer.net/navigating-cancer-care/how-cancer-treated/immunotherapy-and-vaccines/understanding-immunotherapy

American Society of Clinical Oncology. (2016b). Understanding targeted therapy. Retrieved from http://www.cancer.net/navigating-cancer-care/how-cancer-treated/personalized-and-targeted-therapies/understanding-targeted-therapy

Amgen Inc. (2015a). *Neupogen® (filgrastim)* [Package insert]. Thousand Oaks, CA: Author.

Amgen Inc. (2015b). *Vectibix® (panitumumab) injection for intravenous use* [Package insert]. Thousand Oaks, CA: Author.

Amgen Inc. (2016a). *Aranesp® (darbepoetin alfa) for injection* [Package insert]. Thousand Oaks, CA: Author.

Amgen Inc. (2016b). *Epogen® (epoetin alfa) for injection* [Package insert]. Thousand Oaks, CA: Author.

Amgen Inc. (2016c). *Neulasta® (pegfilgrastim)* [Package insert]. Thousand Oaks, CA: Author.

Amgen Inc. (2016d). *Nplate® (romiplostim) for injection, for subcutaneous use* [Package insert]. Thousand Oaks, CA: Author.

Azim, H.A., Jr., Azim, H., & Peccatori, F.A. (2010). Treatment of cancer during pregnancy with monoclonal antibodies: A real challenge. *Expert Review of Clinical Immunology, 6,* 821–826. doi:10.1586/eci.10.77

Barnes, T., & Reinke, D. (2011). Practical management of imatinib in gastrointestinal stromal tumors. *Clinical Journal of Oncology Nursing, 15,* 533–545. doi:10.1188/11.CJON.533-545

Baxby, D. (1999). Edward Jenner's inquiry; A bicentenary analysis. *Vaccine, 17,* 301–307. doi:10.1016/S0264-410X(98)00207-2

Bayer HealthCare Pharmaceuticals Inc. (2014). *Nexavar® (sorafenib)* [Package insert]. Wayne, NJ: Author.

Berg, E.A., Platts-Mills, T.A.E., & Commins, S.P. (2014). Drug allergens and food—The cetuximab and galactose-α-1,3-galactose story. *Annals of Allergy, Asthma and Immunology, 112,* 97–101. doi:10.1016/j.anai.2013.11.014

Bickels, J., Kollender, Y., Merinsky, O., & Meller, I. (2002). Coley's toxin: Historical perspective. *Israel Medical Association Journal, 4,* 471–472. Retrieved from http://www.ima.org.il/FilesUpload/IMAJ/0/55/27870.pdf

Biogen Idec Inc. & Genentech, Inc. (2012). *Rituxan® (rituximab) injection for intravenous use* [Package insert]. South San Francisco, CA: Genentech, Inc.

Bouchie, A. (2013). First microRNA mimic enters clinic. *Nature Biotechnology, 31,* 577. doi:10.1038/nbt0713-577

Bourdeanu, L., & Luu, T. (2013). Nursing perspectives on trastuzumab emtansine for the treatment of metastatic breast cancer [Online exclusive]. *Clinical Journal of Oncology Nursing, 17,* E58–E62. doi:10.1188/13.CJON.E58-E62

Breslin, S. (2007). Cytokine-release syndrome: Overview and nursing implications. *Clinical Journal of Oncology Nursing, 11*(Suppl. 1), 37–42. doi:10.1188/07.CJON.S1.37-42

Bristol-Myers Squibb Co. (2015). *Sprycel® (dasatinib) tablets, for oral use* [Package insert]. Princeton, NJ: Author.

Burhenn, P.S., & Smudde, J. (2015). Using tools and technology to promote education and adherence to oral agents for cancer. *Clinical Journal of Oncology Nursing, 19*(Suppl. 3), 53–59. doi:10.1188/15.S1.CJON.53-59

Celgene Corp. (2010). *Thalomid® (thalidomide) capsules* [Package insert]. Summit, NJ: Author.

Celgene Corp. (2015). *Revlimid® (lenalidomide) capsules for oral use* [Package insert]. Summit, NJ: Author.

Centers for Disease Control and Prevention. (2016). *Recommended adult immunization schedule—United States—2016.* Retrieved from http://www.cdc.gov/vaccines/schedules/downloads/adult/adult-schedule.pdf

Cilloni, D., & Saglio, G. (2012). Molecular pathways: BCR-ABL. *Clinical Cancer Research, 18,* 930–937. doi:10.1158/1078-0432.CCR-10-1613

ClinicalTrials.gov. (2016a, June 12). mTOR inhibitors and cancer [Search results]. Retrieved from https://clinicaltrials.gov/ct2/results?term=mtor+inhibitors+and+cancer&Search=Search

ClinicalTrials.gov. (2016b, October 18). PiRNA and cancer [Search results]. Retrieved from https://clinicaltrials.gov/ct2/results?term=piRNA+and+cancer+&Search=Search

ClinicalTrials.gov. (2016c, October 18). SiRNA and cancer [Search results]. Retrieved from https://clinicaltrials.gov/ct2/results?term=siRNA+and+cancer&Search=Search

ClinicalTrials.gov. (2016d, June 23). Telomerase inhibitor and cancer [Search results]. Retrieved from https://clinicaltrials.gov/ct2/results?term=telomerase+inhibitor+and+cancer&Search=Search

Coley, W.B. (1893). The treatment of malignant tumors by repeated inoculations of erysipelas: With a report of ten original cases. *American Journal of the Medical Sciences, 105,* 487–511. doi:10.1097/00000441-189305000-00001

Collins, F.S., & Varmus, H. (2015). A new initiative on precision medicine. *New England Journal of Medicine, 372,* 793–795. doi:10.1056/NEJMp1500523

Creel, P.A. (2014). Optimizing patient adherence to targeted therapies in renal cell carcinoma: Practical management strategies in the second-line setting. *Clinical Journal of Oncology Nursing, 18,* 694–700. doi:10.1188/14.CJON.694-700

Dawson, M.A., & Kouzarides, T. (2012). Cancer epigenetics: From mechanism to therapy. *Cell, 150,* 12–27. doi:10.1016/j.cell.2012.06.013

Dawson, M.A., Kouzarides, T., & Huntly, B.J.P. (2012). Targeting epigenetic readers in cancer. *New England Journal of Medicine, 367,* 647–657. doi:10.1056/NEJMra1112635

Dienstmann, R., Rodon, J., Serra, V., & Tabernero, J. (2014). Picking the point of inhibition: A comparative review of PI3K/AKT/mTOR pathway inhibitors. *Molecular Cancer Therapeutics, 13,* 1021–1031. doi:10.1158/1535-7163.MCT-13-0639

Dimopoulos, M., Spencer, A., Attal, M., Prince, H.M., Harousseau, J.-L., Dmoszynska, A., … Knight, R.D. (2007). Lenalidomide plus dexamethasone for relapsed or refractory multiple myeloma. *New England Journal of Medicine, 357,* 2123–2132. doi:10.1056/NEJMoa070594

Dispenzieri, A., Rajkumar, S.V., Gertz, M.A., Greipp, P.R., Lacy, M.Q., Kyle, R.A., … Dalton, R.J. (2007). Treatment of newly diagnosed multiple myeloma based on Mayo Stratification of Myeloma and Risk-Adapted Therapy (mSMART): Consensus statement. *Mayo Clinic Proceedings, 82,* 323–341. doi:10.1016/S0025-6196(11)61029-X

Divers, J., & O'Shaughnessy, J. (2015). Stomatitis associated with use of mTOR inhibitors: Implications for patients with invasive breast cancer. *Clinical Journal of Oncology Nursing, 19,* 468–474. doi:10.1188/15.CJON.468-474

Dokmanovic, M., Clarke, C., & Marks, P.A. (2007). Histone deacetylase inhibitors: Overview and perspectives. *Molecular Cancer Research, 5,* 981–989. doi:10.1158/1541-7786.MCR-07-0324

Dutcher, J.P., Schwartzentruber, D.J., Kaufman, H.L., Agarwala, S.S., Tarhini, A.A., Lowder, J.N., & Atkins, M.B. (2014). High dose interleukin-2 (aldesleukin)—Expert consensus on best management practices—2014. *Journal for ImmunoTherapy of Cancer, 2,* 26. doi:10.1186/s40425-014-0026-0

Dyer, M.J.S. (2001). Historical aspects of the development of antibody therapy of B-cell malignancies. In B.D. Cheson (Ed.), *New frontiers in cancer therapy: Monoclonal antibody therapy of hematologic malignancies* (pp. 1–12). Oxfordshire, United Kingdom: Darwin Scientific Publishing.

Easton, J.B., & Houghton, P.J. (2006). mTOR and cancer therapy. *Oncogene, 25,* 6436–6446. doi:10.1038/sj.onc.1209886

Eccles, S.A. (2011). The epidermal growth factor receptor/Erb-B/HER family in normal and malignant breast biology. *International Journal of Developmental Biology, 55,* 685–696. doi:10.1387/ijdb.113396se

Elice, F., Jacoub, J., Rickles, F.R., Falanga, A., & Rodeghiero, F. (2008). Hemostatic complications of angiogenesis inhibitors in cancer patients. *American Journal of Hematology, 83,* 862–870. doi:10.1002/ajh.21277

Eli Lilly & Co. (2014). *Gemzar® (gemcitabine)* [Package insert]. Indianapolis, IN: Author.

Enokida, T., Suzuki, S., Wakasugi, T., Yamazaki, T., & Tahara, M. (2014). Incidence and risk factors of hypomagnesemia in head and neck cancer patients treated with cetuximab [Poster abstract]. *Annals of Oncology, 25,* iv344–iv345.

Ewer, M.S., & Ewer, S.M. (2010). Cardiotoxicity of anticancer treatments: What the cardiologist needs to know. *Nature Reviews Cardiology, 7,* 564–575. doi:10.1038/nrcardio.2010.121

Ewing, J.C. (2014). The wave of the future: Genetic profiling in treatment selection. *Clinical Journal of Oncology Nursing, 18,* 717–718. doi:10.1188/14.CJON.717-718

Faivre, S., Neuzillet, C., & Raymond, E. (2016). Predictive biomarkers of response to mTOR inhibitors. In M. Mita, A. Mita, & E.K. Rowinsky (Eds.), *mTOR inhibition for cancer therapy: Past, present and future* (pp. 217–228). doi:10.1007/978-2-8178-0492-7_10

Falkenberg, K.J., & Johnstone, R.W. (2014). Histone deacetylases and their inhibitors in cancer, neurological diseases and immune disorders. *Nature Reviews Drug Discovery, 13,* 673–691. doi:10.1038/nrd4360

Feitelson, M.A., Arzumanyan, A., Kulathinal, R.J., Blain, S.W., Holcombe, R.F., Mahajna, J., ... Nowsheen, S. (2015). Sustained proliferation in cancer: Mechanisms and novel therapeutic targets. *Seminars in Cancer Biology, 35,* S25–S54. doi:10.1016/j.semcancer.2015.02.006

Frankel, C., & Palmieri, F.M. (2010). Lapatinib side-effect management. *Clinical Journal of Oncology Nursing, 14,* 223–233. doi:10.1188/10.CJON.223-233

Friedländer, M.R., Lizano, E., Houben, A.J.S., Bezdan, D., Báñez-Coronel, M., Kudla, G., ... Estivill, X. (2014). Evidence for the biogenesis of more than 1,000 novel human microRNAs. *Genome Biology, 15,* R57. doi:10.1186/gb-2014-15-4-r57

Gajewski, T.F., Schreiber, H., & Fu, Y.-X. (2013). Innate and adaptive immune cells in the tumor microenvironment. *Nature Immunology, 14,* 1014–1022. doi:10.1038/ni.2703

Genentech, Inc. (n.d.). Frequently asked questions about therapeutic antibodies. Retrieved from http://www.gene.com/patients/disease-education/faq-treatment-lymphoma

Genentech, Inc. (2015). *Avastin® (bevacizumab) for intravenous use* [Package insert]. South San Francisco, CA: Author.

Genentech, Inc. (2016). *Herceptin® (trastuzumab) intravenous infusion* [Package insert]. South San Francisco, CA: Author.

Genzyme Corp. (2014). *Campath® (alemtuzumab) injection for intravenous use* [Package insert]. Cambridge, MA: Author.

Gillette, T.G., & Hill, J.A. (2015). Readers, writers, and erasers: Chromatin as the whiteboard of heart disease. *Circulation Research, 116,* 1245–1253. doi:10.1161/CIRCRESAHA.116.303630

Glass, E., & Viale, P.H. (2013). Histone deacetylase inhibitors. *Clinical Journal of Oncology Nursing, 17,* 34–40. doi:10.1188/13.CJON.34-40

GlaxoSmithKline. (2011). *Cervarix® (human papillomavirus bivalent [types 16 and 18] vaccine, recombinant)* [Package insert]. Research Triangle Park, NC: Author.

GlaxoSmithKline. (2013). *Bexxar® (tositumomab and iodine I 131 tositumomab)* [Package insert]. Research Triangle Park, NC: Author.

GlaxoSmithKline. (2015). *Tykerb® (lapatinib) tablets* [Package insert]. Research Triangle Park, NC: Author.

Goldsmith, S.J. (2010). Radioimmunotherapy of lymphoma: Bexxar and Zevalin. *Seminars in Nuclear Medicine, 40,* 122–135. doi:10.1053/j.semnuclmed.2009.11.002

Greenberg, P., Cox, C., LeBeau, M.M., Fenaux, P., Morel, P., Sanz, G., ... Bennett, J. (1997). International scoring system for evaluating prognosis in myelodysplastic syndromes. *Blood, 89,* 2079–2088. Retrieved from http://www.bloodjournal.org/content/89/6/2079.long

Gubin, M.M., Artyomov, M.N., Mardis, E.R., & Schreiber, R.D. (2015). Tumor neoantigens: Building a framework for personalized cancer immunotherapy. *Journal of Clinical Investigation, 125,* 3413–3421. doi:10.1172/JCI80008

Hammerstrom, A.E., Cauley, D.H., Atkinson, B.J., & Sharma, P. (2011). Cancer immunotherapy: Sipuleucel-T and beyond. *Pharmacotherapy, 31,* 813–828. doi:10.1592/phco.31.8.813

Hanahan, D., & Weinberg, R.A. (2011). Hallmarks of cancer: The next generation. *Cell, 144,* 646–674. doi:10.1016/j.cell.2011.02.013

Hashim, A., Rizzo, F., Marchese, G., Ravo, M., Tarallo, R., Nassa, G., ... Weisz, A. (2014). RNA sequencing identifies specific PIWI-interacting small non-coding RNA expression patterns in breast cancer. *Oncotarget, 5,* 9901–9910. doi:10.18632/oncotarget.2476

Hassan, M.N., & Waller, E.K. (2015). Treating chemotherapy-induced thrombocytopenia: Is it time for oncologists to use thrombopoietin agonists? *Oncology, 29,* 295–296.

Hayes, J., Peruzzi, P.P., & Lawler, S. (2014). MicroRNAs in cancer: Biomarkers, functions and therapy. *Trends in Molecular Medicine, 20,* 460–469. doi:10.1016/j.molmed.2014.06.005

Hennessy, E.J., Parker, A.E., & O'Neill, L.A.J. (2010). Targeting Toll-like receptors: Emerging therapeutics? *Nature Reviews Drug Discovery, 9,* 293–307. doi:10.1038/nrd3203

Hudson, C.C., Liu, M., Chiang, G.G., Otterness, D.M., Loomis, D.C., Kaper, F., ... Abraham, R.T. (2002). Regulation of hypoxia-inducible factor 1α expression and function by the mammalian target of rapamycin. *Molecular and Cellular Biology, 22,* 7004–7014. doi:10.1128/MCB.22.20.7004-7014.2002

ImClone LLC. (2016). *Erbitux® (cetuximab)* [Package insert]. Branchburg, NJ: Author.

Isaacs, A., & Lindenmann, J. (1957). Virus interference. I. The interferon. *Proceedings of the Royal Society of London, Series B, 147,* 258–267. doi:10.1098/rspb.1957.0048

Jacene, H.A., & Wahl, R.L. (2014). Non-Hodgkin lymphoma: Radioimmunotherapy using iodine-131 labeled murine anti-CD20 antibodies (^{131}I-tositumomab and tositumomab, "Bexxar"). In R.P. Baum (Ed.), *Therapeutic nuclear medicine* (pp. 505–525). doi:10.1007/174_2013_943

Janssen Products, L.P. (2016). *Procrit® (epoetin alfa) injection, for intravenous or subcutaneous use* [Package insert]. Horsham, PA: Author.

Jin, B., & Yeo, A.E. (2014). Cancer immunotherapy: Does an increasing arsenal of tools point to more fruitful avenues for research? [Editorial]. *Anti-Cancer Agents in Medicinal Chemistry, 14,* 181–182.

Jubb, A.M., & Harris, A.L. (2010). Biomarkers to predict the clinical efficacy of bevacizumab in cancer. *Lancet Oncology, 11,* 1172–1183. doi:10.1016/S1470-2045(10)70232-1

Kannan, R., Madden, K., & Andrews, S. (2014). Primer on immuno-oncology and immune response. *Clinical Journal of Oncology Nursing, 18,* 311–317. doi:10.1188/14.CJON.311-317

Khan, O., & La Thangue, N.B. (2012). HDAC inhibitors in cancer biology: Emerging mechanisms and clinical applications. *Immunology and Cell Biology, 90,* 85–94.

Kisselev, A.F., van der Linden, W.A., & Overkleeft, H.S. (2012). Proteasome inhibitors: An expanding army attacking a unique target. *Chemistry and Biology, 19,* 99–115. doi:10.1016/j.chembiol.2012.01.003

Köhler, G., & Milstein, C. (1975). Continuous cultures of fused cells secreting antibody of predefined specificity. *Nature, 256,* 495–497. doi:10.1038/256495a0

Kreamer, K., & Riordan, D. (2015). Targeted therapies for non-small cell lung cancer: An update on epidermal growth factor receptor and anaplastic lymphoma kinase inhibitors. *Clinical Journal of Oncology Nursing, 19,* 734–742. doi:10.1188/15.CJON.734-742

Ku, H.-Y., & Lin, H. (2014). PIWI proteins and their interactors in piRNA biogenesis, germline development and gene expression. *National Science Review, 1,* 205–218. doi:10.1093/nsr/nwu014

Kubiczkova, L., Pour, L., Sedlarikova, L., Hajek, R., & Sevcikova, S. (2014). Proteasome inhibitors—Molecular basis and current perspectives in multiple myeloma. *Journal of Cellular and Molecular Medicine, 18,* 947–961. doi:10.1111/jcmm.12279

Lemmon, M.A., & Schlessinger, J. (2010). Cell signaling by receptor tyrosine kinases. *Cell, 141,* 1117–1134. doi:10.1016/j.cell.2010.06.011

Lester, J. (2012). Safe handling and administration considerations of oral anticancer agents in the clinical and home setting [Online exclusive]. *Clinical Journal of Oncology Nursing, 16,* E192–E197. doi:10.1188/12.CJON.E192-E197

Lin, S., & Gregory, R.I. (2015). MicroRNA biogenesis pathways in cancer. *Nature Reviews Cancer, 15,* 321–333. doi:10.1038/nrc3932

List, A., Dewald, G., Bennett, J., Giagounidis, A., Raza, A., Feldman, E., ... Knight, R. (2006). Lenalidomide in the myelodysplastic syndrome with chromosome 5q deletion. *New England Journal of Medicine, 355,* 1456–1465. doi:10.1056/NEJMoa061292

Liu, M.A. (2011). Cancer vaccines. *Philosophical Transactions of the Royal Society B, 366,* 2823–2826. doi:10.1098/rstb.2011.0101

Lyman, G.H., Khorana, A.A., Kuderer, N.M., Lee, A.Y., Arcelus, J.I., Balaban, E.P., ... Falanga, A. (2013). Venous thromboembolism prophylaxis and treatment in patients with cancer: American Society of Clinical Oncology clinical practice guideline update. *Journal of Clinical Oncology, 31,* 2189–2204. doi:10.1200/JCO.2013.49.1118

Maloney, D.G. (2012). Anti-CD20 antibody therapy for B-cell lymphomas. *New England Journal of Medicine, 366,* 2008–2016. doi:10.1056/NEJMct1114348

Marjanovic, N.D., Weinberg, R.A., & Chaffer, C.L. (2013). Cell plasticity and heterogeneity in cancer. *Clinical Chemistry, 59,* 168–179. doi:10.1373/clinchem.2012.184655

Martin-Babau, J., Eusen, Y., Verveur, C., Trouboul, F., Cheneau, C., Le Tallec, V.J., ... Metges, J.-P. (2016). Trastuzumab induced cardiotoxicity in HER2-positive metastatic esogastric cancers. *Journal of Clinical Oncology, 34*(Suppl. 4), Abstract No. 152. Retrieved from http://meetinglibrary.asco.org/content/159989-173

McCance, K.L., & Huether, S.E. (2014). Chapter 6: Innate immunity. In K.L. McCance & S.E. Huether (Eds.), *Pathophysiology: The biologic basis for disease in adults and children* (7th ed.). Atlanta, GA: Elsevier.

Merck & Co., Inc. (2011). *Gardasil® (human papillomavirus quadrivalent [types 6, 11, 16, and 18] vaccine)* [Package insert]. Whitehouse Station, NJ: Author.

Merck & Co., Inc. (2016a). *Gardasil® 9 (human papillomavirus 9-valent vaccine, recombinant)* [Package insert]. Whitehouse Station, NJ: Author.

Merck & Co., Inc. (2016b). *Intron® A (interferon alfa-2b, recombinant) for injection* [Package insert]. Whitehouse Station, NJ: Author.

Millennium Pharmaceuticals, Inc. (2014). *Velcade® (bortezomib)* [Package insert]. Cambridge, MA: Author.

Miller, K., Wang, M., Gralow, J., Dickler, M., Cobleigh, M., Perez, E.A., ... Davidson, N.E. (2007). Paclitaxel plus bevacizumab versus paclitaxel alone for metastatic breast cancer. *New England Journal of Medicine, 357,* 2666–2676. doi:10.1056/NEJMoa072113

Mitsudomi, T., & Yatabe, Y. (2010). Epidermal growth factor receptor in relation to tumor development: *EGFR* gene and cancer. *FEBS Journal, 277,* 301–308. doi:10.1111/j.1742-4658.2009.07448.x

Moreau, P., Richardson, P.G., Cavo, M., Orlowski, R.Z., San Miguel, J.F., Palumbo, A., & Harousseau, J.-L. (2012). Proteasome inhibitors in multiple myeloma: 10 years later. *Blood, 120,* 947–959. doi:10.1182/blood-2012-04-403733

National Cancer Institute. (2013, June). Fact sheet: Biological therapies for cancer. Retrieved from http://www.cancer.gov/cancertopics/factsheet/Therapy/biological

National Cancer Institute. (2015, December). Cancer vaccines. Retrieved from https://www.cancer.gov/about-cancer/causes-prevention/vaccines-fact-sheet#q8

National Comprehensive Cancer Network. (2016). *NCCN Clinical Practice Guidelines in Oncology (NCCN Guidelines®): Cancer- and chemotherapy-induced anemia* [v.2.2017]. Retrieved from http://www.nccn.org/professionals/physician_gls/PDF/anemia.pdf

Novartis Pharmaceuticals Corp. (2012). *Afinitor® (everolimus) tablets for oral administration* [Package insert]. East Hanover, NJ: Author.

Novartis Pharmaceuticals Corp. (2015). *Gleevec® (imatinib mesylate) tablets, for oral use* [Package insert]. East Hanover, NJ: Author.

OSI Pharmaceuticals, Inc., Astellas Oncology, & Genentech, Inc. (2016). *Tarceva® (erlotinib) tablets* [Package insert]. Northbrook, IL: OSI Pharmaceuticals, Inc.

Paolo, I., Eugenia, R., Nicola, M., Paola, D.M., Emilio, T., Fabiola, M., ... Donata, G. (2014). Progressive multifocal leukoencephalopathy and rituximab: Time to better stratify the risk? *Journal of Neurology Research, 4,* 34–36. doi:10.14740/jnr235w

Pazdur, R. (2013). FDA approval for alemtuzumab. Retrieved from http://www.cancer.gov/about-cancer/treatment/drugs/fda-alemtuzumab

Peeters, M., Oliner, K.S., Parker, A., Siena, S., Van Cutsem, E., Huang, J., ... Patterson, S.D. (2013). Massively parallel tumor multigene sequencing to evaluate response to panitumumab in a randomized phase III study of metastatic colorectal cancer. *Clinical Cancer Research, 19*(7), 1902–1912. doi:10.1158/1078-0432.CCR-12-1913

Pencheva, N., & Tavazoie, S.F. (2013). Control of metastatic progression by microRNA regulatory networks. *Nature Cell Biology, 15,* 546–554. doi:10.1038/ncb2769

Pfizer Inc. (2015a). *Neumega® (oprelvekin)* [Package insert]. New York, NY: Author.

Pfizer Inc. (2015b). *Rapamune® (sirolimus)* [Package insert]. New York, NY: Author.

Pfizer Inc. (2015c). *Sutent® (sunitinib malate)* [Package insert]. New York, NY: Author.

Pilotte, A.P., Hohos, M.B., Polson, K.M.O., Huftalen, T.M., & Treister, N. (2011). Managing stomatitis in patients treated with mammalian target of rapamycin inhibitors [Online exclusive]. *Clinical Journal of Oncology Nursing, 15,* E83–E89. doi:10.1188/11.CJON.E83-E89

Polovich, M., Olsen, M., & LeFebvre, K.B. (Eds.). (2014). *Chemotherapy and biotherapy guidelines and recommendations for practice* (4th ed.). Pittsburgh, PA: Oncology Nursing Society.

Prometheus Laboratories Inc. (2012). *Proleukin® (aldesleukin) for injection* [Package insert]. San Diego, CA: Author.

Przybylyski, A., & Esper, P. (2016). Early recognition and management of posterior reversible encephalopathy syndrome: A newly recognized complication in patients receiving tyrosine kinase inhibitors. *Clinical Journal of Oncology Nursing, 20,* 305–308. doi:10.1188/16.CJON.305-308

Puri, N., & Girard, J. (2013). Novel therapeutics targeting telomerase and telomeres. *Journal of Cancer Science and Therapy, 5,* e127. doi:10.4172/1948-5956.1000e127

Rosenberg, S.A., Yang, J.C., Sherry, R.M., Kammula, U.S., Hughes, M.S., Phan, G.Q., ... Dudley, M.E. (2011). Durable complete responses in heavily pretreated patients with metastatic melanoma using T-cell transfer immunotherapy. *Clinical Cancer Research, 17,* 455–457. doi:10.1158/1078-0432.CCR-11-0116

Rovira, C., Güida, M.C., & Cayota, A. (2010). MicroRNAs and other small silencing RNAs in cancer. *IUBMB Life, 62,* 859–868. doi:10.1002/iub.399

Rubin, K.M. (2015). Understanding immune checkpoint inhibitors for effective patient care. *Clinical Journal of Oncology Nursing, 19,* 709–717. doi:10.1188/15.CJON.709-717

Rudnitzki, T., & McMahon, D. (2015). Oral agents for cancer: Safety challenges and recommendations. *Clinical Journal of Oncology Nursing, 19,* 41–46. doi:10.1188/15.S1.CJON.41-46

Sanofi-Aventis U.S., LLC. (2013). *Leukine® (sargramostim)* [Package insert]. Bridgewater, NJ: Author.

Schneider, S.M., Hess, K., & Gosselin, T. (2011). Interventions to promote adherence with oral agents. *Seminars in Oncology Nursing, 27,* 133–141. doi:10.1016/j.soncn.2011.02.005

Schulze, M., Stock, C., Zaccagnini, M., Teber, D., & Rassweiler, J.J. (2014). Temsirolimus. In U.M. Martens (Ed.), *Small molecules in cancer research* (2nd ed., pp. 393–403). Heidelberg, Germany: Springer-Verlag.

Scott, A.M., Wolchok, J.D., & Old, L.J. (2012). Antibody therapy of cancer. *Nature Reviews Cancer, 12,* 278–287. doi:10.1038/nrc3236

Senter, P.D., & Sievers, E.L. (2012). The discovery and development of brentuximab vedotin for use in relapsed Hodgkin lymphoma and systemic anaplastic large cell lymphoma. *Nature Biotechnology, 30,* 631–637. doi:10.1038/nbt.2289

Shuptrine, C.W., Surana, R., & Weiner, L.M. (2012). Monoclonal antibodies for the treatment of cancer. *Seminars in Cancer Biology, 22,* 3–13. doi:10.1016/j.semcancer.2011.12.009

Slingerland, M., Guchelaar, H.-J., & Gelderblom, H. (2014). Histone deacetylase inhibitors: An overview of the clinical studies in solid tumors. *Anti-Cancer Drugs, 25,* 140–149. doi:10.1097/CAD.0000000000000040

Spectrum Pharmaceuticals, Inc. (2013). *Zevalin® (ibritumomab tiuxetan) injection for intravenous use* [Package insert]. Irvine, CA: Author.

Spoelstra, S.L., & Sansoucie, H. (2015). Putting evidence into practice: Evidence-based interventions for oral agents for cancer. *Clinical Journal of Oncology Nursing, 19*(Suppl. 3), 60–72. doi:10.1188/15.S1.CJON.60-72

Stephens, T., & Brynner, R. (2001). *Dark remedy: The impact of thalidomide and its revival as a vital medicine.* Cambridge, MA: Basic Books.

Strebhardt, K., & Ullrich, A. (2008). Paul Ehrlich's magic bullet concept: 100 years of progress. *Nature Reviews Cancer, 8,* 473–480. doi:10.1038/nrc2394

Untch, M., Rezai, M., Loibl, S., Fasching, P.A., Huober, J., Tesch, H., ... von Minckwitz, G. (2010). Neoadjuvant treatment with trastuzumab in HER2-positive breast cancer: Results from the GeparQuattro study. *Journal of Clinical Oncology, 28,* 2024–2031. doi:10.1200/JCO.2009.23.8451

U.S. Food and Drug Administration Center for Drug Evaluation and Research. (2016, February). FDA approves cetuximab (Erbitux) and panitumumab (Vectibix). Retrieved from http://www.fda.gov/AboutFDA/CentersOffices/OfficeofMedicalProductsandTobacco/CDER/ucm172905.htm

Wang, T., Shigdar, S., Al Shamaileh, H., Gantier, M.P., Yin, W., Xiang, D., ... Duan, W. (2017). Challenges and opportunities for siRNA-based cancer treatment. *Cancer Letters, 387,* 77–83. doi:10.1016/j.canlet.2016.03.045

Waters, M.F.R. (1971). An internally-controlled double blind trial of thalidomide in severe erythema nodosum leprosum. *Leprosy Review, 42,* 26–42. doi:10.5935/0305-7518.19710004

Weber, D.M., Chen, C., Niesvizky, R., Wang, M., Belch, A., Stadtmauer, E.A., ... Knight, R.D. (2007). Lenalidomide plus dexamethasone for relapsed multiple myeloma in North America. *New England Journal of Medicine, 357,* 2133–2142. doi:10.1056/NEJMoa070596

Weiner, L.M., Surana, R., & Wang, S. (2010). Monoclonal antibodies: Versatile platforms for cancer immunotherapy. *Nature Reviews Immunology, 10,* 317–327. doi:10.1038/nri2744

Weinhold, B. (2006). Epigenetics: The science of change. *Environmental Health Perspectives, 114,* A160–A167.

West, A.C., & Johnstone, R.W. (2014). New and emerging HDAC inhibitors for cancer treatment. *Journal of Clinical Investigation, 124,* 30–39. doi:10.1172/JCI69738

Wiley, K.E. (2007). Multiple myeloma and treatment-related thromboembolism: Oncology nurses' role in prevention, assessment, and diagnosis. *Clinical Journal of Oncology Nursing, 11,* 847–851. doi:10.1188/07.CJON.847-851

Wyeth Pharmaceuticals Inc. (2015). *Torisel® (temsirolimus) injection, for intravenous infusion* [Package insert]. Philadelphia, PA: Author.

Zhu, Y.X., Kortuem, K.M., & Stewart, A.K. (2013). Molecular mechanism of action of immune-modulatory drugs thalidomide, lenalidomide and pomalidomide in multiple myeloma. *Leukemia and Lymphoma, 54,* 683–687. doi:10.3109/10428194.2012.728597

Chapter 10 Study Questions

1. Patients receiving everolimus should be instructed to avoid the use of concomitant CYP3A4 inducers. Which of the following is safe to take when everolimus is prescribed?
   A. Phenytoin
   B. Grapefruit juice
   C. Tomato juice
   D. Dexamethasone

2. Identify a common adverse event associated with sorafenib.
   A. Hand-foot reaction
   B. Anaphylaxis
   C. Hypomagnesemia
   D. Anemia

3. A decreased left ventricular ejection fraction needs to be monitored in which type of targeted therapy?
   A. Mammalian target of rapamycin inhibitor
   B. Histone deacetylase inhibitor
   C. Lapatinib
   D. Alemtuzumab

4. Rituximab targets the CD20 marker. Which of the following markers of malignancies is most sensitive to rituximab?
   A. HER2-positive breast cancer
   B. B-cell
   C. NK-cell
   D. T-cell
   E. EGFR-positive lung cancer

5. The type of antibody conjugated to the medication can be determined by looking at the ending of the generic name. Which type of antibody ends with "-umab"?
   A. Murine
   B. Chimeric
   C. Humanized
   D. Fully human

CHAPTER

11 Hormone Therapy

Rachelle W. Rodriguez, RN, MSN, FNP-BC,
and Virginia Aguilar, RN, MSN, FNP-BC, AOCNP®

Introduction

Hormone therapy is commonly used to treat hormone-sensitive cancers. Hormones are chemical messengers produced in and secreted from endocrine glands to act on specific target cells of other organs or glands. Sometimes referred to as endocrine therapy, hormone therapy is used to alter the hormone levels in the body, either by stimulating release, inhibiting release, or blocking the effects of hormones to prevent the growth of cancers that are sensitive to or dependent on hormones for proliferation. Hormone-dependent tumors rely on the hormones estrogen, progesterone, or testosterone. This chapter will describe approaches to hormone therapy, including (a) reduction of a specific hormone level in the body to decrease the supply available to malignant cells and (b) reduction of cancer cells' ability to respond to the hormone circulating in the body. Accordingly, hormone therapy is only effective in tumors that require hormone for their growth. Cancers commonly treated with hormone therapy are breast, ovarian, endometrial, and prostate cancers.

Hormone therapy is used concomitantly with other treatment modalities, such as surgery, chemotherapy, and radiation. The National Surgical Adjuvant Breast and Bowel Project implemented the Study of Tamoxifen and Raloxifene (STAR) with the agents tamoxifen and raloxifene to determine which would be more effective in preventing breast cancer in women who were never diagnosed but identified as having a high risk for development of the malignancy. The initial results indicated that both medications were equally effective to reduce invasive breast cancer in the targeted population of high-risk women after an average of 47 months of therapy (Cuzick et al., 2013; National Cancer Institute, 2010). After 81 months, raloxifene decreased the incidence of breast cancer by 38% and tamoxifen reduced breast cancer by almost 50% (National Cancer Institute, 2010). Tamoxifen is now used to prevent breast cancer in women at high risk, based on specific guidelines.

In addition to drug therapy, surgical removal of hormone-producing glands or organs can produce the hormone-suppressive effect needed to help shrink or kill cancer cells. Although this treatment option is very effective, it can limit the reproductive capacity of an individual, as well as potentially cause psychological side effects (Kumar, Barqawi, & Crawford, 2005).

Hormone therapy has made great strides since the late 1800s, when surgeons first recognized that removing the ovaries in premenopausal women helped decrease the tumor size in advanced breast cancer in some patients

(Jordan & Furr, 2002; Nunn, 1882). Nearly 50 years later, scientists discovered that the removal of the testes could lead to remission for men with prostate cancer. Accordingly, in the 1950s and 1960s, the standard therapy for treating advanced breast and prostate cancer was removal of the sex hormone–producing organs (Jordan & Furr, 2002).

In the decades that followed, multiple drugs have been developed, all with the goal of inhibiting hormones from feeding cancer cells. In addition to the drugs that alter the body's production of hormones, there are antihormones, aromatase inhibitors (AIs), and gonadotropin-releasing hormone (GnRH) agonists and antagonists.

Antihormones do not reduce the production of hormones, but rather were designed to block cells' ability to respond to the hormones by competing for receptor sites. Examples in this category include tamoxifen, toremifene, raloxifene, and fulvestrant, which are antiestrogen drugs used in breast cancer. Flutamide, bicalutamide, and nilutamide are antiandrogens used in combination therapy with luteinizing hormone–releasing hormone (LHRH) agonists for treatment in prostate cancer (Madan & Dahut, 2014).

AIs target the enzyme aromatase, which is responsible for the production of estrogen from androgens in postmenopausal women. This inhibits the amount of estrogen produced, thus decreasing plasma estrogen levels. This drug class is not effective in premenopausal women because prior to menopause, the production of estrogen is primarily in the ovaries, and not converted from androgens. Drugs included in this category are anastrozole, letrozole, and exemestane (Epocrates, 2015).

Finally, GnRH agonists and antagonists affect hormone production in the anterior pituitary by signaling the body to either secrete or not secrete them. The hypothalamus secretes releasing hormones that cause the release of more hormones from the anterior pituitary. The releasing hormones can either stimulate or inhibit the anterior pituitary hormones. This therapy works for inhibiting the production of estrogen and progesterone. Drugs in this category include goserelin, leuprolide, triptorelin, and degarelix (Epocrates, 2015) (see Table 11-1).

The hormones secreted from the anterior pituitary either directly affect tissues or act on target tissues, which are organs that also secrete hormones. Hormones that affect target tissues to stimulate secretion of more hormones are known as *tropic hormones* (Copstead-Kirkhorn & Banasik, 2013). Releasing hormones include GnRH, growth hormone–releasing hormone (GHRH), somatostatin (SS), thyroid-releasing hormone (TRH), prolactin-inhibiting hormone (PIH), prolactin-releasing hormone (PRH), and corticotropin-releasing hormone (CRH) (see Figure 11-1).

GnRH acts to stimulate the secretion of follicle-stimulating hormone (FSH) and luteinizing hormone (LH). FSH and LH are tropic hormones that act on the target tissues of the gonads (ovaries and testes), which in turn produce estrogens and testosterone. GHRH causes the anterior pituitary to secrete growth hormone, which causes tissue growth (Copstead-Kirkhorn & Banasik, 2013). SS can have an inhibiting effect on both growth hormone and thyroid-stimulating hormone. TRH causes the anterior pituitary to secrete thyroid-stimulating hormone, which acts on the thyroid gland to secrete T_3 and T_4. TRH also has an agonist effect on the secretion of prolactin, as does PRH, which causes the secretion of prolactin. Prolactin causes breast development and milk production. PIH has an antagonistic effect to inhibit the production of prolactin, thus inhibiting milk production. And finally, CRH causes secretion of adrenocorticotropic hormone, which acts on the target tissues of the adrenal cortex to produce cortisol (Copstead-Kirkhorn & Banasik, 2013).

The posterior pituitary gland secretes only two hormones: oxytocin and vasopressin. Oxytocin stimulates uterine contractions and is released during childbirth and breast-feeding. Vasopressin or antidiuretic hormone is

Table 11-1. Characteristics of Hormone Therapies

Medication Name(s)	Mechanism of Action	Dose and Route	Indications	Side Effects	Nursing Considerations
Estrogen Receptor Agonists (Also Known as Selective Estrogen Receptor Modulators)					
Tamoxifen (Nolvadex®)	Inhibits estrogen effects by competing with estrogen for binding on the ER	10 mg PO BID or 20 mg PO QD Optimal duration is 5 years.	Breast cancer with ER+ metastatic tumors or as adjuvant therapy in ER+ tumors after primary therapy in both premenopausal and postmenopausal women	Hot flashes, atrophy of vaginal lining, menstrual irregularities, vaginal bleeding and discharge, pruritus vulvae, nausea, vomiting, hair loss, dermatitis, peripheral edema, reduction in lipid profile, abnormal LFTs, cataract formation	Monitor CBC monthly for myelosuppression. Obtain baseline LFTs. Monitor for endometrial cancer in women with intact uterus. Educate patients regarding discontinuation of use before elective surgery because of increased risk of thromboembolic events, as well as possible bone pain during first few weeks of therapy.
Toremifene (Fareston®)	Competes with estrogen for binding on the ER and inhibits tumor growth–stimulating effects of estrogen	60 mg PO QD	Breast cancer with ER+ tumors in postmenopausal women	Myelosuppression, nausea, vomiting, hot flashes, dizziness, edema, changes in vaginal secretions, increased liver transaminase levels	Monitor for hypercalcemia, especially if patients are using diuretics that may decrease renal calcium excretion, or in patients with bone metastases. Monitor patients on warfarin for an increased prothrombin time. Monitor LFTs. Educate patients regarding potential hot flashes and altered vaginal secretions.
Raloxifene (Evista®)	Competes with estrogen for binding on the ER and inhibits tumor growth–stimulating effects of estrogen	60 mg PO QD	Breast cancer prevention in postmenopausal women and osteoporosis prevention in postmenopausal women	Hot flashes, thromboembolic events, leg cramps, reduction in lipids profile	Assess for history of venous thromboembolic events; risk is especially increased in first 4 months of therapy. Drug must not be taken by women who are pregnant or may become pregnant, as it may cause fetal harm. Drug decreases levothyroxine absorption. Educate patients regarding signs and symptoms of MI, CVA, DVT, and PE and to call emergency services if symptoms occur.

(Continued on next page)

Table 11-1. Characteristics of Hormone Therapies *(Continued)*

Medication Name(s)	Mechanism of Action	Dose and Route	Indications	Side Effects	Nursing Considerations
Estrogen Receptor Antagonists					
Fulvestrant (Faslodex®)	Competitively binds to ER on tumors, decreases DNA synthesis, and inhibits estrogen effects	250 mg IM monthly	Treatment of hormone receptor–positive metastatic breast cancer in postmenopausal women with progressive disease after antiestrogen therapy	Headache, nausea, vomiting, constipation, diarrhea, abdominal pain, pharyngitis, injection site pain, vasodilation	Monitor for GI symptoms, and treat PRN. Educate patients to report any vaginal bleeding, especially at beginning of therapy.
Antiandrogens					
Flutamide (Eulexin®)	Nonsteroidal antiandrogen that competes with androgens for receptor sites in target tissues	250 mg PO TID	Metastatic prostate cancer in combination therapy with LHRH agonists	Breast tenderness, galactorrhea, gynecomastia, hot flashes, impotence, decreased libido, tumor flare, nausea, vomiting, transient increase of transaminase enzymes	Monitor liver enzymes. Educate patients regarding possible sexual dysfunction, breast swelling, and hot flashes. Drug should be taken on empty stomach, unless patient has GI intolerance. Assess family dynamics and refer to counseling if sexual dysfunction interferes with well-being.
Bicalutamide (Casodex®)	Nonsteroidal antiandrogen that competitively binds to androgen receptors, preventing testosterone stimulation of cell growth in prostate cancer	50 mg PO QD in combination with an LHRH agonist	Metastatic prostate cancer in combination with LHRH agonists	Hot flashes, peripheral edema, pain, nausea, vomiting, constipation, diarrhea, pelvic pain, hematuria, back pain, weakness, dyspnea	Obtain baseline LFTs and monitor during first 4 months of treatment for signs or symptoms of liver dysfunction. Monitor for GI symptoms.

(Continued on next page)

Table 11-1. Characteristics of Hormone Therapies *(Continued)*

Medication Name(s)	Mechanism of Action	Dose and Route	Indications	Side Effects	Nursing Considerations
Aromatase Inhibitors					
Anastrozole (Arimidex®)	Type II nonsteroidal imidazole inhibitor that binds competitively to the aromatase enzyme, decreasing biosynthesis of estrogen	1 mg PO QD	Women with ER+ breast cancer, treatment of postmenopausal women with ER+/PR+ breast cancer, adjuvant treatment of postmenopausal breast cancer	Myelosuppression, asthenia, nausea, vomiting, rash, headache, myalgia, arthralgia, peripheral edema, weight gain, dyspnea, cough, constipation, diarrhea, hot flashes	Drug interacts with warfarin, dextromethorphan, nifedipine, tolbutamide, and phenacetin. Educate patients regarding possible hot flashes. Monitor for GI symptoms. Monitor CBC, edema, and weight. Administer analgesics PRN.
Letrozole (Femara®)	Type II nonsteroidal imidazole inhibitor that binds competitively to the aromatase enzyme, decreasing biosynthesis of estrogen	2.5 mg PO QD	ER+ advanced breast cancer in postmenopausal women with progressive disease after antiestrogen treatment	Hot flashes, musculoskeletal pain, headache, sleepiness, fatigue, dizziness, osteoporosis, fractures, nausea, vomiting, hair thinning	Educate patients regarding possible hot flashes and to use caution when driving or performing other tasks requiring alertness. Administer analgesics PRN.
Exemestane (Aromasin®)	Type I steroidal inactivator that irreversibly inactivates the aromatase enzyme	25 mg PO QD	Advanced ER+ breast cancer in postmenopausal women until disease progression or after treatment with nonsteroidal aromatase inhibitors until disease progression	Arthralgia, diarrhea, muscle cramping, fractures, visual disturbances, irregular vaginal discharges	Educate patients to take after a meal. Patients should also take a calcium and vitamin D supplement to help prevent fractures. Warn patients to not drive or do activities that require good vision until effect of drug is known. Monitor symptoms.

(Continued on next page)

Table 11-1. Characteristics of Hormone Therapies *(Continued)*

Medication Name(s)	Mechanism of Action	Dose and Route	Indications	Side Effects	Nursing Considerations
Gonadotropin-Releasing Hormone Agonists (Includes LHRH Agonists)					
Goserelin (Zoladex®)	Synthetic analog of LHRH that causes an initial increase of LH and FSH, then sustained suppression of pituitary gonadotropins, dropping serum testosterone to castration levels	3.6 mg SC into upper abdomen every 28 days	Palliative treatment of advanced breast and prostate cancers	Headache, depression, insomnia, hot flashes, sexual dysfunction, arrhythmia, CVA, HTN, MI	Apply ice to injection site prior to injection to reduce discomfort. Educate patients regarding possible sexual dysfunction, hot flashes, depression, and insomnia. Symptom management may include analgesics and/or antidepressants. Wearing cool, loose clothing may help provide comfort with hot flashes. Educate patients regarding signs and symptoms of MI and CVA and to call emergency services if symptoms occur.
Leuprolide (Lupron®)	Potent analog of LHRH that inhibits gonadotropin secretion; causes initial rise in LH and FSH, followed by decreased levels of LH and FSH, thereby significantly decreasing estrogen and testosterone to levels of castration	7.5 mg IM every 28 days, 22.5 mg IM every 3 months, or 45 mg IM every 6 months	Palliative treatment of metastatic prostate cancer	Hot flashes, injection site reaction, tumor flare, peripheral edema, sexual dysfunction	Transient increases in testosterone levels occur at start of treatment. Monitor closely for weakness, paresthesias, hematuria, urinary tract obstruction, or peripheral edema in first few weeks of therapy. Educate patients that tumor flare (increasing bone pain) may occur at beginning of treatment. Patients may take analgesics PRN. Monitor for hot flashes. Wearing cool, loose clothing may help. Educate patients that decreased libido and impotence can occur. Assess family dynamics and refer to counseling if sexual dysfunction interferes with well-being.

(Continued on next page)

Table 11-1. Characteristics of Hormone Therapies *(Continued)*

Medication Name(s)	Mechanism of Action	Dose and Route	Indications	Side Effects	Nursing Considerations
Triptorelin (Trelstar®)	Suppression of estrogen and testosterone by decreased levels of LH and FSH	3.75 mg IM every 28 days	Palliative treatment of advanced prostate cancer as alternative to orchiectomy or estrogen administration	Hot flashes, headache, bone pain, peripheral edema, sexual dysfunction, tumor flare	Monitor testosterone levels and PSA. Educate patients regarding possible tumor flare, transient hematuria, or urinary retention during initial treatment, as well as hot flashes.
Degarelix (Firmagon®)	Suppression of testosterone by binding to GnRH receptors in the pituitary, which blocks release of LH and FSH	80 mg SC every 28 days	Palliative treatment of metastatic prostate cancer	Injection site reaction, hot flashes, headache, weight gain, sexual dysfunction, QT prolongation, bone density loss, abnormal LFTs	Monitor LFTs, ECG, and electrolytes at baseline.
Progestins					
Medroxyprogesterone acetate (Provera®, Depo-Provera®)	Inhibits secretion of gonadotropins, prevents follicular maturation and ovulation, and causes endometrial thinning	1,000–1,500 mg IM weekly, 400–800 mg PO twice weekly, or 200 mg PO QD	Advanced/recurrent ER+ and PR+ endometrial cancer	Dizziness, headache, decreased libido, menstrual irregularities, abdominal discomfort, weight gain	Measure baseline weight and monitor. Educate patients regarding menstrual irregularities and sexual disturbances.
Megestrol acetate (Megace®)	Synthetic progestin that interferes with normal estrogen cycle, resulting in lower LH	160 mg PO QD	Advanced/recurrent ER+ and PR+ endometrial cancer	Hypercalcemia with initial therapy, mild fluid retention, abnormal LFTs, menstrual irregularities, improved appetite, weight gain, diarrhea, impotence	Monitor for symptoms of hypercalcemia. Obtain baseline weight, chemistry panel, and LFTs. Educate patients regarding potential weight gain. Monitor weight and LFTs.

BID—twice a day; CBC—complete blood count; CVA—cerebrovascular accident; DVT—deep vein thrombosis; ECG—electrocardiogram; ER+/-—estrogen receptor positive/negative; FSH—follicle-stimulating hormone; GI—gastrointestinal; GnRH—gonadotropin-releasing hormone; HTN—hypertension; IM—intramuscularly; LFT—liver function test; LH—luteinizing hormone; LHRH—luteinizing hormone–releasing hormone; MI—myocardial infarction; PE—pulmonary embolism; PO—by mouth; PR—progesterone receptor; PRN—as needed; PSA—prostate-specific antigen; QD—every day; SC—subcutaneously; TID—three times a day

Note. Based on information from Chabner & Longo, 2014; Govindan & Morgensztern, 2015; Shore, 2013; Solimando, 2007.

Figure 11-1. Hormones of the Anterior Pituitary

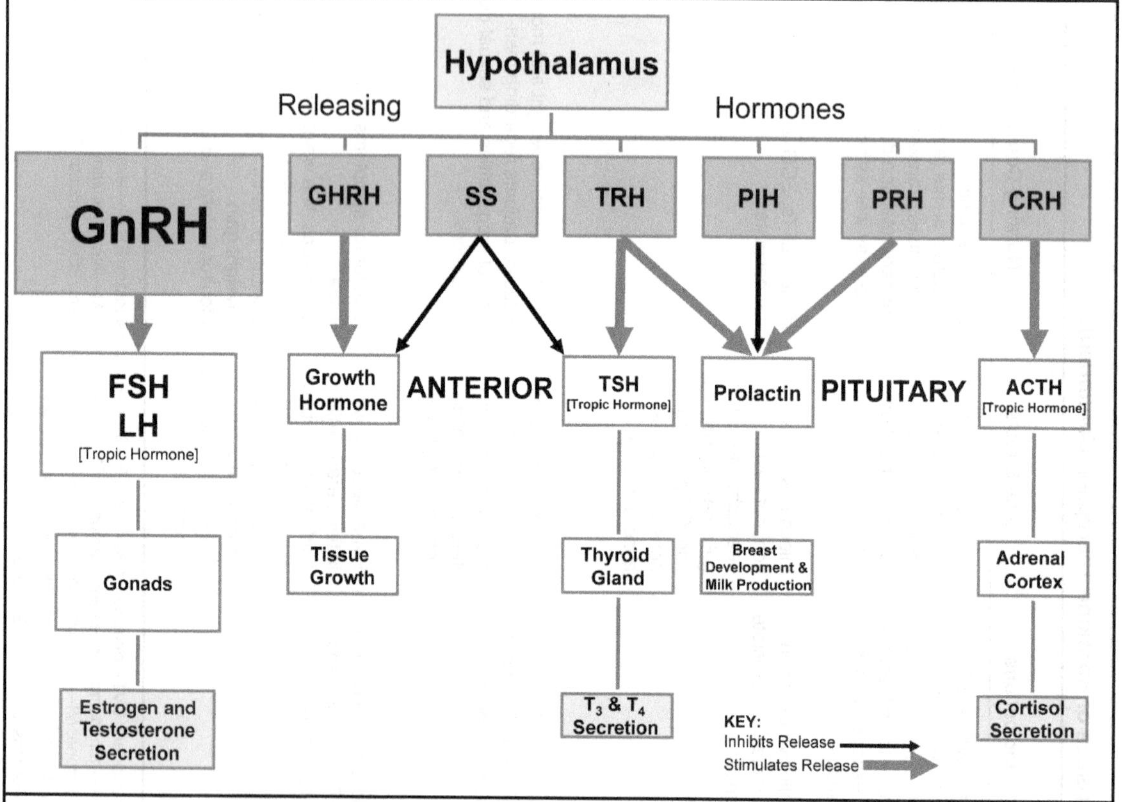

ACTH—adrenocorticotropic hormone; CRH—corticotropin-releasing hormone; FSH—follicle-stimulating hormone; GHRH—growth hormone–releasing hormone; GnRH—gonadotropin-releasing hormone; LH—luteinizing hormone; PIH—prolactin-inhibiting hormone; PRH—prolactin-releasing hormone; SS—somatostatin; TRH—thyroid-releasing hormone; TSH—thyroid-stimulating hormone; T_3—triiodothyronine; T_4—thyroxine

Note. Based on information from Brashers & Jones, 2010.

released when serum osmolality is altered and causes water reabsorption in the renal collecting duct (Copstead-Kirkhorn & Banasik, 2013).

Hormone Therapy in Specific Cancers

Breast Cancer

Breast cancer is the most common cancer in females and the most common cause of cancer deaths in women 45–49 years of age (American Cancer Society [ACS], 2015b) (see also Chapter 5). A majority of breast cancers will require estrogen to enhance the growth of the tumor, otherwise known as *estrogen dependent* (WebMD, 2015). Estrogen-dependent cancer cells produce hormone receptors that have estrogen receptors.

Estrogen is primarily produced in the ovaries until menopause, and then it is produced in the adrenal glands and metabolized in adipose tissue. Estrogen levels are regulated by a negative feedback loop within the hypothalamus. When the hypothalamus detects decreased levels of estrogen in the bloodstream, it secretes GnRH, which stimulates the anterior pituitary gland to release FSH and LH, both of which stimulate the ovaries to produce estrogen (Epocrates, 2015; McCance, 2014) (see Figure 11-2).

Accordingly, ovarian ablation either by surgical resection or radiation therapy is an effective way to decrease estrogen production in the body, thus cutting off the supply to the estrogen-dependent tumor. A woman can also be put into a menopausal state medically with LHRH agonist drugs, such as goserelin by subcutaneous injection or leuprolide by intramuscular injection administered either monthly or biannually, depending on formulation. An oophorectomy, the surgical resection of the ovaries, can make disease management more effective and improve quality of life by eliminating injections and the unfavorable side effects related to the medications. However, LHRH therapy allows for reversible suppression of ovarian function, which may be an important consideration for women of childbearing age (Bush, 2007). Menopause is measured by FSH and estradiol levels, not simply amenorrhea (Bush, 2007).

Figure 11-2. Negative Feedback Loop

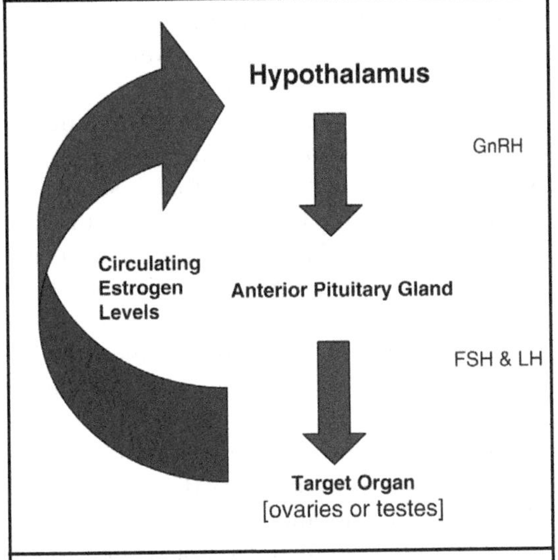

FSH—follicle-stimulating hormone; GnRH—gonadotropin-releasing hormone; LH—luteinizing hormone

The women who benefit from decreased estrogen levels are those with a tumor that has positive estrogen receptor sites. Adjuvant systemic therapy is any additional therapy given after a cancer is surgically removed via mastectomy or lymph node dissection. Adjuvant hormone therapy in breast cancer prevents cancer cells from receiving estrogen. The best known adjuvant drug is tamoxifen, a selective estrogen receptor modulator approved for use in patients with breast cancer (Bush, 2007). This drug prevents estrogen from binding to estrogen receptors on cancer cells, as well as receptors on other estrogen-sensitive organs, such as the endometrium. Undesirable side effects are similar to the symptoms of menopause, which can include hot flashes and vaginal dryness. Others include endometrial cancer, cataract formation, and thromboembolic events (Bush, 2007). Tamoxifen reduces the risk of breast cancer recurrence by 50% and mortality by 28% (Jankowitz & Davidson, 2014). Standard therapy with tamoxifen was initially five years, although treatment has been extended to 10 years as a result of oncology clinical trials research. The American Society of Clinical Oncology Clinical Practice Guidelines note this is due to the associated lower risks of breast cancer recurrence and new lesions in the contralateral breast (Burstein et al., 2014).

Two other selective estrogen receptor modulators, which also compete with estrogen for receptor sites on the tumor, are toremifene and raloxifene. Toremifene is nonsteroidal and approved for treating locally advanced or metastatic breast cancer in postmenopausal women. There is a cross-resistance between tamoxifen and toremifene, so toremifene is ineffective as a second-line agent if tamoxifen has already failed. Another drug, raloxifene, was studied to determine if it was as effective as tamoxifen in women with a high risk of developing breast cancer but never diagnosed with this malignancy. The initial reports from this STAR study found that similar to tamoxifen, raloxifene also reduced the risk of developing invasive breast cancer by 50%, but the side effect profile for raloxifene is significantly improved compared to tamoxifen. Although the risks for stroke, heart attacks, and fractures are the same for both drugs, four-year follow-up data showed 36% fewer uterine cancers and 29% fewer blood clots for the study participants taking raloxifene versus tamoxifen. While useful to prevent breast cancer from developing in never diagnosed, high-risk women older than 35 years of age, raloxifene is not recommended for treatment of hormone sensitive breast cancer (National Comprehensive Cancer Network® [NCCN®], 2016a, 2016b).

Another class of drugs useful in hormone therapy is the AIs, which includes anastrozole, letrozole, and exemestane. These drugs are designed for postmenopausal women only, unlike selective estrogen response modulators, which can be used in both premenopausal and postmenopausal women. After menopause, the adrenal glands are responsible for androgen secretion. These androgens are then converted to estrogen by the enzyme aromatase, which is present in muscles, adipose tissue, and breast tumors. The AIs block the synthesis of estrogen by inhibiting the enzyme aromatase (NCCN, 2016a, 2016b).

AIs do not have agonist effects so there is no increased risk of thromboembolism or endometrial cancer as with tamoxifen. Also, women who have developed a resistance to tamoxifen may be switched to an AI without a cross drug resistant effect. Many research studies have compared tamoxifen and anastrozole in the adjuvant hormone therapy of early breast cancer in postmenopausal women. A double-blind, randomized, phase III study showed that anastrozole provided higher breast cancer–free survival rates, mainly in women younger than age 60, than tamoxifen following ductal carcinoma in situ (Margolese et al., 2016).

Other studies have led to the recommendation for women with a risk of recurrence after chemotherapy to have ovarian function suppression plus adjuvant hormone suppression therapy to significantly reduce the incidence of recurrence (Francis et al., 2015). No formal risk criteria have been developed; however, patients at risk would include those with pathologically involved lymph nodes, large tumor size, high tumor grade, and lymphovascular invasion, as well as patients with a high risk of recurrence based on the genomic assay. Women younger than 35 years old would also be considered high risk.

Estrogen receptor antagonists bind to estrogen receptors but have no agonistic side effects. Fulvestrant is approved for second-line hormone treatment in postmenopausal women with advanced breast cancer after progression on antiestrogen therapy. Fulvestrant destroys the estrogen receptors and reduces progesterone receptors as well. It has no cross-resistance with other hormone treatments (Howell, 2006).

Endometrial Cancer

Endometrial cancer is the most common gynecologic cancer of the Western world; 60,050 new diagnoses and 10,470 deaths were estimated to occur in the United States in 2016 (ACS, 2016a, 2016b). Endometrial cancer type I is another primary cancer that is sensitive to hormone therapy. One of the strongest risk factors for endometrial cancer is a high estrogen state in the body (Ferguson & Herzog, 2004). The estrogen exposure can be from external sources, such as hormone replacement therapy and tamoxifen use, or from internal sources, such as early menarche with late menopause, obesity, polycystic ovary syndrome, and estrogen-secreting tumors in the ovary (Garrett & Quinn, 2008). Type II endometrial cancer is more prevalent in older populations, not related to hormones, and has higher rates of recurrence and metastasis (Lee, Yen, et al., 2014).

As already discussed, unopposed estrogen therapy is one of the main causes of endometrial cancer. Progesterone acts to antagonize the estrogen effects on endometrial carcinoma (Genazzani & Gadducci, 2002), thereby starving the cancer cells of estrogen and inhibiting tumor growth. However, treatment recommendations include surgery, chemotherapy, radiation, or a combination of the three for first-line treatment. Hormone treatment is only used in patients with stage IV recurrent disease and only in endometrioid histology after estrogen receptor and progesterone receptor levels have been checked. In this select population, hormone therapy with either megestrol acetate or medroxyprogesterone acetate produces responses in 15%–30% of patients and is associated with a survival benefit twice as long as nonresponders (Noonan & Annunziata, 2014).

Although most commonly known for its use as a mainstay of therapy for estrogen receptor–positive breast cancer, tamoxifen has been studied as a treatment option for endometrial cancer. Tamoxifen competitively binds to estrogen receptors and causes a decrease in estrogen receptors and an increase in progesterone receptors. Use of tamoxifen has a response rate of 10%–22% when used in advanced endometrial cancer (Rauh-Hain & del Carmen, 2010).

Overall, limited research exists regarding the use of hormone treatment in endometrial cancer. The rationale is that the tumors more likely to respond to hormone therapy are low-grade, hormone receptor–positive cancers, and the most effective management is surgery for total hysterectomy and bilateral salpingo-oophorectomy (Lee, Yen, et al., 2014). The more aggressive tumors, type II endometrial cancer, are more likely to be hormone receptor negative.

Recommendations for adjuvant therapy after surgical resection for endometrial cancer are mixed. Hacker and Friedlander (2010) stated that progesterone administration following surgery has not been shown to prevent recurrence. However, low-grade, hormone receptor–positive tumors seem to respond to progesterone therapy. Endocrine therapy has demonstrated efficacy and can be used before chemotherapy for well-differentiated (grade 1) tumors (Markman, 2014). Additionally, in patients with advanced or recurrent disease, progestins with or without tamoxifen can be used, although the response rate is poor (Lee, Yen, et al., 2014).

Ovarian Cancer

Ovarian cancer is diagnosed in more than 22,000 women each year in the United States and is the fifth leading cause of cancer death in women (ACS, 2016d). Because it usually is not diagnosed early, it has the highest mortality rate of all the gynecologic cancers (ACS, 2016a).

Oral contraceptives, a hormonal form of birth control, have been found to reduce the risk of ovarian cancer by 30%–60%, and the reduction in risk continues for 15 years (Garrett & Quinn, 2008). Other protective factors include tubal ligation, breast-feeding, and progesterone use.

In stage IA or IB ovarian cancer, when the tumors are limited to one or both ovaries, have no detectable abdominal ascites, and are contained within the ovarian capsule, surgery to debulk the tumor is sufficient treatment, carrying a 95% 10-year survival rate (Reed, 2014). Chemotherapy is then administered for higher-grade tumors.

Surgical oophorectomy for early-stage tumors and chemotherapy are the usual treatments for ovarian cancer. Hormone treatment (tamoxifen) is used for either asymptomatic cases with rising CA-125 or cases in which comorbidity excludes more aggressive treatment (Reed, 2014). CA-125 is a serum biomarker that is increased in approximately 50% of early-stage and greater than 90% of advanced-stage ovarian cancers. Unfortunately, its specificity for ovarian cancer is poor, and it can be increased in many benign conditions as well (Lee, de Meritens, Moon, & Kohn, 2014). Because of poor response to therapy, endocrine therapy is only occasionally used in patients with evidence of asymptomatic progression who have hormone-positive receptors. No benefit was shown for endocrine therapy over active surveillance (Birrer & Fujiwara, 2016).

Progesterone use also was proposed for treatment in ovarian cancer. Ovarian cancer cells have hormone receptors, so this therapy seemed plausible. Unfortunately, in the presence of malignant ovarian tumors, the progesterone receptor levels decrease, and tumor response rates were modest at best; therefore, more studies are needed (Williams, Simera, & Bryant, 2010).

Although GnRH receptors are present in 80% of ovarian cancer cells, response rates with GnRH analogs were poor—between 9% and 12% (Duffaud et al., 2001). Accordingly, GnRH analogs are not recommended as part of treatment regimens for ovarian cancer.

Prostate Cancer

Prostate cancer is the second leading cause of cancer death for men in the United States, with approximately 180,890 new diagnoses and 26,120 deaths estimated in 2016 (ACS, 2016c). Autopsies have shown that 30% of men older than age 50 and 70% of men older than age 80 had localized prostate cancer at the time of death (Venkatesh, Strope, & Roth, 2015); most were probably not aware they had the disease.

Androgen deprivation therapy was determined to be an effective treatment for metastatic prostate cancer in 1941 when Nobel laureate Charles Huggins discovered the importance of androgenic influences on the growth of prostate cells (Huggins & Hodges, 1941). Androgen deprivation therapy prolongs survival and decreases bone pain in most patients, but it is still considered palliative therapy. In the early 1980s, high levels of dihydrotestosterone were found in prostate tissue. Dihydrotestosterone increases protein synthesis, which led to the understanding that adrenal androgens were more important than originally believed (ACS, 2016d; Lee & Smith, 2016).

One of the first androgen deprivation therapy drugs developed was diethylstilbestrol (DES), a nonsteroidal estrogen. Estrogens work by a negative feedback to the hypothalamus. High levels of estrogen inhibit the release of LHRH from the hypothalamus, which in turn suppresses the release of LH from the anterior pituitary. This causes the Leyden cells to stop producing testosterone (Copstead-Kirkhorn & Banasik, 2013). The advantages are that in addition to achieving castration levels of testosterone in the body, the estrogen helps prevent bone loss. Unfortunately, it carries significant risk of cardiovascular toxicity, and consequently DES is no longer sold in the United States. Newer GnRH agonists have since been developed that do not have the cardiovascular toxicity found in DES.

Quality-of-life issues play a large part in treatment decisions for prostate cancer, as does the stage of disease at diagnosis. The current trend is to treat according to the patient's serum prostate-specific antigen (PSA). A significant correlation exists among PSA response, time to progression, and overall survival (Hussain et al., 2006). The goal for all prostate cancer therapies is to decrease testosterone levels to those found in castration to inhibit tumor growth (Lee & Smith, 2016).

For localized prostate cancer, treatment options range from expectant management to prostatectomy (laparoscopic radical prostatectomy with or without robotic assistance, or radical retropubic prostatectomy), radiation (external beam or brachytherapy), or cryotherapy (Ward, Vogelzang, & Davis, 2016). Neoadjuvant hormone therapy is used for locally advanced prostate cancer prior to, during, and after external beam radiation therapy (Ward et al., 2016).

The American Society of Clinical Oncology recommends the use of GnRH agonists as part of prostate cancer treatment. GnRH agonists bind to GnRH receptors on pituitary gonadotropin-producing cells, LH, and FSH. Initially, a transient rise of testosterone levels occurs, frequently referred to as *tumor flare*, which may worsen metastatic symptoms such as bone pain, spinal cord compression, and impending ureteric obstruction (Madan & Dahut, 2014). Accordingly, patients with vertebral metastases and urethral obstruction should be closely monitored for weakness, paresthesias, hematuria, and urinary tract obstruction during the first few weeks of therapy (Madan & Dahut, 2014). To prevent the expected flare, combination therapy with an antiandrogen drug such as flutamide, bicalutamide, or nilutamide is commonly used (Madan & Dahut, 2014).

Combined androgen blockade, the term used to describe GnRH agonist therapy plus antiandrogen therapy, is sometimes used for approximately one week prior to the start of GnRH agonist therapy. It is thought to help prevent the initial rise of testosterone in the body. Antiandrogens compete with other androgens in the body by binding to androgen receptors (Chen, Clegg, & Scher, 2009). The benefit of combined androgen blockade as first-line treatment is controversial and has shown limited evidence of clinical benefit, but antiandrogens have a role when used to block the side effects associated with the flare phenomenon at the initiation of androgen deprivation therapy or for long-term treatment to increase the efficacy of androgen deprivation therapy (Shah, Zhu, & Dahut, 2014). Several studies have been designed and implemented that compare combined androgen blocking and GnRH monotherapy, but results have been inconsistent. Meta-analyses of data have shown that a small improvement (1%–5%) may result with combined androgen blockade therapy (Loblaw et al., 2007). Several meta-analyses suggest five-year survival benefits, and in the studies that excluded the steroidal antiandrogen cyproterone acetate for therapy, statistically significant reduction in mortality occurred with combined androgen blockage (Lee & Smith, 2016). Combined androgen therapy is an appropriate option for second-line treatment per NCCN (2016c) guidelines.

An alternative to combined androgen blockade is intermittent androgen deprivation. This refers to the cyclic administration of GnRH agonists plus an antiandrogen, allowing the patient to have periods where the side effects are mitigated. Early studies with overall survival as the endpoint showed no significant difference in disease progression (Crook et al., 2012). However, a later study showed statistically inconclusive results regarding survival but a 10% relative increase in the risk of death with intermittent therapy, and the authors posited that a larger sample size would be needed to show statistical differences. With regard to quality of life, the patients on intermittent therapy showed higher indices at three months but no statistical difference after three months (Hussain et al., 2013). Because the research has not shown a significant difference in survival or quality of life, continuous therapy remains the standard of treatment (Lee & Smith, 2016).

Several formulations of GnRH agonists have been developed and studied. Leuprolide is administered by intramuscular injection and can be dosed once every 28 days or every three, four, or six months. Another form, goserelin, can be injected subcutaneously every 28 days, or a longer-term preparation, the three-month implant, can be injected every 12 weeks (Epocrates, 2015). The physician's preference will play a large part in determining which formulation is used. As already stated, LHRH agonists frequently are used in combination therapy with antiandrogens. Antiandrogens used in combination therapy for initial treatment for metastatic prostate cancer are flutamide, bicalutamide, or nilutamide. However, the benefits for initial long-term combination therapy are not clear for combined androgen blockade, and the side effects must be carefully considered (Lee & Smith, 2016).

An alternative option to exogenous hormone therapy is surgical orchiectomy. It is cost-effective, provides an immediate decrease in circulating testosterone, and minimizes issues of patient compliance. Unfortunately, the negative psychological impact makes this choice very rare. Decreased testosterone, which is the desired therapeutic effect, leads to fatigue, loss of muscle and bone mass, and decreased sexual capacity (Lee & Smith, 2016).

Side Effects of Hormone Therapy

The side effects of hormone therapy in cancer treatment arise from disruption or increase in hormone levels, affecting various parts of the body. Disruption of testosterone in a man leads to a decrease in sexual desire, possible impotence, enlarged breasts (gynecomastia), and symptoms of menopause, including hot flashes, incontinence, and osteoporosis (ACS, 2015a). Eliminating estrogen in a woman will cause menopausal symptoms, including fatigue, hot flashes, mood swings, osteoporosis, and weight gain. Everyone receiving hormone therapy can have nausea and memory problems. Side effects can adversely affect quality of life and can easily cause patients to discontinue therapy. An important nursing consideration when evaluating patients on hormone suppressive therapy is careful assessment of side effects and how well patients are tolerating them (ACS, 2015b).

The Role of Supplements in Hormone-Sensitive Cancers

With an increasing interest in healthy lifestyles and complementary and alternative medicine, the supplement market is ever expanding. Currently, there is little regulation of this industry and little to no standardization of products. Many times, patients believe they are contributing to their health and well-being by treating common ailments with natural supplements. For instance, based on a myth, many individuals take large doses of vitamin C to help treat or prevent a cold (Pauling, 1977). Vitamin E is popular to aid in heart health. Many sports supplements contain a combination of herbal products, anything from flaxseed to androstenedione. Patients often do not consider supplements and herbal remedies to be medications and frequently do not report them to their healthcare team. Unfortunately, some herbal supplements have an estrogenic effect on the body, which can compete with the hormone therapy prescribed by the physician, thereby providing the estrogen needed for cancer cell growth. Not all supplements have this effect, but careful review of all medications and supplements with patients is important to ensure optimal hormone therapy (see Table 11-2).

Treatments on the Horizon

Because of the extraordinary availability of funds for breast cancer research, several potential treatments are being developed. Studies have shown a recurrent mutation in the estrogen receptor 1 (*ESR1*) gene that encodes protein that allows the cancer to acquire resistance to endocrine therapy (Toy et al., 2013). This has led to investigation of selective estrogen receptor downregulators that could inhibit these mutated receptors from producing proteins that promote resistance to endocrine therapy (Chandarlapaty, 2015). Another avenue of exploration is small molecular inhibitor proteins required for the control of gene expression to prevent programmed cell death. New therapies of this type promote apoptosis and antiproliferative effects on the tumor cells (Toy et al., 2013). A third area of development is for estrogen receptor–positive breast cancers deprived of estrogen after prolonged endocrine therapy plus phosphoinositide 3-kinase (PI3K) pathway inhibitors. Mutations in this pathway are seen in estrogen receptor–positive

Table 11-2. Herbal Supplements That Can Interact With Hormone-Sensitive Cancers

Supplement Name	Common Reasons for Taking
Aletris	Rheumatism, female disorders, sedative, laxative, antispasmodic, diuretic
Alfalfa	Diuretic; kidney, bladder, and prostate health; asthma, arthritis, diabetes
Androstenedione	Enhances athletic performance
Anise	Antiflatulent, expectorant
Black tea	Reduce risk of gastrointestinal, ovarian, and breast cancer
Boron	Osteoarthritis, build muscle, increase testosterone levels
Chasteberry	Menstrual and menopausal conditions, acne, miscarriage prevention
Coenzyme Q10	Prevent cardiotoxicity related to chemotherapy
Cohosh	Natural hormone replacement therapy
Deer velvet	Anticancer and anti-inflammatory properties
DHEA	Prevention of heart disease, breast cancer, and diabetes
Dong quai	Gynecologic symptoms
Fennel	Initiation of menstruation
Flaxseed	Constipation, bladder inflammation, prevention of cancer
Ginseng	Atherosclerosis, bleeding disorders, cancer, colitis, rheumatism, memory loss
Glucosamine	Osteoarthritis, weight loss
Hydrazine sulfate	Prevention of weight loss and wasting (cachexia) associated with cancer
Kefir	Improve digestion, hyperlipidemia, and lactose intolerance
Lactobacillus	Diarrhea or digestive conditions
Licorice	Upper respiratory tract conditions, gastrointestinal conditions
Milk thistle	Gastrointestinal and hepatic ailments, treatment of prostate cancer
Pregnenolone	Slowing or reversing of aging
Progesterone	Gynecologic symptoms
Raspberry leaf	Respiratory, cardiovascular, and gastrointestinal disorders
Red clover	Bronchial conditions
Resveratrol	Atherosclerosis, prevention of cancer, lower cholesterol levels
Scarlet pimpernel	Depression, liver and kidney disorders, treatment of cancer
Soy	Prevention of breast or prostate cancer
Star anise	Gastrointestinal and respiratory problems
Vitamin C (high concentrations)	Treatment of the common cold
Vitamin E (high concentrations)	Treatment of cardiovascular conditions and cancer
Wild yam	Used as an estrogen alternative

Note. Based on information from Montbriand, 2004.

breast cancers after prolonged estrogen deprivation and are associated with increased cell proliferation with enhanced survival, growth factor production independent of the cell type and receptor, loss of apoptosis, and resistance to different medications (Janku et al., 2012). Lastly, studies are evaluating endocrine therapy plus CDK4/CDK6 inhibitors to inhibit cellular proliferation and apoptosis associated with the mammalian target of the rapamycin signaling pathway (Baselga et al., 2012).

Conclusion

The goal of hormone therapy in cancer is to prevent the cancer cell from getting the hormone it needs for growth, thereby either halting tumor growth or enhancing the kill of the tumor altogether. Scientific research is continuing to move forward, but much still remains to learn about hormonal influences on cancer cells. Scientists and researchers persistently look for more receptor site–specific therapies to make treatments more effective while decreasing the unpleasant side effects associated with hormone therapies that diminish patients' quality of life during treatment.

Breast cancer has received much national attention and funding. Continued funding is vital for the research necessary to develop new drugs and therapies, as well as the participation of patients in clinical trials. Information for patients is available on multiple websites (see Table 11-3). In this age of technology, most patients and family members will have already done research on the Internet and will have multiple questions about their condition ready for their nurse and the doctor. Nurses need to be not only aware of how and where patients are getting their information, but also educated on the different therapy options available and those available through trial participation so that they are a valuable resource for inquisitive and anxious patients and families.

Table 11-3. Patient Resources

Name	Website
American Cancer Society	www.cancer.org
American Society of Clinical Oncology	www.cancer.net
Breast Cancer Risk Assessment Tool	www.cancer.gov/bcrisktool
Cancer Guide: A Treatment and Facilities Guide for Patients and Their Families; published quarterly	www.patientresource.net
Caregiver Action Network	http://caregiveraction.org
CURE magazine	www.curetoday.com
National Cancer Institute	www.cancer.gov
National Comprehensive Cancer Network®	www.nccn.org
Susan G. Komen	www.komen.org

References

American Cancer Society. (2015a). Hormone (androgen deprivation) therapy for prostate cancer. Retrieved from http://www.cancer.org/cancer/prostatecancer/detailedguide/prostate-treating-hormone-therapy

American Cancer Society. (2015b). Hormone therapy for breast cancer. Retrieved from http://www.cancer.org/cancer/detailedguide/breast-cancer-treating-hormone-therapy

American Cancer Society. (2016a). *Cancer facts and figures 2016.* Atlanta, GA: Author.

American Cancer Society. (2016b). Key statistics for endometrial cancer? Retrieved from https://www.cancer.org/cancer/endometrial-cancer/about/key-statistics.html

American Cancer Society. (2016c). Key statistics for prostate cancer. Retrieved from http://www.cancer.org/cancer/prostatecancer/detailedguide/prostate-cancer-key-statistics

Key Points

- Sometimes referred to as endocrine therapy, hormone therapy is used to alter the hormones in the body, either by stimulating release of hormones, inhibiting the release of hormones, or blocking the effects of hormones to prevent the growth of hormone-sensitive cancers.
- Two methods of hormone therapy use exist: either to reduce a specific hormone level in the body, or to reduce the cancer cells' ability to respond to the hormone.
- In addition to the drugs that alter the body's production of hormones, there are antihormones, AIs, and GnRH agonists and antagonists.
- The hypothalamus secretes releasing hormones that cause the release of more hormones from the anterior pituitary. The released hormones either stimulate or inhibit the anterior pituitary hormones. The anterior pituitary either affects the tissues directly or acts on target tissues. Hormones that target tissues to stimulate secretion of more hormones are known as tropic hormones.
- Tamoxifen is appropriate hormone therapy for premenopausal women with estrogen receptor–positive breast cancer. This drug prevents estrogen from binding to estrogen receptors in the cancer cells.
- Anastrozole and other AIs are appropriate for postmenopausal women because they block the synthesis of estrogen by inhibiting the enzyme aromatase. If they are used in premenopausal women, the reduction in feedback of estrogen to the hypothalamus could increase tumor growth and pituitary by causing increased secretion of estradiol for estrogen-positive tumors.
- Hormone therapy is limited in endometrial cancer and ovarian cancer, for which the mainstay of treatment is surgery, chemotherapy, and radiation.
- The goal for all prostate cancer therapies is to decrease testosterone to castration levels to inhibit tumor growth. This can be achieved surgically (castration) or chemically with androgen deprivation therapy.
- In metastatic prostate cancer, it is important to start a GnRH agonist such as flutamide at least one week prior to the initiation of androgen deprivation therapy (leuprolide) because of the potential for tumor flare.
- Nurses need to ascertain exactly what medications and supplements patients are taking at home. Also, if they are not taking their hormone therapy consistently, try to determine if the nonadherence is due to intolerable side effects.

American Cancer Society. (2016d). What are the key statistics about ovarian cancer? Retrieved from http://www.cancer.org/cancer/ovariancancer/detailedguide/ovarian-cancer-key-statistics

Baselga, J., Campone, M., Piccart, M., Burris, H.A., III, Rugo, H.S., Sahmoud, T., … Hortobagyi, G.N. (2012). Everolimus in postmenopausal hormone-receptor–positive advanced breast cancer. *New England Journal of Medicine, 366,* 520–529. doi:10.1056/NEJMoa1109653

Birrer, M.J., & Fujiwara, K. (2016, July 11). Medical treatment for relapsed epithelial ovarian, fallopian tubal, or peritoneal cancer: Platinum-resistant disease [Literature review current through January 2017]. Retrieved from http://www.uptodate.com/contents/medical-treatment-for-relapsed-epithelial-ovarian-fallopian-tubal-or-peritoneal-cancer-platinum-resistant-disease

Brashers, V.L., & Jones, R.E. (2010). Mechanisms of hormonal regulation. In K.L. McCance & S.E. Huether (Eds.), *Pathophysiology: The biologic basis for disease in adults and children* (6th ed., pp. 696–722). St. Louis, MO: Elsevier Mosby.

Burstein, H.J., Temin, S., Anderson, H., Buchholz, T.A., Davidson, N.E., Gelmon, K.E., … Griggs, J.J. (2014). Adjuvant endocrine therapy for women with hormone receptor–positive breast cancer: American Society of Clinical Oncology clinical practice guideline focused update. *Journal of Clinical Oncology, 32,* 2255–2269. doi:10.1200/jco.2013.54.2258

Bush, N.J. (2007). Advances in hormonal therapy for breast cancer. *Seminars in Oncology Nursing, 23,* 46–54. doi:10.1016/j.soncn.2006.11.008

Chabner, B.A., & Longo, D.L. (Eds.). (2014). *Harrison's manual of oncology* (2nd ed.). New York, NY: McGraw-Hill Education.

Chandarlapaty, S. (2015, September). *Targeting ESR1-mutant breast cancer* (Annual technical report). Fort Detrick, MD: U.S. Army Medical Research and Materiel Command.

Chen, Y., Clegg, N.J., & Scher, H.I. (2009). Anti-androgens and androgen-depleting therapies in prostate cancer: New agents for an established target. *Lancet Oncology, 10,* 981–991. doi:10.1016/S1470-2045(09)70229-3

Copstead-Kirkhorn, L.-E., & Banasik, J. (2013). *Pathophysiology* (5th ed.). St. Louis, MO: Elsevier Saunders.

Crook, J.M., O'Callaghan, C.J., Duncan, G., Dearnaley, D.P., Higano, C.S., Horwitz, E.M., ... Klotz, L. (2012). Intermittent androgen suppression for rising PSA level after radiotherapy. *New England Journal of Medicine, 367,* 895–903. doi:10.1056/NEJMoa1201546

Cuzick, J., Sestak, I., Bonanni, B., Costantino, J.P., Cummings, S., DeCensi, A., ... Wickerham, D.L. (2013). Selective oestrogen receptor modulators in prevention of breast cancer: An updated meta-analysis of individual participant data. *Lancet, 381,* 1827–1834. doi:10.1016/S0140-6736(13)60140-3

Duffaud, F., van der Burg, M., Namer, M., Vergote, I., Willemse, P.B., ten Bokkel Huinink, W., ... Vermorken, J.B. (2001). D-TRP-6-LHRH (triptorelin) is not effective in ovarian carcinoma: An EORTC Gynaecological Cancer Co-operative Group study. *Anti-Cancer Drugs, 12,* 159–162. doi:10.1097/00001813-200102000-00010

Epocrates Online. (2015). Retrieved from http://online.epocrates.com/home

Ferguson, G.G., & Herzog, T.J. (2004). Current research on the use of hormonal therapy in the treatment of advanced or recurrent endometrial cancer. *Women's Oncology Review, 4,* 175–180. doi:10.3109/14733400400009129

Francis, P.A., Regan, M.M., Fleming, G.F., Láng, I., Ciruelos, E., Bellet, M., ... Gelber, R.D. (2015). Adjuvant ovarian suppression in premenopausal breast cancer. *New England Journal of Medicine, 372,* 436–446. doi:10.1056/NEJMoa1412379

Garrett, A., & Quinn, M.A. (2008). Hormonal therapies and gynaecological cancers. *Best Practice and Research: Clinical Obstetrics and Gynaecology, 22,* 407–421. doi:10.1016/j.bpobgyn.2007.08.003

Genazzani, A.R., & Gadducci, A. (2002). Chemoprevention and endocrine therapy of endometrial carcinoma. In A.R. Genazzani (Ed.), *Hormone replacement therapy and cancer: The current status of research and practice* (pp. 125–134). New York, NY: Parthenon.

Govindan, R., & Morgensztern, D. (Eds.). (2015). *The Washington manual of oncology* (3rd ed.). Philadelphia, PA: Wolters Kluwer Health/Lippincott Williams & Wilkins.

Hacker, N.F., & Friedlander, M. (2010). Uterine cancer. In J.S. Berek & N.F. Hacker (Eds.), *Berek and Hacker's gynecologic oncology* (5th ed., pp. 397–442). Philadelphia, PA: Wolters Kluwer Health/Lippincott Williams & Wilkins.

Howell, A. (2006). Fulvestrant ('Faslodex'): Current and future role in breast cancer management. *Critical Reviews in Oncology/Hematology, 57,* 265–273. doi:10.1016/j.critrevonc.2005.08.001

Huggins, C., & Hodges, C.V. (1941). Studies on prostatic cancer. I. The effects of castration of estrogen and of androgen injection on serum phosphatases in metastatic carcinoma of the prostate. *Cancer Research, 1,* 293–297.

Hussain, M., Tangen, C.M., Berry, D.L., Higano, C.S., Crawford, D., Liu, G., ... Thompson, I.M., Jr. (2013). Intermittent versus continuous androgen deprivation in prostate cancer. *New England Journal of Medicine, 368,* 1314–1325. doi:10.1056/NEJMoa1212299

Hussain, M., Tangen, C.M., Higano, C., Schelhammer, P.F., Faulkner, J., Crawford, E.D., ... Raghavan, D. (2006). Absolute prostate-specific antigen value after androgen deprivation is a strong independent predictor of survival in new metastatic prostate cancer: Data from Southwest Oncology Group Trial 9346 (INT-0162). *Journal of Clinical Oncology, 24,* 3984–3990. doi:10.1200/JCO.2006.06.4246

Jankowitz, R.C., & Davidson, N.E. (2014). Breast cancer. In M.M. Boyiadzis, J.N. Frame, D.R. Kohler, & T. Fojo (Eds.), *Hematology-oncology therapy* (2nd ed., pp. 88–190). New York, NY: McGraw-Hill Education.

Janku, F., Wheler, J.J., Westin, S.N., Moulder, S.L., Naing, A., Apostolia, M., ... Kurzrock, R. (2012). PI3K/AKT/mTOR inhibitors in patients with breast and gynecologic malignancies harboring *PIK3CA* mutations. *Journal of Clinical Oncology, 30,* 777–782. doi:10.1200/JCO.2011.36.1196

Jordan, V.C., & Furr, B.J.A. (2002). An introduction to the regulation of sex steroids for the treatment of cancer. In V.C. Jordan & B.J.A. Furr (Eds.), *Hormone therapy in breast and prostate cancer* (pp. 1–16). Totowa, NJ: Humana Press.

Kumar, R.J., Barqawi, A., & Crawford, E.D. (2005). Adverse events associated with hormonal therapy for prostate cancer. *Reviews in Urology,* 7(Suppl. 5), S37–S45. Retrieved from https://www.ncbi.nlm.nih.gov/pmc/articles/PMC1477613

Lee, J.-M., de Meritens, A.B., Moon, D.H., & Kohn, E.C. (2014). Ovarian cancer. In J. Abraham, J.L. Gulley, & C.J. Allegra (Eds.), *The Bethesda handbook of clinical oncology* (4th ed., pp. 233–242). Philadelphia, PA: Wolters Kluwer Health/Lippincott Williams & Wilkins.

Lee, R.J., & Smith, M.R. (2016, July 14). Initial systemic therapy for castration sensitive prostate cancer [Literature review current through January 2017]. Retrieved from http://www.uptodate.com/contents/initial-systemic-therapy-for-castration-sensitive-prostate-cancer

Lee, W.-L., Yen, M.-S., Chao, K.-C., Yuan, C.-C., Ng, H.-T., Chao, H.-T., ... Wang, P.-H. (2014). Hormone therapy for patients with advanced or recurrent endometrial cancer. *Journal of the Chinese Medical Association, 77,* 221–226. doi:10.1016/j.jcma.2014.02.007

Loblaw, D.A., Virgo, K.S., Nam, R., Somerfield, M.R., Ben-Josef, E., Mendelson, D.S., ... Scher, H.I. (2007). Initial hormonal management of androgen-sensitive metastatic, recurrent, or progressive prostate cancer: 2007 update of an American Society of Clinical Oncology practice guideline. *Journal of Clinical Oncology, 25,* 1596–1605. doi:10.1200/JCO.2006.10.1949

Madan, R.A., & Dahut, W. (2014). Prostate cancer. In J. Abraham, J.L. Gulley, & C.J. Allegra (Eds.), *The Bethesda handbook of clinical oncology* (4th ed., pp. 191–207). Philadelphia, PA: Wolters Kluwer Health/Lippincott Williams & Wilkins.

Margolese, R.G., Cecchini, R.S., Julian, T.B., Ganz, P.A., Costantino, J.P., Vallow, L.A., ... Wolmark, N. (2016). Anastrozole versus tamoxifen in postmenopausal women with ductal carcinoma in situ undergoing lumpectomy plus radiotherapy (NSABP B-35): A randomised, double-blind, phase 3 clinical trial. *Lancet, 387,* 849–856. doi:10.1016/S0140-6736(15)01168-X

Markman, M. (2014). Endometrial cancer. In M.M. Boyiadzis, J.N. Frame, D.R. Kohler, & T. Fojo (Eds.), *Hematology-oncology therapy* (2nd ed., pp. 303–311). New York, NY: McGraw-Hill Education.

McCance, K.L. (2014). Cancer epidemiology. In K.L. McCance & S.E. Huether (Eds.), *Pathophysiology: The biologic basis for disease in adults and children* (7th ed., pp. 402–440). St. Louis, MO: Elsevier Mosby.

Montbriand, M.J. (2004). Herbs or natural products that increase cancer growth or recurrence: Part two of a four-part series [Online exclusive]. *Oncology Nursing Forum, 31,* E99–E115. doi:10.1188/04.ONF.E99-E115

National Cancer Institute. (2010, April 19). The Study of Tamoxifen and Raloxifene (STAR): Questions and answers. Retrieved from https://www.cancer.gov/types/breast/research/star-trial-results-qa

National Comprehensive Cancer Network. (2016a). *NCCN Clinical Practice Guidelines in Oncology (NCCN Guidelines®): Breast cancer* [v.2.2016]. Retrieved from https://www.nccn.org/professionals/physician_gls/pdf/breast.pdf

National Comprehensive Cancer Network. (2016b). *NCCN Clinical Practice Guidelines in Oncology (NCCN Guidelines®): Breast cancer risk reduction* [v.1.2017]. Retrieved from https://www.nccn.org/professionals/physician_gls/pdf/breast_risk.pdf

National Comprehensive Cancer Network. (2016c). *NCCN Clinical Practice Guidelines in Oncology (NCCN Guidelines®): Prostate cancer* [v.1.2017]. Retrieved from https://www.nccn.org/professionals/physician_gls/pdf/prostate.pdf

Noonan, A.M., & Annunziata, C.M. (2014). Endometrial cancer. In J. Abraham, J.L. Gulley, & C.J. Allegra (Eds.), *The Bethesda handbook of clinical oncology* (4th ed., pp. 243–251). Philadelphia, PA: Wolters Kluwer Health/Lippincott Williams & Wilkins.

Nunn, T.W. (1882). *On cancer of the breast.* London, England: J. & A. Churchill.

Pauling, L. (1977). *Vitamin C, the common cold and the flu.* New York, NY: W.H. Freeman & Co Ltd.

Rauh-Hain, J.A., & del Carmen, M.G. (2010). Treatment for advanced and recurrent endometrial carcinoma: Combined modalities. *Oncologist, 15,* 852–861. doi:10.1634/theoncologist.2010-0091

Reed, E. (2014). Ovarian cancer. In M.M. Boyiadzis, J.N. Frame, D.R. Kohler, & T. Fojo (Eds.), *Hematology-oncology therapy* (2nd ed., pp. 928–974). New York, NY: McGraw-Hill Education.

Shah, A., Zhu, W., & Dahut, W. (2014). Prostate cancer. In M.M. Boyiadzis, J.N. Frame, D.R. Kohler, & T. Fojo (Eds.), *Hematology-oncology therapy* (2nd ed., pp. 928–974). New York, NY: McGraw-Hill Education.

Shore, N.D. (2013). Experience with degarelix in the treatment of prostate cancer. *Therapeutic Advances in Urology, 5,* 11–24. doi:10.1177/1756287212461048

Solimando, D.A. (2007). *Drug information handbook for oncology: A complete guide to combination chemotherapy regimens* (6th ed.). Hudson, OH: Lexi-Comp.

Toy, W., Shen, Y., Won, H., Green, B., Sakr, R.A., Will, M., ... Chandarlapaty, S. (2013). *ESR1* ligand-binding domain mutations in hormone-resistant breast cancer. *Nature Genetics, 45,* 1439–1445. doi:10.1038/ng.2822

Venkatesh, R., Strope, S., & Roth, B. (2015). Prostate cancer. In R. Govindan & D. Morgensztern (Eds.), *The Washington manual of oncology* (3rd ed., pp. 206–214). Philadelphia, PA: Wolters Kluwer Health/Lippincott Williams & Wilkins.

Ward, J.F., Vogelzang, N., & Davis, B. (2016, June 2). Initial management of regionally localized intermediate, high, and very high-risk prostate cancer [Literature review current through January 2017]. Retrieved from http://www.uptodate.com/contents/initial-management-of-regionally-localized-intermediate-high-and-very-high-risk-prostate-cancer

WebMD. (2015). Types of breast cancer. Retrieved from http://www.webmd.com/breast-cancer/breast-cancer-types-er-positive-her2-positive

Williams, C., Simera, I., & Bryant, A. (2010). Tamoxifen for relapse of ovarian cancer. *Cochrane Database of Systematic Reviews, 2010*(3). doi:10.1002/14651858.CD001034.pub2

Chapter 11 Study Questions

1. A 63-year-old woman was recently diagnosed with stage IV breast carcinoma that is estrogen and progesterone receptor positive and HER2 negative. She completed some chemotherapy and now has been prescribed anastrozole. Is this an appropriate therapy for this patient?
   A. Yes
   B. No

2. What side effects would the oncology nurse tell her to expect?
   A. Hot flashes
   B. Edema
   C. Headaches and fatigue
   D. All of the above

3. A 73-year-old man has just been diagnosed with metastatic prostate adenocarcinoma with metastatic disease noted in his lumbar spine. He has no neurologic deficits at this time. He has leuprolide ordered. Is this appropriate therapy to start him with?
   A. Yes
   B. No

4. What is the goal of hormone (endocrine) therapy in patients with cancer?
   A. Change ratio of hormone levels in the body.
   B. Reduce available hormone or the ability of the cancer cell to respond to the hormone.
   C. Increase availability of the hormone because cancer cell receptors can only "take up" a certain amount and then stimulate programmed cell death.
   D. Alter uptake of hormone by the cancer cells to prevent their growth.

5. Which of the following is true regarding the Study of Tamoxifen and Raloxifene (STAR)?
   A. Result showed that raloxifene could prevent breast cancer at a higher statistical level than tamoxifen.
   B. Tamoxifen should only be used in women with a diagnosis of breast cancer.
   C. Both medications can be used together for the best effect against breast cancer development.
   D. Tamoxifen is more effective than raloxifene to prevent breast cancer.

CHAPTER

12 Clinical Trials

Joan Westendorp, MSN, OCN®, CCRP

Introduction

Clinical trials bring new discoveries and exciting—potentially lifesaving—advances to cancer care. Today's clinical trials are the foundation of tomorrow's cancer cures. They are the heart of all medical advances (National Institutes of Health [NIH], 2016). Approximately 1.7 million new adult cancer cases were diagnosed in the United States in 2016 (American Cancer Society, 2016a), with approximately 3% of adult patients participating in clinical trials (Institute of Medicine, 2010). Pediatric cancer is uncommon, representing 1% of all cancers in the United States. Remarkable progress occurred from 1975 through 2010 with pediatric cancers, resulting in an overall decline of more than 50% in mortality. One reason for this is that more than 90% of U.S. children and adolescents diagnosed with cancer are enrolled in a clinical trial (American Cancer Society, 2014).

Clinical trials look at ways to prevent, detect, diagnose, control, and treat cancer. They allow researchers to study the psychological impact of the disease and ways to improve patient comfort and quality of life. Increased participation in clinical trials will spur the development of better treatments, prevent disease and disability, and ultimately lead to longer, more productive lives for all. Nurses and allied healthcare professionals in oncology are uniquely poised to make a difference by promoting the significance of clinical trials in advancing cancer care and increasing clinical trial participation in their setting. The purpose of this chapter is to help nurses new to oncology and allied healthcare professionals to understand the significance and conduct of clinical trials in the oncology setting.

A Brief History of Clinical Trials

The evolution of clinical research traverses a long and fascinating journey. The journey moves from a study of dietary therapy in patients with scurvy in 1747 to the modern era of drug therapy studies beginning with the first randomized controlled trial of streptomycin in 1946. Since then, a variety of challenges—scientific, ethical, and regulatory—have arisen within the area of clinical trials (Bhatt, 2010). The widespread acceptance of clinical trials is one of the major advances that occurred during the second half of the 20th century. Table 12-1 lists some of the significant events in clinical trials.

Congress appropriated funds in the National Cancer Institute Act of 1937 for the first time to fight a nontransferable epidemic disease—cancer. This act created the National Cancer Institute (NCI). With this landmark legislation, NCI was given a mandate to engage in

Table 12-1. Selected Events in the History of U.S. Oncology Clinical Trials Development

Year	Event
1747	Lind conducts the first documented comparative study on patients with scurvy.
1800s	Drugs and vaccines to treat smallpox, diphtheria, and cholera are developed and tested.
1887	The National Institutes of Health (NIH) is founded.
1900s	Research on prevention and treatment of infectious diseases begins.
1906	The Food and Drug Act, regulating drug purity, safety, and labeling, is signed into law.
1937	The National Cancer Institute Act establishes the National Cancer Institute (NCI).
1938	The Federal Food, Drug, and Cosmetic Act replaces the 1906 Food and Drug Act and requires that drugs be tested for safety before marketing.
1947	The Nuremberg Code establishes a basic code of ethics for experimentation on human subjects.
1962	The Kefauver-Harris Amendment to the Federal Food, Drug, and Cosmetic Act mandates preclinical testing and the provision of informed consent.
1964	The Declaration of Helsinki establishes specific guidelines for physicians conducting human research.
1966	U.S. Surgeon General policy mandates independent review of all research on human subjects, proposing the establishment of institutional review boards.
1971	The National Cancer Act mandates NCI to conduct and apply basic cancer research.
1974	The National Research Act establishes the National Commission for the Protection of Human Subjects of Biomedical and Behavioral Research.
1976	NCI initiates the Cooperative Group Outreach Program.
1979	The Belmont Report outlines ethical principles and guidelines for protection of human subjects.
1981	Laws governing the protection of human subjects in research funded by the U.S. Department of Health and Human Services (DHHS) are added to the Code of Federal Regulations.
1983	NCI funds the Community Clinical Oncology Program (CCOP).
1986	NIH establishes policies for the inclusion of women in clinical trials.
1988	NCI establishes the High-Priority Clinical Trials Program.
1989	The U.S. Food and Drug Administration publishes guidelines for the inclusion of older adult patients in clinical trials.
1990	The Office of Research on Women's Health is created.
1991	Sixteen federal agencies adopt the federal policy for the protection of human subjects, known as the "Common Rule."
1993	The NIH Revitalization Act mandates the inclusion of women and minorities in NIH-sponsored clinical trials.

(Continued on next page)

Table 12-1. Selected Events in the History of U.S. Oncology Clinical Trials Development *(Continued)*

Year	Event
1996	The International Conference on Harmonisation establishes good clinical practice guidelines for human subject research. Congress passes the Health Insurance Portability and Accountability Act (HIPAA).
1997	The Food and Drug Modernization Act mandates establishment of a public resource for information on clinical trials.
1998	NIH Policy and Guidelines on the Inclusion of Children as Participants in Research Involving Human Subjects mandates that children must be included in all NIH-sponsored research except under certain circumstances.
2000	The World Health Organization establishes international guidelines for ethics committees involved in the review of biomedical research.
2002	The Best Pharmaceuticals Act for Children amends the Federal Food, Drug, and Cosmetic Act to improve drug safety and efficacy testing for children.
2003	DHHS implements HIPAA.
2004	The International Committee of Medical Journal Editors issues a statement mandating public registration of clinical trials, including a description of informed consent and ethics committee approval as prerequisites for manuscript publication.
2005	Federalwide Assurance for the Protection of Human Subjects is required for all studies funded or conducted by DHHS that involve human subjects.
2006	NCI initiates phase 0 clinical trials to study the pharmacokinetics and pharmacodynamics of molecular-targeted drugs.
2007	Medicare's Clinical Trials Policy is revised with updated coverage rules for Medicare.
2007	Pilot program of NCI Community Cancer Centers Program (NCCCP) is launched and focuses efforts on cancer research, improving quality cancer care, and survivorship for patients treated at community hospitals.
2010	Enactment of the Patient Protection and Affordable Care Act requires insurers to cover routine costs of participants in clinical trials.
2012	Clinical Trials Cooperative Groups are consolidated to five groups (four adult and one pediatric).
2013	NCI Community Oncology Research Program (NCORP) is created to bring state-of-the-art cancer prevention, control, treatment, and imaging clinical trials, cancer care delivery research, and disparities studies to individuals in their own communities. NCORP replaces the CCOP and NCCCP.
2014	Insurance coverage requirements for clinical trial participation go into effect as mandated by the Patient Protection and Affordable Care Act.

Note. From "History and Background of Oncology Clinical Trials" (pp. 8–9), by K. Donahue and H. Benzel in A.D. Klimaszewski, M. Bacon, J.A. Eggert, E. Ness, J.G. Westendorp, and K. Willenberg (Eds.), *Manual for Clinical Trials Nursing* (3rd ed.), 2016, Pittsburgh, PA: Oncology Nursing Society. Copyright 2016 by Oncology Nursing Society. Adapted with permission.

certain activities: (a) conduct and foster cancer research (clinical trials), (b) review and approve grants to support promising research projects on the causes, prevention, diagnosis, and treatment of cancer, (c) collect, analyze, and disseminate the results of cancer research conducted in the United States and other countries, and (d) provide training and instruction in the diagnosis and treatment of cancer.

In 1971, the National Cancer Act mandated NCI and NIH to significantly expand and advance the national effort against cancer. This act established the President's Cancer Panel; the National Cancer Advisory Board; 15 research, training, and demonstration cancer centers; and cancer control programs. These programs were mandated to speed the application of state-of-the-art cancer care and clinical trials to communities and nonacademic settings. NCI also was instructed to establish "an international cancer research data bank to collect, catalog, store, and disseminate insofar as feasible the results of cancer research undertaken in any country for the use of any person involved in cancer research in any country" (National Cancer Act of 1971, § 407(b)(4)).

In 1983, NCI established the Community Clinical Oncology Program (CCOP) to ensure that patients with cancer have access to clinical trials in their own communities. In 1989, NCI also approved Minority-Based (MB)-CCOPs to increase the involvement of racial and ethnic minority patients in clinical trials. By 2003, NCI was funding 50 CCOPs across 34 states, 11 MB-CCOPs, and 12 research bases, known as clinical trial cooperative groups (NCI, 2004) (see Figure 12-1).

In 2009, NCI requested that the Institute of Medicine (IOM) review the community research programs and the clinical trial cooperative group program. The charge was to make recommendations for changes needed to conduct clinical trials in the United States more efficiently (IOM, 2010).

The clinical trial cooperative group program has been supported by NCI for more than half a century and is an integral part of NIH, but it had remained largely unchanged for those years. IOM recognized that clinical trials must keep pace with advances in scientific knowledge. Therefore, the recommendation was to create a new National Clinical Trials Network (NCTN). The NCTN would improve the speed and efficiency of cancer clinical trials, using fewer but larger groups of research teams and distributing resources. Through NCTN, the clinical trial cooperative group program was consolidated from 12 research bases to four adult groups and one pediatric group (see Figure 12-1). The purpose of the consolidation was to integrate the operations and data management centers, thereby improving the speed and efficiency of cancer clinical trials and distributing resources more effectively (IOM, 2010).

NCI emphasizes the commitment to clinical research in the community, where most patients are treated and followed. That was the rationale for the CCOP grants, which were initiated in 1983. The value of community-based practices for providing access to clinical trials is fundamental to testing promising new interventions in settings in which most patients are seen. Because advances in oncology are occurring rapidly, community-based care must also adapt swiftly, requiring changes in the manner in which clinical trials are conducted in the community. Therefore, upon evaluation by IOM, NCI consolidated its community-based programs into the NCI Community Oncology Research Program (N-CORP). N-CORP was designed to become an integral component of the overall NCTN. It will provide access to studies of cancer control, prevention, screening, treatment, and care delivery in communities (IOM, 2010).

With the new clinical trial infrastructure, NCTN and N-CORP, researchers are better able to implement and complete trials more rapidly than in the past. Important trials are widely available throughout the country, in large cities and small communities.

Figure 12-1. U.S.-Based Clinical Trials Cooperative Group Program Members

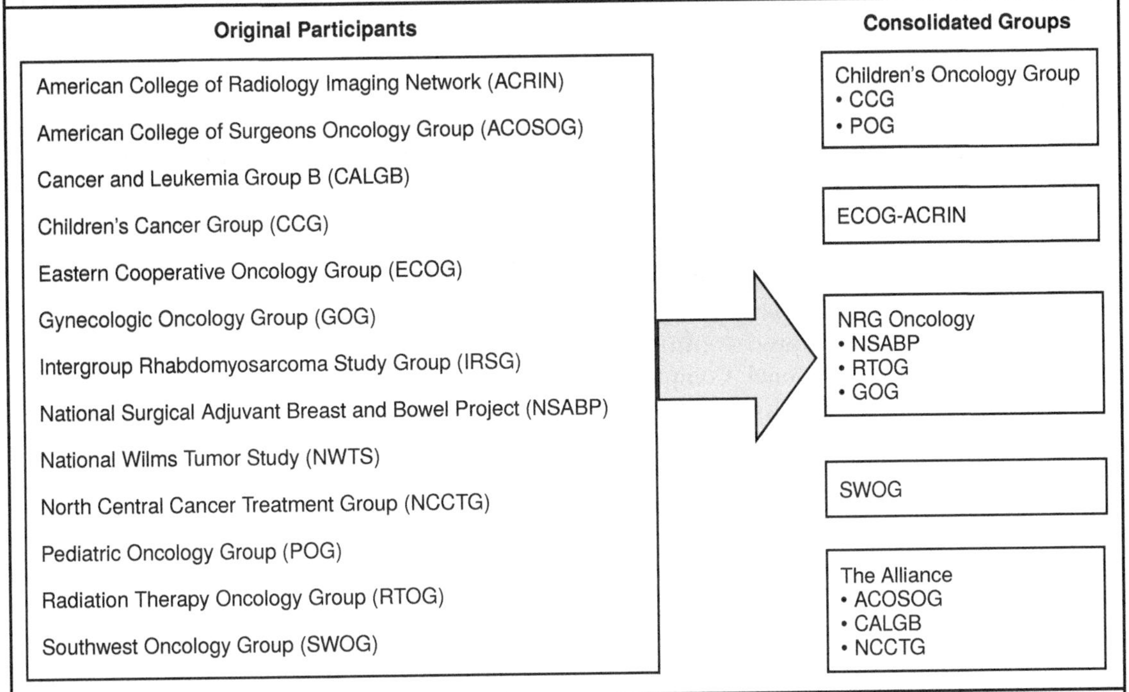
Original Participants
American College of Radiology Imaging Network (ACRIN)
American College of Surgeons Oncology Group (ACOSOG)
Cancer and Leukemia Group B (CALGB)
Children's Cancer Group (CCG)
Eastern Cooperative Oncology Group (ECOG)
Gynecologic Oncology Group (GOG)
Intergroup Rhabdomyosarcoma Study Group (IRSG)
National Surgical Adjuvant Breast and Bowel Project (NSABP)
National Wilms Tumor Study (NWTS)
North Central Cancer Treatment Group (NCCTG)
Pediatric Oncology Group (POG)
Radiation Therapy Oncology Group (RTOG)
Southwest Oncology Group (SWOG)
Consolidated Groups
Children's Oncology Group
• CCG
• POG
ECOG-ACRIN
NRG Oncology
• NSABP
• RTOG
• GOG
SWOG
The Alliance
• ACOSOG
• CALGB
• NCCTG

Note. Based on information from Children's Oncology Group, n.d.; National Cancer Institute, n.d.

Types of Cancer Clinical Trials

Several different types of cancer clinical trials exist. The major types of trials relate to natural history studies, prevention, screening, diagnostic, treatment, and quality of life or supportive care. *Natural history studies* follow a group of people over time who have or are at risk for developing a specific medical condition. These studies are conducted to understand how the medical condition develops and how to treat it (NCI, n.d.). *Prevention trials* look for better approaches to prevent cancer in individuals who have never had cancer or to prevent cancer from recurring. Better approaches may include medicines, vaccines, vitamins, minerals, or lifestyle changes, among other things, that researchers believe may lower the risk of a specific cancer or disease. *Screening trials* test the best way to detect cancer, especially in its early stages when there are no symptoms. *Diagnostic trials* determine better tests or procedures for diagnosing a particular disease condition or cancer. *Treatment trials* test new treatments (such as a new cancer drug, new approaches to surgery or radiation therapy, new combinations of treatments, or new methods such as gene therapy). *Quality-of-life* or *supportive care trials* explore and measure ways to improve the comfort and quality of life of people with a chronic illness, such as cancer (NIH, 2016).

Phases of Cancer Clinical Trials

Trials that involve the testing of a new drug progress in an orderly series of steps, called phases. Most trials also are classified into one of several phases (see Table 12-2). Each phase has different goals and characteristics.

Phase 0

Phase 0 trials are the first clinical trials that target humans. They aim to find out whether the drug reaches the tumor, how the drug acts in the human body, and how cancer cells in the human body respond to the drug. Patients in these studies might need extra biopsies, scans, and blood samples as part of the study process (American Cancer Society, 2016b; National Comprehensive Cancer Network® [NCCN®], n.d.), primarily to determine the pharmacodynamic and pharmacokinetic properties of the drug. *Pharmacodynamic properties* describe the biochemical and physiologic effects of a drug on the body, including how the drug is absorbed, moves throughout the body, binds to various structures, and interacts with certain molecules within target tissues. *Pharmacokinetic properties* describe the activity of a drug in the body over a long period of time. This includes the process by which drugs are absorbed, distributed in the body, localized in the tissues, and excreted. Considered together, data from pharmacodynamic and pharmacokinetic studies help researchers to determine a rational dosage regimen for testing in clinical trials. Furthermore, phase 0 trials expose participants to less toxicity and can be performed in less time and with fewer patients than traditional phase I trials. By conducting a phase 0 trial, researchers can eliminate ineffective agents much more quickly (Takimoto, 2009).

Phase I

A phase I trial aims to find the best dose of a new drug with the fewest side effects. The goal is to find an acceptable dose and schedule with respect to toxicity. Initially, a small group of study participants receive a low dose of the drug. When these individuals tolerate the drug with no or minimal side effects, a higher dose is given to the next set of individuals. This continues until the side effects become severe or the desired effect is seen. Patients who enter phase I trials usually have advanced disease and have failed standard therapies. The new drug may help the individuals, but phase I trials are to test the drug's safety. If it is found to be safe, it can be tested in phase II trials (NCCN, n.d.).

Phase II

The goal of phase II clinical trials is to determine if the treatment has any beneficial effect. Participants in these trials usually have the same type of cancer and are newly diagnosed with advanced disease. Often, new combinations of drugs are tested. Patients are closely watched to see if the drug works. In this phase, the new drug is not usually compared to the standard of care; however, it may be compared to another new drug. If the drug is found to work, it can be tested in a phase III clinical trial (NCCN, n.d.).

Phase III

Phase III clinical trials are comparative studies, whereby one or more experimental treatments are compared with what is known as the current standard therapy. The trials assess the side effects of each drug or combination and which drug or combination works better. Often, these trials are randomized. This means that the patients are placed into treatment groups, called *trial arms*, by chance. Randomization is needed to ensure that the patients in each of the arms are similar. This allows the researchers to know that the results of the trial are due to the treatment and not the differences between the trial arms. A computer program is used to randomly assign participants to trial arms. Neither the patient nor the physician chooses the arms, and both need to accept whichever treatment is assigned. A phase III trial can have anywhere from two to three or more trial arms. The control arm is the one that is considered the standard of care treatment. The other trial arm or arms are considered to be the

Table 12-2. Overview of Phase 0–IV Clinical Trials

Phase	Description	Goals	Subjects	Study Design
0	Exploratory study using small doses of investigational agent (i.e., microdosing for a drug or biologic) Very limited drug exposure with limited duration of dosing (approximately 7 days or less) No therapeutic (or diagnostic) intent	Provide human pharmacokinetic (PK)/pharmacodynamic (PD) data prior to definitive phase I–II testing Determine whether mechanism of action defined in preclinical models can be observed in humans Refine biomarker assay using human tumor tissue and/or surrogate tissue Enhance efficiency and increase chance of success of subsequent development of the agent	Limited number of participants (about 10–15)	Dose escalation Open label Nonrandomized
I	Traditional first-in-human dose-finding study for a single agent Dose-finding study when using multiple agents or multiple interventions (e.g., drug + radiation)	Evaluate the safety and tolerability Determine the maximum tolerated dose (MTD): • Single agent • Combination of agents • Combination of interventions Determine dose-limiting toxicity (DLT) Define optimal biologically active dose Evaluate PK/PD Observe preliminary response (e.g., antitumor activity)	Limited number of subjects (20–100) Healthy volunteer Patient volunteer Usually many cancer types (e.g., solid tumors) Refractory to standard therapy or no remaining standard therapy Adequate organ function (e.g., bone marrow, liver, kidney) Pediatric studies conducted after safety and toxicity evaluation in adults	Dose escalation • Traditional 3 + 3 • Accelerated titration • Adaptive Open label Randomized (healthy volunteer) Nonrandomized (patient volunteer)
II	Phase IIA: Proof of concept study to provide initial information on activity of intervention to justify conducting a larger study Phase IIB: Optimal dosing study to target population	Phase IIA • Demonstrate activity of the intervention in the intended patient condition/targeted population • Establish proof of concept Phase IIB • Establish optimal dosing for the intended patient condition/targeted population to be used in phase III study Evaluate for safety	Moderate number of subjects (80–300) More homogenous population that is deemed likely to respond based on: • Phase I data • Preclinical models and/or mechanisms of action Subject needs to have disease that can be accurately reproduced and measured May limit number of prior treatments	Open label or blinded Nonrandomized or randomized One-stage, two-stage, or crossover Nonstratified or stratified

(Continued on next page)

Table 12-2. Overview of Phase 0–IV Clinical Trials *(Continued)*

Phase	Description	Goals	Subjects	Study Design
III	Randomized controlled study	Compare efficacy of intervention being studied to a control group Evaluate for safety	Large number of subjects (hundreds to thousands) Homogenous population May be used for initial treatment	Open label or blinded Randomized Nonstratified or stratified Multi-institution/multisite
IV	Postmarketing studies	Evaluate safety during postmarketing period May be initiated voluntarily or required by the U.S. Food and Drug Administration Compare the drug to another similar product that is already being marketed Monitor for long-term and additional safety, efficacy, and quality-of-life data Assess drug-food interactions Assess effect in specific populations (e.g., pregnant women, children), or determine cost-effectiveness	Large number of subjects with the labeled indication of the newly marketed drug/biologic	Open label Multi-institution/multisite

Note. Based on information from Doroshow & Kummar, 2009; Kummar et al., 2006; Lertora & Vanevski, 2012.

From "History and Background of Oncology Clinical Trials" (p. 29), by K. Donahue and H. Benzel in A.D. Klimaszewski, M. Bacon, J.A. Eggert, E. Ness, J.G. Westendorp, and K. Willenberg (Eds.), *Manual for Clinical Trials Nursing* (3rd ed.), 2016, Pittsburgh, PA: Oncology Nursing Society.

new treatment. Phase III trials are often needed before the U.S. Food and Drug Administration will approve the use of a new drug for the general public (NCCN, n.d.).

Phase IV

Phase IV trials are postmarketing surveillance studies. After a treatment has been approved by the U.S. Food and Drug Administration, it may be studied in a phase IV trial to identify and assess toxicities that were not apparent in the earlier studies. Some rare side effects may only be found in a large group of individuals. More can be learned about how well the drug works and if it is helpful when used with other treatments or a sequence of treatments. Sometimes, another route may be used to determine if it will offer better quality of life (NCCN, n.d.).

Elements of a Clinical Trial Protocol

Every clinical trial has a written, detailed action plan, called a *protocol.* Every clinical site participating in the trial uses the same protocol, ensuring consistency of procedures and enabling communication among those working on the clinical trial. This uniformity ensures that results from all sites can be combined and compared (Mitchell & Smith, 2016).

NCI's Cancer Therapy Evaluation Program (CTEP) provides guidelines, as well as numerous helpful tools and templates, to facilitate protocol development for the research community. These include an investigator's handbook, a protocol authoring handbook, phase I through III templates, protocol submission worksheet, adverse event guidelines, informed consent guidelines, and treatment assignment instructions and guidelines. All clinical trials will have the basic elements of a protocol, whether it is an NCI- or industry-sponsored trial (NCI CTEP, 2014). Each protocol element has specific information to assist the trial team. Table 12-3 indicates the specific elements of the protocol and what is included in each element of the clinical trial.

Ethical, Legal, and Regulatory Issues

The performance of clinical research is a complex activity. Laws, regulations, and ethics govern research in the protection of human subjects. A comprehensive presentation of this topic is beyond the scope of this chapter; however, key points are discussed. In the area of human subjects and protection of rights, the research team needs to be knowledgeable in three areas: research codes and regulations, local human subject protection, and training of the research investigators and staff.

Research Codes and Regulations

Since 1945, the ethical impact of clinical trials has become increasingly important, resulting in strict regulation of human subject research. Following World War II, leading Nazi doctors who had performed experiments on people in concentration camps were brought to justice (Annas & Grodin, 1995). On December 9, 1946, an international military tribunal at Nuremberg opened criminal proceedings against the doctors for their willing participation in war crimes and crimes against humanity. Experiments had been performed without obtaining informed consent, involving an unacceptable degree of risk (often resulting in death) and without the right of subjects to terminate their involvement. The final verdict from the trial included 10 principles about what constituted legitimate research. These principles later became known as the Nuremberg Code (Nuremberg Code, 1949).

The Nuremburg Code (1949) was the first landmark document in the codification of clinical research ethics, followed by the Declaration of Helsinki in 1964 and the Belmont Report in 1979. These documents provide fundamental guidance for the conduct of teams involved in ethical clinical research.

The Declaration of Helsinki was adopted in 1964 for the medical community by the World Medical Association. It is an important document in the history of research ethics because it was the first significant effort of the medical community to regulate research itself and formed the basis of most subsequent documents in medical research involving human subjects. The declaration developed the 10 principles stated in the Nuremberg Code and tied them to the statement of physicians' ethical duties. It more specifically addressed clinical research, reflecting changes in medical practices in human research and the requirement of consent. Since its inception, it has undergone seven revisions and two clarifications, growing considerably in length from 11 paragraphs in 1964 to 37 in the 2013 version (Carlson, Boyd, & Webb, 2004).

In 1978, the National Commission for the Protection of Human Subjects of Biomedical and Behavioral Research published a report titled *Ethical Principles and Guidelines for the Protection of Human Subjects of Research.* It was named the Belmont Report, for the Belmont Conference Center, where the National Commission met when first drafting the report (National Commission, 1979). The Belmont Report provides the philosophical underpinnings for the current laws gov-

Table 12-3. Elements of a Clinical Trial Protocol

Element	Description
Title page	Includes the title of the protocol, protocol number, primary source of identifying information for the necessary contacts for the protocol, version date, list of participating institutions, and information regarding whether the agents used in the protocol are provided
Schema	Briefly describes the overall treatment plan, including the interventions to be administered and the length of time for each intervention
Objective(s)	Identifies the questions to be answered by the clinical trial and may indicate what can be gained by the clinical trial; may have a primary objective (the main question of the clinical trial) and secondary objective (other items that would like to be gained from the clinical trial, such as quality of life, tumor markers, etc.)
Background and rationale	Presents earlier related studies that led to the development of the present clinical trial and data from those studies in detail with references
Patient eligibility criteria	Includes the unbiased requirements that patients must meet to be enrolled in the study; usually has a section for eligibility criteria and another for ineligibility (exclusion) criteria
Pharmaceutical information	Contains all the details on the agents used in the clinical trial
Treatment plan	Describes what treatment will be given to the patient; includes the dose, route, and schedule of the therapy
Procedures for patient entry on study	Provides detailed requirements needed to enroll patients in the clinical trial, such as if any credentials are required, regulatory requirements, etc.
Adverse events list and reporting requirements	Identifies what side effects have been previously reported with the agents in clinical trials and the specific guidelines for reporting adverse events
Dose modifications for adverse events	Gives guidelines to researchers so that every site is modifying the dose the same according to the adverse events the patients are experiencing
Criteria for response assessment	Provides objective study endpoints, including definitions of complete and partial response, stable disease, and progressive disease
Monitoring of patients	Details the time points and testing required for patients participating in the study
Off-study criteria	Explains the circumstances in which patients should be removed from the clinical trial
Statistical considerations	Provides the rationale for the uniform data method collection, random variation, and generalizability of the study populations, along with the sample size and the statistical power of the sample size
Records to be kept	Specifies all the necessary documents, case report forms, and tissue/blood specimens that need to be submitted, along with the time points of submission

Note. Based on information from Mitchell & Smith, 2016; National Cancer Institute Cancer Therapy Evaluation Program, 2014.

erning human subject research. The Belmont Report established three fundamental ethical principles that are relevant to all research involving human subjects: respect for persons, beneficence, and justice (see Table 12-4).

With respect to regulatory authority, aside from these international codes, nearly every nation that allows research on human subjects has its own set of regulations governing these activities.

Based on the work of the National Commission for the Protection of Human Subjects of Biomedical and Behavioral Research (1974–1978), the U.S. Department of Health and Human Services (DHHS) expanded its regulations for the protection of human subjects, found in the *Code of Federal Regulations* (CFR) at Title 45, Part 46 (45 CFR 46), in the late 1970s and early 1980s. These regulations were enacted for the protection of human subjects and apply to federally funded research. The Office for Human Research Protections protects the rights, welfare, and well-being of subjects involved in research conducted or supported by DHHS and helps to ensure that such research is carried out in accordance with the regulations described in 45 CFR 46.

Local Human Subject Protection

An important process that helps to protect human rights at a local level is the institutional review board (IRB). Federal law requires that every hospital or clinic conducting publicly funded clinical trials have an active IRB committee. The IRB is composed of physicians, pharmacists, nurses, and members of the lay community who critically review the protocol documents for risk to members of the community who may enroll in a trial. A key goal of IRBs is to protect human subjects from physical or psychological

Table 12-4. Application of the Belmont Report

Principle	Application
Respect for persons • Individuals are autonomous agents. • Individuals should be treated with respect. • Persons with diminished autonomy need additional protection.	Informed consent • Participants must be given the opportunity to choose what shall or shall not happen to them. • The consent process must include three elements: – Information sharing – Comprehension – Voluntary participation
Beneficence • Human participants should not be harmed. • Research should maximize possible benefits and minimize possible risks.	Assessment of risks and benefits by investigator and the institutional review board or ethics review committee
Justice • The benefits and burdens of research must be distributed fairly.	Selection of participants • Procedures and outcomes in the selection of research participants should be fair. • Eligibility criteria should include those who may benefit and exclude those who may be harmed.

Note. Based on information from National Commission for the Protection of Human Subjects of Biomedical and Behavioral Research, 1979.

From "Legal, Regulatory, and Legislative Issues" (p. 53), by S. Brown, S. Markus, and C.A. Bales in A.D. Klimaszewski, M. Bacon, J.A. Eggert, E. Ness, J.G. Westendorp, and K. Willenberg (Eds.), *Manual for Clinical Trials Nursing* (3rd ed.), 2016, Pittsburgh, PA: Oncology Nursing Society.

harm, which they attempt to do by reviewing research protocols and related materials. During the review, the IRBs look at the ethical aspects of the clinical trial and its methods. They review whether the prospective subjects are capable of making such choices and seek to maximize the safety of subjects. The IRBs also will make certain that the informed consent is in language that the local community will understand (U.S. Food and Drug Administration, 2016).

Another process to ensure the respect of human rights is informed consent. The Belmont Report (National Commission, 1979) identified informed consent as an ongoing process with three elements: information, comprehension, and voluntariness. The informed consent process consists of many steps, including but not limited to an initial meeting between a potential participant and the physician or a designated member of the research team. The amount of time allotted to the process of consent depends on the nature and complexity of the research and the need to minimize the possibility of coercion or undue influence. An informed consent document is only part of the process, which continues throughout the entire clinical trial, including new information that arises while patients are receiving care. The informed consent may be the most important protection of human subjects. All research personnel should remember the first principle of the Nuremberg Code: "the voluntary consent of the human subject is absolutely essential."

Training of Research Investigators and Staff

One of most frequently used training resources for the research team is the International Council for Harmonisation of Technical Requirements for Pharmaceuticals for Human Use (ICH) Guideline for Good Clinical Practice (GCP), which is an international ethical and scientific quality standard for designing, conducting, recording, and reporting trials that involve the participation of human subjects. Compliance with this standard provides public assurance that the rights, safety, and well-being of trial participants are protected; that trial conduct is consistent with the principles that have their origin in the Declaration of Helsinki; and that the clinical trial data are credible. The objective of ICH GCP guidance is to provide a unified standard for the European Union, Japan, and the United States to facilitate the mutual acceptance of clinical data by the regulatory authorities in these jurisdictions. The principles established in this guidance may be applied to other clinical investigations that may have an impact on the safety and well-being of human subjects (ICH, 1996) (see Figure 12-2). GCP describes the responsibilities and expectations of all participants in the conduct of clinical trials, including investigators, monitors, sponsors, and IRBs. GCP covers aspects of monitoring, reporting, and archiving of clinical trial documents. ICH GCP represents how the research team is to conduct clinical trials in all aspects, from inception to the archival of all documents.

A frequently used training course for most research teams is the NIH Office of Extramural Research's online tutorial, *Protecting Human Research Participants*, which covers all areas of human research protections. It includes review of historical studies, such as the Tuskegee syphilis study, informed consent, and all other vital aspects of human research protection (NIH Office of Extramural Research, n.d.).

Research teams are responsible for conducting trials ethically and according to the regulations and laws for the protection of the individuals enrolling in the study. The Office for Human Research Protections provides leadership in the protection of the rights, welfare, and well-being of individuals involved in research. It provides clarification and guidance to research teams and advice on ethical and regulatory issues. The federal government has a number of systems in place to ensure the safety and well-being of research participants. Many safety nets are in place for research at

Figure 12-2. Principles of Good Clinical Practice

- Clinical trials should be conducted in accordance with the ethical principles that have their origin in the Declaration of Helsinki, and that are consistent with good clinical practice (GCP) and the applicable regulatory requirement(s).
- Before a trial is initiated, foreseeable risks and inconveniences should be weighed against the anticipated benefit for the individual trial subject and society. A trial should be initiated and continued only if the anticipated benefits justify the risks.
- The rights, safety, and well-being of the trial subjects are the most important considerations and should prevail over interests of science and society.
- The available nonclinical and clinical information on an investigational product should be adequate to support the proposed clinical trial.
- Clinical trials should be scientifically sound, and described in a clear, detailed protocol.
- A trial should be conducted in compliance with the protocol that has received prior institutional review board (IRB)/ independent ethics committee (IEC) approval/favorable opinion.
- The medical care given to, and medical decisions made on behalf of, subjects should always be the responsibility of a qualified physician or, when appropriate, of a qualified dentist.
- Each individual involved in conducting a trial should be qualified by education, training, and experience to perform his or her respective task(s).
- Freely given informed consent should be obtained from every subject prior to clinical trial participation.
- All clinical trial information should be recorded, handled, and stored in a way that allows its accurate reporting, interpretation, and verification.
- The confidentiality of records that could identify subjects should be protected, respecting the privacy and confidentiality rules in accordance with the applicable regulatory requirement(s).
- Investigational products should be manufactured, handled, and stored in accordance with applicable good manufacturing practice (GMP). They should be used in accordance with the approved protocol.
- Systems with procedures that assure the quality of every aspect of the trial should be implemented.

Note. From *Guidance for Industry: E6 Good Clinical Practice*: Consolidated Guidance (pp. 8–9), by International Council for Harmonisation of Technical Requirements for Pharmaceuticals for Human Use, 1996, Rockville, MD: U.S. Food and Drug Administration.

the local level also. Research teams are committed to protecting clinical trial participants and increasing the knowledge of treatment for specific diseases. Maintaining the protection of study participants is vital to gain and maintain the public's trust with clinical trials.

Nursing Implications in Cancer Research

Multiple implications exist regarding clinical trials for nurses working with patients with cancer. Oncology clinical trials are important for the improvement of outcomes for individuals with or at risk for cancer. Because of the complexity of oncology clinical trials and the needs of patients with cancer, nurses play a vital role in the clinical trial setting (Lubejko et al., 2011). Research nurses are vital to patients enrolling in a study. Of the total time and effort required to conduct a trial for one patient, the nurses contribute more than 30% of the time, while the physician accounts for only 9% (Baer, Zon, Devine, & Lyss, 2011).

The increasing depth and breadth of the cancer clinical research enterprise has spurred the development of the clinical trial nursing subspecialty. The Oncology Nursing Society (ONS) believes that oncology nurses are essential to the effective conduct of cancer clinical trials. Oncology nurses who work with clinical trials need a background of scientific knowledge, critical-thinking skills, and an understanding of individual and group behavior. Consequently, ONS developed competencies for oncology clinical trial nurses. The competencies are intended to provide a listing of the fundamental knowledge and skills that novice oncology clinical trial nurses should possess or acquire in their role (ONS, 2010).

Nurses new to oncology who are seeking more in-depth information about how to work with cancer clinical trials are encouraged to consult ONS's *Manual for Clinical Trials Nursing* (Klimaszewski et al., 2016). Additional information about the Clinical Trial Nurses ONS Community is available at www.ons.org. Clinical trial resources for healthcare professionals and patients are found in Figure 12-3.

Conclusion

Opportunities exist for nurses and allied healthcare professionals in oncology to make a difference by promoting the significance of clinical trials in advancing cancer care and increasing clinical trial participation. By doing so, advances in cancer care can be more readily achieved, whereby years of human life are not lost, but saved.

Figure 12-3. Clinical Trial Resources

Clinical Trial Databases

CenterWatch Clinical Trials Listing Service™ (www.centerwatch.com): CenterWatch has the largest online database of industry-sponsored global clinical trials actively seeking volunteers.

ClinicalTrials.gov (http://clinicaltrials.gov): ClinicalTrials.gov provides regularly updated information about federally and privately supported clinical research in human volunteers. The National Institutes of Health (NIH), through its National Library of Medicine, developed this site in collaboration with the U.S. Food and Drug Administration. ClinicalTrials.gov contains more than 41,000 clinical studies sponsored by NIH, other federal agencies, and the private industry.

National Cancer Institute (NCI) (www.cancer.gov/about-cancer/treatment/clinical-trials): NCI provides clinical trial information for patients and caregivers and provides the world's most comprehensive database of open and closed clinical trials

World Health Organization International Clinical Trials Registry Platform (ICTRP) (www.who.int/ictrp): ICTRP enables users to search a central database that contains the trial registration data sets provided by primary registers.

Educational Materials

Clinical Trial Staff:

AccrualNet (https://accrualnet.cancer.gov/education/materials_staff?page=6H.WJp1QPkrK1s): Staff education materials include resources for the research team, such as clinical trial workbooks and webinars that teach the basics, sample recruitment plans to help with accrual, online tutorials to help with requirements for human research participant protection training, and more.

Protecting Human Research Participants course (NIH Office of Extramural Research) (https://phrp.nihtraining.com): Online training consists of seven modules, each addressing the principles used to define ethical research using the regulations, policies, and guidance that describe the implementation of those principles.

Patients:

AccrualNet (https://accrualnet.cancer.gov/education/materials_patient#.WJpmpfkRk1s): Patient education materials include clinical trial information for patients in a variety of formats, such as interactive tutorials, videos, and brochures, some of which are available in Spanish.

Dana-Farber Cancer Institute (www.dana-farber.org/Research.aspx): Clinical trial information includes educational material in video and PDF formats.

NCI (www.cancer.gov/about-cancer/treatment/clinical-trials): NCI provides basic information about clinical trials, including information about the benefits and risks, who is responsible for which research costs, and how safety is protected.

NCI Dictionary of Cancer Terms (www.cancer.gov/dictionary): Features thousands of terms related to cancer and medicine. Definitions are in easy-to-understand language for patients.

Professional Membership Organizations

American Society of Clinical Oncology (ASCO) (www.asco.org): ASCO is a nonprofit organization with goals of improving cancer care and prevention and ensuring that all patients with cancer receive the highest quality care. The organization has nearly 25,000 members representing all oncology disciplines and subspecialties. ASCO is committed to advancing oncology education for healthcare professionals, advocating for policies to provide access to high-quality cancer care, and supporting clinical trials and the need for increased clinical and translational research.

(Continued on next page)

Figure 12-3. Clinical Trial Resources *(Continued)*

Professional Membership Organizations *(cont.)*

Association of Clinical Research Professionals (ACRP) (www.acrpnet.org): ACRP is an international association composed of more than 20,000 individuals dedicated to clinical research and development. ACRP is a resource for clinical research professionals in the pharmaceutical, biotechnology, and medical device industries, as well as those in hospitals, academic medical centers, and physician offices.

International Association of Clinical Research Nurses (IACRN) (http://iacrn.memberlodge.org): IACRN is an organization with the purpose of defining, validating, and advancing clinical research nursing—a specialized practice of professional nursing focused on maintaining equilibrium between care of the research participant and fidelity to the research protocol. This specialty practice incorporates human subject protection; care coordination and continuity; contribution to clinical science; clinical practice; and study management throughout a variety of professional roles, practice settings, and clinical specialties.

Oncology Nursing Society (ONS) (www.ons.org): ONS is a professional association of more than 39,000 RNs and other healthcare professionals dedicated to excellence in patient care, teaching, research, administration, and education in the field of oncology. ONS recognizes the value of subspecialty practice and the unique needs of nurses who provide specialized care. ONS offers communities that focus on a particular area (formerly called special interest groups), including the Clinical Trial Nurses ONS Community.

Regulatory Affairs Professionals Society (RAPS) (www.raps.org): RAPS is a worldwide member organization devoted to the health product regulatory profession. With more than 11,000 individual members from industry, government, research, clinical, and academic organizations in more than 50 countries, RAPS develops professional standards for knowledge, competency, and ethics.

Society for Clinical Data Management (SCDM) (www.scdm.org): SCDM is a nonprofit professional society founded to advance the discipline of clinical data management. The interest of all SCDM members is quality clinical data management practices. The society offers certification and publishes a quarterly newsletter.

Society for Clinical Trials (SCT) (www.sctweb.org): SCT is an international professional organization dedicated to the development and dissemination of knowledge about the design and conduct of clinical trials and related healthcare research methodologies.

Society of Clinical Research Associates (SOCRA) (www.socra.org): SOCRA is a nonprofit professional organization dedicated to the advancement and continuing education of clinical research professionals. The society offers certification and publishes a journal, *SOCRA Source*.

Society of Quality Assurance (SQA) (www.sqa.org): SQA is a professional membership organization dedicated to providing a forum for information exchange and utilization of knowledge in research and regulatory quality assurance, enhancing knowledge of regulatory and quality assurance concerns that affect research, and fostering the recognition of the quality assurance profession worldwide.

Other Organizations

Association of Clinical Research Organizations (ACRO) (www.acrohealth.org): ACRO represents clinical research organizations worldwide. ACRO's members provide specialized services that are integral to the development of drugs, biologics, and medical devices. ACRO advances clinical outsourcing to improve the quality, efficiency, and safety of biomedical research.

International Council for Harmonisation of Technical Requirements for Pharmaceuticals for Human Use (ICH) (www.ich.org): ICH brings together the regulatory authorities of Europe, Japan, and the United States and experts from the pharmaceutical industry in the three regions to discuss scientific and technical aspects of product registration.

International Federation of Pharmaceutical Manufacturers and Associations (IFPMA) (www.ifpma.org): IFPMA is a nonprofit, nongovernmental organization representing national industry associations and companies from both developed and developing countries. Member companies of the IFPMA are research-based pharmaceutical, biotechnology, and vaccine companies.

Pharmaceutical Research and Manufacturers of America (PhRMA) (www.phrma.org): PhRMA represents pharmaceutical research and biotechnology companies. It advocates for public policies that encourage discovery of new medicines for patients by pharmaceutical and biotechnology research companies.

Key Points

- Nurses, as part of the research team, are essential to the effective conduct of clinical trials.
- Clinical trials are an avenue for the advancement of clinical management of individuals with cancer and the prevention of cancer.
- Vital historical events in the area of clinical trials include the National Cancer Institute Act of 1937 and the National Cancer Act of 1971, plus the restructure of the NCI clinical trial programs.
- Clinical trial participants are protected in a variety of ways: Nuremberg Code, Declaration of Helsinki, Belmont Report, CFR, local IRBs, and informed consent, along with necessary training of the research staff.

The author would like to acknowledge Heidi E. Deininger, PhD, RN, for her contribution to this chapter that remains unchanged from the first edition of this book.

References

American Cancer Society. (2014). *Cancer facts and figures 2014.* Atlanta, GA: Author.

American Cancer Society. (2016a). *Cancer facts and figures 2016.* Atlanta, GA: Author.

American Cancer Society. (2016b). Clinical trials: What you need to know. Retrieved from http://www.cancer.org/treatment/treatmentsandsideeffects/clinicaltrials/whatyouneedtoknowaboutclinicaltrials

Annas, G.J., & Grodin, M.A. (Eds.). (1995). Introduction. *The Nazi doctors and the Nuremberg Code: Human rights in human experimentation* (pp. 3–12). New York, NY: Oxford University Press.

Baer, A.R., Zon, R., Devine, S., & Lyss, A.P. (2011). The clinical research team. *Journal of Oncology Practice, 7,* 188–192. doi:10.1200/JOP.2011.000276

Bhatt, A. (2010). Evolution of clinical research: A history before and beyond James Lind. *Perspectives in Clinical Research, 1,* 6–10. Retrieved from http://www.picronline.org/text.asp?2010/1/1/6/71839

Carlson, R.V., Boyd, K.M., & Webb, D.J. (2004). The revision of the Declaration of Helsinki: Past, present and future. *British Journal of Clinical Pharmacology, 6,* 695–713. doi:10:111/j.1365-2125.2004.02103x

Doroshow, J.H., & Kummar, S. (2009). Role of phase 0 trials in drug development. *Future Medicinal Chemistry, 1,* 1375–1380. doi:10.4155/fmc.09.117

Institute of Medicine. (2010). *Transforming clinical research in the United States: Challenges and opportunities* (Workshop summary). Washington, DC: National Academies Press.

International Council for Harmonisation of Technical Requirements for Pharmaceuticals for Human Use. (1996, April). *Guidance for industry: E6 good clinical practice: Consolidated guidance.* Retrieved from http://www.fda.gov/downloads/Drugs/.../Guidances/ucm073122.pdf

Klimaszewski, A.D., Bacon, M., Eggert, J.A., Ness, E., Westendorp, J.G., & Willenberg, K. (Eds.). (2016). *Manual for clinical trials nursing* (3rd ed.). Pittsburgh, PA: Oncology Nursing Society.

Kummar, S., Gutierrez, M., Doroshow, J.H., & Murgo, A.J. (2006). Drug development in oncology: Classical cytotoxics and molecularly targeted agents. *British Journal of Clinical Pharmacology, 62,* 15–26. doi:10.1111/j.1365-2125.2006.02713.x

Lertora, J.J.L., & Vanevski, K.M. (2012). Clinical pharmacology and its role in pharmaceutical development. In J.I. Gallin & F.P. Ognibene (Eds.), *Principles and practice of clinical research* (3rd ed., pp. 627–639). doi:10.1016/B978-0-12-382167-6.00043-6

Lubejko, B., Good, M., Weiss, P., Schmieder, L., Leos, D., & Daugherty, P. (2011). Oncology clinical trials nursing: Developing competencies for the novice. *Clinical Journal of Oncology Nursing, 15,* 637–643. doi:10.1188/11.CJON.637-643

Mitchell, W., & Smith, Z. (2016). Elements of a protocol. In A.D. Klimaszewski, M. Bacon, J.A. Eggert, E. Ness, J.G. Westendorp, & K. Willenberg (Eds.), *Manual for clinical trials nursing* (3rd ed., pp. 109–112). Pittsburgh, PA: Oncology Nursing Society.

National Cancer Act of 1971, Pub. L. No. 92-218, 85 Stat. 778 (1971).

National Cancer Institute. (n.d.). *NCI dictionary of cancer terms.* Retrieved from http://www.cancer.gov/publications/dictionaries/cancer-terms

National Cancer Institute. (2004). *Decades of progress: 1983 to 2003. Community Clinical Oncology Program* (NIH Publication No. 04-5562). Retrieved from http://prevention.cancer.gov/sites/default/files/uploads/resources/book.pdf

National Cancer Institute Act of 1937, Pub. L. No. 75-244, 50 Stat. 559 (1937).

National Cancer Institute Cancer Therapy Evaluation Program. (2014). *A handbook for clinical investigators conducting therapeutic clinical trials supported by CTEP, DCTD, NCI* (Version 1.2). Retrieved from http://ctep.cancer.gov/investigatorResources/docs/InvestigatorHandbook.pdf

National Commission for the Protection of Human Subjects of Biomedical and Behavioral Research. (1979, April 18). *The Belmont report: Ethical principles and guidelines for the protection of human subject of research.* Retrieved from http://www.hhs.gov/ohrp/humansubjects/guidance/belmont.html

National Comprehensive Cancer Network. (n.d.). Phases of clinical trials. Retrieved from http://www.nccn.org/patients/resources/clinical_trials/phases.aspx

National Institutes of Health. (2016). NIH clinical research trials and you: The basics. Retrieved from http://www.nih.gov/health/clinicaltrials/basics.htm

National Institutes of Health Office of Extramural Research. (n.d.). *Protecting human research participants* [Online course]. Retrieved from https://phrp.nihtraining.com/users/login.php

Nuremberg Code. (1949). In *Trials of war criminals before the Nuremberg military tribunals under Control Council Law No. 10* (Vol. 2, pp. 181–182). Washington, DC: U.S. Government Printing Office. Retrieved from https://history.nih.gov/research/downloads/nuremberg.pdf

Oncology Nursing Society. (2010). *Oncology clinical trials nurse competencies.* Retrieved from https://www.ons.org/sites/default/files/ctncompetencies.pdf

Takimoto, C.H. (2009). Phase 0 clinical trials in oncology: A paradigm shift for early drug development? *Cancer Chemotherapy and Pharmacology, 63,* 703–709. doi:10.1007/s00280-008-0789-4

U.S. Food and Drug Administration. (2016). Institutional Review Boards frequently asked questions—Information sheet. Retrieved from http://www.fda.gov/RegulatoryInformation/Guidances/ucm126420.htm

Chapter 12 Study Questions

1. Clinical trials that explore and measure ways to improve the comfort and quality of life of individuals with chronic illness are:
   A. Prevention trials.
   B. Natural history studies.
   C. Supportive care studies.
   D. Diagnostic trials.

2. What phase of clinical trial typically enrolls fewer than 300 individuals and has participants with the same type of tumor?
   A. Phase I
   B. Phase II
   C. Phase III
   D. Phase IV

3. Which element of the clinical trial protocol informs the research staff of the time points for required testing during the study?
   A. Records to be kept
   B. Patient eligibility criteria
   C. Treatment plan
   D. Monitoring of patients

4. Which code was created in response to experiments being performed without consent that involved an unacceptable degree of risk and without the right of the subjects to terminate their involvement?
   A. Nuremberg Code
   B. Belmont Report
   C. Declaration of Helsinki
   D. *Code of Federal Regulations*

5. What type of training should the research team undergo?
   A. National Institutes of Health Office of Extramural Research's *Protecting Human Research Participants* course
   B. International Council for Harmonisation of Technical Requirements for Pharmaceuticals for Human Use Good Clinical Practice
   C. A and B

CHAPTER 13

Complementary and Alternative Medicine

Georgia M. Decker, MS, RN, ANP-BC, FAAN

Introduction

Therapeutic interventions based on natural healing (a 19th-century term) or drugless healing (an early 20th-century term) are not new or original in the United States. The history of complementary and alternative medicine (CAM) therapies in the United States dates back to the 1700s. The use of these therapies worldwide dates back to 1200 BC with the first version of Vedic texts and when herbs from India were imported to China (Whorton, 1999). German physician Samuel Hahnemann coined the word *allopathic*, a standard term for conventional or traditional medicine, and founded homeopathy, a system that became popular in the United States in the 1830s. In the late 20th century, an estimated 20% of all medical practice was in the fields of osteopathy, chiropractic, naturopathy, and hydropathy. During this time, contemporary holism emerged, focusing on treating the "whole" patient and promoting the self-care philosophy. This led to the current trend of lifestyle regulation and wellness promotion (Whorton, 1999).

Definitions of CAM have evolved over time. These therapies are now typically termed *integrative*, *integrated*, or *complementary* when combined with conventional approaches and referred to as *alternative* or *unconventional* when the therapy is used instead of conventional approaches. A therapy's intended use also defines it. Miscommunication can occur between healthcare providers as well as between healthcare providers and patients when the terms *complementary* and *alternative* are used interchangeably. Studies have shown that patients with cancer are among the most common consumers of CAM therapies (Mao, Palmer, Healy, Desai, & Amsterdam, 2011). Patients do so for a number of reasons, including symptom management (fatigue, anxiety, nausea) and as another option to fight the cancer (Deng & Cassileth, 2005; van Tonder, Herselman, & Visser, 2009; Verhoef, Balneaves, Boon, & Vroegindewey, 2005). Others report a preference for perceived "natural" or less toxic or nontoxic therapies that can provide a sense of hope and control.

The perception of a decrease in personal attention from conventional medical practitioners and feelings of depersonalization with increased technology in conventional medicine contributes to the appeal of CAM therapies. Imbedded in this perception is the belief that if a product is proclaimed to be natural, it must be safe. Dr. David Eisenberg (2001) coined the phrase "safety trumps efficacy," meaning that even if a particular product or treatment is effective for the reason it is sought, it may not be safe for patients to use under their particular set of circumstances, at that particular time.

The earliest U.S. national survey of the prevalence, cost of use, and pattern of use of CAM was published in 1993. Results revealed that one in three respondents had used at least one "unconventional" therapy within the past year; one-third of the respondents had sought providers for "unconventional" therapy; and CAM users are most likely to be female, well educated, of higher socioeconomic class, and typically using more than one CAM therapy (Eisenberg et al., 1993, 1998). These early CAM surveys were not disease, age, or diagnosis specific. Later studies revealed more about CAM use by patients with cancer, including gender, age, diagnosis, and geography (Ashikaga, Bosompra, O'Brien, & Nelson, 2002; Hedderson et al., 2004; Herron & Glasser, 2003; Najm, Reinsch, Hoehler, & Tobis, 2003; Sparber et al., 2000; Vallerand, Fouladbakhsh, & Templin, 2003). Currently, reports on the use of CAM are updated every few years and provided through a variety of groups including the National Center for Health Statistics and the National Cancer Institute (NCI) Office of Cancer Complementary and Alternative Medicine (OCCAM).

In 2015, Clarke, Black, Stussman, Barnes, and Nahin reported that approximately 34% of U.S. adults reported using complementary health approaches. The most popular approach was nonvitamin, nonmineral supplements. The second most common complementary approach was deep breathing, while the use of yoga, tai chi, and qigong was third. The use of any complementary health approach also differed by selected sociodemographic characteristics, with the most notable differences found by age, ethnicity, and race (Clarke et al., 2015). Figure 13-1 provides a brief CAM timeline.

Figure 13-1. Complementary and Alternative Medicine (CAM) Timeline at a Glance

- Prior to the 19th century, unconventional methods of treatment were considered folk medicine or quackery.
- 1902–1906—The Biologics Control Act (1902) and the Pure Food and Drug Act (1906) formed the foundation of the present-day U.S. Food and Drug Administration.
- 1938—The Food, Drug, and Cosmetic Act required that new drugs have evidence of safety before being put on the market.
- Mid-1970s through 1980s—Consumers continue to seek CAM.
- 1992—The Office of Alternative Medicine (OAM) was established.
- 1994—Under the Dietary Supplement Health and Education Act (DSHEA), a dietary supplement is now defined as a product intended to supplement the diet. DSHEA also created the National Institutes of Health Office of Dietary Supplements to promote, collect, and compile research and maintain a database on supplements and individual nutrients.
- 1998—OAM became the National Center for Complementary and Alternative Medicine (NCCAM). To increase high-quality cancer research and information about CAM use, the National Cancer Institute established the Office of Cancer Complementary and Alternative Medicine.
- 2000—The White House Commission on Complementary and Alternative Medicine Policy was established to address issues of access to and delivery of CAM, priorities for research, and the need to educate consumers and healthcare professionals.
- 2003–2004—The Institute of Medicine of the National Academies (IOM) sponsored meetings to explore scientific, policy, and practice questions caused by the increasing use of CAM by the American public.
- 2005—The final report of the IOM committee was released.
- 2014—NCCAM is renamed the National Center for Complementary and Integrative Health.

Note. Based on information from Decker, 2018.

Levels of Evidence

The gold standard for clinical research is evidence from double-blind, randomized controlled trials (RCTs). Some researchers contend that this is not the best approach to study some CAM therapies, for example, mind–body interventions, because of the complexity of the therapy (Bauer-Wu & Decker, 2012).

Qualitative research provides opportunities to reach a greater understanding of the patient's well-being as well as gather information that can be helpful for future CAM research. While much remains to be learned about CAM therapies, healthcare providers now know far more than when the first surveys were conducted in the early 1990s. The experts do not always agree on how to determine the level of evidence for the research. Clinical trials determine safety and efficacy about a particular product or intervention while providing a foundation of evidence-based medicine and the accepted evidence of efficacy. Effectiveness, as opposed to efficacy, incorporates an evaluation of a clinically meaningful effect and whether the risks outweigh the benefits (Bauer-Wu & Decker, 2012).

Categories of Complementary and Alternative Medicine

The National Institutes of Health National Center for Complementary and Integrative Health (NCCIH, formerly the National Center for Complementary and Alternative Medicine) describes *complementary health approaches* as "a group of diverse medical and health care systems, practices, and products that are not considered to be part of conventional or allopathic medicine," and *integrative medicine* as "a style of practice that places strong emphasis on a holistic approach to patient care while focusing on reduced use of technology," often including complementary health practices (National Institutes of Health NCCIH, 2016, p. 6). NCI's OCCAM defines CAM as "any medical system, practice, or product that is not thought of as standard care" (NCI OCCAM, 2012).

Table 13-1 shows the five CAM categories, their description, and examples as described by NCCIH. NCI OCCAM expanded the NCCIH categories for clarification, adding movement therapy and pharmacologic and biologic treatments with a subcategory of complex natural products (see Table 13-2). It is important to note that the categories overlap, and some therapies may fit into more than one category.

Traditional Chinese Medicine: Acupuncture

In traditional Chinese medicine (TCM), clinical diagnosis and treatment are typically based on the *yin-yang* and *five elements* theories. These theories apply the occurrence and laws of nature to the study of the physiologic activities and pathologic changes of the human body and its interrelationships. Health is a balance of yin and yang (opposite forces present in everyone). Disease or any medical condition is a result of imbalance, usually a result of a blockage or deficiency of energy. Commonly sought TCM therapies include acupuncture, herbal medicine, and qigong exercises. These therapies share the same underlying sets of assumptions and insights regarding the nature of the human body and its place in the universe (Natural Medicines Comprehensive Database, 2015a).

An integral component of TCM is acupuncture. In the United States, it is used alone or as a component of a TCM program. Acupuncture has been used for a variety of health conditions, including pain and other disorders of the musculoskeletal system; headaches; stress; ear, nose, and throat conditions, including sinusitis, tinnitus, and vertigo; allergies; dental pain; addictions; and immune system support, among others. It usually involves insertion of a needle into the skin in specific sites (acupoints) for therapeutic purposes (Natural Medicines Comprehensive Database, 2015a).

Acupoint stimulation may also be achieved via electrical current, laser, moxibustion, pressure, ultrasound, and vibration. There are three types: Japanese, Korean, and Chinese. The underlying principle for all types is that *qi* (pronounced "chee" and translated as meaning *energy*) is present at birth and maintained

Table 13-1. National Institutes of Health National Center for Complementary and Integrative Health Medicine Categories

Category	Description	Examples
Natural products	The most popular form of complementary and alternative medicine among both adults and children	Herbal medicines (botanicals), vitamins, minerals, and other natural products. Some are sold as dietary supplements including probiotics
Mind-body interventions	Mind and body practices focus on the interactions among the brain, mind, body, and behavior, with the intent to use the mind to affect physical functioning and promote health.	Meditation techniques, various types of yoga, acupuncture, deep-breathing exercises, guided imagery, hypnotherapy, progressive relaxation, and tai chi
Manipulative and body-based methods	Focuses on the structures and systems of the body: bones, joints, soft tissues, and circulatory and lymphatic systems	Spinal manipulation, massage
Whole medical systems	Distinct systems of theory and practice that have evolved over time in different cultures	Chinese (or Oriental) medicine, Ayurvedic medicine, homeopathy, naturopathy
Other CAM practices	Movement therapies Practices of traditional healers Energy field manipulation to affect health	Feldenkrais method, Alexander technique, Pilates, Rolfing structural integration, and Trager psychophysical integration Native American healer/medicine man Magnet and light therapies, qi gong, reiki, healing touch, therapeutic touch

Note. From "Integrative Oncology Imperative for Nurses," by S. Bauer-Wu and G.M. Decker, 2012, *Seminars in Oncology Nursing, 28,* p. 4. Copyright 2012 by Elsevier Inc. Reprinted with permission.

throughout life. Qi circulates throughout the body via 12 meridians that provide a major path for the flow of qi. Approximately 350 acupoints exist along the 12 meridians, with additional acupoints that lie outside the meridian pathways (NCI, 2015a).

Acupuncture theory is based on the belief that stimulating the appropriate acupoints aids the body in its ability to correct any imbalance in the flow of energy, thus restoring balance. It also holds that changes in the balance of energy and flow of qi may be identified before disease has developed, and, therefore, acupuncture has a role in the prevention of illness and maintenance of health.

Level of Evidence

More than 400 RCT results are reported in the U.S. National Library of Medicine MEDLINE® database. No scientific evidence supports the physical existence of qi or meridians. However, the effects of acupuncture are reportedly better than placebo in most trials. Efficacy is considered inconclusive by some authors, whereas others suggest the evidence is equivocal or promising for some indications, including addiction, stroke rehabilitation, postoperative and chemotherapy-related nausea and vomiting, tennis elbow, carpal tunnel syndrome, and asthma. The impact of acupuncture on chemotherapy-induced nau-

Table 13-2. National Cancer Institute Office of Cancer Complementary and Integrative Health Medicine Domains of Complementary and Alternative Medicine

Domain	Description	Examples
Alternative medical systems	Systems built upon completed systems of theory and practice	Traditional Chinese medicine, Ayurvedic medicine, homeopathy, naturopathy
Manipulative and body-based methods	Methods based on manipulation and/or movement of parts of the body	Chiropractic, therapeutic massage, osteopathy, reflexology
Energy therapies	Therapies involving the use of energy fields: biofield therapies and bioelectromagnetic-based therapies	Reiki, therapeutic touch, pulsed fields, magnet therapy
Mind-body interventions	Techniques designed to enhance the mind's capacity to affect body function and symptoms	Meditation, hypnosis, art therapy, biofeedback, mental healing, imagery, relaxation therapy, support groups, music therapy, cognitive-behavioral therapy, prayer, dance therapy, aromatherapy, animal-assisted therapy
Movement therapy	Modalities used to improve patterns of body movement	Tai chi, Feldenkrais, hatha yoga, Alexander technique, dance therapy, qi gong, Rolfing, Trager method
Nutritional therapeutics	Assortment of nutrients and non-nutrient and bioactive food components that are used as chemopreventative agents, and the use of specific foods or diets as cancer prevention or treatment strategies	Dietary regimens such as macrobiotics, vegetarian, Gerson therapy, Kelley/Gonzalez regimen, vitamins, dietary macronutrients, supplements, antioxidants, melatonin, selenium, coenzyme Q10, ephedrine, orthomolecular medicine
Pharmacologic and biologic therapies	Includes drugs, vaccines, off-label use of prescription drugs, and other biological interventions not yet accepted in mainstream medicine	Vaccines, off-label use of drugs, antineoplastons, products from honey bees, 714-X, low-dose naltrexone, metencephalin, immunoaugmentative therapy, laetrile, hydrazine sulfate, New Castle Virus, melatonin, ozone therapy, thymus therapy, enzyme therapy, high dose vitamin C
Complex natural products	Subcategory of pharmacologic and biologic treatments consisting of an assortment of plant samples (botanicals), extracts of crude natural substances, and un-fractionate extracts from marine organisms used for healing and treatment of disease	Herbs and herbal extracts, mixtures of tea polyphenols, shark cartilage, essiac tea, Sun Soup, MGN-3

Note. From "Integrative Oncology Imperative for Nurses," by S. Bauer-Wu and G.M. Decker, 2012, *Seminars in Oncology Nursing, 28*, p. 5. Copyright 2012 by Elsevier Inc. Reprinted with permission.

sea and vomiting has been studied for two decades, and the results have been mostly favorable (Bao, 2009; Chandrakantan & Glass, 2011; Ma, 2009).

Contraindications and Side Effects

"Needling" technique is contraindicated in patients with severe bleeding disorders or increased risk for infection, such as those with neutropenia. During the first trimester of pregnancy with the exception of treatment for nausea, patients with cardiac pacemakers should not be treated with electrical stimulation. Caution is advised for the first treatment because some people may become drowsy. Care should be taken if the patient is driving or operating machinery after treatment. Needles should not be reused, and strict asepsis should be mandatory. Potential side effects include bleeding, bruising, pain with needling, and worsening of symptoms (NCI, 2015a; Natural Medicines Comprehensive Database, 2015a). Reported adverse events are rare but include pneumothorax and death (Crew et al., 2007; NCI, 2015a).

Manipulative and Body-Based Methods: Therapeutic Massage

Manipulative and body-based methods use manipulation or movement of body parts. Examples include chiropractic, therapeutic massage, osteopathy, and reflexology.

Various forms of therapeutic manipulation of soft tissue are included in the category of therapeutic massage. Swedish massage is the most common form in the West and provides the core of most types of massage. An important concern regarding massage in cancer care has been whether massage could contribute to metastasis because increased blood and lymph circulation might encourage the spread of cancer. Emphasis on evidence-based practices has led to critical examination of this issue, and the speed of circulation is no longer thought to influence cancer spread (Collinge, MacDonald, & Walton, 2012).

Level of Evidence

Studies consistently demonstrate the potential of massage to improve mood and quality of life. Short-term benefits of massage include improved psychological well-being and in some cases reduced severity of physical symptoms (Collinge et al., 2012; Shin et al., 2016; Walton, 2006). Evidence has suggested that massage can alleviate a wide range of symptoms, including pain, nausea, anxiety, depression, anger, stress, and fatigue (Ernst, 2009; Gansler, Kaw, Crammer, & Smith, 2008). A Cochrane review showed that massage without aromatherapy may provide relief for short-term pain and anxiety in patients with cancer (Shin et al., 2016).

Contraindications and Side Effects

The most common element of massage—pressure—needs to be modified in patients with cancer. For example, patients with a solid tumor should avoid any hand pressure on the area of the solid tumor or surgical site (Walton, 2011). It is acceptable to touch, hold, or stroke using soft hands and to use moderate pressure elsewhere. In the case of known or suspected bone metastasis, including the spine, pressure should be avoided on the area, including jostling or moving the joints. It is all right to use moderate pressure elsewhere on the body (Collinge et al., 2012).

Energy Therapies: Reiki

Energy therapies involve the use of energy fields. Two types exist: biofield therapies and electromagnetic-based therapies. Biofield therapies are intended to affect energy fields that purportedly surround and penetrate the human body. The existence of such fields has not yet been scientifically proven. Examples include qigong, Reiki, and therapeutic touch. Electromagnetic-based therapies involve the nontraditional use of electromagnetic fields, such as pulsed fields, magnetic fields, and alternating current or direct current fields. Examples include pulsed electromagnetic fields and magnet therapy.

Reiki, an ancient form of healing, means "universal life energy." With this form of healing, the practitioner acts as the conduit for the movement of energy. It is the energy, not the healer, that influences healing. Energy travels *through* the healer, not *from* the healer. In this way, Reiki differs from other healing systems. Reiki is said to alleviate physical, emotional, and spiritual blockages. The practitioner gently places his or her hands on or over the client in a particular series of positions, allowing the opening up of blockages (Decker & Potter, 2003). The client remains fully clothed and there is no pressure, massage, or manipulation applied. The environment is kept quiet and soothing. The practitioner spends approximately three to five minutes on each position and treatments last approximately 45 minutes; this may vary based on the needs of the client (Decker & Potter, 2003).

Level of Evidence

There are more than 20 RCTs reported via MEDLINE for Reiki showing it may be helpful in the treatment of pain, mood change, and fatigue. One study tested a standardization procedure for placebo Reiki in an effort to provide a foundation for subsequent randomized and placebo-controlled Reiki efficacy studies (Natural Medicines Comprehensive Database, 2015f).

Contraindications

Reiki does not have antitumor effects and therefore is contraindicated as a primary treatment for cancer (Deng et al., 2009).

Mind–Body Interventions

Mind–body techniques are designed to enhance the mind's capacity to influence body function and symptoms. Examples include meditation, hypnosis, biofeedback, guided imagery, support groups, music therapy, cognitive behavioral therapy, and aromatherapy.

Mindfulness Meditation

Practiced as part of mindfulness-based stress reduction (MBSR), mindfulness meditation is a self-regulatory approach to stress reduction and emotion management. Mindfulness is a state in which an individual is highly aware and focused on the reality of the present moment, including acceptance and acknowledgment. Growing interest in the use of MBSR in cancer care is believed to reflect a desire for a more holistic approach to cancer treatment and acknowledges the links between social, psychological, and physiologic health determinants. MBSR programs are usually six to eight weeks in length and involve daily individual activities and group activities up to several days per week. It is anticipated that individuals will continue to practice the activities for an extended period of time following program completion to obtain full benefit of the intervention (Natural Medicines Comprehensive Database, 2015d; Stafford et al., 2015).

Level of Evidence

Anxiety and emotional control improved in the treatment group as compared to the control group in an RCT assessing the effectiveness of a MBSR program in patients with heart disease. In two RCTs involving patients with cancer, MBSR was effective in decreasing mood disturbance and stress symptoms in both male and female patients (Natural Medicines Comprehensive Database, 2015d).

Contraindications and Side Effects

No contraindications or side effects have been reported (Stafford et al., 2015).

Aromatherapy

Defined as the controlled use of plant essences for therapeutic purposes, aromatherapy uses an *essential oil* from the aromatic essence of a plant in the form of an oil or resin derived from plant leaf, stalk, bark, root, flower, fruit, or seed. The *diluent* is known as the carrier and is used with a concentrated essential oil for application. The *neat* is the direct application of the essential oil compound (essential oil plus carrier) to the skin. The *note* is the unique aromatic variable of an essential oil used when blending combinations of essential oil compounds. Essential oils can be applied directly to the skin through a compressor massage, inhaled via a diffuser or steaming water, or added directly to bath water. Currently, about 150 recognized essential oils exist (NCI, 2015b; Natural Medicines Comprehensive Database, 2015b). The mechanism of action in the use of essential oils begins after sensing the smell. The limbic system is then activated in retrieving learned memories. Essential oils also are absorbed via the dermal route and subcutaneous fat into the bloodstream. Aromatherapy can be practiced with massage. Aromatherapy massage is used in palliative care settings to improve quality of life for patients with cancer (NCI, 2015b, 2015d).

Level of Evidence

Published data on dosing, comparative methods of administration, and therapeutic outcomes in the use of essential oils in aromatherapy are limited. Nearly 40 RCTs were reported in MEDLINE between 1998 and 2014 for the use of aromatherapy in various clinical settings; four involved patients with cancer. Six of the 40 RCTs suggested that aromatherapy massage had a relaxing effect. One study measured the responses of 17 patients with cancer to humidified essential lavender oil. Positive changes were noted in blood pressure, pulse, pain, anxiety, depression, and sense of well-being after both the humidified water treatment and lavender treatments. Another study compared essential oil drop size among six different oils and reported that the bottles differed in their method of delivery. A universal standardization of measure to ensure equity and safety in administration was recommended (Natural Medicines Comprehensive Database, 2015b).

Massage and aromatherapy massage seem to offer short-term benefits for psychological well-being, but limited evidence exists to support the effect on anxiety. Evidence is mixed as to whether aromatherapy enhances the effects of massage. Replication, longer follow-up, and larger trials are needed to accrue the necessary evidence (Natural Medicines Comprehensive Database, 2015b).

Contraindications and Side Effects

Oral entry into the body via the digestive system should be avoided whenever the patient has any of the following: allergy to the oil, pregnancy, contagious disease, epilepsy, venous thrombosis, varicose veins, open wounds or skin sites, or recent surgeries of any type. Essential oils should not be applied to the skin before dilution (Lee, 2003).

Possible adverse events associated with the use of essential oils include photosensitivity, allergic reactions, nausea, and headache. Many essential oils have the potential to either enhance or reduce the effects of prescribed medications, including antibiotics, tranquilizers, antihistamines, anticonvulsants, barbiturates, morphine, and quinidine. Cases of potentially serious reactions involving the use of essential oils have been reported in two individuals without known allergies or sensitivities prior to exposure (Lee, 2003; Maddocks-Jennings, 2004; Natural Medicines Comprehensive Database, 2015b).

Special Considerations

Check resources for safety precautions for each oil before use. Oils should be diluted with a carrier oil such as grape seed or apricot. Check the GRAS (generally regarded as safe) list from the U.S. Food and Drug Administration (FDA), patch test for skin sensitivity, and ascertain if the oil can increase skin sensitivity to sun exposure. Some oils can be hepatotoxic and nephrotoxic with prolonged use, and others can have estrogenic effects that would make it contraindicated for patients with estrogen-sensitive tumors. Some essential oils may compete for receptor sites with chemotherapy; therefore, it is prudent to avoid oils for 9–10 days before or after chemotherapy (Lee, 2003).

Movement Therapies

These types of CAM are used to improve patterns of body movement. Examples include tai chi, hatha yoga, dance therapy, qigong, Rolfing, and Feldenkrais. *Qigong* (chi kung) means "energy cultivation" and refers to movements that are believed to improve health, longevity, and harmony within oneself and the world. There are thousands of such movements, and qigong may include any actions done with the intention of enhancing energy. Qigong is often a component of TCM and is based on four common principles, sometimes referred to as the "secrets" of qigong:

- Mind (the presence of intention)
- Eyes (the focus of intention)
- Movement (the action of intention)
- Breath (the flow of intention)

Numerous styles exist and may include meditation, exercise, and self-massage. Mastery is the achievement of a harmonious existence and action in all situations, but mastery is not exhibited as someone knowing everything, but rather a willingness to continue learning despite level of achievement. Many books and teachers profess to teach the secrets of qigong, but most authors agree that it is actually defined by the person's willingness to practice and experience it (Natural Medicines Comprehensive Database, 2015e).

Level of Evidence

Approximately 100 RCTs are reported in MEDLINE for various conditions. Two trials that provided inspiratory muscle training for patients with cancer and measured relief of breathlessness reported equivocal results (Natural Medicines Comprehensive Database, 2015e).

Contraindications and Side Effects

Psychosis has been reported, but it is not known if there was a latent or undiagnosed psychiatric condition (Natural Medicines Comprehensive Database, 2015e).

Nutritional Therapeutics

A variety of nutrients and non-nutrients, bioactive food components used as chemopreventive agents, and specific foods or diets used as cancer prevention or treatment strategies are included as nutritional therapeutics. Examples include macrobiotic diet, vegetarianism, Gerson therapy, Gonzalez regimen, vitamins, soy phytoestrogens, antioxidants, selenium, and coenzyme Q10.

Gonzalez Regimen

Developed by Dr. Nicholas Gonzalez, the Gonzalez regimen is based on the theory that pancreatic enzymes help the body to rid toxins that lead to cancer. Treatment involves taking nutritional supplements and pancreatic enzymes thought to have anticancer activity, following prescribed diets, and taking coffee enemas. This program purports to facilitate the body's riddance of cancer-causing toxins from the environment and processed foods. It is believed that this balances the autonomic nervous system, affecting body functions and maintaining a healthy immune system.

Key components of the Gonzalez program include a special diet of mainly organic foods; freeze-dried pancreatic enzyme capsules made from pigs and considered to be the primary cancer-fighter in the regimen; large numbers of nutritional supplements (130–160 per day), including magnesium citrate, papaya, vitamins, and other minerals; and coffee enemas twice a day (Gonzalez, 2010).

The nutritional programs used in the Gonzalez regimen are planned for each individual's metabolic type. Metabolic typing is based on a theory that people fall into one of three groups based on the main type of food (protein, carbohydrate, or mixed) that their bodies need to maintain health.

Level of Evidence

Animal studies of the Gonzalez regimen looked at the effect of pancreatic enzymes in cancer treatment, but did not study the regimen as a whole. In 1999, an animal study tested the effect of different doses of pancreatic enzymes taken by mouth on the growth and metastasis of breast cancer in rats. Some of the rats received magnesium citrate in addition to the enzymes. Rats receiving the enzymes were compared to rats that did not receive the enzymes. The results showed that the enzyme did not affect the growth of the primary tumor. Interestingly, the rats that received the highest dose of enzymes had the greatest number of metastases, and the cancer spread to the fewest places in the rats that received the lowest dose of enzymes plus magnesium citrate (NCI, 2015c). Another animal study looked at the effects of pancreatic enzymes on survival rates and tumor growth in rats with pancreatic cancer. Rats in this study receiving the enzyme treatment were more active, lived longer, and had smaller tumors and fewer signs of disease than the control group of rats that did not receive the enzymes (NCI, 2015c).

Nicholas Gonzalez first studied his regimen in 11 patients who had advanced pancreatic cancer. In 1993, he reported results of the study to NCI: patients treated with the Gonzalez regimen lived a median of 17 months, which is longer than usual for patients with this disease; he later published these results (Gonzalez & Isaacs, 1999). Because of the small number of patients in the study, NCI and NCCIH sponsored a second study with a much larger number of patients. This was a seven-year clinical study that included patients who had stage II, stage III, or stage IV nonoperable pancreatic cancer. One group of patients followed the Gonzalez regimen, while another group was given standard chemotherapy treatment (Chabot et al., 2010).

Patients treated with standard chemotherapy survived a median of 14 months, and patients treated with the Gonzalez regimen survived a median of 4.3 months. Patients treated with chemotherapy reported a better quality of life than those treated with only the Gonzalez regimen (Gonzalez, 2010). Gonzalez published comments on his website to express concerns about how the trial was conducted. One of those concerns was how well patients in the Gonzalez regimen group actually followed the regimen (Gonzalez, 2010).

Contraindications and Side Effects

FDA has not approved the Gonzalez regimen or any of its components as a cancer treatment. Side effects reported include gastrointestinal gas, bloating and digestion problems, flu-like symptoms, low-grade fever, muscle aches, and skin rashes. No information is available regarding side effects of the coffee enemas (NCI, 2015c).

Antioxidants

The antioxidant vitamins, vitamins C and E, and beta-carotene are believed to have health-promoting properties. Coenzyme Q10 ubiquinone (CoQ10) is found in all living cells, is involved in the production of energy within cells, and is believed to have powerful antioxidant effects. Researchers consistently report that patients with cancer who take antioxidants typically do so at doses higher than the recommended daily allowances. Antioxidants act by scavenging free radicals. The debate that surrounds antioxidants has focused on cancer therapies such as alkylating agents, antimetabolites, taxanes, and radiation therapy because of the *purposeful* creation of free radicals through cytotoxic mechanisms (Ladas et al., 2004; Prasad & Cole, 2006).

Level of Evidence

The belief and concern that antioxidants may interfere with the efficacy of cancer therapy are not new. Limited research supports the idea that chemotherapy diminishes total antioxidant status, but inconsistencies based on cancer site, cancer therapy, research methodologies, patient populations, dosing, duration of supplementation, and timing of interventions have prevented the formulation of conclusions or consensus (Harvie, 2014). More than 2,000 RCTs involving antioxidants have been reported.

The association between beta-carotene and increased risk of lung cancer in smokers is well known (Albanes et al., 1995). However, it has been suggested that selective inhibition of tumor cell growth is an action of antioxidants and that antioxidants may also promote cellular differentiation with enhanced cytotoxic effects. Researchers have expressed concern that while antioxidants may decrease some kinds of toxicity associated with cancer chemotherapy, the therapeutic benefit of the cancer therapy may be compromised (Harvie, 2014).

Antioxidants may have a role in primary and secondary cancer prevention. Studies have suggested that high vitamin C intake prior to diagnosis of breast cancer may have a positive effect on survival and that vitamin B and E supplements may provide protection against breast cancer among women with a low dietary intake of these vitamins (Dorjgochoo et al., 2008; Harris, Orsini, & Wolk, 2014; Holm et al., 1993; Ingram, 1994; Prasad & Cole, 2006). A meta-analysis assessing the role of vitamin C among women with breast cancer suggested that supplementation with vitamin C after diagnosis may be associated with lower risk of mortality (Harris et al., 2014).

Selenium and vitamin E supplementation was thought to reduce the risk of prostate cancer. Results of the Selenium and Vitamin E Cancer Prevention Trial (SELECT) in 2008 reported that selenium and vitamin E taken alone or together for an average of five and a half years did not prevent prostate cancer, and trial participants were directed to discontinue trial supplements because of lack of benefit. In 2011, updated data revealed that men taking vitamin E had a 17% increase in risk for prostate cancer, compared with men taking the placebo (Klein et al., 2011). These data were again analyzed and updated in 2014, revealing that the men who began the trial with high levels of selenium doubled their risk for developing high-grade prostate cancer by taking selenium supplements and men who had low levels of selenium at the start of the trial doubled their risk of high-grade prostate cancer by taking vitamin E. Variability in doses, duration of supplementation, and timing of interventions has prevented the formulation of conclusions and specific recommendations except in clinical trials (Harvie, 2014).

Contraindications, Side Effects, and Interactions

Specific contraindications exist for certain antioxidants. For example, beta-carotene increases the risk of lung cancer and stomach cancer, and vitamin E increases the risk for prostate cancer and colorectal adenoma (Harvie, 2014; Prasad & Cole, 2006).

Potential interaction examples include the following (Harvie, 2014; Hendler, 2008):

- Vitamin C and aluminum antacids, cyclosporine, statins, calcium channel blockers and protease inhibitors, iron, and vitamin E
- Vitamin E and cholestyramine, colestipol, mineral oil, anticonvulsants, anticoagulants, and verapamil
- Beta-carotene and cholestyramine, colestipol, mineral oil, and orlistat

Pharmacologic and Biologic Therapies

This category includes drugs, vaccines, off-label use of prescription drugs, and other biologic interventions not yet accepted in conventional medicine.

Laetrile

This CAM therapy also is known as amygdalin, apricot almonds, apricot kernel oil, apricot seed, laétrile, prunus kernel, vitamin B_{17}, plus others. It has been taken orally and intravenously as a treatment for cancer (Natural Medicines Comprehensive Database, 2015c).

Level of Evidence

Laetrile is considered to be unsafe when taken orally or intravenously.

Contraindications and Side Effects

An apricot kernel is the source of laetrile, which can cause acute poisoning, with symptoms including dizziness, headache, nausea, vomiting, drowsiness, dyspnea, palpitations, marked hypotension, convulsions, paralysis, coma, and death within 15 minutes. The lethal dose is 50–60 kernels (or equivalent), but the amount can vary. Laetrile also can cause chronic poisoning, with symptoms of increased blood thiocyanate, goiter, thyroid cancer, optic nerve lesions, blindness, ataxia, hypertonia, cretinism, and mental retardation. There are reports of demyelinating lesions and neuromyopathies secondary to chronic exposure, including long-term therapy. FDA sought a permanent injunction against three corporations for unlawfully promoting and marketing laetrile and apricot seeds or kernels for treating cancer on their websites: World Without Cancer, Inc., and The Health World International, Inc., both located in Florida, and Health Genesis Corporation, in Arizona (Natural Medicines Comprehensive Database, 2015c).

714-X

The main ingredient of 714-X is camphor, which comes from the wood and bark of the camphor tree. Nitrogen, water, and salts are added to the camphor. It is purported to help a person's immune system fight cancer. 714-X was developed in the 1960s in Canada, where it is still produced. Its development was based on the theory that there are tiny life forms in the blood called somatids. Some types of somatids are found only in the blood of people who have cancer or other serious diseases. These types of somatids are said to make growth hormones that initiate uncontrolled cell growth. The makers of 714-X state that by looking at the number and type of somatids in the blood, doctors can see if cancer is starting to form or can diagnose cancer and predict where the cancer will spread. The theory states that cancer cells trap nitrogen needed by normal cells and make a toxic substance that weakens the immune system. 714-X is reported to help the body fight cancer cells in specific ways: the camphor is said to prevent cancer cells from taking nitrogen from the body's normal cells and also to help the immune system by increasing the flow of lymph. 714-X is usually given by injection near the lymph nodes in the groin but can be sprayed into the nose using a nebulizer in specific cases. It can be used with conventional treatments. Patients in Canada can get 714-X only from a doctor, for compassionate use. It is used in Mexico and some Western European countries (Natural Medicines Comprehensive Database, 2015c).

Level of Evidence

No clinical study of 714-X has been published in a peer-reviewed scientific journal to show it is safe or effective in treating cancer.

Contraindications and Side Effects

714-X must not be injected into a vein (intravenously) or taken by mouth. Additionally, vitamin B_{12} supplements, vitamin E supplements, shark cartilage, and alcohol should not be used during treatment with 714-X. FDA has not approved 714-X for use in the United States (Kaegi, 1998; NCI, 2015d).

Complex Natural Products

Herbs and herbal extracts are rated by the American Herbal Products Association as follows (McGuffin, Hobbs, Upton, & Goldberg, 1997):

- Class 1: Herbs that can be consumed safely when used appropriately
- Class 2: Herbs for which these restrictions apply, unless otherwise directed by a qualified expert
  - 2a: For external use only
  - 2b: Not to be used during pregnancy
  - 2c: Not to be used while nursing
  - 2d: Other
- Class 3: Herbs for which significant data exist to recommend this labeling are to be used only under the supervision of an expert qualified in the appropriate use of this substance. Labeling must include dosage, contraindications, potential adverse events and drug interactions, and any other relevant information related to the safe use of the substance.
- Class 4: Herbs for which insufficient data are available for classification

See Table 13-3 for commonly used herbs.

Complementary and Alternative Medicine Use

Patients with cancer are among the top consumers of CAM, with a reported 28%–91% using some form. Of concern is that among patients with cancer using CAM, 40%–70% are not reporting their use to healthcare practitioners (Davis, Oh, Butow, Mullan, & Clarke, 2012; Eisenberg et al., 1993). The reasons given for nondisclosure include fear, disapproval, or being dismissed by the provider or practice. Healthcare professionals report that they do not always ask about CAM use because they feel they lack the knowledge to appropriately counsel patients regarding efficacy and safety. Oncology nurses are on the front lines of patient and family education (Bauer-Wu & Decker, 2012). Patients and families expect that their healthcare providers are knowledgeable about cancer and CAM. And yet, many patients remain reluctant to disclose their use of these therapies (Bauer-Wu & Decker, 2012). Surveys have shown that the majority of oncology professionals do not feel prepared to have these discussions with patients (Frenkel, Ben-Arye, & Cohen, 2010). Decker (2005) provided a model that can be used to promote communication (see Figure 13-2). With the increase in demand and evidence, many cancer centers now offer a variety of complementary therapies and some have formal integrative programs.

In 2009, the Society for Integrative Oncology published evidence-based clinical practice guidelines for integrative oncology (Deng et al., 2009). Table 13-4 provides examples of reliable resources for oncology professionals, patients, and families.

Reporting Adverse Effects

Healthcare professionals have an obligation to assist with the process of reporting any adverse effects they believe are related to patient use of CAM therapies. For many of the reasons stated previously, the potential exists for problems to occur from the CAM therapy itself or because of untoward interactions with conventional therapies. Healthcare providers who become aware of unlicensed professionals who are providing alternative and unsubstantiated cancer treatments should report these activities to the proper authorities. Inquiries regarding suspicious CAM treatments and reports of fake cures can be made to FDA (see www.fda.gov/Drugs/DrugSafety/ucm170314.htm). Reports of prod-

Table 13-3. Commonly Used Herbs

Herb	Purported Properties/ Actions	Availability	Potential Side Effects	Precautions/Contraindications	Category*
Aloe *Aloe vera*	Antiseptic Laxative Anti-inflammatory Antiviral Wound healing	Capsules, extract, powder, cream, gel, shampoo, conditioner	May increase risk of hypoglycemia if given concurrently with diabetic agents Risk of hypokalemia if taken concurrently with licorice May alter serum potassium (laxative properties) May decrease serum glucose	Inflammatory bowel disease, fecal impaction, appendicitis, abdominal pain of unknown origin Any spasmodic gastrointestinal complaint, arrhythmia, neuropathy, edema Bone deterioration with long-term use Concurrent use with digoxin can cause digoxin toxicity	2b
Bilberry *Vaccinium myrtillus*	Astringent Tonic Antioxidant and antiseptic Wound healing Antiulcer Vasoprotective	Capsules, fluid extract, fresh berries, dried berries, liquid, tincture, dried root, dried leaves	May cause bleeding, heartburn, hypoglycemia, hypertension May decrease serum glucose	Increased risk of bleeding in individuals who are taking anticoagulants, antiplatelets, thrombolytic agents, or low-molecular-weight heparins	4
Chamomile *Matricaria recutita*	Anxiolytic Mild hypnotic Hypoglycemic effect Estrogen-dependent and estrogen-independent effects Antispasmodic Antimicrobial	Capsules, cream, fluid extract, lotion, shampoo, conditioner, tea, tincture, cosmetics	Topical use: burning of the face, eyes, and mucous membranes Systemic use: hypersensitivity and contact dermatitis, bruising, confusion, drowsiness, anaphylaxis	Increased risk of bleeding with concurrent use with aspirin, antiplatelet agents, heparin, nonsteroidal anti-inflammatory drugs, warfarin, thrombin inhibitors, thrombolytics, darunavir Caution when used concurrently with acetaminophen combination products Increased risk of sedation with benzodiazepines, dextromethorphan/pseudoephedrine combination products, cannabinoids, ethanol, gotu kola, kava, muscle relaxants, all selective serotonin reuptake inhibitors, all sedatives and hypnotics Increased risk of bleeding and sedation with concurrent use with capsaicin, dong quai, primrose oil, fenugreek, feverfew, fish oil, garlic, ginger, ginkgo, ginseng, horse chestnut, licorice, St. John's wort	1

(Continued on next page)

Table 13-3. Commonly Used Herbs *(Continued)*

Herb	Purported Properties/ Actions	Availability	Potential Side Effects	Precautions/Contraindications	Category*
Cinnamon *Cinnamomum cassia*	Antifungal Analgesic Antiseptic Antidiarrheal Antiviral Antidiabetic (insulin potentiator) Also used for • Hypertension • Loss of appetite • Bronchitis	Dried bark, essential oil, leaves, fluid extract, powder, tincture	Flushing, tachycardia, stomatitis, glossitis, gingivitis Increased gastrointestinal mobility, anorexia Allergic dermatitis Shortness of breath Hypersensitivity	Avoid prolonged use in those with intestinal or gastric ulcers	2b
Dong quai (Chinese Angelica) *Angelica sinensis*	Menstrual irregularities and menopausal symptoms Headache Neuralgia Herpes infections Malaria	Capsules, fluid extract, powder, tablets, tea, tincture Primarily a combination product	Nausea, vomiting, diarrhea, anorexia Increased menstrual flow Hypersensitivity reactions Photosensitivity Fever, sweating Bleeding May alter activated partial thromboplastin time (APTT), prothrombin time (PT), and international normalized ratio (INR)	Increased effect of anticoagulants, antiplatelets, estrogens, and hormonal contraceptives Increased risk of bleeding when taken concurrently with chamomile, dandelion, horse chestnut, red clover, St. John's wort Photosensitivity when taken concurrently with St. John's wort Altered PT and INR Increased central nervous system (CNS) depression and muscle relaxation with concurrent use with benzodiazepines Hypoglycemia with concurrent use with tolbutamide	2b

(Continued on next page)

Table 13-3. Commonly Used Herbs *(Continued)*

Herb	Purported Properties/ Actions	Availability	Potential Side Effects	Precautions/Contraindications	Category*
Garlic *Allium sativum*	Antimicrobial Antilipidemic Antitriglyceride Antiplatelet Antioxidant	Capsules, extract, fresh garlic, oil, powder, syrup, tablets, tea	Halitosis Altered coagulation Altered serum glucose Kyolic® garlic has less impact on serum glucose Enteric-coated product lessens halitosis May decrease low-density lipoprotein, triglycerides, and serum lipid profile May increase PT, INR, and serum IgE	Avoid with dacarbazine (CYP2E1 inhibition) Preop/postop (alters coagulation) Caution with other chemotherapy (data are inconclusive)	2b
Ginkgo *Ginkgo biloba*	Cognitive enhancement Peripheral vascular insufficiency Antioxidant Enhances circulation throughout the body Antiarthritic and analgesic	Capsules, fluid extract, tablets, tinctures	Allergic reactions Altered coagulation Anxiety/restlessness Bleeding Gastrointestinal disturbances Insomnia Skin reactions Transient headache May increase C-peptide concentrations and plasma insulin levels	Caution with camptothecin, cyclophosphamide, epidermal growth factor receptor–tyrosine kinase (EGFR-TK) inhibitors, epipodophyllotoxins, taxanes, vinca alkaloids (CYP3A4 and CYP2C19 inhibition) Discourage with alkylating agents, antitumor antibiotics, and platinum analogs (free radical scavenging) Subarachnoid hemorrhage without trauma has been associated with ginkgo One case reported of acute CNS depression in a woman taking trazadone	1

(Continued on next page)

Table 13-3. Commonly Used Herbs *(Continued)*

Herb	Purported Properties/ Actions	Availability	Potential Side Effects	Precautions/Contraindications	Category*
Grapeseed extract *Pycnogel*	Antioxidant Enhances circulation throughout the body Decreases visual stress	Capsules, tablets, drops, liquid concentrate, cream	Dizziness Nausea, anorexia Rash Theoretically: hepatotoxicity	Potential interactions with anticoagulant and antiplatelets (increases risk of bleeding) Caution with camptothecin, cyclophosphamide, EGFR-TK inhibitors, epipodophyllotoxins, vinca alkaloids (CYP3A4 inhibition) Discourage with alkylating agents, antitumor antibiotics, and platinum analogs (free radical scavenging)	4
Kava *Piper methysticum*	Anti-inflammatory	Capsules, beverage, extract, tablets, tincture	Hyper-reflexivity Drowsiness Blurred vision Nausea, vomiting, anorexia, weight loss Potential decrease in platelets, lymphocytes, bilirubin, protein, and albumin Increase in red blood cell volume Hypersensitivity reactions Shortness of breath (pulmonary hypertension) Potential hepatotoxicity May increase hepatic function tests: aspartate aminotransferase (AST), alanine aminotransferase (ALT), and lactate dehydrogenase Chronic use associated with decreased lymphocyte count, decreased platelet	Avoid with antiparkinsonian drugs (increases the symptoms of Parkinson disease) Avoid with antipsychotic medications (may cause neuroleptic movement disorders) Avoid with barbiturates (increases sedation) Avoid with benzodiazepines (increases risk of sedation and/or coma) Avoid with CNS depressants (increases sedation) Avoid with CYP1A2, CYP2C9, CYP2C19, CYP2D6, CYP3A4 substrates (significantly decreases these substrates) Oncology-specific guidelines: Avoid in all patients with existing liver disease, evidence of hepatic damage, herb-induced hepatotoxicity, in combination with hepatotoxic chemotherapy	2b; 2c; 2d

(Continued on next page)

Table 13-3. Commonly Used Herbs *(Continued)*

Herb	Purported Properties/ Actions	Availability	Potential Side Effects	Precautions/Contraindications	Category*
Kava *Piper methysticum (cont.)*			size, and hematuria May decrease albumin, bilirubin, and total protein		
Milk thistle *Silybum marianum*	Hallucinogenic Hepatoprotective Cirrhosis of the liver caused by alcohol or virus Anti-inflammatory Antioxidant Nephroprotective	Tincture, capsules	Headache Nausea, vomiting, diarrhea, anorexia, abdominal bloating, abdominal pain Menstrual changes Hypersensitivity reactions Erectile dysfunction Pruritus Joint pain May decrease aspartate AST, ALT, alkaline phosphatase, and serum glucose	Avoid with warfarin Avoid with combination products involving acetaminophen, dextromethorphan, pseudoephedrine, estrogen/progestin May decrease levels of irinotecan, lorazepam, lovastatin, morphine, meprobamate	1
Purple coneflower *Echinacea purpurea*	Antiviral Immunostimulants Vulvovaginal candidiasis Psoriasis Allergic rhinitis	Capsule, fluid extract, juice, dried powdered extract, sublingual tablets, tea, tincture	Hepatotoxicity Acute asthma attack Anaphylaxis, angioedema May increase ALT, AST, lymphocyte counts, serum IgE, erythrocyte sedimentation rate (ESR)	Do not use in children younger than 2 years old Avoid use in cytochrome P450 3A4 substrates such as immune-modulators (cyclosporine, protease inhibitors, corticosteroids, methotrexate) Altered ALT, AST, lymphocytes, IgG, and ESR	1

(Continued on next page)

Table 13-3. Commonly Used Herbs *(Continued)*

Herb	Purported Properties/ Actions	Availability	Potential Side Effects	Precautions/Contraindications	Category*
Valerian *Valeriana officinalis*	Antianxiety Anti-insomnia	Capsules, brewed herb, extract, tablets, tea, tincture, in combination products with other herbs	Insomnia Headaches Restlessness Nausea, vomiting, anorexia Hepatotoxicity Hypersensitivity reactions Vision changes Palpitations May increase ALT, AST, gamma-glutamyl transferase, total bilirubin, alkaline phosphatase, and urine bilirubin	Increased CNS depression (alcohol, barbiturates, benzodiazepines, opiates, sedatives/hypnotics) Negates therapeutic effects of monoamine oxidase, phenytoin, warfarin Avoid in patients with preexisting liver disease Caution with tamoxifen (CYP2C9 inhibition) Caution with cyclophosphamide, teniposide (CYP2C19)	1

* Classification is for the general population; not cancer-specific.

Note. Based on information from McGuffin et al., 1998; Natural Standard, n.d.; Physicians Desk Reference® for Herbal Medicines, 2007; Skidmore-Roth, 2010.

From *Handbook of Integrative Oncology Nursing: Evidence-Based Practice* (pp. 52–58), by G.M. Decker and C.O. Lee, 2010, Pittsburgh, PA: Oncology Nursing Society.

Table 13-4. Reliable Resources for Cancer Complementary and Alternative Medicine Information

Resource	Website
Organizations	
American Cancer Society	www.cancer.org
American Society of Clinical Oncology	www.asco.org
Cancer Patient Education Network	www.cancerpatienteducation.org
MedlinePlus	https://medlineplus.gov
National Cancer Institute Cancer Information Service	www.cancer.gov/contact/contact-center
National Center for Complementary and Integrative Health	https://nccih.nih.gov
National Institutes of Health	www.nih.gov
Office of Cancer Complementary and Alternative Medicine	https://cam.cancer.gov
Office of Dietary Supplements	http://ods.od.nih.gov
Selected Peer-Reviewed Journals	
Alternative and Complementary Therapies	www.liebertpub.com/act
Clinical Journal of Oncology Nursing	https://cjon.ons.org
Integrative Cancer Therapies	www.sagepub.com/journalsProdDesc.nav?prodId=Journal201510
Journal of Alternative and Complementary Medicine	www.liebertpub.com/publication.aspx?pub_id=26
Journal of Clinical Oncology	http://jco.ascopubs.org
Oncology Nursing Forum	https://onf.ons.org
Seminars in Oncology Nursing	www.journals.elsevier.com/seminars-in-oncology-nursing
Databases	
ClinicalTrials.gov	http://clinicaltrials.gov
Cochrane Collaboration	www.cochrane.org
Micromedex Solutions	http://micromedexsolutions.com
National Cancer Institute Physician's Data Query	www.cancer.gov/publications/PDQ
Natural Medicines Comprehensive Database	http://naturaldatabase.therapeuticresearch.com
PubMed Dietary Supplement Subset	https://ods.od.nih.gov/Research/PubMed_Dietary_Supplement_Subset.aspx
U.S. Food and Drug Administration	www.fda.gov

Note. From "Complementary and Alternative Medicine Therapies in Integrative Oncology" (p. 747), by G. Decker in C.H. Yarbro, D. Wujcik, and B.H. Gobel (Eds.), *Cancer Nursing: Principles and Practice* (8th ed.), 2018, Burlington, MA: Jones & Bartlett Learning. Copyright 2018 by Jones & Bartlett Learning. Adapted with permission.

Figure 13-2. Discussing Complementary and Alternative Medicine (CAM) Therapies With Patients

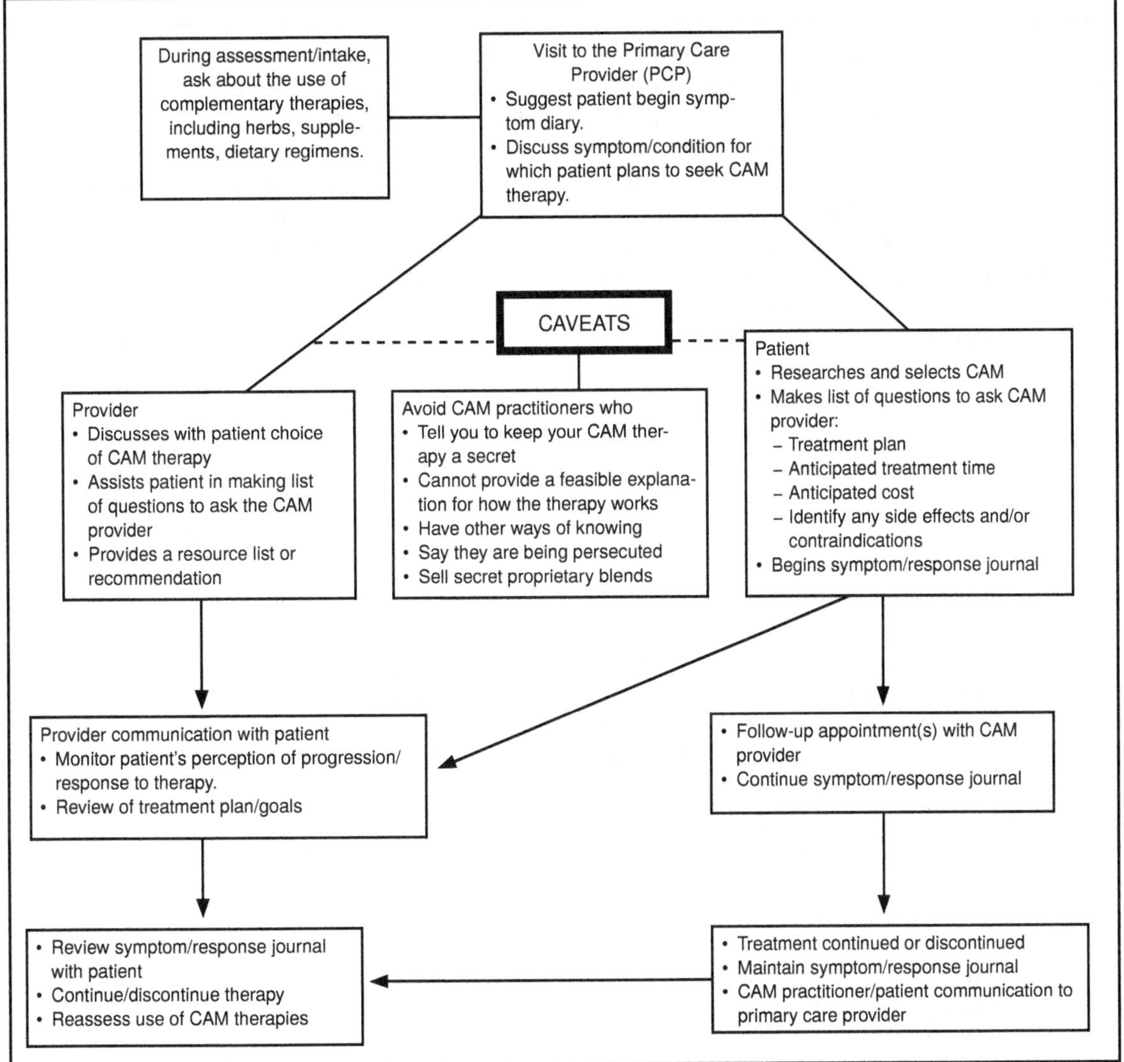

During assessment/intake, ask about the use of complementary therapies, including herbs, supplements, dietary regimens.
Visit to the Primary Care Provider (PCP)
• Suggest patient begin symptom diary.
• Discuss symptom/condition for which patient plans to seek CAM therapy.
CAVEATS
Provider
• Discusses with patient choice of CAM therapy
• Assists patient in making list of questions to ask the CAM provider
• Provides a resource list or recommendation
Avoid CAM practitioners who
• Tell you to keep your CAM therapy a secret
• Cannot provide a feasible explanation for how the therapy works
• Have other ways of knowing
• Say they are being persecuted
• Sell secret proprietary blends
Patient
• Researches and selects CAM
• Makes list of questions to ask CAM provider:
– Treatment plan
– Anticipated treatment time
– Anticipated cost
– Identify any side effects and/or contraindications
• Begins symptom/response journal
Provider communication with patient
• Monitor patient's perception of progression/response to therapy.
• Review of treatment plan/goals
• Follow-up appointment(s) with CAM provider
• Continue symptom/response journal
• Review symptom/response journal with patient
• Continue/discontinue therapy
• Reassess use of CAM therapies
• Treatment continued or discontinued
• Maintain symptom/response journal
• CAM practitioner/patient communication to primary care provider

Note. From "Complementary and Alternative Medicine Therapies in Integrative Oncology" (p. 751), by G. Decker in C.H. Yarbro, D. Wujcik, and B.H. Gobel (Eds.), *Cancer Nursing: Principles and Practice* (8th ed.), 2018, Burlington, MA: Jones & Bartlett Learning. Copyright 2018 by Jones & Bartlett Learning. Adapted with permission.

ucts that are thought to cause more harm than good (e.g., shark cartilage, Essiac® tea) can be made to MedWatch, the FDA Safety Information and Adverse Event Reporting System (www.fda.gov/Safety/MedWatch/default.htm).

Conclusion

Healthcare providers often engage in conversations with patients regarding the role of nutrition, herbal medicine, and complementary approaches in cancer care. Conversations such as these are leading healthcare providers to reconsider their moral, ethical, and legal obligation to remain aware of the best available evidence in CAM, to present evidence-based information in patient-friendly terms, and to address choices from a comprehensive perspective. Ethical struggles in cancer CAM research surrounding informed consent, malpractice, liability, and role of CAM in cancer care are greater than ever, given the rapidly increasing use of such therapies. Although much still remains unknown, there is a great deal that is known. The model for integrated cancer care begins with the nurse, the patient, and other healthcare team members and endorses three core actions: (a) distinguishing fact from fiction, (b) acknowledging misperceptions and biases about CAM, and (c) mixing and unmixing therapies. A baseline knowledge of CAM, beginning with an evaluation of the nurse's personal and professional beliefs, is therefore mandatory.

Oncology curricula in the United States typically guide nurses and other healthcare providers to approach cancer care using the principles and practices of conventional biomedical (Western) medicine. While this is changing, lack of content, misperceptions, and biases surrounding CAM theory and practice within nursing academic programs can leave nurses essentially unprepared to evaluate CAM therapy options. One must ask, do oncology curricula that omit coverage of CAM content inadvertently communicate the belief that CAM has no valid role in health care? Given the widespread availability and affordability of many CAM therapies, integration into cancer care is inevitable.

The American Holistic Nurses Association is the sole nursing body that offers an inclusive certification in the area of CAM. Many nurses choose to undergo training in specific areas of CAM, such as bodywork or aromatherapy, but these certifications focus on a specific modality rather than the broad field. With increasing access to multiple sources of information, oncology nurses can select preferred modes of learning and may, over time, develop a broad knowledge of integrated oncology.

Information from oncology nurses should include reliable resources, assist patients to distinguish fact from fiction, and help them to acknowledge and resolve misperceptions and biases. Additionally, an integrative assessment should be conducted. Evaluation of the nurse's own baseline knowledge and any personal biases is essential.

The law does not provide a definition of CAM that is inclusive or official. Nurses and other healthcare professionals must be aware of any scope of practice issues and vulnerabilities such as the potential for liability when a licensed practitioner refers a patient to an unlicensed practitioner, or a provider who does not have prescriptive authority *prescribes* herbs, vitamins, or supplements. It also is important to consider, in the future, if a healthcare provider fails to offer or include CAM therapies as a treatment or symptom management option, could it be interpreted legally as withholding treatment (Decker, 2018)? The sharing of provider and patient perspectives will help to create unimagined possibilities for evidence-based research and practice (Decker, 2018).

The author would like to acknowledge Rose Mary Carroll-Johnson, MN, RN, for her contribution to this chapter that remains unchanged from the first edition of this book.

References

Albanes, D., Heinonen, O.P., Huttunen, J.K., Taylor, P.R., Virtamo, J., Edwards, B.K., … Palmgren, J. (1995). Effects of alpha-tocopherol and beta-carotene supplements on cancer incidence in the Alpha-Tocopherol Beta-Carotene Cancer Prevention Study. *American Journal of Clinical Nutrition, 62*(Suppl. 6), 1427S–1430S.

Ashikaga, T., Bosompra, K., O'Brien, P., & Nelson, L. (2002). Use of complimentary and alternative medicine by breast cancer patients: Prevalence, patterns and com-

Key Points

- Patients with cancer are among the most common users of complementary and alternative therapies.
- *Complementary* means in addition to traditional therapy, and *alternative* means instead of traditional therapy.
- The more contemporary term, *integrative*, means combining the best evidence-based therapies.
- Early CAM surveys were not disease, age, or diagnosis specific, while contemporary research describes specifics of CAM use by patients with cancer including gender, age, ethnicity, geography, and diagnosis.
- The National Institutes of Health National Center for Complementary and Alternative Medicine was renamed the National Center for Complementary and Integrative Health.
- Oncology nurses should maintain a list of reliable resources for use by healthcare providers, families, and patients.
- It is imperative that nurses discuss the use of CAM therapies with their patients.
- Natural does not mean safe.
- Adverse reactions between herbs, nutritional supplements, medications, and specific cancer therapies are possible.

munication with physicians. *Supportive Cancer in Care, 10,* 542–548. doi:10.1007/s00520-002-0356-1

Bao, T. (2009). Use of acupuncture in the control of chemotherapy-induced nausea and vomiting. *Journal of the National Comprehensive Cancer Network, 7,* 606–612. Retrieved from http://www.jnccn.org/content/7/5/606.long

Bauer-Wu, S., & Decker, G.M. (2012). Integrative oncology imperative for nurses. *Seminars in Oncology Nursing, 28,* 2–9. doi:10.1016/j.soncn.2011.11.002

Chabot, J.A., Tsai, W.-Y., Fine, R.L., Chen, C., Kumah, C.K., … Grann, V.R. (2010). Pancreatic proteolytic enzyme therapy compared with gemcitabine-based chemotherapy for the treatment of pancreatic cancer. *Journal of Clinical Oncology, 28,* 2058–2063. doi:10.1200/JCO.2009.22.8429

Chandrakantan, A., & Glass, P.S.A. (2011). Multimodal therapies for postoperative nausea and vomiting, and pain. *British Journal of Anaesthesia, 107*(Suppl. 1), i27–i40. doi:10.1093/bja/aer358

Clarke, T.C., Black, L.I., Stussman, B.J., Barnes, P.M., & Nahin, R.L. (2015). *Trends in the use of complementary health approaches among adults: United States, 2002–2012.* National Health Statistics Reports; No. 79. Retrieved from http://www.cdc.gov/nchs/data/nhsr/nhsr079.pdf

Collinge, W., MacDonald, G., & Walton, T. (2012). Massage in supportive cancer care. *Seminars in Oncology Nursing, 28,* 45–54. doi:10.1016/j.soncn.2011.11.005

Crew, K.D., Capodice, J.L., Greenlee, H., Apollo, A., Jacobson, J.S., Raptis, G., … Hershman, D.L. (2007). Pilot study of acupuncture for the treatment of joint symptoms related to adjuvant aromatase inhibitor therapy in postmenopausal breast cancer patients. *Journal of Cancer Survivorship, 1,* 283–291. doi:10.1007/s11764-007-0034-x

Davis, E.L., Oh, B., Butow, P.N., Mullan, B.A., & Clarke, S. (2012). Cancer patient disclosure and patient-doctor communication of complementary and alternative medicine use: A systematic review. *Oncologist, 17,* 1475–1481. doi:10.1634/theoncologist.2012-0223

Decker, G.M. (2005). Integrating complementary and alternative medicine therapies into an oncology practice. In P.C. Buchsel & C.H. Yarbro (Eds.), *Oncology nursing in the ambulatory setting: Issues and models of care* (2nd ed., pp. 355–376). Burlington, MA: Jones & Bartlett Learning.

Decker, G.M. (2018). Complementary and alternative medicine therapies in integrating oncology. In C.H. Yarbro, D. Wujcik, & B.H. Gobel (Eds.), *Cancer nursing: Principles and practice* (8th ed., pp. 725–755). Burlington, MA: Jones & Bartlett Learning.

Decker, G.M., & Potter, P. (2003). What are the distinctions between Reiki and therapeutic touch? *Clinical Journal of Oncology Nursing, 7,* 89–91. doi:10.1188/03.CJON.89-91

Deng, G., & Cassileth, B.R. (2005). Integrative oncology: Complementary therapies for pain, anxiety, and mood disturbance. *CA: A Cancer Journal for Clinicians, 55,* 109–116. doi:10.3322/canjclin.55.2.109

Deng, G.E., Frenkel, M., Cohen, L., Cassileth, B.R., Abrams, D.I., Capodice, J.L., … Sagar, S. (2009). Evidence-based clinical practice guidelines for integrative oncology: Complementary therapies and botanicals. *Journal of the Society for Integrative Oncology, 7,* 85–120. Retrieved from https://integrativeonc.org/integrative-oncology-guidelines

Dorjgochoo, T., Shrubsole, M.J., Shu, X.O., Lu, W., Ruan, Z., Zheng, Y., … Zheng, W. (2008). Vitamin supplement use and risk for breast cancer: The Shanghai

Breast Cancer Study. *Breast Cancer Research and Treatment, 111,* 269–278. doi:10.1007/s10549-007-9772-8

Eisenberg, D.M. (2001). *Complementary, alternative and integrative medical therapies: Epidemiology and overview.* Presented at Complementary and Integrative Medicine Clinical Update and Implications for Practice, Copley Hotel, Boston, MA.

Eisenberg, D.M., Davis, R.B., Ettner, S.L., Appel, S., Wilkey, S., Van Rompay, M., & Kessler, R.C. (1998). Trends in alternative medicine use in the United States, 1990–1997: Results of a follow-up national survey. *JAMA, 280,* 1569–1575. doi:10.1001/jama.280.18.1569

Eisenberg, D.M., Kessler, R.C., Foster, C., Norlock, F.E., Calkins, D.R., & Delbanco, T.L. (1993). Unconventional medicine in the United States—Prevalence, costs, and patterns of use. *New England Journal of Medicine, 328,* 246–252. doi:10.1056/NEJM199301283280406

Ernst, E. (2009). Massage therapy for cancer palliation and supportive care: A systematic review of randomised clinical trials. *Supportive Care in Cancer, 17,* 333–337. doi:10.1007/s00520-008-0569-z

Frenkel, M., Ben-Arye, E., & Cohen, L. (2010). Communication in cancer care: Discussing complementary and alternative medicine. *Integrative Cancer Therapies, 9,* 177–185. doi:10.1177/1534735410363706

Gansler, T., Kaw, C., Crammer, C., & Smith, T. (2008). A population-based study of prevalence of complementary methods use by cancer survivors: A report from the American Cancer Society's studies of cancer survivors. *Cancer, 113,* 1048–1057. doi:10.1002/cncr.23659

Gonzalez, N.J. (2010). The truth about the NCI-NCCAM clinical study. Retrieved from http://www.dr-gonzalez.com/jco_rebuttal.htm

Gonzalez, N.J., & Isaacs, L.L. (1999). Evaluation of pancreatic proteolytic enzyme treatment of adenocarcinoma of the pancreas, with nutrition and detoxification support. *Nutrition and Cancer, 33,* 117–124.

Harris, H.R., Orsini, N., & Wolk, A. (2014). Vitamin C and survival among women with breast cancer: A meta-analysis. *European Journal of Cancer, 50,* 1223–1231. doi:10.1016/j.ejca.2014.02.013

Harvie, M. (2014). Nutritional supplements and cancer: Potential benefits and proven harms. *American Society of Clinical Oncology Educational Book, 2014,* e478–e486. doi:10.14694/edbook_am.2014.34.e478

Hedderson, M.M., Patterson, R.E., Neuhouser, M.L., Schwartz, S.M., Bowen, D.J., Standish, L.J., & Marshall, L.M. (2004). Sex differences in motives for use of complementary and alternative medicine among cancer patients. *Alternative Therapies in Health and Medicine, 10*(5), 58–64.

Hendler, S.S. (with Rorvik, D.). (2008). *PDR® for nutritional supplements* (2nd ed.). Montvale, NJ: Physicians' Desk Reference.

Herron, M., & Glasser, M. (2003). Use of and attitudes toward complementary and alternative medicine among family practice patients in small rural Illinois communities. *Journal of Rural Health, 19,* 279–284. doi:10.1111/j.1748-0361.2003.tb00574.x

Holm, L.E., Nordevang, E., Hjalmar, M.L., Lidbrink, E., Callmer, E., & Nilsson, B. (1993). Treatment failure and dietary habits in women with breast cancer. *Journal of the National Cancer Institute, 85,* 32–36. doi:10.1093/jnci/85.1.32

Ingram, D. (1994). Diet and subsequent survival in women with breast cancer. *British Journal of Cancer, 69,* 592–595.

Klein, E.A., Thompson, I.M., Jr., Tangen, C.M., Crowley, J.J., Lucia, M.S., Goodman, P.J., ... Baker, L.H. (2011). Vitamin E and the risk of prostate cancer: The Selenium and Vitamin E Cancer Prevention Trial (SELECT). *JAMA, 306,* 1549–1556. doi:10.1001/jama.2011.1437

Kaegi, E. (1998). Unconventional therapies for cancer: 6. 714-X. *Canadian Medical Association Journal, 158,* 1621–1624. Retrieved from http://www.cmaj.ca/content/158/12/1621.reprint

Ladas, E.J., Jacobson, J.S., Kennedy, D.D., Teel, K., Fleischauer, A., & Kelly, K.M. (2004). Antioxidants and cancer therapy: A systematic review. *Journal of Clinical Oncology, 22,* 517–528. doi:10.1200/JCO.2004.03.086

Lee, C.O. (2003). Clinical aromatherapy part II: Safe guidelines for integration into clinical practice. *Clinical Journal of Oncology Nursing, 7,* 597–598. doi:10.1188/03.CJON.597-598

Ma, L. (2009). Acupuncture as a complementary therapy in chemotherapy-induced nausea and vomiting. *Proceedings (Baylor University Medical Center), 22,* 138–141.

Maddocks-Jennings, W. (2004). Critical incident: Idiosyncratic allergic reactions to essential oils. *Complementary Therapies in Nursing and Midwifery, 10,* 58–60. doi:10.1016/S1353-6117(03)00084-2

Mao, J.J., Palmer, C.S., Healy, K.E., Desai, K., & Amsterdam, J. (2011). Complementary and alternative medicine use among cancer survivors: A population-based study. *Journal of Cancer Survivorship, 5,* 8–17. doi:10.1007/s11764-010-0153-7

McGuffin, M., Hobbs, C., Upton, R., & Goldberg, A. (1997). Herb listing by classification. In M. McGuffin, C. Hobbs, R. Upton, & A. Goldberg (Eds.), *American Herbal Products Association's botanical safety handbook* (pp. 181–190). Boca Raton, FL: CRC Press.

Najm, W., Reinsch, S., Hoehler, F., & Tobis, J. (2003). Use of complementary and alternative medicine among the ethnic elderly. *Alternative Therapies in Health and Medicine, 9,* 50–57.

National Cancer Institute. (2015a). Acupuncture (PDQ®) [Health professional version]. Retrieved from https://

www.cancer.gov/about-cancer/treatment/cam/hp/acupuncture-pdq

National Cancer Institute. (2015b). Aromatherapy and essential oils (PDQ®) [Health professional version]. Retrieved from http://www.cancer.gov/about-cancer/treatment/cam/hp/aromatherapy-pdq

National Cancer Institute. (2015c). Gonzalez regimen (PDQ®) [Patient version]. Retrieved from http://www.cancer.gov/about-cancer/treatment/cam/patient/gonzalez-pdq

National Cancer Institute. (2015d). Topics in integrative, alternative, and complementary therapies (PDQ®) [Health professional version]. Retrieved from https://www.cancer.gov/about-cancer/treatment/cam/hp/cam-topics-pdq

National Cancer Institute Office of Cancer Complementary and Alternative Medicine. (2012, November 9). CAM definitions. Retrieved from https://cam.cancer.gov/health_information/cam_definitions.htm

National Institutes of Health National Center for Complementary and Integrative Health. (2016). *2016 strategic plan: Exploring the science of complementary and integrative health* (NIH Publication No. 16-AT-7643). Retrieved from https://nccih.nih.gov/sites/nccam.nih.gov/files/NCCIH_2016_Strategic_Plan.pdf

Natural Medicines Comprehensive Database. (2015a). Acupuncture. Retrieved from https://naturalmedicines.therapeuticresearch.com

Natural Medicines Comprehensive Database. (2015b). Aromatherapy. Retrieved from https://naturalmedicines.therapeuticresearch.com

Natural Medicines Comprehensive Database. (2015c). Laetrile. Retrieved from https://naturalmedicines.therapeuticresearch.com

Natural Medicines Comprehensive Database. (2015d). Mindfulness meditation. Retrieved from https://naturalmedicines.therapeuticresearch.com

Natural Medicines Comprehensive Database. (2015e). Qi gong. Retrieved from https://naturalmedicines.therapeuticresearch.com

Natural Medicines Comprehensive Database. (2015f). Reiki. Retrieved from https://naturalmedicines.therapeuticresearch.com

Natural Standard Database. (n.d.). Retrieved from http://www.3rdparty.naturalstandard.com/frameset.asp

PDR® for herbal medicines (4th ed.). (2007). Montvale, NJ: Thomson Healthcare.

Prasad, K.N., & Cole, W.C. (2006). Antioxidants in cancer therapy [Letter to the editor]. *Journal of Clinical Oncology, 24*(6), e8–e9. doi:10.1200/JCO.2005.04.1327

Shin, E.-S., Seo, K.-H., Lee, S.-H., Jang J.-E., Jung, Y.-M., Kim, M.-J., & Yeon, J.-Y. (2016). Massage with or without aromatherapy for symptom relief in people with cancer. *Cochrane Database of Systematic Reviews, 2016*(6). doi:10.1002/14651858.CD009873.pub3

Skidmore-Roth, L. (2010). *Mosby's handbook of herbs and natural supplements* (4th ed.). St. Louis, MO: Elsevier Mosby.

Sparber, A., Bauer, L., Curt, G., Eisenberg, D., Levin, T., Parks, S., ... Wootton, J. (2000). Use of complementary medicine by adult patients participating in cancer clinical trials. *Oncology Nursing Forum, 27,* 623–630.

Stafford, L., Thomas, N., Foley, E., Judd, F., Gibson, P., Komiti, A., ... Kiropoulos, L. (2015). Comparison of the acceptability and benefits of two mindfulness-based interventions in women with breast or gynecologic cancer: A pilot study. *Supportive Care in Cancer, 23,* 1063–1071. doi:10.1007/s00520-014-2442-6

Vallerand, A.H., Fouladbakhsh, J.M., & Templin, T. (2003). The use of complementary/alternative medicine therapies for the self-treatment of pain among residents of urban, suburban, and rural communities. *American Journal of Public Health, 93,* 923–925. doi:10.2105/AJPH.93.6.923

van Tonder, E., Herselman, M.G., & Visser, J. (2009). The prevalence of dietary-related complementary and alternative therapies and their perceived usefulness among cancer patients. *Journal of Human Nutrition and Dietetics, 22,* 528–535. doi:10.1111/j.1365-277X.2009.00986.x

Verhoef, M.J., Balneaves L.G., Boon, H.S., & Vroegindewey, A. (2005). Reasons for and characteristics associated with complementary and alternative medicine use among adult cancer patients: A systematic review. *Integrative Cancer Therapies, 4,* 274–286. doi:10.1177/1534735405282361

Walton, T. (2006). Part 2. Cancer and massage therapy: Contraindications and cancer treatment. *Massage Therapy Journal, 45,* 119–134. Retrieved from https://www.amtamassage.org/uploads/cms/documents/CE_Cancer_Care_Part2.pdf

Walton, T. (2011). *Medical conditions and massage therapy: A decision tree approach.* Philadelphia, PA: Wolters Kluwer Health/Lippincott Williams & Wilkins.

Whorton, J.C. (1999). The history of complementary and alternative medicine. In M.B. Jonas & J.S. Levin (Eds.), *Essentials of complementary and alternative medicine* (pp. 16–30). Philadelphia, PA: Lippincott Williams & Wilkins.

Chapter 13 Study Questions

1. The U.S. Food and Drug Administration MedWatch program depends on reports of adverse events from healthcare professionals and the public.
   A. True
   B. False

2. Integrative medicine is composed of the best evidence-based therapies from traditional and nontraditional medicine.
   A. True
   B. False

3. Most complementary and alternative medicine (CAM) therapies lack evidence of effectiveness.
   A. True
   B. False

4. The healthcare professional at the forefront of patient and family education is which of the following?
   A. Physician
   B. Nurse
   C. Patient advocate
   D. Resident

5. The law does not provide an inclusive, official definition of CAM. Therefore, which of the following statements is **most true**?
   A. Nurses should not ask patients about CAM use because they can be held legally responsible for the answer.
   B. Nurses should not refer to a CAM practitioner because they are not qualified to do so.
   C. Nurses are responsible for knowing and understanding any scope of practice issues related to CAM.
   D. Nurses are in the trenches and should not discuss anything with their patients that might upset patients or their families.

CHAPTER 14

Hematopoietic Stem Cell Transplantation

Stephanie Jacobson Gregory, FNP-C, BMTCN®

Introduction

Hematopoietic stem cell transplantation (HSCT) is a potentially curative method of treatment used for a variety of malignant and nonmalignant diseases. According to the Center for International Blood and Marrow Transplant Research (Pasquini & Zhu, 2015), more than 11,000 autologous and 8,000 allogeneic transplants were performed in the United States in 2013 alone. HSCT is the transplantation of hematopoietic progenitor cells (HPCs, also called hematopoietic stem cells [HSCs]); these cells proliferate and replenish the bone marrow with blood cells and other cells responsible for immunity (Niess, 2013). HSCT can be performed using multiple techniques, including different types of transplant, supportive therapies, stem cell collection processes, and with either myeloablative or nonmyeloablative regimens as preparative therapy. HSCT can be either *autologous*, in which a patient's own cells are used, or *allogeneic*, in which donor stem cells are used, which can be derived from a multitude of possible sources.

Malignant indications for HSCT include leukemia, lymphoma, multiple myeloma, and high-risk solid tumors such as neuroblastoma and germ cell tumors such as testicular cancer (Be The Match, n.d.-a). HSCT also is indicated for disorders such as aplastic anemia, sickle-cell disease, and thalassemia and has been studied as treatment for autoimmune disorders such as systemic lupus erythematosus (Be The Match, n.d.-a). Many factors affect HSCT outcomes, including patient- and disease-related variables such as age, comorbidities, prior therapies, diagnosis, and disease stage. Donor factors and transplant types also play a role in outcomes: human leukocyte antigen (HLA) and gender match, conditioning regimen, stem cell source, and graft-versus-host disease (GVHD) prophylaxis.

This chapter will describe the types of stem cell treatments available, stem cell collection and processing procedures, and acute and chronic complications associated with HSCT. The chapter will conclude with discussion on future directions in HSCT. The term *HSCT* will be used throughout this chapter to refer to any source of stem cells, including bone marrow, peripheral blood, and umbilical cord blood (UCB).

The History of Transplantation

Serious interest in bone marrow transplantation began in reaction to the threats of nuclear bombs in the 1950s when scientists began studying it as a method of treating patients exposed to radiation. Radiation exposure in high doses can severely damage a person's bone marrow function; therefore, studies were conducted to evaluate the effectiveness of bone marrow transplant in replacing damaged bone marrow (Gupta, n.d.). Research conducted by Leon Jacobson and his colleagues in the early 1950s demonstrated that mice could recover from lethal doses of radiation if given an injection of cells from the spleen, further fueling interest in bone marrow transplant as a form of treatment (Niess, 2013). In the late 1950s, Dr. E. Donnall Thomas performed the first successful bone marrow transplant using an identical twin as a donor. His pioneering work in transplant science led to his receiving the Nobel Prize in Physiology or Medicine in 1990 (Fred Hutchinson Cancer Research Center, n.d.). The development of HLA typing in the 1960s improved understanding of donor compatibility, and in 1968, the first successful allogeneic transplant for leukemia was performed at the University of Minnesota using a sibling who was not an identical twin (Niess, 2013). As a result of further research and increasing knowledge about HSCT, the first successful full HLA-matched, unrelated transplant was performed in 1973. With the growing interest in bone marrow transplant, research expanded into alternative methods of collecting HSCs. Prior to the 1980s, the only way to collect stem cells was through a bone marrow harvest, which meant inserting a large-bore needle directly into the bone marrow and withdrawing cells for transplant. The first successful peripheral blood stem cell (PBSC) collection and transplant was performed in the 1980s and is now the most common method of HSC collection (Niess, 2013). UCB transplants gained popularity in the late 1980s when the first successful cord blood transplant was performed, thereby expanding options for stem cell sources (Niess, 2013). Recent advances in research have made the use of haploidentical donors possible with significant strides in improving options for patients in need of HSCT.

Hematopoietic and Immunologic Concepts of Transplantation

To understand the concepts of HSCT as treatment for many blood disorders and cancers, a basic understanding of hematopoiesis and immunology is necessary. Diseases such as acute myeloid leukemia, aplastic anemia, multiple myeloma, and numerous others interfere with the normal process of hematopoiesis, or blood cell growth, division, and differentiation (Mak & Saunders, 2011). The basic concept of HSCT is that by treating the bone marrow with high doses of chemotherapy followed by transplant with immature, bone marrow–stimulating cells, the bone marrow function can potentially be restored to normal. All cells within the human hematopoietic system begin as pluripotent stem cells, also called HSCs, which are capable of dividing and producing either more stem cells or further differentiating into HPCs that can become cells within the myeloid or lymphoid lineages (Barrett, 2009).

The myeloid lineage consists of cells that produce neutrophils, basophils, megakaryocytes, dendritic cells, and other myeloid cells, whereas the lymphoid lineage consists of precursors for B and T lymphocytes as well as natural killer (NK) lineages (Devine, 2013). Each HSC expresses surface proteins that help to distinguish cell function; for example, CD34 is a known marker of the HSC. The cluster of differentiation (CD) system was developed to help classify and identify cells and their specific roles in the hematopoietic system (Devine, 2013). As HSCs differentiate, they acquire markers more specific to lineage. T cells acquire CD4 or CD8, while B cells acquire immunoglobulins (Mak & Saunders, 2011).

Many factors assist the process of hematopoietic cell proliferation and division, including proteins such as cell adhesion molecules, cytokines, and chemokines, which have many functions, including serving as communication signals for cells. These proteins mobilize cells into the bone marrow, facilitate cell growth, and even play a role in transmission of information between cells (Massberg, Khandoga, & von Andrian, 2013). Cytokines are polypeptide hormones that can stimulate or inhibit cell activities and play a significant role in the proliferation and differentiation of HPCs. The main cytokines that have activity related to hematopoiesis are interleukin (IL)-1, IL-3, IL-6, granulocyte–colony-stimulating factor (G-CSF), erythropoietin, and stem cell factor (Massberg et al., 2013). G-CSF is an important cytokine in the later stages of neutrophil maturation. Synthetically produced growth factors, including granulocyte macrophage–colony-stimulating factor (GM-CSF), G-CSF, and erythropoietin, are used to stimulate hematopoietic cell proliferation as a method of stem cell collection for HSCT recipients. Chemokines (chemotactic cytokines) play a role in adaptive immune response as well as regulation of HPCs; they are a key component in the process of stem cell mobilization (Massberg et al., 2013). Figure 14-1 shows the specific delineation of cell lines within the process of hematopoiesis and cytokines associated with cell types.

The myeloid and lymphoid lineages also play distinct roles in the process of immunity. The myeloid cells are the "first responders" to infection but have nonspecific function, whereas the lymphoid cells, with the assistance of antigen-presenting cells and cytokines, have more specific functions, including the production of memory T cells, which help to recognize, target, and bind to antigens (Powell, Chung, & Baum, 2013). B cells help with the production of immunoglobulins, an important part of humoral immunity. T cells, however, can only function by recognizing antigens displayed on cells and determining those antigens to be either "self" or "nonself." Foreign invaders can be recognized and destroyed by T cells with the help of major histocompatibility antigen complexes (MHCs), molecules that present the antigen on the surface of a cell in order for the T cell to identify the type of cell (Abbas, Lichtman, & Pillai, 2015). MHCs are an important component of the immune system and autoimmunity but also contain genes that code for HLAs. HLA differences between donor and recipient are a major determinant for graft rejection and other post-HSCT complications (Abbas et al., 2015). HLAs will be discussed further in the next section. Prior to HSCT, the bone marrow is depleted significantly to allow for regeneration of normally functioning bone marrow processes. After HSCT, both humoral and cell-mediated immunity can be altered for a prolonged period of time, leaving patients susceptible to opportunistic and viral infections for months in the case of autologous transplants and for months to years after allogeneic transplants.

Human Leukocyte Antigen Matching in Allogeneic Transplantation

HLAs (see Figure 14-2) are unique to each individual and present foreign antigens to immune cells for destruction. They play a significant role in the recognition of self and nonself. HLAs are involved with transplant rejection, GVHD, and acceptance of the donor graft (Devine, 2013). Determining the HLA alleles for each individual is termed *HLA typing* and is the method used to determine appropriate donors for HSCT. HLA typing can help predict outcomes of cell, tissue, and organ transplantation using serologic and molecular methods. Serologic testing can identify the phenotype of the individual, but molecular testing is

Figure 14-1. Hematopoiesis and Cytokine Delineation

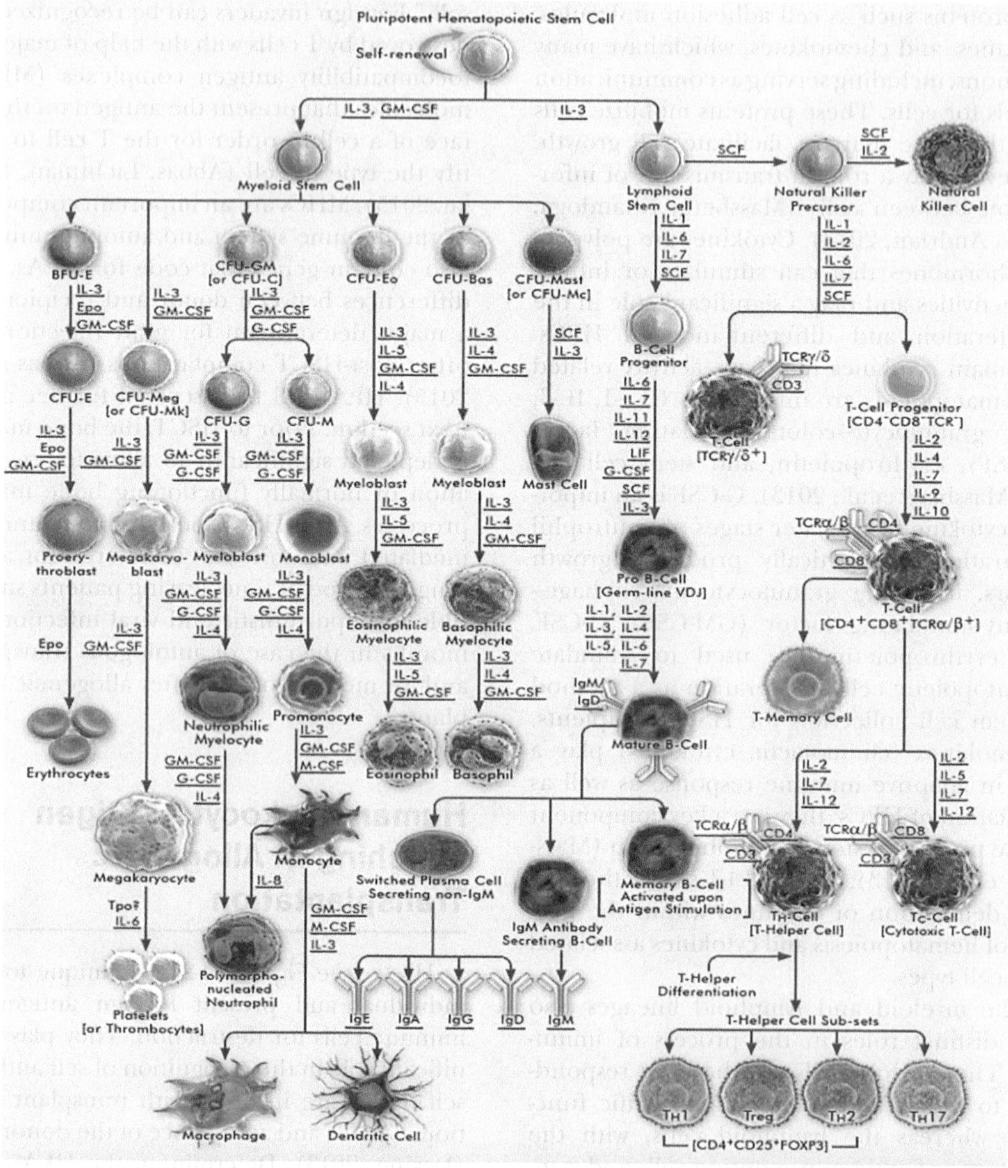

BFU-E—burst-forming unit–erythroid; CD—cluster of differentiation; CFU-Bas—colony-forming unit–basophil; CFU-C—colony-forming unit in culture; CFU-E—colony-forming unit–erythroid; CFU-Eo—colony-forming units–eosinophil; CFU-G—colony-forming unit granulocyte; CFU-GM—colony-forming unit–granulocyte/macrophage; CFU-M—colony-forming unit macrophage; CFU-Mast—colony-forming unit–mast; CFU-Meg—colony-forming unit–megakaryocyte; Epo—erythropoietin; G-CSF—granulocyte–colony-stimulating factor; GM-CSF—granulocyte macrophage–colony-stimulating factor; Ig—immunoglobulin; IL—interleukin; LIF—leukemia inhibitory factor; M-CSF—macrophage colony-stimulating factor; SCF—stem cell factor; TCR—T-cell receptor; Tpo—thrombopoietin

Note. Copyright 2012 by Affymetrix. Retrieved from https://www.thermofisher.com/us/en/home/life-science/antibodies/antibodies-learning-center/antibodies-resource-library/cell-signaling-pathways/hematopoiesis-pluripotent-stem-cells.html. Used with permission.

required to identify the genotype (Mickelson & Petersdorf, 2009). The HLA loci are located on chromosome 6 and typically are inherited as complete haplotypes, or a set of alleles that are linked on the same chromosome (Genetics Home Reference, 2009).

The HLA region within the MHC is divided into subgroups; however, class I and II HLA subgroups are the most important for determining HLA compatibility for HSCT. Class I (HLA-A, HLA-B, and HLA-C) are found in every cell and are responsible for presenting antigens to cytotoxic T (Tc) cells for recognition. Class II (HLA-DR, HLA-DQ, HLA-DP) are found on B cells, macrophages, and dendritic cells and present antigens to helper T (Th) cells (Abbas et al., 2015). GVHD and graft failure incidences typically increase with increasing HLA disparity between donor and recipient (Mickelson & Petersdorf, 2009). Monozygotic twins share an identical HLA genotype, whereas full siblings have a 25% chance of having an identical HLA haplotype. With improvements in HLA typing methods, outcomes for disease-free survival have improved for HSCT performed with unrelated donors, although rates of GVHD and nonrelapse mortality are still higher in these patients. Common HLA alleles are present in all populations, but some ethnic tendencies in HLA inheritance make finding an unrelated match among certain ethnic groups more difficult. According to the National Marrow Donor Program (NMDP), people of African American background have only a 20% likelihood of finding a full donor match (Be The Match, n.d.-b). UCB transplantation can allow for a higher degree of HLA disparity because of the immaturity of the donor immune system, but better HLA matches are still associated with improved outcomes (Antin & Raley, 2013; Mickelson & Petersdorf, 2009).

Figure 14-2. Human Leukocyte Antigen Locus on Chromosome 6

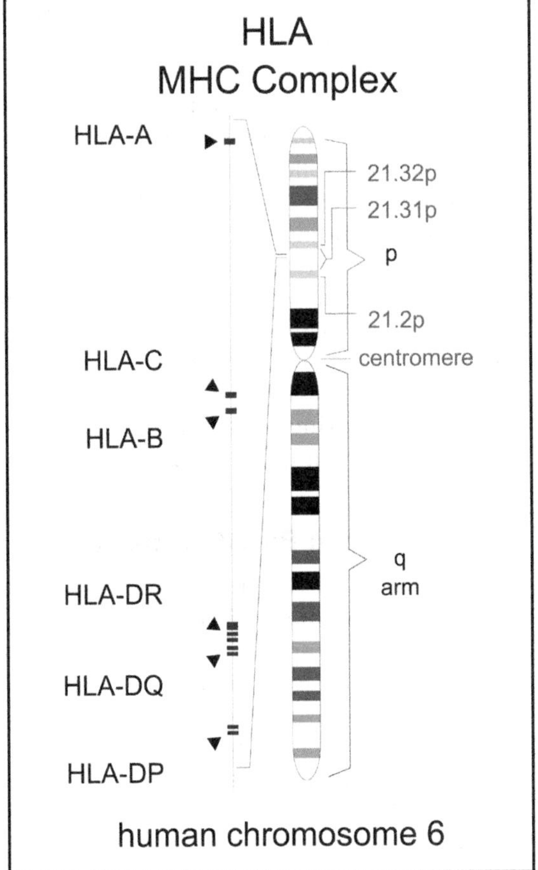

Note. Public domain image by Pdeitiker. Retrieved from https://commons.wikimedia.org/wiki/File:HLA.svg.

Types of Transplants

Multiple methods for performing HSCT exist. An allogeneic HSCT is performed with the cells of a donor other than the recipient and can be performed using a number of different donor sources. This form of transplant is preferred in patients with diseases such as myelodysplastic syndrome, acute leukemias, chronic myeloid leukemia, and aplastic anemia. An autologous transplant is performed using a patient's own previously collected stem cells and is used primarily in diseases such as multiple myeloma, lymphomas, and testicular cancer.

Allogeneic Transplant

With allogeneic transplant, high-dose chemotherapy is administered to suppress the recipient's immune system. Donor marrow is infused to restore the bone marrow, and allogeneic transplant also has the benefit of graft-versus-tumor (GVT) effect. This is the process in which the donor cells recognize any residual leukemia/tumor cells as foreign and destroy them (Bacigalupo et al., 2009). However, allogeneic transplant also has the potential risk of severe forms of GVHD, in which the donor immune system attacks the recipient tissues, causing damage to the skin, liver, gut, and other organ systems. Some research has indicated that patients who developed some form of GVHD experienced significantly less disease relapse than patients who had no GVHD (Cutler & Antin, 2006).

Allogeneic transplants can be performed with multiple different donor sources. A syngeneic HSCT is performed with the use of cells from an identical twin. Syngeneic transplants have shown inferior outcomes with higher rates of relapse. HLA-matched siblings (nonidentical) are the preferred source for a donor, as post-transplant complications have been reported less frequently with less chance of failure to engraft. However, according to NMDP, approximately 70% of patients in need of an allogeneic transplant will not have an HLA-matched donor in the family (Be The Match, 2014). Recent studies have indicated similar survival outcomes in patients who received sibling donor transplants and those who received matched unrelated donor transplants (Ho et al., 2011). Unrelated donors are obtained from the NMDP's Be The Match registry, the world's largest and most diverse registry of volunteer donors. This program connects patients in need with potential donors within its registry and through connections with international registries for marrow, peripheral blood, and cord blood sources of stem cells for HSCT (Be The Match, 2014). Although the registry has significantly improved patient access to potential donors, approximately 30% of patients may not have an HLA match on the donor registry. A critical need exists for minority volunteers within the donor registry, and community outreach and education to recruit donors is essential. See Table 14-1 for the composition of Be The Match registry donors.

Autologous Transplant

The goal of an autologous transplant is to administer high doses of chemotherapy with HSCT as a "rescue" of the bone marrow. Chemotherapy affects all cells within the bone marrow, not just the abnormal cells; therefore, at very high doses, chemotherapy causes severe myelotoxicity. The autologous transplant serves as a way to assist with the recovery of the depleted bone marrow after chemotherapy. Because the autologous transplant is from "self," immune suppression therapy is not needed following transplant because no GVHD risk exists. Also, no HLA testing is required for finding a donor, which can be a lengthy process. However, autologous HSCT carries the potential for damage to the stem cells from the patient's prior chemotherapy treatments, the possibility of contamination of the stem cell product with tumor from the patient's underlying disease, and a higher risk of relapse (Bacigalupo et al., 2009).

Umbilical Cord Blood Transplant

Cord blood transplants are another option for patients without a sibling or a matched unrelated donor option. Limitations to cord blood transplants are significant, as cord blood is a finite source. Once the cells are used, more cells cannot be obtained from the donor source if there is graft failure or a need for donor lymphocyte infusion (DLI) (Brunstein & Laughlin, 2010). The amount of cells is typically much smaller in a cord blood unit, and two different matched cords typically are needed for transplant in adult patients. Additionally, recovery of white blood cells after transplant takes longer in patients after cord blood transplant than from any other source, thus increasing a patient's risk of infection and other severe complications (Brunstein & Laughlin, 2010).

Table 14-1. Breakdown of Be The Match Registry Members by Race/Ethnicity

Race/Ethnicity	Total Number/% of Total
African American or Black	Nearly 775,000/ 6%
American Indian/Alaska Native	More than 131,000/ 1%
Asian	More than 792,000/ 6%
Chinese	More than 135,000/ 1%
Filipino	More than 68,000/ 0.5%
Japanese	More than 36,000/ 0.3%
Korean	More than 95,000/ 0.8%
South Asian	Nearly 236,000/ 2%
Vietnamese	More than 55,000/ 0.4%
All other Asian (includes people who select more than one Asian subgroup)	Nearly 166,000/ 1%
Hispanic or Latino (total number of indicating Hispanic or Latino ethnicity or race)	Nearly 1.2 million/ 10%
Multiple races	More than 493,000/ 4%
Native Hawaiian or Other Pacific Islander	More than 18,000/ 0.1%
White	Nearly 7.6 million/ 61%

Note. Table courtesy of Be The Match. Used with permission.

Haploidentical Transplant

Preliminary studies into the transplantation of haploidentical cells—those with a one haplotype match—have recently been showing success using donors with as few as 6/12 loci matched (Kasamon et al., 2013). This is promising for the 30% of patients who may not have an HLA-matched donor in the registry because it improves options for HSCT recipients who may not have otherwise been eligible for transplant due to lack of a full-matched donor. Haploidentical (half-matched) donors can be any first-degree relative (siblings, children, and parents) with at least a half HLA match. Current research has shown that survival outcomes of haploidentical transplants are similar to those of full HLA-matched transplants and that incidence of complications such as GVHD is not significantly increased (Bashey et al., 2013).

Methods of Hematopoietic Cell Collection

Multiple factors, including the type of transplant planned, determine the method of cell collection. The goal of the collection is to obtain adequate numbers of HPCs to achieve engraftment. *Engraftment* is the term used for the process in which the donor stem cells make their way to the recipient bone marrow and begin producing healthy blood cells. Engraftment is indicated by the recovery of neutrophil counts to 500/mm^3 (Horowitz, 2009). The minimum number of HPCs required for engraftment has not yet been established (Antin & Raley, 2013).

Hematopoietic Progenitor Cell, Marrow

Initially, hematopoietic progenitor cell, marrow (HPC-M) was the primary method of stem cell collection. Bone marrow harvest requires placing the donor under general anesthesia and performing multiple needle aspirations of marrow from either the anterior or posterior iliac crests or from the sternum. The marrow is then mixed with anticoagulant and filtered for removal of bone, fat cells, blood clots, and other cellular debris (Antin & Raley, 2013). This method is advantageous in that it can be performed as an outpatient procedure and completed in several hours. Typically, the procedure is well tolerated, and this method decreases rates of GVHD. HPC-M can be modified as well to remove red blood cells if the donor and recipient are not blood type (ABO) compatible, thus reducing the potential for red cell lysis. This method carries the risk of infection, bleeding, and possible bone damage, in addition to requiring general or epidural anesthesia (Nuss, Barnes, Fisher, Olson, & Skeens, 2011).

Hematopoietic Progenitor Cell, Apheresis

An alternative method of stem cell collection is that of obtaining PBSCs via an apheresis procedure, known as hematopoietic progenitor cell, apheresis (HPC-A). This method was primarily used for autologous HSCT but has increased in frequency for allogeneic transplant and is now the most common method of stem cell collection. The process of PBSC collection is called *mobilization*; with this method, stem cells are "mobilized," or pushed out of the bone marrow into the peripheral blood using mobilization regimens that consist of either chemotherapy alone, chemotherapy combined with G-CSF, G-CSF or GM-CSF alone, or G-CSF in combination with plerixafor hydrochloride (Shea & DiPersio, 2009). The cells can be collected with apheresis machines that use centrifugation to remove stem cells from the blood while returning the remaining blood components to the donor.

Apheresis can be performed using large-bore peripheral IVs or with the placement of either tunneled or nontunneled apheresis catheters. The number of stem cells collected can be calculated by determining the number of cells that have the stem cell marker CD34 (Schmit-Pokorny, 2013). The procedure may be completed in as little as one collection but may require several days of collection with each procedure lasting several hours (Schmit-Pokorny, 2013). Potential complications of the apheresis procedure include hypocalcemia, hypovolemia, and thrombocytopenia. Hypocalcemia is caused by the anticoagulant citrate dextrose solution, formula A (known as ACD-A) used during the procedure, which binds to calcium in the body and can cause symptoms of hypocalcemia, including numbness, tingling, nausea, and vomiting (Szczepiorkowski et al., 2010). Hypovolemia and thrombocytopenia are related to the procedure itself as the blood volume is processed by the apheresis machine. Early intervention for these complications can prevent or minimize them. For example, donors may receive calcium supplements to prevent severe hypocalcemia and may receive IV fluids during the procedure as well. Transfusions of platelets and packed red blood cells may be needed following the collection process (Szczepiorkowski et al., 2010).

PBSC collection can be performed as an outpatient procedure, does not require anesthesia, and typically is well tolerated by donors of all ages. Cells collected in this manner are more mature and therefore can engraft more quickly than cells obtained through bone marrow harvest. This is important because it decreases the amount of time that an HSCT recipient is thrombocytopenic, reducing bleeding risk; this also reduces the length of neutropenia, thereby decreasing the risk of major infection (Schmit-Pokorny, 2013). A disadvantage associated with the use of peripherally collected stem cells is an increase in chronic GVHD (cGVHD) compared to bone marrow transplant (Bensinger, 2012). Apheresis procedures also introduce the risk of central line–associated infections and other central line complications, such as thrombosis and pneumothorax (Schmit-Pokorny, 2013). Patients undergoing PBSC mobilization also may fail to collect adequate numbers of stem cells; this is primarily seen in autologous donors who have had multiple previous courses of chemotherapy (Shea & DiPersio, 2009).

Hematopoietic Progenitor Cell, Cord

Hematopoietic progenitor cell, cord (HPC-C) harvesting requires collection of stem cells from the umbilical cord and the placenta at the time of delivery. The cord blood is HLA-typed, cryopreserved, and stored immediately, thus enabling much faster availability of stem cell product to the recipient. This method can be performed quickly with no risk to the mother or infant. HPC-C transplants have decreased rates of viral transmission but also the potential for passing genetic diseases to the recipient (Schmit-Pokorny, 2013). As with all forms of collection, the stem cell product can be depleted of red cells and plasma. Often the cell dose in one UCB unit is not enough for adults and combining two products is preferred; however, this increases the risk of acute GVHD (aGVHD) (Antin & Raley, 2013). Additional disadvantages with this cell source include delayed engraftment and delayed post-transplant immune reconstitution (Schmit-Pokorny, 2013).

Cell Processing and Storage

Cell processing begins with quantifying the number of stem cells (CD34+ cells) collected. Each medical center has a goal for CD34+ cells per kilogram of recipient weight. Higher doses of cell infusions are associated with faster engraftment (Rosselet, 2013). The HPC product is tested for sterility, tumor or other contamination, mononuclear cell counts, and cell viability. The product also is evaluated for infectious diseases and blood type to ensure product safety and compatibility. Often, the volume of HPC product is reduced to decrease the cryoprotectant dosage required for storage because increased amounts of cryoprotectant are associated with increased clinical toxicity at the time of reinfusion (Schmit-Pokorny, 2013). If tumor contamination is noted within autologous product, purging of the cells may occur. Methods to purge tumor from cells include using chemotherapy and monoclonal antibodies. Other techniques, such as sorting devices and magnetic cells, may be used to separate the stem cells from the HPC product. The decision to purge the stem cell product must be made judiciously, as manipulation can harm cells and result in delayed or failed engraftment (Schmit-Pokorny, 2013).

Allogeneic HPC products also can be depleted of red blood cells or plasma if ABO incompatibility exists. Cells for autologous and UCB transplants are cryopreserved (frozen) and stored for later use. Allogeneic products can be infused immediately following processing without freezing or can be frozen if there will be time between product collection and the planned reinfusion. During the freezing process, a cryoprotectant, most commonly dimethyl sulfoxide (DMSO), is added to the product to prevent cell lysis during freezing or thawing. Finally, the product is placed into long-term storage freezers using liquid nitrogen or the vapor phase of liquid nitrogen until ready for use (Schmit-Pokorny, 2013). Further research is being conducted in improving stem cell grafts, ex vivo expansion of stem cell products for HSCT, and gene manipulation as a means of modifying or tracing specific cells (Schmit-Pokorny, 2013).

Donor and Recipient Evaluation

Donors undergoing stem cell collection, including both autologous and allogeneic donors, must be evaluated before beginning the collection process to verify they are eligible to undergo collection. Regulating bodies, such as the U.S. Food and Drug Administration (FDA) and the Foundation for the Accreditation of Cellular Therapy (FACT), set standards for how donors and recipients should be evaluated for eligibility to undergo the collection and HSCT process (Antin & Raley, 2013). Donors should be evaluated to ensure that the product collected will be safe for the recipient and to verify that the donation process is not likely to cause harm to the donor. Donors also should understand what they will be asked to do and be made aware of all risks associated with the donation process. Informed consent must be obtained and documented after the donor has been made aware of possible risks and complications of the collection process (Schmit-Pokorny, 2013). Donor evaluation should include a complete physical, assessment for the need for central line placement, and any contraindications to the mobilization process. A complete history and physical should be performed, including assessment for high-risk behaviors such as recreational drug use, alcohol consumption, blood transfusions, and pregnancies. Testing to determine eligibility includes basic laboratory work evaluating organ function such as kidneys and liver, as well as a complete blood count. Donors also undergo blood typing, HLA testing, pregnancy testing for females of childbearing potential, and infectious disease testing as dictated by regulating bodies (Antin & Raley, 2013).

HSCT recipient evaluation prior to transplant should include determination of the patient's physical capability to withstand the transplant process. Physical examination and a complete history, including assessment for high-risk behaviors, should be obtained. Age, comorbidities, type of disease, stage of disease, and performance status all play a role in treatment decisions and selection of transplant type. As with donor evaluation, laboratory work should be performed, as well as infectious disease testing. Recipients should have baseline organ function evaluated, including creatinine clearance, echocardiogram, electrocardiogram, chest x-ray, pulmonary function tests, and any restaging of their underlying disease as deemed appropriate per program guidelines and provider discretion. Additionally, any needed consults for dental examination, fertility preservation, radiation therapy, nutrition, and psychiatric evaluation should be completed prior to transplant (Antin & Raley, 2013). Psychosocial evaluations should be performed on all recipients to evaluate psychological needs as well as caregiver support and any possible financial strain, as the transplant process is time consuming and requires adequate caregiver support. HSCT has a high risk of treatment-related morbidity and mortality, and patients choosing to undergo this process should be made aware of potential outcomes. Informed consent should be obtained from the patient after explanation of all risks of the transplant procedure (Antin & Raley, 2013).

Transplant Program Standards

FACT was founded in 1996 by the International Society for Cellular Therapy and the American Society for Blood and Marrow Transplantation in an effort to establish quality standards within the field of cellular therapy (FACT, n.d.). FACT is an international voluntary inspection and accreditation program whose standards apply to all phases of hematopoietic cell collection, processing, and transplant. FACT outlines standards for aspects of transplant programs, including staff training, donor evaluation, cell collection, cell processing, and cellular therapy infusion. Currently, more than 200 programs are accredited for adult or pediatric transplant, cell collection, or cell processing. A center can achieve accreditation for autologous, allogeneic, or both types of transplants (FACT, n.d.). In addition to FACT accreditation, cell processing facilities also are regulated by FDA with guidelines on how cells may or may not be manipulated for use (U.S. FDA, 2014).

Transplant Regimen

Once collection of HPC product is completed and the patient is deemed eligible to move forward with the HSCT process, a conditioning therapy is selected. Patients receive the conditioning therapy prior to the HSC infusion. In the early post-transplant period, the focus is on prevention and management of complications related to conditioning and the HSCT.

Conditioning

The preparative, or conditioning, regimen is the first step of the transplant course. The primary goal of the conditioning regimen is to prepare the body to receive new blood-forming cells (HSCs). The conditioning regimen consists of high doses of chemotherapy to eliminate any remaining malignant cells in the body. In allogeneic transplants, chemotherapy also is used to suppress the recipient's immune system to prevent graft rejection and allow new cells to form (Be The Match, n.d.-a). A variety of conditioning regimens exist, and each is selected based on the type of transplant, the disease type, and the goal of therapy.

Regimens can be myeloablative or nonmyeloablative (reduced-intensity). Myeloablative regimens use very high doses of chemotherapy that ablate the bone marrow of the recipient to the point that without HSCT, the marrow would not recover on its own (McAdams & Burgunder, 2013). Nonmyeloablative regimens use lower doses of chemotherapy designed to suppress the recipient's immune system enough to allow donor engraftment of HPCs and induce a graft-versus-leukemia effect in which the donor cells attack and destroy any remaining tumor cells (McAdams & Burgunder, 2013). Reduced-intensity regimens are generally used for specific populations, such as those of older age or with significant comorbidities, who would otherwise be ineligible for myeloablative chemotherapy.

Total Body Irradiation

Some regimens contain high-dose chemotherapy plus total body irradiation (TBI). TBI involves treatment of the entire body with radiation. This approach can be useful as a part of HSCT because it contributes to immunosuppression and can eliminate tumor cells by reaching areas of the body, such as the central nervous system, testes, and ovaries, that are a safe harbor for tumor cells. TBI toxicities are more intense when the radiation is delivered in one dose; therefore, TBI doses often are split over a number of days (McAdams & Burgunder, 2013). Table 14-2 provides examples of common conditioning regimens.

Prevention of Toxicities Related to Conditioning

Some recognized practices exist for the prevention of commonly seen toxicities related to specific conditioning regimens. Hydration is used to manage any urinary bleeding with regimens containing cyclophosphamide. Busulfan lowers seizure threshold, and using an antiseizure medication prophylactically has been shown to reduce this complication. Additionally, cryotherapy may be used for drugs, primarily melphalan, that are well known for causing stomatitis and mucositis (Antin & Raley, 2013; Ezzone, 2013). Cryotherapy is the practice of having the patient eat ice, popsicles, and other cold products before, during, and shortly after the chemotherapy infusion in order to vasoconstrict the vessels in the oral cavity, with the goal of decreased drug perfusion to this area to reduce the severity of mucositis. Although no clear guidelines are available that direct the frequency and timing of cryotherapy for these patients, some documented evidence has shown it is beneficial in preventing or minimizing the toxicities from mucositis (Batlle et al., 2014).

Table 14-2. Conditioning Regimens*

Acronym/Regimen	Indications	Common Side Effects/Toxicity
Cy/TBI—cyclophosphamide + TBI	Leukemias, NHL, MDS	Myelosuppression, nausea/vomiting, hemorrhagic cystitis, cardiovascular toxicity, pulmonary toxicity
BEAM—carmustine, etoposide, cytarabine, melphalan	HL, NHL	Stomatitis/mucositis, nausea/vomiting, cardiovascular toxicity, myelosuppression, nephrotoxicity
Bu/Cy with or without TBI—busulfan (PO or IV), cyclophosphamide	Leukemias, MDS	Myelosuppression, neurotoxicity—busulfan lowers seizure threshold, nausea/vomiting, diarrhea, stomatitis, hepatitis, HSOS, cardiovascular toxicity, hemorrhagic cystitis, pulmonary toxicity
Flu/Bu with or without TBI—fludarabine, busulfan	Leukemias, MDS	Myelosuppression, neurotoxicity—busulfan lowers seizure threshold, nausea/vomiting, diarrhea, stomatitis, hepatitis, HSOS
ATG usually in combination with other listed drugs	Aplastic anemia	Immediate allergic reaction: fever, chills, hypotension, pulmonary edema; may have delayed skin rash, joint pain
Flu/Mel—fludarabine, melphalan	MM	Myelosuppression, nausea/vomiting, diarrhea, stomatitis/mucositis
Flu/TBI—fludarabine, low-dose TBI	MM	Myelosuppression, nausea/vomiting, diarrhea
CBV—cyclophosphamide, carmustine (BCNU), etoposide (VP-16)	HL, NHL	Myelosuppression, nausea/vomiting, pulmonary toxicity, nephrotoxicity, hemorrhagic cystitis, skin rash, cardiovascular toxicity

* Table is not all inclusive.

ATG—antithymocyte globulin; HL—Hodgkin lymphoma; HSOS—hepatic sinusoidal obstruction syndrome; IV—intravenously; MDS—myelodysplastic syndrome; MM—multiple myeloma; NHL—non-Hodgkin lymphoma; PO—by mouth; TBI—total body irradiation

Note. Based on information from Antin & Raley, 2013; McAdams & Burgunder, 2013.

Stem Cell Infusion

The process of cell infusion is similar to a blood transfusion. Premedications such as antiemetics, antihistamine, acetaminophen, and sometimes corticosteroids (hydrocortisone or methylprednisolone) typically are given to prevent transfusion-related hemolytic reactions (Antin & Raley, 2013). After identification of the product and recipient, the stem cells are infused. The length of time for reinfusion depends on the volume of product to be reinfused. Cryopreserved cells are thawed by immersion in a sterile saline or sterile water bath. Administration of cryopreserved cells over a longer period may help to minimize the effects of DMSO (McAdams & Burgunder, 2013). Infusion toxicities can occur due to the blood product administration or the DMSO used to cryopreserve frozen products. Infusion-related reactions may include fevers, chills, fluid overload, and, rarely, acute hemolytic transfusion reactions. DMSO causes many of the immediate complications related to infusion, such as nausea and vomiting, erythema, headaches, dizziness, and changes in blood pressure (Antin & Raley, 2013). DMSO excretes a unique odor described as garlic-like that can be noted around the patient's room for about 24 hours after transplant (McAdams & Burgunder, 2013). During infusion of cell products, vital signs are monitored at frequent intervals, with some patients placed on continuous telemetry monitoring. Aggressive hydration is initiated to maintain renal perfusion with careful monitoring of the volume status. Emergency medications should be readily available in case of severe hypersensitivity reactions (McAdams & Burgunder, 2013).

Complications of Hematopoietic Stem Cell Transplantation

Early Complications

Following transplant and prior to engraftment, patients are at high risk for developing complications due to the preparative chemotherapy and to the prolonged myelosuppression causing an increased risk for severe infection. This section outlines the most common side effects and their management during the post-transplant neutropenic phase. Engraftment generally is indicated by the recovery of absolute neutrophil count, typically 9–25 days after infusion of stem cells. Timing of engraftment depends on the type of transplant performed and the amount of chemotherapy the patient received prior to HSCT, as well as the use of growth factor such as G-CSF. Cord blood transplants typically take the longest to achieve engraftment. Some reports indicate recipients can take as long as 40 days after transplant to recover their absolute neutrophil count (Antin & Raley, 2013).

Infection

Following HSCT, patients have a high risk of developing infection. This is due to multiple factors, such as severe myelosuppression from the chemotherapy, as well as additional immunosuppression used in allogeneic transplants. HSCT recipients experience one to four weeks of neutropenia; even after neutrophil recovery, it can take anywhere from three months to two years for complete immune reconstitution in some allogeneic transplant recipients (Tomblyn et al., 2009). Because hematopoietic growth factors G-CSF or GM-CSF stimulate the growth of granulocytes and macrophages, they may be used to decrease the period of neutropenia, thus causing a decrease in infection rates. Several recommendations exist for post-transplant prophylaxis with antibiotic, antifungal, and antiviral medications. The use of these recommended agents or alternative prophylactic agents is determined by individual centers, and local epidemiology reports may assist in the decision. Vaccinations also must be readministered after allogeneic transplant as antibody titers decline. It is not recommended to revaccinate until B- and T-cell immune function has recovered and the patient is off of immunosuppression medications (Antin & Raley, 2013).

Infection following HSCT can occur either early or late, with certain infection types more likely to occur at specific time frames after HSCT. The highest risk for infection for an autologous HSCT recipient is pre-engraftment and immediately following engraftment. Because of continued immunosuppression following engraftment and the time required for a donor's cells to fully reconstitute a functioning immune system, allogeneic HSCT recipients will have a prolonged period of infection risk (McAdams & Burgunder, 2013). Early onset of infection during the pre-engraftment phase is most commonly due to gram-positive and gram-negative bacteria secondary to mucosal injury related to the conditioning regimen. Severe viral and fungal infections also can be seen after transplant as a result of prolonged immunosuppression including the use of steroids for GVHD complications (Antin & Raley, 2013).

Techniques for infection prevention are highly encouraged. Proper hand washing is a critical component to prevent the spread of infection. Many programs utilize private rooms that have HEPA filters capable of removing infectious particles from the air and controlling the flow of air particles within the transplant units (Antin & Raley, 2013). Catheter sites, impaired skin or mucosal barriers, pulmonary status, mental status, and laboratory values should be assessed and monitored frequently. Following transplant and once patients are discharged home, instructions for infection prevention should include proper hand washing and avoidance of large crowds and individuals with a known infection. HSCT recipients should be made aware of risks associated with gardening, diaper changing, or contact with animal feces (Antin & Raley, 2013). Dietary restrictions are also recommended to prevent infection, such as avoidance of raw and undercooked meats and eggs, as well as avoidance of fruits and vegetables with thin skins unless cooked thoroughly (Antin & Raley, 2013).

Early identification and immediate intervention are imperative in the care of HSCT recipients. Vital signs, including temperature, must be monitored frequently. A temperature of 38°C (100.4°F) is the limit to define neutropenic fever and must be reported to a provider for urgent action. A full fever workup typically includes blood and urine cultures; throat and sputum cultures may be indicated as well. A chest x-ray may be indicated for upfront evaluation if the patient displays symptoms that may indicate a pulmonary source of infection. Broad-spectrum IV antibiotics must be administered immediately. If fever continues for several days, coverage should be broadened, and antifungal and antiviral agents added (Tomblyn et al., 2009).

Myelosuppression

As a result of the conditioning regimen, patients experience more dramatic immune dysfunction with pancytopenia. In addition to the neutropenia described previously, anemia and thrombocytopenia are expected. Patients may require blood product support, such as red blood cells and platelets (Antin & Raley, 2013). Generally, blood products are only required early in the transplant process, but some patients may require transfusions for long periods as a side effect of medications used in treatment. It is typically recommended that blood products be irradiated and leukoreduced to minimize infection, alloimmunization, and transfusion reaction. Patients are monitored closely for signs of bleeding and may require platelet transfusions. Some may receive red cell transfusions for severe fatigue, shortness of breath, or hypotension (Antin & Raley, 2013).

Gastrointestinal Complications

Gastrointestinal (GI) toxicities related to the conditioning regimen are caused by the chemotherapy, which targets rapidly dividing cells, such as mucous membrane cells of the GI tract beginning in the oral cavity and extending to the rectum. The chemotherapy causes tissue damage, which leads to GI symptoms such as mucositis, nausea, vomiting, and diarrhea. The chemotherapy also causes myelosuppression; therefore, the mucous membranes need time to restore function and heal the damaged mucosa. Nausea and vomiting are common after HSCT, with exacerbation due to a number of reasons. Many chemotherapy drugs, as well as TBI, used in conditioning regimens are highly emetogenic. Patients may experience nausea and vomiting related to other medications, such as antibiotics, immunosuppressants, and opioids. Symptoms also may be due to the DMSO used to preserve stem cells.

Additionally, infections such as herpes simplex virus, cytomegalovirus (CMV), and adenovirus can contribute to symptoms of nausea and vomiting. Upper GI GVHD can manifest as nausea, and it is typically delayed nausea that occurs after engraftment (Antin & Raley, 2013). Medications are given prophylactically according to the emetogenic potential of the specific conditioning regimen. Multiple agents often are used in combination for added benefit in preventing nausea and vomiting. After chemotherapy, antiemetics may continue as scheduled around the clock or as needed. Relaxation and distraction techniques, dietary modifications, and timing of antiemetic administration prior to meals are all methods of decreasing nausea in HSCT recipients (Ezzone, 2013).

Diarrhea following transplant can have multiple etiologies, including chemotherapy, infection such as *Clostridium difficile* or CMV infection, or other medications, such as antibiotics. Diarrhea due to GVHD typically occurs after engraftment, and diagnosis can be confirmed with endoscopy for biopsies (Antin & Raley, 2013). Treatment for diarrhea is targeted at the underlying cause. Antidiarrheal medications can be used for noninfectious diarrhea. Depending on symptom severity, gut rest may be warranted by placing the patient on a nothing by mouth (NPO) diet. Many programs have developed individualized GVHD diet phases for those with severe diarrhea symptoms. These start with NPO and gradually advance the diet as tolerated. Lactose intolerance is common following transplant as well, and patients may need to be advised to avoid lactose products for symptom improvement (Antin & Raley, 2013).

Mucositis

Mucositis, characterized by inflammation of the mucous membranes, can lead to tissue damage and ulcerations, causing significant pain and difficulty swallowing. It is a frequent side effect of conditioning regimens and has been reported to occur in nearly 71% of HSCT recipients (Vagliano et al., 2011). Mucositis can affect the post-transplant course in many ways, including increased pain, risk of malnutrition, dehydration, and increased risk of infection. The damage to the lining of the GI tract/mucosa allows normal microbial flora found in the body to enter the bloodstream, causing systemic infection. Severe mucositis may require opioid analgesia and parenteral nutrition as well. Patients can expect symptoms to persist until neutrophil recovery occurs, at which time the immune system can begin to heal the damaged tissue (Ezzone, 2013).

Nursing care should focus on prevention of mucositis and other oral complications during the HSCT process. Patients should have a thorough dental evaluation prior to undergoing transplant to identify and resolve any potential areas of concern that may lead to infectious complication once the patient is immunocompromised. Good dental and oral hygiene throughout the HSCT process should be encouraged several times a day to reduce the amount of microbial flora in the oral cavity, minimize pain and bleeding, and decrease infection risk. Patients should be instructed to avoid injury to the oral mucosa, which may increase risk of developing mucositis; using a soft-bristle toothbrush and avoiding excessively hot beverages or food are some methods of prevention that can be taught to patients. A multitude of oral hygiene agents have been tried and vary across transplant programs, although the use of these agents is not well studied and evidence supporting their use for prevention or treatment is not strong (Ezzone, 2013). The use of cryotherapy during administration of mucotoxic conditioning therapies was discussed previously in the section on conditioning regimens. Nursing interventions include encouragement of good oral hygiene. Patients should undergo frequent oral assessments for tissue damage or pain. They also should be assessed for difficulty swallowing medications or food. Any abnormal findings should be reported for early intervention and symptom management.

Hepatic Complications

HSCT can lead to hepatic complications, including elevated liver function tests resulting from medications such as prophylactic antifungals. Hepatitis can result as a manifestation of the high-dose chemotherapy regimen or as a reactivation of hepatitis infection if the patient had a known hepatitis diagnosis prior to the transplant process. Additionally, conditioning regimens, particularly those containing busulfan, cyclophosphamide, and TBI, can lead to hepatic sinusoidal obstruction syndrome (HSOS), also known as veno-occlusive disease (Moreb, 2009). Chemotherapy causes damage to the endothelial lining of hepatic sinusoids, which leads to sloughing off of the injured tissue and obstruction of the venous pathways, resulting in fluid retention, weight gain, hyperbilirubinemia, and, in some cases, hepatomegaly. Most commonly, HSOS occurs within the first 30 days following conditioning therapy. Doppler studies of the liver help to rule out other potential etiologies of abnormal liver tests, such as infection or abscess, gallbladder disease, or venous thrombosis. Liver biopsy and measurement of hepatic pressure gradients can confirm a diagnosis of HSOS but generally are not performed because of thrombocytopenia following chemotherapy (Moreb, 2009). Figure 14-3 lists patient risk factors that increase the likelihood of developing HSOS.

Prevention and timely treatment of HSOS is imperative, although approximately 70% of HSOS cases have been reported to spontaneously resolve without residual complications. Severe HSOS has been reported as fatal in as many as 20%–50% of patients who develop it following HSCT (Anderson-Reitz & Clancy, 2013; Chao, 2014). Studies on the effectiveness of prophylactic agents such as heparin, ursodiol, and antithrombin III in preventing HSOS have conflicting results, but these agents may still be used in some transplant programs. In mild cases of HSOS, no treatment is needed. Patients with moderate to severe HSOS require fluid volume management and avoidance of nephrotoxic or hepatotoxic medications. Defibrotide has shown promise in the treatment of severe HSOS and was approved by FDA in 2016 for the treatment of adults and children with HSOS with renal or pulmonary dysfunction following HSCT (U.S. FDA, 2016) (see also Chapter 23 for more detailed information on HSCT).

Figure 14-3. Hepatic Sinusoidal Obstruction Syndrome Risk Factors

- Conditioning regimen (busulfan, cyclophosphamide, total body irradiation)
- History of abdominal radiation
- History of hepatitis or prior liver disease
- Bone marrow versus peripheral blood stem cell transplant
- Unrelated or human leukocyte antigen–mismatched donor
- Advanced disease

Note. Based on information from Moreb, 2009.

Neurologic Complications

HSCT also carries the risk of neurologic complications associated with a variety of causes. Infections involving the central nervous system can be seen post-transplant, with the most common infecting organisms being toxoplasmosis and fungal infections. Some viruses also may cause central nervous system effects, such as human herpesvirus 6, John Cunningham virus, and reactivation of herpes simplex or varicella zoster viruses (Antin & Raley, 2013). Additionally, neurotoxicities related to medications can occur. Busulfan, a common agent used in conditioning regimens, has been associated with seizures.

Calcineurin inhibitors (CNIs) such as cyclosporine and tacrolimus are used in allogeneic transplant recipients as a form of immunosuppression and may cause tremors, somnolence, nystagmus, and confusion. Posterior reversible encephalopathy syndrome (PRES) has been connected to the use of CNIs and usually is accompanied by rapid onset of hypertension. Radiologic findings for PRES are consistent with white matter edema within the posterior circulation of the brain. Discontinuing the agent causing the problem generally reverses the problem, although it may take time for the encephalopathy to completely resolve (Antin & Raley, 2013). Electrolyte disturbances related to chemotherapy also place patients at risk for complications such as seizures and muscle spasms. Aggressive replacement of low electrolytes should be encouraged. Steroid-induced myopathy can be a difficult thing to manage in patients who require long-term steroids for GVHD treatment and may require intensive physical and occupational therapy. Neurologic changes should be reported if noted on assessment so that rapid interventions can be initiated (Antin & Raley, 2013).

Pulmonary Complications

Pulmonary complications occur in approximately one-third of patients who undergo transplantation and are associated with significant morbidity and mortality (Chi, Soubani, White, & Miller, 2013). Post-HSCT pulmonary issues can be either infectious or noninfectious. Infectious complications arise as a result of myelosuppression from conditioning therapy and, in the case of allogeneic HSCT, the additional use of immunosuppression therapy; they are the most common form of post-transplant lung injury. Bacterial, fungal, and viral pneumonia all may potentially develop following HSCT. Many organizations, such as the Infectious Diseases Society of America, provide recommendations for prophylactic use of antimicrobials in hopes of preventing certain uncommon infections that have occurred in the transplant population, for example, *Nocardia* and *Pneumocystis*. Fungal infections noted in the HSCT course include *Aspergillus* and Zygomycetes forms such as *Mucor*. Fungal prophylaxis is generally recommended following HSCT and for the duration of immunosuppressive therapy. This recommendation is the same for antiviral prophylaxis (Chi et al., 2013). Viral pneumonia can also be noted following HSCT; CMV monitoring is typically recommended in allogeneic transplant recipients. The majority of viral pneumonia infections that are not related to CMV can be attributed to respiratory syncytial virus, influenza, and parainfluenza (Chi et al., 2013).

Noninfectious complications after HSCT include diffuse alveolar hemorrhage, typically seen within the first month of HSCT. Risk factors include conditioning chemotherapy including TBI. It is seen more frequently in allogeneic versus autologous transplants. Diffuse hemorrhagic secretions are seen on bronchoalveolar lavage. Treatment is controversial but typically includes platelet transfusions in the case of thrombocytopenia plus high-dose steroids (Antin & Raley, 2013).

Idiopathic pneumonia syndrome (IPS) is a noninfectious pneumonia more commonly seen in allogeneic transplant recipients. The etiology of IPS is not well understood but is theorized to be related to injury from conditioning therapy with associated cytokine damage to the pulmonary vasculature and endothelial cells. As with diffuse alveolar hemorrhage, treatment is high-dose steroids. However, etanercept, a tumor necrosis factor blocker, may be used to decrease cytokine activity associated with IPS (Antin & Raley, 2013).

Bronchiolitis obliterans syndrome (BOS) is another problem that may arise primarily in allogeneic transplant recipients and is associated with poor prognosis. This syndrome is characterized by a slow, progressive narrowing of airways, leading to obstruction and air trapping. It often is associated with GVHD of the lung as well (Antin & Raley, 2013). The American Society for Blood and Marrow Transplantation recommends lung evaluation with pulmonary function tests at six months after transplant and then annually (Chi et al., 2013). Treatment for BOS is high-dose steroids, immunosuppressive therapy, and supportive measures such as oxygen support (Chi et al., 2013).

Cryptogenic organizing pneumonia (COP), formerly known as bronchiolitis obliterans organizing pneumonia, is a distinct and separate entity from BOS. COP can occur in both autologous and allogeneic transplant recipients and features small airway fibrosis and interstitial and alveolar inflammation (Chi et al., 2013). Symptoms progress over days to weeks, and fever can sometimes develop because of inflammatory changes. However, it is important to note that COP is a noninfectious process (Antin & Raley, 2013). As with other noninfectious etiologies for pulmonary complications, treatment for COP is primarily high-dose steroids (Chi et al., 2013).

Renal Complications

Renal dysfunction can occur in the period following transplant as a result of chemotherapy, infection, antibiotic therapy, cyclosporine, tacrolimus, or other medications used in the HSCT course. Acute renal failure (ARF) is associated with a two to three times higher mortality rate in patients who develop it following HSCT (Anderson-Reitz & Clancy, 2013). Nursing intervention should focus on closely monitoring fluid status, blood pressure, and laboratory values, in addition to patient mental status and medications. Diuretics, volume replacement, correcting electrolyte imbalances, reducing use of nephrotoxic agents, and hemodialysis are methods of medical management that may be implemented in patients who have developed or are at risk for renal failure (Antin & Raley, 2013). Sepsis is another risk factor for the development of ARF; therefore, swift identification of signs of infection and prompt action are important in prevention(Anderson-Reitz & Clancy, 2013).

Hemorrhagic cystitis also can occur following transplant. It may be related to conditioning chemotherapy agents, such as ifosfamide and cyclophosphamide, or viral infections, such as BK virus and adenovirus (Bubalo, 2015; Strasfeld, 2015). Clinical manifestations of hemorrhagic cystitis include dysuria, frequency, urgency, and frank hematuria. Prophylactic measures are initiated in the case of chemotherapy-related cystitis and include mesna and aggressive fluid hydration during and after chemotherapy administration. Treatment is focused on symptom management and supportive care and includes pain management, antispasmodic medications, platelet transfusions in the case of thrombocytopenia, and, in severe cases, continuous bladder irrigation (Bubalo, 2015; Strasfeld, 2015).

Cardiovascular Complications

Chemotherapy- and radiation-induced toxicity to the cardiac tissue can lead to problems such as myopericarditis, cardiomyopathy, pericardial tamponade, pulseless electrical activity, congestive heart failure, and myocardial edema. Conditioning therapies such as cyclophosphamide, anthracyclines such as daunorubicin, and TBI are most commonly associated with cardiotoxicity (Stephens, 2013). Arrhythmia also may manifest following HSCT. Risk factors include advanced age, high-dose anthracyclines, and low ejection fraction. Some drugs are also known to be associated with arrhythmias, including voriconazole, a commonly used antifungal medication, and DMSO, the cryopreservative used to process stem cell products (Stephens, 2013). Additionally, hypertensive crisis can be seen and usually is related to medications such as CNIs used for immunosuppression in allogeneic transplant recipients. Uncontrolled hypertension may also be seen in patients on long-term steroid therapy (Antin & Raley, 2013).

Late Complications

The majority of late complications seen in HSCT recipients are related to long-term immunosuppression therapy in allogeneic transplant recipients: osteoporosis, avascular bone necrosis, infection, and secondary malignancy.

Skeletal Complications

Osteoporosis, a condition of severe bone loss and degeneration, occurs with increased frequency in HSCT recipients because of corticosteroid use, gonadal failure related to conditioning therapy such as TBI, and long-term immunosuppression. Bone density scanning to assess for bone disease should be performed regularly, and vitamin D and calcium supplementation should be considered. Nearly 50% of patients are found to have low bone density after HSCT (Tichelli & Socié, 2012). In some HSCT recipients, bisphosphonate therapy has been used as a method of reducing post-transplant bone loss (Tierney & Robinson, 2013). Avascular necrosis (AVN) of bones, most commonly occurring in weight-bearing bones, can occur as a result of corticosteroid treatment as well as immunosuppressive therapy and is more commonly seen in men and patients diagnosed with Hodgkin lymphoma or multiple myeloma. AVN is characterized by decreased blood flow to the bones resulting in ischemic bone damage and has been reported to affect 4%–10% of patients (Tichelli & Socié, 2012). Patients with AVN may experience pain and limited range of motion, most commonly in the hips, shoulders, and knees. Treatment options include physical therapy, pain management, and, in severe cases, joint replacement. Avoidance of further corticosteroids also is recommended (Tichelli & Socié, 2012).

Ocular Complications

Ocular complications related to HSCT include microvascular retinopathy, hemorrhagic complications, infectious retinitis, cataracts, and sicca syndrome. Cataracts are most commonly associated with corticosteroids and TBI; incidence is reported as greater than 80% in those who receive unfractionated TBI compared to those who receive fractionated doses (Tichelli & Socié, 2012). Sicca syndrome occurs in approximately 20% of HSCT recipients, but incidence increases to 40% in patients with cGVHD (Tierney & Robinson, 2013). Sicca syndrome has several manifestations, including reduced lacrimation, eye discomfort, conjunctivitis, corneal ulceration, and retinal hemorrhage (Tichelli, 2012). Treatment for sicca syndrome may include topical lubricants, topical cyclosporine, or topical retinoic acid (Tierney & Robinson, 2013). Microvascular retinopathy caused by immunosuppressants and TBI conditioning is described as cotton-wool spots and optic disk edema. Once the immunosuppressive therapy is discontinued, microvascular retinopathy is typically reversible (Tierney & Robinson, 2013). HSCT recipients should be encouraged to have regular ophthalmologic evaluations to monitor for these potential complications.

Secondary Malignancies

Secondary malignancies are a potential complication of HSCT because of the agents used in the treatment of the patient's primary malignant condition. Therapy-related myelodysplastic syndrome/acute myeloid leukemia has been reported in up to 36% of patients (Tichelli & Socié, 2012). Alkylating agents and TBI have been associated with a higher incidence of secondary malignancy. Methods of prevention include tapering immunosuppressive therapy as soon as possible (Tichelli & Socié, 2012). HSCT recipients are also at risk for developing solid tumors and should be educated to perform self-examinations and undergo recommended screening. Maintenance of a healthy weight, regular exercise, sun protection, and smoking cessation are methods that should be encouraged in patients as well (Shannon, 2013). Post-transplant lymphoproliferative disorder is an aggressive and often fatal disorder characterized by the overproliferation of donor lymphoid cells. The disorder is categorized into four subtypes with individual features and outcome measures. In general, treatment involves the tapering of immunosuppression if present, and chemotherapy is typically required. These are often associated with Epstein-Barr virus (EBV). Many programs monitor EBV load in patients after HSCT, and some preemptively initiate therapy if EBV loads are noted to be rising (Shannon, 2013).

Graft Rejection and Failure

Graft rejection refers to the process in which the residual host immune system rejects the donor hematopoietic system and donor cells fail to regenerate within the host marrow. This is more common in patients with aplastic anemia, those who receive reduced-intensity conditioning, and those who undergo unrelated or mismatched transplants (Antin & Raley, 2013). Alternatively, *graft failure* is not immune mediated and typically is related to inadequate stem cell numbers or poor stem cell viability. This can be seen where there is full donor chimerism but the patient fails to achieve hematopoietic recovery. Medications that can be myelotoxic may contribute as well; examples are sulfamethoxazole-trimethoprim, valganciclovir, and mycophenolate mofetil (Antin & Raley, 2013). Infections such as CMV, human herpesvirus 6, and varicella zoster virus also may depress blood counts. Primary graft failure is seen in less than 5% of HSCT recipients with a hematologic malignancy (Rosselet, 2013). If graft failure or rejection occurs, treatment involves another infusion of stem cell product. If chimerism shows few or no donor cells present, the patient will require further conditioning therapy. Graft rejection and failure after HSCT can be traumatic for patients and their families, as mortality is high (Antin & Raley, 2013).

Disease Relapse

Multiple factors play a role in relapse risk following HSCT. Of patients who relapse after HSCT, the majority will do so within the first three years (Shannon, 2013). Prognosis for patients who relapse is typically poor. For autologous transplant recipients, the goal of HSCT is potentially curative for some diseases, but for diseases such as multiple myeloma and mantle cell lymphoma, the primary goal is to achieve and maintain remission for as long as possible. In general, those in remission or with minimal residual disease going into transplant are less likely to relapse than those with residual disease (Shannon, 2013). Research aimed at preventing relapse for autologous transplant recipients is an active area, and strategies include determining the optimal timing of transplant, purging cells, and administering immunologic agents. Allogeneic transplant following relapse from autologous HSCT may be considered in some patients if a donor is available (Shannon, 2013).

Although recipients of allogeneic HSCT benefit from the GVT effect in addition to the ablative effect of high-dose chemotherapy, relapse can still occur. Risk factors include disease type, conditioning regimen, and risk profile of the underlying malignancy. Relapse for allogeneic recipients may be systemic or found in extramedullary sites (outside the medulla of the bone) such as the testes, skin, eyes, and central nervous system (Solh, DeFor, Weisdorf, & Kaufman, 2012). Treatment for allogeneic recipients may involve withdrawing immunosuppressive agents to invoke graft-versus-leukemia effects with the additional use of DLI. DLI involves readministering donor immunocompetent T and NK cells to provide additional activity against disease. It can be given as a single large dose or in small divided doses over several weeks. A major complication of DLI is the development of GVHD; therefore, patients with significant GVHD from HSCT are not eligible for DLI (Antin & Raley, 2013). In cases where a cure is not possible, supportive care should be offered (Shannon, 2013).

Fertility and Sexuality

The high doses of chemotherapy and radiation used in transplant conditioning regimens have the potential to decrease or eliminate reproductive function in both male and female patients. Busulfan, cyclophosphamide, and TBI are associated with gonadal dysfunction, with ovaries typically being more vulnerable than testes (Tichelli & Socié, 2012). Age at the time of transplant is a significant factor, as the younger the patient, the more likely that reproductive function will recover. Following HSCT, effects of the conditioning therapy can manifest as erectile dysfunction and low libido in men and menopause-like symptoms in women. The potential of the conditioning therapy to cause infertility and sterility should be discussed with patients considering HSCT. Sperm and embryo preservation methods can be discussed as well. However, these methods have major barriers, including cost and timing (Tichelli & Socié, 2012).

Sexual function and satisfaction can be negatively affected following HSCT. Many women experience premature menopause related to ovarian failure and hormonal changes, which can lead to vaginal dryness and hot flashes. Many transplant survivors experience sexual problems such as lack of libido and impotence. TBI and cGVHD are risk factors associated with decreased sexual satisfaction linked to decreased desire and arousal. Wong et al. (2013) described a prospective study evaluating men and women with cGVHD or who received TBI as part of the conditioning regimen, and all cohorts reported significantly decreased sexual satisfaction, with women describing less satisfaction than men. In some patients, these effects are related to hormonal changes or due to gonadal effects of TBI. GVHD can cause thinning of the vaginal tissue as well as dryness, leading to pain or discomfort during intercourse. Some changes in sexuality occur because of body appearance changes related to transplant, such as hair loss, weight gain or loss, and skin changes (Antin & Raley, 2013). Patients may feel embarrassed to speak with their provider about these concerns, and clinical assessment of these issues is important.

Graft-Versus-Host Disease

GVHD is an immune-mediated response in which the donor-derived T cells launch an attack on the host cells that are recognized as foreign. This releases inflammatory cytokines, leading to tissue damage. Other cells involved in GVHD include Th cells, Tc cells, NK cells, lymphokine-activated killer cells, and antigen-presenting cells (Mitchell, 2013). GVHD depends on differences in histocompatibility between donor and recipient; these differences can be minor antigens or MHC antigens if HLA incompatibility is present (Antin & Raley, 2013). This is a phenomenon seen in allogeneic HSCT recipients and can occur in anywhere from 20%–80% of patients. The risk is higher in unrelated and mismatched donor transplants than in matched sibling transplants (Martin et al., 2012).

Severe GVHD has been associated with higher morbidity and mortality; however, alloreactive donor T cells involved in the development of GVHD have also been shown to be beneficial when involved in the GVT effect. With the GVT effect, the alloreactive donor T cells and NK cells seek and attack any remaining tumor cells that may not have been eradicated with the conditioning regimen. The presence of GVHD in allogeneic transplant recipients has been associated with lower risk of recurrent disease and less graft failure (Warren, 2009). Therefore, the focus of GVHD prophylaxis and treatment has shifted from eliminating GVHD completely to preventing severe forms of GVHD while still allowing for some GVT effect with the goal of preventing disease relapse (Mitchell, 2013).

GVHD can be designated as either acute (aGVHD) or chronic (cGVHD). Classification of GVHD historically had been based on timing of symptom development. Previously, any manifestation before day 100 was considered aGVHD, and any occurrence after day 100 was cGVHD. However, classification is now based on clinical manifestations of the disease. Both forms can occur before or after day 100, and an overlap syndrome exists that has features of both (Antin & Raley, 2013).

Acute GVHD typically develops in the first several weeks after transplant and is a major cause of morbidity and mortality following allogeneic HSCT. Risk factors include increased age of donor, female donor to male recipient, female donors who are multiparous, herpes simplex virus or CMV seropositivity, disparity at class I or class II HLA loci, and use of DLI (Antin & Raley, 2013). Classic presentation of aGVHD involves one or more of the skin, liver, or GI tract systems. Clinical manifestations of aGVHD include maculopapular rash, jaundice, nausea, vomiting, anorexia, and diarrhea. Confirmation of aGVHD diagnosis can be done by performing a biopsy of affected tissue for evaluation (Antin & Raley, 2013). Two widely accepted staging and grading systems for aGVHD exist. The Glucksberg scale, first developed in 1975 and modified according to different transplant programs, is most commonly used. The International Bone Marrow Transplant Registry severity index is used to assess severity of aGVHD (Rowlings et al., 1997). These scales have demonstrated a correlation between severity of GVHD and risk of transplant-related mortality and treatment failure (Antin & Raley, 2013; Thomas et al., 1975).

The pathogenesis of cGVHD is not well understood but is believed to include all aspects of aGVHD pathogenesis in addition to autoimmune reactions of the donor cells. T lymphocytes recognize both minor and major histocompatibility antigens as foreign (Mitchell, 2013). Risk factors for cGVHD include increased donor and recipient age, prior aGVHD, female donor to male recipient, PBSC source versus bone marrow source, disparity at class I or class II HLA loci, and use of DLI (Antin & Raley, 2013; Mitchell, 2013). Incidence of cGVHD depends on stem cell source, degree of HLA mismatch, type of transplant, and other factors but has been reported to occur in up to 85% of allogeneic HSCT recipients (Mitchell, 2013).

Clinical manifestations of cGVHD may occur in any body system, including the skin, liver, eyes, oral cavity, lungs, GI system, female genitalia, and neuromuscular system. The National Institutes of Health (NIH) Working Group has published recommendations for the diagnosis of cGVHD based on diagnostic and distinctive manifestations. For a diagnosis of cGVHD, the NIH Working Group recommends that at least one diagnostic manifestation or at least one distinctive manifestation be present, as well as a biopsy confirming cGVHD in the same or another organ (Filipovich et al., 2005). See Table 14-3 for more details on the most common cGVHD manifestations. In addition to those listed in the table, other potential but far less common presentations of cGVHD include serositis, peripheral neuropathy, myasthenia gravis, nephritic syndrome, and cardiac involvement (Antin & Raley, 2013). In 2005, the NIH Working Group also developed a grading/scoring system to classify cGVHD as mild, moderate, or severe. Mild cGVHD involves one or two organs without significant functional impairment. Moderate cGVHD is determined by at least one organ site with significant but not major functional impairment, or a maximum score of 2 in any affected organ, or three or more organs involved without significant functional impairment, or cGVHD of the lung with a score of 1. Severe cGVHD is diagnosed if a score of 3 is present in any organ with major disability, or cGVHD of the lung is present with a score of 2 or higher. Increased severity scores of cGVHD are associated with decreased overall survival and increased nonrelapse mortality (Filipovich et al., 2005). More research is needed to further understand the pathophysiology of cGVHD in order to develop new methods for prevention and treatment.

Prevention and treatment of GVHD has been limited, as the complete mechanism and pathogenesis of GVHD are not yet understood. Immunosuppressive agents are the mainstay of prevention and are administered immediately before HSCT and continued for several months following allogeneic HSCT. A multitude of therapies are used for prevention and treatment, and both aGVHD and cGVHD are treated with the same methods. The goal of immunosuppression is to partially suppress the donor's immunity to prevent or manage GVHD while allowing the benefits of the GVT effect. Upfront prophylaxis for GVHD often includes agents such as CNIs and methotrexate, often used in combination (Mitchell, 2013). Doses of prophylactic immunosuppressants are slowly tapered during the months after transplant, as tolerated by the patient. T-cell depletion of the stem cell graft is another method that has been researched and used to prevent GVHD. Several approaches have been developed to remove the donor T cells from the HPC product, including

Table 14-3. Chronic Graft-Versus-Host Disease Clinical Manifestations

Organ System	Diagnostic Manifestations	Distinctive Manifestations	Diagnostic Tools	Findings
Skin/nails	Poikiloderma, lichen planus–like eruptions, deep sclerotic features, morphea-like superficial sclerotic features, lichen sclerosis–like lesions Nails: Longitudinal ridging, splitting, brittleness, onycholysis, pterygium unguis, dystrophy, nail loss	Depigmentation, sweat impairment, temperature intolerance, erythema, maculopapular rash, pruritus, diffuse mottling, reduction in hair, alopecia	Skin biopsy	–
Oral/mucous membranes	Lichen planus–like changes, hyperkeratotic plaques (leukoplakia), decreased oral range of motion	Xerostomia, mucoceles, mucosal atrophy, pseudomembranes, pain, ulcers	–	–
Eyes	Sicca syndrome, keratoconjunctivitis sicca	New-onset dry, gritty, painful eyes; cicatricial conjunctivitis; confluent areas of punctate keratopathy; photophobia, periorbital hyperpigmentation; corneal abrasions	Schirmer test, slit-lamp examination	Low Schirmer test (both eyes ≤ 5 mm)
Genitals	Lichen planus–like features, vaginal scarring or stenosis, narrowed introitus due to scar tissue, hair loss	Dryness, fissures, burning, dyspareunia, ulcers	N/A	Diagnosis is based on symptoms and physical findings.
Gastrointestinal tract	Esophageal web and strictures/stenosis Hepatic: hyperbilirubinemia, elevated alkaline phosphatase	Anorexia, nausea, vomiting, diarrhea, weight loss, failure to thrive, wasting syndrome, sometimes acute hepatitis	Biopsies by endoscopy from duodenum, stomach, and esophagus; biopsies from colon, rectum, and liver	Endoscopy findings: mucosal edema and erythema, focal erosions Histologic findings: apoptotic epithelial cells and crypt cell dropout Liver biopsy: focal portal inflammation with bile duct obliteration or sclerosis

(Continued on next page)

Table 14-3. Chronic Graft-Versus-Host Disease Clinical Manifestations *(Continued)*

Organ System	Diagnostic Manifestations	Distinctive Manifestations	Diagnostic Tools	Findings
Lung	Bronchiolitis obliterans syndrome is the only diagnostic feature of pulmonary graft-versus-host disease.	Dyspnea on exertion, shortness of breath, cough, wheeze, chronic asymptomatic rales	Pulmonary function tests (including FEV_1 and DLCO), radiologic testing	$FEV_1/FVC < 0.7$ and $FEV_1 < 75\%$, evidence of air trapping, small airway thickening on radiologic tests, pathologic confirmation of constrictive bronchiolitis
Hematologic/immune system	Cytopenias, refractory thrombocytopenia, eosinophilia, lymphopenia, hypogammaglobulinemia	N/A	N/A	Cytopenias are commonly seen in chronic graft-versus-host disease but not used to establish diagnosis.
Musculoskeletal	Fascial involvement, fasciitis presenting with stiffness, decreased range of motion, edema, dimpling skin, joint contractures	Clinical myositis: tender muscles Arthralgia, arthritis	Electromyography, creatinine phosphokinase, aldolase, muscle biopsy	–

DLCO—diffusing capacity of the lungs for carbon monoxide; FEV_1—forced expiratory volume in one second; FVC—forced vital capacity; N/A—not applicable

Note. Based on information from Mitchell, 2013.

physical and immunologic separation methods. Although T-cell depletion has been shown to decrease the incidence of GVHD, this process has been shown to increase engraftment failures, delay immune reconstitution, and increase the risk of disease relapse and infections (Mitchell, 2013). Treatment of aGVHD flares and cGVHD typically includes corticosteroids, CNIs, and a number of other possible options, including polyclonal or monoclonal antibodies, IV immunoglobulin and other systemic therapies, phototherapy, and topical therapy. Table 14-4 indicates the drugs used to prevent and treat GVHD. Management of aGVHD and cGVHD can be very difficult and places the patient at higher risk for infections and complications accompanied by a significant increase in mortality.

Survivorship and Quality of Life

HSCT has evolved into a standard method of treatment for multiple hematologic malignancies; therefore, the frequency of HSCT has increased over the past several years. Advances in the field have significantly improved post-HSCT survival rates. However, the procedure carries inherent risks and complications that can be severe and cause major limitations, in some cases for years following the transplant. As HSCT has become a more common method

Table 14-4. Drugs Used to Treat Graft-Versus-Host Disease

Drug	Adverse Effects	Nursing Considerations
Calcineurin Inhibitors		
Cyclosporine, tacrolimus	Hypertension, glucose intolerance, headache, microangiopathic hemolytic anemia, seizures, confusion, nephrotoxicity, tremor, hirsutism, electrolyte imbalances, posterior reversible encephalopathy syndrome	Many cytochrome P450-related drug interactions are possible. Avoid grapefruit juice. Drug levels must be monitored closely, and IV administration should be done through a dedicated line. Both are cleared through hepatic metabolism; liver dysfunction may occur.
Corticosteroids		
Methylprednisolone	Hyperglycemia, insomnia, cataracts, hypertension, osteopenia, infection risk, muscle wasting, fluid retention	High-dose steroids must be tapered.
Monoclonal Antibodies		
Alemtuzumab Basiliximab Daclizumab Infliximab Rituximab	Headache, nausea/vomiting, hypersensitivity and infusion reactions, infection risk, elevated transaminase concentrations	Fever, rigors, and hypotension may occur. Follow administration protocols to minimize infusion reactions.
Polyclonal Antibodies		
Antithymocyte globulin Thymoglobulin/ATGAM, ATG	Hypersensitivity and infusion reactions, serum sickness, fever, chills, rash, joint pain	Risk for anaphylaxis; follow administration protocols to minimize infusion reactions.
Other		
Etanercept Pentostatin	Hypersensitivity reactions, infection risk, myelosuppression, nausea/vomiting	Agents are investigative.
Methotrexate	Mucositis, delayed engraftment, hepatotoxicity	Drug is administered on days +1, +3, +6, and +11. 50%–100% renally excreted Patient should be evaluated for pleural and pericardial effusions, ascites, and third spacing prior to dosing.
Mycophenolate mofetil (MMF)	Nausea/vomiting, diarrhea, mild myelosuppression	MMF levels must be monitored closely.
Phototherapy: Psoralen and UVA irradiation and extracorporeal photopheresis (ECP)	Hypotension, photosensitivity	Wear sun protective gear and sunscreen. Avoid high-fat diet prior to ECP procedure.

(Continued on next page)

Table 14-4. Drugs Used to Treat Graft-Versus-Host Disease *(Continued)*

Drug	Adverse Effects	Nursing Considerations
Sirolimus	Hyperlipidemia, hypertriglyceridemia, cytopenias	Metabolized by liver and cytochrome P450 enzymes. Drug levels need to be monitored. Increases risk of veno-occlusive disease/ hepatic sinusoidal obstruction syndrome.

Note. Based on information from Mitchell, 2013.

of treatment and patients are surviving longer, the focus on research has shifted to not only evaluate survival and relapse rates but also to evaluate quality of life (QOL). QOL measures are subjective and multidimensional and typically include physical, psychological, social, and spiritual assessments (Kiviat, 2013). Frequently reported issues include fatigue, fertility and sexuality concerns, inability to assume social roles, and difficult family relationships and caregiver support problems. Many QOL measurement tools have been developed to provide valuable information to the treatment team. Information about QOL should be provided to patients and families during the transplant decision-making process (Kiviat, 2013). Nurses have an important role related to assessing QOL, providing education, performing symptom management, and providing referrals for community support. Rehabilitation programs, counseling, and support groups may be beneficial for patients and their families when dealing with the sequelae of HSCT.

Conclusion

Developments and advances in HSCT continue to be studied. The use of nonmyeloablative regimens, for example, has quickly increased in popularity, and ongoing research is being performed to determine optimal chemotherapy combinations and appropriate patient selection. Other areas of research include gene therapy, post-transplant immune reconstitution methods, and methods to maximize GVT effects, as well as ways to reduce relapse and infectious complications (Antin & Raley, 2013; Burcat, 2013). The use of mismatched donors for transplantation is another growing research area that is showing promise in increasing donor options for transplant recipients without increasing GVHD potential. Improvements in patient selection, GVHD therapy, and infection prevention have the potential to make HSCT a more tolerable therapy for larger numbers of patients.

HSCT is a complex process that requires management for years following the transplant in many cases; patients depend on nursing support for education, compassion, and timely assessment and interventions to assist in achieving the best possible outcomes. Figure 14-4 lists some helpful resources for clinicians, patients, and their families. Nurses should remain up to date on current methods of HSCT treatment, including symptom management, immunosuppression guidelines, and goals of care. Nursing staff often are the frontline resource for patients and are relied on to provide accurate and dependable education. Nursing assessments for clinical signs and symptoms that may indicate serious complications are imperative and can allow for quick and effective intervention.

The author would like to acknowledge Debra J. Harris, BA, MSN, RN, OCN®, for her contribution to this chapter that remains unchanged from the first edition of this book.

Figure 14-4. Internet Resources

- American Cancer Society: www.cancer.org
- American Society for Blood and Marrow Transplantation: www.asbmt.org
- Bone Marrow Donors Worldwide: www.bmdw.org
- Center for International Blood and Marrow Transplant Research: www.cibmtr.org
- International Society for Cellular Therapy: www.celltherapysociety.org
- National Bone Marrow Transplant Link: www.nbmtlink.org
- National Institutes of Health: www.nih.gov
- National Marrow Donor Program—Be The Match: https://bethematch.org

Key Points

- The basic concept of HSCT is that by treating the bone marrow with high doses of chemotherapy followed by transplant with immature, bone marrow–stimulating cells, the bone marrow function can potentially be restored to normal.
- HSCT can be performed using cells from a multitude of sources, including a patient's own stem cells, a related donor, an unrelated donor, or a cord blood donor.
- The type of transplant chosen for a patient and the conditioning regimen are based on many factors including disease type, age, and performance status.
- Although white blood cell count engraftment is achieved within the first few weeks of HSCT, humoral and cell-mediated immunity can take up to a year to recover.
- Early complications of HSCT include nausea, vomiting, diarrhea, mucositis, myelosuppression, and liver and renal toxicity. Acute GVHD can occur in allogeneic transplant recipients, typically within the first few weeks of transplant, and is a major cause of morbidity and mortality.
- Late complications can include cGVHD and pulmonary complications such as cryptogenic organizing pneumonia. Focused assessments on the eyes, skin, and GI tract should be performed. Long-term issues such as fertility and sexuality should also be discussed.

References

Abbas, A.K., Lichtman, A.H., & Pillai, S. (2015). *Cellular and molecular immunology* (8th ed.). Philadelphia, PA: Elsevier Saunders.

Anderson-Reitz, L., & Clancy, C. (2013). Hepatorenal complications. In S.A. Ezzone (Ed.), *Hematopoietic stem cell transplantation: A manual for nursing practice* (2nd ed., pp. 191–199). Pittsburgh, PA: Oncology Nursing Society.

Antin, J.H., & Raley, D.Y. (2013). *Manual of stem cell and bone marrow transplantation* (2nd ed.). New York, NY: Cambridge University Press.

Bacigalupo, A., Ballen, K., Rizzo, D., Giralt, S., Lazarus, H., Ho, V., … Horowitz, M. (2009). Defining the intensity of conditioning regimens: Working definitions. *Biology of Blood and Marrow Transplantation, 15,* 1628–1633. doi:10.1016/j.bbmt.2009.07.004

Barrett, A.J. (2009). Essential biology of stem cell transplantation. In J. Treleaven & A.J. Barrett (Eds.), *Hematopoietic stem cell transplantation in clinical practice* (pp. 9–22). Philadelphia, PA: Elsevier Churchill Livingstone.

Bashey, A., Zhang, X., Sizemore, C.A., Manion, K., Brown, S., Holland, H.K., … Solomon, S.R. (2013). T-cell–replete HLA-haploidentical hematopoietic transplantation for hematologic malignancies using post-transplantation cyclophosphamide results in outcomes equivalent to those of contemporaneous HLA-matched related and unrelated donor transplantation. *Journal of Clinical Oncology, 31,* 1310–1360. doi:10.1200/JCO.2012.44.3523

Batlle, M., Morgades, M., Vives, S., Ferrà, C., Oriol, A., Sancho, J.-M., … Ribera, J.-M. (2014). Usefulness and safety of oral cryotherapy in the prevention of oral mucositis after conditioning regimens with high-dose melphalan for autologous stem cell transplantation for lymphoma and myeloma. *European Journal of Haematology, 93,* 487–491. doi:10.1111/ejh.12386

Bensinger, W.I. (2012). Allogeneic transplantation: Peripheral blood vs. bone marrow. *Current Opinion in Oncology, 24,* 191–196. doi:10.1097/CCO.0b013e32834f5c27

Be The Match. (n.d.-a). Disease-specific HCT indications and outcomes data. Retrieved from https://bethematchclinical.org/transplant-indications-and-outcomes/disease-specific-indications-and-outcomes

Be The Match. (n.d.-b). Likelihood of finding a match for patients. Retrieved from https://bethematchclinical.org/Transplant-Therapy-and-Donor-Matching/Donor-or-Cord-Blood-Search-Process/Likelihood-of-Finding-a-Match

Be The Match. (2014). *Together we deliver cures for blood cancer: 2014 report to the community.* Retrieved from http://bethematch.org/WorkArea/DownloadAsset.aspx?id=7521

Brunstein, C.G., & Laughlin, M.J. (2010). Extending cord blood transplant to adults: Dealing with problems and results overall. *Seminars in Hematology, 47,* 86–96. doi:10.1053/j.seminhematol.2009.10.010

Bubalo, J.S. (2015). Conditioning regimens. In R.T. Maziarz & S.S. Slater (Eds.), *Blood and marrow transplant handbook: Comprehensive guide for patient care* (2nd ed., pp. 67–80). New York, NY: Springer.

Burcat, S. (2013). Current research and future directions. In S.A. Ezzone (Ed.), *Hematopoietic stem cell transplantation: A manual for nursing practice* (2nd ed., pp. 293–319). Pittsburgh, PA: Oncology Nursing Society.

Chao, N. (2014). How I treat sinusoidal obstruction syndrome. *Blood, 123,* 4023–4026. doi:10.1182/blood-2014-03-551630

Chi, A.K., Soubani, A.O., White, A.C., & Miller, K.B. (2013). An update on pulmonary complications of hematopoietic stem cell transplantation. *Chest, 144,* 1913–1922. doi:10.1378/chest.12-1708

Cutler, C., & Antin, J.H. (2006). Chronic graft-versus-host disease. *Current Opinion in Oncology, 18,* 126–131. doi:10.1097/01.cco.0000208784.07195.84

Devine, H. (2013). Overview of hematopoiesis and immunology: Implications for hematopoietic stem cell transplantation. In S.A. Ezzone (Ed.), *Hematopoietic stem cell transplantation: A manual for nursing practice* (2nd ed., pp. 1–11). Pittsburgh, PA: Oncology Nursing Society.

Ezzone, S.A. (2013). Gastrointestinal complications. In S.A. Ezzone (Ed.), *Hematopoietic stem cell transplantation: A manual for nursing practice* (2nd ed., pp. 173–190). Pittsburgh, PA: Oncology Nursing Society.

Filipovich, A.H., Weisdorf, D., Pavletic, S., Socie, G., Wingard, J.R., Lee, S.J., … Flowers, M.E.D. (2005). National Institutes of Health consensus development project on criteria for clinical trials in chronic graft-versus-host disease: I. Diagnosis and Staging Working Group report. *Biology of Blood and Marrow Transplantation, 11,* 945–956. doi:10.1016/j.bbmt.2005.09.004

Foundation for the Accreditation of Cellular Therapy. (n.d.). About FACT. Retrieved from http://www.factwebsite.org/AboutFACT

Fred Hutchinson Cancer Research Center. (n.d.). History of transplantation. Retrieved from https://www.fredhutch.org/en/treatment/long-term-follow-up/FAQs/transplantation.html

Genetics Home Reference. (2009). Human leukocyte antigens. Retrieved from http://ghr.nlm.nih.gov/genefamily/hla

Gupta, S. (n.d.). Human stem cells at Johns Hopkins: A forty year history. Retrieved from http://www.hopkinsmedicine.org/stem_cell_research/cell_therapy/human_stem_cells_johns_hopkins.html

Ho, V.T., Kim, H.T., Aldridge, J., Liney, D., Kao, G., Armand, P., … Alyea, E.P. (2011). Use of matched unrelated donors compared with matched related donors is associated with lower relapse and superior progression-free survival after reduced-intensity conditioning hematopoietic stem cell transplantation. *Biology of Blood and Marrow Transplantation, 17,* 1196–1204. doi:10.1016/j.bbmt.2010.12.702

Horowitz, M. (2009, November). *Neutrophil recovery: The first step in posttransplant recovery.* Presentation at the 2009 Center for International Blood and Marrow Transplant Research's Clinical Research Professionals/Data Management Conference, Minneapolis, MN. Retrieved from http://www.cibmtr.org/meetings/materials/crpdmc/pages/fall09horowitz.aspx

Kasamon, Y.L., Prince, G., Bolaños-Meade, J., Tsai, H.-L., Luznik, L., Ambinder, R.F., … Jones, R.J. (2013). Encouraging outcomes in older patients (Pts) following nonmyeloablative (NMA) haploidentical blood or marrow transplantation (haploBMT) with high-dose posttransplantation cyclophosphamide (PT/Cy). *Blood, 122*(21), Abstract 158. Retrieved from http://www.bloodjournal.org/content/122/21/158

Kiviat, J. (2013). Quality-of-life issues. In S.A. Ezzone (Ed.), *Hematopoietic stem cell transplantation: A manual for nursing practice* (2nd ed., pp. 283–291). Pittsburgh, PA: Oncology Nursing Society.

Mak, T.W., & Saunders, M.E. (2011). *Primer to the immune response* (Academic Cell update ed.). Burlington, MA: Elsevier Academic Press.

Martin, P.J., Rizzo, J.D., Wingard, J.R., Ballen, K., Curtin, P.T., Cutler, C., … Carpenter, P.A. (2012). First- and second-line systemic treatment of acute graft-versus-host disease: Recommendations of the American Society of Blood and Marrow Transplantation. *Biology of Blood and Marrow Transplantation, 18,* 1150–1163. doi:10.1016/j.bbmt.2012.04.005

Massberg, S., Khandoga, A.G., & von Andrian, U.H. (2013). Hematopoietic cell trafficking and chemokines. In R. Hoffman, E.J. Benz Jr., L.E. Silberstein, H.E. Heslop, J.I.

Weitz, & J. Anastasi (Eds.), *Hematology: Basic principles and practice* (6th ed., pp. 105–116). Philadelphia, PA: Elsevier Saunders.

McAdams, F.W., & Burgunder, M.R. (2013). Transplant treatment course and acute complications. In S.A. Ezzone (Ed.), *Hematopoietic stem cell transplantation: A manual for nursing practice* (2nd ed., pp. 47–66). Pittsburgh, PA: Oncology Nursing Society.

Mickelson, E., & Petersdorf, E.W. (2009). Histocompatibility. In F.R. Appelbaum, S.J. Forman, R.S. Negrin, & K.G. Blume (Eds.), *Thomas' hematopoietic cell transplantation* (4th ed., pp. 145–162). West Sussex, United Kingdom: Wiley-Blackwell.

Mitchell, S.A. (2013). Acute and chronic graft-versus-host disease. In S.A. Ezzone (Ed.), *Hematopoietic stem cell transplantation: A manual for nursing practice* (2nd ed., pp. 103–153). Pittsburgh, PA: Oncology Nursing Society.

Moreb, J.S. (2009). Liver disease after hematopoietic stem cell transplant. In J.R. Wingard, D.A. Gastineau, H.L. Leather, Z.M. Szczepiorkowski, & E.L. Snyder (Eds.), *Hematopoietic stem cell transplantation: A handbook for clinicians* (pp. 365–375). Bethesda, MD: AABB.

Niess, D. (2013). Basic concepts of transplantation. In S.A. Ezzone (Ed.), *Hematopoietic stem cell transplantation: A manual for nursing practice* (2nd ed., pp. 13–16). Pittsburgh, PA: Oncology Nursing Society.

Nuss, S., Barnes, Y., Fisher, V., Olson, E., & Skeens, M. (2011). Hematopoietic cell transplantation. In C. Baggott, D. Fochtman, G.V. Foley, & K.P. Kelly (Eds.), *Nursing care of children and adolescents with cancer and blood disorders* (4th ed., pp. 405–466). Glenview, IL: Association of Pediatric Hematology/Oncology Nurses.

Pasquini, M.C., & Zhu, X. (2015). *Current uses and outcomes of hematopoietic stem cell transplantation: CIBMTR summary slides, 2015.* Retrieved from https://www.cibmtr.org/ReferenceCenter/SlidesReports/SummarySlides/Pages/index.aspx

Powell, L.D., Chung, P., & Baum, L.G. (2013). Overview and compartmentalization of the immune system. In R. Hoffman, E.J. Benz Jr., L.E. Silberstein, H.E. Heslop, J.I. Weitz, & J. Anastasi (Eds.), *Hematology: Basic principles and practice* (6th ed., pp. 172–181). Philadelphia, PA: Elsevier Saunders.

Rosselet, R.M. (2013). Hematologic effects. In S.A. Ezzone (Ed.), *Hematopoietic stem cell transplantation: A manual for nursing practice* (2nd ed., pp. 155–172). Pittsburgh, PA: Oncology Nursing Society.

Rowlings, P.A., Przepiorka, D., Klein, J.P., Gale, R.P., Passweg, J.R., Henslee-Downey, P.J., … Horowitz, M.M. (1997). IBMTR Severity Index for grading acute graft-versus-host disease: Retrospective comparison with Glucksberg grade. *British Journal of Haematology, 97,* 855–864. doi:10.1046/j.1365-2141.1997.1112925.x

Schmit-Pokorny, K. (2013). Stem cell collection. In S.A. Ezzone (Ed.), *Hematopoietic stem cell transplantation: A manual for nursing practice* (2nd ed., pp. 23–46). Pittsburgh, PA: Oncology Nursing Society.

Shannon, S.P. (2013). Relapse and secondary malignancies. In S.A. Ezzone (Ed.), *Hematopoietic stem cell transplantation: A manual for nursing practice* (2nd ed., pp. 245–249). Pittsburgh, PA: Oncology Nursing Society.

Shea, T., & DiPersio, J. (2009). Mobilization of autologous peripheral blood hematopoietic cells for cellular therapy. In F.R. Appelbaum, S.J. Forman, R.S. Negrin, & K.G. Blume (Ed.), *Thomas' hematopoietic cell transplantation* (4th ed., pp. 590–604). West Sussex, United Kingdom: Wiley-Blackwell.

Solh, M., DeFor, T.E., Weisdorf, D.J., & Kaufman, D.S. (2012). Extramedullary relapse of acute myelogenous leukemia after allogeneic hematopoietic stem cell transplantation: Better prognosis than systemic relapse. *Biology of Blood and Marrow Transplantation, 18,* 106–112. doi:10.1016/j.bbmt.2011.05.023

Stephens, J.M.L. (2013). Cardiopulmonary complications. In S.A. Ezzone (Ed.), *Hematopoietic stem cell transplantation: A manual for nursing practice* (2nd ed., pp. 201–229). Pittsburgh, PA: Oncology Nursing Society.

Strasfeld, L. (2015). Infectious complications. In R.T. Maziarz & S.S. Slater (Eds.), *Blood and marrow transplant handbook: Comprehensive guide for patient care* (2nd ed., pp. 201–222). New York, NY: Springer.

Szczepiorkowski, Z.M., Winters, J.L., Bandarenko, N., Kim, H.C., Linenberger, M.L., Marques, M.B., … Shaz, B.H. (2010). Guidelines on the use of therapeutic apheresis in clinical practice—Evidence-based approach from the apheresis applications committee of the American Society for Apheresis. *Journal of Clinical Apheresis, 25,* 83–177. doi:10.1002/jca.20240

Thomas, E.D., Storb, R., Clift, R.A., Fefer, A., Johnson, F.L., Neiman, P.E., … Buckner, C.D. (1975). Bone-marrow transplantation (second of two parts). *New England Journal of Medicine, 292,* 895–902. doi:10.1056/NEJM197504242921706

Tichelli, A., & Socié, G. (2012). Late effects in patients treated with HSCT. In J. Apperley, E. Carreras, E. Gluckman, & T. Masszi (Eds.), *The ESH-EBMT handbook on haematopoietic stem cell transplantation* (6th ed., pp. 248–269). Leiden, Netherlands: European Society for Blood and Marrow Transplantation.

Tierney, D.K., & Robinson, T. (2013). Long-term care of hematopoietic cell transplant survivors. In S.A. Ezzone (Ed.), *Hematopoietic stem cell transplantation: A manual for nursing practice* (2nd ed., pp. 251–267). Pittsburgh, PA: Oncology Nursing Society.

Tomblyn, M., Chiller, T., Einsele, H., Gress, R., Sepkowitz, K., Storek, J., … Boeckh, M.A. (2009). Guidelines for preventing infectious complications among hematopoietic cell transplantation recipients: A global perspective. *Biology of Blood and Marrow Transplantation, 15,* 1143–1238. doi:10.1016/j.bbmt.2009.06.019

U.S. Food and Drug Administration. (2014). *Minimal manipulation of human cells, tissues, and cellular and tissue-based products: Draft guidance.* Retrieved from http://www.fda.gov/BiologicsBloodVaccines/GuidanceComplianceRegulatoryInformation/Guidances/CellularandGeneTherapy/ucm427692.htm

U.S. Food and Drug Administration. (2016). Defitelio (defibrotide sodium). Retrieved from http://www.fda.gov/Drugs/InformationOnDrugs/ApprovedDrugs/ucm493278.htm

Vagliano, L., Feraut, C., Gobetto, G., Trunfio, A., Errico, A., Campani, V., … Dimonte, V. (2011). Incidence and severity of oral mucositis in patients undergoing haematopoietic SCT—Results of a multicentre study. *Bone Marrow Transplantation, 46,* 727–732. doi:10.1038/bmt.2010.184

Warren, E.H., III. (2009). The human graft-versus-tumor response—and how to exploit it. In F.R. Appelbaum, S.J. Forman, R.S. Negrin, & K.G. Blume (Eds.), *Thomas' hematopoietic cell transplantation: Stem cell transplantation* (4th ed., pp. 232–247). West Sussex, United Kingdom: Wiley-Blackwell.

Wong, F.L., Francisco, L., Togawa, K., Kim, H., Bosworth, A., Atencio, L., … Bhatia, S. (2013). Longitudinal trajectory of sexual functioning after hematopoietic cell transplantation: Impact of chronic graft-versus-host disease and total body irradiation. *Blood, 122,* 3973–3981. doi:10.1182/blood-2013-05-499806

Chapter 14 Study Questions

1. Which of the following is NOT a manifestation of acute graft-versus-host disease?
   A. Diarrhea
   B. Skin rash
   C. Hyperbilirubinemia
   D. Dry eyes

2. The term used for the process in which the donor stem cells make their way to the recipient bone marrow and begin producing healthy blood cells resulting in rising white blood cell count is:
   A. Engraftment.
   B. Hematopoiesis.
   C. Myeloablation.
   D. None of the above.

3. All of the following are methods of preventing or treating mucositis due to conditioning chemotherapy EXCEPT:
   A. Cryotherapy.
   B. Alcohol-based mouth rinse.
   C. Avoidance of extremely hot beverages/foods.
   D. Good oral hygiene.

4. Full siblings who are not identical twins have what percent chance of having an identical human leukocyte antigen haplotype?
   A. 50%
   B. 75%
   C. 33%
   D. 25%

5. Which of the following classes of drugs is used as an immunosuppressive agent to prevent or treat graft-versus-host disease?
   A. Alkylating agents
   B. Calcineurin inhibitors
   C. Antimetabolites
   D. Beta-blockers

SECTION III

Symptom Management

CHAPTER

15 Alopecia

Denise Portz, MSN, RN, ACNS-BC, AOCNS®

Introduction

Hair is an important aspect of a person's body image. Unfortunately, during many cancer treatments, hair loss, or alopecia, can occur. The incidence of alopecia is extremely high, and it can be profoundly distressing—some patients may even refuse cancer treatment for fear of hair loss (Camp-Sorrell, 2018).

A healthy scalp has about 100,000 hairs; on average, 60%–90% of hair follicles are dividing and being replaced every 24 hours (Dowd, 1993). Alopecia signifies a diffuse amount of hair shedding. Approximately 50% of hair is lost before it becomes noticeable (Callaghan & Cooper, 2014). Alopecia most commonly occurs on the scalp; however, it can occur anywhere on the body, including facial (beards, eyebrows, eyelashes), axillary, and pubic hair (Polovich, Olsen, & LeFebvre, 2014). Causes of alopecia can include congenital factors, dermatitis, childbirth, aging, stress, and trauma. It also may be drug induced, such as by chemotherapy, or radiation induced, as a side effect of treatment for cancer. Hair loss is a transient and usually, although not always, reversible consequence of cancer therapy (Payne, 2015).

Significant progress has been made during the past 20 years for many of the side effects associated with cancer treatment, including emesis, pancytopenia, xerostomia, mucositis, infection, pain, and thrombosis. Chemotherapy-induced alopecia, however, remains understudied, even though efforts in prevention and treatment have been ongoing for several decades.

Alopecia has been cited by 47%–58% of women with cancer as the most disturbing anticipated aspect of receiving chemotherapy. In a study by McGarvey, Baum, Pinkerton, and Rogers (2001), 8% of women were found to be at risk for avoiding treatment because the idea of baldness was too difficult for them to tolerate. Another report indicated that the hair loss was harder to conceptualize than the loss of a breast in some patients (Batchelor, 2001). Both men and women still consider alopecia to be one of the most devastating side effects. In young adults aged 18–38, men and women reported equally negative experiences related to chemotherapy-induced alopecia (Hilton, Hunt, Emslie, Salinas, & Ziebland, 2008).

Oncology nurses need to understand that for patients receiving chemotherapy, hair loss is a serious physical and quality-of-life side effect. Teaching patients about alopecia and how to manage it must be a priority in their plan of care. This chapter will discuss chemotherapy- and radiation-induced alopecia.

Pathophysiology

Alopecia is a common side effect of both chemotherapy and radiation therapy, and its pathophysiology is largely unknown. Cells responsible for hair growth have high mitotic and metabolic rates. Certain cytotoxic agents disrupt the proliferative phase of hair growth. Approximately 90% of hair follicles on the scalp are in the anagen (growth) phase of the hair cycle at any given time (Trüeb, 2010). Chemotherapy and radiation are known to target rapidly dividing cells, with side effects resulting because certain normal cells are also rapidly dividing.

Two major types of chemotherapy-induced alopecia exist: telogen effluvium and anagen effluvium (Yeager & Olsen, 2011). Telogen effluvium involves less than 50% of the scalp and results in hair thinning. Hair enters the telogen, or resting, phase and results in shedding three to four months after drug administration. Cytotoxic drugs that can cause this type of alopecia are methotrexate, 5-fluorouracil, and retinoids (Yeager & Olsen, 2011). Anagen effluvium is the most common form of chemotherapy-induced alopecia. Most hair follicles are in the growth phase, and chemotherapy damages these rapidly growing cells, leading to damage of the inner root sheath cells or the hair shaft integrity. The hair shaft is no longer anchored and falls out easily or breaks off at the scalp. Hair falls out spontaneously or during washing or combing. Chemotherapy agents such as cyclophosphamide, daunorubicin, doxorubicin, etoposide, ifosfamide, and paclitaxel are associated with this type of damage. The hairs remain in the telogen phase after damage occurs until the chemotherapy is completed, at which time they can enter the anagen phase again and hair regrowth resumes (Yeager & Olsen, 2011).

Incidence and Risk

As many as 65% of patients receiving chemotherapy will experience some degree of alopecia (Trüeb, 2010). The incidence and severity is dependent on several factors, including the mechanism of action of the drug, administration route, drug dose, serum half-life, duration (e.g., bolus versus continuous infusion), response of the patient, use of combination chemotherapy, and condition of the hair prior to treatment (Chon, Champion, Geddes, & Rashid, 2012).

Molecularly targeted agents such as monoclonal antibodies, which target the epidermal growth factor receptor (EGFR) (e.g., cetuximab), and small molecular inhibitors of EGFR (e.g., erlotinib) have been associated with diffuse alopecia that is generally reversible (Chon et al., 2012; Donovan, Ghazarian, & Shaw, 2008). Multitargeted tyrosine kinase inhibitors (e.g., sorafenib, sunitinib) are also associated with alopecia.

Irreversible alopecia has been reported after high-dose chemotherapy and hematopoietic stem cell transplantation (HSCT), especially related to conditioning regimens containing busulfan and cyclophosphamide; however, the overall incidence is not known (Machado, Moreb, & Khan, 2007). Machado et al. (2007) conducted a retrospective study to identify patients with chemotherapy-induced permanent alopecia after HSCT. Among 760 patients transplanted between 1997 and 2004, six patients showed that permanent alopecia is a significant long-term side effect of HSCT (Machado et al., 2007). Permanent alopecia also can occur with long-term use of EGFR inhibitors and after treatment with taxanes (Donovan et al., 2008; Miteva et al., 2011; Tallon, Blanchard, & Goldberg, 2010).

Alopecia begins about two weeks after the initiation of chemotherapy, can be either a gradual thinning or rapid loss, and may continue for two months after cessation of chemotherapy (Polovich et al., 2014). Hair regrowth may be visible four to six weeks after the drugs are stopped, but complete regrowth may take one to two years (Camp-Sorrell, 2018). The first hair to regrow may be downy in appearance. For many people, the color and texture of their hair will be different than it was before treatment. The shade of the hair may be lighter or darker than its original color, and it is often curlier as it regrows (McGarvey et al., 2011).

Radiation-induced alopecia can be just as troubling for patients. The extent of body hair loss experienced by patients receiving radiation treatment can be unpredictable but is related to dose. Generally, as the doses of radiation increase, the probability of alopecia increases and the possibility of hair regrowth diminishes. Doses as low as 2 Gy in a single fraction have been shown to cause temporary alopecia. Radiation doses greater than 40 Gy may cause permanent hair loss in the radiation treatment field (Lawenda et al., 2014). When the hair loss is only temporary, hair in the treatment field will fall out two to three weeks after the first radiation treatment and will grow back three to six months after completion of radiation therapy (Lawenda et al., 2004).

It is important to emphasize that reasons other than cancer treatment can cause alopecia. Hormonal factors, including hypothyroidism, poor nutrition, and genetic factors can result in alopecia, including a family history of hair loss. Certain noncytotoxic drugs such as propranolol hydrochloride, heparin sodium, lithium carbonate, prednisone, vitamin A, and androgen preparations can cause alopecia. Stress can induce hair loss, and patients undergoing cancer treatment experience a great deal of stress both physically and emotionally. And finally, hair care behaviors can result in alopecia. Overhandling and overprocessing hair will contribute to alopecia when treatment begins because the hair shafts become fragile, brittle, and break easily (Camp-Sorrell, 2018; Polovich et al., 2014).

Assessment

During an initial encounter with a patient who is newly diagnosed with cancer and scheduled for treatment, the nurse needs to assess for all of the physical and emotional factors related to the probability of alopecia. When taking a medical history, the nurse should note any comorbidities or medications that may already be causing alopecia (Polovich et al., 2014). Assessment also includes the patient's nutritional status and family history related to hair loss. The nurse should review the patient's treatment regimen and whether he or she is having combination therapy, chemotherapy concurrently with radiation, radiation to a large field where hair grows, and the potential of the chemotherapy drugs for causing alopecia. After gathering this information, the oncology nurse will know whether to proceed further with an assessment of the patient's emotional response to hair loss and assessment of coping skills.

Scalp dryness, soreness, pruritus, and rash can occur before, during, or after hair loss (Polovich et al., 2014). The National Cancer Institute's Cancer Therapy Evaluation Program (NCI CTEP, 2010) has established grading criteria for adverse events related to cancer treatments. The criteria provide a means for all nurses to both assess the degree of alopecia experienced by a patient at each clinic visit and to consistently document that assessment. The NCI CTEP system considers grade 1 to be a hair loss of up to 50% that is noticeable only on close inspection and for which a different hairstyle may be required; a wig or hairpiece is not required. Grade 2 is a hair loss of greater than 50% that is readily apparent and for which a wig or hairpiece is required if the patient wants to camouflage the loss. Grade 2 alopecia is associated with psychosocial impact (NCI CTEP, 2010).

Treatment

Alopecia is a constant reminder of disease and greatly affects patients' sense of self. Since the 1970s, a number of preventive measures have been proposed and tried, including scalp cooling, scalp tourniquets, and minoxidil (Cigler et al., 2015; Payne, 2015; Trüeb, 2009; Yeager & Olsen, 2011). Of these, scalp cooling has been the most used and studied, more frequently in Europe and Canada (Cigler et al., 2015; Grevelman & Breed, 2005).

Scalp cooling is accomplished with either cooling agents applied via a cooling cap that is changed several times or by continuous cooling of the scalp with cold air or liquid. Scalp cooling is said to work by (a) reducing the blood flow via vasoconstriction to hair follicles during peak plasma concentration of the chemotherapy agent, reducing its cellular uptake, or (b) by reducing the biochemical activity, making the hair follicles less vulnerable to the damage of chemotherapy agents (Cigler et al., 2015; Trüeb, 2009). The most common side effects of scalp cooling include headaches, excessive coldness, and feelings of claustrophobia (Trüeb, 2010). The success of scalp cooling for preventing or reducing chemotherapy-induced alopecia is highly variable among patients and chemotherapy regimens. Positive results were most evident when anthracyclines or taxanes were the chemotherapy agents (Komen, Smorenburg, van den Hurk, & Nortier, 2013). Recent clinical performance of both the DigniCap System (Rugo et al., 2015) and Penguin Cold Cap (Cigler et al., 2015) has showed effectiveness in reducing chemotherapy-induced alopecia with a meaningful benefit among patients with cancer receiving chemotherapy.

Despite the history of effective use in Europe and Canada, scalp cooling has been slow to gain popularity in the United States, perhaps because of the concern that reducing circulation to the scalp through vasoconstriction may create a sanctuary site for malignant cells, resulting in scalp metastasis (Cigler et al., 2015; Roe, 2014). Studies to date, however, indicate that rates of scalp metastasis between scalp-cooled and non-cooled patients with solid tumor malignancies are virtually identical, and no long-term risks have been identified (Cigler et al., 2015).

At present, no approved pharmacologic treatment exists for chemotherapy-induced alopecia. Multiple classes of agents with different mechanisms of action have been and are being evaluated for the prevention and treatment of alopecia, such as epidermal growth factor, keratinocyte growth factor, cytokines, antioxidants, and apoptosis inhibitors (Yeager & Olsen, 2011). Among the few agents that have been evaluated in humans, the immune modulator AS101 and the hair growth–promoting agent minoxidil show promise in reducing the severity or shortening the duration of alopecia, but could not prevent it altogether (Chon et al., 2012; Trüeb, 2009).

In many cases, healthcare professionals still underestimate the impact of alopecia for patients with cancer. Interventions such as scalp cooling or minoxidil can be an effective alternative for some patients; however, more randomized and larger studies with longer-term follow-up are needed (Breed, van den Hurk, & Peerbooms, 2011).

Patient Education

Hair loss is unavoidable for many patients receiving cancer treatment. It is important that healthcare providers prepare patients for hair loss through education. Teaching about hair loss is most appropriate prior to the first treatment. Providing accurate and specific information about the management of hair loss can offer a psychological benefit (see Figure 15-1). Exploring the meaning and significance of hair loss to each patient will help guide the development of individualized coping strategies. Hair loss will begin approximately two weeks after the initiation of chemotherapy and radiation. It is a priority to spend time assessing, teaching, and planning with the patient before the hair loss begins (Borsellino & Young, 2010).

Figure 15-1. Patient Education Tips for Alopecia

- Protect the scalp from the sun and cold.
- Wear sunscreen.
- Try cotton head coverings because they will not slip off.
- Wear sunglasses in bright sun, and use eye drops to keep eyes moist and clean.
- Shampoo twice a week with mild shampoo.
- Use a soft hairbrush, and brush minimally.
- Use the low setting when using a hair dryer.
- Avoid perms, dyes, electric curlers, curling and straightening irons, and hairspray.
- Consider changing to a short hairstyle or shaving the head.
- Be aware that new hair that grows after therapy completion may differ from the original hair in color or texture.

Note. Based on information from Polovich et al., 2014.

The emotional experience of hair loss varies, but for most patients, alopecia is an additional stressor at a time when life is already very serious. Hair loss is a visible reminder of their diagnosis and robs them of their privacy about having cancer. They feel as though they "look" like a patient with cancer and are perceived by others in this way. Hair loss can create a sense of loss of identity because the person in the mirror no longer looks like "self" (Frith, Harcourt, & Fussell, 2007). Hairstyle can be perceived as an important part of personal identity. Alopecia has been studied within varied frameworks, including self-esteem, body image, and self-perception (Borsellino & Young, 2010). Understanding the unique psychosocial impact of alopecia on each individual assists the healthcare provider in developing a management plan.

In preparing for hair loss, patients must first decide if they will appear bald or use a head covering. Some first prepare by having their hair cut shorter in the hope that it will minimize the trauma of losing their long hair. Additionally, when the hair begins to regrow, it takes less time to reach the shorter hairstyle. Some people will shave their head at the first sign of alopecia. For those who choose to wear a head covering, multiple choices are available. For some patients, alopecia is an opportunity to experiment with new looks offered by the many choices in wigs. It is optimal for patients to choose a wig before the hair loss begins, especially if they want to match their natural hair color. Providing pictures or preserving a portion of normal hair prior to complete hair loss also can help the stylist match color and texture. Nurses need to be mindful that wigs are not an immediate and easy solution to the problem of alopecia. Some patients find them very uncomfortable and feel as though they are "covering" up their illness. The changed appearance that may result from wearing a wig has the potential to create an even bigger problem than the alopecia (Williams, Wood, & Cunningham-Warburton, 1999). Head coverings include wigs, hats, scarves, and turbans. Patients should be instructed to check with their insurance carrier about coverage for part or all of the cost of a head covering (Camp-Sorrell, 2018). Having a prescription for a "cranial prosthesis" may provide some insurance carriers with the necessary documentation for allowing insurance coverage. Cotton head coverings are optimal because they allow the scalp to breathe. A non-profit patient service of the American Cancer Society (ACS), TLC Tender Loving Care®, provides an array of wigs and head coverings that are affordable and available by catalog (ACS, n.d.). Patients should be encouraged to check with their local ACS office for donated wigs and head coverings or assistance in obtaining them. Local hair stylists can help patients find a wig that closely matches their natural hair color and style. To do so, however, patients must consult the stylist before any significant hair loss. Wigs can be synthetic or made of actual human hair. Salons or stores that specialize in wigs can provide a discussion of the pros and cons of each type of wig with the patient. Synthetic wigs may be damaged by excessive heat during styling. If a wig is purchased prior to hair loss, it should be adjustable so that the size can be decreased as hair loss occurs (Look Good Feel Better, n.d.).

Patients should also be taught about local resources for support. Look Good Feel Better is a local program offered by the Personal Care Products Council, the Professional Beauty Association, and ACS to provide guidance and support regarding wigs and other head coverings, makeup, and skin care (Personal Care Products Council, n.d.). Some cancer centers also offer these services within their own organizations. Figure 15-2 provides a list of Internet resources for patients and healthcare professionals.

It is easy to forget that at one time, hair served an important function in survival, and this biologic inheritance continues to serve humans well. Eyelashes protect the eyes from foreign bodies and dust; the eyebrows protect against rain and sweat; and scalp hair protects against sunlight and cold (Hansen, 2007). Patients need to be taught to protect the scalp from the sun by wearing a head covering and using sunscreen with SPF 15 or higher. Patients who experience the loss of all body hair, including the eyebrows and eyelashes, will need to wear sunglasses to protect the eyes from the effects of the sun and use moisturizing eye drops to keep the eyes clean and moist. Patients who live in a cold climate will need to be taught to protect the scalp from the cold, as hair prevents the loss of body heat from the top of the head.

Figure 15-2. Internet Resources for Patients and Healthcare Professionals

- American Cancer Society (www.cancer.org): Provides basic information on hair loss and how to handle it
- Cancer*Care* (www.cancercare.org): Offers one-page fact sheets on a wide range of topics, including tips for hair loss
- Look Good Feel Better (www.lookgoodfeelbetter.org): Provides resources to help women offset appearance-related changes from cancer treatment
- TLC Tender Loving Care® (www.tlcdirect.org): Provides an array of wigs and head coverings that are affordable and available by catalog

Caps and hats will protect the head from the cold and the resulting loss of body heat. Sometimes patients find it is more comfortable for them to wear a soft cap or turban while sleeping (Batchelor, 2001; Chon et al., 2012; Hesketh et al., 2004).

Recommended guidelines exist for hair and scalp care during cancer treatment and during hair regrowth. During both time periods, the hair will be fragile and will break easily with excessive handling and the use of harsh shampoos or chemicals. Teach patients to limit washing their hair to twice a week and to use a mild shampoo without detergents, menthol, salicylic acid, alcohol, or heavy perfumes (Batchelor, 2001; Chon et al., 2012; Hesketh et al., 2004; Polovich et al., 2014). Baby shampoo is a perfect substitute. They should be advised to use a soft hairbrush and to style hair gently, limiting the amount of hard brushing. During cancer treatment and hair regrowth, patients should avoid blow-drying with high heat and should completely forgo the use of chemical products on their hair for curling, straightening, or coloring. When hair begins to regrow after treatment ends, it will initially be fine and prone to breaking. Hair coloring should not be used for at least three months after treatment ends, and curling or straightening with chemicals should be avoided until the hair is at least three inches long. Patients should also be advised that new hair growth might differ from their original hair in color or texture (Batchelor, 2001; Chon et al., 2012; Hesketh et al., 2004; Polovich et al., 2014).

When nurses take the time to listen and teach, patients undergoing cancer treatment will be able to move through the potentially devastating experience of alopecia with more ease.

Conclusion

Alopecia consistently ranks as one of the most distressing treatment-related side effects that cancer survivors experience. It is the responsibility of oncology nurses to understand the significance of hair loss for patients and to help them to prepare for this loss. Alopecia is a physical side effect that affects quality of life. Caregivers must incorporate this into their plan of care and teach the patient about risk factors and management. The plan of care must include taking the time to understand the emotional implications of alopecia for each patient and assisting in planning interventions to minimize the emotional impact.

The author would like to acknowledge Wanda Jo Johnson, MA, RN, BSN, OCN®, for her contribution to this chapter that remains unchanged from the first edition of this book.

References

American Cancer Society. (n.d.). TLC Tender Loving Care®. Retrieved from http://www.tlcdirect.org

Batchelor, D. (2001). Hair and cancer chemotherapy: Consequences and nursing care—A literature study. *European Journal of Cancer Care, 10,* 147–163. doi:10.1046/j.1365-2354.2001.00272.x

Borsellino, M., & Young, M.M. (2010). Anticipatory coping: Taking control of hair loss. *Clinical Journal of Oncology Nursing, 15,* 311–315. doi:10.1188/11.CJON.311-315

Breed, W.P.M., van den Hurk, C.J.G., & Peerbooms, M. (2011). Presentation, impact and prevention of chemotherapy-induced hair loss: Scalp cooling potentials and limitations. *Expert Review of Dermatology, 6,* 109–125. doi:10.1586/edm.10.76

Callaghan, M., & Cooper, A. (2014). Alopecia. In C.H. Yarbro, D. Wujcik, & B.H. Gobel (Eds.), *Cancer symptom management* (4th ed., pp. 495–505). Burlington, MA: Jones & Bartlett Learning.

Camp-Sorrell, D. (2018). Chemotherapy toxicities and management. In C.H. Yarbro, D. Wujcik, & B.H. Gobel (Eds.), *Cancer nursing: Principles and practice* (8th ed., pp. 497–554). Burlington, MA: Jones & Bartlett Learning.

Chon, S.Y., Champion, R.W., Geddes, E.R., & Rashid, R.M. (2012). Chemotherapy-induced alopecia. *Journal of the American Academy of Dermatology, 67,* e37–e47. doi:10.1016/j.jaad.2011.02.026

Cigler, T., Isseroff, D., Fiederlein, B., Schneider, S., Chuang, E., Vahdat, L., & Moore, A. (2015). Efficacy of scalp cooling in preventing chemotherapy-induced alopecia in breast cancer patients receiving adjuvant docetaxel and cyclophosphamide chemotherapy. *Clinical Breast Cancer, 15,* 332–334. doi:10.1016/j.clbc.2015.01.003

Donovan, J.C., Ghazarian, D.M., & Shaw, J.C. (2008). Scarring alopecia associated with use of the epidermal growth factor receptor inhibitor gefitinib. *Archives of Dermatology, 144,* 1524–1525. doi:10.1001/archderm.144.11.1524

Dowd, I. (1993). Coping with alopecia. *Cancer Care, 2,* 232–233.

Frith, H., Harcourt, D., & Fussell, A. (2007). Anticipating an altered appearance: Women undergoing chemotherapy treatment for breast cancer. *European Journal of Oncology Nursing, 11,* 385–391. doi:10.1016/j.ejon.2007.03.002

Key Points

- Alopecia is a common side effect of cancer treatment.
- Hair is not only lost from the head but also from the face (including eyebrows, eyelashes, and beards), arms, legs, underarms, and pubic areas; hair loss normally occurs approximately one to two weeks after beginning cancer treatment.
- The incidence and severity of alopecia with cancer treatments depend on the types of agents, combination of agents, and dose of radiation.
- Scalp cooling is currently the best method to reduce the incidence of chemotherapy-induced alopecia.
- Although not life threatening, alopecia can have a great impact on a patient's self-esteem and quality of life.
- Nurses need to assess the likelihood of alopecia and pay particular attention to a patient's emotional response to hair loss and ability to cope.
- Patients need to be provided information about resources early in the treatment decision-making process.

Grevelman, E.G., & Breed, W.P.M. (2005). Prevention of chemotherapy-induced hair loss by scalp cooling. *Annals of Oncology, 16,* 352–358. doi:10.1093/annonc/mdi088

Hansen, H.P. (2007). Hair loss induced by chemotherapy: An anthropological study of women, cancer and rehabilitation. *Anthropology and Medicine, 14,* 15–26. doi:10.1080/13648470601106335

Hesketh, P.J., Batchelor, D., Golant, M., Lyman, G.H., Rhodes, N., & Yardley, D. (2004). Chemotherapy-induced alopecia: Psychosocial impact and therapeutic approaches. *Supportive Care in Cancer, 12,* 543–549.

Hilton, S., Hunt, K., Emslie, C., Salinas, M., & Ziebland, S. (2008). Have men been overlooked? A comparison of young men and women's experiences of chemotherapy-induced alopecia. *Psycho-Oncology, 17,* 577–583. doi:10.1002/pon.1272

Komen, M.M.C., Smorenburg, C.H., van den Hurk, C.J.G., & Nortier, J.W.R. (2013). Factors influencing the effectiveness of scalp cooling in the prevention of chemotherapy-induced alopecia. *Oncologist, 18,* 885–891. doi:10.1634/theoncologist.2012-0332

Lawenda, B.D., Gagne, H.M., Gierga, D.P., Niemierko, A., Wong, W.M., Tarbell, N.J., ... Loeffler, J.S. (2004). Permanent alopecia after cranial irradiation: Dose–response relationship. *International Journal of Radiation Oncology, Biology, Physics, 60,* 879–887. doi:10.1016/j.ijrobp.2004.04.031

Look Good Feel Better. (n.d.). Beauty guide: New hair looks. Retrieved from http://lookgoodfeelbetter.org/programs/beauty-guide/new-hair-looks/#main

Machado, M., Moreb, J.S., & Khan, S.A. (2007). Six cases of permanent alopecia after various conditioning regimens commonly used in hematopoietic stem cell transplantation. *Bone Marrow Transplantation, 40,* 979–982. doi:10.1038/sj.bmt.1705817

McGarvey, E.L., Baum, L.D., Pinkerton, R.C., & Rogers, L.M. (2001). Psychological sequelae and alopecia among women with cancer. *Cancer Practice, 9,* 283–289. doi:10.1111/j.1523-5394.2001.96007.pp.x

Miteva, M., Misciali, C., Fanti, P.A., Vincenzi, C., Romanelli, P., & Tosti, A. (2011). Permanent alopecia after systemic chemotherapy: A clinicopathological study of 10 cases. *American Journal of Dermatopathology, 33,* 345–350. doi:10.1097/DAD.0b013e3181fcfc25

National Cancer Institute Cancer Therapy Evaluation Program. (2010). *Common terminology criteria for adverse events* [v.4.03]. Retrieved from http://evs.nci.nih.gov/ftp1/CTCAE/About.html

Payne, A.S. (2015, February 4). Chemotherapy-induced alopecia [Literature review current through January 2017]. Retrieved from http://www.uptodate.com/contents/chemotherapy-induced-alopecia

Personal Care Products Council. (n.d.). Look Good Feel Better. Retrieved from http://www.personalcarecouncil.org/public-information/look-good-feel-better

Polovich, M., Olsen, M., & LeFebvre, K.B. (Eds.). (2014). *Chemotherapy and biotherapy guidelines and recommendations for practice* (4th ed.). Pittsburgh, PA: Oncology Nursing Society.

Roe, H. (2014). Scalp cooling: Management option for chemotherapy-induced alopecia. *British Journal of Nursing, 23*(Suppl. 16), S4–S11. doi:10.12968/bjon.2014.23.Sup16.S4

Rugo, H.S., Klein, P., Melin, S.A., Hurvitz, S.A., Melisko, M.E., Moore, A., ... Cigler, T. (2015). Clinical performance of the DigniCap system, a scalp hypothermia system, in preventing chemotherapy-induced alopecia. *Journal of Clinical Oncology, 33*(Suppl.), Abstract 9518. Retrieved from http://meetinglibrary.asco.org/content/149240-156

Tallon, B., Blanchard, E., & Goldberg, L.J. (2010). Permanent chemotherapy-induced alopecia: Case report and review of the literature. *Journal of the American Academy of Dermatology, 63,* 333–336. doi:10.1016/j.jaad.2009.06.063

Trüeb, R.M. (2009). Chemotherapy-induced alopecia. *Seminars in Cutaneous Medicine and Surgery, 28,* 11–14. doi:10.1016/j.sder.2008.12.001

Trüeb, R.M. (2010). Chemotherapy-induced alopecia. *Current Opinion in Supportive and Palliative Care, 4,* 281–284. doi:10.1097/SPC.0b013e3283409280

Williams, J., Wood, C., & Cunningham-Warburton, P. (1999). A narrative study of chemotherapy-induced alopecia. *Oncology Nursing Forum, 26,* 1463–1468.

Yeager, C.E., & Olsen, E.A. (2011). Treatment of chemotherapy-induced alopecia. *Dermatologic Therapy, 24,* 432–442. doi:10.1111/j.1529-8019.2011.01430.x

Chapter 15 Study Questions

1. A patient is starting her first chemotherapy regimen that includes doxorubicin and cyclophosphamide. She states she is very worried about losing her hair and having everyone stare at her. What would be the nurse's best response?
   A. Provide her with a referral to Look Good Feel Better and encourage her family to be supportive.
   B. Discuss accurate and specific information about management of hair loss before it begins and acknowledge that hair loss can be a very personal and emotional experience.
   C. Assure her that hair loss is only temporary and that she is on the road to being cancer free.
   D. Emphasize the multiple resources that are available, as hair loss often makes others uncomfortable.

2. A patient is scheduled to start a chemotherapy regimen that includes paclitaxel and carboplatin. She states she is very worried about losing her hair. She heard about scalp cooling and would like to try it. What would be the nurse's best response?
   A. The efficacy of scalp cooling to prevent alopecia depends on the chemotherapy agents, dosages, and duration and the patient's liver function. Scalp cooling may be an option.
   B. The patient should not be concerned about hair loss because it is temporary, and she should focus on optimal treatment results, not appearance.
   C. The patient should shave her head as soon as possible and consider head coverings (e.g., wigs, scarves, turbans), which should counterbalance her concerns about hair loss.
   D. Using a scalp tourniquet and minoxidil would be a better option.

3. Chemotherapy-induced hair loss normally occurs how soon after receiving treatment?
   A. 1–2 months
   B. 1–2 days
   C. 1–2 weeks
   D. 12 weeks

4. Patients who receive high doses of chemotherapy for hematopoietic stem cell transplantation are at risk for which of the following?
   A. Permanent hair loss
   B. Temporary hair loss
   C. Minimal hair loss
   D. No hair loss

5. A patient is scheduled to receive radiation therapy for cancer that will include a portion of the head and is concerned about hair loss. What dose will most likely cause permanent hair loss in the area that is treated?
   A. Greater than 16 Gy
   B. Greater than 20 Gy
   C. Greater than 30 Gy
   D. Greater than 40 Gy

CHAPTER

16 Cardiotoxicity

Anecita Fadol, PhD, RN, FNP-BC, FAANP, and Courtney L. Meuth, PharmD, BCPS

Introduction

Cancer treatment has progressed tremendously in the recent years with the development of novel, effective anticancer therapies. However, with the addition of several new agents to the therapeutic armamentarium, cardiotoxicity has become an increasing concern not only for conventional chemotherapy agents (i.e., anthracyclines), but also for novel targeted therapies (i.e., trastuzumab).

Cardiotoxicity is defined by the National Cancer Institute (n.d.) as "toxicity that affects the heart." This definition encompasses a broad range of cardiovascular side effects related to cancer therapy (i.e., heart failure [HF], cardiomyopathy [CMP], arrhythmias, ischemia, valvular disease, pericardial disease, hypertension, or thrombosis). The precise magnitude of the problem is undefined because of the increasing number of cardiotoxic anticancer drugs entering the pipeline; the significant improvement in the life expectancy of patients with cancer, thus requiring long-term monitoring; and the similarities between cancer and cardiovascular diseases in terms of incidence, risk factors, and pathogenesis (Raschi & De Ponti, 2012). Anticancer drug–induced cardiotoxicity represents a rapidly evolving field with clinical implications for clinicians, including primary care physicians, advanced practice nurses, and clinical nurses who play a pivotal role in managing practical issues (i.e., hypertension) of cancer survivors. This chapter will discuss the emerging cardiovascular toxicities associated with anticancer agents, focusing on left ventricular dysfunction (LVD)/HF, hypertension, acute coronary syndromes, and QT prolongation, by offering a concise review on cardiotoxicity associated with anticancer agents and recommendations for effective patient management, including detection, treatment, and monitoring of cardiovascular side effects.

Left Ventricular Dysfunction/ Heart Failure

Cardiotoxicity in patients with cancer is most often associated with the development of LVD/HF. From the clinical standpoint, the Cardiac Review and Evaluation Committee (CREC) supervising trastuzumab clinical trials defined drug-related cardiotoxicity as one or more of the following: (a) CMP characterized by a decrease in left ventricular ejection fraction (LVEF), either global or more severe in the septum, (b) symptoms associated with congestive heart failure (CHF), (c) signs associated with CHF (e.g., S_3 gallop, tachycardia or both), or (d) a reduction in LVEF from baseline of less than 5% to less than 55% with accompanying signs or symptoms of CHF, or a reduction in LVEF of greater than 10% to less than 55% without accompanying signs or symptoms (Raschi & De Ponti, 2012).

Several anticancer treatments have been implicated in causing LVD/HF (see Table 16-1). Chemotherapy-induced LVD/HF has been described with anthracyclines; however, recent data have suggested that cardiotoxicity caused by some of the targeted agents is generated through mechanisms distinct from that of anthracyclines. These findings have led some to propose the terms *type I* and *type II* cardiotoxicity (Suter & Ewer, 2013).

Anthracyclines, which demonstrate type I cardiotoxicity, are associated with irreversible damage to the cardiomyocyte that is dependent on the cumulative dose. Even after withdrawal of anthracyclines and initiation of HF therapy, LVD/HF may be irreversible. Therefore, rechallenge with anthracycline therapy is not always possible (Ewer & Lippman, 2005; Le, Cao, & Yang, 2014). On microscopy, myocardial damage is characterized by vacuoles, myofibrillar disarray, and necrosis. Oxidative stress via free radical formation is generally accepted as the main mechanism by which anthracyclines cause cardiotoxicity (Ewer & Lippman, 2005; Le et al., 2014). However, doxorubicin also may cause cardiotoxicity through its interference with topoisomerase II beta (Zhang et al., 2012).

In contrast, type II cardiotoxicity, which is modeled by trastuzumab, is associated with reversible cardiomyocyte dysfunction, and LVD/HF typically recovers after discontinuation of the targeted agent and initiation of HF therapy. No apparent structural abnormalities are seen on microscopy; it does not appear to be dependent on cumulative dose; and rechallenge with the targeted treatment often is tolerated after recovery (Ewer & Lippman, 2005; Le et al., 2014). The mechanisms in which the monoclonal antibodies and small molecule tyrosine kinase inhibitors (TKIs) cause cardiotoxicity are typically related to their individual targets of action for cancer therapy. While these agents are highly effective in targeting the cancer cells on- and off-target, adverse reactions such as LVD/HF can occur.

Table 16-1. Cancer Therapy Associated With Left Ventricular Dysfunction Heart Failure

Chemotherapy Agents	Examples
Anthracyclines	Doxorubicin (Adriamycin®) Epirubicin (Ellence®) Idarubicin (Idamycin PFS®)
Alkylating agents	Cyclophosphamide (Cytoxan®) Ifosfamide (Ifex®)
Antimetabolite	Decitabine (Dacogen®)
Antimicrotubule agents	Docetaxel (Taxotere®) Ixabepilone (Ixempra®)
Angiogenesis inhibitor	Lenalidomide (Revlimid®)
Monoclonal antibody–based tyrosine kinase inhibitors	Ado-trastuzumab emtansine (Kadcyla®) Bevacizumab (Avastin®) Pertuzumab (Perjeta®) Trastuzumab (Herceptin®)
Proteasome inhibitors	Bortezomib (Velcade®) Carfilzomib (Kyprolis®)
Small molecule tyrosine kinase inhibitors	Afatinib (Gilotrif®) Axitinib (Inlyta®) Dabrafenib (Tafinlar®) Dasatinib (Sprycel®) Imatinib mesylate (Gleevec®) Lapatinib (Tykerb®) Pazopanib (Votrient®) Ponatinib (Iclusig®) Sorafenib (Nexavar®) Sunitinib (Sutent®) Trametinib (Mekinist®) Vandetanib (Caprelsa®)
Miscellaneous	Tretinoin (Vesanoid®)

Note. Based on information from Micromedex 2.0, n.d.; Yeh & Bickford, 2009.

Diagnosis of Heart Failure in a Patient With Cancer

Establishing a correct diagnosis is the first essential step in the management of HF in a patient with cancer and relies mainly on clinical judgment based on patient history, physical examination, and appropriate investigations. It is a complex process because of the heterogeneous presentation and the overlap of HF and cancer symptoms. For example, the cardinal signs of HF—fatigue, shortness of breath, and lower extremity edema—also can be a manifestation of cancer (e.g., lung cancer), chemotherapy, radiation therapy, and other comorbid conditions (e.g., renal failure). Identification of the causes of HF is important because some of these precipitating conditions are potentially treatable or reversible. Diagnostic tests used to confirm the diagnosis of HF are listed in Table 16-2.

Assessment of LVEF by echocardiography has become the most common screening method for cardiotoxic effects. Echocardiography is noninvasive and can be performed at the bedside and allows for assessment of changes in systolic and diastolic function, as well as ruling out pericardial effusion and pulmonary hypertension. Walker et al. (2010) tested the accuracy of the conventional echocardiography and multigated acquisition scan with three-dimensional echocardiography and cardiac magnetic resonance imaging in a breast cancer population receiving adjuvant trastuzumab and anthracycline. These researchers found that echocardiography is as accurate as conventional methods for LVEF measurements.

Other imaging modalities have been proposed for the early detection of cardiotoxicity, including tissue Doppler imaging and speckle-tracking strain echocardiography. Tissue Doppler imaging can detect markers of underlying diastolic function (e.g., deformation [strain] and deformation rate [strain rate] of ventricular walls) for early detection of chemotherapy-related cardiotoxicity. Stress echocardiography is a technique that can assess the myocardium contractile reserve.

Table 16-2. Diagnostic Tests for Heart Failure

Diagnostic Test	Purpose
Echocardiogram	To detect a decrease in left ventricular dysfunction, valvular problems, and wall motion abnormalities
MUGA scan	To evaluate cardiac function
Chest x-ray	To rule out pulmonary causes of symptoms (e.g., pulmonary edema, pleural effusion)
Endomyocardial biopsy	To diagnose anthracycline-induced CMP, endomyocardial biopsies demonstrate sarcoplasmic reticulum dilation, vacuole formation, myofibrillar dropout, and necrosis.
Cardiac biomarkers (TnI, N-terminal proBNP)	Elevated TnI and BNP levels signal myocardial damage after chemotherapy, and are associated with increased incidence of cardiac events. Elevated BNP levels indicate volume overload.
Thyroid function	To evaluate for hyperthyroidism/hypothyroidism as HF etiology
Viral titers	To evaluate viral etiology for HF (i.e., myocarditis, endocarditis, and pericarditis)
Blood cultures	To define organisms in sepsis-related HF
Iron studies	To evaluate for hemochromatosis resulting in HF

BNP—brain natriuretic peptide; CMP—cardiomyopathy; HF—heart failure; MUGA—multigated acquisition; TnI—troponin I

Prevention and Treatment

Appropriate management should include early detection of those patients at risk (see Figure 16-1), development of preventive strategies, and early treatment of cardiotoxicity when it occurs. In clinical practice, no specific guidelines are available for patients with cancer with cardiotoxicity, although a number of recommendations have been proposed to manage cardiotoxicity, especially for trastuzumab in early breast cancer (Carver, 2010). When pharmacologic treatment is required, the patient should be managed with the standardized pharmacologic armamentarium as recommended per clinical guidelines (see Table 16-3). Agent selection should be based on clinical judgment, the patient's needs, and side effects.

Early intervention can have a positive impact on cardiac function. Cardinale, Colombo, Torrisi, et al. (2010) demonstrated that in patients with anthracycline-induced CMP, early treatment (within two months from the end of anthracycline therapy) with an angiotensin-converting enzyme (ACE) inhibitor (and possibly a beta-blocker) allows complete recovery of LVEF. Responders often show a lower rate of cumulative cardiac events. However, many cancer survivors with asymptomatic decreased

Figure 16-1. Risk Factors for the Development of Heart Failure in a Patient With Cancer

- Hypertension
- Ischemic heart disease
- Cardiotoxic agents (e.g., anthracyclines, trastuzumab, small molecule tyrosine kinase inhibitors)
- Diabetes mellitus/metabolic syndrome
- Obesity
- Familial history/genetic markers
- Low ejection fraction (left ventricular ejection fraction < 50%)
- Impaired diastolic function
- Left ventricular hypertrophy
- Radiation treatment to left side of the chest

Note. Based on information from Carver et al., 2007; Swain et al., 2003.

Table 16-3. Recommended Medications for Treatment of Heart Failure

Drug	Dosage Range
Angiotensin-Converting Enzyme Inhibitors	
Captopril (Capoten®)	6.25–50 mg 3x/day
Enalapril (Vasotec®)	2.5–20 mg 2x/day
Fosinopril (Monopril®)	5–40 mg/day
Lisinopril (Prinivil®, Zestril®)	2.5–20 mg/day
Perindopril (Aceon®)	2–16 mg/day
Quinapril (Accupril®)	5–20 mg 2x/day
Ramipril (Altace®)	1.25–10 mg/day
Trandolapril (Mavik®)	1–4 mg/day
Angiotensin Receptor Blockers	
Candesartan (Atacand®)	4–32 mg/day
Losartan (Cozaar®)	25–150 mg/day
Valsartan (Diovan®)	20–160 mg 2x/day
Aldosterone Antagonists	
Eplerenone (Inspra®)	25–50 mg/day
Spironolactone (Aldactone®)	12.5–25 mg/day
Beta-Blockers	
Bisoprolol (Zebeta®)	1.25–10 mg/day
Carvedilol (Coreg®)	3.125–25 mg 2x/day (50 mg 2x/day if > 85 kg)
Carvedilol phosphate (Coreg CR®)	10–80 mg/day
Metoprolol succinate (Toprol XL®)	12.5–200 mg 2x/day
Direct-Acting Vasodilator	
Hydralazine and isosorbide dinitrate (BiDil®)	37.5 mg hydralazine/20 mg isosorbide dinitrate 3x/day–75 mg hydralazine/40 mg isosorbide dinitrate 3x/day

Note. Based on information from Yancy et al., 2013.

LVEF are neither receiving standard HF treatment nor referred to an HF specialist for consultation (Yoon et al., 2010).

Monitoring for Cardiotoxicity

Despite the lack of consensus about the strategy to evaluate cardiotoxicity (Altena, Perik, van Veldhuisen, de Vries, & Gietema, 2009), periodic evaluation of LVEF should be carried out before, during, and after treatment with cytotoxic or targeted agents known to induce HF in order to detect subclinical cardiac damage (Driver, Djoussé, Logroscino, Gaziano, & Kurth, 2008). Close monitoring is essential for early detection and treatment of cardiovascular disease induced by antineoplastic treatment. This policy minimizes serious acute and chronic cardiac consequences. Antineoplastic drugs should be discontinued in cases of a significant decrease in LVEF (Driver et al., 2008) based on the CREC criteria (Raschi & De Ponti, 2012). Other potential causes, such as electrolyte disturbances or coronary artery disease, should be studied and treated.

Cardioprotection

The American Society of Clinical Oncology guidelines recommend that dexrazoxane treatment should be considered only in patients with metastatic breast cancer who have received the minimum of 300 mg/m^2 of anthracycline and would benefit from continued anthracycline-based therapy (Hensley et al., 2009). Several trials were conducted to determine the efficacy of cardioprotective medications such as ACE inhibitors and beta-blockers for the prevention of chemotherapy-induced cardiomyopathy (Cardinale, Colombo, Lamantia, et al., 2010; Kalay et al., 2006). None of the patients receiving ACE inhibitors while on high-dose chemotherapy developed HF, compared to 24% of the control patients (Cardinale et al., 2006). In addition, none of the patients receiving an ACE inhibitor experienced a decline in LVEF, compared to 43% of the control group. Similarly, Kalay et al. (2006) found that prophylactic use of carvedilol in patients receiving anthracycline-based chemotherapy may protect both systolic and diastolic functions of the left ventricle.

Hypertension

Hypertension (HTN) is the most frequent comorbid condition reported in cancer registries (Piccirillo, Tierney, Costas, Grove, & Spitznagel, 2004). Rates of HTN observed in the oncology population prior to chemotherapy are reported to be 28%–29%, which is similar to the general population (Jain & Townsend, 2007; Maitland et al., 2010). The incidence of HTN increases up to 80% in patients with cancer with the addition of newer targeted cancer therapies that disrupt angiogenesis (Lankhorst, Saleh, Danser, & van den Meiracker, 2015). The most common chemotherapy agents known to cause HTN include several of the angiogenesis inhibitors commonly known as vascular signaling pathway inhibitors. These drugs include the vascular endothelial growth factor (VEGF) inhibitors and other small molecule TKIs (Lankhorst et al., 2015). Table 16-4 highlights cancer therapies associated with clinically significant HTN.

The mechanism of HTN is not fully understood; however, for the monoclonal antibody–based TKIs and small molecule TKIs that target VEGF, it is thought to be directly related to the inhibition of VEGF signaling. Blocking VEGF leads to decreased nitric oxide bioavailability, causing vasoconstriction, an increase in systemic vascular resistance, and blood pressure. Evidence also indicates that antiangiogenic drugs can lead to chronic remodeling of the capillary beds throughout the body, a process referred to as *capillary rarefaction.* Other proposed mechanisms include activation of the endothelin pathway, renal function impairment, and salt sensitivity, as well as alterations

Table 16-4. Cancer Therapy Associated With Hypertension

Classification	Examples
Antimetabolites	Decitabine (Dacogen®)
Monoclonal antibodies	Alemtuzumab (Campath®) Ibritumomab (Zevalin®) Ofatumumab (Arzerra®) Rituximab (Rituxan®)
Monoclonal antibody–based tyrosine kinase inhibitors	Ado-trastuzumab emtansine (Kadcyla®) Bevacizumab (Avastin®)
Proteasome inhibitors	Bortezomib (Velcade®) Carfilzomib (Kyprolis®)
Small molecule tyrosine kinase inhibitors	Axitinib (Inlyta®) Cabozantinib (Cometriq®) Ibrutinib (Imbruvica®) Nilotinib (Tasigna®) Pazopanib (Votrient®) Ponatinib (Iclusig®) Ramucirumab (Cyramza®) Regorafenib (Stivarga®) Sorafenib (Nexavar®) Sunitinib (Sutent®) Tofacitinib (Xeljanz®) Trametinib (Mekinist®) Vandetanib (Caprelsa®) Ziv-aflibercept (Zaltrap®)

in activity of the renin–angiotensin–aldosterone system and sympathetic nervous system (Lankhorst et al., 2015).

Management of Hypertension

Adequately diagnosing and managing HTN in patients with cancer is critical because HTN is well established as a risk factor for chemotherapy-induced cardiotoxicity. Poorly controlled HTN can significantly influence cancer management and even result in discontinuation of certain therapies.

Before starting treatment with VEGF inhibitors, a careful screening for cardiovascular risk is recommended. The purpose of this initial assessment is not to exclude patients from receiving therapy, but rather to provide a baseline patient risk level to guide surveillance. Risk factors include age greater than 50 years, borderline LVEF, preexisting HTN, and history of cardiovascular disease. Patients with preexisting HTN and on multiple antihypertensive agents should be evaluated for renal function and proteinuria. Underlying glomerular disease can result in worsening HTN in patients receiving VEGF inhibitors (Robinson, Khankin, Karumanchi, & Humphreys, 2010).

Monitoring During Treatment

Monitoring of blood pressure while patients are receiving VEGF inhibitors is recommended, especially during the first cycle of chemotherapy, when most patients experience an elevation in blood pressure. Patients should be instructed to measure blood pressure while at home and keep a log. Measurement may be carried out either with home or office nursing monitoring on a regular basis, especially during the first week of treatment because the magnitude of blood pressure elevation is unpredictable. Target blood pressure should be based on Joint National Committee 8 classification and guidelines (James et al., 2014). It is important to maintain or start antihypertensive therapy with a blood pressure goal of less than 150/90 mm Hg for hypertensive persons aged 60 years and older. These thresholds should be adjusted accordingly to associated comorbidities (e.g., less than 140/90 mm Hg in patients with diabetes or chronic kidney disease) (James et al., 2014).

The selection of the most appropriate antihypertensive medications should be based on two main considerations: (a) pharmacokinetic aspects of the drug (e.g., drug–drug interactions) that can cause potential cardiotoxicity of the chemotherapy and antihypertensive medications, and (b) specific indications and contraindications related to the drug, preexisting comorbidities, and the patient's needs (e.g., calcium channel blockers for calcineurin-induced HTN, diuretics for steroid-related HTN, ACE inhibitors for diabetic patients due to the positive effect on the underlying proteinuria) (Mancia & Grassi, 2013; Wang et al., 2008).

When choosing an antihypertensive agent, clinicians should observe caution when administering CYP3A4 inhibitors (e.g., diltiazem, verapamil) in patients receiving sunitinib and pazopanib because concomitant administration of these agents can lead to increased levels of the chemotherapy agents. Lastly, monitoring of thyroid and liver function, complete blood counts, and electrolyte imbalances, especially hypokalemia and hypomagnesemia, is important during therapy.

Myocardial Ischemia

Chest pain is a common cardiac event experienced by patients with cancer, often requiring a workup for myocardial ischemia. Many anticancer treatments, including radiation and chemotherapy, are associated with an increased risk of coronary artery disease or acute coronary syndrome (Yeh & Bickford, 2009). Chemotherapy agents implicated in the development of myocardial infarction (MI) and ischemia are listed in Table 16-5.

The most common cancer therapies associated with myocardial ischemia are 5-fluorouracil and capecitabine. Although the mechanism of cardiotoxicity associated with these agents is unknown, coronary artery thrombosis, arteritis, or vasospasm have been proposed as the most likely underlying pathophysiology (Kosmas et al., 2008). Myocardial ischemia attributed to antimicrotubule agents, such as paclitaxel, is thought to be multifactorial in etiology, with other drugs and underlying heart disease as possible contributing factors. The Kolliphor® EL, formerly Cremophor® EL, vehicle in which paclitaxel is formulated in, which induces histamine release, also may be responsible for its cardiac toxicity (Rowinsky et al., 1991; Wang et al., 2008).

Arterial thromboembolic events associated with the monoclonal antibody–based TKIs (e.g., bevacizumab) and small molecule TKIs are thought to be directly related to the inhibition of VEGF signaling. Blocking VEGF may cause endothelial cell apoptosis; disturb platelet–endothelial cell homeostasis, causing platelet aggregation; and result in exposure of the extracellular matrix to blood cells—all increasing the risk for thrombotic events (Chen & Cleck, 2009). In addition, inhibiting VEGF may reduce nitric oxide and prostacyclin production and increase erythropoietin production, which may predispose patients to an increased risk of thromboembolic events (Kamba & McDonald, 2007).

Proteasome inhibitors, such as carfilzomib, may cause adverse effects on the cardiovascular system via proteasome inhibition leading

Table 16-5. Cancer Therapy Associated With Myocardial Infarction/Ischemia

Classification	Examples
Angiogenesis inhibitors	Lenalidomide (Revlimid®) Thalidomide (Thalomid®)
Antimetabolites	Capecitabine (Xeloda®) Fluorouracil (Adrucil®)
Antimicrotubule agents	Docetaxel (Taxotere®) Ixabepilone (Ixempra®) Paclitaxel (Taxol®)
Monoclonal antibody–based tyrosine kinase inhibitor	Bevacizumab (Avastin®)
Proteasome inhibitor	Carfilzomib(Kyprolis®)
Small molecule tyrosine kinase inhibitors	Erlotinib (Tarceva®) Imatinib (Gleevec®) Nilotinib (Tasigna®) Pazopanib (Votrient®) Ponatinib (Iclusig®) Ramucirumab (Cyramza®) Regorafenib (Stivarga®) Sorafenib (Nexavar®) Ziv-aflibercept (Zaltrap®)

to changes in endothelial nitric oxide synthase activity and nitric oxide levels (Baz et al., 2005). Lastly, thalidomide- and lenalidomide-induced thromboembolism may involve its direct action on endothelial cells, interaction between platelets and the endothelium, or increased platelet aggregation and von Willebrand factor (Baz et al., 2005; Rodeghiero & Elice, 2003; Zangari, Elice, Fink, & Tricot, 2007).

Diagnostic Criteria

The diagnosis of acute coronary syndromes or MI is based on a combination of symptoms, elevated biomarkers, and positive diagnostic testing. The World Health Organization's definition of MI involves at least two of the following criteria: (a) a history of ischemic-type chest pain symptoms, (b) evolutionary electrocardiogram (ECG) changes, and (c) a rise and fall in serial cardiac biomarkers (Antman, 2012). The 2014 American College of Cardiology (ACC) and American Heart Association (AHA) guideline update for the management of patients with non–ST-elevation acute coronary syndrome combines unstable angina and non–ST-elevation myocardial infarction (NSTEMI) into a new classification, known as non–ST-elevation acute coronary syndromes (NSTE-ACS), on the basis that these patient populations are not always distinguishable with their clinical manifestation (Amsterdam et al., 2014).

The cardiac biomarkers used in the diagnosis of acute coronary syndrome include creatine kinase-MB (CK-MB) and troponin I levels. CK-MB is an isoenzyme of creatine kinase found in the highest concentration in the myocardium and is released into the bloodstream with injury. After myocardial infarct, the CK-MB will be elevated in three hours, peak in 12–24 hours, and return to normal within 1–3 days (Anderson et al., 2013). Troponin I begins to elevate 3–12 hours after the onset of an infarct and peaks in 12–24 hours. It remains elevated for 7–14 days, so it can be helpful in the diagnosis if the patient complains of angina symptoms that occurred several days prior (Antman, 2012). Troponin I is more specific than CK-MB, as its degree of elevation correlates with patient's prognosis (Anderson et al., 2013).

Treatment

Currently, no clinical guideline exists specific for the management of acute coronary syndrome in patients with cancer. The treatment options available for these patients are based on studies done in the general population. Patients with cancer have been largely excluded from all acute coronary syndrome trials; hence, the evidence-based treatment regimen for MI in this group of patients is unknown. Until specific guidelines are available, patients with suspected acute coronary syndrome should be managed according to the guidelines established by ACC and AHA (Anderson et al., 2013). The foundation of acute coronary syndrome treatment includes percutaneous coronary intervention and medications such as antiplatelets and anticoagulants (Anderson et al., 2013); however, all of these may pose challenges to patients with cancer with thrombocytopenia or recent surgery. One of the first studies evaluating the efficacy and safety of aspirin therapy in patients with cancer with thrombocytopenia and acute coronary syndrome showed aspirin use significantly improved seven-day survival without increasing the bleeding risk (Sarkiss et al., 2007). In addition, a recent retrospective review of patients with cancer with MI demonstrated that medical therapy with aspirin and beta-blockers was associated with improved survival (Stegeman, Bossuyt, Yu, Boyd, & Puhan, 2015).

QT Prolongation

QT prolongation is a measure of delayed ventricular repolarization and can predispose patients to ventricular arrhythmias, specifically torsades de pointes (TdP). Oftentimes, QT prolongation is caused by medications, including chemotherapy agents (see Table 16-6). However, patients with cancer are at an increased risk for the development of QT prolongation for several reasons. First, 16% of patients with cancer have a prolonged QT interval at baseline, and 36% have baseline ECG abnormalities (Strevel, Ing, & Siu, 2007; Yusuf, Razeghi, & Yeh, 2008). Furthermore, patients with cancer receive concomitant QT-prolonging medications, such as antiemetics, azole antifungal agents, fluoroquinolone antibiotics, antihistamines, and antidepressants, or suffer from electrolyte abnormalities due to nausea, vomiting, diarrhea, constipation, poor oral intake, and renal dysfunction, which can all increase the likelihood of QT prolongation (Kowey, VanderLugt, & Luderer, 1996; Rowinsky et al., 1991).

The mechanism by which cancer therapies cause QT prolongation remains unknown. However, drug-induced QT prolongation generally is thought to be related to blockade of delayed return of potassium to the inside of the cell (delayed rectifier potassium current). In addition, one or more risk factors in the presence of underlying long QT syndrome may lead to significant QT interval prolongation (Vorchheimer, 2005; Yeh & Bickford, 2009).

Table 16-6. Cancer Therapy Associated With QT Prolongation

Classification	Examples
Histone deacetylase inhibitors	Belinostat (Beleodaq®) Romidepsin (Istodax®) Vorinostat (Zolinza®)
Miscellaneous	Arsenic trioxide (Trisenox®)
Small molecule tyrosine kinase inhibitors	Bosutinib (Bosulif®) Ceritinib (Zykadia®) Crizotinib (Xalkori®) Dabrafenib (Tafinlar®) Dasatinib (Sprycel®) Lapatinib (Tykerb®) Nilotinib (Tasigna®) Pazopanib (Votrient®) Sorafenib (Nexavar®) Sunitinib (Sutent®) Trametinib (Mekinist®) Vandetanib (Caprelsa®) Vemurafenib (Zelboraf®)

QT Monitoring

A corrected QT interval is considered normal if it is 440 msec or shorter. It is considered prolonged if it is greater than 450 msec in men and greater than 470 msec in women. Increases of 60 msec or more from baseline or more than 500 msec after administration of a medication raise concern about the potential risk of an arrhythmia (Vorchheimer, 2005). As a general rule, it is recommended that a baseline ECG should be performed prior to starting anticancer agents that could potentially cause QT prolongation. In addition, avoidance of drug–drug interactions and correction of electrolyte abnormalities, such as hypomagnesemia and hypokalemia, should be completed prior to initiation of anticancer agents that prolong the QT interval. AHA and ACC published the scientific statement on the prevention of TdP in the hospital setting. QT monitoring is recommended with (a) initiation of a drug known to cause TdP, (b) overdose from a potentially proarrhythmic agent, (c) new-onset bradyarrhythmia, and (d) severe electrolyte imbalance, including hypokalemia or hypomagnesemia (Epstein et al., 2008).

Treatment

Prior to administration of anticancer agents that could potentially produce QT prolongation, a comprehensive review of the patient's concomitant medications and correction of electrolyte disturbances is recommended. A serum potassium level of 4.5–5 mmol/L is recommended because it has been shown to shorten the QT interval (Bisinov, Mitchell, & January, 2003; Choy et al., 1997; Kim & Ewer, 2014).

Currently, no consistent guidelines are available for the treatment of chemotherapy-induced QT prolongation. However, baseline and periodic ECG monitoring should be performed for cancer therapies that may prolong the QT interval, and dose adjustments or discontinuation of therapy may be necessary in the face of QT prolongation (Ederhy et al., 2009). If evidence of TdP is present, magnesium sulfate should be administered promptly (Ederhy et al., 2009). IV magnesium has been shown to suppress TdP even in the presence of normal serum magnesium. In the presence of hemodynamic compromise, emergent direct-current cardioversion should be performed. Second-line therapy may include medical treatment with isoproterenol or temporary atrial and ventricular pacing to a heart rate of 70 beats per minute in drug-induced recurrent TdP. High-risk patients should be referred for evaluation for an implantable cardiac defibrillator when they have recurrent syncope despite medical therapy, sustained ventricular arrhythmias, or have been resuscitated from an episode of impending sudden cardiac death (Epstein et al., 2008).

Conclusion

Cardiotoxicity associated with anticancer therapy represents a multifaceted and multidisciplinary issue requiring a collaborative approach. Prevention, early detection, timely

Key Points

- Several chemotherapy agents have detrimental effects on the heart. Although cardiotoxicity is often used to describe LVD/HF, it also encompasses a variety of other complications, including HTN, MI, and QT prolongation.
- Chemotherapy-induced cardiotoxicity can be classified into two types. Type I is exemplified by anthracycline-induced cardiac dysfunction and causes cumulative dose-dependent cardiac damage. Type II cardiotoxicity is exemplified by trastuzumab and is not dose dependent.
- Various mechanisms have been proposed regarding the pathophysiology of chemotherapy-related cardiotoxicity. However, the type of chemotherapy and its mechanism of action seem to play an essential role in the development of cardiotoxicity.
- Establishing a correct diagnosis is the first essential step in the management of HF in a patient with cancer. It is a complex process because of the heterogeneous presentation and overlap of HF and cancer symptoms.
- Currently, no guidelines have been developed specifically for the treatment of chemotherapy-induced cardiotoxicity. Until then, guidelines for the treatment of the specific disease states mentioned (i.e., HF, HTN, MI, and QT prolongation) should be followed.
- Appropriate management of cardiotoxicity in patients with cancer should include early detection of those patients at risk, the development of preventive strategies, and early initiation of treatment of cardiotoxicity when it occurs.
- Selection of the most appropriate antihypertensive medication for HTN induced by anticancer agents should be based on the pharmacokinetic aspects of the drug, specific indications and contraindications related to the drug, and preexisting comorbidities and the patient's needs.
- Radiation therapy, particularly on the left side of the chest, is associated with an increased risk of early-onset coronary artery disease and valvular problems.
- Optimal management of cardiac risk factors and cardiovascular disease before, during, and after antineoplastic treatment is essential to reduce morbidity and mortality in patients with cancer and cancer survivors.
- Cardiotoxicity associated with anticancer therapy requires a multifaceted and multidisciplinary collaborative approach between oncology and cardiology to improve patient outcomes.

reporting, and initiation of recommended medications should be promoted to mitigate cardiac dysfunction associated with cardiovascular toxicity. Teamwork is of paramount importance and should be strengthened to improve clinical outcomes. Optimal management of cardiovascular disease before, during, and after antineoplastic treatment is essential to reduce morbidity and mortality in patients with cancer and cancer survivors.

The authors would like to acknowledge Dawn Camp-Sorrell, RN, MSN, FNP, AOCN®, for her contribution to this chapter that remains unchanged from the first edition of this book.

References

Altena, R., Perik, P.J., van Veldhuisen, D.J., de Vries, E.G., & Gietema, J.A. (2009). Cardiovascular toxicity caused by cancer treatment: Strategies for early detection. *Lancet Oncology, 10,* 391–399. doi:10.1016/S1470-2045(09)70042-7

Amsterdam, E.A., Wenger, N.K., Brindis, R.G., Casey, D.E., Jr., Ganiats, T.G., Holmes, D.R., Jr., ... Zieman, S.J. (2014). 2014 AHA/ACC guideline for the management of patients with non–ST-elevation acute coronary syndromes: Executive summary. A report of the American College of Cardiology/American Heart Association Task Force on Practice Guidelines. *Circulation, 130,* 2354–2394. doi:10.1161/CIR.0000000000000133

Anderson, J.L., Adams, C.D., Antman, E.M., Bridges, C.R., Califf, R.M., Casey, D.E., Jr., ... Wright, R.S. (2013). 2012 ACCF/AHA focused update incorporated into the ACCF/AHA 2007 guidelines for the management of patients with unstable angina/non-ST-elevation myocardial infarction: A report of the American College of Cardiology Foundation/American Heart Association Task Force on Practice Guidelines. *Journal of the American College of Cardiology, 61,* e179–e347. doi:10.1016/j.jacc.2013.01.014

Antman, E.M. (2012). ST-segment elevation myocardial infarction: Pathology, pathophysiology, and clinical features. In R.O. Bonow, D.L. Mann, D.P. Zipes, & P. Libby (Eds.), *Braunwald's heart disease: A textbook of cardiovascular medicine* (9th ed., pp. 1087–1109). Philadelphia, PA: Elsevier Saunders.

Baz, R., Li, L., Kottke-Marchant, K., Srkalovic, G., McGowan, B., Yiannaki, E., ... Hussein, M.A. (2005). The role of aspirin in the prevention of thrombotic complications of thalidomide and anthracycline-based chemotherapy for multiple myeloma. *Mayo Clinic Proceedings, 80,* 1568–1574. doi:10.4065/80.12.1568

Bisinov, E., Mitchell, J.H., & January, C.T. (2003). Potassium and long QT syndrome: A new look at an old therapy. *Journal of the American College of Cardiology, 42,* 1783–1784. doi:10.1016/j.jacc.2003.08.015

Cardinale, D., Colombo, A., Lamantia, G., Colombo, N., Civelli, M., De Giacomi, G., ... Cipolla, C.M. (2010). Anthracycline-induced cardiomyopathy: Clinical relevance and response to pharmacologic therapy. *Journal of the American College of Cardiology, 55,* 213–220. doi:10.1016/j.jacc.2009.03.095

Cardinale, D., Colombo, A., Sandri, M.T., Lamantia, G., Colombo, N., Civelli, M., ... Cipolla, C.M. (2006). Prevention of high-dose chemotherapy-induced cardiotoxicity in high-risk patients by angiotensin-converting enzyme inhibition. *Circulation, 114,* 2474–2481. doi:10.1161/CIRCULATIONAHA.106.635144

Cardinale, D., Colombo, A., Torrisi, R., Sandri, M.T., Civelli, M., Salvatici, M., ... Cipolla, C.M. (2010). Trastuzumab-induced cardiotoxicity: Clinical and prognostic implications of troponin I evaluation. *Journal of Clinical Oncology, 28,* 3910–3916. doi:10.1200/JCO.2009.27.3615

Carver, J.R. (2010). Management of trastuzumab-related cardiac dysfunction. *Progress in Cardiovascular Diseases, 53,* 130–139. doi:10.1016/j.pcad.2010.07.001

Carver, J.R., Shapiro, C.L., Ng, A., Jacobs, L., Schwartz, C., Virgo, K.S., ... Vaughn, D.J. (2007). American Society of Clinical Oncology clinical evidence review on the ongoing care of adult cancer survivors: Cardiac and pulmonary late effects. *Journal of Clinical Oncology, 25,* 3991–4008. doi:10.1200/JCO.2007.10.9777

Chen, H.X., & Cleck, J.N. (2009). Adverse effects of anticancer agents that target the VEGF pathway. *Nature Reviews Clinical Oncology, 6,* 465–477. doi:10.1038/nrclinonc.2009.94

Choy, A.M., Lang, C.C., Chomsky, D.M., Rayos, G.H., Wilson, J.R., & Roden, D.M. (1997). Normalization of acquired QT prolongation in humans by intravenous potassium. *Circulation, 96,* 2149–2154. doi:10.1161/01.CIR.96.7.2149

Driver, J.A., Djoussé, L., Logroscino, G., Gaziano, J.M., & Kurth, T. (2008). Incidence of cardiovascular disease and cancer in advanced age: Prospective cohort study. *BMJ, 337,* a2467. doi:10.1136/bmj.a2467

Ederhy, S., Cohen, A., Dufaitre, G., Izzedine, H., Massard, C., Meuleman, C., ... Soria, J.-C. (2009). QT interval prolongation among patients treated with angiogenesis inhibitors. *Targeted Oncology, 4,* 89–97. doi:10.1007/s11523-009-0111-3

Epstein, A.E., DiMarco, J.P., Ellenbogen, K.A., Estes, N.A.M., Freedman, R.A., Gettes, L.S., ... Sweeney, M.O.

(2008). ACC/AHA/HRS 2008 guidelines for device-based therapy of cardiac rhythm abnormalities: A report of the American College of Cardiology/American Heart Association Task Force on Practice Guidelines (Writing Committee to Revise the ACC/AHA/NASPE 2002 Guideline Update for Implantation of Cardiac Pacemakers and Antiarrhythmia Devices): Developed in collaboration with the American Association for Thoracic Surgery and Society of Thoracic Surgeons. *Circulation, 117,* e350–e408. doi:10.1161/CIRCUALTIONAHA.108.189742

Ewer, M.S., & Lippman, S.M. (2005). Type II chemotherapy-related cardiac dysfunction: Time to recognize a new entity. *Journal of Clinical Oncology, 23,* 2900–2902. doi:10.1200/JCO.2005.05.827

Hensley, M.L., Hagerty, K.L., Kewalramani, T., Green, D.M., Meropol, N.J., Wasserman, T.H., ... Schuchter, L.M. (2009). American Society of Clinical Oncology 2008 clinical practice guideline update: Use of chemotherapy and radiation therapy protectants. *Journal of Clinical Oncology, 27,* 127–145. doi:10.1200/JCO.2008.17.3627

Jain, M., & Townsend, R.R. (2007). Chemotherapy agents and hypertension: A focus on angiogenesis blockade. *Current Hypertension Reports, 9,* 320–328. doi:10.1007/s11906-007-0058-7

James, P.A., Oparil, S., Carter, B.L., Cushman, W.C., Dennison-Himmelfarb, C., Handler, J., ... Ortiz, E. (2014). 2014 evidence-based guideline for the management of high blood pressure in adults: Report from the panel members appointed to the Eighth Joint National Committee (JNC 8). *JAMA, 311,* 507–520. doi:10.1001/jama.2013.284427

Kalay, N., Basar, E., Ozdogru, I., Er, O., Cetinkaya, Y., Dogan, A., ... Ergin, A. (2006). Protective effects of carvedilol against anthracycline-induced cardiomyopathy. *Journal of the American College of Cardiology, 48,* 2258–2262. doi:10.1016/j.jacc.2006.07.052

Kamba, T., & McDonald, D.M. (2007). Mechanisms of adverse effects of anti-VEGF therapy for cancer. *British Journal of Cancer, 96,* 1788–1795. doi:10.1038/sj.bjc.6603813

Kim, P.Y., & Ewer, M.S. (2014). Chemotherapy and QT prolongation: Overview with clinical perspective. *Current Treatment Options in Cardiovascular Medicine, 16,* 303. doi:10.1007/s11936-014-0303-8

Kosmas, C., Kallistratos, M.S., Kopterides, P., Syrios, J., Skopelitis, H., Mylonakis, N., ... Tsavaris, N. (2008). Cardiotoxicity of fluoropyrimidines in different schedules of administration: A prospective study. *Journal of Cancer Research and Clinical Oncology, 134,* 75–82. doi:10.1007/s00432-007-0250-9

Kowey, P.R., VanderLugt, J.T., & Luderer, J.R. (1996). Safety and risk/benefit analysis of ibutilide for acute conversion of atrial fibrillation/flutter. *American Journal of Cardiology, 78*(8, Suppl. 1), 46–52. doi:10.1016/S0002-9149(96)00566-8

Lankhorst, S., Saleh, L., Danser, A.H.J., & van den Meiracker, A.H. (2015). Etiology of angiogenesis inhibition-related hypertension. *Current Opinion in Pharmacology, 21,* 7–13. doi:10.1016/j.coph.2014.11.010

Le, D.L., Cao, H., & Yang, L.X. (2014). Cardiotoxicity of molecular-targeted drug therapy. *Anticancer Research, 34,* 3243–3249.

Maitland, M.L., Bakris, G.L., Black, H.R., Chen, H.X., Durand, J.-B., Elliott, W.J., ... Tang, W.H.W. (2010). Initial assessment, surveillance, and management of blood pressure in patients receiving vascular endothelial growth factor signaling pathway inhibitors. *Journal of the National Cancer Institute, 102,* 596–604. doi:10.1093/jnci/djq091

Mancia, G., & Grassi, G. (2013). Individualization of antihypertensive drug treatment. *Diabetes Care, 36*(Suppl. 2), S301–S306. doi:10.2337/dcS13-2013

Micromedex 2.0. (n.d.). Greenwood Village, CO: Truven Health Analytics. Retrieved from http://www.micromedexsolutions.com

National Cancer Institute. (n.d.). Cardiotoxicity. In *NCI dictionary of cancer terms.* Retrieved from https://www.cancer.gov/publications/dictionaries/cancer-terms?CdrID=44004

Piccirillo, J.F., Tierney, R.M., Costas, I., Grove, L., & Spitznagel, E.L., Jr. (2004). Prognostic importance of comorbidity in a hospital-based cancer registry. *JAMA, 291,* 2441–2447. doi:10.1001/jama.291.20.2441

Raschi, E., & De Ponti, F. (2012). Cardiovascular toxicity of anticancer-targeted therapy: Emerging issues in the era of cardio-oncology. *Internal and Emergency Medicine, 7,* 113–131. doi:10.1007/s11739-011-0744-y

Robinson, E.S., Khankin, E.V., Karumanchi, S.A., & Humphreys, B.D. (2010). Hypertension induced by vascular endothelial growth factor signaling pathway inhibition: Mechanisms and potential use as a biomarker. *Seminars in Nephrology, 30,* 591–601. doi:10.1016/j.semnephrol.2010.09.007

Rodeghiero, F., & Elice, F. (2003). Thalidomide and thrombosis. *Pathophysiology of Haemostasis and Thrombosis, 33*(Suppl. 1), 15–18. doi:10.1159/000073282

Rowinsky, E.K., McGuire, W.P., Guarnieri, T., Fisherman, J.S., Christian, M.C., & Donehower, R.C. (1991). Cardiac disturbances during the administration of taxol. *Journal of Clinical Oncology, 9,* 1704–1712.

Sarkiss, M.G., Yusuf, S.W., Warneke, C.L., Botz, G., Lakkis, N., Hirch-Ginsburg, C., ... Durand, J.-B. (2007). Impact of aspirin therapy in cancer patients with thrombocytopenia and acute coronary syndromes. *Cancer, 109,* 621–627. doi:10.1002/cncr.22434

Stegeman, I., Bossuyt, P.M., Yu, T., Boyd, C., & Puhan, M.A. (2015). Aspirin for primary prevention of cardiovascular disease and cancer: A benefit and harm analysis. *PLOS ONE, 10,* e0127194. doi:10.1371/journal.pone.0127194

Strevel, E.L., Ing, D.J., & Siu, L.L. (2007). Molecularly targeted oncology therapeutics and prolongation of the QT interval. *Journal of Clinical Oncology, 25,* 3362–3371. doi:10.1200/JCO.2006.09.6925

Suter, T.M., & Ewer, M.S. (2013). Cancer drugs and the heart: Importance and management. *European Heart Journal, 34,* 1102–1111. doi:10.1093/eurheartj/ehs181

Swain, S.M., Whaley, F.S., & Ewer, M.S. (2003). Congestive heart failure in patients treated with doxorubicin: A retrospective analysis of three trials. *Cancer, 97,* 2869–2879. doi:10.1002/cncr.11407

Vorchheimer, D.A. (2005). What is QT interval prolongation? *Journal of Family Practice,* 56(Suppl.), S4–S7.

Walker, J., Bhullar, N., Fallah-Rad, N., Lytwyn, M., Golian, M., Fang, T., ... Jassal, D.S. (2010). Role of three-dimensional echocardiography in breast cancer: Comparison with two-dimensional echocardiography, multiple-gated acquisition scans, and cardiac magnetic resonance imaging. *Journal of Clinical Oncology, 28,* 3429–3436. doi:10.1200/JCO.2009.26.7294

Wang, Y., Zhou, L., Dutreix, C., Leroy, E., Yin, Q., Sethuraman, V., ... Shen, Z.-X. (2008). Effects of imatinib (Glivec) on the pharmacokinetics of metoprolol, a CYP2D6 substrate, in Chinese patients with chronic myelogenous leukaemia. *British Journal of Pharmacology, 65,* 885–892. doi:10.1111/j.1365-2125.2008.03150.x

Yancy, C.W., Jessup, M., Bozkurt, B., Butler, J., Casey, D.E., Jr., Drazner, M.H., ... Wilkoff, B.L. (2013). 2013 ACCF/AHA guideline for the management of heart failure: A report of the American College of Cardiology Foundation/American Heart Association Task Force on Practice Guidelines. *Circulation, 128,* e240–e327. doi:10.1161/CIR.0b013e31829e8776

Yeh, E.T.H., & Bickford, C.L. (2009). Cardiovascular complications of cancer therapy: Incidence, pathogenesis, diagnosis, and management. *Journal of the American College of Cardiology, 53,* 2231–2247. doi:10.1016/j.jacc.2009.02.050

Yoon, G.J., Telli, M.L., Kao, D.P., Matsuda, K.Y., Carlson, R.W., & Witteles, R.M. (2010). Left ventricular dysfunction in patients receiving cardiotoxic cancer therapies: Are clinicians responding optimally? *Journal of the American College of Cardiology, 56,* 1644–1650. doi:10.1016/j.jacc.2010.07.023

Yusuf, S.W., Razeghi, P., & Yeh, E.T. (2008). The diagnosis and management of cardiovascular disease in cancer patients. *Current Problems in Cardiology, 33,* 163–196. doi:10.1016/j.cpcardiol.2008.01.002

Zangari, M., Elice, F., Fink, L., & Tricot, G. (2007). Thrombosis in multiple myeloma. *Expert Review of Anticancer Therapy, 7,* 307–315. doi:10.1586/14737140.7.3.307

Zhang, S., Liu, X., Bawa-Khalfe, T., Lu, L.-S., Lyu, Y.L., Liu, L.F., & Yeh, E.T.H. (2012). Identification of the molecular basis of doxorubicin-induced cardiotoxicity. *Nature Medicine, 18,* 1639–1642. doi:10.1038/nm.2919nm.2919

Chapter 16 Study Questions

1. Which of the following characteristics is true regarding type II cardiotoxicity associated with cancer therapies?
   A. Type II cardiotoxicity is associated with irreversible cardiomyocyte dysfunction.
   B. Type II cardiotoxicity is associated with cumulative dose of the chemotherapy.
   C. Structural abnormalities are seen on microscopy.
   D. Heart failure typically recovers after treatment discontinuation of the chemotherapy agent and initiation of heart failure therapy.

2. Which of the following anticancer therapies is associated with heart failure, hypertension, myocardial infarction, and QT prolongation?
   A. Doxorubicin
   B. Sorafenib
   C. Nilotinib
   D. Ponatinib

3. Which of the following cardiac biomarkers is frequently measured for early detection and diagnosis of acute myocardial infarction?
   A. B-type natriuretic peptide (BNP)
   B. Creatine kinase–MM (CK-MM)
   C. Creatine kinase–BB (CK-BB)
   D. Troponin I

4. Which of the following tests is considered a gold standard for establishing the diagnosis of anthracycline-induced cardiomyopathy/heart failure?
   A. Echocardiogram
   B. Multigated acquisition scan
   C. Endomyocardial biopsy
   D. Cardiac biomarkers

5. It has been observed in clinical practice that patients with chemotherapy-induced heart failure can potentially improve their cardiac function with heart failure medications recommended in clinical guidelines. The recommended pharmacologic therapy includes which of the following medications?
   A. Angiotensin-converting enzyme inhibitor
   B. Angiotensin receptor blocker
   C. Beta-blocker
   D. Nondihydropyridine calcium channel blockers
   E. A, B, and C
   F. B, C, and D

CHAPTER

17 Cognitive Changes

Catherine Jansen, PhD, RN, AOCNS®

Introduction

Of the many symptoms associated with cancer and cancer treatment, cognitive changes are the least understood. Cognition has been defined as thinking skills that include language use, calculation, perception, memory, awareness, reasoning, judgment, learning, intellect, social skills, and imagination (Venes, 2014). Patients describe cognitive problems as the following:

- Trouble concentrating
- Memory lapses
- Inability to focus on tasks
- Difficulty following instructions
- Decreased ability to handle personal finances
- Disorganized behavior or thinking
- Loss of initiative
- Difficulty with remembering common words (or the accurate use of words and word meanings)
- Inability to recognize familiar objects
- Altered perception
- Taking longer to learn new things

These problems become more apparent when an individual is multitasking and affect quality of life by hindering one's performance in activities of daily living, employment, and social activities (Myers, 2013). This is especially pertinent in patients with cancer who are undergoing treatment, as normal cognitive functioning is essential for self-care and adherence to treatment regimens. It is important to note that survivors often reenter the workplace with a sense of decreased confidence in their abilities because of cognitive concerns (Cheung et al., 2012; Collins, Gehrke, & Feuerstein, 2013; Munir, Burrows, Yarker, Kalawsky, & Bains, 2010; Myers, 2013; Von Ah, Habermann, Carpenter, & Schneider, 2013). At times, loss of employment results (Myers, 2012).

Cognitive function is a multidimensional concept that encompasses multiple domains (i.e., attention and concentration, executive function, information processing speed, language, motor function, visuospatial skill, learning, and memory) that are regulated by the brain (Jansen, Miaskowski, Dodd, Dowling, & Kramer, 2005). These cognitive domains and their definitions are listed in Table 17-1.

Risk Factors

Individual characteristics, or risk factors, that influence cognitive function and are unrelated to cancer include intelligence and education levels, age, gender, menopausal status, psychological factors, genetics, comorbidities, and medications. Intelligence and education levels have strong, positive relationships with neuropsychological test performances and are thought to be protective (Lezak, Howieson, Bigler, & Tranel, 2012). In contrast, cognitive

Table 17-1. Domains of Cognitive Function

Domain	Description
Attention and concentration	Ability to triage relevant inputs, thoughts, or actions while ignoring those that distract or are irrelevant Ability to maintain attention toward a stimulus for a more extended time period
Executive function	Ability to initiate and generate hypotheses, plan, and make decisions
Information processing speed	Ability to rapidly and efficiently process simple and complex information
Language	Ability to comprehend and communicate symbolic information, either verbally or in writing
Motor function	Refers to motor performance, such as speed, strength, and coordination
Visuospatial skill	Ability to process and interpret visual information about where things are in space
Learning and memory	Ability to acquire new information Ability to acquire, store, and recall learned information, differentiated as working (short term) or semantic (long term)

Note. From "Potential Mechanisms for Chemotherapy-Induced Impairments in Cognitive Function," by C. Jansen, C.E. Miaskowski, M.A. Dodd, G.J. Dowling, and J.A. Kramer, 2005, *Oncology Nursing Forum, 32,* p. 1152. Copyright 2005 by Oncology Nursing Society. Adapted with permission.

functioning declines with increasing age; however, most neuropsychological tests are corrected for age and education level.

Gender differences exist in cognitive functioning for specific domains (Lezak et al., 2012). Hormonal levels differ depending on menopausal status and therefore may influence cognition. However, because menopause occurs as women age, it is difficult to differentiate whether cognitive decline is due to aging or decreased estrogen associated with menopause (Lobo, 2014). Psychological factors, such as stress and depression, can reduce performance on neuropsychological testing, whereas anxiety may either improve or diminish neuropsychological test performance.

Several gene variations have been identified that link cognitive decline with aging, head trauma, and Alzheimer disease, which may play a role in increasing a patient's susceptibility to cognitive changes related to cancer or its treatment (Mandelblatt, Jacobsen, & Ahles, 2014). Comorbidities that are known to affect cognition include neurologic illnesses (e.g., stroke, Alzheimer disease, developmental disorders), cardiovascular diseases, metabolic diseases, diabetes mellitus, hypertension, head injury, thyroid dysfunction, drug or alcohol abuse, nutritional deficiencies, fatigue, and psychiatric illnesses. Medications that have been shown to influence cognition include but are not limited to analgesics, antidepressants, antiemetics, antiepileptics, anxiolytics, antipsychotics, anesthesia, immunosuppressants, and steroids.

The most obvious cancer-related risk factor for cognitive changes is the presence of a brain tumor. Central nervous system (CNS) tumors include primary cancers (gliomas, CNS lymphoma), metastatic disease, and leptomeningeal disease. However, even cancers outside the CNS, when advanced, can cause cognitive changes because of the systemic effects of hypercalcemia, metabolic disturbances, infections, or multisystem failure. In addition, many treatments, regardless of tumor location, have similar risk factors for causing cognitive changes.

Cancer therapies that have been associated with cognitive changes include surgery, radiation therapy, chemotherapy, hormone therapy, and immunotherapy. Factors related to cancer treatments include therapy delivered directly to the CNS, the specific regimen or regimens used, the dose, and cumulative effects. Because most patients receive multimodal therapy, it is difficult to determine which regimens promote higher incidences of cognitive changes. The influence of surgery on cognitive function may be caused by structural changes from the removal of the CNS disease or even from the lingering effects of anesthesia. Cognitive changes in patients receiving cranial irradiation are related to the total dose received, with patients receiving whole brain irradiation having the highest risk (Bohan, 2013; Greene-Schloesser & Robbins, 2012).

Although it is probable that the risk for cognitive changes caused by chemotherapy increases with higher doses (i.e., dose intensity), as well as cumulative cycles, the evidence in this area is less clear. Regardless of an individual's risk factors, each domain of cognitive function depends heavily on intact connections between various neuroanatomic regions, as well as the functioning of multiple brain regions. To fully comprehend the complex relationships involved in cognitive function, a basic understanding of the anatomy and organization of the brain is essential (see Figure 17-1).

Pathophysiology

The human brain is made up of nervous tissue, glial cells, and blood vessels. The basic fundamental element of the brain is the neuron, which consists of a cell body, dendrites (branches that receive and conduct impulses to the cell body), and axons (which conduct impulses out of the cell). Approximately 100 billion neurons are involved in the transmission and processing of information between various areas of the brain, and they comprise cognitive function (Kandel, Barres, & Hudspeth, 2013). Neurons are supported by glial cells (i.e., oligodendrocytes, microglia, and astrocytes).

Oligodendrocytes produce myelin, a white, fatty substance that surrounds and insulates the axons to increase the effectiveness of informational delivery to other parts of the CNS. The function of microglia is to clean up and remove damaged cells. The functions of astrocytes are not fully understood, but they are known to have a role in covering endothelial cells to form a barrier between neuronal tissue and its blood supply (Cardoso, Brites, & Brito, 2010). This barrier, known as the blood-brain barrier (BBB), is crucial for brain functioning. The BBB is an anatomic and physiologic complex that controls the movement of substances from the extracellular fluids of the body to the extracellular fluids of the brain (Vanderah & Gould, 2015). Substances are not able to readily diffuse across the BBB if they are hydrophilic (i.e., have poor lipid solubility) or are of molecular weights greater than 200 daltons (Mrugala, Supko, & Batchelor, 2011).

The main structural components of the brain are the brain stem, cerebellum, and cerebral cortex. The brain stem (incorporating the medulla, pons, and midbrain) connects the right and left cerebral hemispheres with the spinal cord. The cerebellum interrelates with the brain stem and the cerebral cortex to execute various motor functions (e.g., maintaining posture, coordination) and also has a role in language (Amaral & Strick, 2013; Lisberger & Thach, 2013). The cerebral cortex, the focal area for cognitive function, is divided into four lobes: frontal, temporal, parietal, and occipital (Amaral & Strick, 2013).

The frontal lobe is responsible for the initiation of muscle contraction, the coordination and execution of movements, the control of gross or postural movements, and voluntary eye movements—all of which are essential for efficient psychomotor functioning. Also essential in formulating language, the frontal lobe combines speech sounds into complete sentences and controls the affective and motor control of speech production (Filley, 2011). Finally, the frontal lobe is well known for its role with higher intellectual function (i.e., executive function), as well as aspects of memory and emotion (Pearl & Emsellem, 2014).

The temporal lobe is associated with language, memory, and complex visuospatial functions. Although the temporal lobe receives auditory input, its primary role is in mediating

Figure 17-1. Anatomic Correlates of Cognitive Function

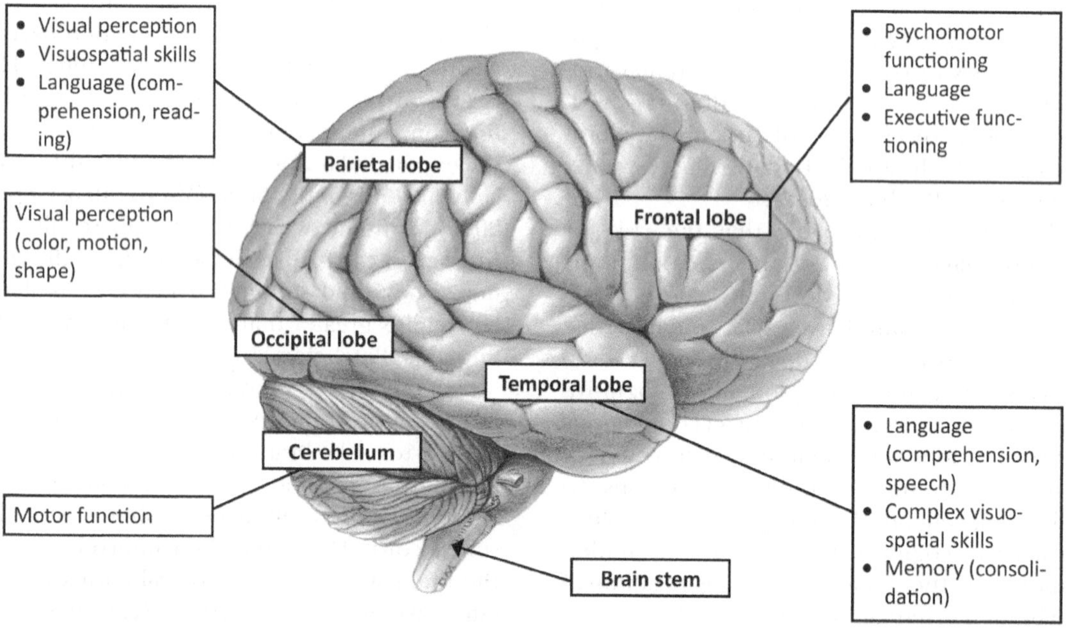

Note. Based on information from Filley, 2011; Gazzaniga et al., 2014; Lisberger & Thach, 2013; Olson & Colby, 2013; Pearl & Emsellem, 2014.

the comprehension of language and the normal rhythm, melody, and articulation of speech (Filley, 2011; Pearl & Emsellem, 2014). The hippocampus and amygdala are important components of the temporal lobe and are crucial for the laying down, strengthening, and storage (or consolidation) of new memories, as well as the expression of emotions (Olson & Colby, 2013). One reason for the complexity of memory is the influence of the closely connected limbic system, which is involved in emotional processing, learning, and memory (Gazzaniga, Ivry, & Mangun, 2014; Olson & Colby, 2013).

The parietal lobe integrates visual perception with motor processes and is central to spatial attention (Gazzaniga et al., 2014; Olson & Colby, 2013). This lobe often is associated with visual attention, proprioception, sensory perception, calculations, and visuospatial perception and construction. In addition, the parietal lobe receives tactile input from somatosensory relays of the thalamus; processes information regarding touch, changes in temperature, the presence of pain and limb proprioception, and the mediation of visuospatial competence; and subserves reading and calculation skills (Filley, 2011; Gazzaniga et al., 2014). Both language comprehension and auditory functions are important functions that occur via the parietal lobe (Pearl & Emsellem, 2014). The multiple connections within the parietal lobe integrate visual perception with motor processes, thus facilitating the ability to draw, write, and perform mathematical operations and constructional tasks (Pearl & Emsellem, 2014).

The occipital lobe is the smallest and most posterior lobe in the brain It receives primary visual input and mediates perception of visual material, before further processing occurs in more anterior regions (Filley, 2011; Olson & Colby, 2013). Other responsibilities include the processing of color, motion, and shape (Pearl & Emsellem, 2014).

However, despite clearly identified roles in cognitive functioning for the various areas of the brain, the underlying pathophysiology of cognitive changes related to cancer and its treatment is complex and poorly understood. CNS tumors cause changes by direct extension into the brain or by disruption of pathways that connect different areas of the brain. Although location is important in predicting which cognitive domains will be affected, CNS tumors with high growth rates can cause pressure and displacement of other brain structures, inducing further cognitive changes (Bohan, 2013). In addition, evidence of cognitive impairment has been found in approximately 40% of patients without tumor involvement of the CNS prior to treatment (Wefel, Kesler, Noll, & Schagen, 2015).

Identifying cognitive changes related to cancer and its treatments is challenging, as causes are most likely multifactorial, and patients also may have many of the risk factors discussed earlier. Although the science defining the phenomenon and its mechanisms is ongoing, experts have suggested several potential mechanisms (e.g., DNA damage, direct neurotoxic effects, leukoencephalopathy, cytokines, anemia, changes in hormonal levels) for cognitive changes related to cancer and its treatment.

DNA damage has been linked to neurocognitive disorders (e.g., Alzheimer disease, mild cognitive impairment, Parkinson disease) in addition to cancer (Ahles & Saykin, 2007; Mandelblatt et al., 2014). Some classes of chemotherapy drugs are known to work by causing direct injury to cellular DNA. Historically, it was thought that most chemotherapy agents were unable to cross the BBB because of their molecular weight and poor lipid solubility. But many chemotherapy drugs can cause CNS changes, and it has been speculated that chemotherapy damages blood vessels and eventually the BBB, thereby allowing chemotherapy to have a direct adverse neurotoxic effect on brain tissue and neurotransmitters (Ahles, 2012; Merriman, Von Ah, Miaskowski, & Aouizerat, 2013). Direct cytotoxic effects on the CNS resulting in neural cell damage, increased cell death (Monje & Dietrich, 2012), and cognitive changes have been reported in animal studies (Seigers & Fardell, 2011; Seigers, Schagen, Van Tellingen, & Dietrich, 2013; Winocur et al., 2012).

Leukoencephalopathy is structural alteration in the cerebral white matter, especially myelin (responsible for nerve insulation and facilitating neurotransmission). Generalized disruptions in brain function can occur with cranial irradiation acutely, within two weeks, because of the edema associated with treatment, or one to six months after the completion of therapy (Bohan, 2013). Leukoencephalopathy has also been reported with various chemotherapy agents, and imaging studies of cancer survivors have found structural changes in white and gray matter (Holohan, Von Ah, McDonald, & Saykin, 2013; Koppelmans et al., 2014). Regardless of the cause, cognitive deficits caused by leukoencephalopathy are dependent on the degree of myelin and axonal damage (Jansen et al., 2005).

Cytokines are proteins that have a role in neural function and repair, as well as in the metabolism of neurotransmitters, and therefore have the potential to cause cognitive changes (Seruga, Zhang, Bernstein, & Tannock, 2008). Evidence for treatment-related increases in cytokine levels exists for standard-dose chemotherapy (Merriman et al., 2013), although it is more limited for biologics, such as interferon alpha (Bender & Thelen, 2013; Capuron, Ravaud, & Dantzer, 2001; Scheibel, Valentine, O'Brien, & Meyers, 2004). Increased levels also have been found prior to treatment (Myers, 2010).

Red blood cells are essential for the transport of oxygen to the brain, as well as to the rest of the body. Insufficient brain oxygenation has been associated with decreased mental alertness, poor concentration, memory problems, decreased motor function, and mental flexibility problems (Lezak et al., 2012). Anemia can be related to decreased red blood cell production caused by iron deficiency or low erythropoietin levels, tumor involvement of the bone marrow, primary or metastatic disease in the bones, radiation therapy to areas of actively producing marrow, chemotherapy, or any combination of these. It is ultimately associated with cognitive changes due to lack of oxygenation.

Reproductive hormones have a relevant role in CNS development and are responsible for gender differences in cognitive test performance. Estrogen receptors exist in multiple locations throughout the brain, especially in regions involved with attention, memory, and learning, such as the cerebral cortex, hippocampus, and amygdala (Boss, Kang, Marcus, & Bergstrom, 2014; Lobo, 2014; Toffoletto, Lanzenberger, Gingnell, Sundström-Poromaa, & Comasco, 2014). Androgen receptors also are present in similar areas of the brain (Boss et al., 2014).

Because hormone therapy is aimed at reducing levels of these kinds of hormones, it is not surprising that cognitive changes occur. Although the cognitive effects of hormone therapy have been more extensively studied in patients with breast and prostate cancers, the evidence is still inconsistent (Batalo, Nagaiah, & Abraham, 2011; Ganz et al., 2014; McGinty et al., 2014). Chemotherapy is known to cause more rapid drops in estrogen than women would normally experience during natural menopause. However, the implication of this accelerated decrease in relation to cognitive function is still not clear (Conroy, McDonald, Ahles, West, & Saykin, 2013; Vearncombe et al., 2011).

Assessment

Identifying cognitive changes caused by cancer and its treatments is challenging, as standardized assessment guidelines are lacking, and various factors independent of cancer and its corresponding treatments can influence cognitive function. Assessing cognition should therefore be done in concert with a thorough evaluation of the presenting complaint, general and cancer-specific risk factors, coexisting medical conditions, current medications, pertinent laboratory values, and social history, as well as any potential influencing factors as described in Table 17-2 (Jansen, 2013). A physical examination should note any potential sensory deficits (e.g., hearing, vision), which may influence neuropsychological test performance. Laboratory testing should include complete blood count, electrolytes (e.g., calcium, sodium), thyroid level, and liver function. A complete social history should include the patient's current living situation and level of social functioning, as well as educational and occupational accomplishments or failures (Lezak et al., 2012). Family members are a valuable source of information when noting subtle changes in the patient's social activities and work habits. Evaluation of cognitive function requires the use of standardized scaled tests and discrete activities within a neuropsychological examination to assess specific domains (Lezak et al., 2012).

Test selection should be based on the following factors: specific cognitive domain to be measured, appropriateness of the test for the domain being studied, reliability and validity of the test and availability of normative data, sensitivity and specificity for measuring cancer treatment–related cognitive changes, availability of parallel forms or resistance to practice effects for use with repeated measures, and feasibility of instrument for clinical use (Lezak et al., 2012).

Although a variety of neuropsychological tests have been used to measure cognitive changes in patients with cancer, most of these tests were originally designed to assess patients with significant brain damage (e.g., brain tumors, stroke, Alzheimer disease). Information regarding tests that are sensitive and spe-

Table 17-2. Pertinent Components of a Comprehensive Clinical Assessment

Component	Specific Information to Evaluate
Presenting complaint	Duration of problem, primary symptoms, changes over time, impact on daily functioning
Cancer-specific risk factors	Cancer type, staging, disease trajectory Presence or absence of paraneoplastic syndromes Treatment history—surgery (duration, post-operative complications), radiation to CNS (fraction size, total volume), chemotherapy (specific drugs, dose intensity, route, duration of treatment), hormonal therapy, biologicals and/or targeted therapies Treatment-related toxicities
Co-morbidities	Chronic fatigue syndrome Degenerative disorders (e.g., multiple sclerosis) Dementias (e.g., Alzheimer's disease, Huntington's disease, MCI) Heart disease Infection (e.g., herpes simplex encephalitis, HIV) Metabolic and/or endocrine disorders (e.g., diabetes, liver disease, thyroid dysfunction) Traumatic brain injury Vascular disorders (e.g., epilepsy, hypertension, migraines, stroke)
Medications	Assess current prescriptions for analgesics (or presence of pain), antidepressants, antiemetics, anti-epileptics, anti-psychotics, immunosuppressants, steroids Changes in regimens (e.g., drug, dose), drug–drug interactions
Pertinent laboratory values	CBC (e.g., anemia) Electrolytes (e.g., calcium, sodium) Liver function laboratory tests Thyroid level
Social history	Basic demographics (e.g., age, culture, linguistic ability) Current living situation and level of social functioning Highest educational accomplishments or failures (e.g., attentional disorders, learning disabilities) Lifestyle factors (e.g., alcohol or drug abuse, fatigue, insomnia, nutritional deficiencies [thiamine, vitamin E]) Occupational experience

CBC—complete blood count; CNS—central nervous system; HIV—human immunodeficiency virus; MCI—mild cognitive impairment

Note. From "Cognitive Changes Associated With Cancer and Cancer Therapy: Patient Assessment and Education," by C.E. Jansen, 2013, *Seminars in Oncology Nursing, 29,* p. 271. Copyright 2013 by Elsevier Inc. Reprinted with permission.

cific to measure subtle cancer- and cancer treatment–related cognitive changes is limited (Jansen, 2013; Jansen, Miaskowski, Dodd, & Dowling, 2007).

Baseline neuropsychological assessment prior to the initiation of treatment is necessary to determine if changes occur after treatment. However, changes may be difficult to assess because they may be subtle (e.g., patients test within normal limits but lower than non-chemotherapy-treated patients). Preexisting risk factors also may influence results. The currently available neuropsychological tests may not assess functional ability or the impact of cognitive changes or provide clinically significant results.

Other testing considerations are the length of time needed to complete comprehensive batteries and the effects of practice due to repeated testing (Lezak et al., 2012). Because many self-report instruments lack validated data on psychometric appraisal, they may be more practical for the clinic setting, provide insight into patients' perception of their cognitive functioning, and elucidate the impact on their everyday functioning (Jansen, 2013).

Symptom Management

As much as possible, identification, prevention, and treatment of underlying causes (e.g., anemia, depression, fatigue, hypertension) should be promoted. The use of steroids to reduce swelling, as well as minimally invasive surgery and more precise radiation therapy, may manage the cognitive effects of CNS tumors. Although researchers have evaluated many medications (e.g., donepezil, erythropoietin, memantine, methylphenidate, modafinil), no proven pharmacologic interventions are currently available to prevent or treat cognitive changes (see Figure 17-2). Consequently, several nonpharmacologic interventions have been suggested.

Interventional studies have been directed toward evaluating the impact of antioxidants, cognitive training, compensatory strategies, health promotion (e.g., moderate exercise), neurofeedback, structured rehabilitation, and restorative activities on cognitive functioning. Thus far, however, only cognitive training programs (provided either in a group format or individualized) are likely to be effective in improving cognitive function in cancer survivors (Von Ah, Jansen, & Allen, 2014; Von Ah, Storey, Jansen, & Allen, 2013).

Patients should be informed that cognitive changes are possible side effects of treatment and, although little is known, studies elucidating this phenomenon, its mechanisms, and potential interventions are ongoing. Listening to, acknowledging, and validating patient reports regarding cognitive changes can be

Figure 17-2. Research on Cognitive Impairment Interventions in Cancer Survivors

Likely to Be Effective
- Cognitive training: group (Hassler et al., 2010; Poppelreuter et al., 2009; Von Ah et al., 2012)
- Cognitive training: individual (Gehring et al., 2009; Kesler et al., 2013; Miotto et al., 2013; Zucchella et al., 2013)

Effectiveness Not Established
- Cognitive-behavioral training (Cherrier et al., 2013; Ferguson et al., 2007, 2012; Goedendorp et al., 2014; Locke et al., 2008; McDougall, 2001; McDougall et al., 2011; Sherer et al., 1997)
- Electroencephalography or neurofeedback (Alvarez et al., 2013)
- Exercise (Baumann et al., 2011; Korstjens et al., 2006; Reid-Arndt et al., 2012; Schwartz et al., 2002)
- Meditation (Milbury et al., 2013)
- Mindfulness-based stress reduction (Hoffman et al., 2012)
- Natural restorative environmental (Cimprich, 1993; Cimprich & Ronis, 2003)
- Qigong (Oh et al., 2012)
- Structured rehabilitation (Rottmann et al., 2012)
- Vitamin E (Chan et al., 2004; Jatoi et al., 2005)
- Pharmacologic approaches
  - Methylphenidate (Bruera et al., 1992; Butler et al., 2007; Escalante et al., 2014; Gagnon et al., 2005; Gehring et al., 2012; Gong et al., 2014; Lower et al., 2009; Mar Fan et al., 2008; Meyers et al., 1998; Schwartz et al., 2002; Stone & Minton, 2011)
  - Memantine (Brown et al., 2013)
  - Modafinil (Blackhall et al., 2009; Gehring et al., 2012; Kohli et al., 2009; Lundorff et al., 2009)
  - Donepezil (Jatoi et al., 2005; Shaw et al., 2006)

Effectiveness Unlikely
- Ginkgo biloba (Attia et al., 2012; Barton et al., 2013)

Not Recommended for Practice
- Erythropoiesis-stimulating agents (Chang et al., 2004; Iconomou et al., 2008; Mancuso et al., 2006; Mar Fan et al., 2009; Massa et al., 2006; O'Shaughnessy, 2002; O'Shaughnessy et al., 2005)

Note. From "Evidence-Based Interventions for Cancer- and Treatment-Related Cognitive Impairment," by D. Von Ah, C.E. Jansen, and D.H. Allen, 2014, *Clinical Journal of Oncology Nursing, 18*(Suppl. 6), p. 19.

therapeutic and reduce distress. As discussed earlier, medical personnel should thoroughly assess for and address any underlying conditions that may affect cognitive functioning.

It may be helpful to share positive coping strategies with patients, such as ensuring adequate sleep and rest, pursuing stress-reduction activities (e.g., physical activity, meditation, yoga), engaging in brain-stimulating activities (e.g., learning new skills, working on puzzles), developing routines, using reminders (e.g., daily planner, notes), and asking for help (Myers, 2013; Von Ah, 2015). Referral to a neuropsychologist may be indicated if cognitive changes are interfering with everyday functioning (Jansen, 2013).

Conclusion

Cognitive function and its corresponding neuroanatomic correlates, as well as individual risk factors unrelated to cancer, are well understood. However, the complexity of cancer- and cancer treatment–related cognitive changes (with the exception of CNS tumors) is still unclear. Further investigation of this phenomenon is ongoing, including identifying its characteristics (e.g., prevalence, onset, duration) and establishing which neurologic tests are valid, reliable, sensitive, and specific enough to detect these changes. Although the etiology of cognitive changes related to cancer and its treatment is most likely multifactorial, knowledge of these mechanisms is crucial to the development of strategies to prevent and manage cognitive changes. In the meantime, patients' concerns should continue to be addressed with thorough clinical assessments, screening for risk factors, management of underlying causes, and practical suggestions to combat cognitive issues.

References

Ahles, T.A. (2012). Brain vulnerability to chemotherapy toxicities. *Psycho-Oncology, 21,* 1141–1148. doi:10.1002/pon.3196

Ahles, T.A., & Saykin, A.J. (2007). Candidate mechanisms for chemotherapy-induced cognitive changes. *Nature Reviews Cancer, 7,* 192–201. doi:10.1038/nrc2073

Alvarez, J., Meyer, F.L., Granoff, D.L., & Lundy, A. (2013). The effect of EEG biofeedback on reducing postcancer cognitive impairment. *Integrative Cancer Therapies, 12,* 475–487. doi:10.1177/1534735413477192

Amaral, D.G., & Strick, P.L. (2013). The organization of the central nervous system. In E.R. Kandel, J.H. Schwartz, T.M. Jessell, S.A. Siegelbaum, & A.J. Hudspeth (Eds.), *Principles of neural science* (5th ed., pp. 337–355). New York, NY: McGraw-Hill.

Attia, A., Rapp, S.R., Case, L.D., D'Agostino, R., Lesser, G., Naughton, M., … Shaw, E.G. (2012). Phase II study of *Ginkgo biloba* in irradiated brain tumor patients: Effect on cognitive function, quality of life, and mood. *Journal of Neuro-Oncology, 109,* 357–363. doi:10.1007/s11060-012-0901-9

Barton, D.L., Burger, K., Novonty, P.J., Fitch, T.R., Kohli, S., Soori, G., … Loprinzi, C.L. (2013). The use of *Ginkgo*

Key Points

- Cognitive function is a multidimensional concept that encompasses multiple domains regulated by the brain.
- Each structural component of the brain has clearly identified roles in cognitive functioning.
- Risk factors influencing cognitive functioning can be related to individual characteristics, psychological factors, genetic mutations, cancer, and cancer therapies.
- The mechanisms for cancer- and cancer treatment–related cognitive impairments are multifactorial.
- Assessing patients for cognitive impairment should incorporate a comprehensive evaluation of the presenting complaint and pertinent history.

biloba for the prevention of chemotherapy-related cognitive dysfunction in women receiving adjuvant treatment for breast cancer, N00C9. *Supportive Care in Cancer, 21,* 1185–1192. doi:10.1007/s00520-012-1647-9

Batalo, M., Nagaiah, G., & Abraham, J. (2011). Cognitive dysfunction in postmenopausal breast cancer patients on aromatase inhibitors. *Expert Review of Anticancer Therapy, 11,* 1277–1282. doi:10.1586/era.11.112

Baumann, F.T., Drosselmeyer, N., Leskaroski, A., Knicker, A., Krakowski-Roosen, H., Zopf, E.M., & Bloch, W. (2011). 12-week resistance training with breast cancer patients during chemotherapy: Effects on cognitive abilities. *Breast Care, 6,* 142–143. doi:10.1159/000327505

Bender, C.M., & Thelen, B.D. (2013). Cancer and cognitive changes: The complexity of the problem. *Seminars in Oncology Nursing, 29,* 232–237. doi:10.1016/j.soncn.2013.08.003

Blackhall, L., Petroni, G., Shu, J., Baum, L., & Farace, E. (2009). A pilot study evaluating the safety and efficacy of modafinal for cancer-related fatigue. *Journal of Palliative Medicine, 12,* 433–439. doi:10.1089/jpm.2008.0230

Bohan, E.M. (2013). Cognitive changes associated with central nervous system malignancies and treatment. *Seminars in Oncology Nursing, 29,* 238–247. doi:10.1016/j.soncn.2013.08.004

Boss, L., Kang, D.-H., Marcus, M., & Bergstrom, N. (2014). Endogenous sex hormones and cognitive function in older adults: A systematic review. *Western Journal of Nursing Research, 36,* 388–426. doi:10.1177/0193945913500566

Brown, P.D., Pugh, S., Laack, N.N., Wefel, J.S., Khuntia, D., Meyers, C.A., ... Watkins-Bruner, D. (2013). Memantine for the prevention of cognitive dysfunction in patients receiving whole-brain radiotherapy: A randomized, double-blind, placebo-controlled trial. *Neuro-Oncology, 15,* 1429–1437. doi:10.1093/neuonc/not114

Bruera, E.J., Miller, M.J., Macmillan, K., & Kuehn, N. (1992). Neuropsychological effects of methylphenidate in patients receiving a continuous infusion of narcotics for cancer pain. *Pain, 48,* 163–166. doi:10.1016/0304-3959(92)90053-E

Butler, J.M., Jr., Case, L.D., Atkins, J., Frizzell, B., Sanders, G., Griffin, P., ... Shaw, E.G. (2007). A phase III, double-blind, placebo-controlled prospective randomized clinical trial of d-threo-methylphenidate HCl in brain tumor patients receiving radiation therapy. *International Journal of Radiation Oncology, Biology, Physics, 69,* 1496–1501. doi:10.1016/j.ijrobp.2007.05.076

Capuron, L., Ravaud, A., & Dantzer, R. (2001). Timing and specificity of the cognitive changes induced by interleukin-2 and interferon-alpha treatments in cancer patients. *Psychosomatic Medicine, 63,* 376–386. doi:10.1097/00006842-200105000-00007

Cardoso, F.L., Brites, D., & Brito, MA. (2010). Looking at the blood–brain barrier: Molecular anatomy and possible investigation approaches. *Brain Research Reviews, 64,* 328–363. doi:10.1016/j.brainresrev.2010.05.003

Chan, A.S., Cheung, M.-C., Law, S.C., & Chan, J.H. (2004). Phase II study of alpha-tocopherol in improving the cognitive function of patients with temporal lobe radionecrosis. *Cancer, 100,* 398–401. doi:10.1002/cncr.11885

Chang, J., Couture, F.A., Young, S.D., Lau, C.Y., & McWatters, K.L. (2004). Weekly administration of epoetin alfa improves cognition and quality of life in patients with breast cancer receiving chemotherapy. *Supportive Cancer Therapy, 2,* 52–58. doi:10.3816/SCT.2004.n.023

Cherrier, M.M., Anderson, K., David, D., Higano, C.S., Gray, H., Church, A., & Willis, S.L. (2013). A randomized trial of cognitive rehabilitation in cancer survivors. *Life Sciences, 93,* 617–622. doi:10.1016/j.lfs.2013.08.011

Cheung, Y.T., Shwe, M., Tan, Y.P., Fan, G., Ng, R., & Chan, A.S. (2012). Cognitive changes in multiethnic Asian breast cancer patients: A focus group study. *Annals of Oncology, 23,* 2547–2552. doi:10.1093/annonc/mds029

Cimprich, B. (1993). Development of an intervention to restore attention in cancer patients. *Cancer Nursing, 16,* 83–92. doi:10.1097/00002820-199304000-00001

Cimprich, B., & Ronis, D.L. (2003). An environmental intervention to restore attention in women with newly diagnosed breast cancer. *Cancer Nursing, 26,* 284–292. doi:10.1097/00002820-200308000-00005

Collins, C., Gehrke, A., & Feuerstein, M. (2013). Cognitive tasks challenging brain tumor survivors at work. *Journal of Occupational and Environmental Medicine, 55,* 1426–1430. doi:10.1097/JOM.0b013e3182a64206

Conroy, S.K., McDonald, B.C., Ahles, T.A., West, J.D., & Saykin, A.J. (2013). Chemotherapy-induced amenorrhea: A prospective study of brain activation changes and neurocognitive correlates. *Brain Imaging and Behavior, 7,* 491–500. doi:10.1007/s11682-013-9240-5

Escalante, C.P., Meyers, C., Reuben, J.M., Wang, X., Qiao, W., Manzullo, E., ... Cleeland, C. (2014). A radomized, double-blind, 2-period, placebo-controlled crossover trial of a sustained-release methylphenidate in the treatment of fatigue in cancer patients. *Cancer Journal, 20,* 8–14. doi:10.1097/PPO.0000000000000018

Ferguson, R.J., Ahles, T.A., Saykin, A.J., McDonald, B.C., Furstenberg, C.T., Cole, B.F., & Mott, L.A. (2007). Cognitve-behavioral management of chemotherapy-related cognitive change. *Psycho-Oncology, 16,* 772–777. doi:10.1002/pon.1133

Ferguson, R.J., McDonald, B.C., Rocque, M.A., Furstenberg, C.T., Horrigan, S., Ahles, T.A., & Saykin, A.J. (2012). Development of CBT for chemotherapy-related cognitive change: Results of a waitlist control trial. *Psycho-Oncology, 21,* 176–186. doi:10.1002/pon.1878

Filley, C.M. (2011). *Neurobehavioral anatomy* (3rd ed.). Boulder, CO: University Press of Colorado.

Gagnon, B., Low, G., & Schreier, G. (2005). Methylphenidate hydrochloride improves cognitive function in patients with advanced cancer and hypoactive delirium: A prospective clinical study. *Journal of Psychiatry and Neuroscience, 30,* 100–107.

Ganz, P.A., Petersen, L., Castellon, S.A., Bower, J.E., Silverman, D.H.S., Cole, S.W., ... Belin, T.R. (2014). Cognitive function after the initiation of adjuvant endocrine therapy in early-stage breast cancer: An observational cohort study. *Journal of Clinical Oncology, 32,* 3559–3567. doi:10.1200/JCO.2014.56.1662

Gazzaniga, M.S., Ivry, R.B., & Mangun, G.R. (2014). *Cognitive neuroscience: The biology of the mind* (4th ed.). New York, NY: W.W. Norton and Company.

Gehring, K., Patwardhan, S.Y., Collins, R., Groves, M.D., Etzel, C.J., Meyers, C.A., & Wefel, J.S. (2012). A randomized trial on the efficacy of methylphenidate and modafinil for improving cognitive functioning and symptoms in patients with a primary brain tumor. *Journal of Neuro-Oncology, 107,* 165–174. doi:10.1007/s11060-011-0723-1

Gehring, K., Sitskoorn, M.M., Gundy, C.M., Sikkes, S.A.M., Klein, M., Postma, T.J., ... Aaronson, N.K. (2009). Cognitive rehabilitation in patients with gliomas: A randomized, controlled trial. *Journal of Clinical Oncology, 27,* 3712–3722. doi:10.1200/JCO.2008.20.5765

Goedendorp, M.M., Knoop, H., Gielissen, M.F.M., Verhagen, C., & Bleijenberg, G. (2014). The effects of cognitive behavorial therapy for postcancer fatigue on perceived cognitive disabilities and neuropsychological test performance. *Journal of Pain and Symptom Management, 47,* 35–44. doi:10.1016/j.jpainsymman.2013.02.014

Gong, S., Sheng, P., Jin, H., He, H., Qi, E., Chen, W., ... Hou, L. (2014). Effect of methylphenidate in patients with cancer-related fatigue: A systematic review and meta-analysis. *PLOS ONE, 9,* e84391. doi:10.1371/journal.pone.0084391

Greene-Schloesser, D., & Robbins, M.E. (2012). Radiation-induced cognitive impairment—from bench to bedside. *Neuro-Oncology, 14*(Suppl. 4), iv37–iv44. doi:10.1093/neuonc/nos196

Hassler, M.R., Elandt, K., Preusser, M., Lehrner, J., Binder, P., Dieckmann, K., ... Marosi, C. (2010). Neurocognitive training in patients with high-grade glioma: A pilot study. *Journal of Neuro-Oncology, 97,* 109–115. doi:10.1007/s11060-009-0006-2

Hoffman, C.J., Ersser, S.J., Hopkinson, J.B., Nicholls, P.G., Harrington, J.E., & Thomas, P.W. (2012). Effectiveness of mindfulness-based stress reduction in mood, breast- and endocrine-related quality of life, and well-being in stage 0 to III breast cancer: A randomized, controlled trial. *Journal of Clinical Oncology, 30,* 1335–1342. doi:10.1200/JCO.2010.34.0331

Holohan, K.N., Von Ah, D., McDonald, B.C., & Saykin, A.J. (2013). Neuroimaging, cancer, and cognition: State of the knowledge. *Seminars in Oncology Nursing, 29,* 280–287. doi:10.1016/j.soncn.2013.08.008

Iconomou, G., Koutras, A., Karaivazoglou, K., Kalliolias, G.D., Assimakopoulos, K., Argyriou, A.A., ... Kalofonos, H.P. (2008). Effect of epoetin alfa therapy on cognitive function in anaemic patients with solid tumours undergoing chemotherapy. *European Journal of Cancer Care, 17,* 535–541. doi:10.1111/j.1365-2354.2007.00857.x

Jansen, C.E. (2013). Cognitive changes associated with cancer and cancer therapy: Patient assessment and education. *Seminars in Oncology Nursing, 29,* 270–279. doi:10.1016/j.soncn.2013.08.007

Jansen, C.E., Miaskowski, C.A., Dodd, M.J., Dowling, G.A., & Kramer, J. (2005). Potential mechanisms for chemotherapy-induced impairments in cognitive function. *Oncology Nursing Forum, 32,* 1151–1163. doi:10.1188/05.ONF.1151-1163

Jansen, C.E., Miaskowski, C.A., Dodd, M.J., & Dowling, G.A. (2007). A meta-analysis of the sensitivity of various neuropsychological tests used to detect chemotherapy-induced cognitive impairment in patients with breast cancer. *Oncology Nursing Forum, 34,* 997–1005. doi:10.1188/07.ONF.997-1005

Jatoi, A., Kahanic, S.P., Frytak, S., Schaefer, P., Foote, R.L., Sloan, J., & Petersen, R.C. (2005). Donepezil and vitamin E for preventing cognitive dysfunction in small cell lung cancer patients: Preliminary results and suggestions for future study designs. *Supportive Care in Cancer, 13,* 66–69. doi:10.1007/s00520-004-0696-0

Kandel, E.R., Barres, B.A., & Hudspeth, A.J. (2013). Nerve cells, neural circuitry, and behavior. In E.R. Kandel, J.H. Schwartz, T.M. Jessell, S.A. Siegelbaum, & A.J. Hudspeth (Eds.), *Principles of neural science* (5th ed., pp. 21–38). New York, NY: McGraw-Hill.

Kesler, S., Hadi Hosseini, S.M., Heckler, C., Janelsins, M., Palesh, O., Mustian, K., & Morrow, G. (2013). Cognitive training for improving executive function in chemotherapy-treated breast cancer survivors. *Clinical Breast Cancer, 13,* 299–306. doi:10.1016/j.clbc.2013.02.004

Kohli, S., Fisher, S.G., Tra, Y., Adams, M.J., Mapstone, M.E., Wesnes, K.A., ... Morrow, G.R. (2009). The effect of modafinil on cognitive function in breast cancer survivors. *Cancer, 115,* 2605–2616. doi:10.1002/cncr.24287

Koppelmans, V., de Groot, M., de Ruiter, M.B., Boogerd, W., Seynaeve, C., Vernooij, M.W., ... Breteler, M.M. (2014). Global and focal white matter integrity in breast cancer survivors 20 years after adjuvant chemotherapy. *Human Brain Mapping, 35,* 889–899. doi:10.1002/hbm.22221

Korstjens, I., Mesters, I., van der Peet, E., Gijsen, B., & van den Borne, B. (2006). Quality of life of cancer survivors after physical and psychosocial rehabilitation. *European*

Journal of Cancer Prevention, 15, 541–547. doi:10.1097/01.cej.0000220625.77857.95

Lezak, M.D., Howieson, D.B., Bigler, E.D., & Tranel, D. (2012). *Neuropsychological assessment* (5th ed.). New York, NY: Oxford University Press.

Lisberger, S.G., & Thach, W.T. (2013). The cerebellum. In E.R. Kandel, J.H. Schwartz, T.M. Jessell, S.A. Siegelbaum, & A.J. Hudspeth (Eds.), *Principles of neural science* (5th ed., pp. 960–981). New York, NY: McGraw-Hill.

Lobo, R.A. (2014). Menopause and aging. In J.F. Strauss III & R.L. Barbieri (Eds.), *Yen & Jaffe's reproductive endocrinology* (7th ed., pp. 308–339.e8). doi:10.1016/B978-1-4557-2758-2.00015-9

Locke, D.E., Cerhan, J.H., Wu, W., Malec, J.F., Clark, M.M., Rummans, T.A., & Brown, P.D. (2008). Cognitive rehabilitation and problem-solving to improve quality of life of patients with primary brain tumors: A pilot study. *Journal of Supportive Oncology, 6,* 383–391.

Lower, E.E., Fleishman, S., Cooper, A., Zeldis, J., Faleck, H., Yu, Z., & Manning, D. (2009). Efficacy of dexmethylphenidate for the treatment of fatigue after cancer chemotherapy: A randomized clinical trial. *Journal of Pain and Symptom Management, 38,* 650–662. doi:10.1016/j.jpainsymman.2009.03.011

Lundorff, L.E., Jønsson, B.H., & Sjøgren, P. (2009). Modafinil for attentional and psychomotor dysfunction in advanced cancer: A double-blind, randomised, cross-over trial. *Palliative Medicine, 23,* 731–738. doi:10.1177/0269216309106872

Mancuso, A., Migliorino, M., De Santis, S., Saponiero, A., & De Marinis, F. (2006). Correlation between anemia and functional/cognitive capacity in elderly lung cancer patients treated with chemotherapy. *Annals of Oncology, 17,* 146–150. doi:10.1093/annonc/mdj038

Mandelblatt, J.S., Jacobsen, P.B., & Ahles, T.A. (2014). Cognitive effects of cancer systemic therapy: Implications for care of older patients and survivors. *Journal of Clinical Oncology, 32,* 2617–2626. doi:10.1200/JCO.2014.55.1259

Mar Fan, H.G., Clemons, M., Xu, W., Chemerynsky, I., Breunis, H., Braganza, S., & Tannock, I.F. (2008). A randomised, placebo-controlled, double-blind trial of the effects of d-methylphenidate on fatigue and cognitive dysfunction in women undergoing adjuvant chemotherapy for breast cancer. *Supportive Care in Cancer, 16,* 577–583. doi:10.1007/s00520-007-0341-9

Mar Fan, H.G., Park, A., Xu, W., Yi, Q.-L., Braganza, S., Chang, J., … Tannock, I.F. (2009). The influence of erythropoietin on cognitive function in women following chemotherapy for breast cancer. *Psycho-Oncology, 18,* 156–161. doi:10.1002/pon.1372

Massa, E., Madeddu, C., Lusso, M.R., Gramignano, G., & Mantovani, G. (2006). Evaluation of the effectiveness of treatment with erythropoietin on anemia, cognitive functioning and functions studied by comprehensive geriatric assessment in elderly cancer patients with anemia related to cancer chemotherapy. *Critical Reviews in Oncology/Hematology, 57,* 175–182. doi:10.1016/j.critrevonc.2005.06.001

McDougall, G.J., Jr. (2001). Memory improvement program for elderly cancer survivors. *Geriatric Nursing, 22,* 185–190. doi:10.1067/mgn.2001.117916

McDougall, G.J., Jr., Becker, H., Acee, T.W., Vaughan, P.W., & Delville, C.L. (2011). Symptom management of affective and cognitive disturbance with a group of cancer survivors. *Archives of Psychiatric Nursing, 25,* 24–35. doi:10.1016/j.apnu.2010.05.004

McGinty, H.L., Phillips, K.M., Jim, H.S.L., Cessna, J.M., Asvat, Y., Cases, M.G., … Jacobsen, P.B. (2014). Cognitive functioning in men receiving androgen deprivation therapy for prostate cancer: A systematic review and meta-analysis. *Supportive Care in Cancer, 22,* 2271–2280. doi:10.1007/s00520-014-2285-1

Merriman, J.D., Von Ah, D., Miaskowski, C., & Aouizerat, B.E. (2013). Proposed mechanisms for cancer- and treatment-related cognitive changes. *Seminars in Oncology Nursing, 29,* 260–269. doi:10.1016/j.soncn.2013.08.006

Meyers, C.A., Weitzner, M.A., Valentine, A.D., & Levin, V.A. (1998). Methylphenidate therapy improves cognition, mood, and function of brain tumor patients. *Journal of Clinical Oncology, 16,* 2522–2527.

Milbury, K., Chaoul, A., Biegler, K.A., Wangyal, T., Spelman, A., Meyers, C.A., … Cohen, L. (2013). Tibetan sound meditation for cognitive dysfunction: Results of a randomized controlled pilot trial. *Psycho-Oncology, 22,* 2354–2363. doi:10.1002/pon.3296

Miotto, E.C., Savage, C.R., Evans, J.J., Wilson, B.A., Martin, M.G.M., Balardin, J.B., … Amaro, E., Jr. (2013). Semantic strategy training increases memory performance and brain activity in patients with prefrontal cortex lesions. *Clinical Neurology and Neurosurgery, 115,* 309–316. doi:10.1016/j.clineuro.2012.05.024

Monje, M., & Dietrich, J. (2012). Cognitive side effects of cancer therapy demonstrate a functional role for adult neurogenesis. *Behavioral Brain Research, 227,* 376–379. doi:10.1016/j.bbr.2011.05.012

Mrugala, M.M., Supko, J.G., & Batchelor, T.T. (2011). Delivering anticancer drugs to brain tumors. In B.A. Chabner & D.L. Longo (Eds.), *Cancer chemotherapy and biotherapy: Principles and practice* (5th ed., pp. 62–79). Philadelphia, PA: Wolters Kluwer Health/Lippincott Williams & Wilkins.

Munir, F., Burrows, J., Yarker, J., Kalawsky, K., & Bains, M. (2010). Women's perceptions of chemotherapy-induced cognitive side affects on work ability: A focus group study. *Journal of Clinical Nursing, 19,* 1362–1370. doi:10.1111/j.1365-2702.2009.03006.x

Myers, J.S. (2010). The possible role of cytokines in chemotherapy-induced cognitive deficits. In R.B. Raffa & R.J. Tallarida (Eds.), *Advances in experimental medicine and biology: Chemo fog: Cancer chemotherapy-related cognitive impairment* (Vol. 678, pp. 119–123). doi:10.1007/978-1-4419-6306-2_15

Myers, J.S. (2012). Chemotherapy-related cognitive impairment: The breast cancer experience [Online exclusive]. *Oncology Nursing Forum, 39,* E31–E40. doi:10.1188/12.ONF.E31-E40

Myers, J.S. (2013). Cancer- and chemotherapy-related cognitive changes: The patient experience. *Seminars in Oncology Nursing, 29,* 300–307. doi:10.1016/j.soncn.2013.08.010

Oh, B., Butow, P.N., Mullan, B.A., Clarke, S.J., Beale, P.J., Pavlakis, N., ... Vardy, J. (2012). Effect of medical Qigong on cognitive function, quality of life, and a biomarker of inflammation in cancer patients: A randomized controlled trial. *Supportive Care in Cancer, 20,* 1235–1242. doi:10.1007/s00520-011-1209-6

Olson, C.R., & Colby, C.L. (2013). The organization of cognition. In E.R. Kandel, J.H. Schwartz, T.M. Jessell, S.A. Siegelbaum, & A.J. Hudspeth (Eds.), *Principles of neural science* (5th ed., pp. 392–411). New York, NY: McGraw-Hill.

O'Shaughnessy, J.A. (2002). Effects of epoetin alfa on cognitive function, mood, asthenia, and quality of life in women with breast cancer undergoing adjuvant chemotherapy. *Clinical Breast Cancer, 3*(Suppl. 3), S116–S120. doi:10.3816/CBC.2002.s.022

O'Shaughnessy, J.A., Vukelja, S.J., Holmes, F.A., Savin, M., Jones, M., Royall, D., ... Von Hoff, D. (2005). Feasibility of quantifying the effects of epoetin alfa therapy on cognitive function in women with breast cancer undergoing adjuvant or neoadjuvant chemotherapy. *Clinical Breast Cancer, 5,* 439–446. doi:10.3816/CBC.2005.n.002

Pearl, P.L., & Emsellem, H.A. (2014). *Neuro-logic: A primer on localization.* New York, NY: Demos Medical Publishing.

Poppelreuter, M., Weis, J., & Bartsch, H.H. (2009). Effects of specific neuropsychological training programs for breast cancer patients after adjuvant chemotherapy. *Journal of Psychosocial Oncology, 27,* 274–296. doi:10.1080/07347330902776044

Reid-Arndt, S.A., Matsuda, S., & Cox, C.R. (2012). Tai chi effects on neuropsychological, emotional, and physical functioning: A pilot study. *Complementary Therapies in Clinical Practice, 18,* 26–30. doi:10.1016/j.ctcp.2011.02.005

Rottmann, N., Dalton, S.O., Bidstrup, P.E., Würtzen, H., Høybye, M.T., Ross, L., ... Johansen, C. (2012). No improvement in distress and quality of life following psychosocial cancer rehabilitation. *Psycho-Oncology, 21,* 505–514. doi:10.1002/pon.1924

Scheibel, R.S., Valentine, A.D., O'Brien, S., & Meyers, C.A. (2004). Cognitive dysfunction and depression during treatment with interferon alpha and chemotherapy. *Journal of Neuropsychiatry and Clinical Neurosciences, 16,* 185–191. doi:10.1176/jnp.16.2.1854

Schwartz, A.L., Thompson, J.A., & Masood, N. (2002). Interferon-induced fatigue in patients with melanoma: A pilot study of exercise and methylphenidate [Online exclusive]. *Oncology Nursing Forum, 29,* E85–E90. doi:10.1188/02.ONF.E85-E90

Seigers, R., & Fardell, J.E. (2011). Neurological basis of chemotherapy-induced cognitive impairment: A review of rodent research. *Neuroscience and Biobehavioral Reviews, 35,* 729–741. doi:10.1016/j.neubiorev.2010.09.006

Seigers, R., Schagen, S.B., Van Tellingen, O., & Dietrich, J. (2013). Chemotherapy-related cognitive dysfunction: Current animal studies and future directions. *Brain Imaging and Behavior, 7,* 453–459. doi:10.1007/s11682-013-9250-3

Seruga, B., Zhang, H.B., Bernstein, L.J., & Tannock, I.F. (2008). Cytokines and their relationship to the symptoms and outcome of cancer. *Nature Reviews Cancer, 8,* 887–899. doi:10.1038/nrc2507

Shaw, E.G., Rosdhal, R., D'Agostino, R.B., Jr., Lovato, J., Naughton, M.J., Robbins, M.E., & Rapp, S.R. (2006). Phase II study of donepezil in irradiated brain tumor patients: Effect on cognitive function, mood, and quality of life. *Journal of Clinical Oncology, 24,* 1415–1420. doi:10.1200/JCO.2005.03.3001

Sherer, M., Meyers, C.A., & Bergloff, P. (1997). Efficacy of postacute brain injury rehabilitation for patients with primary malignant brain tumors. *Cancer, 80,* 250–257. doi:10.1002/(SICI)1097-0142(19970715)80:2<250::AID-CNCR13>3.0.CO;2-T

Stone, P., & Minton, O. (2011). European Palliative Care Research collaborative pain guidelines. Central side-effects management: What is the evidence to support best practice in the management of sedation, cognitive impairment and myoclonus? *Palliative Medicine, 25,* 431–441. doi:10.1177/0269216310380763

Toffoletto, S., Lanzenberger, R., Gingnell, M., Sundström-Poromaa, I., & Comasco, E. (2014). Emotional and cognitive functional imaging of estrogen and progesterone effects in the female human brain: A systematic review. *Psychoneuroendocrinology, 50,* 28–52. doi:10.1016/j.psyneuen.2014.07.025

Vanderah, T., & Gould, D. (2015). *Nolte's the human brain: An introduction to its functional anatomy* (7th ed.). Philadelphia, PA: Elsevier Mosby.

Vearncombe, K.J., Rolfe, M., Andrew, B., Pachana, N.A., Wright, M., & Beadle, G. (2011). Cognitive effects of chemotherapy-induced menopause in breast cancer. *Clinical Neuropsychologist, 25,* 1295–1313. doi:10.1080/13854046.2011.631586

Venes, D. (Ed.). (2014). *Taber's cyclopedic medical dictionary* (22nd ed.). Philadelphia, PA: F.A. Davis.

Von Ah, D. (2015). Cognitive changes associated with cancer and cancer treatment: State of the science. *Clinical Journal of Oncology Nursing, 19,* 47–56. doi:10.1188/15.CJON.19-01AP

Von Ah, D., Carpenter, J.S., Saykin, A., Monahan, P.O., Wu, J., Yu, M., ... Unverzagt, F. (2012). Advanced cognitive training for breast cancer survivors: A randomized controlled trial. *Breast Cancer Research and Treatment, 135,* 799–809. doi:10.1007/s10549-012-2210-6

Von Ah, D., Habermann, B., Carpenter, J.S., & Schneider, B.L. (2013). Impact of perceived cognitive impairment in breast cancer survivors. *European Journal of Oncology Nursing, 17,* 236–241. doi:10.1016/j.ejon.2012.06.002

Von Ah, D., Jansen, C.E., & Allen, D.H. (2014). Evidence-based interventions for cancer- and treatment-related cognitive impairment. *Clinical Journal of Oncology Nursing, 18*(Suppl. 6), 17–25. doi:10.1188/14.CJON.S3.17-25

Von Ah, D., Storey, S., Jansen, C.E., & Allen, D.H. (2013). Coping strategies and interventions for cognitive changes in patients with cancer. *Seminars in Oncology Nursing, 29,* 288–299. doi:10.1016/j.soncn.2013.08.009

Wefel, J.S., Kesler, S.R., Noll, K.R., & Schagen, S.B. (2015). Clinical characteristics, pathophysiology, and management of noncentral nervous system cancer-related cognitive impairment in adults. *CA: A Cancer Journal for Clinicians, 65,* 123–138. doi:10.3322/caac.21258

Winocur, G., Henkelman, M., Wojtowicz, J.M., Zhang, H., Binns, M.A., & Tannock, I.F. (2012). The effects of chemotherapy on cognitive function in a mouse model: A prospective study. *Clinical Cancer Research, 18,* 3112–3121. doi:10.1158/1078-0432.CCR-12-0060

Zucchella, C., Capone, A., Codella, V., De Nunzio, A.M., Vecchione, C., Sandrini, G., ... Bartolo, M. (2013). Cognitive rehabilitation for early post-surgery inpatients affected by primary brain tumor: A randomized controlled trial. *Journal of Neuro-Oncology, 14,* 93–100. doi:10.1007/s11060-013-1153-z

Chapter 17 Study Questions

1. All of the following conditions are known to affect cognitive function EXCEPT:
   A. Diabetes mellitus.
   B. Psychiatric illnesses.
   C. Drug or alcohol abuse.
   D. Vitamin C deficiency.

2. What intervention has been shown to be unlikely to be effective in treating cancer-related cognitive impairment?
   A. Ginkgo biloba
   B. Vitamin E
   C. Methylphenidate
   D. Erythropoietin

3. Neuropsychological test performance may be negatively influenced by all of the following EXCEPT:
   A. Stress.
   B. Depression.
   C. Anxiety.
   D. Genetic mutations.

4. What part of the brain is responsible for the consolidation of memories?
   A. Frontal lobe
   B. Temporal lobe
   C. Parietal lobe
   D. Occipital lobe

5. A patient with cancer has been continuing to work as a store manager during chemotherapy and complains of difficulty making decisions. He is demonstrating a deficit in:
   A. Attention.
   B. Information processing.
   C. Executive functioning.
   D. Memory.

CHAPTER

18 Dermatologic Complications

Pamela Hallquist Viale, RN, MS, CS, ANP

Introduction

Chemotherapy is a common treatment for patients with cancer and is associated with a variety of side effects. Many of the side effects and toxicities may be considered dose limiting for some agents or specific to individual therapies; dermatologic or cutaneous reactions can range from mild to dose limiting as well. These cutaneous toxicities can be general in nature or very specific and can present in many different forms. Although graft-versus-host disease and Stevens-Johnson syndrome may be considered serious dermatologic adverse events, they are not common toxicities. The most common toxicities include hyperpigmentation and photosensitivity, radiation recall effects, hand-foot syndrome (HFS) or palmar-plantar erythrodysesthesia (PPE), hypersensitivity reactions (HSRs, i.e., wheals or rash), hair and nail changes, and extravasation of chemotherapy agents into skin (Viale, 2006). The rapidly increasing number of targeted therapies has produced dermatologic toxicities that are unique in both their presentation and management. This chapter will cover the most frequently seen cutaneous toxicities encountered in the oncology practice setting, as well as symptom management strategies.

Pathophysiology

Most conventional chemotherapy agents are directed toward rapidly dividing cell lines, creating the commonly seen side effects of myelosuppression and mucositis. Therefore, because skin, hair, and nail cells also can divide rapidly, these tissues are affected by the chemotherapy agents as well (Kyllo & Anadkat, 2014). Alopecia, or sudden hair loss or spot baldness, occurs with a variety of chemotherapy and targeted therapy treatments (see Chapter 15). Exposure to the sun can create photosensitivity reactions, which are linked to many different chemotherapy agents. Additionally, sun exposure can worsen the rash associated with targeted therapy agents. Although many agents can cause rash, the epidermal growth factor receptor (EGFR) rash is related to the EGFR inhibitor class of drugs and is specific for them alone. Nail changes can range from inflammatory effects to total loss of the nail (onycholysis). HSRs are primarily caused by the massive release of histamine after exposure to an antigen, with skin reactions ranging from the appearance of characteristic wheals and rash to anaphylaxis. Finally, cutaneous reactions are varied and can be general or specific to certain treatments (Kyllo & Anadkat, 2014).

Side Effects

Radiation Recall and Enhancement

Radiation recall (the "recalling" of a previous radiation skin reaction initiated by the administration of certain drugs) and radiation enhancement are two different skin entities (Hird et al., 2008; Kyllo & Anadkat, 2014). Presentation of this skin reaction varies but can generally occur at any time after cessation of radiation therapy (Kyllo & Anadkat, 2014). Traditional chemotherapy agents implicated in radiation recall include anthracyclines, cisplatin, taxanes, and gemcitabine and capecitabine; however, newer agents, such as vemurafenib and pemetrexed, have been reported to cause this side effect as well (Boesmans, Decoster, & Schallier, 2014; Forschner et al., 2014). In approximately one-third of cases, recall reactions may occur in skin sites differing from prior radiation sites, particularly with gemcitabine (Burris & Hurtig, 2010). Radiation enhancement occurs when radiation therapy and certain chemotherapy agents are given within close periods of time, usually one week (Kyllo & Anadkat, 2014). Many agents have been implicated in radiation enhancement, including bleomycin, doxorubicin, 5-fluorouracil (5-FU), and methotrexate (Chan et al., 2014; Salvo et al., 2010). Treatment is largely symptomatic, with attempts to carefully schedule therapies to minimize effects.

Alopecia

Nonscarring alopecia occurs as two different entities: telogen effluvium and anagen effluvium. Telogen effluvium is most frequently seen in patients receiving treatment with 5-FU and methotrexate (Kyllo & Anadkat, 2014). *Effluvium* is hair shedding and refers to a loss of more than 100 hairs a day over a shorter time period versus alopecia, considered a marked reduction in the density of hair, usually 30% (Kanwar & Narang, 2013). Acute telogen effluvium usually refers to hair loss lasting less than six months, whereas chronic telogen effluvium refers to shedding lasting longer than six months. Chemotherapy can cause anagen effluvium, with profound hair loss caused by the agents' impairment of mitotic activity of the hair follicle (Kanwar & Narang, 2013). This type of hair loss usually occurs within two to four weeks of drug exposure (Kyllo & Anadkat, 2014; Yun & Kim, 2007). Hair changes can present as thinning (as may be seen with EGFR inhibitor therapy) to complete hair loss (as experienced by patients receiving anthracycline or paclitaxel therapy) and generally are considered reversible, but hair regrowth may be different in color or texture (Kyllo & Anadkat, 2014). Changes in hair growth also can occur with targeted therapy agents, and color and texture can be altered (Choi, 2014). See Chapter 15 for a detailed discussion of alopecia.

Hyperpigmentation and Photosensitivity

Hyperpigmentation occurs commonly with many chemotherapy agents, appearing as focused skin color changes or diffuse changes throughout the skin (Kyllo & Anadkat, 2014). Hyperpigmentation can involve the nail beds, oral mucosa, and hands and feet, or can even trace along the vein path itself. Most hyperpigmentation skin effects will resolve within several months after treatment, and time to onset varies with different drugs (Kyllo & Anadkat, 2014). Agents most frequently implicated in hyperpigmentation include mitotic inhibitors, alkylating agents, and antitumor antibiotics (Viale, 2006). Exposure to the sun (and photosensitivity) can enhance hyperpigmentation changes and occurs with many agents, including EGFR inhibitors. Patients should be instructed to avoid sun exposure, particularly after treatment with 5-FU, doxorubicin, bleomycin, dactinomycin, dacarbazine, hydroxyurea, and vinblastine. Severe skin reactions can occur after high-dose methotrexate as well

(Viale, 2006). Patients should be encouraged to wear protective clothing and a hat and to use sunscreen to provide additional protection.

Palmar-Plantar Erythrodysesthesia

PPE and HFS essentially refer to the same phenomenon. Symptoms of PPE usually consist of a painful, erythematous skin change to the soles of the feet and palms of the hands, with localized areas of painful hyperkeratosis in areas associated with pressure or friction (Kyllo & Anadkat, 2014). PPE usually presents as areas of localized hyperkeratosis with necrosis of keratinocytes and lymphohistiocytic infiltrates (Lacouture, Reilly, Gerami, & Guitart, 2008). The changes then can proceed to desquamation with blisters and skin breakdown, necessitating drug cessation or dose reduction for some patients (see Figures 18-1 and 18-2). Although the pathophysiology of PPE is not completely understood, it is commonly thought to be related to capillary rupture occurring while walking or during other weight-bearing activity. This creates an inflammatory reaction in the affected area, possibly related to the release of chemotherapy in those locations (Wilkes & Doyle, 2005). The use of capecitabine, an oral fluoropyrimidine, provides a longer exposure time of tissues to drug (similar to continuous infusion of 5-FU), which causes a higher incidence of PPE (Madi et al., 2012). PPE is a dose-limiting side effect of both capecitabine and liposomal doxorubicin, and careful assessment and management are needed, often requiring dose adjustment or cessation.

Targeted therapies may cause dermatologic complications, including PPE. Sorafenib, a multitargeted tyrosine kinase inhibitor therapy, is known to cause PPE, albeit with more significant peeling than the symptoms associated with capecitabine or other therapies. Desquamation is more frequently seen with sunitinib (Lacouture et al., 2008). Both sorafenib and sunitinib can produce hyperkeratosis, but the phenom-

Figure 18-1. Grade 2 Hand-Foot Syndrome Reaction—Plantar

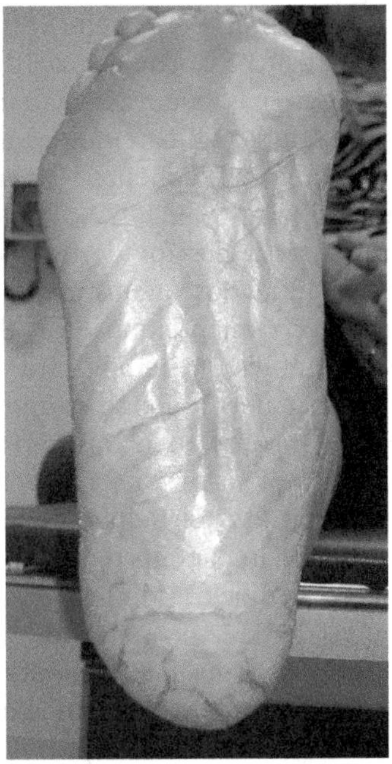

Note. Image courtesy of Laura Zitella. Used with permission.

Figure 18-2. Grade 2 Hand-Foot Syndrome Reaction—Palmar

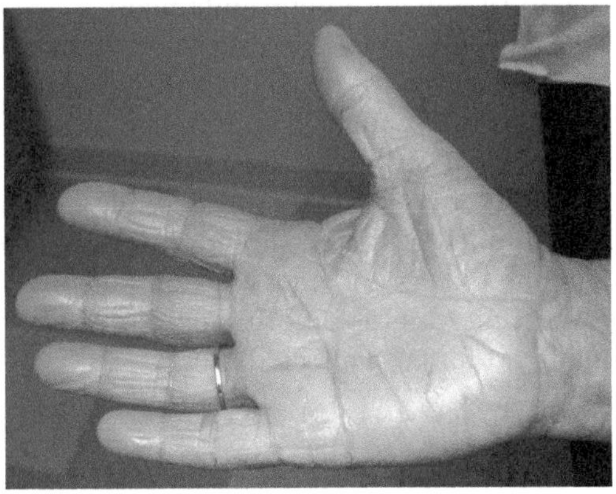

Note. Image courtesy of Pamela Viale. Used with permission.

enon is more common with sorafenib (Escudier et al., 2007). Vemurafenib, a *BRAF* inhibitor, has also produced dermatologic toxic effects similar to sorafenib-associated PPE (Huang, Hepper, Anadkat, & Cornelius, 2012). In addition, this agent has been associated with the onset of squamous cell carcinomas when used in the treatment of patients with metastatic melanoma (Huang et al., 2012).

Treatment strategies for dermatologic complications include dose adjustments or cessations, with recommendations for the generous use of emollient therapy and avoidance of activities that may increase symptoms (such as increased pressure to palms and soles and immersion in hot water). Local application of ice packs was found to be helpful to decrease the incidence of PPE in patients receiving pegylated liposomal doxorubicin (Mangili et al., 2008). Topical steroids have been recommended for some patients to reduce inflammation. Different pharmacologic treatments, such as pyridoxine (vitamin B_6), have been employed with varying successes, and most evidence is from either small trials or case reports only (Kyllo & Anadkat, 2014; Rossi & Catalano, 2007). In most cases, symptoms will resolve within three to four weeks after cessation of treatment. Chavarri-Guerra and Soto-Perez-de-Celis (2015) recently reported an unusual case in which a woman receiving capecitabine and bevacizumab lost the fingerprints of her thumb and fingers.

Oncology nurses are crucial for educating patients regarding the signs and symptoms of PPE and the particular importance of prompt reporting of symptoms while on oral therapies, as these effects often appear while patients are at home. Nurses should carefully assess patients' palms and the soles of their feet at each clinic visit, as differing grades of toxicity may exist for both affected sites.

Nail Changes

Many chemotherapy agents and certain targeted therapies are known to cause changes to the nail or nail bed. The nail is made of the nail plate, bed, hyponychium, and proximal and lateral nail folds (Hinds & Thomas, 2008). The plate is normally affixed to the nail bed to the level of the hyponychium, and the proximal and lateral nail folds form a barrier to infections and provide protection. Normal fingernail growth takes 6 months, versus 12 months for toenail formation (Hinds & Thomas, 2008). Interruption of nail bed growth can cause the appearance of white lines across the nail beds, called Mees' lines, or grooves and lines, called Beau's lines, which may be cosmetically uncomfortable but usually are not painful (Kyllo & Anadkat, 2014). Complete onycholysis (loss of the nail) can occur, as well as hyperpigmentation changes and subungual hemorrhages (bleeding under the nail bed) (Hinds & Thomas, 2008). Onycholysis can occur with anthracyclines, taxanes, and topical 5-FU (Brant, Marrs, & Newton, 2004). The taxanes (docetaxel and paclitaxel) are associated with hemorrhagic onycholysis and nail loss; ixabepilone can cause this type of damage as well (Capriotti et al., 2015). The documented incidence of nail toxicities with taxanes is 0%–44% (Minisini et al., 2003). The incidence of brittle nails and nail color changes in patients receiving vemurafenib has been reported as 7% (Choi, 2014).

Changes in the proximal nail fold can occur with taxanes, methotrexate, mitoxantrone, and EGFR inhibitor agents. Paronychia (erythema, inflammation, and pain in the nail folds) has been noted in approximately 12%–16% of patients taking EGFR inhibitor therapy and can be exudative in nature (Kyllo & Anadkat, 2014). The syndrome generally takes approximately eight weeks to manifest. Topical steroids, mupirocin, and doxycycline have been employed in the treatment of paronychia, reducing inflammation and infectious sequelae (Gilbar, Hain, & Peereboom, 2009). Paronychia also responds to drug cessation, with many patients successfully rechallenged without recurrence of the side effect. Chemotherapy-induced nail changes are common and can affect patients' quality of life (Miller, Gorcey, & McLellan, 2014). The use of cryotherapy (using frozen gloves or socks) has been studied in patients receiving taxanes and has been found to be helpful in prevention of nail toxicity (Gilbar et al., 2009). Although cryotherapy has demonstrated reduction in nail adverse effects, the use of scalp cooling for hair loss has not been widely accepted because of concern over scalp metastasis (Komen, Smorenburg, Van Den Hurk, & Nortier, 2013). Oncology nurses play important roles in the assessment and management of nail bed toxicities by promoting prevention of infection and educating patients regarding the natural timing of these effects.

Rash

General skin rashes may appear as mild, acne-like eruptions to more serious, even life-threatening, presentations with many different chemotherapy agents (Rosen et al., 2014). Purpuric rashes have been reported with bortezomib therapy in case reports, and erythema multiforme has occurred with specific agents as well (Viale, 2006). The BRAF inhibitors (vemurafenib and dabrafenib) are noted to have significant cutaneous side effects (Choi, 2014). Patients receiving vemurafenib have experienced rash, usually pruritic in nature and maculopapular in appearance (Lacouture et al., 2013). Vemurafenib-associated dermatologic events usually are manageable and rarely require dose interruptions (Lacouture et al., 2013). Management strategies include steroid creams, oral antihistamines, oral steroids for grade 2 rash, and pain control as appropriate (Lacouture et al., 2013). Squamoproliferative and keratinocytic lesions are seen with BRAF inhibitors, where 49%–85% of patients reportedly experience benign keratinocytic growths (Choi, 2014). More concerning, squamoproliferative growths occur in 4%–31% of patients receiving therapy with vemurafenib, requiring removal and ongoing skin surveillance examinations to monitor for further involvement (Choi, 2014).

Ipilimumab is an anti–cytotoxic T-lymphocyte antigen-4 (CTLA-4) immune-checkpoint molecule used in melanoma treatment. However, this agent produces dermatologic toxicity in the form of maculopapular rash in 10%–50% of patients (Scarpati et al., 2014). This rash can be pruritic in nature, and treatment with topical or systemic corticosteroids may be appropriate. Patients are urged to avoid sun exposure and use broad-spectrum sunscreen prophylactically. With severe presentation, a dermatology consult with consideration of biopsy is recommended (Fecher, Agarwala, Hodi, & Weber, 2013). In some patients, rash with dermal ulceration (or Stevens-Johnson syndrome) has occurred, requiring permanent cessation of the drug (Scarpati et al., 2014). The larger class of EGFR inhibitor agents can produce the EGFR inhibitor–associated rash, which is considered a significant side effect of treatment with those agents. EGFR inhibitor–associated rash can be dose limiting in its severity.

Dermatologic toxicities are extremely common with EGFR inhibitor agents. Dermatologic events associated with EGFR inhibitors are not limited to rash and may include dry skin (or xerosis), periungual inflammations (or paronychia), and alopecia of the scalp with abnormal growth of the eyelashes (Lynch et al., 2007). However, papulopustular rash represents a potential marker of patient response to therapy and usually manifests early after initiation of therapy. As the EGFR inhibitors exert their antitumor effects, they interfere with the normal activity of the follicular and interfollicular epidermal growth signaling pathway, creating the dermatologic toxicities specific to this class of therapy. Patients receiving EGFR inhibitors experience changes in epidermal-derived tissues, causing damaged keratinocytes, and changes in the expression of chemokines. These changes lead to recruitment of inflammatory cells and cause injury to the cutaneous tissue, producing rash and periungual inflammation (Melosky et al., 2015).

Assessment and grading of the EGFR inhibitor–associated rash is critical for nurses to strategize potential treatments. The most commonly used grading system for acneform rash is the National Cancer Institute's Common Terminology Criteria for Adverse Events (National Cancer Institute Cancer Therapy Evaluation Program, 2010). The development of photo libraries can aid clinicians in accurate identification of the phases of EGFR inhibitor–associated rash.

Because EGFR inhibitor–associated rash may be considered a surrogate marker of efficacy, its appearance is important. However, because therapy must be interrupted or dose reduced with a continued severity of rash, it must be managed to reduce symptoms and keep patients on therapy as long as response to treatment is noted. Although no identified "gold standard" therapeutic approach exists for EGFR inhibitor–associated rash, many therapies have been used to treat this side effect (Heidary, Naik, & Burgin, 2008). Figure 18-3 outlines possible management strategies. A proactive approach has been proposed by several clinicians, and the National Comprehensive Cancer Network® has released a task force paper reporting on possible management strategies for decreasing the severity of skin rash (Burtness et al., 2009; Lynch et al., 2007). Protection against the sun with maximal SPF products and moisturizers is critical to reduce symptoms related to EGFR inhibitor–induced rash, and these strategies should be employed early in treatment. Application of alcohol- and perfume-free emollient creams twice daily is recommended as a preventive strategy (Melosky et al., 2015).

Colloidal oatmeal lotion can be effective in reduction of symptoms associated with the rash, and a randomized, double-blinded trial confirmed that minocycline (a tetracycline analog) was effective in reducing the number of facial lesions associated with cetuximab rash (Alexandrescu, Vaillant, & Dasanu, 2007; Scope et al., 2007). The 2008 STEPP (Skin Toxicity Evaluation Protocol With Panitumumab) trial included 95 patients and reported efficacy with doxycycline given proactively versus reactively for treatment of EGFR inhibitor–associated rash (Amgen Inc., 2008). The addition of a topical steroid, moisturizer, and sun protectant also was noted to be helpful in the trial participants. Proactive therapy reduced the incidence of grade 2 or higher skin toxicities by approximately 50% compared to patients treated reactively (Amgen Inc., 2008). The recommended dose of oral minocycline is 100 mg twice daily for four weeks (Melosky et al., 2015). Lacouture et al. (2011) recommended doxycycline as the preferred therapy for patients with renal impairment; minocycline is considered less photosensitizing.

Patients receiving radiation and EGFR inhibitor therapy may experience increased incidences of radiation dermatitis, progressing from erythema and desquamation to skin necrosis or ulceration (Lacouture et al., 2011). Keeping the irradiated area clean and dry is essential, with gentle cleansing of the area. High-potency topical corticosteroids may also be beneficial. Prompt recognition and management of suspected infection is critical (Lacouture et al., 2011).

Oncology nurses are vital to the assessment and management of patients with EGFR inhibitor–associated rash. A significant financial impact is associated with the diagnosis and treatment of this rash (Eaby-Sandy, Grande, & Viale, 2012). Therefore, education regarding appropriate treatment strategies, coupled with support, can help patients maintain therapy. Early intervention is essential and may keep patients on therapy for longer periods of time (Lacouture et al., 2011; Melosky et al., 2015).

Extravasation

Oncology nurses are specially trained in the administration of chemotherapy agents.

Figure 18-3. Suggested Management Strategies for Epidermal Growth Factor Receptor (EGFR) Rash

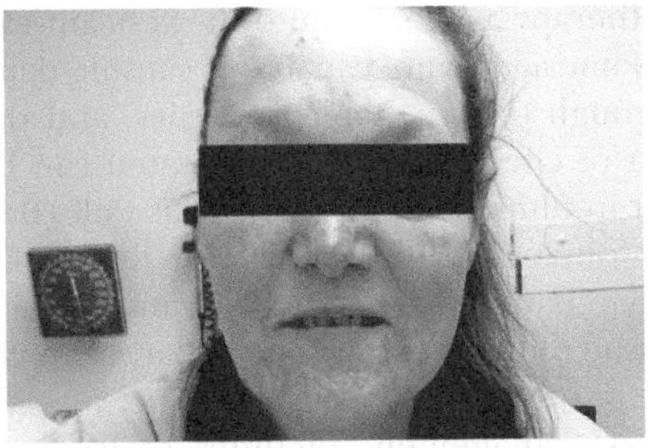

Figure A. Mild EGFR Rash

Possible care strategies
- Mild soaps
- Protective sun cream
- Emollients
- Clindamycin gel
- If necessary, steroid cream
- Tetracycline analogs (doxycycline or minocycline); proactive treatment suggested
- Colloidal oatmeal lotion

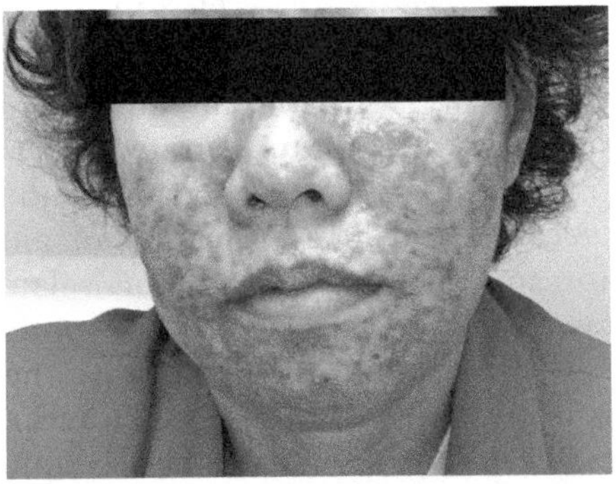

Figure B. Moderate EGFR Rash

Possible care strategies
- Mild soaps
- Protective sun cream
- Emollients
- Clindamycin gel
- If necessary, steroid cream
- Tetracycline analogs (doxycycline or minocycline)
- Colloidal oatmeal lotion

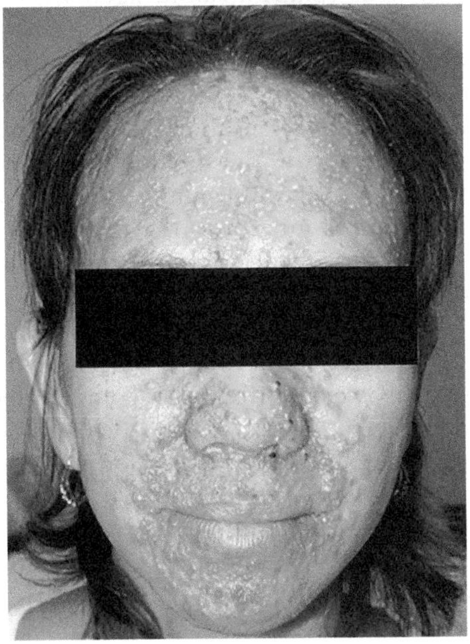

Figure C. Severe EGFR Rash

Possible care strategies
- Mild soaps
- Protective sun cream
- Emollients
- Clindamycin gel
- If necessary, steroid cream or consideration of short course of oral steroids
- Tetracycline analogs (doxycycline or minocycline)
- Colloidal oatmeal lotion

Note. Based on information from Alexandrescu et al., 2007; Amgen Inc., 2008; Lynch et al., 2007; Scope et al., 2007.

Images courtesy of Pamela Viale. Used with permission.

The Oncology Nursing Society (ONS) guidelines specifically note optimal administration methods for chemotherapy and management strategies for extravasation (Polovich, Olsen, & Lefebvre, 2014). Avoidance of extravasation is extremely important, as many agents can injure the skin if they leak out of the vessel into the surrounding skin (see Figure 18-4). Despite use of appropriate administration techniques, extravasation can occur. The importance of informing patients regarding the risk of vesicant chemotherapy and the possibility of extravasation has been recognized in court decisions; therefore, oncology nurses should include extravasation in their patient education regarding chemotherapy treatment (Schulmeister, 2008). Although the incidence of extravasation in patients receiving chemotherapy has been estimated to be approximately 0.1%–7%, this estimate may be lower than the actual numbers because it is thought that many cases are not reported (Pérez Fidalgo et al., 2012).

Tissue damage may be related to the agent extravasated. Risk factors also include a limited vein selection, the size and type of vein chosen for the infusion of drug, comorbid conditions, and an alteration in mental status of the patient (Polovich et al., 2014). Although many chemotherapy agents fall into the vesicant category, some agents are capable of causing damage through their irritant properties, and the amount of chemotherapy extravasated can be a factor in ultimate tissue damage as well (Barbee, Owonikoko, & Harvey, 2014). Taxanes in particular have the potential to cause significant tissue injury if extravasated (Barbee et al., 2014).

Figure 18-4. Extravasation of Vinblastine

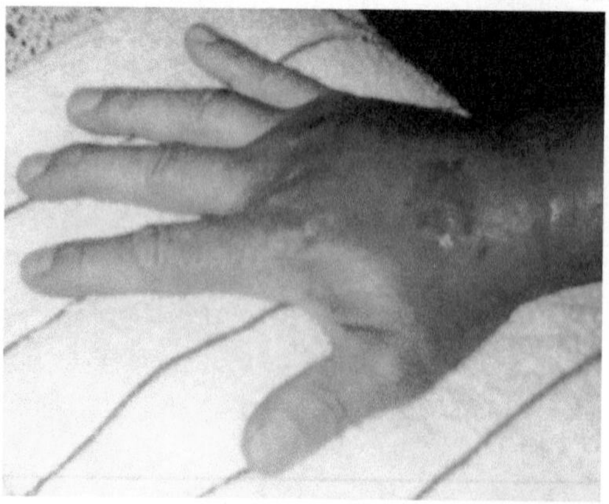

Note. Image courtesy of Pamela Viale. Used with permission.

Initial management includes early treatment, and an extravasation kit with appropriate materials should be considered (Pérez Fidalgo et al., 2012). Discontinuation of drug infusion and an attempt to aspirate the drug from tissue, if possible, are recommended (Kyllo & Anadkat, 2014). The use of antidotes for amelioration of symptoms related to extravasation is controversial, but cooling of the site combined with conservative therapy has been used for some agents (anthracyclines), whereas others require the application of heat (plant alkaloid agents). The U.S. Food and Drug Administration approval of dexrazoxane for the treatment of anthracycline extravasation offers an additional treatment strategy to minimize the potential damage that can occur with this side effect (Schulmeister, 2008). Although the mechanism of action is unknown, the therapy is a three-day treatment infused over one to two hours each day and given in a large vein in an area away from the site of the original extravasation (Schulmeister, 2008). Subcutaneous corticosteroids are not recommended (Pérez Fidalgo et al., 2012). European guidelines report benefit in the use of sodium thiosulfate for mechlorethamine extravasation and topical dimethyl sulfoxide was found to be helpful in the treatment of anthracycline extravasation (Pérez Fidalgo et al., 2012). Hyaluronidase has been used for extravasation of plant alkaloids (Schulmeister, 2008). The use of best practices is recommended to avoid extravasation, but inadvertent extravasation may occur despite this. Prompt recognition and early intervention are important to reduce potential tissue damage. Accurate and thorough documentation of the event by oncology nurses is essential (Gonzalez, 2013).

Hypersensitivity Reactions

Almost any chemotherapy agent has the potential to cause an HSR. Hypersensitivity can be termed as either an *anaphylactic* or an *anaphylactoid* reaction. Anaphylaxis is systemic with an immediate HSR reaction from immunoglobulin E (IgE) and mast cell interactions, resulting in an antigen–antibody reaction with a massive release of histamine (Gobel, 2005). Anaphylactoid reactions are not mediated by IgE and are related to the release of cytokines. This reaction is most often associated with monoclonal antibodies (Kang & Saif, 2007). The nurse's response to both is essentially the same, and the physical manifestations can be the same as well. Rechallenge often is possible with mild to moderate monoclonal antibody reactions. The general incidence of a severe HSR is approximately 5%, but individual agents may have much higher incidences (Lenz, 2007).

The timing of HSRs can vary as well. Platinum agents typically cause reactions after repeated doses of therapy, whereas taxanes almost always produce reactions on the first or second infusion (Lenz, 2007). Ixabepilone, approved in the treatment of metastatic breast cancer, has a 1% incidence of severe HSR, including anaphylaxis (Bristol-Myers Squibb Co., 2015). Some patients can be retreated with appropriate premedication. Kolliphor® EL (formerly Cremopher EL®), the diluent used with paclitaxel for solubility, frequently causes severe HSRs. Patients with a history of reaction to this agent should avoid using it again.

Monoclonal antibodies, which are made from fully murine (mouse), partial murine (either chimeric or humanized), or fully human sources, frequently produce HSRs on the first exposure to the agent. The mechanism of action for infusion reactions associated with monoclonal antibodies is not entirely clear, but the degree of antibody humanization affects the frequency of infusion reactions, with mouse and chimeric antibodies most often implicated (Thompson et al., 2014). Trastuzumab is an important part of the armamentarium for breast cancer, but the literature reports a 0.7%–40% incidence of infusion-related reactions in patients receiving the agent (Thompson et al., 2014).

Infusion-related HSRs can be fatal for some patients; therefore, it is not surprising that oncology nurses are frightened of having patients experience one (Winkeljohn & Polovich, 2006). Different strategies to identify patients at risk for HSRs include the use of skin prick tests or intradermal skin testing (Liccardi et al., 2006). Desensitization protocols have been used with success reported in certain populations of patients receiving platinum agents (Confino-Cohen, Fishman, Altaras, & Goldberg, 2004). Monoclonal antibody infusion reactions often can be managed by slowing the infusion rate and administering medications to treat the reaction (Kang & Saif, 2007). Although signs of hypersensitivity can include the appearance of wheals or skin rash, a patient suffering an HSR may experience myriad symptoms, including respiratory symptoms (stridor and wheezing), cardiovascular symptoms (hypotension, hypovolemia, intravascular volume loss), and gastrointestinal symptoms (pain, vomiting, diarrhea) (American Heart Association, 2005). The ONS guidelines call for specific management of HSRs, including cessation of chemotherapy, maintenance of IV fluids, and monitoring of vital signs with appropriate resuscitative equipment nearby (Polovich et al., 2014). Administration of oxygen and emergency medications and maintenance of airway are important components of the reaction of the oncology nurses

(Gobel, 2005; Lenz, 2007). Documentation of events is crucial.

Conclusion

Oncology nurses encounter a variety of dermatologic side effects when caring for patients receiving chemotherapy and targeted therapy agents. Recognition of these events is vital for their proper identification and treatment. Early intervention with appropriate clinical care strategies is essential to reduce the symptoms of many dermatologic or cutaneous side effects and may contribute to patients' ability to stay on therapy, as well as to reducing the discomfort associated with EGFR inhibitor–associated rash or even limiting the damage from extravasation. Because cutaneous side effects usually are visible, photo libraries of these effects (such as those recommended with EGFR inhibitor–associated rash) could aid clinicians in identifying and grading commonly occurring toxicities (Viale, 2006). Oncology nurses play an important role in the management of dermatologic effects related to cancer treatment.

References

Alexandrescu, D.T., Vaillant, J.G., & Dasanu, C.A. (2007). Effect of treatment with a colloidal oatmeal lotion on the acneform eruption induced by epidermal growth factor receptor and multiple tyrosine-kinase inhibitors. *Clinical and Experimental Dermatology, 32,* 71–74. doi:10.1111/j.1365-2230.2006.02285.x

American Heart Association. (2005). Part 10.6: Anaphylaxis. *Circulation, 112*(Suppl. 24), IV-143–IV-145. doi:10.1161/CIRCULATIONAHA.105.166568

Amgen Inc. (2008, June 26). *New data show preemptive treatment may significantly reduce skin toxicities in patients receiving Vectibix® (panitumumab)* [News release]. Retrieved from http://www.amgen.com/media/media_pr_detail.jsp?releaseID=1169981

Barbee, M.S., Owonikoko, T.K., & Harvey, R.D. (2014). Taxanes: Vesicants, irritants, or just irritating? *Therapeutic Advances in Medical Oncology, 6,* 16–20. doi:10.1177/1758834013510546

Boesmans, S., Decoster, L., & Schallier, D. (2014). Pemetrexed-induced radiation recall dermatitis of the breast. *Anticancer Research, 24,* 1179–1182.

Key Points

- Dermatologic complications are commonly seen in patients receiving chemotherapy agents.
- These may include skin reactions, HSRs (wheals or rash), hair and nail changes, and extravasation of chemotherapy agents into the skin.
- Hyperpigmentation and photosensitivity are very common with chemotherapy administration, and patient education is essential to provide strategies to protect the skin.
- Palmar-plantar erythrodysesthesia can be a dose-limiting side effect of chemotherapy.
- Nail changes require nursing assessment to promote infection prevention.
- Although general skin rashes can occur with chemotherapy administration, EGFR inhibitor–associated rash can be dose limiting and lead to infection, requiring careful assessment and management.
- Early intervention and management of EGFR inhibitor–associated rash is essential and may help keep patients on therapy.
- Extravasation of some chemotherapy agents can be injurious; careful administration and management is crucial to help limit damage.
- HSRs may occur with almost any chemotherapy agent. Oncology nurses must be vigilant and manage reactions quickly and appropriately.

Brant, J.M., Marrs, J., & Newton, S. (2004). Chemotherapy-induced nail changes: An unsightly nuisance. *Clinical Journal of Oncology Nursing, 8,* 527–528. doi:10.1188/04.CJON.527-528

Bristol-Myers Squibb Co. (2015). *Ixempra® (ixabepilone)* [Package insert]. Retrieved from http://packageinserts.bms.com/pi/pi_ixempra.pdf

Burris, H.A., III, & Hurtig, J. (2010). Radiation recall with anticancer agents. *Oncologist, 15,* 1227–1237. doi:10.1634/theoncologist.2009-0090

Burtness, B., Anadkat, M., Basti, S., Hughes, M., Lacouture, M.E., Myskowski, P.L., ... Spencer, S. (2009). NCCN Task Force report: Management of dermatologic and other toxicities associated with EGFR inhibition in patients with cancer. *Journal of the National Comprehensive Cancer Network, 7*(Suppl. 1), S5–S21.

Capriotti, K., Capriotti, J.A., Lessin, S., Wu, S., Goldfarb, S., Belum, V.R., & Lacouture, M.E. (2015). The risk of nail changes with taxane chemotherapy: A systematic review of the literature and meta-analysis. *British Journal of Dermatology, 173,* 842–845. doi:10.1111/bjd.13743

Chan, R.J., Webster, J., Chung, B., Marquart, L., Ahmed, M., & Garantziotis, S. (2014). Prevention and treatment of acute radiation-induced skin reactions: A systematic review and meta-analysis of randomized controlled trials. *BMC Cancer, 14,* 53. doi:10.1186/1471-2407-14-53

Chavarri-Guerra, Y., & Soto-Perez-de-Celis, E. (2015). Loss of fingerprints. *New England Journal of Medicine, 372,* e22. doi:10.1056/NEJMicm1409635

Choi, J.N. (2014). Dermatologic adverse events to chemotherapeutic agents, part 2: BRAF inhibitors, MEK inhibitors, and ipilimumab. *Seminars in Cutaneous Medicine and Surgery, 33,* 40–48. doi:10.12788/j.sder.0061

Confino-Cohen, R., Fishman, A., Altaras, M., & Goldberg, A. (2004). Successful carboplatin desensitization in patients with proven carboplatin allergy. *Cancer, 104,* 640–643. doi:10.1002/cncr.21168

Eaby-Sandy, B., Grande, C., & Viale, P.H. (2012). Dermatologic toxicities in epidermal growth factor receptor and multikinase inhibitors. *Journal of the Advanced Practitioner in Oncology, 3,* 138–150. doi:10.6004/jadpro.2012.3.3.2

Escudier, B., Eisen, T., Stadler, W.M., Szczylik, C., Oudard, S., Siebels, M., ... Bukowski, R.M. (2007). Sorafenib in advanced clear-cell renal-cell carcinoma. *New England Journal of Medicine, 356,* 125–134. doi:10.1056/NEJMoa060655

Fecher, L.A., Agarwala, S.S., Hodi, F.S., & Weber, J.S. (2013). Ipilimumab and its toxicities: A multidisciplinary approach. *Oncologist, 18,* 733–743. doi:10.1634/theoncologist.2012-0483

Forschner, A., Zips, D., Schraml, C., Röcken, M., Iordanou, E., Leiter, U., ... Meier, F. (2014). Radiation recall dermatitis and radiation pneumonitis during treatment with vemurafenib. *Melanoma Research, 24,* 512–516. doi:10.1097/CMR.0000000000000078

Gilbar, P., Hain, A., & Peereboom, V.-M. (2009). Nail toxicity induced by cancer chemotherapy. *Journal of Oncology Pharmacy Practice, 15,* 143–155. doi:10.1177/1078155208100450

Gobel, B.H. (2005). Chemotherapy-induced hypersensitivity reactions. *Oncology Nursing Forum, 32,* 1027–1035. doi:10.1188/05.ONF.1027-1035

Gonzalez, T. (2013). Chemotherapy extravasations: Prevention, identification, management, and documentation. *Clinical Journal of Oncology Nursing, 17,* 61–66. doi:10.1188/13.CJON.61-66

Heidary, N., Naik, H., & Burgin, S. (2008). Chemotherapeutic agents and the skin: An update. *Journal of the American Academy of Dermatology, 58,* 545–570. doi:10.1016/j.jaad.2008.01.001

Hinds, G., & Thomas, V.D. (2008). Malignancy and cancer treatment-related hair and nail changes. *Dermatologic Clinics, 26,* 59–68. doi:10.1016/j.det.2007.08.003

Hird, A.E., Wilson, J., Symons, S., Sinclair, E., Davis, M., & Chow, E. (2008). Radiation recall dermatitis: Case report and review of the literature. *Current Oncology, 15,* 53–62. doi:10.3747/co.2008.201

Huang, V., Hepper, D., Anadkat, M., & Cornelius, L. (2012). Cutaneous toxic effects associated with vemurafenib and inhibition of the BRAF pathway. *Archives of Dermatology, 148,* 628–633. doi:10.1001/archdermatol.2012.125

Kang, S.P., & Saif, M.W. (2007). Infusion-related and hypersensitivity reactions of monoclonal antibodies used to treat colorectal cancer—Identification, prevention, and management. *Journal of Supportive Oncology, 5,* 451–457.

Kanwar, A.J., & Narang, T. (2013). Symposium—Hair disorders. *Indian Journal of Dermatology, Venereology and Leprology, 79,* 604–612. doi:10.4103/0378-6323.116728

Komen, M.M.C., Smorenburg, C.H., Van Den Hurk, C.J.G., & Nortier, J.W.R. (2013). Factors influencing the effectiveness of scalp cooling in the prevention of chemotherapy-induced alopecia. *Oncologist, 18,* 885–891. doi:10.1634/theoncologist.2012-0332

Kyllo, R.L., & Anadkat, M.J. (2014). Dermatologic adverse events to chemotherapeutic agents, part 1: Cytotoxic agents, epidermal growth factor inhibitors, multikinase inhibitors, and proteasome inhibitors. *Seminars in Cutaneous Medicine and Surgery, 33,* 28–39. doi:10.12788/j.sder.0060

Lacouture, M.E., Anadkat, M.J., Bensadoun, R.-J., Bryce, J., Chan, A., Epstein, J.B., ... Murphy, B.A. (2011). Clinical practice guidelines for the prevention and treatment of EGFR inhibitor–associated dermatologic toxicities. *Supportive Care in Cancer, 19,* 1079–1095. doi:10.1007/s00520-011-1197-6

Lacouture, M.E., Duvic, M., Hauschild, A., Prieto, V.G., Robert, C., Schadendorf, D., ... Joe, A.K. (2013). Analysis of dermatologic events in vemurafenib-treated patients with melanoma. *Oncologist, 18,* 314–322. doi:10.1634/theoncologist.2012-0333

Lacouture, M.E., Reilly, L.M., Gerami, P., & Guitart, J. (2008). Hand foot skin reaction in cancer patients treated with the multikinase inhibitors sorafenib and sunitinib. *Annals of Oncology, 19,* 1955–1961. doi:10.1093/annonc/mdn389

Lenz, H.-J. (2007). Management and preparedness for infusion and hypersensitivity reactions. *Oncologist, 12,* 601–609. doi:10.1634/theoncologist.12-5-601

Liccardi, G., D'Amato, G., Canonica, G.W., Salzillo, A., Piccolo, A., & Passalacqua, G. (2006). Systemic reactions from skin testing: Literature review. *Journal of Investigational Allergology and Clinical Immunology, 16,* 75–78.

Lynch, T.J., Jr., Kim, E.S., Eaby, B., Garey, J., West, D.P., & Lacouture, M.E. (2007). Epidermal growth factor receptor inhibitor-associated cutaneous toxicities: An evolving paradigm in clinical management. *Oncologist, 12,* 610–621. doi:10.1634/theoncologist.12-5-610

Madi, A., Fisher, D., Wilson, R.H., Adams, R.A., Meade, A.M., Kenny, S.L., ... Maughan, T.S. (2012). Oxaliplatin/capecitabine vs oxaliplatin/infusional 5-FU in advanced colorectal cancer: The MRC COIN trial. *British Journal of Cancer, 107,* 1037–1043. doi:10.1038/bjc.2012.384

Mangili, G., Petrone, M., Gentile, C., De Marzi, P., Viganó, R., & Rabaiotti, E. (2008). Prevention strategies in palmar-plantar erythrodysesthesia onset: The role of regional cooling. *Gynecologic Oncology, 108,* 332–335. doi:10.1016/j.ygyno.2007.10.021

Melosky, B., Leighl, N.B., Rothenstein, J., Sangha, R., Stewart, D., & Papp, K. (2015). Management of EGFR TKI-induced dermatologic adverse events. *Current Oncology, 22,* 123–132. doi:10.3747/co.22.2430

Miller, K.K., Gorcey, L., & McLellan, B.N. (2014). Chemotherapy-induced hand-foot syndrome and nail changes: A review of clinical presentation, etiology, pathogenesis, and management. *Journal of the American Academy of Dermatology, 71,* 787–794. doi:10.1016/j.jaad.2014.03.019

Minisini, A.M., Tosti, A., Sobrero, A.F., Mansutti, M., Piraccini, B.M., Sacco, C., & Puglisi, F. (2003). Taxane-induced nail changes: Incidence, clinical presentation and outcome. *Annals of Oncology, 14,* 333–337. doi:10.1093/annonc/mdg050

National Cancer Institute Cancer Therapy Evaluation Program. (2010). *Common terminology criteria for adverse events* [v.4.03]. Retrieved from http://evs.nci.nih.gov/ftp1/CTCAE/CTCAE_4.03_2010-06-14_QuickReference_5x7.pdf

Pérez Fidalgo, J.A., Fabregat, L.G., Cervantes, A., Margulies, A., Vidall, C., & Roila, F. (2012). Management of chemotherapy extravasation: ESMO-EONS clinical practice guidelines. *Annals of Oncology, 23*(Suppl. 7), vii167–vii173. doi:10.1093/annonc/mds294

Polovich, M., Olsen, M., & LeFebvre, K.B. (Eds.). (2014). *Chemotherapy and biotherapy guidelines and recommendations for practice* (4th ed.). Pittsburgh, PA: Oncology Nursing Society.

Rosen, A.C., Balagula, Y., Raisch, D.W., Garg, V., Nardone, B., Larsen, N., ... Lacouture, M.E. (2014). Life-threatening dermatologic adverse events in oncology. *Anti-Cancer Drugs, 25,* 225–234. doi:10.1097/CAD.0000000000000032

Rossi, D., & Catalano, G. (2007). Pyridoxine as prophylactic therapy for palmar-plantar erythrodysesthesia associated with administration of pegylated liposomal doxorubicin (Caelyx): A single-center experience. *Oncology, 73,* 277–278. doi:10.1159/000127427

Salvo, N., Barnes, E., van Draanen, J., Stacey, E., Mitera, G., Breen, D., ... De Angelis, C. (2010). Prophylaxis and management of acute radiation-induced skin reactions: A systematic review of the literature. *Current Oncology, 17,* 94–112.

Scarpati, G.D.V., Fusciello, C., Perri, F., Sabbatino, F., Ferrone, S., Carlomagno, C., & Pepe, S. (2014). Ipilimumab in the treatment of metastatic melanoma: Management of adverse events. *OncoTargets and Therapy, 7,* 203–209. doi:10.2147/OTT.S57335

Schulmeister, L. (2008). Managing vesicant extravasations. *Oncologist, 13,* 284–288. doi:10.1634/theoncologist.2007-0191

Scope, A., Agero, A.L.C., Dusza, S.W., Myskowski, P.L., Lieb, J.A., Saltz, L., ... Halpern, A.C. (2007). Randomized double-blind trial of prophylactic oral minocycline and topical tazarotene for cetuximab-associated acne-like eruption. *Journal of Clinical Oncology, 25,* 5390–5396. doi:10.1200/JCO.2007.12.6987

Thompson, L.M., Eckmann, K., Boster, B.L., Hess, K.R., Michaud, L.B., Esteva, F.J., ... Barnett, C.M. (2014). Incidence, risk factors, and management of infusion-related reactions in breast cancer patients receiving trastuzumab. *Oncologist, 19,* 228–234. doi:10.1634/theoncologist.2013-0286

Viale, P.H. (2006). Chemotherapy and cutaneous toxicities: Implications for oncology nurses. *Seminars in Oncology Nursing, 22,* 144–151. doi:10.1016/j.soncn.2006.04.007

Wilkes, G.M., & Doyle, D. (2005). Palmar-plantar erythrodysesthesia. *Clinical Journal of Oncology Nursing, 9,* 103–106. doi:10.1188/05.CJON.103-106

Winkeljohn, D., & Polovich, M. (2006). Carboplatin hypersensitivity reactions. *Clinical Journal of Oncology Nursing, 10,* 595–598. doi:10.1188/06.CJON.595-598

Yun, S.J., & Kim, S.-J. (2007). Hair loss pattern due to chemotherapy-induced anagen effluvium: A cross-sectional observation. *Dermatology, 215,* 36–40. doi:10.1159/000102031

Chapter 18 Study Questions

1. Dermatologic complications range from distressing and uncomfortable to unsightly or fatal. Palmar-plantar erythrodysesthesia (PPE, hand-foot syndrome) is a painful, erythematous skin change seen on the soles of the feet and the palms of the hands. Although uncomfortable, PPE often improves with:
   A. The use of foot soaks in hot water.
   B. Oral steroid treatment.
   C. Complete bed rest.
   D. Emollient therapy and avoidance of pressure-bearing activities.

2. Which of the following statements is true?
   A. Nail toxicities occur 100% of the time in patients receiving taxanes.
   B. The appearance of white lines or grooves in the fingernails and toenails of patients receiving chemotherapy signals that complete loss of the nail will occur.
   C. *Paronychia* refers to bloody collections under the nail beds.
   D. Normal fingernail growth takes 6 months, versus 12 months for toenail formation.

3. Dermatologic events associated with epidermal growth factor receptor (EGFR) inhibitor agents are not limited to rash; practitioners also may see:
   A. Dry skin (xerosis).
   B. Periungual inflammations.
   C. Alopecia of the scalp.
   D. Abnormal growth of the eyelashes.
   E. All of the above.

4. The best treatment for an EGFR inhibitor–associated rash is to:
   A. Treat the rash as soon as it appears.
   B. Protect the skin with an SPF 15 product.
   C. Apply a perfumed lotion to moisturize dry skin.
   D. Treat patients proactively to reduce symptoms and keep patients on therapy as long as necessary.

5. *Extravasation* refers to the accidental infusion of a substance out of the vessel into the surrounding skin. Despite best practices, accidental extravasation can occur. The nurse should:
   A. Initially manage an extravasation with early treatment.
   B. Have an extravasation kit readily available.
   C. Use antidotes for specific drug extravasations, although the practice is still considered controversial.
   D. Use cooling for anthracycline extravasations as appropriate.
   E. Thoroughly document the event.
   F. All of the above.

CHAPTER

19 Fatigue

Lanell M. Bellury, PhD, RN, AOCNS®, OCN®, and Jane C. Clark, PhD, RN, AOCN®, OCN®, GNP-BC

Introduction

Fatigue, like other cancer-related symptoms, is a subjective phenomenon commonly experienced by both ill and healthy people. Many illnesses, from the common cold to congestive heart failure, are associated with the experience of fatigue, and in some illnesses (e.g., anemia, chronic fatigue syndrome), fatigue is a presenting and diagnostic symptom. Additionally, interventions to treat many diseases, from surgery to drug therapy, result in fatigue. Consequently, nurses are familiar with fatigue from both personal experiences and from providing care to patients across specialties and settings. Because of the universal experience of fatigue and the severity of other acute symptoms related to cancer treatment, cancer-related fatigue (CRF) was generally ignored by oncology clinicians and patients for many years (Stasi, Abriani, Beccaglia, Terzoli, & Amadori, 2003). Additionally, CRF has been consistently underreported and therefore undertreated because of a lack of consensus and empirically based evidence related to methods to measure, define, and effectively treat it (Minton & Stone, 2009).

The Oxford dictionary defines *fatigue* as "extreme tiredness typically resulting from mental or physical exertion or illness." The term is derived from the Latin *fatigare*, meaning to tire out ("Fatigue," n.d.). Winningham (2000) noted that "fatigue is perceived as a loss, a deficit, a lack or inability as the result of an exertion or excess, a response to a stimulus" (p. 38). Both definitions imply a temporal relationship between exertion and fatigue, in which fatigue is present *after* exertion. CRF is different. The purpose of this chapter is to delineate the difference between the more ubiquitous experience of fatigue and that experienced by individuals diagnosed with cancer.

CRF is the most common and most distressing symptom reported by patients with cancer, even more distressing than pain (Barsevick et al., 2010; Weis & Horneber, 2015). CRF is often debilitating, relentless, misinterpreted, frustrating, and discouraging. Patients have described CRF as different from previous experiences with fatigue in its intensity, severity, sudden onset, and physical, social, emotional, and cognitive impact (Scott, Lasch, Barsevick, & Piault-Louis, 2011). For example, Barsevick, Whitmer, and Walker (2001) quoted a patient's description of the experience: "The fatigue was so debilitating that there are days that to turn the pages of the newspaper was more than I could do" (p. 1367). Similarly, Wu and McSweeney (2007) reported a patient describing CRF:

> I couldn't overcome it. I couldn't force myself . . . the fatigue was overwhelming . . . I couldn't make myself do things anyway during cer-

> tain phases of it. So it was just overwhelming and it . . . kind of took over my life. (p. 121)

Despite these poignant descriptions from patients with cancer, CRF is still routinely overlooked and undertreated by clinicians (Mitchell et al., 2014; Weis & Horneber, 2015). Patients consider CRF "a symptom to be endured" (Vogelzang et al., 1997) and do not perceive that healthcare providers are able to help them deal with CRF (Mitchell et al., 2014; Wu & McSweeney, 2007). This chapter will detail the definition, prevalence, etiology, pathophysiology, assessment, and treatment of CRF, as well as the role of oncology nurses in the identification and modification of the CRF experience.

Definition

Part of the complexity of identifying and managing CRF results from the lack of consensus regarding the definition of CRF. The National Comprehensive Cancer Network® (NCCN®, 2015) defines CRF as a "distressing, persistent, subjective sense of physical, emotional, and/or cognitive tiredness or exhaustion related to cancer or cancer treatment that is not proportional to recent activity and interferes with usual functioning" (p. FT-1). This definition recognizes four significant components of CRF. The first component is the quality of CRF, described as distressing and persistent. The quality of CRF is distinctly different from fatigue experienced by healthy people. Second, CRF, experienced as tiredness or exhaustion that can be physical, emotional, or cognitive, must be related to cancer. The next component of the NCCN definition identifies a key difference from other fatigue in that CRF is not proportional to activity. CRF has been noted to arise suddenly and unexpectedly at times and to be persistent despite rest. The last component of the definition specifies that CRF interferes with functioning.

Although the NCCN definition is comprehensive and commonly accepted, other definitions include additional components, and some discrepancies exist (see Table 19-1). For example, the National Cancer Institute (NCI) definition adds the acute versus chronic nature of CRF (NCI, n.d.). Stone and Minton (2008) reported that patients with cancer and survivors may report persistent fatigue and yet continue to function, which according to the NCCN definition would exclude them from a CRF diagnosis. The Common Terminology Criteria for Adverse Events (CTCAE) omits several components found in most CRF definitions, and the grading criteria include fatigue relieved by rest, a criterion inconsistent with most definitions of CRF, and activity interference (NCI Cancer Therapy Evaluation Program, 2010), which would again eliminate those who experience CRF yet continue to function. An alternate diagnostic criteria proposed by the Fatigue Coalition requires experience of fatigue that lasts for at least two weeks as a result from cancer or cancer treatment, is not related to psychiatric conditions, and includes at least 5 of 10 reported symptoms, including weakness; problems with concentration, motivation, and sleep; emotional reactions to fatigue; difficulty completing or beginning tasks; memory problems; and malaise (Weis & Horneber, 2015).

CRF generally is considered a subjective symptom, such as nausea, pain, insomnia, and depression, but it is undeniably multidimensional and multifactorial (Barsevick et al., 2010; Stone & Minton, 2008; Wang, 2008). Regardless of how it is defined, CRF is one of the "most prevalent and distressing long-term effects of cancer treatment, significantly affecting patients' quality of life" (Bower et al., 2014, p. 1842).

Prevalence

Establishing the prevalence of CRF is complicated because of the lack of a consistent definition, the variety of methods used to measure

Table 19-1. Definitions of Cancer-Related Fatigue

Organization/Source	Definitions
Cancer.Net (2016)	"A persistent feeling of physical, emotional, or mental tiredness or exhaustion related to cancer and/or its treatment"
Common Terminology Criteria for Adverse Events [v.4.03] (National Cancer Institute Cancer Therapy Evaluation Program, 2010, p. 22)	"A disorder characterized by a state of generalized weakness with a pronounced inability to summon sufficient energy to accomplish daily activities"
European Association of Palliative Care (Radbruch et al., 2008, p. 13)	"A subjective feeling of tiredness, weakness or lack of energy"
National Cancer Institute (n.d.)	"A condition marked by extreme tiredness and inability to function due to lack of energy. Fatigue may be acute or chronic."
National Comprehensive Cancer Network (2016, p. FT-1)	"A distressing, persistent, subjective sense of physical, emotional, and/or cognitive tiredness or exhaustion related to cancer or cancer treatment that is not proportional to recent activity and interferes with usual functioning"
Stone and Minton (2008, p. 1097)	"A subjective sensation that is disproportional to the widely recognized feeling of being tired. . . . It is characterized by being pervasive and not relieved by rest."
Weis and Horneber (2015, p. 3)	"A self-recognized phenomenon that is subjective in nature and experienced as a feeling of tiredness or lack of energy that varies in degree, frequency, and duration, which is not proportional to physical activities, and not relieved by sleep or rest"

CRF, and differences related to the patient experience of CRF across the cancer experience. When compared to the general population, patients with cancer, even patients without anemia, experience significantly more fatigue (Cella, Lai, Chang, Peterman, & Slavin, 2002). Four systematic reviews (Abrahams et al., 2016; Prue, Rankin, Allen, Gracey, & Cramp, 2006; Servaes, Verhagen, & Bleijenberg, 2002; Stasi et al., 2003) and a meta-analysis (Kreissl et al., 2016) reported CRF prevalence. When compared to healthy controls, patients with cancer report significantly higher frequency and severity of fatigue (Prue et al., 2006; Servaes et al., 2002). Prevalence during cancer treatment ranged from 39% reporting significant fatigue to 50%–90% reporting the experience of fatigue (Kreissl et al., 2016; Prue et al., 2006). The prevalence of severe post-treatment fatigue was 27% in breast cancer survivors (Abrahams et al., 2016), and prevalence of post-treatment fatigue in patients with Hodgkin lymphoma was 34%–76% (Kreissl et al., 2016). Most studies with baseline measures of fatigue found significantly more fatigue mid-treatment and post-treatment compared to pretreatment levels (Servaes et al., 2002); however, fatigue in patients with lymphoma was higher at baseline (76%–83%) than at the end of treatment (36%–47%) or after treatment (Kreissl et al., 2016).

Cancer-Related Fatigue Across the Cancer Experience

CRF occurs in all stages of cancer survivorship, beginning with fatigue as an initial symptom leading to diagnosis and continuing through end-of-life care (Weis & Horneber, 2015). Estimates of CRF prevalence varies by stage of survivorship, with highest prevalence reported during active treatment (see Table 19-2). Although CRF is expected during cancer treatment, levels of fatigue may fluctuate over the course of treatment (de Jong, Kester, Schouten, Abu-Saad, & Courtens, 2006; Prue et al., 2006; Weis & Horneber, 2015). CRF during treatment also predicts post-treatment fatigue. CRF has been found to persist for many years after treatment (Weis & Horneber, 2015), but the number of years it persists is difficult to approximate because of the relatively short follow-up in most studies. A longitudinal study of breast cancer survivors found that 34% of participants reported elevated fatigue persisting 5–10 years after treatment (Bower et al., 2006). A 2002 literature review reporting on 13 studies (mean time since treatment of 9 months to 12 years) demonstrated persistent CRF in multiple diagnostic groups (Servaes et al., 2002). CRF is also highly prevalent in palliative and end-of-life settings (Keeney & Head, 2011). Wide individual variation and even diurnal patterns of CRF have been reported (Dhruva et al., 2010), as well as a model that depicts a linear progression of CRF occurring in stages of tiredness, fatigue, and exhaustion (Olson, Krawchuk, & Quddusi, 2007).

Table 19-2. Reported Prevalence of Cancer-Related Fatigue by Stage of Cancer Survivorship

Stage of Survivorship	Reported Prevalence (%)
Diagnosis (Stasi et al., 2003)	50–75
Treatment (Stone & Minton, 2008)	90
• Chemotherapy (Stasi et al., 2003)	80–96
• Radiation (Stasi et al., 2003)	60–93
Post-treatment (Stone & Minton, 2008)	19–38
• Long-term survivorship (Weis & Horneber, 2015)	25–35
Palliative care (Stone & Minton, 2008)	78

CRF occurs throughout the cancer experience and affects a significant number of patients. The distressing and prevalent experience of CRF requires the attention of clinicians to teach patients to recognize CRF and to monitor changes in CRF, to assess for CRF at each patient encounter even during long-term survivorship, and to consistently inquire about patient adherence to and efficacy of suggested treatments.

Etiology

CRF etiology models involve complex, multifactorial processes that include physical, emotional, and cognitive components (Horneber, Fischer, Dimeo, Rüffer, & Weis, 2012). Commonly identified components include comorbidities, stress, sleep disorders, tumor mediation, treatment modalities, metabolic or hormonal changes, mood disorders, anemia, inflammation, or deconditioning (Barsevick et al., 2010; Weis & Horneber, 2015). For example, depression is associated with fatigue in people who are healthy, people diagnosed with cancer, and people diagnosed with other chronic illnesses. But while treatment with antidepressants has shown improvements in mood, antidepressant therapy has not demonstrated effectiveness in the treatment of CRF (Mitchell et al., 2014; Stone & Minton, 2008). Similarly, sleep disorders, including sleep apnea, periodic limb movement, or frequent nighttime awakening, may be caused by comorbid conditions in patients with cancer or may be a result of cancer treatment (e.g., frequent awakening due to hydrating treatment protocols), but CRF is not simply caused by insomnia because in some studies improvement in sleep did not necessarily relieve fatigue (Stone & Minton, 2008).

The exact etiology of CRF is unknown, and a rational approach to treatment will be elusive until the causes are clarified. However, an understanding of factors found to increase the risk of CRF and the suspected underlying pathophysiology of CRF offer clues to causation and will be discussed in the following section.

Risk Factors

Risk factors have been identified that contribute to the experience of CRF. These risk factors should be considered when developing effective treatment strategies for patients experiencing CRF and include emotional distress (e.g., depression, anxiety, fear of recurrence), sleep disturbances, nutritional deficits, decreased physical function, anemia, and pain (Bower et al., 2014). Pretreatment fatigue is strongly associated with CRF, and accumulating research implicates genetic risk factors related to genes involved in inflammation (Bower, 2014).

In a systematic review (Prue et al., 2006), no association was found between CRF and stage of disease (except for lung cancer), age, gender, ethnicity, marital status, occupation, education, or income. In post-treatment cancer survivors, no association has been demonstrated with CRF and diagnosis, tumor size, time since diagnosis, stage of disease, or treatment; however, in all of the reviewed studies, psychological symptoms and sleep were associated with CRF. Multiple symptoms (anxiety, depression, pain, nausea, dyspnea, symptom distress, and decreased appetite), poor performance status, and inactivity have also been associated with CRF (Prue et al., 2006).

Pathophysiology

The pathophysiology underlying the patient experience of CRF is unclear. Several possible explanations of CRF are presented in this section; however, a detailed discussion of these mechanisms is beyond the scope of this chapter. More in-depth discussion of pathophysiology can be found in the publications by Wang (2008) and Barsevick et al. (2010).

The most predominant physiologic pathways implicated in CRF include dysregulation of proinflammatory cytokines, the hypothalomic–pituitary–adrenal (HPA) axis (cortisol), 5-hydroxytryptamine (5-HT, or serotonin) dysregulation, circadian rhythm disturbance, and changes in genes that regulate these cellular functions (Barsevick et al., 2010; Horneber et al., 2012). Others have suggested causal pathways related to mood and sleep disorders, sickness behavior syndrome, or increased energy expenditure due to accelerated tumor metabolism or increased expression of growth factors (Wang, 2008; Weis & Horneber, 2015). As a multidimensional syndrome, CRF is likely caused by all or combinations of these processes. Additionally, the progression of fatigue may indicate the effect of cumulative or sequential physiologic pathway involvement occurring over time (Barsevick et al., 2010). In fact, many of these pathways are interconnected, so the discovery of a single physiologic cause of CRF seems unlikely, and dysregulation of one pathway will cause changes in the other related pathways (Berger, Mitchell, Jacobsen, & Pirl, 2015).

Proinflammation Cytokines

Cytokines are proteins produced by the immune system to regulate the immune response. Increased expression of proinflammatory cytokines, such as interleukins, interferon, and tumor necrosis factor, is found in tumor cells (Barsevick et al., 2010; Berger et al., 2015). Additionally, increased levels of cytokines are seen in patients receiving chemotherapy and radiation therapy (Weis & Horneber, 2015). Treatment with interferon may cause fatigue in as many as 70% of patients, and breast cancer survivors with persistent CRF also were found to have increased levels of proinflammatory cytokines (Barsevick et al., 2010; Wang, 2008).

Cytokines are thought to play a role in sickness behavior, which parallels flu-like symptoms that result from biologic response modifiers. Finally, in advanced cancer, interleukin-6 and tumor necrosis factor-alpha are related to tissue catabolism, resulting in cachexia (Wang, 2008), which has also been associated with the development of CRF. Cytokine activity in cancer as a result of the disease or treatment is strongly implicated in the pathogenesis of CRF.

Hypothalamic–Pituitary–Adrenal Axis Dysfunction

The HPA axis is an integrated system that regulates the steroid hormone cortisol produced by the adrenal gland in response to stressors (e.g., physical exertion, emotional stress, infection, injury). Cancer and its treatment may cause alterations in the HPA axis. For example, hormone ablation therapy for prostate cancer that alters gonadotropin (a part of the HPA axis) has been shown to significantly increase CRF (Wang, 2008). Interestingly, some proinflammatory cytokines can stimulate the HPA axis, and conversely, cortisol inhibits the development of immune cells and cytokine production (Barsevick et al., 2010; Wang, 2008). Reduced HPA activity and low levels of cortisol have been associated with CRF (Barsevick et al., 2010; Wang, 2008).

5-Hydroxytryptamine Dysregulation

Serotonin, or 5-HT, is a neurotransmitter produced in the central nervous system and gastrointestinal system. It is widely distributed in cells and influences a variety of body functions (Ryan et al., 2007). The serotonin pathway is interrelated with both the proinflammatory cytokines and the HPA axis such that an increase in proinflammatory cytokines caused by the tumor or treatment might, in turn, increase 5-HT levels, which modifies the HPA axis and culminates in fatigue (Barsevick et al., 2010). Serotonin levels also are associated with depression, and because depression and fatigue commonly co-occur in both healthy and cancer populations, the supposition that the two conditions share a common pathway is logical. However, as mentioned previously, while treatment with serotonin uptake inhibitors resulted in improved depression symptoms during cancer treatment, no subsequent reduction in CRF occurred (Roscoe et al., 2005).

Additional theories that may play a part in CRF include growth factors (e.g., vascular endothelial growth factor, epidermal growth factor); anemia; disturbances in the circadian sleep-wake cycle related to melatonin regulation, which also impacts cortisol levels; activation of vagal-afferent nerves through stimulation of neuroactive substances; and disruption of adenosine triphosphate metabolism (Wang, 2008). Clinical features of cancer or its treatment, including postoperative fatigue, nausea, diarrhea, vomiting, infections, malnutrition, pain, distress, comorbidity, and organ failure, play a role in the physiologic development of CRF (Berger et al., 2015; Stasi et al., 2003; Wang, 2008).

Multiple risk factors for CRF have been identified, and several physiologic mechanisms have been implicated in its development, but the exact pathways and causes of CRF remain unknown. Knowledge of all of the suggested pathways will help nurses to understand the complexity of the human body's response to cancer and its treatment and to be alert to the extensive sequelae, signs, and symptoms associated with a cancer diagnosis. Another significant challenge for patients and nurses alike is the clustering of symptoms.

Symptom Clusters

Symptom clusters are generally defined as three or more symptoms that occur together but may not share similar etiology (Honea, Brant, & Beck, 2007). Symptom cluster research began because the common practice of focusing on one symptom, usually the most problematic one for the patient or treatment regimen, resulted in lack of attention to other symptoms. Studies have demonstrated that multiple symptoms have an additive, synergistic effect on each other, and patients who experience multiple, co-occurring symptoms are at risk for poor quality of life, declining physical function, and poor overall outcomes (Barsevick, 2007; Given, Given, Sikorskii, & Hadar, 2007).

Clustered symptoms may be interrelated. For example, pain has been shown to have a direct and indirect effect on sleep, fatigue, and depression (Honea et al., 2007). The identification of symptom clusters can focus assessment and treatment on commonly unmanaged symptoms that might efficiently improve patient outcomes (Given et al., 2007).

Empirical data support CRF as a component of several identified symptom clusters. The fatigue, pain, depression, and sleep disturbance cluster has been commonly described across diagnosis and treatment types (Barsevick, 2007) and was called the "cross-cutting symptom cluster" in patients undergoing treatment (Honea et al., 2007, p. 144). A cluster of pain, fatigue, and insomnia was reported in 18% of patients with breast cancer, 16% of patients with colon cancer, and 29% of patients with lung cancer; at least two of the three symptoms co-occurred in approximately half of these patients (Given et al., 2007). Fatigue, dyspnea, drowsiness, and pain were identified as one of four clusters commonly occurring in patients with advanced cancer (Dong, Butow, Costa, Lovell, & Agar, 2014). Treatment of one clustered symptom can have positive or negative effects on other symptoms. For example, treatment for pain may increase the experience of fatigue because of central nervous system depression from opioids.

Pain and fatigue have been identified as sentinel symptoms—a symptom that should prompt immediate assessment for other frequently co-occurring symptoms (Barsevick, 2007; Given et al., 2007). CRF is an important symptom, as demonstrated by its prevalence as an individual symptom, its presence in the common symptom clusters discussed in the literature, and its identification as a sentinel symptom. Therefore, routine nursing assessments need to include the presence and degree of CRF in addition to the presence of other clustered symptoms.

Assessment

Assessment of a subjective symptom relies on the patient's ability to describe the phenomena that he or she is experiencing, as well as the interest of the care provider in hearing and interpreting what the patient describes. In the case of CRF, as with many subjective symptoms, barriers exist to accurate assessment.

First, if symptom effects are not observed in the clinical setting, the care provider may not be cued to ask the patient about the symptom. Evidence indicates that providers are hesitant to ask about CRF because of a lack of understanding about the symptom, lack of awareness about available treatment, and belief that little can be done to manage the experience (Borneman et al., 2010; Nail, 2002; NCCN, 2016). Patients often are reluctant to report CRF because of beliefs that fatigue associated with cancer and treatment is inevitable, concern that reporting fatigue may influence the medical care provided, and fear that the presence or worsening of fatigue is an indicator that the cancer is not responding to the treatment (Borneman et al., 2010). Therefore, if healthcare providers are reluctant to ask and patients are reluctant to report, CRF often is unrecognized, underdiagnosed, and undertreated.

The assessment of CRF, therefore, begins at the first patient encounter and relies on both patient and provider awareness of CRF prevalence, assessment, and treatment. Assessment can be accomplished through careful screening, a detailed patient history with qualitative descriptors and open-ended discussions, and quantitative instruments.

Screening for Cancer-Related Fatigue

Because of the ubiquitous nature of CRF and evidence that CRF continues well after completion of active cancer treatment, patients should be screened for the presence and severity of CRF at each encounter (NCCN, 2016). The recommended measure for CRF screening in the clinical area is the 1-item, 11-point, self-report visual analog scale (0 = no fatigue; 10 = worst possible fatigue) (see Figure 19-1) (NCCN, 2016). This self-reported measure provides information on both the presence and perceived severity of primarily the physical component of CRF.

Although NCCN (2016) guidelines indicate that a mandatory comprehensive assessment should occur when the patient reports fatigue severity of greater than 4 (moderate CRF) on a 0–10 scale, the clinician should consider asking the patient to define the level of fatigue that would be acceptable or tolerable. Any difference between the actual and acceptable level of fatigue would trigger a more comprehensive assessment and initiation of appropriate interventions. Early intervention may inhibit the exacerbation of CRF.

Another common measurement instrument used as a screening assessment of fatigue, especially for patients enrolled in NCI clinical trials, is the CTCAE (NCI Cancer Therapy Evaluation Program, 2010). This instrument evaluates the effectiveness of a single alleviating factor (rest) and the impact of the fatigue on activities of daily living (see Table 19-3).

The CTCAE (version 4.03) grades the presence of an adverse event on a scale from 1 (mild change) to 5 (death) and is used in cancer research to make clinical decisions related to treatment delays, dose reductions, and discontinuation of treatment. The CTCAE has limited reliability and validity estimates specific to individuals diagnosed with cancer. An additional limitation of the CTCAE for fatigue is that the grade 3 rating indicates that the patient is not capable of performing the basic activities of daily living of feeding, dressing, bathing, etc. A grade 3 rating, therefore, should signal safety concerns for a patient living independently and should result in interventions to prevent falls and other safety concerns. Finally, the scale has no descriptors for grade 4 and grade 5, which in the evaluation of other toxicities would generally be used to make treatment decisions (NCI Cancer Therapy Evaluation Program, 2010).

Figure 19-1. Self-Report, 11-Point Fatigue Scale

Energetic No Fatigue										Worst Possible Fatigue
0	1	2	3	4	5	6	7	8	9	10
No Fatigue	Mild Fatigue				Moderate Fatigue				Severe Fatigue	

Note. Based on information from National Comprehensive Cancer Network, 2016.

Table 19-3. Common Terminology Criteria for Adverse Events Grading for Fatigue

Grade	Descriptors
1	Fatigue relieved by rest
2	Fatigue not relieved by rest, limiting instrumental ADL
3	Fatigue not relieved by rest, limiting self-care ADL
4	–
5	–

ADL—activities of daily living

Note. From *Common Terminology Criteria for Adverse Events* [v.4.03], by National Cancer Institute Cancer Therapy Evaluation Program, 2010. Retrieved from http://evs.nci.nih.gov/ftp1/CTCAE/CTCAE_4.03_2010-06-14_QuickReference_5x7.pdf.

Comprehensive Assessment of Cancer-Related Fatigue

Multiple methods for conducting a comprehensive assessment of CRF are available. NCCN (2016) guidelines for CRF recommend that the assessment include a complete history and evaluation of disease status, assessment of treatable contributing factors, laboratory studies, and imaging, as indicated. The oncology nurse can contribute to the comprehensive assessment by evaluating the history of CRF and assessing for contributing factors.

The nurse, through the use of open-ended questions, can assess the onset, pattern, and duration of CRF, factors from the patient's perspective that aggravate and alleviate CRF, previous self-care strategies the patient has used to address CRF and their perceived effectiveness, and the effect of CRF on instrumental and self-care activities of daily living and quality of life (see Figure 19-2). Given that patients often report CRF as a component of a symptom cluster across the cancer experience (Aktas, Walsh, & Rybicki, 2010), the assessment should also include an evaluation for pain, sleep disturbance, and depression.

In addition to this more qualitative, open-ended approach to assessment, a number of quantitative measurement instruments are available to assess CRF (see Table 19-4). These instruments have been applied to the assessment of CRF in both medical and nursing research among patients with cancer. However, adoption of the use of these instruments has been limited in the clinical setting, although acceptable reliability and validity estimates have been established for the instruments. Barriers to use include lack of agreement on a "gold" standard for clinical use, the limited components of fatigue measured, the time burden on the patient and staff for completion and analysis of results, and the lack of a clear understanding of how the assessment results drive decisions about potential interventions.

To plan effective care for patients experiencing CRF, nurses, in collaboration with the healthcare team, must take the initiative to assess for the presence of CRF on a regular basis throughout the cancer experience. The use of a common method of assessment that

Figure 19-2. Instrumental and Self-Care Activities of Daily Living

Instrumental Activities of Daily Living	Self-Care Activities of Daily Living
Measure the patient's ability to perform tasks needed to live in the community independently (Graf, 2013): • Managing finances • Using transportation (driving or navigating public transit) • Shopping • Food preparation • Ability to use communication devices (i.e., telephone) • Managing medications • Housework and basic home maintenance, laundry	Measure the patient's ability to perform self-care activities of daily living independently (Shelkey & Wallace, 2012): • Feeding • Bathing • Dressing • Toileting • Transferring • Maintaining continence

Table 19-4. Selected Quantitative Measurement Instruments for Assessing Cancer-Related Fatigue

Instrument	Number of Items	Components Measured
Brief Fatigue Inventory (Mendoza et al., 1999)	9	Physical functioning
European Organisation for Research and Treatment of Cancer Quality of Life Questionnaire (EORTC QLQ-C30), fatigue subscale (Aaronson et al., 1993)	3	Fatigue and need for rest
Fatigue Symptom Inventory (Hann et al., 2000)	13	Physical and mental functioning
Functional Assessment of Cancer Therapy–Fatigue (Yellen et al., 1993)	9	Physical functioning
Lee's Visual Analogue Scale for Fatigue (Lee et al., 1999)	18	Fatigue and energy
Multidimensional Fatigue Symptom Inventory–Short Form (Stein et al., 2004)	30	Global, somatic, cognitive, affective, and behavioral
Profile of Mood States Fatigue/Inertia Subscale (McNair et al., 1971)	7	Physical functioning
Revised Piper Fatigue Scale (Piper et al., 1998)	22	Behavioral, severity, affective meaning, sensory, and cognitive/mood
Revised Schwartz Cancer Fatigue Scale (Schwartz, 1998)	6	Physical and perceptual

has established reliability and validity estimates among patients diagnosed with cancer and that bases the assessment on the perceptions of the patient is imperative for consistency in evaluation and planning of effective care. In the following section, evidence-based strategies for management of CRF will be discussed.

Planning Care for Patients at Risk for Cancer-Related Fatigue

Expectations of patients diagnosed with cancer and the relationships they develop with healthcare providers are contributing factors to outcomes of care. In planning care for patients at risk for CRF, oncology nurses work collaboratively with the healthcare team to develop a therapeutic, trusting, and supportive relationship with patients from the initial encounter.

One of the most important roles for the oncology nurse is in assisting patients to manage their expectations of CRF through providing evidence-based information about the incidence, onset, pattern, and duration of fatigue associated with specific treatments. Many resources are available to assist oncology nurses in providing information about CRF to patients (see Figure 19-3).

For example, patients receiving active treatment with chemotherapy commonly describe the onset and pattern of CRF as increasing in

Figure 19-3. Cancer-Related Fatigue Resources for Patients

- American Cancer Society: https://www.cancer.org/treatment/treatments-and-side-effects/physical-side-effects/fatigue.html
- Cancer.Net: www.cancer.net/navigating-cancer-care/side-effects/fatigue
- Livestrong Foundation: www.livestrong.org/we-can-help/finishing-treatment/fatigue
- National Cancer Institute: https://www.cancer.gov/about-cancer/treatment/side-effects/fatigue/fatigue-pdq
- National Comprehensive Cancer Network: www.nccn.org/patients/resources/life_with_cancer/managing_symptoms/fatigue.aspx
- Oncology Nursing Society Putting Evidence Into Practice—Patient Education: Fatigue, pages 44–45 in Mitchell et al., 2014: https://cjon.ons.org/cjon/18/6/supplement/putting-evidence-practice-update-evidence-based-interventions-cancer-related

severity immediately after receiving the treatment. CRF usually abates to some degree over the following weeks prior to the next course of treatment. Over time, the level of CRF increases and the recovery between treatments decreases, resulting in an increase in overall perceived severity unless an effective intervention is recommended and the patient adheres to the recommendation. Understanding these patterns of CRF can help patients have realistic expectations and effectively manage life during treatment.

Even after active chemotherapy treatment, CRF can continue to be a problem for patients for varying lengths of time. Patients should be encouraged to report fatigue that they experience, as well as any associated signs and symptoms that may contribute to CRF, at each encounter with the healthcare team. Patients also should report the impact of CRF on both instrumental (e.g., managing finances and medications, shopping, housework, maintenance, laundry) and self-care (e.g., feeding, bathing, toileting) activities of daily living (Graf, 2013; Shelkey & Wallace, 2012), quality of life, and the perceived effectiveness of recommended CRF-reducing strategies (see Figure 19-4).

The impact of CRF on activities of daily living requires assessment of the functional status of the patient and activity limitations. A CRF assessment also serves as a baseline for treatment planning and a measurement of the outcomes of CRF-reducing strategies. Ultimately, effective assessments will provide an evaluation of the patient's ability to safely maintain an independent living environment.

Interventions

Two basic categories of interventions for CRF exist: nonpharmacologic and pharmacologic. Recent systematic, meta-analytic reviews of the literature have detailed evidence on the effectiveness of selected interventions (Berger et al., 2015; Mitchell et al., 2014), which informed the Oncology Nursing Society Putting Evidence Into Practice recommendations (see www.ons.org/practice-resources/pep/fatigue).

Nonpharmacologic Interventions

Numerous research studies have been conducted on the use of nonpharmacologic strategies to modify the CRF experience among individuals with cancer. These interventions are particularly attractive for implementation by nurses in

Figure 19-4. Topics to Be Discussed With Patients When Assessing Cancer-Related Fatigue

- Onset, pattern, and duration
- Aggravating factors
- Alleviating factors
- Self-care strategies used and perceived effectiveness
- Impact on activities of daily living and instrumental activities of daily living
- Impact on quality of life

that they do not require prescriptive authority and have minimal associated adverse events. For nonpharmacologic interventions, the key issues in successful implementation are access to providers with specific skill sets to deliver the interventions, coverage of visits by third-party payers to allow mastery of the required self-care interventions, willingness of the patient to learn the associated self-care techniques, and commitment of the patient to adhere to the recommended program of care across the cancer experience until CRF abates to a tolerable level or resolves.

Physical Activity/Exercise

Implementation of a generalized activity/exercise intervention to manage CRF has been consistently recommended as effective across the cancer experience based on empirical evidence (e.g., NCCN guidelines, American Cancer Society recommendations). Although somewhat counterintuitive, activity/exercise helps to prevent deconditioning, especially during the active treatment period, and improves tolerance and endurance after treatment is completed. However, specificity in the recommended activity/exercise intervention continues to be problematic for clinicians as efforts are made to translate this evidence into practice (Berger et al., 2015; Mitchell et al., 2014; NCCN, 2016).

A number of different types of physical activity/exercise modalities have been prescribed and evaluated among patients with a variety of cancers, including breast, colon, and prostate cancer. The most common types of physical activity/exercise that have been evaluated are walking, swimming, cycling, and resistive exercises (Berger et al., 2015). Unfortunately, a lack of data to support the superior benefits of one type over another remains an issue for cancer care clinicians and researchers to determine. In addition, questions still remain regarding the frequency, duration, and intensity of physical activity/exercise that is optimal for individuals diagnosed with cancer (Berger et al., 2015; Mitchell et al., 2014). Multiple ongoing clinical trials are evaluating physical therapies to modify the effects of CRF (search for trials at https://clinicaltrials.gov).

One of the concerns in current clinical practice is the lack of referrals to experts within healthcare institutions and the community to manage CRF. Key to the initiation of any physical activity/exercise program for patients diagnosed with cancer is an evaluation of their current status (activity, tolerance, and endurance), which is best accomplished through a consultation with a physical therapist (NCCN, 2016). During the consultation, the physical therapist also can assess the types of activity the patient is most likely to adhere to; establish a progressive program starting with small, achievable goals; and gradually increase the duration and intensity of the physical activity/exercise over time. Once the plan is in place, the physician or nurse can evaluate the patient's adherence to the plan, as well as the perceived effectiveness of the intervention over time. If the patient has adhered to the plan but did not perceive it to be effective in modifying CRF, then reevaluation of the factors contributing to CRF is warranted.

The following nonpharmacologic CRF-reducing strategies have been the topics of numerous research studies: energy conservation, mind–body techniques, and psychoeducational interventions. Because of the lack of use of conceptual or theoretical CRF models, inconsistencies in conceptual and operational definitions of CRF, methodologic flaws, convenience sampling, small sample sizes, lack of control groups, and limited follow-up, consistency of the outcomes has been mixed. Therefore, these interventions have been categorized as likely to be effective (Mitchell et al., 2014).

Energy Conservation

Energy conservation techniques are another nonpharmacologic strategy that may be effective in modifying the experience of CRF. Such strategies include balancing activity and rest, setting priorities according to which activities are most important, delegating tasks, scheduling activities when energy levels are the greatest, and asking for help when needed (Mitchell et al., 2014). In addition to these general energy conservation techniques, consultation with occupational therapy may extend the specific strategies required to meet instrumental and self-care activities of daily living and promote independence.

Mind–Body Techniques

Mind–body techniques, such as the use of progressive muscle relaxation, relaxation breathing, guided imagery, meditation, mindfulness-based stress reduction, and hypnosis have been evaluated in multiple research studies and are likely to be effective in modifying CRF and a variety of contributing factors, such as depression, sleep disturbances, and pain (Berger et al., 2015; Mitchell et al., 2014). Mastery of teaching these techniques to patients is generally not included in undergraduate curricula in schools of nursing. Therefore, consultation with healthcare team members with this expertise, such as psychologists, physical and occupational therapists, and advanced practice nurses with specialized training, is warranted. Application of these interventions requires a commitment by the patient to learn and practice the new skills and ongoing evaluation as to the effectiveness of the techniques in modifying the CRF experience.

Psychoeducational Interventions

A number of psychoeducational interventions have been evaluated for modifying CRF (Berger et al., 2015; Mitchell et al., 2014). Many of the psychoeducational studies have included combined interventions such as anticipatory guidance, CRF management self-care such as energy conservation, goal setting, managing activity/rest balance, nutrition, and exercise. These educational interventions also focused on provision of coaching, emotional support, praise, and encouragement. Successful implementation requires individuals with adequate time and specific skills in conducting group and individual psychoeducational interventions. Referrals to appropriate members of the healthcare team are warranted.

Outcomes of psychoeducational interventions on modifying CRF have been mixed. Factors that limit overall assessment of the benefits include the use of multiple strategies, lack of detailed descriptions of the interventions, length of time for the interventions, short-term follow-up, lack of use of conceptual or theoretical models, and inconsistencies in the primary focus of the interventions on CRF. As with other nonpharmacologic strategies, these interventions have been evaluated as likely to be effective (Berger et al., 2015; Mitchell et al., 2014).

Other nonpharmacologic therapies have been evaluated for which insufficient evidence exists to support their use in modifying CRF. These include acupuncture, acupressure, massage, therapeutic touch, expressive writing, animal therapy, aromatherapy, reflexology, bright light therapy, tai chi, and qigong (Mitchell et al., 2014).

Pharmacologic Interventions

The use of pharmacologic interventions to manage CRF has been studied extensively. Agents evaluated have been grouped into three basic categories: agents to manage concurrent, contributing signs and symptoms associated with CRF (i.e., sleep deprivation, depression, pain, and anemia), psychostimulants, and anti-inflammatory agents. Because of the limited empirical data generated on the use of pharmacologic agents, inconsistent outcomes in modifying CRF, potential exacerbation of other signs and symptoms in the CRF symptom cluster (noted in italics in Table 19-5), and concerns about the risk-benefit ratio for use of selected agents (see Table 19-5), no pharmacologic agents have been evaluated as effective in treating CRF (Berger et al., 2015; Mitchell et al., 2014). To date, no pharmacologic agents have been approved by the U.S. Food and Drug Administration specifically for the treatment of CRF.

Other pharmacologic and nutritional agents have been evaluated and lack sufficient evidence to support their use to modify CRF. These agents include paroxetine, sertraline, venlafaxine, donepezil, bupropion, etanercept, infliximab, celecoxib, high-dose vitamin C, multiple vitamins, valerian, omega-3 fatty acid and protein supplements, and mistletoe (Mitchell et al., 2014).

Table 19-5. Risk-Benefit Concerns for Pharmacologic Agents to Modify Cancer-Related Fatigue

Type of Agent	Side Effects	Safety Concerns
Erythropoiesis-stimulating agents	Myalgia and arthralgia *Nausea* *Vomiting*	Hypertension Red cell aplasia Thrombosis • Stroke • Myocardial infarction Tumor progression
Glucocorticoids • Dexamethasone • Megestrol acetate • Prednisone	Chest pain *Depression* Dizziness Hypokalemia Hyperglycemia Hypertension Impotence *Insomnia* Irregular heart beat *Nausea* Peripheral edema Sudden numbness or weakness (unilateral) *Vomiting* Weight gain	Adrenal insufficiency Birth defects Drug interactions Glucose intolerance Thrombotic events
Psychostimulants • Dexmethylphenidate • Methylphenidate • Modafinil	*Agitation* Anorexia *Anxiety* Dry mouth Headache *Insomnia* *Nausea* *Nightmares* *Vomiting*	Cardiovascular events • Hypertension • Tachycardia Decreased efficacy of birth control pills Psychological dependence Psychoses

Note. Italics indicate cancer-related fatigue symptom cluster.

Patient-Centered Outcomes

Nurses have an important role in assessing, teaching, monitoring, supporting, and evaluating patients at risk for or experiencing CRF. Nurses across cancer care settings are able to assist patients to perform the following:

- Identify personal risk factors for experiencing CRF (disease, treatment, concurrent symptoms, lifestyle choices, socioeconomic and psychological factors).
- Describe the expected onset and pattern of CRF based on empirical data determined by disease, treatment modality, and phase of the cancer experience.
- Report the incidence, severity, concurrent symptoms, and impact of CRF on activities of daily living and quality of life at each encounter with the healthcare team.
- Commit to adherence to CRF-relieving self-care recommendations suggested by the multidisciplinary healthcare team (physicians, nurses, physical and occupational therapists, psychologists, social workers, palliative care team).
- Report on adherence to and the perceived effectiveness of CRF-relieving self-care strategies recommended by the healthcare team at each encounter.
- Access appropriate institutional and community resources to address identified needs and services to manage CRF, obtain assistance with activities of daily living, manage concurrent symptoms, and relieve suffering.

Conclusion

Cancer-related fatigue is a common problem experienced by a majority of patients diagnosed with cancer both during and after treatment. CRF is underreported, underdiagnosed, and undertreated. Patients should be encouraged to describe their experience of CRF and its effects on their ability to perform instrumental and self-care activities of daily living at each encounter with the healthcare team. Healthcare professionals should include a screening question about the presence and severity of CRF at each patient encounter. As the experience of CRF is subjective, the patient becomes the expert at diagnosing CRF, and based on that diagnosis, the healthcare team should attempt to elicit a comprehensive assessment of fatigue and intervene to modify the experience.

Limiting the ability to rationally approach the management of CRF is the lack of consensus related to a definition of CRF and knowledge regarding the etiology and pathophysiology of CRF. A variety of nonpharmacologic and pharmacologic approaches have been studied, yet only a single intervention, physicial activity/exercise, has been consistently determined to be effective in modifying the CRF experience among patients with cancer. A number of other nonpharmacologic approaches have been identified as likely to be effective, including energy conservation, mind–body techniques, and psychoeducational interventions. No pharmacologic interventions have shown consistent effectiveness in modifying CRF, and no agents are currently approved by the U.S. Food and Drug Administration for use in modifying CRF. In addition, many of the agents that have been evaluated have significant side effects and safety concerns that should be considered in a risk-benefit analysis before using in patients with CRF.

Continued research is needed to provide empirical data to identify the mechanisms of CRF and the effectiveness of both nonpharmacologic and pharmacologic interventions to modify the CRF experience among individuals with cancer. Use of conceptual and theoretical models of CRF and consistency in conceptual and operational definitions of CRF, research design, sampling methods, sample size, detailed descriptions of interventions, duration of interventions, and length of follow-up for effectiveness are recommended.

Finally, oncology nurses hold key positions in health care with potential to improve patient outcomes related to CRF. Beginning with the initial patient encounter and the development of a trusting nurse–patient relationship, nurses can provide consistent assessment of CRF and other cancer-related symptoms, provide education to meet the information needs of patients, evaluate adherence to and perceived effectiveness of CRF-modifying treatment regimens, and guide patients through the complexities of the CRF experience.

Key Points

- CRF is highly prevalent and distressing. It is also suspected to be underreported and poorly managed.
- The cause of CRF is currently unknown, but multiple pathways may be involved.
- Patient education regarding the anticipated pattern of CRF is critical in helping patients to manage expectations about the experience.
- Because CRF is a subjective phenomenon, patients are the experts in evaluating the symptom and its impact on activities of daily living and quality of life.
- Oncology nurses should include an assessment of CRF at each encounter during treatment and long-term survivorship.
- Adherence to a program that includes physical activity (cardiovascular, muscle strengthening, and stretching) is critical to ameliorate the effects of CRF.
- Access to multidisciplinary resources, such as physical and occupational therapists, nutritionists, and social workers, may be helpful to patients in managing CRF.

References

Aaronson, N.K., Ahmedzai, S., Bergman, B., Bullinger, M., Cull, A., Duez, N.J., ... Takeda, F. (1993). The European Organization for Research and Treatment of Cancer QLQ-C30: A quality-of-life instrument for use in international clinical trials in oncology. *Journal of the National Cancer Institute, 85,* 365–376. doi:10.1093/jnci/85.5.365

Abrahams, H.J.G., Gielissen, M.F.M., Schmits, I.C., Verhagen, C.A.H.H.V.M., Rovers, M.M., & Knoop, H. (2016). Risk factors, prevalence, and course of severe fatigue after breast cancer treatment: A meta-analysis involving 12 327 breast cancer survivors. *Annals of Oncology, 27,* 965–974. doi:10.1093/annonc/mdw099

Aktas, A., Walsh, D., & Rybicki, L. (2010). Review: Symptom clusters: Myth or reality? *Palliative Medicine, 24,* 373–385. doi:10.1177/0269216310367842

Barsevick, A.M. (2007). The concept of symptom cluster. *Seminars in Oncology Nursing, 23,* 89–98. doi:10.1016/j.soncn.2007.01.009

Barsevick, A.M., Frost, M., Zwinderman, A., Hall, P., Halyard, M., & GENEQOL Consortium. (2010). I'm so tired: Biological and genetic mechanisms of cancer-related fatigue. *Quality of Life Research, 19,* 1419–1427. doi:10.1007/s11136-010-9757-7

Barsevick, A.M., Whitmer, K., & Walker, L. (2001). In their own words: Using the common sense model to analyze patient descriptions of cancer-related fatigue. *Oncology Nursing Forum, 28,* 1363–1369.

Berger, A.M., Mitchell, S.A., Jacobsen, P.B., & Pirl, W.F. (2015). Screening, evaluation, and management of cancer-related fatigue: Ready for implementation to practice? *CA: A Cancer Journal for Clinicians, 65,* 190–211. doi:10.3322/caac.21268

Borneman, T., Koczywas, M., Sun, G.-Y., Piper, B.F., Uman, G., & Ferrell, B. (2010). Reducing patient barriers to pain and fatigue management. *Journal of Pain and Symptom Management, 39,* 486–501. doi:10.1016/j.jpainsymman.2009.08.007

Bower, J.E. (2014). Cancer-related fatigue: Mechanism, risk factors, and treatments. *Nature Reviews Clinical Oncology, 11,* 597–609. doi:10.1038/nrclinonc.2014.127

Bower, J.E., Bak, K., Berger, A., Breitbart, W., Escalante, C.P., Ganz, P.A., ... Jacobsen, P.B. (2014). Screening, assessment, and management of fatigue in adult survivors of cancer: An American Society of Clinical Oncology clinical practice guideline adaptation. *Journal of Clinical Oncology, 32,* 1840–1850. doi:10.1200/JCO.2013.53.4495

Bower, J.E., Ganz, P.A., Desmond, K.A., Bernaards, C., Rowland, J.H., Meyerowitz, B.E., & Belin, T.R. (2006). Fatigue in long-term breast carcinoma survivors. *Cancer, 106,* 751–758. doi:10.1002/cncr.21671

Cancer.Net. (2016). Fatigue. Retrieved from http://www.cancer.net/navigating-cancer-care/side-effects/fatigue

Cella, D., Lai, J., Chang, C., Peterman, A., & Slavin, M. (2002). Fatigue in cancer patients compared with fatigue in the general United States population. *Cancer, 94,* 528–538. doi:10.1002/cncr.10245

de Jong, N., Kester, A.D.M., Schouten, H.C., Abu-Saad, H.H., & Courtens, A.M. (2006). Course of fatigue between two cycles of adjuvant chemotherapy in breast cancer patients. *Cancer Nursing, 29,* 467–477. doi:10.1097/00002820-200611000-00007

Dhruva, A., Dodd, M., Paul, S.M., Cooper, B.A., Lee, K., West, C., ... Miaskowski, C. (2010). Trajectories of fatigue in patients with breast cancer before, during, and after radiation therapy. *Cancer Nursing, 33,* 201–212. doi:10.1097/NCC.0b013e3181c75f2a

Dong, S.T., Butow, P.N., Costa, D.S.J., Lovell, M.R., & Agar, M. (2014). Symptom clusters in patients with advanced cancer: A systematic review of observational studies. *Journal of Pain and Symptom Management, 48,* 411–450. doi:10.1016/j.jpainsymman.2013.10.027

Fatigue. (n.d.). In *Oxford dictionaries.* Retrieved from http://www.oxforddictionaries.com/us/definition/american_english/fatigue

Given, B.A., Given, C.W., Sikorskii, A., & Hadar, N. (2007). Symptom clusters and physical function for patients receiving chemotherapy. *Seminars in Oncology Nursing, 23,* 121–126. doi:10.1016/j.soncn.2007.01.005

Graf, C. (2013). The Lawton Instrumental Activities of Daily Living (IADL) Scale. *Try This: Best Practices in Nursing Care to Older Adults.* Retrieved from https://consultgeri.org/try-this/general-assessment/issue-23

Hann, D.M., Denniston, M.M., & Baker, F. (2000). Measurement of fatigue in cancer patients: Further validation of the Fatigue Symptom Inventory. *Quality of Life Research, 9,* 847–854. doi:10.1023/A:1008900413113

Honea, N., Brant, J., & Beck, S.L. (2007). Treatment-related symptom clusters. *Seminars in Oncology Nursing, 23,* 142–151. doi:10.1016/j.soncn.2007.01.002

Horneber, M., Fischer, I., Dimeo, F., Rüffer, J.U., & Weis, J. (2012). Cancer-related fatigue: Epidemiology, pathogenesis, diagnosis, and treatment. *Deutsches Arzteblatt International, 109,* 161–172. doi:10.3238/arztebl.2012.0161

Keeney, C.E., & Head, B.A. (2011). Palliative nursing care of the patient with cancer-related fatigue. *Journal of Hospice and Palliative Nursing, 13,* 270–280. doi:10.1097/njh.0b013e318221aa36

Kreissl, S., Mueller, H., Goergen, H., Mayer, A., Brillant, C., Behringer, K., ... Borchmann, P. (2016). Cancer-related fatigue in patients with and survivors of Hodgkin's lymphoma: A longitudinal study of the German Hodgkin Study Group. *Lancet Oncology, 17,* 1453–1462. doi:10.1016/S1470-2045(16)30093-6

Lee, K.A., Hicks, G., & Nino-Murcia, G. (1991). Validity and reliability of a scale to assess fatigue. *Psychiatry Research, 36,* 291–298. doi:10.1016/0165-1781(91)90027-M

McNair, D.M., Lorr, M., & Droppelman, L.F. (1971). *Manual for the Profile of Mood States.* San Diego, CA: Educational and Industrial Testing Service.

Mendoza, T.R., Wang, X.S., Cleeland, C.S., Morrissey, M., Johnson, B.A., Wendt, J.K., & Huber, S.L. (1999). The rapid assessment of fatigue severity in cancer patients: Use of the Brief Fatigue Inventory. *Cancer, 85,* 1186–1196. doi:10.1002/(SICI)1097-0142(19990301)85:5<1186::AID-CNCR24>3.0.CO;2-N

Minton, O., & Stone, P. (2009). A systematic review of the scales used for the measurement of cancer-related fatigue (CRF). *Annals of Oncology, 20,* 17–25. doi:10.1093/annonc/mdn537

Mitchell, S.A., Hoffman, A.J., Clark, J.C., DeGennaro, R.M., Poirier, P., Robinson, C.B., & Weisbrod, B.L. (2014). Putting evidence into practice: An update of evidence-based interventions for cancer-related fatigue during and following treatment. *Clinical Journal of Oncology Nursing, 18,* 38–58. doi:10.1188/14.CJON.S3.38-58

Nail, L.M. (2002). Fatigue in patients with cancer. *Oncology Nursing Forum, 29,* 537–546. doi:10.1188/ONF.537-546

National Cancer Institute. (n.d.). Fatigue. In *NCI dictionary of cancer terms.* Retrieved from https://www.cancer.gov/publications/dictionaries/cancer-terms?CdrID=321374

National Cancer Institute Cancer Therapy Evaluation Program. (2010). *Common terminology criteria for adverse events* [v.4.03]. Retrieved from http://evs.nci.nih.gov/ftp1/CTCAE/CTCAE_4.03_2010-06-14_QuickReference_8.5x11.pdf

National Comprehensive Cancer Network. (2016). *NCCN Clinical Practice Guidelines in Oncology (NCCN Guidelines®): Cancer-related fatigue* [v.1.2017]. Retrieved from https://www.nccn.org/professionals/physician_gls/pdf/fatigue.pdf

Olson, K., Krawchuk, A., & Quddusi, T. (2007). Fatigue in individuals with advanced cancer in active treatment and palliative settings. *Cancer Nursing, 30*(4), E1–E10. doi:10.1097/01.NCC.0000281736.25609.74

Piper, B.F., Dibble, S.L., Dodd, M.J., Weiss, M.C., Slaughter, R.E., & Paul, S.M. (1998). The revised Piper Fatigue Scale: Psychometric evaluation in women with breast cancer. *Oncology Nursing Forum, 25,* 677–684.

Prue, G., Rankin, J., Allen, J., Gracey, J., & Cramp, F. (2006). Cancer-related fatigue: A critical appraisal. *European Journal of Cancer, 42,* 846–863. doi:10.1016/j.ejca.2005.11.026

Radbruch, L., Strasser, F., Elsner, F., Gonçalves, J.F., Løge, J., Kaasa, S., ... Research Steering Committee of the European Association for Palliative Care (EAPC). (2008). Fatigue in palliative care patients—An EAPC approach. *Palliative Medicine, 22,* 13–32. doi:10.1177/0269216307085183

Roscoe, J.A., Morrow, G.R., Hickok, J.T., Mustian, K.M., Griggs, J.J., Matteson, S.E., ... Smith, B. (2005). Effect of paroxetine hydrochloride (Paxil®) on fatigue and depression in breast cancer patients receiving chemotherapy. *Breast Cancer Research and Treatment, 89,* 243–249. doi:10.1007/s10549-004-2175-1

Ryan, J.L., Carroll, J.K., Ryan, E.P., Mustian, K.M., Fiscella, K., & Morrow, G.R. (2007). Mechanisms of cancer-related fatigue. *Oncologist, 12*(Suppl. 1), 22–34. doi:10.1634/theoncologist.12-S1-22

Schwartz, A.L. (1998). The Schwartz Cancer Fatigue Scale: Testing reliability and validity. *Oncology Nursing Forum, 25,* 711–717.

Scott, J.A., Lasch, K.E., Barsevick, A.M., & Piault-Louis, E. (2011). Patients' experiences with cancer-related fatigue: A review and synthesis of qualitative research [Online exclusive]. *Oncology Nursing Forum, 38,* E191–E203. doi:10.1188/11.ONF.E191-E203

Servaes, P., Verhagen, C., & Bleijenberg, B. (2002). Fatigue in cancer patients during and after treatment: Prevalence, correlates and interventions. *European Journal of Cancer, 38,* 27–43. doi:10.1016/S0959-8049(01)00332-X

Shelkey, M., & Wallace, M. (2012). The Katz Index of Independence in Activities of Daily Living (ADL). *Try This: Best Practices in Nursing Care to Older Adults.* Retrieved from https://consultgeri.org/try-this/general-assessment/issue-2

Stasi, R., Abriani, L., Beccaglia, P., Terzoli, E., & Amadori, S. (2003). Cancer-related fatigue: Evolving concepts in evaluation and treatment. *Cancer, 98,* 1786–1801. doi:10.1002/cncr.11742

Stein, K.D., Jacobsen, P.B., Blanchard, C.M., & Thors, C. (2004). Further validation of the Multidimensional Fatigue Symptom Inventory–Short Form. *Journal of Pain and Symptom Management, 27,* 14–23. doi:10.1016/j.jpainsymman.2003.06.003

Stone, P.C., & Minton, O. (2008). Cancer-related fatigue. *European Journal of Cancer, 44,* 1097–1104. doi:10.1016/j.ejca.2008.02.037

Vogelzang, N.J., Breitbart, W., Cella, D., Curt, G.A., Groopman, J.E., Horning, S.J., ... Portenoy, R.K. (1997). Patient, caregiver, and oncologist perceptions of cancer-related fatigue: Results of a tripart assessment survey. The Fatigue Coalition. *Seminars in Hematology, 34*(3, Suppl. 2), 4–12.

Wang, X.S. (2008). Pathophysiology of cancer-related fatigue. *Clinical Journal of Oncology Nursing, 12*(Suppl. 5), 11–20. doi:10.1188/08.CJON.S2.11-20

Weis, J., & Horneber, M. (2015). *Cancer-related fatigue.* doi:10.1007/978-1-907673-76-4

Winningham, M.L. (2000). The puzzle of fatigue: How do you nail pudding to the wall? In M.L. Winningham &

M. Barton-Burke (Eds.), *Fatigue in cancer: A multidimensional approach* (pp. 3–29). Burlington, MA: Jones & Bartlett Learning.

Wu, H.-S., & McSweeney, M. (2007). Cancer-related fatigue: "It's so much more than just being tired." *European Journal of Oncology Nursing, 11,* 117–125. doi:10.1016/j.ejon.2006.04.037

Yellen, S.B., Cella, D.F., Webster, K., Blendowski, C., & Kaplan, E. (1997). Measuring fatigue and other anemia-related symptoms with the Functional Assessment of Cancer Therapy (FACT) measurement system. *Journal of Pain and Symptom Management, 13,* 63–74. doi:10.1016/S0885-3924(96)00274-6

Chapter 19 Study Questions

1. Cancer-related fatigue (CRF) is different from fatigue commonly experienced during both health and illness because:
   A. CRF occurs only after exertion.
   B. CRF is not related temporally to exertion.
   C. CRF is caused by cytokine dysregulation, which is not a fatigue pathway during health.
   D. CRF is only experienced during or immediately after cancer treatment.

2. The definition of CRF:
   A. Is clear and consistently understood among healthcare providers.
   B. Is based on rigorous research and a common measurement strategy.
   C. Varies based on the organization, but is consistently multidimensional and subjective.
   D. Always relates CRF to decreased functional status.

3. Based on currently available empirical evidence, the presence of which of the following signs and symptoms would the oncology nurse include in a comprehensive assessment of CRF?
   A. Fear
   B. Depression
   C. Anorexia
   D. Dyspnea

4. The oncology nurse is evaluating a patient who experienced CRF during a six-week course of radiation therapy. The patient states that he is worried about the effectiveness of the radiation because his fatigue has not improved since completing the treatment. Which of the following responses from the oncology nurse would be most appropriate?
   A. "Let's speak with the doctor about your continued fatigue after treatment."
   B. "Are you continuing your exercise program after completing the radiation?"
   C. "It is common for fatigue to continue after treatment, and many experience fatigue as a long-term effect."
   D. "Are there circumstances that make the fatigue worse?"

5. The oncology nurse is counseling a patient receiving cytotoxic therapy for lung cancer. Which of the following energy conservation recommendations may be recommended to address CRF?
   A. Wear clothing that closes with buttons versus a zipper.
   B. Take a tub bath rather than a shower each day.
   C. Wear shoes that lace and tie versus slip on.
   D. Ask for help with important instrumental activities of daily living.

CHAPTER

20 Gastrointestinal Symptoms

Elizabeth Prechtel Dunphy, DNP, CRNP, BC, AOCN®, and Suzanne Walker, CRNP, MSN, AOCN®, BC

Introduction

The gastrointestinal (GI) tract encompasses a large portion of the human body, extending from the mouth to the anus. Consequently, this organ system provides a vast surface area for cancer-related complications to occur. GI symptoms may develop in patients with cancer for a variety of reasons, including the underlying cancer or as treatment-related sequelae. This chapter will explore commonly occurring GI toxicities in patients with cancer, including prevention and management strategies.

Xerostomia

Xerostomia is defined as a dry mouth due to reduced or absent saliva caused by damage to the salivary glands (Bhide, Miah, Harrington, Newbold, & Nutting, 2009). It can be caused by treatments such as surgery, chemotherapy, and radiation. Xerostomia can affect patients' quality of life. The impact will vary with the degree of dryness (Carr, 2018). To understand the implications of and treatments for xerostomia, it helps to understand its pathophysiology.

Pathophysiology

Saliva is an important host defense component of the oral cavity. Major salivary glands (the parotid, submandibular, and sublingual glands) contribute to most of the secretion volume and electrolyte content of saliva, accounting for 90% of saliva production, whereas minor salivary glands contribute little secretion volume (Dalton & Gosselin, 2014; Pinna, Campus, Cumbo, Mura, & Milia, 2015). Ninety percent of saliva is composed of water. Saliva has antimicrobial, digestive, antacid, lubricating, and homeostatic properties. Saliva aids in the clearance of sugars and carbohydrates, inhibits enamel decalcification, and provides an excretory route for blood-borne urea, uric acid, ammonia, and thiocyanate (Bruce, 2004). Figure 20-1 summarizes the functions of saliva. The parotid cells have a low mitotic rate. This, along with the parotid being a radiosensitive gland, contributes to the permanent damage that can be caused by radiation, leading to little or no saliva production. Salivary flow decreases

Figure 20-1. Functions of Saliva

- Antifungal activity
- Antimicrobial activity
- Buffering activity
- Digestion
- Homeostatic activity
- Inhibition of enamel decalcification
- Lubrication

Note. Based on information from Bruce, 2004.

by 50%–70% from baseline after 10–16 Gy of radiation (Bhide et al., 2009).

Signs and Symptoms

Oral dryness can cause functional alterations, such as speech and swallowing difficulties, taste alterations, glossodynia (burning sensation of the tongue), and cheilitis (inflamed lips and tongue). Dry mouth can cause a gagging sensation with fear of choking for the patient and difficulty or painful swallowing. Xerostomia can cause periodontal disease. Halitosis can occur because of food stagnation, drug therapy, or oral tissue damage. Xerostomia also can promote oral infections (Dalton & Gosselin, 2014; Pinna et al., 2015). These factors can cause reduced nutritional intake, weight loss, and significantly altered general health and quality of life. Acute xerostomia often results from chemotherapy, whereas permanent xerostomia is a result of surgery or radiation therapy.

Assessment and Diagnosis

The oral mucosa should be carefully inspected for infection, quality of saliva, cheilitis, and dental caries. Two grading scales can be used to assess and describe xerostomia: the National Cancer Institute (NCI) Cancer Therapy Evaluation Program's (CTEP's) Common Terminology Criteria for Adverse Events (CTCAE) and the Radiation Therapy Oncology Group (RTOG) scale. NCI CTEP uses the CTCAE grading criteria for adverse events related to cancer treatments. These grading criteria provide a means for all nurses and providers to assess the degree of xerostomia experienced by a patient at each clinic visit and to consistently document that assessment. The CTCAE defines dry mouth as "a disorder characterized by reduced salivary flow in the oral cavity" (NCI CTEP, 2010, p. 33). Grade 1 dry mouth is where the patient is symptomatic with dry or thick saliva without significant dietary alteration, and unstimulated saliva flow is greater than 0.2 ml/min. With grade 2 dry mouth, the patient experiences moderate symptoms and has oral intake alterations, such as copious water, other lubricants, and diet limited to pureed or soft, moist foods, with unstimulated saliva flow of 0.1–0.2 ml/min. Grade 3 dry mouth often leads to the inability to adequately take oral nutrition; tube feeding or total parenteral nutrition is indicated, and unstimulated saliva flow is less than 0.1 ml/min (NCI CTEP, 2010).

The RTOG scale also is often used to describe xerostomia (Cox, Stetz, & Pajak, 1995). The RTOG scale grades reactions from 0 to 4. Grade 0 xerostomia indicates no change in baseline salivary production or characteristics. Grade 1 xerostomia is characterized by mild mouth dryness, slightly thickened saliva, and a slight alteration in taste, but no alteration in baseline oral intake. Grade 2 xerostomia is described as moderate to complete oral dryness; thick, sticky saliva; and markedly altered taste. No description is given for grade 3 xerostomia. Grade 4 xerostomia results in acute salivary gland necrosis.

Management

Therapies to prevent radiation-induced xerostomia include the use of cytoprotectants, sialagogues, and salivary gland–sparing radiation therapy techniques.

Amifostine (Ethyol®) is approved by the U.S. Food and Drug Administration (FDA) to decrease the rate and severity of acute and chronic xerostomia (Brizel et al., 2000; Cumberland Pharmaceuticals Inc., 2016). It is a cytoprotectant, a free radical scavenger that is metabolized to free thiol. Amifostine is administered intravenously to reduce the incidence of moderate to severe dry mouth in patients undergoing postoperative radiation therapy for head and neck cancer where the radiation treatment field (port) includes a substantial portion of the parotid glands.

The American Society of Clinical Oncology (ASCO) clinical practice guidelines (Hensley et al., 2009) recommend amifostine to decrease the incidence of acute and late xerostomia in patients undergoing fractionated radiation therapy alone for head and neck cancer. However, the current data do not support the routine use of amifostine with concurrent radiation therapy and platinum-based chemotherapy for head and neck cancer. The approved dose of amifostine is 910 mg/m^2 IV given over 15 minutes. Common toxicities associated with amifostine include acute hypotension, nausea, vomiting, and allergic reactions (Bhide et al., 2009).

Sialagogues increase the flow of saliva and require residual salivary function (Guchelaar, Vermes, & Meerwaldt, 1997). These saliva substitutes are designed to mimic the lubricating, hydrating, and antimicrobial properties of natural saliva (Radvansky, Pace, & Siddiqui, 2013). Pilocarpine is a sialagogic agent that is FDA-approved for radiation-induced xerostomia. Pilocarpine acts as a muscarinic-cholinergic agonist with mild beta-adrenergic activity. Witsell, Stinnett, and Chambers (2012) randomized patients receiving radiation therapy to the head and neck (greater than 40 Gy and including at least three major salivary glands) to receive cevimeline 30 mg or placebo three times daily for six weeks. They found no statistically significant differences in oral health or quality of life; however, during the six weeks of the study, the severity of xerostomia decreased from baseline in the cevimeline group. Pilocarpine is also used in a topical preparation, a lozenge. The lozenge had fewer systemic side effects than the oral tablets (Lovelace, Fox, Sood, Nguyen, & Day, 2014). Pilocarpine is associated with more side effects than the artificial saliva.

Furness, Worthington, Bryan, Birchenough, and McMillan (2011) reviewed interventions for the management of dry mouth, specifically topical therapies. Both integrated mouth care systems (toothpaste plus gel plus mouthwash) and oral reservoir devices showed promising results, but evidence was insufficient to recommend their use. Chewing gum was associated with increased saliva production in the majority of those with residual capacity, but no evidence demonstrated that gum was more or less effective than saliva substitutes (Furness et al., 2011).

Three-dimensional (3-D) intensity-modulated radiation therapy can provide a dose distribution that more accurately conforms to the 3-D configuration of the target volume, delivering a higher dose to the target area and sparing normal tissue. This potentially can deliver a lower dose of radiation to the parotid glands, decreasing the severity of xerostomia (Bhide et al., 2009). Furness, Bryan, McMillan, Birchenough, and Worthington (2013) conducted a systematic review evaluating acupuncture in treatment of patients with salivary hypofunction. They determined that low-quality evidence supported that acupuncture is no different from placebo in improving dry mouth symptoms.

Nursing Implications

Nurses should advise patients to receive dental care before the initiation of radiation therapy to the head and neck areas. They should teach patients with residual salivary gland function to drink fluids or try other agents that may stimulate salivary secretion, such as sugarless gums or lozenges. Patients should be instructed to avoid mouth-drying medications, such as tricyclic antidepressants, selective serotonin reuptake inhibitors, antihistamines, and narcotic analgesics. Other measures to manage radiation-induced xerostomia include the use of prescription fluoride to maximize oral hygiene, antimicrobials to prevent caries and infection, and saliva substitutes to relieve dryness.

Xerostomia associated with chemotherapy generally is temporary, whereas xerostomia associated with radiation often is permanent. ASCO recommendations (Hensley et al., 2009) for the treatment of radiation-induced xerostomia can be used to help affected patients. Currently, no guidelines exist for the treatment of chemotherapy-induced xerostomia. Further research is needed to develop more effective treatment strategies.

Mucositis

Mucositis can affect the mucous membranes of the GI tract from the mouth through the rectum. Oral mucositis, also known as *stomatitis,* is an inflammation and ulcerative reaction of the oral cavity mucosa. Mucositis that occurs in the esophagus is termed *esophagitis. Gastroenteritis* is mucositis that occurs in the intestine. This section will focus on oral mucositis or stomatitis. Oral mucositis can lead to chemotherapy and radiation therapy dose reductions and delays in treatment that can affect a patient's response to therapy. Oral mucositis disrupts the function and integrity of the oral cavity, which affects functional status and quality of life. The incidence and severity vary among patient populations. The mucositis from radiation can vary with the location treated, the depth and volume treated, the number of treatments, and the frequency of the treatment (Lalla, Bowen, et al., 2014; Wujcik, 2014).

Pathophysiology

The mucosal membranes proliferate with a high turnover rate, which makes them at risk for trauma or injury. Sonis et al. (2004) proposed that oral mucositis develops as a result of microvascular injury and connective tissue damage to the submucosa. This is followed by damage to the epithelial stem cells of the oral cavity caused by chemotherapy and radiation therapy. Many chemotherapy agents cause damage at the cellular level and are not able to differentiate between normal cells and cancer cells. Table 20-1 lists the chemotherapy agents, biologics, and targeted therapies that can cause mucositis.

Sonis (2007) described five phases of mucosal injury: initiation, upregulation with the generation of messengers, signaling and

Table 20-1. Chemotherapy, Biologics, and Targeted Therapies That Can Cause Mucositis

Type of Agent	Agent
Chemotherapy	Bleomycin Busulfan Capecitabine Cyclophosphamide Cytarabine Decitabine Docetaxel Doxorubicin Doxorubicin hydrochloride liposome injection Epirubicin hydrochloride Eribulin mesylate 5-Fluorouracil Floxuridine Gemcitabine hydrochloride Idarubicin Methotrexate Mitomycin Mitoxantrone Nelarabine Paclitaxel Pemetrexed Temozolomide Thioguanine Vinblastine Vinorelbine
Targeted therapy	Ado-trastuzumab emtansine Cabozantinib Cetuximab Crizotinib Erlotinib Everolimus Ibrutinib Panitumumab Ponatinib Temsirolimus Trametinib
Biologic therapy	Aldesleukin (interleukin-2) Interferon alfa

Note. Based on information from Wilkes & Barton-Burke, 2016.

amplification, ulceration with inflammation, and healing. In the initiation phase, chemotherapy and radiation therapy initiate mucositis directly by causing DNA strand breaks, and generation of reactive oxygen species (ROS) occurs. ROS directly damage cells, tissues, and blood vessels by causing DNA damage, which can lead to cell death. Stimulation of transcription factors in response to the ROS also occurs. During the second phase, multiple events occur simultaneously. Transcription factors, such as nuclear factor-κB, are activated in response to the ROS. Upregulation of genes occurs, which produces proinflammatory cytokines, such as tumor necrosis factor-alpha, that cause cellular injury and apoptosis. The upregulation of other genes activates the cyclooxygenase-2 pathway, leading to angiogenesis. In the third phase, signaling and amplification, proinflammatory cytokines amplify the injury started by the chemotherapy and radiation, biologically altering the tissue even though it may appear normal. The development of an ulcer occurs in the fourth phase, and angiogenesis and bacterial colonization can occur. Other consequences of this phase are further cytokine amplification, inflammation, and pain. The fifth, and last, phase is healing. Healing occurs with a signal from the extracellular matrix and leads to a renewal of epithelial proliferation, differentiation, and the reestablishment of local microbial flora.

Signs and Symptoms

Patient risk factors for developing oral mucositis include the patient's age, malignancy type (patients with head and neck cancer and esophageal cancer are at highest risk), oral condition prior to treatment, current oral hygiene practices, exposure to tobacco and alcohol, and nutritional status (Wujcik, 2014). Other risk factors include sex (women have a greater risk than men) (Sonis & Fey, 2002), genetic predisposition, and comorbidities. Treatment factors include the location of the head and neck mucosa being irradiated, the surface area and volume of treatment, the fractionation of radiation, and the concurrent chemotherapy agent and schedule (Wujcik, 2014).

Physical symptoms of oral mucositis may vary and can include the following (Wujcik, 2014):

- A change in mucosa color: pallor, erythema, white patches, and discolored lesions or ulcers
- A change in the moistness of the oral cavity, or change in the saliva texture and quantity
- Foul odor and a change in the color of the teeth
- Changes in the integrity of the oral mucosa: cracks, fissures, ulcers, or blisters
- A change in taste
- A change in the voice quality (hoarseness), tone, and strength
- Difficulty swallowing, pain, burning, or stinging

Assessment and Diagnosis

Nurses should do a thorough job of assessing patients before treatment begins and as it continues. Various scales are used to assess and grade mucositis (see Table 20-2).

Oral assessment using a validated tool should be conducted regularly in patients who are at risk for or already experiencing mucositis. McGuire, Correa, Johnson, and Wienandts (2006), as part of the Mucositis Study Group of the Multinational Association of Supportive Care in Cancer (MASCC) and the International Society of Oral Oncology (ISOO), recommended that a multidisciplinary approach involving the nurse, the physician, a dentist, a dental hygienist, a dietitian, and a pharmacist would be the most effective and comprehensive way to manage patients with oral mucositis. Most assessment tools use a variety of scales to grade the toxicity of mucositis but do not include measures of the effectiveness of interventions. Additional assessments of patients with cancer with mucositis include vital signs (heart rate, blood pressure, temperature, and pain) and a complete blood count (CBC). Initially, patients present with erythema of the oral mucosa. This can progress to erosion and frank ulceration. It typically occurs 7–14 days after initiation of chemotherapy and heals within a few weeks after the end of chemotherapy. In patients receiving radiation for the head and neck, the onset of mucositis occurs by the second or third week of therapy. Severity can

Table 20-2. Common Mucositis Assessment and Grading Scales

Title/Year	Rating Scale
Common Terminology Criteria for Adverse Events (National Cancer Institute Cancer Therapy Evaluation Program, 2010)	Mucositis oral definition: "A disorder characterized by inflammation of the oral mucosa" (p. 45) 1 = Asymptomatic or mild symptoms; intervention not indicated 2 = Moderate pain; not interfering with oral intake; modified diet indicated 3 = Severe pain; interfering with oral intake 4 = Life-threatening consequences; urgent intervention indicated 5 = Death
Oral Assessment Guide (Eilers et al., 1988)	1 = Normal 2 = Altered, but no loss of function or barrier breakdown 3 = Loss of function or barrier breakdown
Oral Mucosa Rating Scale (Kolbinson et al., 1988)	0 = Normal 3 = Severe Evaluates atrophy, erythema, ulceration, and pseudomembranous, hyperkeratotic, lichenoid, and edematous changes
Oral Mucositis Assessment Scale (Sonis et al., 1999)	0 = No erythema 2 = Severe erythema, ulceration, pseudomembrane formation Includes measurement of lesions from 0 (no lesion) to 3 (more than 3 cm lesion)
Oral Mucositis Index (McGuire et al., 2002; Schubert et al., 1992)	0 = None 3 = Severe Evaluates atrophy, ulceration, erythema, and edema
Radiation Therapy Oncology Group (Cox et al., 1995)	0 = No change over baseline 1 = Injection; may experience mild pain not requiring analgesic 2 = Patchy mucositis that may produce an inflammatory serosanguinous discharge; may experience moderate pain requiring analgesia 3 = Confluent fibrinous mucositis; may include severe pain requiring narcotics 4 = Ulceration, hemorrhage, or necrosis
Western Consortium for Cancer Nursing Research stomatitis staging system (Colson et al., 1998)	0 = No lesions; pink mucosa; no bleeding 1 = 1–4 lesions; slightly red mucosa; no bleeding 2 = More than 4 lesions; moderately red mucosa; bleeding occurs with eating and performing oral hygiene 3 = Lesions are coalescing; very red mucosa; spontaneous bleeding
World Health Organization (1979) grading scale	0 = None 1 = Soreness with or without erythema 2 = Erythema, ulcers; able to swallow food 3 = Ulcers with extensive erythema; cannot swallow food 4 = Oral intake not possible

worsen with continued therapy. Oral mucositis occurring with radiation therapy usually lasts for several weeks after therapy completion (Lalla, Saunders, & Peterson, 2014).

Complications of Mucositis

Complications of mucositis include pain, infection, and bleeding. The major complaint of patients with mucositis is pain. The pain can affect a patient's oral hygiene because the patient may not be able to perform adequate mouth care. Impaired swallowing affects the patient's nutritional status and ability to take oral medications. Patients may need to be given their medications via alternate routes and may require both topical and systemic treatments for the pain associated with mucositis. Mucositis pain often is treated with opioids. Patients who have difficulty swallowing because of mucositis may benefit from transdermal fentanyl.

Bar et al. (2010) evaluated the use of gabapentin for the treatment of pain syndrome related to radiation-induced mucositis in patients with head and neck cancer treated with chemoradiation. Gabapentin was initiated in the second week of radiation, and opiates were prescribed in addition to gabapentin as clinically indicated to obtain adequate pain control. They found that only 33% of the patients receiving gabapentin required additional low-dose narcotic medications for pain control during the third and fourth week of treatment, despite exhibiting a grade 2 or higher mucositis. One patient required a treatment interruption during the trial. The use of gabapentin is promising in reducing the need for high total doses of opioids and avoiding unplanned treatment interruptions for patients with head and neck malignancies treated with concurrent chemoradiation who develop mucositis.

A second complication is infection. Prevention is most effective to avoid infection. Bacterial, viral, or fungal infections can occur. A patient should have a culture of the suspicious lesion or area if an infection is suspected. In patients who are neutropenic, fever may be an unusual presentation. Cultures allow the offending agent to be identified and treated accordingly. Antibiotics effective against the offending bacteria should be administered. Fungal infections that commonly occur include *Candida* and *Aspergillus*. Viral infections, including herpes simplex (HSV) and cytomegalovirus, also may develop, with HSV occurring most frequently. *Candida* and HSV infections occur most frequently in patients with oral mucositis (Lalla, Saunders, et al., 2014).

Management

The management of mucositis can vary greatly. Eilers et al. (2016) reviewed the literature as part of the Putting Evidence Into Practice (PEP) initiative of the Oncology Nursing Society (ONS). They developed evidence-based interventions for the management of oral mucositis. They noted that oral care is the foundation for maintaining mucosal health, function, and integrity. They reviewed the basic components of an oral care regimen/protocol, assessment, patient education, and treatment strategies. The core elements described by the ONS PEP team were recommendations that clinicians collaborate with a multidisciplinary team in all phases of treatment, conduct a systematic assessment daily or at each patient visit (in the outpatient setting, this includes teaching patients to perform a daily assessment and report findings to the clinician), provide written instruction and education to patients regarding oral care, and verify patients' understanding. The ONS PEP recommendations for practice include cryotherapy, low-level laser therapy, oral care protocols, palifermin, and sodium bicarbonate rinses (Eilers et al., 2016). These will be reviewed further in this section. The most current practice recommendations can be found at www.ons.org/practice-resources/pep/mucositis.

In 2014, MASCC and ISOO published guidelines for the treatment of oral mucositis in patients with cancer (Lalla, Bowen, et al., 2014). They recommended the following preventive interventions for oral mucositis, suggesting that strong evidence supports their effectiveness:

- Thirty minutes of oral cryotherapy in patients receiving bolus 5-fluorouracil
- Palifermin for three days prior to conditioning treatment and three days after transplant for patients receiving high-dose chemotherapy and total body irradiation followed by autologous hematopoietic stem cell transplantation (HSCT) for a hematologic malignancy
- Low-level laser therapy in patients receiving HSCT conditioned with high-dose chemotherapy with or without total body irradiation
- Patient-controlled analgesia with morphine to treat pain due to oral mucositis in patients undergoing HSCT
- Benzydamine mouthwash in patients with head and neck cancer receiving moderate-dose radiation (up to 50 Gy) without concomitant chemotherapy

They provided the following preventive interventions for oral mucositis, suggesting that effective but weaker evidence supports their effectiveness:

- Oral care products in all age groups and across all cancer treatment modalities
- Oral cryotherapy in patients receiving high-dose melphalan with or without total body irradiation as conditioning for HSCT
- Low-level laser therapy in patients undergoing radiation therapy with or without concomitant chemotherapy for head and neck cancer
- Transdermal fentanyl to treat pain in patients receiving conventional or high-dose chemotherapy with or without total body irradiation
- 2% morphine mouthwash to treat pain
- 0.5% doxepin mouthwash to treat pain
- Systemic zinc supplement administered orally in patients with oral cancer who are receiving radiation therapy or chemoradiation

Palifermin is recommended for practice per the most recent ONS PEP guidelines (Eilers et al., 2016). Palifermin is a recombinant human keratinocyte growth factor-1. It binds to the receptor found on epithelial cells, including the tongue and buccal mucosa. It stimulates the proliferation, differentiation, and migration of epithelial cells. Palifermin decreases the incidence and duration of severe mucositis in patients with hematologic malignancies who undergo high-dose chemotherapy and radiation therapy with stem cell rescue. The dose is 60 mcg/kg/day as an IV bolus for three consecutive days before and three days after myelotoxic therapy for a total of six doses. The third pretreatment dose should be given 24–48 hours before therapy. The first post-treatment dose is given on the same day stem cell infusion is completed and at least four days after the most recent administration of palifermin (Wilkes & Barton-Burke, 2016).

Cryotherapy is also recommended for practice per the most recent ONS PEP guidelines (Eilers et al., 2016). It involves the use of ice chips. The ice chips cause local vasoconstriction, causing a decreased exposure of the oral mucosa to cytotoxic agents. A Cochrane review by Riley et al. (2015) indicated that ice chips may be beneficial in preventing or reducing the severity of mucositis in patients treated with 5-fluorouracil given as a bolus because of its short half-life. In the trials reviewed in the Cochrane report, ice chips were given before, during, and after chemotherapy administration. The duration of cryotherapy has not been defined and needs further evaluation. This can often be difficult to use when patients are receiving oxaliplatin with the bolus 5-fluorouracil because of the cold dysesthesia associated with oxaliplatin.

Low-level laser therapy involves the use of a handheld infrared laser in an attempt to affect cells and physical symptoms often related to inflammation. Carvalho et al. (2011) evaluated the use of low-level laser therapy in prevention and treatment of radiation-induced mucositis in patients with head and neck cancer. They found that the low-dose laser therapy delayed the development of mucositis and decreased the severity and pain associated with mucositis. Arbabi-Kalati, Arbabi-Kalati, and Moridi (2013) evaluated the effect of a low-level laser on prevention of chemotherapy-induced mucositis. They found that 8.3% of patients treated in the laser group experienced grade 2 mucositis, whereas 91.6% of those in the control group developed grade 2 or higher mucositis. In addition, the pain levels were lower in the treatment group. Additional research needs to be done to determine the most effective schedule and dose for low-level laser therapy.

Rinses are recommended to remove loose debris and aid with oral hydration. Bland rinses include 0.9% saline rinses (normal saline), sodium bicarbonate, and a saline and sodium bicarbonate mixture. Patients should rinse, swish solution in the oral cavity, and expectorate four times a day. Although oral hygiene should include brushing, flossing, and rinsing, commercial mouthwashes with alcohol should be avoided because they can be drying (Eilers, Harris, Henry, & Johnson, 2014).

Other interventions for mucositis for which effectiveness has not been established include allopurinol, anti-inflammatory rinses, antimicrobial agents, flurbiprofen tooth patches, granulocyte–colony-stimulating factor, granulocyte macrophage–colony-stimulating factor, immunoglobulin, L-alanyl-L-glutamine, low-level laser therapy, multiagent ("magic" or "miracle") rinses, oral aloe vera, pilocarpine, oral povidone-iodine, and tetracaine. A complete list of interventions for mucositis for which the effectiveness has not been established can be found at www.ons.org/practice-resources/pep/mucositis (Eilers et al., 2016).

Nursing Implications

After reviewing the literature, McGuire et al. (2006), as part of the MASCC Oral Care Study Group, identified three main topics in the management of oral care and clinical practice principles: pain management, oral assessment and oral care, and dental care. In addition, they made two other recommendations based on expert opinion. The first is that patients and families should receive education in all areas of oral care. Second, outcome assessment using quality improvement processes should be included to evaluate the recommended oral care protocols on a regular basis.

MASCC, ISOO, ASCO, and ONS have published guidelines to prevent and treat oral mucositis as outlined previously. Good oral hygiene is the basic tenet to prevent and decrease the incidence of oral mucositis. Interventions to treat mucositis are often palliative in nature—barrier protectants, topical antimicrobials, analgesics, and ice.

Patient education is key to the management of mucositis (see Figure 20-2). Patients need to be provided with information about mucositis, its cause, and its relation to chemotherapy and radiation therapy. They also need to be taught the importance of oral hygiene and maintenance of mucous membrane integrity. Oral hygiene during and after radiation therapy will reduce the risk for dental complications, including caries, infections, gingivitis, and osteoradionecrosis.

Dysphagia

Dysphagia is the medical term used to describe any difficulty that people experience when swallowing. It often is subjective. Dysphagia is described as the sensation of delay in passage of a food bolus within 10 seconds of swallowing (Javle et al., 2006; Johnson, 2001). Three different types of dysphagia exist: transfer, transit, and obstructive. Transfer dysphagia occurs with alteration in oral–pharyngeal bolus transfer. Transit dysphagia is classified by the absence of primary and secondary esophageal peristalsis. Obstructive dysphagia results from mechanical stenosis in the pharynx, esophagus, or esophagogastric junction. Esophageal stricture can result from extrinsic or intrinsic tumor compression. Intrinsic narrowing can

Figure 20-2. ONS Putting Evidence Into Practice Patient Education: Mouth Care During Cancer Treatment

The mouth, also called the oral cavity, is often the site of changes from cancer and cancer treatment. These changes can vary from minimal to severe and painful.

One of these changes is called "mucositis" (mu – ko – si – tis). The term *mucositis* means an inflammation of the mucous membranes. It can occur in the mouth and the rest of the gastrointestinal tract. This includes your esophagus, stomach, bowel, and rectum. You may see or feel changes. These changes can include the following.

- Deep or raspy voice: may be like when you have a sore throat or loss of your voice
- Pain when you swallow: may be mild to severe
- Dry or cracked lips: may include bleeding
- Coated and/or shiny tongue: may blister or crack
- Altered taste in your mouth and as you eat
- Thick or rope-like saliva and/or loss of saliva
- Reddened tender mouth: may have no sores or open sores with bleeding
- Swollen gums or bleeding

You may have some but not all of these changes. Also, how intense each of the changes is may vary.

What You Can Do to Make a Difference

Care of your mouth is important during cancer treatment. It can help to prevent and treat problems.
Good mouth care includes:

- Brush your teeth at least two times per day.
- Brush all tooth surfaces for at least 90 seconds using a soft toothbrush.
- Allow your toothbrush to dry before storing.
- Continue to floss your teeth at least daily. Speak with your nurse if you have not been doing this.
- Rinse your mouth at least four times per day.
- Use a bland, alcohol-free rinse.
- You may use a mixture of a little salt and baking soda in a cup of warm water for your rinse.
- Rinse your mouth more often (every two hours while awake) if you have sores or other problems.
- Keep your lips moist using a lip moisturizer of your choice. Avoid petroleum-based products or products that cause your lips to burn or feel dry. Select a moisturizing lip balm available "over the counter" through your local pharmacy.
- Avoid tobacco, alcohol, and irritating foods (hot, rough, acidic, or spicy).

If you develop problems:

- Tell your doctor or nurse.
- Continue to brush your teeth with a soft toothbrush if you can.
- Use a soft foam toothette to clean the entire inside of your mouth. Dip these in the salt and baking soda mixture.
- Take your pain medications as ordered by your doctor.

When to call your doctor or nurse:

- If you have symptoms of an infection such as fever, chills, or white patches in your mouth
- If you develop new or more severe mouth pain
- If you are not able to eat or drink
- Before you go to the dentist or have dental work done

A limited number of other treatments may be available, so check with your doctor or nurse. Always check with them before using any "natural" or other product you can purchase without a specific order.

Note. From "Evidence-Based Interventions for Cancer Treatment–Related Mucositis: Putting Evidence Into Practice," by J. Eilers, D. Harris, K. Henry, and L.A. Johnson, 2014, *Clinical Journal of Oncology Nursing, 18*(Suppl. 6), p. 87. Copyright 2014 by Oncology Nursing Society. Reprinted with permission.

be caused by tumor or can be a result of treatment, including radiation and surgery. Extrinsic compression can be caused by lymphadenopathy or tumor (Camp-Sorrell, 2014).

Obstructive dysphagia is seen most often in patients with cancer, especially esophageal cancer. In esophageal cancer, the tumor often blocks the esophageal lumen, preventing the passage of food (Camp-Sorrell, 2014). Obstructive dysphagia also can result from treatment-induced fibrosis or a postoperative stricture. In patients with esophageal cancer, dysphagia occurs late, when 80%–90% of the lumen is occluded (Javle et al., 2006). After esophagectomy, fibrotic strictures can develop that cause dysphagia. Patients who experience obstructive dysphagia are at risk for weight loss, malnutrition, and aspiration. Dysphagia is a distressing symptom for patients and can greatly affect their quality of life (Camp-Sorrell, 2014).

Pathophysiology

Dysphagia occurs as a result of interruption in the phases of swallowing. The phases of swallowing include the oral preparatory phase, the oral phase, the pharyngeal phase, and the esophageal phase. The oral preparatory phase occurs while processing the food bolus for swallowing. It is followed by the oral phase, in which the food from the oral cavity is propelled into the oropharynx with the tongue. The pharyngeal phase involves overlapping events starting with the swallowing reflex. The soft palate elevates the hyoid bone, the larynx moves upward and forward, the vocal cords move to midline, the epiglottis folds backward to protect the airway, and the tongue pushes backward and downward into the pharynx to propel the food bolus forward. The upper esophageal sphincter relaxes, opens, and closes after the food passes. The final phase is the esophageal phase. In the esophageal phase, the food bolus moves downward by a peristaltic motion beginning at the pharynx with the swallow reflex and continuing into the esophagus. The lower esophageal sphincter relaxes and the food bolus is propelled into the stomach, which completes the swallowing process (Camp-Sorrell, 2014).

Risk factors are associated with the development of dysphagia. These include head and neck cancer, esophageal cancer, radiation to the salivary glands causing xerostomia, infection (fungal, bacterial, or viral), cranial nerve neuropathy from tumor or chemotherapy, tracheotomy, odynophagia, stroke, poor dentition, achalasia, goiter, and esophageal stenosis (Camp-Sorrell, 2014).

Signs and Symptoms

It is important to elicit from the patient the history of dysphagia, including the duration and associated symptoms. The symptoms of dysphagia depend on which phase of swallowing is affected. When the oral/pharyngeal phase is affected, patients often present with cough or choking with swallowing, difficulty initiating swallowing, poor bolus control, pooling of secretions, food sticking in the throat, drooling, and trismus. When the esophageal phase is affected, patients often report food "sticking" in the chest, or regurgitation, heartburn, indigestion, and belching. Other symptoms that do not necessarily correlate with a phase of swallowing include weight loss, change in dietary habits, recurrent pneumonia, and pain with swallowing (Camp-Sorrell, 2014).

Assessment and Diagnosis

The physical assessment of dysphagia includes an assessment of the patient's weight; visual assessment of the oropharynx (including the lips, oral cavity, tongue, and jaw); observation of the movement of the tongue (including evaluation of the tongue's range of motion); evaluation of dentition, strength and symmetry of jaw and facial movements, cranial nerves, and cough and gag reflexes; assessment for abnormal voice or articulation and cervical/neck adenopathy; and auscultation of the lungs (Camp-Sorrell, 2014).

NCI CTEP's (2010) CTCAE describes the grading of dysphagia from 1 to 5. In grade 1 dysphagia, patients are symptomatic but able to eat. In grade 2 dysphagia, patients are symptomatic with altered eating and swallowing. IV fluids may be indicated. Grade 3 dysphagia is described as symptoms causing severely altered eating and swallowing, with inadequate oral caloric and fluid intake, requiring IV fluids, tube feedings, total parenteral nutrition, or hospitalization. Grade 4 dysphagia has life-threatening consequences, such as obstruction or perforation, that require urgent intervention. Grade 5 is characterized by death (NCI CTEP, 2010).

The goal of the evaluation of dysphagia is to determine the likely cause of the problem as well as the correct management. A diagnostic workup for dysphagia should include a barium swallow examination, esophagogastroduodenoscopy, and computed tomography of the chest, abdomen, and pelvis (Javle et al., 2006). Endoscopy is used most often to determine the cause of dysphagia. Biopsy and esophageal dilation can be done during an endoscopy. Videofluorographic swallowing studies are the standard diagnostic tool used to study swallowing. A barium swallow study may be used to identify anatomic abnormalities (Camp-Sorrell, 2014).

Management

The goals of therapy for dysphagia are to decrease the risk of aspiration, improve swallowing, and optimize nutrition. Anticipation of this complication from cancer and its treatment is key in the management of dysphagia. Patients should be evaluated and treated by a multidisciplinary team including a nutritionist and speech therapist. Nutritional support monitors patients' nutritional intake. The speech therapist determines the appropriate consistency of food for patients (Camp-Sorrell, 2014).

If patients are unable to swallow because of an esophageal stricture, they may be a candidate for esophageal dilation. This is frequently required after a patient has surgery or radiation to the esophageal and head and neck areas. Esophageal dilation may be performed during endoscopy, and balloons or rigid dilators often are used. For patients who have strictures that are causing dysphagia, esophageal stents can be considered. The stents typically are metal with wire mesh or coils.

Dilation is used frequently in the postoperative setting. The normal lumen of the esophagus is 25 mm, and symptoms of dysphagia occur when the size of the lumen decreases to 13 mm. Often, an endoscopy is done for initial evaluation of a patient with dysphagia. Endoscopic balloon dilation or a wire-guided procedure can provide temporary relief. The relief obtained from dilation is short-lived, and a repeat dilation may be needed. Self-dilation is used for benign and postoperative strictures (Javle et al., 2006).

The goals of stenting in malignant dysphagia are to minimize symptoms and improve oral food, water, and medication intake, seal fistulas or anastomotic leaks following surgery, and improve quality of life. Self-expanding esophageal metal stents (SEMS) were created to decrease the complication rate and increase the ease of insertion compared to the older metal mesh stents. Ell and May (1997) reported that the major disadvantages of SEMS were cost, tumor growth, chest pain, stent migration, fistulization, airway obstruction, and hemorrhage. The location of the stent can be associated with complications. Stents placed in the gastroesophageal junction may cause intractable reflux symptoms, whereas stents placed in the proximal esophagus may cause a sensation of a foreign body or respiratory compromise. Self-expanding plastic stents (SEPS) are a more recent addition used in the palliation of dysphagia. They are similar to SEMS but are larger and less flexible. The advantage of SEPS is that they can be removed or repositioned if needed (Javle et al., 2006).

Laser therapy can also be used in the management of dysphagia. It causes localized coagulation of abnormal tissues. This may be used in the treatment of malignancy. The laser vaporizes the tumor, recannulating the lumen and restoring lumen patency. It has few systemic effects and can be done in an outpatient setting. Treatment is done every other day for three to four sessions (Camp-Sorrell, 2014).

Photodynamic therapy (PDT) can be used to treat tissue overgrowth or ingrowth in patients who have undergone esophageal stenting, patients with early-stage disease who are high-risk surgical candidates, or those who refuse surgery. With PDT, porfimer is given to cause damage to the vasculature of the tumor, leading to ischemia. The porfimer accumulates in the malignant cells. The area is exposed to a low-power laser, which causes a photochemical reaction leading to tumor necrosis. The most common side effects with PDT are chest pain, worsening dysphagia, fever, pleural effusion, leukocytosis, and skin photosensitivity (Javle et al., 2006). The treatment can be cost prohibitive.

Enteral feedings using a jejunostomy or gastrostomy tube should be considered for long-term treatment. Selection of an enteral formulation should factor in the product's calorie content and cost to the patient. Feedings can be bolus or continuous.

Speech pathologists are intimately involved in the management of patients experiencing dysphagia. They make recommendations based on safe swallowing strategies that avoid aspiration, therapeutic postures and exercises that may improve swallowing function over time, and dietary modifications that ensure adequate, safe oral intake. Swallowing therapy or rehabilitation before and after surgery in patients with head and neck cancer is important. Techniques used include postural maneuvers, exercises to strengthen swallowing muscles, and exercises to perform while swallowing. Oromotor exercises improve bolus manipulation, voluntary swallow, and triggering of the swallow reflex. Laryngeal closure exercises improve airway protection. Other direct strategies include posturing and positioning. These techniques aid in bolus placement, manipulation, and transit in the oral cavity (Camp-Sorrell, 2014).

Complications of Dysphagia

Complications of dysphagia include dehydration, weight loss, fistula formation, airway compromise, aspiration pneumonia, and bronchial irritation (Camp-Sorrell, 2014; Murphy & Gilbert, 2009). Aspiration can occur during different phases of swallowing and usually manifests by a cough or clearing of the throat before, during, or after swallowing. Patients with dysphagia are at risk for malnutrition. Late effects of dysphagia can result in long-term or permanent feeding tube placement (Murphy & Gilbert, 2009). A comprehensive nutritional evaluation and early involvement of a nutritionist in patients' care is imperative. A diary or 24-hour dietary recall with anthropometric measurements should be done at initial evaluation and at designated intervals. Anthropometric measurements include height, weight, and skinfold measurements. Laboratory tests such as folate and B_{12} levels, CBC, iron studies, and albumin levels will assist in patient assessment.

Nursing Implications

Dysphagia often is not relieved or palliated effectively. The previous discussion summarized treatments that are available for dysphagia in the hope of improving patients' quality of life. Dysphagia is best treated by a multidisciplinary team approach involving the physician, nurse, nurse practitioner, and nutritionist, among others.

Nausea and Vomiting

Nausea and vomiting are common symptoms in the oncology population. More than 20% of patients with advanced cancer experience vomiting (Kirkova, Rybicki, Walsh, & Aktas, 2012; Portenoy et al., 1994), and up to 68% of patients with advanced cancer report nausea (Solano, Gomes, & Higginson, 2006). The etiology of nausea and vomiting in patients with cancer may be multifactorial, including medications such as chemotherapy or opioids, radiation, central nervous system causes such as increased intracranial pressure from tumor, metabolic abnormalities including uremia and hypercalcemia, vestibular dysfunction, or gastrointestinal problems such as bowel obstruction, constipation, or impaired gastric motility (Gordon, LeGrand, & Walsh, 2013). In one study, the most common causes of nausea and vomiting in patients with advanced cancer were impaired gastric emptying, primarily from tumor or hepatomegaly, chemical causes such as a metabolic source or a medication, and bowel obstruction (Stephenson & Davies, 2006). The impact of nausea and vomiting may be significant, leading to impaired quality of life and higher rates of distress (Pirri et al., 2013). Therefore, oncology nurses must not only be familiar with the various causes of nausea and vomiting in patients with cancer, but also must be skilled in the assessment, prevention, and treatment of this condition.

Definition

Although nausea and vomiting often are associated with one another, they are distinct entities that may not always occur together. Nausea involves a subjective sensation of imminent vomiting, with associated symptoms including tachycardia, sweating, pallor, dizziness, and excessive salivation. It may or may not result in vomiting. Nausea is controlled by the autonomic nervous system (Camp-Sorrell, 2018). Vomiting is a protective mechanism for eliminating noxious stimuli and is controlled by the respiratory muscles (Hornby, 2001).

Chemotherapy-Induced Nausea and Vomiting

Chemotherapy is a common culprit of nausea and vomiting in patients with cancer. Even in the modern era with the addition of neurokinin-1 receptor antagonists such as aprepitant, approximately one-third of patients receiving chemotherapy do not achieve complete control of nausea and vomiting (Majem et al., 2011). Perhaps more importantly, healthcare providers such as physicians and nurses have been shown to either over- or underestimate how well chemotherapy-induced nausea and vomiting (CINV) is controlled in this population (Majem et al., 2011). Furthermore, national evidence-based guidelines may not always be followed in clinical practice, with Gilmore et al. (2014) reporting that just over half of patients receive prophylaxis consistent with guidelines. In addition to adversely affecting patients' quality of life and daily functioning (Fernández-Ortega et al., 2012; Haiderali, Menditto, Good, Teitelbaum, & Wegner, 2011; Hilarius et al., 2012), CINV may negatively influence treatment adherence and, potentially, overall survival (Neymark & Crott, 2005). It also has been associated with malnutrition (Davidson et al., 2012). From an economic standpoint, CINV may result in higher costs and the use of more healthcare resources (Burke, Wisniewski, & Ernst, 2011; Shih, Xu, & Elting, 2007), with one study estimating those costs to be 30% higher (Shih et al., 2007). CINV therefore remains a significant problem for patients with cancer, and further work is needed to improve outcomes.

Pathophysiology

CINV was once thought to be regulated by a single region in the medulla known as the vomiting center. Current hypotheses, however, postulate that several neuronal areas exist in the medulla to receive sensory input and ultimately control emesis (Hornby, 2001). Researchers have referred to this area as the central pattern generator (Koga & Fukuda, 1992). Sensory input to the medulla may be received through either peripheral pathways, including the vagus nerve from GI tract stimuli, or centrally, from areas such as the chemoreceptor trigger zone located in the area postrema (Aapro, Jordan, & Feyer, 2013). Chemotherapy agents primarily initiate CINV through the GI pathway via release of 5-hydroxytryptamine (5-HT), also known as serotonin, from the enterochromaffin cells of the GI tract (Hesketh, 2008). The released serotonin subsequently binds to serotonin receptors along the vagus nerve in the GI tract (Hesketh, 2008). Serotonin appears to primarily be involved in the development of acute nausea and vomiting (Hesketh et al., 2003), with the 5-HT_3 receptor representing the most important serotonin receptor in acute CINV (Aapro et al., 2013).

In addition to serotonin, the neurotransmitter substance P has been implicated in CINV (Saito, Takano, & Kamiya, 2003). Substance P binds to neurokinin-1 receptors located throughout the central nervous system, ultimately producing emesis. Delayed nausea and vomiting are most likely regulated by substance P (Hesketh et al., 2003). Additional chemicals thought to be involved in CINV include dopamine and cholecystokinin (Hesketh, 2008) (see Figure 20-3).

Classification

CINV may be classified according to the timing of its development as either acute or delayed. Acute CINV typically is defined as CINV that occurs within the first 24 hours following chemotherapy. Delayed CINV may occur beyond the initial 24-hour time period and persist for up to five days (Kris et al., 1985). The risk factors for experiencing either acute or delayed CINV are multifactorial and will be discussed in the following paragraphs. Anticipatory CINV is a conditioned response in which certain stimuli may provoke episodes of nausea or vomiting prior to or during the administration of chemotherapy. The incidence of anticipatory CINV, however, has diminished in the era of more effective prophylaxis (Roila et al., 2016).

Risk Factors and Assessment

Numerous risk factors have been identified for the development of CINV. The most important risk factor is the level of emetogenicity of the chemotherapy agents (Hesketh, 2008). Chemotherapy agents are typically classified as having a minimal, low, moderate, or high risk of emesis, with cisplatin being considered the prototype for highly emetogenic agents (see National Comprehensive Cancer Network® [NCCN®], 2017, for emetic classifications of specific chemotherapy agents).

Additional contributing factors to CINV include female gender, younger age, low alcohol intake, prior history of emesis (i.e., CINV, motion sickness, or pregnancy), anxiety, pain, and type of antiemetic prescription (Chan et al., 2015; Molassiotis, Stamataki, & Kontopantelis, 2013; Sekine, Segawa, Kubota, & Saeki, 2013; Warr, 2013). In 2013, Molassiotis and colleagues developed a risk prediction model that may assist clinicians in targeting antiemetic prescriptions more effectively. The tool is freely available at www.cinvrisk.org. An area of future research that may be promising includes the role of pharmacogenomics and genetic polymorphisms, which may have implications for selection of antiemetic therapy. For now, careful assessment of identifiable risk factors should be performed before the initiation of chemotherapy, with antiemetic regimens adjusted routinely and appropriately based on findings.

Assessment of CINV is a necessary yet complex process. Specifically, the nursing assessment of chemotherapy-related symptoms, including CINV, may positively influence patient care (Braud et al., 2003). Unfortunately, few reliable and validated CINV assess-

Figure 20-3. Production of Emesis

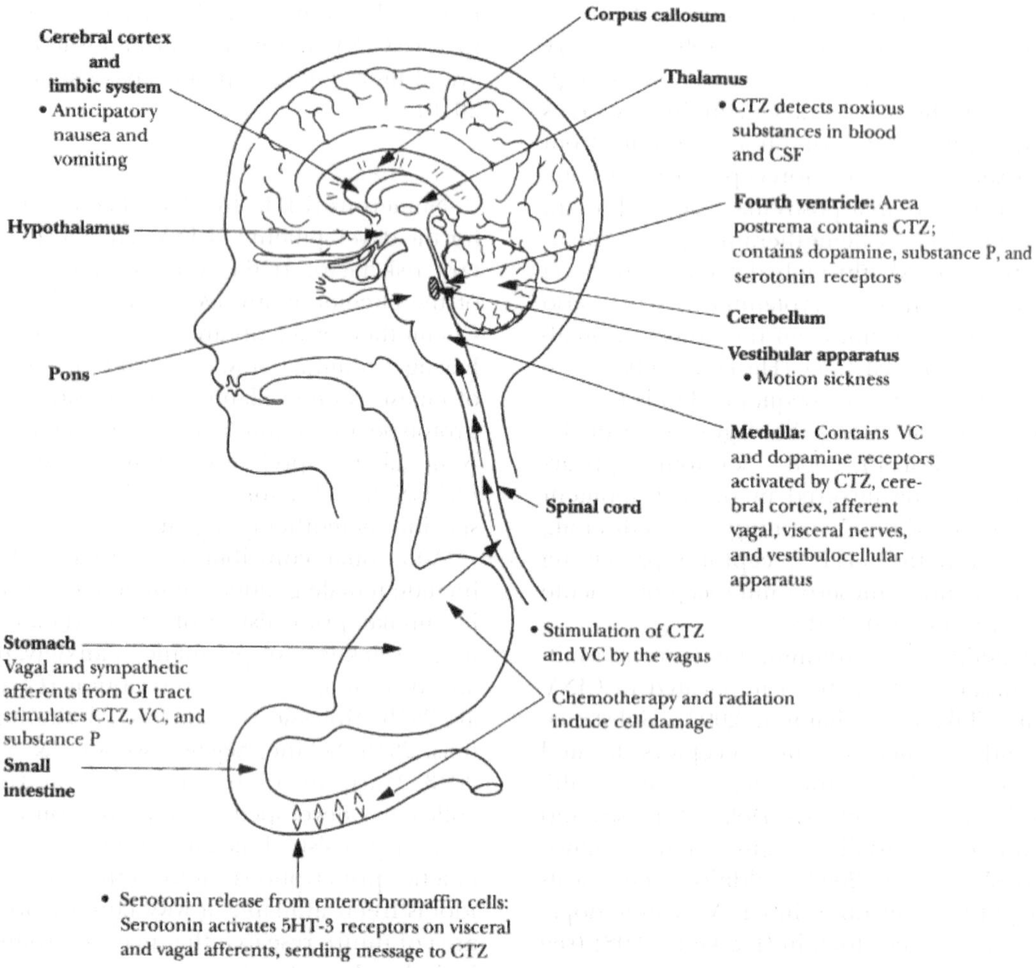
Corpus callosum
Cerebral cortex and limbic system
• Anticipatory nausea and vomiting
Thalamus
• CTZ detects noxious substances in blood and CSF
Fourth ventricle: Area postrema contains CTZ; contains dopamine, substance P, and serotonin receptors
Hypothalamus
Cerebellum
Vestibular apparatus
• Motion sickness
Pons
Medulla: Contains VC and dopamine receptors activated by CTZ, cerebral cortex, afferent vagal, visceral nerves, and vestibulocellular apparatus
Spinal cord
• Stimulation of CTZ and VC by the vagus
Stomach
Vagal and sympathetic afferents from GI tract stimulates CTZ, VC, and substance P
Chemotherapy and radiation induce cell damage
Small intestine
• Serotonin release from enterochromaffin cells: Serotonin activates 5HT-3 receptors on visceral and vagal afferents, sending message to CTZ

CSF—cerebrospinal fluid; CTZ—chemotherapy trigger zone; GI—gastrointestinal; VC—vomiting center

Note. From "Chemotherapy Toxicities and Management" (p. 517), by D. Camp-Sorrell in C.H. Yarbro, D. Wujcik, and B.H. Gobel (Eds.), *Cancer Nursing: Principles and Practice* (8th ed.), 2011, Burlington, MA: Jones & Bartlett Learning. Copyright 2018 by Jones & Bartlett Learning. Reprinted with permission.

ment tools exist (Brearley, Clements, & Molassiotis, 2008). Molassiotis et al. (2007), however, have developed the MASCC Antiemesis Tool to better assess this phenomenon. The tool is patient friendly and needs to be completed only once per chemotherapy cycle. Nurses are in a key position to assess CINV and therefore should be familiar with the various resources available.

Pharmacologic Management

Because of the ramifications of uncontrolled CINV, proper prevention and management of this untoward side effect are necessary. Several organizations, including ASCO, MASCC, NCCN, and ONS, have published guidelines with evidence-based recommendations for prevention and treatment of CINV. The importance of guideline adherence should not be underestimated. Both Aapro et al. (2012) and Gilmore et al. (2014) demonstrated significant improvements in CINV incidence when evidence-based guidelines were followed. See Table 20-3 for a comparison of guideline recommendations.

5-HT_3 receptor antagonists: The 5-HT_3 receptor antagonists (RAs) are the cornerstone of CINV prevention. These agents, developed in the early 1990s, are believed to prevent the binding of 5-HT to the 5-HT_3 receptor (Endo et al., 2000). Currently approved 5-HT_3 RAs in the United States include ondansetron, granisetron, dolasetron, and palonosetron. All are available in both oral and IV formulations, with the exception of dolasetron, which is only available in an oral formulation. Ondansetron is also available as an orally disintegrating tablet, and granisetron has a transdermal formulation as well. Also, no difference was observed in efficacy among the three older 5-HT_3 RAs: ondansetron, dolasetron, and granisetron (Jordan et al., 2007). Palonosetron is a 5-HT_3 RA that has a longer half-life and a higher binding affinity for the 5-HT_3 receptor than the other 5-HT_3 RAs (Naeim et al., 2008). A meta-analysis and a pooled analysis of palonosetron in highly and moderately emetogenic regimens demonstrated superiority over first-generation 5-HT_3 RAs for prevention of CINV in both the acute and delayed settings without differences in toxicity (Jin et al., 2013; Schwartzberg et al., 2014). Although palonosetron is classified as a 5-HT_3 RA, its efficacy in prevention of delayed CINV is likely due to inhibition of substance P (Rojas et al., 2010). The older, shorter-acting 5-HT_3 RAs, however, are not effective for use in delayed CINV and are costlier than other available agents, such as dexamethasone (Geling & Eichler, 2005). Side effects of 5-HT_3 RAs generally are mild and may include headache, dizziness, constipation, and, rarely, prolonged QT interval (Jin et al., 2013). The prolonged QT interval occurs less frequently with palonosetron than with first-generation 5-HT_3 RAs (Jin et al., 2013; Popovic et al., 2014).

Neurokinin-1 receptor antagonists: Aprepitant was the first FDA-approved neurokinin-1 receptor antagonist (NK_1 RA) in the United States. It is available in both an oral preparation and an IV form (fosaprepitant). Aprepitant is approved for the prevention of CINV in patients receiving either moderately or highly emetogenic chemotherapy as part of a regimen that includes a corticosteroid and a 5-HT_3 RA. It also is approved for the prevention of postoperative nausea and vomiting. Aprepitant acts as an antagonist for the substance P/NK_1 receptors located throughout the central nervous system (Merck & Co., Inc., 2006). Aprepitant is universally recommended for use with highly emetogenic regimens and in select populations receiving moderately emetogenic regimens (Basch et al., 2011; NCCN, 2017; Roila et al., 2016). The recommended dosing of aprepitant for highly emetogenic regimens is 125 mg PO on day 1 in conjunction with a 5-HT_3 RA and dexamethasone and 80 mg PO on days 2 and 3. Patients also should receive dexamethasone orally on days 2–4. For moderately emetogenic chemotherapy regimens, the regimen is similar; however, corticosteroids may be eliminated for days 2–4 (Merck & Co., Inc., 2006). The IV form of aprepitant, fosaprepitant, may be substituted for the oral dose on day 1. The recommended dose is 115 mg. Aprepitant is well tolerated, with side effects including asthenia, diarrhea, and hiccups (Merck & Co., Inc., 2006). The potential for drug interactions with aprepitant exists, however, because of the enzymatic pathway of elimination of this drug. The concentrations of concomitant medications such as dexamethasone, warfarin, and certain chemotherapy agents may be affected (Merck & Co., Inc., 2006).

In 2014, FDA approved a combination oral agent consisting of netupitant, a highly selec-

Table 20-3. Comparison of Recommendations for the Treatment of Nausea and Vomiting

	Level of Emetogenicity				
Guideline	**High**	**Moderate**	**Low**	**Minimal**	**Breakthrough**
ASCO	Day 1 NK_1 RA (aprepitant or fosaprepitant*) + 5-HT_3 RA (palonosetron preferred) or netupitant/palonosetron + dexamethasone Days 2–4 NK_1 RA (aprepitant) + dexamethasone[†] Note: An NK_1 RA is not required on days 2–3 if fosaprepitant or netupitant was used.	Day 1 Palonosetron[‡] + dexamethasone Days 2–3 Dexamethasone	Day 1 Single dose of dexamethasone 8 mg	No antiemetic prophylaxis is necessary.	No specific recommendations; if uncontrolled emesis occurs despite optimal prophylaxis, consider addition of lorazepam, alprazolam, olanzapine, or a dopamine antagonist, and consider substitution of high-dose IV metoclopramide for the 5-HT_3 RA.
MASCC	Day 1 NK_1 RA (aprepitant, fosaprepitant, rolapitant, or netupitant*) + 5-HT_3 RA + dexamethasone Days 2–3 Aprepitant + dexamethasone or metoclopramide + dexamethasone Note: An NK_1 RA is not needed on days 2 and 3 if rolapitant, fosaprepitant, or netupitant were given on day 1. Day 4 Dexamethasone + metoclopramide (if metoclopramide used on days 2 and 3)	**AC regimen:** Day 1 NK_1 RA (aprepitant, netupitant, rolapitant, or fosaprepitant*) + 5-HT_3 RA + dexamethasone Days 2–3 NK_1 RA (aprepitant) or dexamethasone Note: An NK_1 RA is not given if fosaprepitant, rolapitant, or netupitant were used on day 1. **Non-AC regimens:** Day 1 5-HT_3 RA + dexamethasone Days 2–3 Dexamethasone may be considered with selected agents. **Carboplatin:** See Roila et al., 2016.	Day 1 Single agent such as dexamethasone, 5-HT_3 RA, or dopamine RA	Routine prophylaxis is not recommended.	Add an antiemetic with a different mechanism of action than that of those used previously.

(Continued on next page)

Table 20-3. Comparison of Recommendations for the Treatment of Nausea and Vomiting *(Continued)*

Guideline	Level of Emetogenicity: High	Moderate	Low	Minimal	Breakthrough
NCCN	Day 1 NK_1 RA (aprepitant, rolapitant, or fosaprepitant*) + 5-HT_3 RA + dexamethasone Days 2–3 NK_1 RA (aprepitant) + dexamethasone Note: No NK_1 RA on days 2–4 is needed if rolapitant, fosaprepitant, or netupitant was used on day 1. Day 4 Dexamethasone Or Day 1 Netupitant/palonosetron + dexamethasone Days 2–4 Dexamethasone Or Day 1 Olanzapine + palonosetron + dexamethasone Days 2–4 Olanzapine	Day 1 5-HT_3 RA + dexamethasone ± NK_1 RA Days 2–3 Dexamethasone ± NK_1 RA; or dexamethasone single agent; or 5-HT_3 RA if NK_1 RA not given **Alternative options:** Day 1 Netupitant/palonosetron + dexamethasone Days 2–3 +/- Dexamethasone Or Day 1 Olanzapine + palonosetron + dexamethasone Days 2–3 Olanzapine Note: All regimens ± lorazepam or H_2 blocker/PPI days 1–4 as needed	Day 1 Dexamethasone; or prochlorperazine; or metoclopramide; or 5-HT_3 RA; ± lorazepam or H_2 blocker/PPI days 1–4 as needed Delayed: N/A	No routine prophylaxis is required.	Add an agent from a different drug class to the current regimen.

* Fosaprepitant is only required day 1.

† Dexamethasone may also be given on day 4.

‡ First-generation 5-HT_3 RA may be considered if palonosetron unavailable; consideration could be given to use of aprepitant for which limited evidence supports its use; if using aprepitant, can use any one of the 5-HT_3 RAs.

AC—doxorubicin (Adriamycin®) + cyclophosphamide; ASCO—American Society of Clinical Oncology; 5-HT_3—5-hydroxytryptamine-3 (serotonin); H_2—histamine-2; MASCC—Multinational Association of Supportive Care in Cancer; N/A—not applicable; NCCN—National Comprehensive Cancer Network; NK_1—neurokinin-1; PPI—proton pump inhibitor; RA—receptor antagonist

Note. Based on information from Basch et al., 2011; Hesketh et al., 2016; National Comprehensive Cancer Network, 2017; Roila et al., 2016.

tive NK_1 inhibitor, and palonosetron, a $5\text{-}HT_3$ RA. It is indicated for the prevention of acute and delayed nausea and vomiting associated with cancer chemotherapy, including but not limited to highly emetogenic chemotherapy (Eisai Inc. & Helsinn Therapeutics Inc., 2015). The combination of netupitant and palonosetron is recognized by NCCN (2017) as a viable option for CINV prevention with both highly and moderately emetogenic chemotherapy regimens. It should be given with dexamethasone on days 1–4 for highly emetogenic regimens; however, for moderately emetogenic regimens, dexamethasone is only required on day 1. The side effect profile is similar to palonosetron, with headache and constipation being the most common (Aapro et al., 2014).

Corticosteroids: Corticosteroids such as dexamethasone are effective in the prevention of both acute and delayed CINV (Ioannidis, Hesketh, & Lau, 2000). They typically are used in combination with a $5\text{-}HT_3$ RA and NK_1 RA for the prevention of acute CINV in highly or moderately emetogenic regimens, but they also are recommended as a single agent for the prevention of CINV in mildly emetogenic regimens and for delayed emesis (Basch et al., 2011; NCCN, 2017; Roila et al., 2016). The exact mechanism of action of corticosteroids in the prevention of CINV is unknown. Dexamethasone is the most widely studied corticosteroid, is readily available, and is inexpensive. The dosing and schedule for dexamethasone are variable and dependent on several factors, including emetogenic potential of the chemotherapy regimen and whether it is being used in combination with aprepitant (see Table 20-3). A shorter course of dexamethasone has been studied in combination with palonosetron in moderately emetogenic regimens and in regimens containing an anthracycline/cyclophosphamide, and a single dose versus a three-day course appears to be equally efficacious (Aapro et al., 2010; Celio et al., 2011). These findings could have implications for patients who may have poor tolerability to corticosteroids or in certain populations, such as patients with diabetes. Although corticosteroids have many short- and long-term side effects, the most commonly occurring ones in patients taking dexamethasone for prophylaxis of delayed emesis include insomnia, indigestion, agitation, increased appetite and weight gain, and acne (Vardy, Chiew, Galica, Pond, & Tannock, 2006).

Cannabinoids: Cannabinoids such as dronabinol and nabilone are approved for treatment of refractory CINV when other conventional antiemetics are ineffective. These agents activate cannabinoid receptors, which are located throughout the central and peripheral nervous systems, and either directly or indirectly inhibit the release of neurotransmitters involved in emesis (Davis, Maida, Daeninck, & Pergolizzi, 2007). Major guidelines such as NCCN (2016a) include cannabinoids as an option for breakthrough or refractory CINV. Although these agents have some efficacy in the treatment of CINV, their usefulness may be limited by significant side effects, such as sedation, drowsiness, dizziness, dysphoria, and depression (Rocha, Stéfano, Haiek, Oliveira, & Da Silveira, 2008; Tramèr et al., 2001).

Dopamine receptor antagonists: Dopamine RAs include the phenothiazines, butyrophenones (i.e., haloperidol), and metoclopramide, a substituted benzamide. Examples of phenothiazines include prochlorperazine, promethazine, and chlorpromazine. Both phenothiazines and metoclopramide may be used as premedication with chemotherapy regimens of low emetogenic potential (NCCN, 2017). Additionally, they may be prescribed for treatment of breakthrough CINV. Possible side effects include drowsiness, hypotension, dystonia, and extrapyramidal effects (Monthly Prescribing Reference, 2016).

Benzodiazepines: Benzodiazepines may be helpful as adjuncts for breakthrough or refractory CINV. Lorazepam is the prototypical benzodiazepine that has been endorsed by various national guidelines for breakthrough/refractory or anticipatory CINV (Basch et al., 2011;

NCCN, 2017; Roila et al., 2016). The exact mechanism of action of benzodiazepines for CINV is not clearly elucidated, but they appear to work primarily on the limbic system (Malik et al., 1995). Benzodiazepines have also been shown to confer amnesic properties (Malik et al., 1995; Semrad, Leuchter, Townsend, Wade, & Lagasse, 1984), making these agents very useful in the CINV setting.

Atypical antipsychotics: Olanzapine, a thienobenzodiazepine, is an atypical antipsychotic drug that interferes with both dopamine and 5-HT receptors. It has activity in prevention of CINV with moderately and highly emetogenic chemotherapy, as well as in treatment of breakthrough CINV (Navari, Nagy, & Gray, 2013). Olanzapine appears to be well tolerated, with no significant adverse effects identified in several studies (Navari et al., 2005, 2007, 2013). Additionally, because it is available in a generic formulation, olanzapine may offer a cost-effective option for managing CINV. National guidelines such as NCCN, ASCO, MASCC/European Society for Medical Oncology (ESMO), and ONS include olanzapine as an option for the management of breakthrough CINV. NCCN (2017) also endorses olanzapine in combination with palonosetron and dexamethasone for the prevention of CINV with moderately and highly emetogenic regimens.

Nonpharmacologic Management

Nonpharmacologic management may be considered for some patients with uncontrolled or anticipatory CINV. There continues to be some discordance, however, with recommendations. For example, Cassileth et al. (2007) recommended consideration of acupuncture for uncontrolled CINV; however, ONS PEP guidelines (Lee et al., 2017) did not endorse this option. In a Cochrane review, Ezzo et al. (2006) reported limitations in acupuncture and acupressure studies, including lack of a sham control in some of the studies, as well as a lack of concurrent modern antiemetics. According to Naeim et al. (2008), accessing a quality provider of acupuncture, particularly electroacupuncture (electrical stimulation plus needles), may be challenging.

Hypnosis is recommended by NCCN, ONS, and MASCC/ESMO as a modality for managing anticipatory CINV. In addition to hypnosis, muscle relaxation training and systematic desensitization may be effective behavioral techniques for treating anticipatory CINV (Roila et al., 2016).

Numerous other nonpharmacologic therapies have been studied but for which effectiveness has not been established. Examples include acupressure, massage, exercise, ginger, herbal medicine, and psychoeducational interventions (Lee et al., 2017).

Although not as much strong evidence exists for the use of nonpharmacologic measures as for pharmacologic therapies, the risks associated with them are low. Nonpharmacologic therapies may be considered as adjunctive therapies to pharmacologic treatments for some patients.

Radiation-Induced Nausea and Vomiting

Radiation-induced nausea and vomiting (RINV) occurs in more than one-quarter of all patients receiving radiation therapy (Maranzano et al., 2010). The likelihood of developing RINV is dependent on the anatomic site of radiation and the dose and size of the radiation field. Of these, treatment field is a major consideration: total body irradiation has the highest risk for developing RINV; the upper abdomen and craniospinal area are moderate risk; the cranium, head and neck, thorax region, and pelvis are low risk; and the extremities and breast are minimal risk (Roila et al., 2016). The pathophysiology of RINV is thought to be similar to that of CINV—controlled by 5-HT_3 receptors and the chemoreceptor trigger zone (Feyer, Jahn, & Jordan, 2014; Horiot, 2004). Management of RINV is dependent on the level of risk; patients considered to be at high risk should receive prophylaxis with a 5-HT_3 RA prior to each fraction of radiation and continuing for a minimum of 24 hours beyond the final treatment. Moderate-risk patients should also receive a 5-HT_3 RA prior to each fraction of radiation, but therapy does not need to continue beyond the final radiation dose. A five-day course of corticosteroids during days 1–5 could be considered. A 5-HT_3 RA may be considered for low-risk patients as either prophylaxis or rescue, and for minimal-risk patients, either a 5-HT_3 RA or a dopamine RA is appropriate for a rescue antiemetic (Basch et al., 2011).

Miscellaneous Causes of Nausea and Vomiting in Patients With Cancer

As discussed earlier, nausea and vomiting may have numerous etiologies in patients with cancer. In addition to CINV and RINV, other causes include increased intracranial pressure resulting from tumor involvement, bowel obstruction, underlying renal disease, electrolyte disturbances, vestibular dysfunction, anxiety, and medications such as opioids (NCCN, 2017). In fact, nearly 50% of patients with advanced cancer may experience nausea while not receiving chemotherapy or radiation (Komurcu, Nelson, Walsh, Ford, & Rybicki, 2002). Therapeutic interventions may be based on treating the underlying cause of nausea and vomiting or simply palliating the symptom. For example, in patients with nausea and vomiting caused by increased intracranial pressure from central nervous system involvement, an appropriate intervention would include corticosteroids and radiation therapy. In patients with advanced cancer with nonspecific nausea and vomiting, the evidence to support one specific antiemetic agent is limited; however, a systematic review by Davis and Hallerberg (2010) found modest evidence to support the use of metoclopramide as a first-line agent. A 5-HT_3 RA or phenothiazine could be considered as well (Davis & Hallerberg, 2010). In patients with malignant bowel obstructions, pharmacologic management may include the use of butyrophenones or phenothiazines, an anticholinergic, or octreotide (Davis & Hallerberg, 2010). See Table 20-4 for treatment recommendations for miscellaneous causes of nausea and vomiting in patients with cancer.

Nursing Implications

Nausea and vomiting in patients with cancer continues to represent a prevalent issue for this vulnerable population. Nurses should be routinely assessing for this symptom and making appropriate evidence-based recommendations for its management. Nurses involved in the care of patients with cancer also should continue to play a leading role in nausea and vomiting research.

Constipation

Constipation is a common problem among patients with cancer, affecting anywhere from 39% (Goodman, Low, & Wilkinson, 2005) to more than 70% (Droney et al., 2008). It is particularly prevalent among patients receiving opioid therapy (Abramowitz et al., 2013; Bell et al., 2009; Droney et al., 2008). Constipation may affect a patient's quality of life (Abramowitz et al., 2013; Bell et al., 2009), as well as result in life-threatening complications such as bowel obstruction or intestinal perforation. It also may have economic implications, including additional expenditures for pharmacy costs and hospitalizations (Dik et al., 2014). In fact, the number of hospitalizations for patients with constipation has more than doubled since 1997 (Sethi et al., 2014). Proper assessment and management of this symptom, therefore, are imperative.

Constipation is categorized as either functional (primary) or secondary, with secondary sources typically arising from medications or

Table 20-4. Etiology and Management of Nausea and Vomiting in Patients With Cancer

Etiology	Intervention
Gastrointestinal	
• Dyspepsia	Metoclopramide
• Gastric stasis	Prokinetic agent
• Constipation	Laxatives, disimpaction, enemas
• Bowel obstruction	Corticosteroids, octreotide, anticholinergics, surgical intervention, endoscopic stent placement, decompression with nasogastric or gastrostomy tube
• Gastric outlet obstruction	Corticosteroids, proton pump inhibitor, metoclopramide, endoscopic stent placement, decompression with gastrostomy tube
• Gastritis/gastroesophageal reflux disease	Proton pump inhibitor; H_2 blocker
Metabolic/chemical	
• Hypercalcemia	Hydration, bisphosphonates, prochlorperazine, haloperidol
• Uremia	Treatment of underlying cause, hydration, prochlorperazine, haloperidol
• Opioids	Opioid rotation, prochlorperazine, haloperidol
• Miscellaneous medications	Discontinuation or dose reduction; consideration of prochlorperazine or haloperidol
Central nervous system (increased intracranial pressure)	Corticosteroids, radiation therapy, possible surgical intervention
• Vestibular	Prochlorperazine, promethazine, cyclizine
• Psychological	Anxiolytics, consideration of psychiatric referral
• Unknown/miscellaneous	Dopamine receptor antagonists (metoclopramide, haloperidol, prochlorperazine); 5-HT_3 receptor antagonists; olanzapine, chlorpromazine

Note. Based on information from Ang et al., 2010; Cherny, 2004; Glare et al., 2004, 2008; Lichter, 1996; National Comprehensive Cancer Network, 2017.

medical conditions (Jamshed, Lee, & Olden, 2011). According to the Rome III Criteria, developed by an expert panel of gastroenterologists, functional constipation is defined as persistently difficult or infrequent stools, or incomplete evacuation of stool, which do not meet criteria for irritable bowel syndrome (Longstreth et al., 2006). Diagnostic criteria include straining during defecation, lumpy or hard stools, a sensation of incomplete evacuation or anorectal obstruction, or manual maneuvers to facilitate defecation on at least 25% of occasions. At least two of these criteria must be met to diagnose the condition (Longstreth et al., 2006).

Constipation may be further classified as either normal-transit, slow-transit, or defecation disorders. Normal-transit constipation is the most commonly seen type (Andrews & Storr, 2011). It is associated with a perceived difficulty with defecation or the presence of hard stools (Lembo & Camilleri, 2003). Slow-transit constipation typically starts at puberty and may be described as a delay in stool transit time (Rao, 2007). Symptoms may include infrequent bowel movements, bloating, and abdominal discomfort (Lembo & Camilleri, 2003). Finally, defecation disorders typically are secondary to irregularities of the pelvic floor or anal sphincter (Lembo & Camilleri, 2003).

Pathophysiology

Constipation may occur because of a disruption in either structural, mechanical, metabolic, or functional capabilities of the colon, rectum, or anus (Rao, 2007). The pathophysiology of constipation is complex and may involve both physical and psychological components (Chan et al., 2005; Hertig, Cain, Jarrett, Burr, & Heitkemper, 2007). In the human body, defecation involves both voluntary and involuntary reflexes and is regulated by the central nervous and peripheral nervous systems (McCrea, Miaskowski, Stotts, Macera, & Varma, 2008). Stool collection and transit occurs in the colon, with the rectosigmoid portion responsible for stool evacuation (Rao, 2007). Filling of the rectum precipitates evacuation, which triggers autonomic neurons to cause internal sphincter relaxation (McCrea et al., 2008). Relaxation of the external anal sphincter is a voluntary process that permits the individual to ultimately control defecation when convenient (McCrea et al., 2008). Factors involved in defecation include the consistency and volume of stool. A variety of neurotransmitters are involved in this process, including serotonin, acetylcholine, calcitonin gene-related peptide, and substance P (Rao, 2007). Additionally, opioid receptors that are present in the GI tract are responsible for opioid-induced constipation (Tavani, Bianchi, Ferretti, & Manara, 1980).

Etiology and Risk Factors

Of the numerous proposed causes of constipation in patients with cancer, opioid use is the most common (Solomon & Cherny, 2006). In addition to opioids, other medications such as serotonin antagonists, antidepressants, iron supplements, and diuretics may contribute to constipation. Common over-the-counter analgesics such as acetaminophen, aspirin, and nonsteroidal anti-inflammatory medications have been associated with constipation (Chang, Locke, Schleck, Zinsmeister, & Talley, 2007). Chemotherapy drugs, including vinca alkaloids, cisplatin, and thalidomide, are culprits, and electrolyte disturbances, such as hypercalcemia and hyponatremia, may produce constipation. Constipation in patients with cancer may be a manifestation of neurologic complications, such as spinal cord compression. Primary GI or pelvic tumors, which cause colonic obstruction, may cause constipation through mechanical forces. According to Leung (2007), literature is scarce to support many previously implicated causes, such as decreased physical activity, inadequate fluid intake, and low dietary fiber consumption. In the non-oncology population, risk factors for constipation include advanced age, female gender, and lower socioeconomic status (Suares & Ford, 2011).

Assessment and Diagnosis

Proper diagnosis of constipation requires a thorough assessment and physical examination. Various assessment scales and tools have been developed. Examples include the Bristol Stool Form Scale (Longstreth et al., 2006), the Constipation Assessment Scale (McMillan & Williams, 1989), the Patient Assessment of Constipation Symptoms (Frank, Kleinman, Farup, Taylor, & Miner, 1999), and the Constipation Visual Analogue Scale (Goodman et al., 2005). According to Izumi (2014), the Patient Assessment of Constipation Symptoms and the Constipation Assessment Scale may be the most useful assessment tools for nurses.

Physical examination should include an abdominal examination, which may reveal lower quadrant tenderness in constipation (Heitkemper & Wolff, 2007). A digital rectal examination may reveal the presence of impacted stool or hemorrhoids, which may be indicators of constipation. No evidence exists to support the use of diagnostic studies such as laboratory tests, x-rays, or endoscopy in patients without alarm features of a serious underlying medical condition (Rao, Ozturk, & Laine, 2005).

Pharmacologic Management

The management of constipation in the cancer population primarily revolves around the use of laxative therapy. More than half of patients receiving palliative care may be using laxatives (Noguera, Centeno, Librada, & Nabal, 2010; Riechelmann, Krzyzanowska, O'Carroll, & Zimmermann, 2007). Although a paucity of studies have been dedicated to the management of constipation in patients with cancer, both NCCN and ONS have developed guidelines to assist clinicians in dealing with this common problem. NCCN (2016) stresses prevention of constipation with the use of a stimulant laxative, such as senna, with or without a stool softener, such as docusate. ONS PEP guidelines report that this combination is likely to be effective. Additional laxatives that are likely to be effective include polyethylene glycol (PEG), alvimopan, and amidotrizoate (Thorpe, Byar, Conley, Davis, Drapek, Hays, ... Ramsdell, 2017).

Treatment of persistent constipation or failure after frontline therapy may involve the use of additional laxatives, such as bisacodyl, lactulose, magnesium citrate, magnesium hydroxide, or PEG. Metoclopramide may also be added. For opioid-induced constipation, consideration may be given to the use of methylnaltrexone (NCCN, 2016). The ONS PEP resource also recommends methylnaltrexone for management of opioid-induced constipation. Additional strategies that are recommended for practice by ONS PEP includes the selection of less constipating opioids, such as transdermal fentanyl or the combination of oxycodone and naloxone, in select patients. The use of prophylactic laxatives for opioid therapy is also likely to be an effective strategy to minimize constipation (Thorpe, Byar, Conley, Davis, Drapek, Hays, ... Ramsdell, 2016). A brief discussion of the various classes of laxatives follows.

Bulk Agents

Bulk agents include cellulose or psyllium. They work by increasing stool bulk and water content (Mancini & Bruera, 1998). These agents have few side effects, but because they require adequate concomitant fluid intake, they may not be appropriate for many patients with cancer. Also, little evidence exists to support their use for managing constipation (Canadian Agency for Drugs and Technologies in Health, 2014). The risk of intestinal obstruction may be present for certain patients with underlying delayed GI transit times (Xing & Soffer, 2001). Consequently, NCCN (2016) advises against the use of psyllium for opioid-induced constipation.

Osmotic Laxatives

Osmotic agents, which include sorbitol, lactulose, and polyethylene glycol, act to increase the fluid content in the bowel and may increase peristalsis (Belsey, Geraint, & Dixon, 2010). PEG is an osmotic laxative that has efficacy for chronic constipation in patients without cancer (DiPalma, Cleveland, McGowan, & Herrera, 2007b), as well as in patients who are taking medications known to cause constipation (DiPalma, Cleveland, McGowan, & Herrera, 2007a). PEG, most often used in the form of PEG 3350, is well tolerated with no statistically significant difference in side effects compared with placebo (DiPalma et al., 2007a, 2007b). In the general population, it is superior for treatment of constipation when compared with lactulose (Belsey et al., 2010; Lee-Robichaud, Thomas, Morgan, & Nelson, 2010). It has also been shown to be more effective in the cancer population (Wirz, Nadstawek, Elsen, Junker, & Wartenberg, 2012). According to the ONS PEP resource (Thorpe, Byar, Conley, Davis, Drapek, Hays, ... Ramsdell, 2017), amidotrizoate is another osmotic laxative that is likely to be effective for the management of constipation in patients with cancer. It has been studied in patients for whom other laxatives have been ineffective and was found to produce a bowel movement within 10 hours in nearly half of patients (Mercadante, Ferrera, & Casuccio, 2011). Other symptoms, such as nausea, early satiety, and appetite, were improved as well. Amidotrizoate is well tolerated, with mild diarrhea as the main adverse effect (Mercadante et al., 2011). It may be a useful option for patients who have not had successful outcomes with other laxatives, but additional studies are required to confirm these findings.

Saline Laxatives

The saline laxatives include magnesium salts, such as magnesium hydroxide and magnesium citrate, and sodium salts, such as sodium phosphate. These laxatives act by increasing water absorption into the bowel, along with increasing intestinal transit time. Saline laxatives should be used with caution in patients with underlying cardiac or renal disease (Lembo & Camilleri, 2003).

Stimulant Laxatives

Stimulant laxatives include the diphenylmethanes (bisacodyl) and anthraquinones (senna, cascara). Their mechanism of action is through increasing GI motility and fecal water content through both motor and secretory pathways (Twycross, Sykes, Mihalyo, & Wilcock, 2012). Despite concern to the contrary, stimulant laxatives appear to be safe for chronic use (Wald, 2003). Both NCCN (2016) and ONS PEP guidelines (Thorpe, Byar, Conley, Davis, Drapek, Hays, ... Ramsdell, 2017) include stimulant laxatives, such as senna, in their recommendations for prophylaxis of constipation.

Prokinetic Agents

Metoclopramide is a prokinetic agent that has serotonin agonist and antidopaminergic properties (Tack, 2008). It may be useful in cases of persistent constipation (NCCN, 2016). Side effects include drowsiness, extrapyramidal effects, dizziness, and hypertension (Monthly Prescribing Reference, 2016).

Peripheral Opioid Antagonists

Peripheral opioid antagonists, such as methylnaltrexone and alvimopan, selectively block the mu-opioid receptors involved in opioid-induced constipation (Jansen et al., 2011; Yuan, 2007). Methylnaltrexone effectively relieves opioid-induced constipation in patients with advanced illness, including cancer, without compromising the efficacy of opioid therapy (Candy, Jones, Goodman, Drake, & Tookman, 2011; Thomas et al., 2008). It works quickly, with a median time to laxation of just over six hours in one study (Thomas et al., 2008). Side effects include abdominal pain and flatulence (Thomas et al., 2008). Potential drawbacks of methylnaltrexone include that it is only available as a subcutaneous (SC) injection, as well as the cost. Although alvimopan is currently approved for accelerating GI recovery time in patients who have undergone partial bowel resections with anastomoses (Merck & Co., Inc., 2015), it also has demonstrated efficacy in the management of opioid-induced constipation in the non-oncology setting (Jansen et al., 2011; Webster et al., 2008).

Chloride Channel Activators

Lubiprostone is a chloride channel activator that increases the release of chloride-rich fluid into the intestine, subsequently increasing intestinal motility (Sucampo Pharma Americas, LLC, & Takeda Pharmaceuticals America, Inc., 2015). It is approved for use in chronic idiopathic constipation, as well as in irritable bowel syndrome with constipation in adult women and opioid-induced constipation in adults with chronic non-cancer pain (Sucampo Pharma Americas, LLC, & Takeda Pharmaceuticals America, Inc., 2015). Lubiprostone has clearly demonstrated efficacy in chronic idiopathic constipation, including for long-term use of up to 48 weeks (Barish, Drossman, Johanson, & Ueno, 2010; Lembo et al., 2011). It has also proved effective in opioid-induced constipation in non-cancer patients (Cryer, Katz, Vallejo, Popescu, & Ueno, 2014; Jamal, Adams, Jansen, & Webster, 2015). Side effects include nausea, headache, abdominal distention, abdominal pain, and diarrhea (Lembo et al., 2011).

Various suppositories and enemas, including glycerin, mineral oil, phosphate, and bisacodyl, are available to stimulate laxation. NCCN guidelines (2016) recommend the use of glycerin suppositories with or without mineral oil enemas for patients with stool impaction. Tap water enemas could also be considered (NCCN, 2016); however, rectal manipulation typically is contraindicated in patients who are neutropenic or thrombocytopenic.

Nonpharmacologic Management

A nonpharmacologic intervention that practitioners have historically recommended for the management of constipation is to increase dietary fiber intake. However, the data are inconclusive to support this recommendation (Thorpe, Byar, Conley, Davis, Drapek, Hays, ... Ramsdell, 2017). Exercise also has not been proved effective for constipation in patients with cancer (Lofti-Jam et al., 2008). Interestingly, a systematic review of prune therapy revealed promising activity, with evidence of improvements in stool frequency and consistency when compared with psyllium (Lever, Cole, Scott, Emery, & Whelan, 2014). Additional nonpharmacologic interventions for which efficacy has not been established include aromatherapy, massage therapy, biofeedback, fresh baker's yeast, and herbal supplements (Thorpe, Byar, Conley, Davis, Drapek, Hays, ... Ramsdell, 2017).

Nursing Implications

Constipation is a common symptom in patients with cancer. Proper assessment and management are key to alleviating this distressing problem in the oncology population. Nurses can play a pivotal role in assisting patients to navigate the numerous pharmacologic options, as well as the unsubstantiated nonpharmacologic ones. It is important for nurses to keep abreast of the current literature and guideline recommendations for this prevalent symptom. Oncology nurses have significant ongoing contact with patients with cancer and play a pivotal role in the assessment and management of constipation in this population. Despite this, constipation continues to be underassessed and poorly managed by healthcare providers. Johnson, Moore, and Fortner (2007) found that only 15% of patients with cancer were assessed for risk of constipation before beginning chemotherapy. Furthermore, in patients who subsequently reported a problem with constipation, a documented assessment occurred in just less than half of patients. Only 14% of patients who experienced constipation had documented evidence of constipation management (Johnson et al., 2007). Recommendations for oncology nurses to improve symptom management include performing a pretreatment risk assessment, ongoing symptom assessment, patient education regarding the symptom, and evidence-based management of the symptom (Johnson et al., 2007).

Diarrhea

Diarrhea can be a significant problem in patients receiving chemotherapy and radiation therapy. Patients who experience diarrhea while on treatment may require a dose reduction or treatment interruptions. This puts those patients at risk for negative outcomes as a result of not receiving full-dose therapy in the prescribed time frame.

Diarrhea is the passage of abnormally liquid or unformed stool at an increased frequency. The definition of diarrhea is greater than 200 g/day of fecal output, with a volume of 300 ml that is 70%–90% water, and more than three stools per day (Muehlbauer & Lopez, 2014). Because of individual variability, stool consistency and number are commonly used to quantify diarrhea. It is not always practical to be able to measure stool volume or weight.

Diarrhea can be acute or chronic. Acute diarrhea occurs within 24–48 hours of contact with an agent and resolves within 7–14 days or earlier with intervention. Chronic diarrhea can have a late onset, last for two to three weeks, and occur as the result of an unidentified agent or as the result of tissue injury related to a treatment modality that interferes with normal bowel functioning. Radiation-induced diarrhea typically occurs within two weeks of beginning radiation therapy (Muehlbauer & Lopez, 2014).

Pathophysiology

Seven types of diarrhea exist: osmotic, secretory, exudative, dysmotility associated, chemotherapy induced (including biotherapy and targeted therapy), radiation induced, and decreased absorptive surface (malabsorptive).

Osmotic diarrhea is caused by a mechanical disturbance in which a large volume influx of fluid into the intestinal lumen overwhelms the absorptive capacity. Secretory diarrhea is characterized by intestinal hypersecretion that is stimulated by endogenous mediators that increase the intestinal transport of water and electrolytes, exceeding the absorptive capacity. Exudative diarrhea is caused by compromised intestinal epithelium allowing mucus, protein, blood, and serum to escape into the GI tract, causing inflammation. Dysmotility-associated diarrhea occurs when there is an uncoordinated control of intestinal propulsion with a rapid transit of stool through the small and large intestines. Malabsorptive diarrhea occurs when there is incomplete digestion or absorption of macronutrients, resulting in a high volume of hyperosmolar substances entering the colon (Muehlbauer & Lopez, 2014).

Chemotherapy-induced diarrhea is a combination of mechanical and biochemical disturbances caused by the chemotherapy's effect on the bowel mucosa. It can occur when an imbalance exists between absorption and secretion in the small bowel (Camp-Sorrell, 2018). Chemotherapy-induced diarrhea is a cascade of events starting with the mitotic arrest of intestinal epithelial crypt cells, followed by superficial necrosis and inflammation of the bowel wall causing the production of leukotrienes, cytokines, and free radicals, which stimulate the oversecretion of intestinal water and electrolytes. The influx of fluid leads to the decreased absorptive capacity of the bowel, leading to diarrhea (Andreyev et al., 2014; Muehlbauer & Lopez, 2014).

Targeted therapy and biotherapy also can cause diarrhea. The exact mechanism is not clear. Diarrhea associated with tyrosine kinase inhibitors often occurs within the first three weeks of starting therapy. Multikinase inhibitors are associated with a higher incidence of diarrhea. Certain biologic agents also can cause diarrhea. Ipilimumab is a monoclonal antibody that can lead to immune-related colitis. Beck et al. (2006) identified on pathology neutrophilic inflammation with cryptitis and crypt cell abscesses in patients treated with ipilimumab.

Radiation-induced diarrhea is caused by acute damage to the epithelial crypt cells of the GI tract. The damage results in cell death, inflammation, and ulceration of the intestinal mucosa. These mechanisms cause the loss of absorptive surface in the bowel, leading to diarrhea. The incidence and severity of radiation-induced diarrhea are dependent on the site of radiation, the size of the radiation field, and the dose per fraction being administered. The highest incidence of radiation-induced diarrhea occurs in patients receiving abdominal and pelvic irradiation (Muehlbauer & Lopez, 2014). The addition of chemotherapy to radiation increases the incidence of diarrhea.

Patients undergoing HSCT can have diarrhea caused by the conditioning regimen, graft-versus-host disease (GVHD), or an infection related to immunosuppressive therapy. Recipients of allogeneic stem cell transplants also can develop GVHD, which starts three weeks or longer after transplantation. The diarrhea associated with acute GVHD is characterized by voluminous watery diarrhea and abdominal cramping. It is secretory and can be bloody (Davila & Bresalier, 2008).

Dihydropyrimidine dehydrogenase (DPD) is an enzyme involved in the catabolism of 5-fluorouracil and other fluoropyrimidines. A small number of patients may have a DPD deficiency. These patients have profound toxicities once given 5-fluorouracil, including diarrhea, neutropenia, and mucositis. Patients can be tested for DPD deficiency through a serum laboratory test. Treatment would include discontinuation of the fluoropyrimidine or significant dose reductions. Another special circumstance in which diarrhea may be amplified is in patients with a UGT1A1 deficiency. Irinotecan has a metabolite, SN-38, which is conjugated by UGT1A1 and secreted in the bile. In these patients, irinotecan is not adequately conjugated and secreted, causing severe toxicities, including diarrhea and neutropenia. Clinicians test for this deficiency and adjust irinotecan doses accordingly (Patel & Papachristos, 2015).

Signs and Symptoms

Each type of diarrhea has distinctive characteristics. Osmotic diarrhea is a large volume that resolves with fasting or when the provoking factor is eliminated. Malabsorptive diarrhea often is large volume with foul-smelling, oily, or frothy stool associated with cramping, bloating, gas, and weight loss. Secretory diarrhea is large volume, which persists despite fasting. Exudative diarrhea occurs more than six times a day, is of variable volume, and can be associated with hypoalbuminemia and anemia. Dysmotility-associated diarrhea is characterized by small, frequent, semisolid to liquid stools of variable volume and frequency. Chemotherapy-induced diarrhea often occurs within 24–96 hours after chemotherapy administration and consists of frequent, watery to semisolid stools. Severe diarrhea can lead to dehydration, electrolyte abnormalities, and renal insufficiency (Muehlbauer & Lopez, 2014).

Diarrhea can alter patients' quality of life. Patients frequently are anxious when eating for fear of diarrhea as a consequence. This may lead to weight loss. Patients' fears of incontinence can be quite distressing. Patients may alter their lifestyle habits to accommodate the chronic diarrhea, which can lead to social isolation. Nocturnal stooling can interrupt sleep habits, leading to fatigue. Altered body image, depression, and avoidance of intimacy are additional issues associated with chronic diarrhea (Muehlbauer & Lopez, 2014; Pessi et al., 2014).

Assessment and Diagnosis

Nurses play a key role in the assessment and education of patients at risk for diarrhea and in the management of patients who develop diarrhea. Nurses can work with the physician and nurse practitioner to develop a management plan for patients based on their risk factors, prior treatment, and planned treatment. Nurses often are the caregivers who provide education for patients with and at risk for diarrhea.

Nurses should document a detailed bowel history that includes the onset and timing of symptoms, the nature of bowel movements, frequency, the consistency and character of the stool, aggravating and alleviating symptoms, the patient's normal bowel habits, the change in bowel habits related to diagnosis and therapy, comorbid conditions, and associated symptoms that affect quality of life. They should inquire about what treatments the patients have tried for the diarrhea, what results they have had, and what concurrent medications they are using, including herbal supplements (Gwede, 2003). ASCO guidelines concur with rigorous assessment of diarrhea symptoms, including the duration and severity of symptoms, number of stools over baseline, and stool composition, as well as nocturnal diarrhea. ASCO also recommended to include fever, orthostatic symptoms, dizziness, abdominal pain, cramping, weakness, and hydration status. Stool volume is helpful but is unlikely to be obtained in most clinical settings (Benson et al., 2004).

Patients who are at risk for diarrhea are those with carcinoid tumors, those undergoing HSCT, those receiving radiation therapy to the abdomen and pelvic area, and those receiving certain chemotherapies such as fluoropyrimidines, topoisomerase inhibitors, epidermal growth factor receptor antibodies, and tyrosine kinase inhibitors. A list of agents that can cause diarrhea can be found in Table 20-5. Other patients who are at risk include patients with bowel obstruction, ischemic colitis, or enzyme deficiency; those who have had surgical procedures; those receiving certain supportive therapies such as parenteral nutritional formulas; and those experiencing narcotic withdrawal (Andreyev et al., 2014; Muehlbauer & Lopez, 2014; Pessi et al., 2014).

The CTCAE (NCI CTEP, 2010) is used commonly in the assessment of diarrhea. It describes five grades of diarrhea. Grade 1 is described as an increase of less than four stools per day over baseline or a mild increase in ostomy output compared to baseline. Grade 2 is an increase of four to six stools per day over baseline or a moderate increase in ostomy output compared to baseline. Grade 3 is characterized by an increase of more than seven stools per day over baseline, incontinence, the need for hospitalization, a severe increase in ostomy output compared to baseline, and limitation in performing self-care activities of daily living. Grade 4 diarrhea has life-threatening consequences, such as hemodynamic collapse, that require urgent intervention. Grade 5 diarrhea results in death (NCI CTEP, 2010).

Another tool used to assess diarrhea is the RTOG toxicity criteria, which is graded from 0 to 4 (Cox et al., 1995). Grade 0 indicates no change in bowel habits. Grade 1 is an increased frequency or a change in the quality of bowel habits but not requiring medication, or rectal discomfort not requiring analgesics. Grade 2 diarrhea requires parasympatholytic intervention (e.g., diphenoxylate hydrochloride with atropine sulfate), rectal or abdominal pain is present, requiring analgesics, and a mucous discharge occurs that does not require san-

Table 20-5. Common Chemotherapy, Biologics, and Targeted Therapies That Can Cause Diarrhea

Type of Agent	Examples
Chemotherapy	Arsenic trioxide, azacitidine, bendamustine hydrochloride, cabazitaxel, capecitabine, carboplatin, cladribine, clofarabine, cyclophosphamide, dactinomycin, daunorubicin, docetaxel, doxorubicin, enzalutamide, eribulin mesylate, fludarabine, 5-fluorouracil, gemcitabine, irinotecan, ixabepilone, mechlorethamine hydrochloride, methotrexate, mitotane, nelarabine, omacetaxine mepesuccinate, oxaliplatin, paclitaxel, paclitaxel protein-bound particles, pemetrexed, pentostatin, pralatrexate, temozolomide, topotecan hydrochloride, trimetrexate
Biologics	Aldesleukin (interleukin-2), interferon alfa, interferon alfa-2b, interferon gamma, peginterferon alfa-2b
Targeted therapies	Ado-trastuzumab, afatinib, axitinib, belinostat, bortezomib, bosutinib, brentuximab vedotin, cabozantinib, carfilzomib, ceritinib, cetuximab, crizotinib, dasatinib, denileukin diftitox, erlotinib, everolimus, ibrutinib, idelalisib, imatinib mesylate, ipilimumab, lapatinib, lenalidomide, nilotinib, panitumumab, pazopanib, pembrolizumab, pertuzumab, pomalidomide, regorafenib, romidepsin, sorafenib, sunitinib, temsirolimus, trametinib, tretinoin, vandetanib, vemurafenib, vorinostat, ziv-aflibercept

Note. Based on information from Wilkes & Barton-Burke, 2016.

itary pads. Grade 3 diarrhea requires parenteral support and includes symptoms of severe mucous or bloody discharge necessitating sanitary pads, or abdominal distention. Grade 4 diarrhea is reported as acute or subacute obstruction, fistula, abdominal perforation, GI bleeding requiring transfusion, or tenesmus requiring tube decompression or bowel diversion.

ASCO guidelines reported by Benson et al. (2004) classified patients' symptoms as complicated or uncomplicated. Patients with uncomplicated symptoms are those with grade 1 or 2 diarrhea (based on the CTCAE) and no other symptoms. ASCO recommended that these patients be managed conservatively. If a patient with a grade 1 or 2 diarrhea has additional risk factors, such as moderate to severe cramping, grade 2 vomiting, fever, neutropenia, bleeding, or dehydration, the diarrhea is classified as complicated and would require aggressive treatment. Any case of grade 3 or 4 diarrhea is automatically classified as complicated.

Complications of diarrhea include the loss of fluid and electrolytes, with persistent or severe diarrhea resulting in life-threatening dehydration, renal insufficiency, and electrolyte imbalances that can lead to cardiovascular collapse. The risk of infection can be increased in patients with concomitant chemotherapy-induced neutropenia (Benson et al., 2004).

Physical examination should include an assessment for dehydration, including an evaluation of skin turgor and mucous membranes. Blood pressure, heart rate, and urine output, along with weight loss, should be evaluated. A thorough examination of the abdomen, including palpation, auscultation of bowel sounds, and a rectal examination (in non-neutropenic patients), should be performed. In addition, assessment of the skin in the perianal area or peristomal area should be performed and documented (Andreyev et al., 2014).

Stool testing for infection, such as *Clostridium difficile*, ova and parasites, fecal blood, and fecal leukocytes should be done with new-onset diarrhea to rule out an infectious etiology. Laboratory studies including electrolytes (serum albumin, potassium, creatinine, blood urea nitrogen, magnesium) should be performed. Testing that is used in patients with negative stool testing and persistent symptoms includes endoscopy, computed tomography scan, and biopsy as needed. In patients with carcinoid tumors, a 24-hour urine collection for 5-HIAA (5-hydroxyindoleacetic acid) is obtained to assess the disease (Andreyev et al., 2014).

Management

Early prevention of diarrhea is paramount in the care of patients with cancer. If diarrhea is left untreated, it can cause treatment delays, dose reductions, or discontinuation, which may interfere with patients' response to treatment. ONS PEP recommendations can be found at www.ons.org/practice-resources/pep/diarrhea/chemotherapy-induced-diarrhea for chemotherapy-induced diarrhea and www.ons.org/practice-resources/pep/diarrhea/radiation-induced-diarrhea for radiation-induced diarrhea.

Patients need to take care of irritated skin in the perirectal area, especially if they are neutropenic or otherwise immunocompromised. Nurses should assess patients for dehydration (Andreyev et al., 2014). Current radiation treatment planning techniques, such as 3-D treatment planning, can reduce the involvement of normal tissue in the treatment fields, thus lowering the incidence of radiation-induced diarrhea.

Patient education needs to start early. Nurses should emphasize the importance of accurate and timely reporting of diarrhea, along with a review of the potential complications of diarrhea. Patients should be instructed to keep a detailed log of their diarrhea, including any associated symptoms. The records will assist the clinician with management strategies. Patients should be instructed to keep hydrated and adhere to dietary modifications. Patients should be educated about the signs and symptoms that need to be reported to their healthcare provider, such as fever, dizziness, excessive thirst, bloody stool, intense cramping, or refractory diarrhea (Muehlbauer & Lopez, 2014).

Dietary changes are recommended when diarrhea begins. The BRAT diet (bananas, rice, applesauce, and toast) should be recommended. A list of dietary restrictions is found in Figure 20-4. Medications can antagonize diarrhea, including antibiotics, laxatives, cytoprotectants, magnesium-containing medications, promotility agents, stool softeners, and herbal supplements (Muehlbauer & Lopez, 2014).

Four types of medications are used to treat chemotherapy-induced diarrhea: intestinal transport inhibitors, intraluminal agents, proabsorptive agents, and antisecretory agents. Intestinal transport inhibitors work to prolong transit time through the bowel and increase fluid absorption. Intraluminal agents decrease water in the gut by absorption, increasing the bulk of the stool and protecting the intestinal mucosa. Proabsorptive agents act as intraluminal absorbent agents. Antisecretory agents work to decrease the fluid secretion of gut hormones, slow transit time, and improve water regulation (Ippoliti, 1998; Stern & Ippoliti, 2003). Intestinal transport inhibitors include loperamide, diphenoxylate with atropine, and tincture of opium.

Figure 20-4. Foods and Substances to Be Avoided With Diarrhea

- Spicy foods
- High-fat foods
- High-fiber foods
- Caffeine
- Alcohol
- Hyperosmotic liquids
- Foods containing lactose

Note. Based on information from Muehlbauer & Lopez, 2014.

Interventions for chemotherapy-induced diarrhea classified as likely be effective are loperamide hydrochloride and octreotide treatment (Thorpe, Byar, Conley, Davis, Drapek, Hays, ... Wolles, 2016). Loperamide hydrochloride decreases intestinal motility by affecting the smooth muscles of the intestinal wall, increasing stool bulk and viscosity. The recommended dose of loperamide is 4 mg with the initial loose bowel movement, followed by 2 mg with each loose bowel movement thereafter for a maximum of 16 mg a day. Patients should be instructed to follow the same directions if diarrhea persists to a second day (Andreyev et al., 2014; Muehlbauer & Lopez, 2014; Muehlbauer et al., 2009; Stern & Ippoliti, 2003).

Octreotide acetate is an analog of somatostatin that has multiple actions. It is an antisecretory agent that enhances water and electrolyte absorption, decreases splanchnic blood flow, decreases intestinal motility, and inhibits secretion across the gut wall. It can be dosed as a continuous infusion, subcutaneously, or by intramuscular injection. It is dosed at 100 mcg SC three times a day. The maximum dose is 500 mcg daily. Patients may use a long-acting formulation once they have achieved control with the short-acting formulation. The long-acting medication is given intramuscularly every 28 days and takes 10–14 days to achieve therapeutic drug levels (Andreyev et al., 2014; Stern & Ippoliti, 2003).

For diarrhea that is refractory to loperamide, diphenoxylate hydrochloride and atropine often are used. This combination of agents inhibits intestinal peristalsis and decreases the defecation reflex. The dose is 2.5 mg diphenoxylate hydrochloride with 0.025 mg of atropine sulfate dosed four times a day, with a maximum of eight tablets a day (Stern & Ippoliti, 2003).

Atropine is an anticholinergic agent. It is used to treat acute diarrhea associated with irinotecan. The dose is 0.25–1 mg SC or IV given before or when symptoms occur. The total daily dose should not exceed 1.2 mg (Andreyev et al., 2014; Muehlbauer & Lopez, 2014; Stern & Ippoliti, 2003). It works by controlling the cholinergic effects of irinotecan.

Tincture of opium is an opium antidiarrheal agent. It increases GI smooth muscle tone and inhibits GI motility, delaying the movement of intestinal contents. It is dosed at 5 ml every three to four hours as needed. It can have a bad taste and can be administered with juice to disguise the taste (Muehlbauer & Lopez, 2014; Stern & Ippoliti, 2003).

Opioids can mask symptoms of perforation and should be used with caution. The immunotherapy monoclonal antibody ipilimumab can cause diarrhea. If a patient develops grade 1 diarrhea, the drug should be stopped, loperamide should be started, and electrolytes should be replaced if needed. If grade 2 diarrhea develops, corticosteroids should be administered. Diarrhea persisting longer should be evaluated for infection or inflammatory bowel disease (Muehlbauer & Lopez, 2014).

In the 2004 ASCO diarrhea management guidelines, Benson et al. recommended aggressive management for complicated diarrhea cases. This includes IV hydration; octreotide starting at 100–150 mcg SC three times a day, or 25–50 mcg/hr IV if the patient is severely dehydrated, with dose escalation up to 500 mcg IV or SC three times a day until diarrhea is controlled; and the administration of antibiotics. Treatment is recommended until the patient has been diarrhea free for 24 hours. Hospitalization may be considered. The treatment of moderate to mild diarrhea should include dietary modifications and instructions to keep a thorough record of the number of stools and associated symptoms. Loperamide can be started at a dose of 4 mg. If symptoms resolve, the patient should continue dietary recommendations and can discontinue loperamide when diarrhea free for 12 hours. In mild diarrhea induced by radiation therapy, loperamide should be continued because of repeated intestinal mucosal injury. If mild to moderate diarrhea persists for more than 24 hours, the dose of loperamide should be increased to 2 mg every two hours, and oral antibiotics may be started for infection prophylaxis. If mild to moderate diarrhea persists for more than 48 hours on loperamide, it should be discontinued and the patient should be started on SC octreotide or another second-line agent, such as tincture of opium.

Nursing Implications

The goals of treatment of diarrhea are to restore normal bowel function, minimize the risk of complications and associated medical problems, and maintain patient function, comfort, and quality of life. Prompt intervention is important to prevent serious consequences. Patient education is paramount for early detection and intervention of chemotherapy- and radiation-induced diarrhea.

Conclusion

Patients with cancer may experience GI-related symptoms for numerous reasons, such as the cancer itself or as a result of cancer therapy. Oncology nurses need to be familiar with commonly occurring GI complications so that they can promptly recognize these symptoms and intervene appropriately. Several evidence-based guidelines are available for nurses to use when managing GI toxicities in patients with cancer, and oncology nurses should recognize that such resources are invaluable tools for providing these patients with the most current recommendations. Oncology nurses are on the forefront of symptom assessment and management, and they must remain abreast of changing therapies.

Key Points

- Xerostomia is defined as a dry mouth due to reduced or absent saliva caused by damage to the salivary glands. It can significantly affect a patient's quality of life. It can occur with radiation and chemotherapy.
- Mucositis affects the mucous membranes of the GI tract. It can occur as a result of chemotherapy and radiation. Patients should be assessed for mucositis before, during, and after therapy. Good oral hygiene is the basic tenet to prevent and decrease the incidence of oral mucositis.
- Obstructive dysphagia is seen most often in patients with cancer. It can result from treatment-induced fibrosis or a postoperative stricture. Patients who experience obstructive dysphagia are at risk for weight loss, malnutrition, and aspiration.
- Nausea and vomiting are common symptoms in the oncology population and may be a consequence of chemotherapy, radiation, or other sources.
- Uncontrolled nausea and vomiting may negatively influence quality of life, patient adherence, and healthcare costs.
- CINV is the most frequent cause of nausea and vomiting in the cancer setting, and national guidelines have been published to assist clinicians with prophylaxis and management of this problem.
- Constipation occurs commonly in the cancer population, with opioid-induced constipation being the most frequent culprit.
- Although limited data exist to support the use of specific laxatives in patients with cancer, experts agree that prophylaxis of opioid-induced constipation with laxatives is likely to be an effective strategy for managing this symptom.
- Diarrhea is a significant problem in patients receiving chemotherapy and radiation therapy. Early prevention of diarrhea is paramount in the care of patients with cancer.

References

Aapro, M., Fabi, A., Nolè, F., Medici, M., Steger, G., Bachmann, C., ... Roila, F. (2010). Double-blind, randomised, controlled study of the efficacy and tolerability of palonosetron plus dexamethasone for 1 day with or without dexamethasone on days 2 and 3 in the prevention of nausea and vomiting induced by moderately emetogenic chemotherapy. *Annals of Oncology, 21,* 1083–1088. doi:10.1093/annonc/mdp584

Aapro, M., Jordan, K., & Feyer, P. (2013). *Prevention of nausea and vomiting in cancer patients.* doi:10.1007/978-1-907673-58-0_2

Aapro, M., Molassiotis, A., Dicato, M., Peláez, I., Rodríguez-Lescure, A., Pastorelli, D., ... Roila, F. (2012). The effect of guideline-consistent antiemetic therapy on chemotherapy-induced nausea and vomiting (CINV): The Pan European Emesis Registry (PEER). *Annals of Oncology, 23,* 1986–1992. doi:10.1093/annonc/mds021

Aapro, M., Rugo, H., Rossi, G., Rizzi, G., Borroni, M.E., Bondarenko, I., ... Grunberg, S. (2014). A randomized phase III study evaluating the efficacy and safety of NEPA, a fixed-dose combination of netupitant and palonosetron, for prevention of chemotherapy-induced nausea and vomiting following moderately emetogenic chemotherapy. *Annals of Oncology, 25,* 1328–1333. doi:10.1093/annonc/mdu101

Abramowitz, L., Béziaud, N., Labreze, L., Giardina, V., Caussé, C., Chuberre, B., ... Perrot, S. (2013). Prevalence and impact of constipation and bowel dysfunction induced by strong opioids: A cross-sectional survey of 520 patients with cancer pain: DYONISOS study. *Journal of Medical Economics, 16,* 1423–1433. doi:10.3111/13696998.2013.851082

Andrews, C.N., & Storr, M. (2011). The pathophysiology of chronic constipation. *Canadian Journal of Gastroenterology, 25*(Suppl. B), 16B–21B. doi:10.1155/2011/715858

Andreyev, J., Ross, P., Donellan, C., Lennan, E., Leonard, P., Waters, C., ... Ferry, D. (2014). Guidance on the management of diarrhea during cancer chemotherapy. *Lancet, 15,* e447–e460. doi:10.1016/S1470-2045(14)70006-3

Ang, S.K., Shoemaker, L.K., & Davis, M.P. (2010). Nausea and vomiting in advanced cancer. *American Journal of Hospice and Palliative Medicine, 27,* 219–225. doi:10.1177/1049909110361228

Arbabi-Kalati, F., Arbabi-Kalati, F., & Moridi, T. (2013). Evaluation of the effect of low level laser on prevention of chemotherapy-induced mucositis. *Acta Medica Iranica, 51,* 157–162. Retrieved from http://acta.tums.ac.ir/index.php/acta/article/view/4471

Bar, V., Weinstein, G., Dutta, P.R., Dosoretz, A., Chalian, A., Both, S., & Quon, H. (2010). Gabapentin for the treatment of pain syndrome related to radiation-induced mucositis in patients with head and neck cancer treated with concurrent chemoradiotherapy. *Cancer, 116,* 4206–4213. doi:10.1002/cncr.25274

Barish, C.F., Drossman, D., Johanson, J.F., & Ueno, R. (2010). Efficacy and safety of lubiprostone in patients with chronic constipation. *Digestive Diseases and Sciences, 55,* 1090–1097. doi:10.1007/s10620-009-1068-x

Basch, E., Prestrud, A.A., Hesketh, P.J., Kris, M.G., Feyer, P.C., Somerfield, M.R., ... Lyman, G.H. (2011). Antiemetics: American Society of Clinical Oncology clinical practice guideline update. *Journal of Clinical Oncology, 29,* 4189–4198. doi:10.1200/JCO.2010.34.4614

Beck, K.E., Blansfield, J.A., Tran, K.Q., Feldman, A.L., Hughes, M.S., Royal, R.E., ... Yang, J.C. (2006). Enterocolitis in patients with cancer after antibody blockade of cytotoxic T-lymphocyte–associated antigen 4. *Journal of Clinical Oncology, 24,* 2283–2289. doi:10.1200/JCO.2005.04.5716

Bell, T.J., Panchal, S.J., Miaskowski, C., Bolge, S.C., Milanova, T., & Williamson, R. (2009). The prevalence, severity, and impact of opioid-induced bowel dysfunction: Results of a US and European patient survey (PROBE 1). *Pain Medicine, 10,* 35–42. doi:10.1111/j.1526-4637.2008.00495.x

Belsey, J.D., Geraint, M., & Dixon, T.A. (2010). Systematic review and meta analysis: Polyethylene glycol in adults with non-organic constipation. *International Journal of Clinical Practice, 64,* 944–955. doi:10.1111/j.1742-1241.2010.02397.x

Benson, A.B., III, Ajani, J.A., Catalano, R.B., Engelking, C., Kornblau, S.M., Martenson, J.A., Jr., ... Wadler, S. (2004). Recommended guidelines for the treatment of cancer treatment-induced diarrhea. *Journal of Clinical Oncology, 22,* 2918–2926. doi:10.1200/JCO.2004.04.132

Bhide, S.A., Miah, A.B., Harrington, K.J., Newbold, K.L., & Nutting, C.M. (2009). Radiation-induced xerostomia: Pathophysiology, prevention and treatment. *Clinical Oncology, 21,* 737–744. doi:10.1016/j.clon.2009.09.002

Braud, A.-C., Genre, D., Leto, C., Nemer, V., Cailhol, J.-F., Macquart-Moulin, G., ... Viens, P. (2003). Nurses' repeat measurement of chemotherapy symptoms: Feasibility, resulting information, patient satisfaction. *Cancer Nursing, 26,* 468–475. doi:10.1097/00002820-200312000-00006

Brearley, S.G., Clements, C.V., & Molassiotis, A. (2008). A review of patient self-report tools for chemotherapy-induced nausea and vomiting. *Supportive Care in Cancer, 16,* 1213–1229. doi:10.1007/s00520-008-0428-y

Brizel, D.M., Wasserman, T.H., Henke, M., Strnad, V., Rudat, V., Monnier, A., ... Sauer, R. (2000). Phase III randomized trial of amifostine as a radioprotector in head and neck cancer. *Journal of Clinical Oncology, 18,* 3339–3345. doi:10.1200/JCO.2000.18.19.3339

Bruce, S.D. (2004). Radiation-induced xerostomia: How dry is your patient? *Clinical Journal of Oncology Nursing, 8,* 61–67. doi:10.1188/04.CJON.61-67

Burke, T.A., Wisniewski, T., & Ernst, F.R. (2011). Resource utilization and costs associated with chemotherapy-induced nausea and vomiting (CINV) following highly or moderately emetogenic chemotherapy administered in the US outpatient hospital setting. *Supportive Care in Cancer, 19,* 131–140. doi:10.1007/s00520-009-0797-x

Camp-Sorrell, D. (2014). Dysphagia. In C.H. Yarbro, D. Wujcik, & B.H. Gobel (Eds.), *Cancer symptom management* (4th ed., pp. 385–402). Burlington, MA: Jones & Bartlett Learning.

Camp-Sorrell, D. (2018). Chemotherapy toxicities and management. In C.H. Yarbro, D. Wujcik, & B.H. Gobel (Eds.), *Cancer nursing: Principles and practice* (8th ed., pp. 497–554). Burlington, MA: Jones & Bartlett Learning.

Canadian Agency for Drugs and Technologies in Health. (2014). *Treatments for constipation: A review of systematic reviews.* Retrieved from https://www.cadth.ca/treatments-constipation-review-systematic-reviews

Candy, B., Jones, L., Goodman, M.L., Drake, R., & Tookman, A. (2011). Laxatives or methylnaltrexone for the management of constipation in palliative care patients. *Cochrane Database of Systematic Reviews, 2011*(1). doi:10.1002/14651858.CD003448.pub3

Carr, E. (2018). Head and neck malignancies. In C.H. Yarbro, D. Wujcik, & B.H. Gobel (Eds.), *Cancer nursing: Principles and practice* (8th ed., pp. 1573–1598). Burlington, MA: Jones & Bartlett Learning.

Carvalho, P.A., Jaguar, G.C., Pellizzon, A.C., Prado, J.D., Lopes, R.N., & Alves, F.A. (2011). Evaluation of low-level laser therapy in the prevention and treatment of radiation-induced mucositis: A double-blind randomized study in head and neck cancer patients. *Oral Oncology, 47,* 1176–1181. doi:10.1016/j.oraloncology.2011.08.021

Cassileth, B.R., Deng, G.E., Gomez, J.E., Johnstone, P.A.S., Kumar, N., & Vickers, A.J. (2007). Complementary therapies and integrative oncology in lung cancer: ACCP evidence-based clinical practice guidelines (2nd ed.). *Chest, 132*(Suppl. 3), 340S–354S. doi:10.1378/chest.07-1389

Celio, L., Frustaci, S., Denaro, A., Buonadonna, A., Ardizzoia, A., Piazza, E., ... Bajetta, E. (2011). Palonosetron in combination with 1-day versus 3-day dexamethasone for prevention of nausea and vomiting following moderately emetogenic chemotherapy: A randomized, multicenter, phase III trial. *Supportive Care in Cancer, 19,* 1217–1225. doi:10.1007/s00520-010-0941-7

Chan, A.O.O., Cheng, C., Hui, W.M., Hu, W.H.C., Wong, N.Y.H., Lam, K.F., ... Wong, B.C.Y. (2005). Differing coping mechanisms, stress level and anorectal physiology in patients with functional constipation. *World Journal of Gastroenterology, 11,* 5362–5366. doi:10.3748/wjg.v11.i34.5362

Chan, A.O.O., Kim, H.-K., Hsieh, R.K., Yu, S., de Lima Lopes, G., Jr., Su, W.-C., … Keefe, D.M.K. (2015). Incidence and predictors of anticipatory nausea and vomiting in Asia Pacific clinical practice—A longitudinal analysis. *Supportive Care in Cancer, 23,* 283–291. doi:10.1007/s00520-014-2375-0

Chang, J.Y., Locke, G.R., Schleck, C.D., Zinsmeister, A.R., & Talley, N.J. (2007). Risk factors for chronic constipation and a possible role of analgesics. *Neurogastroenterology and Motility, 19,* 905–911. doi:10.1111/j.1365-2982.2007.00974.x

Cherny, N.I. (2004). Taking care of the terminally ill cancer patient: Management of gastrointestinal symptoms in patients with advanced cancer. *Annals of Oncology, 15*(Suppl. 4), iv205–iv213.

Cox, J.D., Stetz, J., & Pajak, T.F. (1995). Toxicity criteria of the Radiation Therapy Oncology Group (RTOG) and the European Organization for Research and Treatment of Cancer (EORTC). *International Journal of Radiation Oncology, Biology, Physics, 31,* 1341–1346. doi:10.1016/0360-3016(95)00060-C

Cryer, B., Katz, S., Vallejo, R., Popescu, A., & Ueno, R. (2014). A randomized study of lubiprostone for opioid-induced constipation in patients with chronic noncancer pain. *Pain Medicine, 15,* 1825–1834. doi:10.1111/pme.12437

Cumberland Pharmaceuticals Inc. (2016). *Ethyol® (amifostine) for injection* [Package insert]. Nashville, TN: Author.

Dalton, K.A., & Gosselin, T.K. (2014). Xerostomia. In C.H. Yarbro, D. Wujcik, & B.H. Gobel (Eds.), *Cancer symptom management* (4th ed., pp. 421–434). Burlington, MA: Jones & Bartlett Learning.

Davidson, W., Teleni, L., Muller, J., Ferguson, M., McCarthy, A.L., Vick, J., & Isenring, E. (2012). Malnutrition and chemotherapy-induced nausea and vomiting: Implications for practice [Online exclusive]. *Oncology Nursing Forum, 39,* E340–E345. doi:10.1188/12.ONF.E340-E345

Davila, M., & Bresalier, R.S. (2008). Gastrointestinal complications of oncologic therapy. *Nature Reviews Gastroenterology and Hepatology, 5,* 682–696. doi:10.1038/ncpgasthep1277

Davis, M.P., & Hallerberg, G. (2010). A systematic review of the treatment of nausea and/or vomiting in cancer unrelated to chemotherapy or radiation. *Journal of Pain and Symptom Management, 39,* 756–767. doi:10.1016/j.jpainsymman.2009.08.010

Davis, M.P., Maida, V., Daeninck, P., & Pergolizzi, J. (2007). The emerging role of cannabinoid neuromodulators in symptom management. *Supportive Care in Cancer, 15,* 63–71. doi:10.1007/s00520-006-0180-0

Dik, V.K., Siersema, P.D., Joseph, A., Hodgkins, P., Smeets, H.M., & van Oijen, M.G.H. (2014). Constipation-related direct medical costs in 16 887 patients newly diagnosed with chronic constipation. *European Journal of Gastroenterology and Hepatology, 26,* 1260–1266. doi:10.1097/MEG.0000000000000167

DiPalma, J.A., Cleveland, M.B., McGowan, J., & Herrera, J.L. (2007a). A comparison of polyethylene glycol laxative and placebo for relief of constipation from constipating medications. *Southern Medical Journal, 100,* 1085–1090. doi:10.1097/SMJ.0b013e318157ec8f

DiPalma, J.A., Cleveland, M.B., McGowan, J., & Herrera, J.L. (2007b). A randomized, multicenter, placebo-controlled trial of polyethylene glycol laxative for chronic treatment of chronic constipation. *American Journal of Gastroenterology, 102,* 1436–1441. doi:10.1111/j.1572-0241.2007.01199.x

Droney, J., Ross, J., Gretton, S., Welsh, K., Sato, H., & Riley, J. (2008). Constipation in cancer patients on morphine. *Supportive Care in Cancer, 16,* 453–459. doi:10.1007/s00520-007-0373-1

Eilers, J.G., Asakura, Y., Blecher, C.S., Burgoon, D., Burns, B.R., Chiffelle, R., … Valinski, S. (2016, November 2). ONS Putting Evidence Into Practice: Mucositis. Retrieved from https://www.ons.org/practice-resources/pep/mucositis

Eilers, J.G., Berger, A.M., & Petersen, M.C. (1988). Development, testing, and application of the oral assessment guide. *Oncology Nursing Forum, 15,* 325–330.

Eilers, J.G., Harris, D., Henry, K., & Johnson, L.A. (2014). Evidence-based interventions for cancer treatment–related mucositis: Putting evidence into practice. *Clinical Journal of Oncology Nursing, 18*(Suppl. 6), 80–96. doi:10.1188/14.CJON.S3.80-96

Eisai Inc. & Helsinn Therapeutics Inc. (2015). *Akynzeo® (netupitant/palonosetron)* [Package insert]. Woodcliff Lake, NJ: Eisai Inc.

Ell, C., & May, A. (1997). Self-expanding metal stents for palliation of stenosing tumors of the esophagus and cardia: A critical review. *Endoscopy, 29,* 392–398. doi:10.1055/s-2007-1004222

Endo, T., Minami, M., Hirafuji, M., Ogawa, T., Akita, K., Nemoto, M., … Parvez, S.H. (2000). Neurochemistry and neuropharmacology of emesis—The role of serotonin. *Toxicology, 153,* 189–201. doi:10.1016/S0300-483X(00)00314-0

Ezzo, J., Richardson, M.A., Vickers, A., Allen, C., Dibble, S., Issell, B.F., … Zhang, G. (2006). Acupuncture-point stimulation for chemotherapy-induced nausea or vomiting. *Cochrane Database of Systematic Reviews, 2006*(2). doi:10.1002/14651858.CD002285.pub2

Fernández-Ortega, P., Caloto, M.T., Chirveches, E., Marquilles, R., San Francisco, J., Quesada, A., … Llombart-Cussac, A. (2012). Chemotherapy-induced nausea and vomiting in clinical practice: Impact on patients' quality of life. *Supportive Care in Cancer, 20,* 3141–3148. doi:10.1007/s00520-012-1448-1

Feyer, P., Jahn, F., & Jordan, K. (2014). Radiation induced nausea and vomiting. *European Journal of Pharmacology, 722,* 165–171. doi:10.1016/j.ejphar.2013.09.069

Frank, L., Kleinman, L., Farup, C., Taylor, L., & Miner, P., Jr. (1999). Psychometric validation of a constipation symptom assessment questionnaire. *Scandinavian Journal of Gastroenterology, 34,* 870–877.

Furness, S., Bryan, G., McMillan, R., Birchenough, S., & Worthington, H.V. (2013). Interventions for the management of dry mouth: Non-pharmacological interventions. *Cochrane Database of Systematic Reviews, 2013*(9). doi:10.1002/14651858.CD009603.pub3

Furness, S., Worthington, H.V., Bryan, G., Birchenough, S., & McMillan, R. (2011). Interventions for the management of dry mouth: Topical therapies. *Cochrane Database of Systematic Reviews, 2011*(12). doi:10.1002/14651858.CD008934.pub2

Geling, O., & Eichler, H.-G. (2005). Should 5-hydroxytryptamine-3 receptor antagonists be administered beyond 24 hours after chemotherapy to prevent delayed emesis? Systematic re-evaluation of clinical evidence and drug cost implications. *Journal of Clinical Oncology, 23,* 1289–1294. doi:10.1200/JCO.2005.04.022

Gilmore, J.W., Peacock, N.W., Gu, A., Szabo, S., Rammage, R., Sharpe, J., ... Burke, T.A. (2014). Antiemetic guideline consistency and incidence of chemotherapy-induced nausea and vomiting in US community oncology practice: INSPIRE study. *Journal of Oncology Practice, 10,* 68–74. doi:10.1200/JOP.2012.000816

Glare, P.A., Dunwoodie, D., Clark, K., Ward, A., Yates, P., Ryan, S., & Hardy, J.R. (2008). Treatment of nausea and vomiting in terminally ill cancer patients. *Drugs, 68,* 2575–2590. doi:10.2165/0003495-200868180-00004

Glare, P.A., Pereira, G., Kristjanson, L.J., Stockler, M., & Tattersall, M. (2004). Systematic review of the efficacy of antiemetics in the treatment of nausea in patients with far-advanced cancer. *Supportive Care in Cancer, 12,* 432–440. doi:10.1007/s00520-004-0629-y

Goodman, M., Low, J., & Wilkinson, S. (2005). Constipation management in palliative care: A survey of practices in the United Kingdom. *Journal of Pain and Symptom Management, 29,* 238–244. doi:10.1016/j.jpainsymman.2004.06.013

Gordon, P., LeGrand, S.B., & Walsh, D. (2013). Nausea and vomiting in advanced cancer. *European Journal of Pharmacology, 722,* 187–191. doi:10.1016/j.ejphar.2013.10.010

Guchelaar, H.J., Vermes, A., & Meerwaldt, J.H. (1997). Radiation-induced xerostomia: Pathophysiology, clinical course and supportive treatment. *Supportive Care in Cancer, 5,* 281–288.

Gwede, C.K. (2003). Overview of radiation- and chemoradiation-induced diarrhea. *Seminars in Oncology Nursing, 19*(4, Suppl. 3), 6–10. doi:10.1053/j.soncn.2003.09.008

Haiderali, A., Menditto, L., Good, M., Teitelbaum, A., & Wegner, J. (2011). Impact on daily functioning and indirect/direct costs associated with chemotherapy-induced nausea and vomiting (CINV) in a US population. *Supportive Care in Cancer, 19,* 843–851. doi:10.1007/s00520-010-0915-9

Heitkemper, M., & Wolff, J. (2007). Challenges in chronic constipation management. *Nurse Practitioner, 32*(4), 36–42. doi:10.1097/01.NPR.0000266512.55726.e0

Hensley, M.L., Hagerty, K.L., Kewalramani, T., Green, D.M., Meropol, N.J., Wasserman, T.H., ... Schuchter, L.M. (2009). American Society of Clinical Oncology 2008 clinical practice guideline update: Use of chemotherapy and radiation therapy protectants. *Journal of Clinical Oncology, 27,* 127–145. doi:10.1200/JCO.2008.17.2627

Hertig, V.L., Cain, K.C., Jarrett, M.E., Burr, R.L., & Heitkemper, M.M. (2007). Daily stress and gastrointestinal symptoms in women with irritable bowel syndrome. *Nursing Research, 56,* 399–406. doi:10.1097/01.NNR.0000299855.60053.88

Hesketh, P.J. (2008). Chemotherapy-induced nausea and vomiting. *New England Journal of Medicine, 358,* 2482–2494. doi:10.1056/NEJMra0706547

Hesketh, P.J., Bohlke, K., Lyman, G.H., Basch, E., Chesney, M., Clark-Snow, R.A., ... Kris, M.G. (2016). Antiemetics: American Society of Clinical Oncology focused guideline update. *Journal of Clinical Oncology, 34,* 381–386. doi:10.1200/JCO.2015.64.3635

Hesketh, P.J., Van Belle, S., Aapro, M., Tattersall, F.D., Naylor, R.J., Hargreaves, R., ... Horgan, K.J. (2003). Differential involvement of neurotransmitters through the time course of cisplatin-induced emesis as revealed by therapy with specific receptor antagonists. *European Journal of Cancer, 39,* 1074–1080. doi:10.1016/S0959-8049(02)00674-3

Hilarius, D.L., Kloeg, P.H., van der Wall, E., van den Heuvel, J.J.G., Gundy, C.M., & Aaronson, N.K. (2012). Chemotherapy-induced nausea and vomiting in daily clinical practice: A community hospital-based study. *Supportive Care in Cancer, 20,* 107–117. doi:10.1007/s00520-010-1073-9

Horiot, J.-C. (2004). Prophylaxis versus treatment: Is there a better way to manage radiotherapy-induced nausea and vomiting? *International Journal of Radiation Oncology, Biology, Physics, 60,* 1018–1025. doi:10.1016/j.ijrobp.2004.07.722

Hornby, P.J. (2001). Central neurocircuitry associated with emesis. *American Journal of Medicine, 111*(Suppl. 1), 106S–112S. doi:10.1016/S0002-9343(01)00849-X

Ioannidis, J.P.A., Hesketh, P.J., & Lau, J. (2000). Contribution of dexamethasone to control of chemotherapy-induced nausea and vomiting: A meta-analysis of randomized evidence. *Journal of Clinical Oncology, 18,* 3409–3422.

Ippoliti, C. (1998). Antidiarrheal agents for the management of treatment-related diarrhea in cancer patients. *American Journal of Health-System Pharmacy, 55,* 1573–1580.

Izumi, K. (2014). The measures to evaluate constipation: A review article. *Gastroenterology Nursing, 37,* 137–146. doi:10.1097/SGA.0000000000000034

Jamal, M.M., Adams, A.B., Jansen, J.P., & Webster, L.R. (2015). A randomized, placebo-controlled trial of lubiprostone for opioid-induced constipation in chronic noncancer pain. *American Journal of Gastroenterology, 110,* 725–732. doi:10.1038/ajg.2015.106

Jamshed, N., Lee, Z.-E., & Olden, K.W. (2011). Diagnostic approach to chronic constipation in adults. *American Family Physician, 84,* 299–306.

Jansen, J.-P., Lorch, D., Langan, J., Lasko, B., Hermanns, K., Kleoudis, C.S., … Mortensen, E.R. (2011). A randomized, placebo-controlled phase 3 trial (Study SB-767905/012) of alvimopan for opioid-induced bowel dysfunction in patients with non-cancer pain. *Journal of Pain, 12,* 185–193. doi:10.1016/j.jpain.2010.06.012

Javle, M., Ailawadhi, S., Yang, G.Y., Nwogu, C.E., Schiff, M.D., & Nava, H.R. (2006). Palliation of malignant dysphagia in esophageal cancer: A literature-based review. *Journal of Supportive Oncology, 4,* 365–373, 379.

Jin, Y., Sun, W., Gu, D., Yang, J., Xu, Z., & Chen, J. (2013). Comparative efficacy and safety of palonosetron with the first 5-HT3 receptor antagonists for the chemotherapy-induced nausea and vomiting: A meta-analysis. *European Journal of Cancer Care, 22,* 41–50. doi:10.1111/j.1365-2354.2012.01353.x

Johnson, G.D., Moore, K., & Fortner, B. (2007). Baseline evaluation of the AIM Higher Initiative: Establishing the mark from which to measure. *Oncology Nursing Forum, 34,* 729–734. doi:10.1188/07.ONF.729-734

Johnson, M.C. (2001). The esophagus. *Primary Care, 28,* 459–485. doi:10.1016/S0095-4543(05)70048-8

Jordan, K., Hinke, A., Grothey, A., Voigt, W., Arnold, D., Wolf, H.-H., & Schmoll, H.-J. (2007). A meta-analysis comparing the efficacy of four 5-HT_3-receptor antagonists for acute chemotherapy-induced emesis. *Supportive Care in Cancer, 15,* 1023–1033. doi:10.1007/s00520-006-0186-7

Kirkova, J., Rybicki, L., Walsh, D., & Aktas, A. (2012). Symptom prevalence in advanced cancer: Age, gender, and performance status interactions. *American Journal of Hospice and Palliative Medicine, 29,* 139–145. doi:10.1177/1049909111410965

Koga, T., & Fukuda, H. (1992). Neurons in the nucleus of the solitary tract mediating inputs from emetic vagal afferents and the area postrema to the pattern generator for the emetic act in dogs. *Neuroscience Research, 14,* 166–179. doi:10.1016/0168-0102(92)90078-Q

Kolbinson, D.A., Schubert, M.M., Flournoy, N., & Truelove, E.L. (1988). Early oral changes following bone marrow transplantation. *Oral Surgery, Oral Medicine, Oral Pathology, 66,* 130–138. doi:10.1016/0030-4220(88)90080-1

Komurcu, S., Nelson, K.A., Walsh, D., Ford, R.B., & Rybicki, L.A. (2002). Gastrointestinal symptoms among inpatients with advanced cancer. *American Journal of Hospice and Palliative Medicine, 19,* 351–355. doi:10.1177/104990910201900513

Kris, M.G., Gralla, R.J., Clark, R.A., Tyson, L.B., O'Connell, J.P., Wertheim, M.S., & Kelsen, D.P. (1985). Incidence, course, and severity of delayed nausea and vomiting following the administration of high-dose cisplatin. *Journal of Clinical Oncology, 3,* 1379–1384.

Lalla, R.V., Bowen, J., Barasch, A., Elting, L., Epstein, J., Keefe, D.M., … Mucositis Guidelines Leadership Group of the Multinational Association of Supportive Care in Cancer and International Society of Oral Oncology (MASCC/ISOO). (2014). MASCC/ISOO clinical practice guidelines for the management of mucositis secondary to cancer therapy. *Cancer, 120,* 1453–1461. doi:10.1002/cncr.28592

Lalla, R.V., Saunders, D.P., & Peterson, D.E. (2014). Chemotherapy or radiation-induced oral mucositis. *Dental Clinics of North America, 58,* 341–349. doi:10.1016/j.cden.2013.12.005

Lee, J., Cherwin, C., Czaplewski, L.M., Dabbour, R., Doumit, M., Duran, B., … Whiteside, S. (2017, January 2). ONS PEP resource: Chemotherapy-induced nausea and vomiting. Retrieved from https://www.ons.org/practice-resources/pep/chemotherapy-induced-nausea-and-vomiting

Lee-Robichaud, H., Thomas, K., Morgan, J., & Nelson, R.L. (2010). Lactulose versus polyethylene glycol for chronic constipation. *Cochrane Database of Systematic Reviews, 2010*(7). doi:10.1002/14651858.CD007570.pub2

Lembo, A.J., & Camilleri, M. (2003). Chronic constipation. *New England Journal of Medicine, 349,* 1360–1368. doi:10.1056/NEJMra020995

Lembo, A.J., Johanson, J.F., Parkman, H.G., Rao, S.S., Miner, P.B., Jr., & Ueno, R. (2011). Long-term safety and effectiveness of lubiprostone, a chloride channel (ClC-2) activator, in patients with chronic idiopathic constipation. *Digestive Diseases and Sciences, 56,* 2639–2645. doi:10.1007/s10620-011-1801-0

Leung, F.W. (2007). Etiologic factors of chronic constipation: Review of the scientific evidence. *Digestive Diseases and Sciences, 52,* 313–316. doi:10.1007/s10620-006-9298-7

Lever, E., Cole, J., Scott, S.M., Emery, P.W., & Whelan, K. (2014). Systematic review: The effect of prunes on gastrointestinal function. *Alimentary Pharmacology and Therapeutics, 40,* 750–758. doi:10.1111/apt.12913

Lichter, I. (1996). Nausea and vomiting in patients with cancer. *Hematology/Oncology Clinics of North America, 10,* 207–220.

Lofti-Jam, K., Carey, M., Jefford, M., Schofield, P., Charleson, C., & Aranda, S. (2008). Nonpharmacologic strategies for managing common chemotherapy adverse effects: A systematic review. *Journal of Clinical Oncology, 26,* 5618–5629. doi:10.1200/JCO.2007.15.9053

Longstreth, G.F., Thompson, W.G., Chey, W.D., Houghton, L.A., Mearin, F., & Spiller, R.C. (2006). Functional bowel disorders. *Gastroenterology, 130,* 1480–1491. doi:10.1053/j.gastro.2005.11.061

Lovelace, T.L., Fox, N.F., Sood, A.J., Nguyen, S.A., & Day, T.A. (2014). Management of radiotherapy-induced salivary hypofunction and consequent xerostomia in patients with oral or head and neck cancer: Meta-analysis and literature review. *Oral Surgery, Oral Medicine, Oral Pathology and Oral Radiology, 117,* 595–607. doi:10.1016/j.oooo.2014.01.229

Majem, M., Moreno, M.E., Calvo, N., Feliu, A., Pérez, J., Mangues, M.A., & Barnadas, A. (2011). Perception of healthcare providers versus patient reported incidence of chemotherapy-induced nausea and vomiting after the addition of NK-1 receptor antagonists. *Supportive Care in Cancer, 19,* 1983–1990. doi:10.1007/s00520-010-1042-3

Malik, I.A., Khan, W.A., Qazilbash, M., Ata, E., Butt, A., & Khan, A. (1995). Clinical efficacy of lorazepam in prophylaxis of anticipatory, acute, and delayed nausea and vomiting induced by high doses of cisplatin. *American Journal of Clinical Oncology, 18,* 170–175. doi:10.1097/00000421-199504000-00017

Mancini, I., & Bruera, E. (1998). Constipation in advanced cancer patients. *Supportive Care in Cancer, 6,* 356–364. doi:10.1007/s005200050177

Maranzano, E., De Angelis, V., Pergolizzi, S., Lupattelli, M., Frata, P., Spagnesi, S., ... Di Gennaro, D. (2010). A prospective observational trial on emesis in radiotherapy: Analysis of 1020 patients recruited in 45 Italian radiation oncology centres. *Radiotherapy and Oncology, 94,* 36–41. doi:10.1016/j.radonc.2009.11.001

McCrea, G.L., Miaskowski, C., Stotts, N.A., Macera, L., & Varma, M.G. (2008). Pathophysiology of constipation in the older adult. *World Journal of Gastroenterology, 14,* 2631–2638. doi:10.3748/wjg.14.2631

McGuire, D.B., Correa, M.E., Johnson, J., & Wienandts, P. (2006). The role of basic oral care and good clinical practice principles in the management of oral mucositis. *Supportive Care in Cancer, 14,* 541–547. doi:10.1007/s00520-006-0051-8

McGuire, D.B., Peterson, D.E., Muller, S., Owen, D.C., Slemmons, M.F., & Schubert, M.M. (2002). The 20 item oral mucositis index: Reliability and validity in bone marrow and stem cell transplant patients. *Cancer Investigation, 20,* 893–903. doi:10.1081/CNV-120005902

McMillan, S.C., & Williams, F.A. (1989). Validity and reliability of the Constipation Assessment Scale. *Cancer Nursing, 12,* 183–188. doi:10.1097/00002820-198906000-00012

Mercadante, S., Ferrera, P., & Casuccio, A. (2011). Effectiveness and tolerability of amidotrizoate for the treatment of constipation resistant to laxatives in advanced cancer patients. *Journal of Pain and Symptom Management, 41,* 421–425. doi:10.1016/j.jpainsymman.2010.04.022

Merck & Co., Inc. (2006). *Emend®* (aprepitant) [Package insert]. Whitehouse Station, NJ: Author.

Merck & Co., Inc. (2015). *Entereg® (alvimopan)* [Package insert]. Whitehouse Station, NJ: Author.

Molassiotis, A., Coventry, P.A., Stricker, C.T., Clements, C., Eaby, B., Velders, L., ... Gralla, R.J. (2007). Validation and psychometric assessment of a short clinical scale to measure chemotherapy-induced nausea and vomiting: The MASCC Antiemesis Tool. *Journal of Pain and Symptom Management, 34,* 148–159. doi:10.1016/j.jpainsymman.2006.10.018

Molassiotis, A., Stamataki, Z., & Kontopantelis, E. (2013). Development and preliminary validation of a risk prediction model for chemotherapy-related nausea and vomiting. *Supportive Care in Cancer, 21,* 2759–2767. doi:10.1007/s00520-013-1843-2

Monthly Prescribing Reference. (2016). Retrieved from http://www.empr.com

Muehlbauer, P.M., & Lopez, R.C. (2014). Diarrhea. In C.H. Yarbro, D. Wujcik, & B.H. Gobel (Eds.), *Cancer symptom management* (4th ed., pp. 185–212). Burlington, MA: Jones & Bartlett Learning.

Muehlbauer, P.M., Thorpe, D., Davis, A., Drabot, R., Rawlings, B.L., & Kiker, E. (2009). Putting evidence into practice: Evidence-based interventions to prevent, manage and treat chemotherapy- and radiotherapy-induced diarrhea. *Clinical Journal of Oncology Nursing, 13,* 336–341. doi:10.1188/09.CJON.336-341

Murphy, B.A., & Gilbert, J. (2009). Dysphagia in head and neck cancer patients treated with radiation: Assessment, sequelae, and rehabilitation. *Seminars in Radiation Oncology, 19,* 35–42. doi:10.1016/j.semradonc.2008.09.007

Naeim, A., Dy, S.M., Lorenz, K.A., Sanati, H., Walling, A., & Asch, S.M. (2008). Evidence-based recommendations for cancer nausea and vomiting. *Journal of Clinical Oncology, 26,* 3903–3910. doi:10.1200/JCO.2007.15.9533

National Cancer Institute Cancer Therapy Evaluation Program. (2010). *Common terminology criteria for adverse events* [v.4.03]. Retrieved from https://evs.nci.nih.gov/ftp1/CTCAE/CTCAE_4.03_2010-06-14_QuickReference_5x7.pdf

National Comprehensive Cancer Network. (2016). *NCCN Clinical Practice Guidelines in Oncology (NCCN Guidelines®): Palliative care* [v.1.2016]. Retrieved from https://

www.nccn.org/professionals/physician_gls/pdf/palliative.pdf

National Comprehensive Cancer Network. (2017). *NCCN Clinical Practice Guidelines in Oncology (NCCN Guidelines®): Antiemesis* [v.2.2017]. Retrieved from http://www.nccn.org/professionals/physician_gls/pdf/antiemesis.pdf

Navari, R.M., Einhorn, L.H., Loehrer, P.J., Sr., Passik, S.D., Vinson, J., McClean, J., ... Johnson, C.S. (2007). A phase II trial of olanzapine, dexamethasone, and palonosetron for the prevention of chemotherapy-induced nausea and vomiting: A Hoosier Oncology Group study. *Supportive Care in Cancer, 15,* 1285–1291. doi:10.1007/s00520-007-0248-5

Navari, R.M., Einhorn, L.H., Passik, S.D., Loehrer, P.J., Sr., Johnson, C., Mayer, M.L., ... Pletcher, W. (2005). A phase II trial of olanzapine for the prevention of chemotherapy-induced nausea and vomiting: A Hoosier Oncology Group study. *Supportive Care in Cancer, 13,* 529–534. doi:10.1007/s00520-004-0755-6

Navari, R.M., Nagy, C.K., & Gray, S.E. (2013). The use of olanzapine versus metoclopramide for the treatment of breakthrough chemotherapy-induced nausea and vomiting in patients receiving highly emetogenic chemotherapy. *Supportive Care in Cancer, 21,* 1655–1663. doi:10.1007/s00520-012-1710-6

Neymark, N., & Crott, R. (2005). Impact of emesis on clinical and economic outcomes of cancer therapy with highly emetogenic chemotherapy regimens: A retrospective analysis of three clinical trials. *Supportive Care in Cancer, 13,* 812–818. doi:10.1007/s00520-005-0803-x

Noguera, A., Centeno, C., Librada, S., & Nabal, M. (2010). Clinical use of oral laxatives in palliative care services in Spain. *Supportive Care in Cancer, 18,* 1491–1494. doi:10.1007/s00520-010-0956-0

Olson, K., Davies, B.L., Degner, L., Neufiled, K., Plummer, H., Thurston, N., ... Dyek, S. (1998). Assessing stomatitis: Refinement of the Western Consortium for Cancer Nursing Research (WCCNR) stomatitis staging system. *Canadian Oncology Nursing Journal, 8,* 160–165. doi:10.5737/1181912x83160162

Patel, J.N., & Papachristos, A. (2015). Personalizing chemotherapy dosing using pharmacological methods. *Cancer Chemotherapy and Pharmacology, 76,* 879–896. doi:10.1007/s00280-015-2849-x

Pessi, M.A., Zilembo, N., Haspinger, E.R., Molino, L., Di Cosimo, S., Garassino, M., & Ripamonti, C.I. (2014). Targeted therapy-induced diarrhea: A review of the literature. *Critical Reviews in Oncology/Hematology, 90,* 165–179. doi:10.1016/j.critrevonc.2013.11.008

Pinna, R., Campus, G., Cumbo, E., Mura, I., & Milia, E. (2015). Xerostomia induced by radiotherapy: An overview of the physiopathology, clinical evidence, and management of the oral damage. *Therapeutics and Clinical Risk Management, 11,* 171–188. doi:10.2147/TCRM.S70652

Pirri, C., Bayliss, E., Trotter, J., Olver, I.N., Katris, P., Drummond, P., & Bennett, R. (2013). Nausea still the poor relation in antiemetic therapy? The impact on cancer patients' quality of life and psychological adjustment of nausea, vomiting and appetite loss, individually and concurrently as part of a symptom cluster. *Supportive Care in Cancer, 21,* 735–748. doi:10.1007/s00520-012-1574-9

Popovic, M., Warr, D.G., DeAngelis, C., Tsao, M., Chan, K.K.W., & Poon, M. (2014). Efficacy and safety of palonosetron for the prophylaxis of chemotherapy-induced nausea and vomiting (CINV): A systematic review and meta-analysis of randomized controlled trials. *Supportive Care in Cancer, 22,* 1685–1697. doi:10.1007/s00520-014-2175-6

Portenoy, R.K., Thaler, H.T., Kornblith, A.B., Lepore, J.M., Friedlander-Klar, H., Coyle, N., ... Scher, H. (1994). Symptom prevalence, characteristics and distress in a cancer population. *Quality of Life Research, 3,* 183–189.

Radvansky, L.J., Pace, M.B., & Siddiqui, A. (2013). Prevention and management of radiation-induced dermatitis, mucositis and xerostomia. *American Journal of Health-System Pharmacy, 70,* 1025–1032. doi:10.2146/ajhp120467

Rao, S.S.C. (2007). Constipation: Evaluation and treatment of colonic and anorectal motility disorders. *Gastroenterology Clinics of North America, 36,* 687–711. doi:10.1016/j.gtc.2007.07.013

Rao, S.S.C., Ozturk, R., & Laine, L. (2005). Clinical utility of diagnostic tests for constipation in adults: A systematic review. *American Journal of Gastroenterology, 100,* 1605–1615. doi:10.1111/j.1572-0241.2005.41845.x

Riechelmann, R.P., Krzyzanowska, M.K., O'Carroll, A., & Zimmermann, C. (2007). Symptom and medication profiles among cancer patients attending a palliative care clinic. *Supportive Care in Cancer, 15,* 1407–1412. doi:10.1007/s00520-007-0253-8

Riley, P., Glenny, A.-M., Worthington, H.V., Littlewood, A., Clarkson, J.E., & McCabe, M.G. (2015). Interventions for preventing oral mucositis in patients with cancer receiving treatment: Oral cryotherapy. *Cochrane Database of Systematic Reviews, 2015*(12). doi:10.1002/14651858.CD011552.pub2

Rocha, F.C.M., Stéfano, S.C., Haiek, R.D.C., Oliveira, L.M.Q.R., & Da Silveira, D.X. (2008). Therapeutic use of *Cannabis sativa* on chemotherapy-induced nausea and vomiting among cancer patients: Systematic review and meta-analysis. *European Journal of Cancer Care, 17,* 431–443. doi:10.1111/j.1365-2354.2008.00917.x

Roila, F., Molassiotis, A., Herrstedt, J., Aapro, M., Gralla, R.J., Bruera, E., ... van der Wetering, M. (2016). 2016 MASCC and ESMO guideline update for the prevention of chemotherapy- and radiotherapy-induced nausea and vomiting and of nausea and vomiting in advanced cancer patients. *Annals of Oncology, 27*(Suppl. 5), v119–v133. doi:10.1093/annonc/mdw270

Rojas, C., Li, Y., Zhang, J., Stathis, M., Alt, J., Thomas, A.G., ... Slusher, B.S. (2010). The antiemetic 5-HT$_3$ receptor antagonist palonosetron inhibits substance P-mediated responses in vitro and in vivo. *Journal of Pharmacology and Experimental Therapeutics, 335,* 362–368. doi:10.1124/jpet.110.166181

Saito, R., Takano, Y., & Kamiya, H.-O. (2003). Roles of substance P and NK$_1$ receptor in the brainstem in the development of emesis. *Journal of Pharmacological Sciences, 91,* 87–94. doi:10.1254/jphs.91.87

Schubert, M.M., Williams, B.E., Lloid, M.E., Donaldson, G., & Chapko, M.K. (1992). Clinical assessment scale for the rating of oral mucosal changes associated with bone marrow transplantation. Development of an oral mucositis index. *Cancer, 69,* 2469–2477. doi:10.1002/1097-0142(19920515)69:10<2469::AID-CNCR2820691015>3.0.CO;2-W

Schwartzberg, L., Barbour, S.Y., Morrow, G.R., Ballinari, G., Thorn, M.D., & Cox, D. (2014). Pooled analysis of phase III clinical studies of palonosetron versus ondansetron, dolasetron, and granisetron in the prevention of chemotherapy-induced nausea and vomiting (CINV). *Supportive Care in Cancer, 22,* 469–477. doi:10.1007/s00520-013-1999-9

Sekine, I., Segawa, Y., Kubota, K., & Saeki, T. (2013). Risk factors of chemotherapy-induced nausea and vomiting: Index for personalized antiemetic prophylaxis. *Cancer Science, 104,* 711–717. doi:10.1111/cas.12146

Semrad, N.F., Leuchter, R.S., Townsend, D.E., Wade, M.E., & Lagasse, L.D. (1984). A pilot study of lorazepam-induced amnesia with *cis*-platinum-containing chemotherapy. *Gynecologic Oncology, 17,* 277–280. doi:10.1016/0090-8258(84)90211-7

Sethi, S., Mikami, S., LeClair, J., Park, R., Jones, M., Wadhwa, V., ... Lembo, A. (2014). Inpatient burden of constipation in the United States: An analysis of national trends in the United States from 1997 to 2010. *American Journal of Gastroenterology, 109,* 250–256. doi:10.1038/ajg.2013.423

Shih, Y.-C.T., Xu, Y., & Elting, L.S. (2007). Costs of uncontrolled chemotherapy-induced nausea and vomiting among working-age cancer patients receiving highly or moderately emetogenic chemotherapy. *Cancer, 110,* 678–685. doi:10.1002/cncr.22823

Solano, J.P., Gomes, B., & Higginson, I.J. (2006). A comparison of symptom prevalence in far advanced cancer, AIDS, heart disease, chronic obstructive pulmonary disease and renal disease. *Journal of Pain and Symptom Management, 31,* 58–69. doi:10.1016/j.jpainsymman.2005.06.007

Solomon, R., & Cherny, N.I. (2006). Constipation and diarrhea in patients with cancer. *Cancer Journal, 12,* 355–364. doi:10.1097/00130404-200609000-00005

Sonis, S.T. (2007). Pathobiology of oral mucositis: Novel insights and opportunities. *Journal of Supportive Oncology, 5*(9, Suppl. 4), 3–11.

Sonis, S.T., Eilers, J.P., Epstein, J.B., LeVeque, F.G., Liggett, W.H., Jr., Mulagha, M.T., ... Wittes, J.P. (1999). Validation of a new scoring system for the assessment of clinical trial research of oral mucositis induced by radiation or chemotherapy. *Cancer, 85,* 2103–2113. doi:10.1002/(SICI)1097-0142(19990515)85:10<2103::AID-CNCR2>3.0.CO;2-0

Sonis, S.T., Elting, L.S., Keefe, D., Peterson, D.E., Schubert, M., Hauer-Jensen, M., ... Rubenstein, E.B. (2004). Perspectives on cancer therapy-induced mucosal injury: Pathogenesis, measurement, epidemiology, and consequences for patients. *Cancer, 100,* 1995–2025. doi:10.1002/cncr.20162

Sonis, S.T., & Fey, E.G. (2002). Oral complications of cancer therapy. *Oncology, 16,* 680–686.

Stephenson, J., & Davies, A. (2006). An assessment of aetiology-based guidelines for the management of nausea and vomiting in patients with advanced cancer. *Supportive Care in Cancer, 14,* 348–353. doi:10.1007/s00520-005-0897-1

Stern, J., & Ippoliti, C. (2003). Management of acute cancer treatment-induced diarrhea. *Seminars in Oncology Nursing, 19*(Suppl. 3), 11–16. doi:10.1053/j.soncn.2003.09.009

Suares, N.C., & Ford, A.C. (2011). Prevalence of, and risk factors for, chronic idiopathic constipation in the community: Systematic review and meta-analysis. *American Journal of Gastroenterology, 106,* 1582–1591. doi:10.1038/ajg.2011.164

Sucampo Pharma Americas, LLC, & Takeda Pharmaceuticals America, Inc. (2015). *Amitiza® (lubiprostone) capsules* [Package insert]. Bethesda, MD, and Deerfield, IL: Authors.

Tack, J. (2008). Prokinetics and fundic relaxants in upper functional GI disorders. *Current Opinion in Pharmacology, 8,* 690–696. doi:10.1016/j.coph.2008.09.009

Tavani, A., Bianchi, G., Ferretti, P., & Manara, L. (1980). Morphine is most effective on gastrointestinal propulsion in rats by intraperitoneal route: Evidence for local action. *Life Sciences, 27,* 2211–2217. doi:10.1016/0024-3205(80)90386-0

Thomas, J., Karver, S., Cooney, G.A., Chamberlain, B.H., Watt, C.K., Slatkin, N.E., ... Israel, R.J. (2008). Methylnaltrexone for opioid-induced constipation in advanced illness. *New England Journal of Medicine, 358,* 2332–2343. doi:10.1056/NEJMoa0707377

Thorpe, D.M., Byar, K.L., Conley, S., Davis, A.B., Drapek, L., Hays, A., ... Ramsdell, M.J. (2017, February 27). ONS Putting Evidence Into Practice: Constipation. Retrieved from https://www.ons.org/practice-resources/pep/constipation

Thorpe, D.M., Byar, K.L., Conley, S., Davis, A.B., Drapek, L., Hays, A., ... Wolles, B. (2016, September 9). ONS PEP resource: Diarrhea. Retrieved from https://www.ons.org/practice-resources/pep/diarrhea

Tramèr, M.R., Carroll, D., Campbell, F.A., Reynolds, D.J.M., Moore, R.A., & McQuay, H.J. (2001). Cannabinoids for control of chemotherapy induced nausea and vomiting: Quantitative systematic review. *BMJ, 323,* 16–21. doi:10.1136/bmj.323.7303.16

Twycross, R., Sykes, N., Mihalyo, M., & Wilcock, A. (2012). Stimulant laxatives and opioid-induced constipation. *Journal of Pain and Symptom Management, 43,* 306–313. doi:10.1016/j.jpainsymman.2011.12.002

Vardy, J.L., Chiew, K.S., Galica, J., Pond, G.R., & Tannock, I.F. (2006). Side effects associated with the use of dexamethasone for prophylaxis of delayed emesis after moderately emetogenic chemotherapy. *British Journal of Cancer, 94,* 1011–1015. doi:10.1038/sj.bjc.6603048

Wald, A. (2003). Is chronic use of stimulant laxatives harmful to the colon? *Journal of Clinical Gastroenterology, 36,* 386–389. doi:10.1097/00004836-200305000-00004

Warr, D. (2013). Prognostic factors for chemotherapy induced nausea and vomiting. *European Journal of Pharmacology, 722,* 192–196. doi:10.1016/j.ejphar.2013.10.015

Webster, L., Jansen, J.P., Peppin, J., Lasko, B., Irving, G., Morlion, B., ... Carter, E. (2008). Alvimopan, a peripherally acting mu-opioid receptor (PAM-OR) antagonist for the treatment of opioid-induced bowel dysfunction: Results from a randomized, double-blind, placebo-controlled, dose-finding study in subjects taking opioids for chronic non-cancer pain. *Pain, 137,* 428–440. doi:10.1016/j.pain.2007.11.008

Wilkes, G.M., & Barton-Burke, M. (2016). *2016 Oncology nursing drug handbook* (20th ed.). Burlington, MA: Jones & Bartlett Learning.

Wirz, S., Nadstawek, J., Elsen, C., Junker, U., & Wartenberg, H.C. (2012). Laxative management in ambulatory cancer patients on opioid therapy: A prospective, open-label investigation of polyethylene glycol, sodium picosulphate and lactulose. *European Journal of Cancer Care, 21,* 131–140. doi:10.1111/j.1365-2354.2011.01286.x

Witsell, D.L., Stinnett, S., & Chambers, M.S. (2012). Effectiveness of cevimeline to improve oral health in patients with postradiation xerostomia. *Head and Neck, 34,* 1136–1142. doi:10.1002/hed.21894

World Health Organization. (1979). *WHO handbook for reporting results of cancer treatment.* Geneva, Switzerland: Author.

Wujcik, D. (2014). Mucositis. In C.H. Yarbro, D. Wujcik, & B.H. Gobel (Eds.), *Cancer symptom management* (4th ed., pp. 385–402). Burlington, MA: Jones & Bartlett Learning.

Xing, J.-H., & Soffer, E.E. (2001). Adverse effects of laxatives. *Diseases of the Colon and Rectum, 44,* 1201–1209. doi:10.1007/BF02234645

Yuan, C.-S. (2007). Methylnaltrexone mechanisms of action and effects on opioid bowel dysfunction and other opioid adverse effects. *Annals of Pharmacotherapy, 41,* 984–993. doi:10.1345/aph.1K009

Chapter 20 Study Questions

1. Which of the following interventions is used to prevent radiation-induced xerostomia?
   A. Brachytherapy
   B. Glycerin swabs
   C. Sialagogues
   D. Lidocaine mouthwash

2. The most common infections associated with mucositis are:
   A. *Aspergillus* and *Candida.*
   B. Cytomegalovirus and herpes simplex.
   C. Herpes simplex and *Aspergillus.*
   D. *Candida* and herpes simplex.

3. Which test is done most often to identify the cause of dysphagia?
   A. Endoscopy
   B. Computed tomography scan
   C. Positron-emission tomography–computed tomography scan
   D. Colonoscopy

4. The most significant complication of diarrhea associated with cancer therapy is:
   A. Dehydration.
   B. Aspiration.
   C. Hypocalcemia.
   D. Rhabdomyolysis.

5. Patients who are receiving highly emetogenic chemotherapy should receive prophylaxis with which of the following?
   A. Dopamine antagonist and dexamethasone
   B. 5-HT_3 receptor antagonist, dexamethasone, and an NK_1 receptor antagonist
   C. Cannabinoid and dexamethasone
   D. 5-HT_3 receptor antagonist and dexamethasone

CHAPTER

21 Genitourinary Symptoms

Amy Y. Zhang, PhD

Introduction

The term *genitourinary (GU) cancer* is commonly used to describe cancers of the bladder, kidney (renal), penis, testicle, and prostate. The incidence of individual GU cancers varies widely. Although penile and testicular cancers rarely occur, an estimated 76,960 new cases of bladder cancer and 180,890 new cases of prostate cancer were projected to occur in the United States in 2016 (American Cancer Society, 2016).

Urinary continence relies on the bladder, which maintains constant detrusor pressures during filling, and both internal and external sphincter muscles, which provide urethral resistance to the detrusor pressures in the bladder (Foote, Yun, & Leach, 1991). Continence is maintained as long as the pressure in the urethra remains higher than the pressure in the bladder (Palmer, Fogarty, Somerfield, & Powel, 2003). Unfortunately, current treatments for specific types and stages of bladder, cervical, rectal, and prostate cancer involve compromising the nerves and muscles that maintain continence. For example, prostatectomy can lead to damage to the urinary sphincter and cause temporary or permanent incontinence. This chapter provides an overview of urinary incontinence (UI) that occurs as a result of treatment for a GU cancer, with an emphasis on UI that begins after prostate cancer treatment.

Overview of Urinary Incontinence

UI is broadly defined by the International Continence Society as "the complaint of any involuntary leakage of urine" (Abrams et al., 2002, p. 168). The *Gale Encyclopedia of Medicine* defined UI as "unintentional loss of urine that is sufficient enough in frequency and amount to cause physical and/or emotional distress in the person experiencing it" (as cited in "Urinary Incontinence," n.d.).

Some existing clinical trials use "daily pad use" to screen patients' incontinence status for a research study. Other clinical trials use "occasional use of pad" as an eligibility criterion.

Because minor leakage (e.g., dripping) is common among patients with persistent UI, and it imposes physical and mental burdens and can progress without adequate care, those who experience minor (as well as major) symptoms may be considered for treatment irrespective of pad use.

Symptoms of urinary infection, including fever, sweats, dark urine, pain, and confusion, or urinary retention, including distended bladder, trouble starting urination, and decreased urine volume, worsen the condition of UI. Patients experiencing symptoms of urinary infection or retention need to see a physician for further examination prior to receiving a UI diagnosis.

Assessment

A commonly used UI assessment tool for men in the United States is the American Urological Association Symptom Index (or symptom score, referred to as the AUASS). This instrument has seven items that measure UI symptoms in men on a six-point scale (Barry et al., 1992). Another screening tool for men, recommended by the International Consultation on Incontinence, is the International Continence Society Short-Form Male Questionnaire, the ICSmaleSF. The ICSmaleSF has two subscales, the ICSmaleIS, which assesses stress and urge incontinence on six items, and the ICSmaleVS, which assesses voiding problems on five items. In addition, the ICSmaleSF has a single item assessing the extent to which UI interferes with the patient's life, with 0 indicating no interference at all and 3 indicating a lot of interference (Donovan et al., 2000).

A brief and robust screening tool for UI in both men and women is the International Consultation on Incontinence Questionnaire Short Form (ICIQ-SF). The scale has three scored items that assess the frequency, severity, and perceived impact of incontinence and an unscored self-diagnostic item. It has been widely studied and has established satisfactory psychometric properties. The ICIQ-SF is internationally known and can be used in various patient populations (Avery et al., 2004).

Pathophysiology of Urinary Incontinence After Prostatectomy

In the case of prostate cancer, when the prostate is surgically resected, the internal sphincter muscles are excised, leaving the maintenance of urinary continence to the external sphincter muscles alone. A weakened external sphincter following surgery leads to sphincter insufficiency—the inability to resist increased detrusor pressure—resulting in *stress incontinence*, which is urinary leakage during stressful events such as coughing, stooping, or lifting. Furthermore, patients with prostate cancer tend to compensate with more frequent bladder contractions for the obstruction caused by malignant prostatic enlargement. When the prostate is surgically removed, the bladder contractions persist, and this overactive bladder, or so-called detrusor instability, results in urge incontinence, which is the frequent urge or pressure to urinate (Harris, 1997). Patients with urge incontinence cannot withstand increasing detrusor pressure, and they often leak urine suddenly and uncontrollably. The type of surgery (open radical, laparoscopic, or robotic prostatectomy) does not significantly affect the rate of postsurgical UI (Jacobsen, Moore, Estey, & Voaklander, 2007; Romero & Martinez-Salamanca, 2007). Radiation therapy also can weaken sphincter muscles and cause UI.

Incidence of Postprostatectomy Urinary Incontinence

The incidence of UI after radical prostatectomy has been reported as 2%–90.3%, depending on the definition of UI and the methodology of studies (Novara et al., 2010; Peterson & Chen, 2012). A strict definition of UI is total incontinence (i.e., uncontrollable leakage). The six-month post-treatment prevalence of total incontinence was reported to be 6%, but when counting mild incontinence, for which an "occasional" pad was used, the prevalence of UI rose to 40% (Penson et al., 2008).

UI after prostatectomy recedes gradually over time (Lepor, Kaci, & Xue, 2004; Peyromaure, Ravery, & Boccon-Gibod, 2002; Smither, Guralnick, Davis, & See, 2007). One study reported that by the end of 12 months, 40% of patients used pads daily and 74% had some degree of leakage (Holm, Fosså, Hedlund, Schultz, & Dahl, 2014). *Delayed incontinence*, defined as the persistence of urine leakage one year after surgery (Peyromaure et al., 2002), was reported for 42% of patients who dripped (Lepor et al., 2004) and 30% of patients who wore pads at 24 months (Penson et al., 2008). The Prostate Cancer Outcomes Study reported that 14% of patients continued to have frequent urinary leakage five years after surgery (Penson et al., 2008; Potosky et al., 2004). The prevalence of lifelong postprostatectomy incontinence requiring daily use of protective pads has been estimated, in some reports, to be as high as 45% (Poon et al., 2000).

The incidence of UI is lower in patients treated with external beam radiation therapy (Nicolaisen, Müller, Patel, & Hanssen, 2014) and interstitial radioisotope seed implant (brachytherapy) (Bradley, Bissonette, & Theodorescu, 2004; Downs et al., 2003; Raabe, Normann, & Lilleby, 2015), but both can result in muscle damage and irritative voiding symptoms (Quek & Penson, 2005). Most studies estimated the rate of UI as 5%–10% for both treatments (de Reijke & Laguna, 2003; Fontaine, Ben Mouelli, Thomas, Otmezguine, & Beurton, 2004; Liu et al., 2005; Locke, Ellis, Wallner, Cavanagh, & Blasko, 2002; Madalinska et al., 2001; Potosky et al., 2000; Reis, Netto, Reinato, Thiel, & Zani, 2004). However, one study found that 35% of patients were incontinent and 6% still used pads three years after external beam radiation therapy (Little, Kuban, Levy, Zagars, & Pollack, 2003). Talcott, Clark, Stark, and Mitchell (2001) noted that 45% of patients receiving brachytherapy were incontinent. In short, UI is prevalent in patients with prostate cancer over time and across treatment modalities, thus constituting a serious clinical problem for these patients.

Urinary Incontinence in Patients With Other Cancers

Emerging evidence supports that UI among women with cervical cancer and patients with other cancers appears to be common. A study of 319 Norwegian women who survived gynecologic cancer reported that 34.3% suffered from total UI 12 years after initial treatment (Skjeldestad & Hagen, 2008). Another study conducted urodynamic testing in 28 Italian patients with gynecologic cancer and reported that 32% and 24% of patients were incontinent at 3 months and 12 months, respectively, after surgery (Angioli et al., 2007). Hysterectomy to treat cervical cancer can damage urethral sphincter muscles and reduce intraurethral pressure, resulting in UI (Axelsen, Bek, & Petersen, 2007). Zullo, Plotti, Calcagno, Angioli, and Panici (2008) reported that 21%–53% of women who underwent radical hysterectomy experienced UI. Other recent studies support the finding of worsening UI following radical hysterectomy (Ceccaroni et al., 2012; de Noronha, de Figueiredo, Franco, Cândido, & Silva-Filho, 2013; Donovan, Boyington, Judson, & Wyman, 2014). Bladder dysfunction following radical hysterectomy has been estimated to range from 8% to 80% (Plotti et al., 2011). Evidence also suggests that surgery plus radiation therapy is associated with more severe incontinent symptoms than surgery without radiation therapy or radiation therapy alone (Erekson, Sung, DiSilvestro, & Myers, 2009; Hazewinkel et al., 2010).

Other cancers, such as bladder and rectal cancers, also may require surgery that compromises pelvic nerves and muscles, resulting in UI. Researchers conducting a study of 315 patients with bladder cancer at the University of Michigan reported that patients undergoing cystectomy had significantly poorer urinary function and quality of life than patients receiving other treatment (Gilbert et al., 2007). Another study found that 82.4% of 121 women who had undergone radical cystectomy for bladder cancer continued experiencing UI at a median follow-up of 56 months (Jentzmik et al., 2012). In patients with rectal cancer, Contin et al. (2014) reported that 51.2% of 225 patients experienced UI after rectal cancer surgery. Panjari et al. (2012) found in a systematic literature review study that 60% of women undergoing rectal cancer treatment had concerns about incontinence. UI was found to be worse at 12 months after rectal cancer surgery (Varpe et al., 2011). Curative surgeries for rectal cancer including total mesorectal excision are reported to be associated with long-term UI at a rate of 38% (Lange et al., 2008). Nevertheless, evidence on UI pathology and its effect on quality of life is insufficient at this time to accurately estimate the severity of urinary problems in these populations. Future clinical trials need to study treatment approaches for efficacy among both men and women diagnosed with cervical, bladder, and rectal cancers.

UI is one of the common symptoms of menopause, and cancer treatment can lead to early menopause. However, research is lacking regarding the prevalence and severity of UI as a result of treatment-induced menopause in patients with cancer.

Consequences of Urinary Incontinence

Unresolved temporary and permanent UI is costly to both individuals and society and has adverse physical, social, and emotional consequences (Ko & Sawatzky, 2008; Palmer et al., 2003; Stothers, Thom, & Calhoun, 2005). Patients with UI may experience physical discomfort of irritation, sores, and reddening of the skin, as well as rashes from protective briefs (Ko & Sawatzky, 2008; Nahon, Waddington, Dorey, & Adams, 2009). Their daily functioning (Martin et al., 2011; Weber, Roberts, Chumbler, Mills, & Algood, 2007) and routine physical exercise such as walking (Butler, Downe-Wamboldt, Marsh, Bell, & Jarvi, 2000; Kyrdalen, Dahl, Hernes, Småstuen, & Fosså, 2013; Petry et al., 2004) may be restricted or eliminated.

Studies of patients with prostate cancer shed light on this issue. Men treated for prostate cancer were forced to rearrange their lives to suit urgent needs for access to a restroom (Jakobsson, Hallberg, & Lovén, 2000). They had to avoid traveling long distances, doing yard work, golfing, dancing, playing tennis, or having sex for fear of urinary leakage (Fan, Heyes, & King, 2012; Hedestig, Sandman, Tomic, & Widmark, 2005; Kirschner-Hermanns & Jakse, 2002; Palmer et al., 2003; Weber et al., 2007).

Men with UI using pads were five times as likely to be bothered as opposed to those who had no need to use a pad (Wallerstedt et al., 2012). Significant bother was present even when one pad was required daily for a minor leakage (Cooperberg, Master, & Carroll, 2003; Wallerstedt et al., 2012).

Frequent use of pads brought about social stigma (Elstad, Taubenberger, Botelho, & Tennstedt, 2010; Higa, Lopes, & D'Ancona, 2013; Paterson, 2000), isolation (Ko & Sawatzky, 2008; Palmer et al., 2003), feelings of being embarrassed (Ko & Sawatzky, 2008) or burdened (Waller & Pattison, 2013), anger over a loss of control (Burt, Caelli, Moore, & Anderson, 2005; Rondorf-Klym & Colling, 2003; Waller & Pattison, 2013), and loss of self-worth (O'Shaughnessy & Laws, 2010). In some cases, patients became depressed (Ko & Sawatzky, 2008; Weber, Roberts, Mills, Chumbler, & Algood, 2008). In short, UI had significant adverse effects on the quality of life of patients receiving prostate cancer treatment (Hoyland, Vasdev, Abrof, & Boustead, 2014; Katz, 2007; Walsh & Hegarty, 2010).

Furthermore, 74% of patients who had undergone postprostatectomy considered UI to be an important problem to resolve (Palmer et al., 2003; Smith, Shaw, & Rashid, 2009) and viewed it as more bothersome than sexual dysfunction (Weber et al., 2007). UI significantly inflates hardship for the family (McCorkle, Siefert, Dowd, Robinson, & Pickett, 2007). Men with UI typically rely on women in the family as the primary caregivers, usually a wife or a daughter who is likely an older adult herself or a caretaker of children (Harden et al., 2002; Lobchuk & Rosenberg, 2014). The stress associated with a cancer diagnosis and treatment has already strained these women, and taking care of catheters or pad changes further taxes their energy (Shelby, Taylor, Kerner, Coleman, & Blum, 2002) and increases the restrictions in their lives (Harden et al., 2002). In fact, UI is more highly associated with spousal distress than patient distress (Couper et al., 2006; Resendes & McCorkle, 2006). As patients' urinary frequency increases and quality of life decreases, the spouses' quality of life significantly worsens (McCorkle et al., 2007).

UI places a tremendous burden on society (Coyne et al., 2014). In addition to the patient's need for personal care (e.g., dressing, using the toilet), domestic activities (e.g., cooking, shopping, housework) and professional services (e.g., respite care, visit by a healthcare professional), utilization of medical services was significantly higher among those suffering from incontinence (Tang et al., 2014). Based on 2007 statistics, the annual total cost of UI in the United States was $65.9 billion, with an estimated cost of $76.2 billion in 2015 and $82.6 billion in 2020 (Coyne et al., 2014). The cost covers expenditures for diagnosis, evaluation, treatment, complications (skin breakdown or urinary tract infections), routine care, and the loss of work.

Pelvic Floor Muscle Exercise

Pharmacologic and surgical treatments of postprostatectomy incontinence are costly and unpopular because of their intrusiveness, side effects, and possibility of failure (Resel-Folkersma, Salinas-Casado, & Moreno-Sierra, 2014). Pelvic floor muscle exercise (PFME), a behavioral approach proposed by Arnold Kegel in the late 1940s (Kegel, 1948), namely Kegel exercises, is a learned technique of muscle contraction and relaxation and has been used to treat women with UI from a variety of causes for decades. The underlying assumption is that regular and repeated muscle contractions can strengthen a voluntary muscle, thus causing the muscle to grow in size (Ocampo-Trujillo et al., 2014). PFME strengthens pelvic sphincter muscles and may improve urethral sphincter closure during periods of increased intravesical pressure (Filocamo et al., 2005).

Previous research has documented the effectiveness of PFME in treating women with incontinence (Hersh & Salzman, 2013; Kocaöz, Eroğlu, & Sivaslıoğlu, 2013; Stafne, Salvesen, Romundstad, Torjusen, & Mørkved, 2012). A study of the anatomy of the urethral sphincter complex in both sexes using histologic and three-dimensional imaging technique reported that the urinary sphincter morphology is analogous in both sexes (Yucel & Baskin, 2004), supporting the feasibility of PFME for men with UI. Increased strength of the external sphincter muscles is expected to increase urethral resistance to mitigate both stress and urge incontinence.

Effect in Early Postsurgical or Preoperative Patients

Evidence for efficacy of PFME in treating men following prostatectomy was encouraging initially but remains inconclusive in recent years. Based on a systematic literature review of nine randomized controlled trials, the Cochrane Incontinence Group in 2004 concluded that the five clinical trials of PFME with biofeedback provided evidence for better continence outcomes in early postoperative months than no treatment or the placebo control (Hunter, Moore, Cody, & Glazener, 2004). However, the same group reached a more conservative conclusion in 2015. Based on a review of 50 studies, they concluded that the effect of conservative management of postprostatectomy UI up to 12 months remained "uncertain" and there was "insufficient evidence to demonstrate a beneficial effect of pelvic floor muscle training" (Anderson et al., 2015). Fernández et al. (2015), however, conducted a meta-analysis of eight selected studies. They reported a significantly improved continence rate in the short ($p \leq 0.001$), medium ($p =$

0.001), and long term (p = 0.002) due to pelvic floor muscle training.

Van Kampen et al. (2000) conducted the first randomized study of 102 patients who received either biofeedback PFME treatment or placebo after catheter removal. At three months after surgery, the treatment group had 32% more participants achieving continence and significantly shorter duration of incontinence than the control group based on 1- and 24-hour pad tests. The group difference in the return of continence was 14% at 12 months. Van Kampen (2006) further reported that a session of biofeedback training in PFME plus daily PFME produced a significant reduction in severe incontinence (odds ratio [OR] = 0.29, 95% confidence interval [CI] [0.09, 0.94]) and pad use (OR = 0.44, 95% CI [0.24, 0.99]), as well as a faster return to continence (mean time = 3.5 months vs. more than 6 months), compared to no PFME treatment at six months in a sample of 125 subjects.

Filocamo et al. (2005) randomized 300 patients to either PFME treatment or control after catheter removal. Significantly more patients in the treatment group than the control group achieved continence at one month (19% vs. 8%) and six months (94.6% vs. 65%) using 1- and 24-hour pad tests.

Porru et al. (2001) reported that biofeedback PFME significantly increased the grade of muscle strength from 2.8 to 3.8 points after four weeks of exercise, but muscle strength remained unchanged (2.5 to 2.4 points) in the control group without PFME training. The PFME treatment group reported significantly fewer incontinent episodes and less leakage than the control group at weeks 1, 2, and 3 after catheter removal.

However, a number of randomized studies failed to find a significant effect from PFME. For example, Robinson, Bradway, Nuamah, Pickett, and McCorkle (2008) randomized 126 participants to either an intervention group that received four weeks of PFME training following catheter removal or a control group. The researchers assessed participants at 3, 6, and 12 months following radical prostatectomy. Their findings showed no significant group difference in UI and quality of life.

Glazener et al. (2011) conducted two parallel trials of men undergoing radical prostatectomy or transurethral resection and experiencing UI six weeks after surgery. The participants were randomized to an intervention group that received four sessions of PFME training from a therapist or to a control group of standard care plus lifestyle advice. Incontinence outcome was assessed using the participants' self-report. No difference in the continence rate was observed between the intervention (76% and 65% in trial one and two, respectively) and the control group (77% and 62%, respectively) at 12 months. The authors concluded that one-to-one sessions of PFME training for men with incontinence after prostate surgery were unlikely to be effective.

Some studies have examined the preoperative effect of PFME on UI, and the results are inconclusive. Parekh et al. (2003) randomized 38 surgical patients to receive biofeedback PFME training or control prior to prostatectomy. Patients who received PFME training preoperatively had regained continence (defined as less than one pad daily) significantly better than those without PFME training (68% vs. 37%) at three months after surgery.

Burgio et al. (2006) randomized 125 patients to preoperative biofeedback PFME or a control arm. They reported significantly quicker return of continence and fewer patients with severe or continual leakage in the treatment group than the control group (5.9% vs. 19.6%) at six months after surgery.

Centemero et al. (2010) randomized 118 men who were undergoing radical prostatectomy to start PFME preoperatively and continue postoperatively or to start PFME postoperatively. They reported that the group starting PFME preoperatively had a significantly higher rate of continence at one month (44.1% vs. 20.3%) and three months (59.3% vs. 37.3%)

than those in the postoperative PFME group ($p \leq 0.05$).

Moreover, Tienforti et al. (2012) studied 32 patients randomized to a preoperative group and a postoperative PFME group. They reported that the preoperative PFME group showed a significantly higher rate of continence at one ($p = 0.02$), three ($p = 0.01$), and six ($p = 0.002$) months, better self-reported urinary function, and fewer incontinence episodes or less pad use per week than the postoperative PFME group.

Geraerts et al. (2013) studied 180 men who were randomized to receive PFME training three weeks prior to radical prostatectomy or to start PFME after surgery. They did not observe a significant group difference in the mean time to continence and the leakage amount based on a one-hour pad test. Further, a meta-analysis of five selected studies concluded that preoperative PFME did not improve UI after radical prostatectomy at early (3 months), interim (6 months), or late (12 months) recovery stages (Wang, Huang, Liu, & Mao, 2014).

Evidence suggests that some patients have difficulty identifying the correct muscles with verbal instruction on PFME, thus affecting its outcome (Floratos et al., 2002). Studies have provided supporting evidence of superior PFME outcomes based on biofeedback over verbal instruction (Hunter et al., 2004; Ribeiro et al., 2010). Although a few studies failed to find a difference between the two instruction approaches (Floratos et al., 2002; MacDonald, Fink, Huckabay, Monga, & Wilt, 2007), existing evidence generally favors biofeedback training.

Effect in Patients With Persistent Urinary Incontinence

Persistent UI that lasts 12 months or longer is difficult to treat, and evidence supporting the effect of PFME on persistent UI is scarce. However, two recent studies provided promising results. In a trial of 208 men with incontinence for 1–17 years after radical prostatectomy, study participants were randomized to three groups: (a) eight weeks of behavioral therapy (PFME training and bladder control strategies), (b) behavioral therapy plus in-office biofeedback and daily electrical stimulation at home, and (c) delayed treatment as a control group. It was reported that the mean number of incontinence episodes was significantly reduced in the behavioral therapy and behavioral therapy plus biofeedback and electrical stimulation groups (55% and 51% reduction, respectively) compared to the control group (24% reduction) at eight weeks ($p = 0.001$). No significant difference was observed between the two intervention groups. The researchers concluded that eight weeks of behavioral therapy with or without electrical stimulation can reduce the frequency of incontinence episodes (Goode et al., 2011).

In another clinical trial of 244 men with an average of two to three years of incontinence after prostatectomy and/or radiation therapy, study participants were randomized to three groups: (a) biofeedback PFME plus six sessions of a support group, (b) biofeedback PFME plus six sessions of telephone contact, and (c) usual care that continued with routine medical care without any exposure to the intervention (Zhang et al., 2015). The biofeedback PFME was a 60-minute session of biofeedback training in PFME. The problem-solving therapy delivered symptom management skills through a peer support group or telephone contacts with a therapist over six biweekly sessions. Participants were assessed at baseline, three months, and six months. The researchers found that both intervention groups had significantly fewer incontinence episodes daily than the control group at the end of the three-month study intervention period but not at the six-month follow-up, and that participants in the biofeedback PFME plus support group study arm had a reduction of 13.3 g of urine at six months, significantly lower than the control group. The researchers concluded that the intervention of biofeedback PFME plus symptom management skills can significantly improve urinary function and quality of life in men with persistent incontinence after prostate cancer treatment and that the intervention needs to extend beyond three months to achieve greater improvement in these patients (Zhang et al., 2015). Furthermore, Zhang and Fu (2016) compared the direct and indirect costs, as well as intervention effectiveness, of these study participants in the three groups with a group of eligible patients who had declined participation in the intervention study. They reported that the incremental cost-effectiveness ratios were $16,759 per quality-adjusted-life-year (QALY) and $12,561/QALY for the peer support and telephone groups compared to the nonparticipating group; therefore, the interventions were cost-effective in consideration of eligible patients who had declined the interventions (Zhang & Fu, 2016).

Nursing Implications

Despite inconsistent findings in the current literature, evidence suggests that immediate provision of biofeedback PFME training to patients with prostate cancer after postoperative catheter removal reduces UI symptoms and facilitates an early return of continence. Initial evidence also suggests that biofeedback PFME combined with behavioral modification, such as a support group, promotes adherence to PFME and recovery from persistent UI. The clinical implication is that provision of biofeedback PFME training and follow-up care may be considered complementary care for patients with prostate cancer. However, additional research is needed before generalizing this statement to all forms of UI resulting from GU cancer or resulting from interventions for gynecologic and rectal cancers. Practicing PFME individually or in a group can be a practical and useful management approach to temporary and persistent symptoms of UI.

UI symptoms resulting from muscle damage can be aggravated by a range of conditions, including inadequate fluid intake, which can induce urinary tract infection; caffeine or alcohol intake, which stimulates bladder contraction; constipation or obesity, which adds pressure on the bladder; and certain medications or diseases (e.g., diabetes) that worsen UI (Registered Nurses' Association of Ontario, 2011).

A common practice in nursing care for women with UI involves teaching self-care management of fluid intake, voiding, constipation, physical activity, and medication. Studies of women with UI have shown the effect of self-management of incontinent symptoms. In a systematic review of 12 randomized controlled trials, Du Moulin, Hamers, Paulus, Berendsen, and Halfens (2005) found evidence that supports nursing intervention in women with UI. The Registered Nurses' Association of Ontario (2011) best practice guideline recommends a comprehensive approach to UI symptoms in the belief that appropriate self-management alleviates UI symptoms, thus complementing PFME that aims to eradicate UI through muscle building.

Future Research

The future direction of nonsurgical management of UI symptoms points at the integration of PFME and self-management, as well as various behavioral modifications. The application of this strategy to patients with other cancers and other diseases that result in UI also requires further investigation.

Conclusion

UI can be caused by compromised integrity of the pelvic floor nerves and muscles. This occurs commonly in the treatment of some GU cancers, such as prostate cancer, as well as gynecologic and rectal cancers and other noncancer diseases. Numerous clinical trials evaluating PFME as a way to decrease or eliminate UI in patients who have undergone prostatectomy show promise for all patients affected by UI. The conflicting findings in the current literature may reflect the complexity of research methods, sample selection, measurement, and other research issues that have yet to be applied with a recommended guideline based on gained knowledge.

Improvement of persistent incontinence is contingent upon adherence to PFME and self-management. Several critical behavioral intervention elements can reinforce behavioral adherence (Duncan & Pozehl, 2002), including goal setting, self-monitoring, physiologic feedback about performance, multiple contacts, social support, and problem-solving strategies to overcome barriers.

A decade of literature shows that these elements significantly predict exercise adherence across diverse patient populations (Dubbert, 1992; Rhodes & Fiala, 2009). Various treatment modalities, including group, individual, and telephone-based approaches, can deliver these critical intervention elements and should be considered in the future for the benefit of patients with cancer who develop UI.

References

Abrams, P., Cardozo, L., Fall, M., Griffiths, D., Rosier, P., Ulmsten, U., … Wein, A. (2002). The standardisation of terminology of lower urinary tract function: Report from the standardisation sub-committee of the International Continence Society. *Neurourology and Urodynamics, 21,* 167–178. doi:10.1002/nau.10052

American Cancer Society. (2016). *Cancer facts and figures 2016.* Atlanta, GA: Author.

Anderson, C.A., Omar, M.I., Campbell, S.E., Hunter, K.F., Cody, J.D., & Glazener, C.M.A. (2015). Conservative management for postprostatectomy urinary incontinence. *Cochrane Database of Systematic Reviews, 2015*(1). doi:10.1002/14651858.cd001843.pub5

Angioli, R., Zullo, M.A., Plotti, F., Bellati, F., Basile, S., Damiani, P., … Panici, P.B. (2007). Urologic function and urodynamic evaluation of urinary diversion (rome pouch) over time in gynecologic cancer patients. *Gynecologic Oncology, 107,* 200–204. doi:10.1016/j.ygyno.2007.06.020

Avery, K., Donovan, J., Peters, T.J., Shaw, C., Gotoh, M., & Abrams, P. (2004). ICIQ: A brief and robust measure for evaluating the symptoms and impact of urinary incontinence. *Neurourology and Urodynamics, 23,* 322–330. doi:10.1002/nau.20041

Axelsen, S.M., Bek, K.M., & Petersen, L.K. (2007). Urodynamic and ultrasound characteristics of incontinence after radical hysterectomy. *Neurourology and Urodynamics, 26,* 794–799. doi:10.1002/nau.20431

Barry, M.J., Fowler, F.J., Jr., O'Leary, M.P., Bruskewitz, R.C., Holtgrewe, H.L., Mebust, W.K., & Cockett, A.T. (1992). The American Urological Association symptom index for benign prostatic hyperplasia. The Measurement Committee of the American Urological Association. *Journal of Urology, 148,* 1549–1557.

Key Points

- UI is common among people who have undergone treatments for prostate, cervical, bladder, and rectal cancers.
- The incidence of UI after radical prostatectomy has been reported as high as 90%. More than 30% of patients continued to leak 12 months after prostatectomy and 15% continued to leak after 5 years.
- Unresolved temporary and permanent UI is costly to individuals and society and has adverse physical, social, and emotional consequences.
- PFME has been commonly used to treat postprostatectomy UI. However, evidence for the effect of PFME on UI is mixed.
- Persistent postprostatectomy UI is especially difficult to treat. Initial, encouraging evidence supports that PFME plus self-management of UI symptoms improves urinary function and reduces UI problems.
- Evidence regarding UI in patients diagnosed with cervical, bladder, and rectal cancers is emerging. Evidence is lacking about how to treat UI in these patients. More research is needed in this area.

Bradley, E.B., Bissonette, E.A., & Theodorescu, D. (2004). Determinants of long-term quality of life and voiding function of patients treated with radical prostatectomy or permanent brachytherapy for prostate cancer. *BJU International, 94,* 1003–1009. doi:10.1111/j.1464-410X.2004.05094.x

Burgio, K.L., Goode, P.S., Urban, D.A., Umlauf, M.G., Locher, J.L., Bueschen, A., & Redden, D.T. (2006). Preoperative biofeedback assisted behavioral training to decrease post-prostatectomy incontinence: A randomized, controlled trial. *Journal of Urology, 175,* 196–201. doi:10.1016/S0022-5347(05)00047-9

Burt, J., Caelli, K., Moore, K., & Anderson, M. (2005) Radical prostatectomy: Men's experiences and postoperative needs. *Journal of Clinical Nursing, 14,* 883–890. doi:10.1111/j.1365-2702.2005.01123.x

Butler, L., Downe-Wamboldt, B., Marsh, S., Bell, D., & Jarvi, K. (2000). Behind the scenes: Partners' perceptions of quality of life post radical prostatectomy. *Urologic Nursing, 20,* 254–258.

Ceccaroni, M., Roviglione, G., Spagnolo, E., Casadio, P., Clarizia, R., Peiretti, M., ... Aletti, G. (2012). Pelvic dysfunctions and quality of life after nerve-sparing radical hysterectomy: A multicenter comparative study. *Anticancer Research, 32,* 581–588. Retrieved from http://ar.iiarjournals.org/content/32/2/581.long

Centemero, A., Rigatti, L., Giraudo, D., Lazzeri, M., Lughezzani, G., Zugna, D., ... Guazzoni, G. (2010). Preoperative pelvic floor muscle exercise for early continence after radical prostatectomy: A randomised controlled study. *European Urology, 57,* 1039–1044. doi:10.1016/j.eururo.2010.02.028

Contin, P., Kulu, Y., Bruckner, T., Sturm, M., Welsch, T., Müller-Stich, B.P., ... Ulrich, A. (2014). Comparative analysis of late functional outcome following preoperative radiation therapy or chemoradiotherapy and surgery or surgery alone in rectal cancer. *International Journal of Colorectal Disease, 29,* 165–175. doi:10.1007/s00384-013-1780-z

Cooperberg, M.R., Master, V.A., & Carroll, P.R. (2003). Health related quality of life significance of single pad urinary incontinence following radical prostatectomy. *Journal of Urology, 170,* 512–515. doi:10.1097/01.ju.0000074941.27370.c4

Couper, J., Bloch, S., Love, A., Macvean, M., Duchesne, G.M., & Kissane, D. (2006). Psychosocial adjustment of female partners of men with prostate cancer: A review of the literature. *Psycho-Oncology, 15,* 937–953. doi:10.1002/pon.1031

Coyne, K.S., Wein, A., Nicholson, S., Kvasz, M., Chen, C.-I., & Milsom, I. (2014). Economic burden of urgency urinary incontinence in the United States: A systematic review. *Journal of Managed Care and Specialty Pharmacy, 20,* 130–140. doi:10.18553/jmcp.2014.20.2.130

de Noronha, A.F., de Figueiredo, E.M., Franco, T.M.R.D.F., Cândido, E.B., & Silva-Filho, A.L. (2013). Treatments for invasive carcinoma of the cervix: What are their impacts on the pelvic floor functions? *International Brazilian Journal of Urology, 39,* 46–54. doi:10.1590/S1677-5538.IBJU.2013.01.07

de Reijke, T.M., & Laguna, M.P. (2003). Long-term complications of brachytherapy in local prostate cancer. *BJU International, 92,* 869–873. doi:10.1046/j.1464-410X.2003.04497.x

Donovan, J.L., Peters, T.J., Abrams, P., Brookes, S.T., de la Rosette, J.J., & Schäfer, W. (2000). Scoring the Short Form ICSmaleSF questionnaire. *Journal of Urology, 164,* 1948–1955. doi:10.1016/S0022-5347(05)66926-1

Donovan, K.A., Boyington, A.R., Judson, P.L., & Wyman, J.F. (2014). Bladder and bowel symptoms in cervical and endometrial cancer survivors. *Psycho-Oncology, 23,* 672–678. doi:10.1002/pon.3461

Downs, T.M., Sadetsky, N., Pasta, D.J., Grossfeld, G.D., Kane, C.J., Mehta, S.S., ... Lubeck, D.P. (2003). Health related quality of life patterns in patients treated with interstitial prostate brachytherapy for localized prostate cancer—Data from CaPSURE. *Journal of Urology, 170,* 1822–1827. doi:10.1097/01.ju.0000091426.55735.f0

Dubbert, P.M. (1992). Exercise in behavioral medicine. *Journal of Consulting and Clinical Psychology, 60,* 613–618. doi:10.1037/0022-006X.60.4.613

Du Moulin, M.F., Hamers, J.P., Paulus, A., Berendsen, C., & Halfens, R. (2005). The role of the nurse in community continence care: A systematic review. *International Journal of Nursing Studies, 42,* 479–492. doi:10.1016/j.ijnurstu.2004.08.002

Duncan, K.A., & Pozehl, B. (2002). Staying on course: The effects of an adherence facilitation intervention on home exercise participation. *Progress in Cardiovascular Nursing, 17,* 59–65, 71. doi:10.1111/j.0889-7204.2002.01229.x

Elstad, E.A., Taubenberger, S.P., Botelho, E.M., & Tennstedt, S.L. (2010). Beyond incontinence: The stigma of other urinary symptoms. *Journal of Advanced Nursing, 66,* 2460–2470. doi:10.1111/j.1365-2648.2010.05422.x

Erekson, E.A., Sung, V.W., DiSilvestro, P.A., & Myers, D.L. (2009). Urinary symptoms and impact on quality of life in women after treatment for endometrial cancer. *International Urogynecology Journal, 20,* 159–163. doi:10.1007/s00192-008-0755-z

Fan, X., Heyes, S., & King, L. (2012). Men's experiences of urinary incontinence after prostatectomy: A literature review by Xiaojing Fan and colleagues of patients' post-surgical problems identified long- and short-term effects and, importantly, the need for nurses to offer more education and information to help men cope. *Cancer Nursing Practice, 11*(9), 29–34. doi:10.7748/cnp2012.11.11.9.29.c9409

Fernández, R.A., García-Hermoso, A., Solera-Martínez, M., Correa, M.T., Morales, A.F., & Martínez-Vizcaíno, V. (2015). Improvement of continence rate with pelvic floor muscle training post-prostatectomy: A meta-analysis of randomized controlled trials. *Urologia Internationalis, 94,* 125–132. doi:10.1159/000368618

Filocamo, M.T., Marzi, V.L., Del Popolo, G., Cecconi, F., Marzocco, M., Tosto, A., & Nicita, G. (2005). Effectiveness of early pelvic floor rehabilitation treatment for post-prostatectomy incontinence. *European Urology, 48,* 734–738. doi:10.1016/j.eururo.2005.06.004

Floratos, D.L., Sonke, G.S., Rapidou, C.A., Alivizatos, G.J., Deliveliotis, C., Constantinides, C.A., & Theodorou, C. (2002). Biofeedback vs. verbal feedback as learning tools for pelvic muscle exercises in the early management of urinary incontinence after radical prostatectomy. *BJU International, 89,* 714–719. doi:10.1046/j.1464-410X.2002.02721.x

Fontaine, E., Ben Mouelli, S., Thomas, L., Otmezguine, Y., & Beurton, D. (2004). Urinary continence after salvage radiation therapy following radical prostatectomy, assessed by a self-administered questionnaire: A prospective study. *BJU International, 94,* 521–523. doi:10.1111/j.1464-410X.2004.04995.x

Foote, J., Yun, S., & Leach, G.E. (1991). Postprostatectomy incontinence: Pathophysiology, evaluation, and management. *Urologic Clinics of North America, 18,* 229–241.

Geraerts, I., Van Poppel, H., Devoogdt, N., Joniau, S., Van Cleynenbreugel, B., De Groef, A., & Van Kampen, M. (2013). Influence of preoperative and postoperative pelvic floor muscle training (PFMT) compared with postoperative PFMT on urinary incontinence after radical prostatectomy: A randomized controlled trial. *European Urology, 64,* 766–772. doi:10.1016/j.eururo.2013.01.013

Gilbert, S.M., Wood, D.P., Dunn, R.L., Weizer, A.Z., Lee, C.T., Montie, J.E., & Wei, J.T. (2007). Measuring health-related quality of life outcomes in bladder cancer patients using the Bladder Cancer Index (BCI). *Cancer, 109,* 1756–1762. doi:10.1002/cncr.22556

Glazener, C., Boachie, C., Buckley, B., Cochran, C., Dorey, G., Grant, A., ... N'Dow, J. (2011). Urinary incontinence in men after formal one-to-one pelvic-floor muscle training following radical prostatectomy or transurethral resection of the prostate (MAPS): Two parallel randomised controlled trials. *Lancet, 378,* 328–337. doi:10.1016/S0140-6736(11)60751-4

Goode, P.S., Burgio, K.L., Johnson, T.M., Clay, O.J., Roth, D.L., Markland, A.D., ... Lloyd, L.K. (2011). Behavioral therapy with or without biofeedback and pelvic floor electrical stimulation for persistent postprostatectomy incontinence: A randomized controlled trial. *JAMA, 305,* 151–159. doi:10.1001/jama.2010.1972

Harden, J., Schafenacker, A., Northouse, L., Mood, D., Smith, D., Pienta, K., ... Baranowski, K. (2002). Couples' experiences with prostate cancer: Focus group research. *Oncology Nursing Forum, 29,* 701–709. doi:10.1188/02.ONF.701-709

Harris, J.L. (1997). Treatment of postprostatectomy urinary incontinence with behavioral methods. *Clinical Nurse Specialist, 11,* 159–166. doi:10.1097/00002800-199707000-00007

Hazewinkel, M.H., Sprangers, M.A.G., van der Velden, J., van der Vaart, C.H., Stalpers, L.J.A., Burger, M.P.M., & Roovers, J.P.W.R. (2010). Long-term cervical cancer survivors suffer from pelvic floor symptoms: A cross-sectional matched cohort study. *Gynecologic Oncology, 117,* 281–286. doi:10.1016/j.ygyno.2010.01.034

Hedestig, O., Sandman, P.O., Tomic, R., & Widmark, A. (2005). Living after radical prostatectomy for localized prostate cancer: A qualitative analysis of patient narratives. *Acta Oncologica, 44,* 679–686. doi:10.1080/02841860500326000

Hersh, L., & Salzman, B. (2013). Clinical management of urinary incontinence in women. *American Family Physician, 87,* 634–640.

Higa, R., Lopes, M.H.B.D.M., & D'Ancona, C.A.L. (2013). Male incontinence: A critical review of the literature. *Texto and Contexto Enfermagem, 22,* 231–238. doi:10.1590/S0104-07072013000100028

Holm, H.V., Fosså, S.D., Hedlund, H., Schultz, A., & Dahl, A.A. (2014). How should continence and incontinence after radical prostatectomy be evaluated? A prospective study of patient ratings and changes with time. *Journal of Urology, 192,* 1155–1161. doi:10.1016/j.juro.2014.03.113

Hoyland, K., Vasdev, N., Abrof, A., & Boustead, G. (2014). Post-radical prostatectomy incontinence: Etiology and prevention. *Reviews in Urology, 16,* 181–188.

Hunter, K.F., Moore, K.N., Cody, D.J., & Glazener, C.M.A. (2004). Conservative management for postprostatectomy urinary incontinence. *Cochrane Database of Systematic Reviews, 2004*(2). doi:10.1002/14651858.CD001843.pub2

Jacobsen, N.-E., Moore, K.N., Estey, E., & Voaklander, D. (2007). Open versus laparoscopic radical prostatectomy: A prospective comparison of postoperative urinary incontinence rates. *Journal of Urology, 177,* 615–619. doi:10.1016/j.juro.2006.09.022

Jakobsson, L., Hallberg, I.R., & Lovén, L. (2000). Experiences of micturition problems, indwelling catheter treatment and sexual life consequences in men with prostate cancer. *Journal of Advanced Nursing, 31,* 59–67. doi:10.1046/j.1365-2648.2000.01259.x

Jentzmik, F., Schrader, A.J., de Petriconi, R., Hefty, R., Mueller, J., Doetterl, J., ... Schrader, M. (2012). The ileal neobladder in female patients with bladder cancer: Long-term clinical, functional, and oncological outcome. *World Journal of Urology, 30,* 733–739. doi:10.1007/s00345-012-0837-x

Katz, A. (2007). Quality of life for men with prostate cancer. *Cancer Nursing, 30,* 302–308. doi:10.1097/01.NCC.0000281726.87490.f2

Kegel, A.H. (1948). The nonsurgical treatment of genital relaxation: Use of the perineometer as an aid in restoring anatomic and functional structure. *Annals of Western Medicine and Surgery, 2,* 213–216.

Kirschner-Hermanns, R., & Jakse, G. (2002). Quality of life following radical prostatectomy. *Critical Reviews in Oncology/Hematology, 43,* 141–151. doi:10.1016/S1040-8428(02)00026-4

Ko, W.F.Y., & Sawatzky, J.-A.V. (2008). Understanding urinary incontinence after radical prostatectomy: A nursing framework. *Clinical Journal of Oncology Nursing, 12,* 647–654. doi:10.1188/08.CJON.647-654

Kocaöz, S., Eroğlu, K., & Sivaslıoğlu, A.A. (2013). Role of pelvic floor muscle exercises in the prevention of stress urinary incontinence during pregnancy and the postpartum period. *Gynecologic and Obstetric Investigation, 75,* 34–40. doi:10.1159/000343038

Kyrdalen, A.E., Dahl, A.A., Hernes, E., Småstuen, M.C., & Fosså, S.D. (2013). A national study of adverse effects and global quality of life among candidates for curative treatment for prostate cancer. *BJU International, 111,* 221–232. doi:10.1111/j.1464-410X.2012.11198.x

Lange, M.M., Maas, C.P., Marijnen, C.A.M., Wiggers, T., Rutten, H.J., Kranenbarg, E.K., & van de Velde, C.J.H. (2008). Urinary dysfunction after rectal cancer treatment is mainly caused by surgery. *British Journal of Surgery, 95,* 1020–1028. doi:10.1002/bjs.6126

Lepor, H., Kaci, L., & Xue, X. (2004). Continence following radical retropubic prostatectomy using self-reporting instruments. *Journal of Urology, 171,* 1212–1215. doi:10.1097/01.ju.0000110631.81774.9c

Little, D.J., Kuban, D.A., Levy, L.B., Zagars, G.K., & Pollack, A. (2003). Quality-of-life questionnaire results 2 and 3 years after radiotherapy for prostate cancer in a randomized dose-escalation study. *Urology, 62,* 707–713. doi:10.1016/S0090-4295(03)00504-1

Liu, M., Pickles, T., Berthelet, E., Agranovich, A., Kwan, W., Tyldesley, S., ... Prostate Cohort Initiative. (2005). Urinary incontinence in prostate cancer patients treated with external beam radiotherapy. *Radiotherapy and Oncology, 74,* 197–201. doi:10.1016/j.radonc.2004.09.016

Lobchuk, M.M., & Rosenberg, F. (2014). A qualitative analysis of individual and family caregiver responses to the impact of urinary incontinence on quality of life. *Journal of Wound, Ostomy and Continence Nursing, 41,* 589–596. doi:10.1097/WON.0000000000000064

Locke, J., Ellis, W., Wallner, K., Cavanagh, W., & Blasko, J. (2002). Risk factors for acute urinary retention requiring temporary intermittent catheterization after prostate brachytherapy: A prospective study. *International Journal of Radiation Oncology, Biology, Physics, 52,* 712–719. doi:10.1016/S0360-3016(01)02657-8

MacDonald, R., Fink, H.A., Huckabay, C., Monga, M., & Wilt, T.J. (2007). Pelvic floor muscle training to improve urinary incontinence after radical prostatectomy: A systematic review of effectiveness. *BJU International, 100,* 76–81. doi:10.1111/j.1464-410X.2007.06913.x

Madalinska, J.B., Essink-Bot, M.L., de Koning, H.J., Kirkels, W.J., van der Maas, P.J., & Schröder, F.H. (2001). Health-related quality-of-life effects of radical prostatectomy and primary radiotherapy for screen-detected or clinically diagnosed localized prostate cancer. *Journal of Clinical Oncology, 19,* 1619–1628.

Martin, A.D., Nakamura, L.Y., Nunez, R.N., Wolter, C.E., Humphreys, M.R., & Castle, E.P. (2011). Incontinence after radical prostatectomy: A patient centered analysis and implications for preoperative counseling. *Journal of Urology, 186,* 204–208. doi:10.1016/j.juro.2011.02.2698

McCorkle, R., Siefert, M.L., Dowd, M.F., Robinson, J.P., & Pickett, M. (2007). Effects of advanced practice nursing on patient and spouse depressive symptoms, sexual function, and marital interaction after radical prostatectomy. *Urologic Nursing, 27,* 65–77.

Nahon, I., Waddington, G.S., Dorey, G., & Adams, R. (2009). Assessment and conservative management of post-prostatectomy incontinence after radical prostatectomy. *Australian and New Zealand Continence Journal, 15,* 70–77.

Nicolaisen, M., Müller, S., Patel, H.R., & Hanssen, T.A. (2014). Quality of life and satisfaction with information after radical prostatectomy, radical external beam radiotherapy and postoperative radiotherapy: A long-term follow-up study. *Journal of Clinical Nursing, 23,* 3403–3414. doi:10.1111/jocn.12586

Novara, G., Ficarra, V., D'elia, C., Secco, S., Cioffi, A., Cavalleri, S., & Artibani, W. (2010). Evaluating urinary continence and preoperative predictors of urinary continence after robot assisted laparoscopic radical prostatectomy. *Journal of Urology, 184,* 1028–1033. doi:10.1016/j.juro.2010.04.069

Ocampo-Trujillo, Á., Carbonell-González, J., Martínez-Blanco, A., Díaz-Hung, A., Muñoz, C.A., & Ramírez-Vélez, R. (2014). Pre-operative training induces changes in the histomorphometry and muscle function of the pelvic floor in patients with indication of radical prostatectomy. *Actas Urológicas Españolas (English Edition), 38,* 378–384. doi:10.1016/j.acuroe.2014.02.017

O'Shaughnessy, P., & Laws, T. (2010). Australian men's long term experiences following prostatectomy: A qualitative descriptive study. *Contemporary Nurse, 34,* 98–109. doi:10.5172/conu.2009.34.1.098

Palmer, M.H., Fogarty, L.A., Somerfield, M.R., & Powel, L.L. (2003). Incontinence after prostatectomy: Coping with incontinence after prostate cancer surgery.

Oncology Nursing Forum, 30, 229–238. doi:10.1188/03.ONF.229-238

Panjari, M., Bell, R.J., Burney, S., Bell, S., McMurrick, P.J., & Davis, S.R. (2012). Sexual function, incontinence, and wellbeing in women after rectal cancer—A review of the evidence. *Journal of Sexual Medicine, 9,* 2749–2758. doi:10.1111/j.1743-6109.2012.02894.x

Parekh, A.R., Feng, M.I., Kirages, D., Bremner, H., Kaswick, J., & Aboseif, S. (2003). The role of pelvic floor exercises on post-prostatectomy incontinence. *Journal of Urology, 170,* 130–133. doi:10.1097/01.ju.0000072900.82131.6f

Paterson, J. (2000). Stigma associated with postprostatectomy urinary incontinence. *Journal of Wound, Ostomy and Continence Nursing, 27,* 168–173. doi:10.1016/s1071-5754(00)90054-8

Penson, D.F., McLerran, D., Feng, Z., Li, L., Albertsen, P.C., Gilliland, F.D., ... Stanford, J.L. (2008). 5-year urinary and sexual outcomes after radical prostatectomy: Results from the Prostate Cancer Outcomes Study. *Journal of Urology, 179*(Suppl. 5), S40–S44. doi:10.1016/j.juro.2008.03.136

Peterson, A.C., & Chen, Y. (2012). Patient reported incontinence after radical prostatectomy is more common than expected and not associated with the nerve sparing technique: Results from the Center for Prostate Disease Research (CPDR) database. *Neurourology and Urodynamics, 31,* 60–63. doi:10.1002/nau.21189

Petry, H., Berry, D.L., Spichiger, E., Kesselring, A., Gasser, T.C., Sulser, T., & Kiss, A. (2004). Responses and experiences after radical prostatectomy: Perceptions of married couples in Switzerland. *International Journal of Nursing Studies, 41,* 507–513. doi:10.1016/j.ijnurstu.2003.11.005

Peyromaure, M., Ravery, V., & Boccon-Gibod, L. (2002). The management of stress urinary incontinence after radical prostatectomy. *BJU International, 90,* 155–161. doi:10.1046/j.1464-410X.2002.02824.x

Plotti, F., Angioli, R., Zullo, M.A., Sansone, M., Altavilla, T., Antonelli, E., ... Panici, P.B. (2011). Update on urodynamic bladder dysfunctions after radical hysterectomy for cervical cancer. *Critical Reviews in Oncology/Hematology, 80,* 323–329. doi:10.1016/j.critrevonc.2010.12.004

Poon, M., Ruckle, H., Bamshad, B.R., Tsai, C., Webster, R., & Lui, P. (2000). Radical retropubic prostatectomy: Bladder neck preservation versus reconstruction. *Journal of Urology, 163,* 194–198. doi:10.1016/S0022-5347(05)68003-2

Porru, D., Campus, G., Caria, A., Madeddu, G., Cucchi, A., Rovereto, B., ... Usai, E. (2001). Impact of early pelvic floor rehabilitation after transurethral resection of the prostate. *Neurourology and Urodynamics, 20,* 53–59. doi:10.1002/1520-6777(2001)20:1<53::AID-NAU7>3.0.CO;2-B

Potosky, A.L., Davis, W.W., Hoffman, R.M., Stanford, J.L., Stephenson, R.A., Penson, D.F., & Harlan, L.C. (2004). Five-year outcomes after prostatectomy or radiotherapy for prostate cancer: The Prostate Cancer Outcomes Study. *Journal of the National Cancer Institute, 96,* 1358–1367. doi:10.1093/jnci/djh259

Potosky, A.L., Legler, J., Albertsen, P.C., Stanford, J.L., Gilliland, F.D., Hamilton, A.S., ... Harlan, L.C. (2000). Health outcomes after prostatectomy or radiotherapy for prostate cancer: Results from the Prostate Cancer Outcomes Study. *Journal of the National Cancer Institute, 92,* 1582–1592. doi:10.1093/jnci/92.19.1582

Quek, M.L., & Penson, D.F. (2005). Quality of life in patients with localized prostate cancer. *Urologic Oncology, 23,* 208–215. doi:10.1016/j.urolonc.2005.03.003

Raabe, N.K., Normann, M., & Lilleby, W. (2015). Low-dose-rate brachytherapy for low-grade prostate cancer. *Tidsskrift for den Norske Laegeforening: Tidsskrift for Praktisk Medicin, ny Raekke, 135,* 548–552. doi:10.4045/tidsskr.13.1404

Registered Nurses' Association of Ontario. (2011). *Best practice guideline: Promoting continence using prompted voiding (guideline supplement).* Retrieved from http://rnao.ca/sites/rnao-ca/files/storage/related/7719_BPG_Continence-Supplement-Only-2011.pdf

Reis, F., Netto, N.R., Jr., Reinato, J.A.S., Thiel, M., & Zani, E. (2004). The impact of prostatectomy and brachytherapy in patients with localized prostate cancer. *International Urology and Nephrology, 36,* 187–190. doi:10.1023/B:UROL.0000034686.55747.a5

Resel-Folkersma, L., Salinas-Casado, J., & Moreno-Sierra, J. (2014). Post-prostatectomy stress urinary incontinence: A review of contemporary surgical treatments. *Reviews in Clinical Gerontology, 24,* 191–204. doi:10.1017/S0959259814000069

Resendes, L.A., & McCorkle, R. (2006). Spousal responses to prostate cancer: An integrative review. *Cancer Investigation, 24,* 192–198. doi:10.1080/07357900500524652

Rhodes, R.E., & Fiala, B. (2009). Building motivation and sustainability into the prescription and recommendations for physical activity and exercise therapy: The evidence. *Physiotherapy Theory and Practice, 25,* 424–441. doi:10.1080/09593980902835344

Ribeiro, L.H.S., Prota, C., Gomes, C.M., de Bessa, J., Jr. Boldarine, M.P., Dall'Oglio, M.F., ... Srougi, M. (2010). Long-term effect of early postoperative pelvic floor biofeedback on continence in men undergoing radical prostatectomy: A prospective, randomized, controlled trial. *Journal of Urology, 184,* 1034–1039. doi:10.1016/j.juro.2010.05.040

Robinson, J.P., Bradway, C.W., Nuamah, I., Pickett, M., & McCorkle, R. (2008). Systematic pelvic floor training for lower urinary tract symptoms post-prostatectomy: A randomized clinical trial. *International Journal of Urological Nursing, 2,* 3–13. doi:10.1111/j.1749-771X.2007.00033.x

Romero, O.J., & Martínez-Salamanca, J.I. (2007). Critical comparative analysis between open, laparoscopic and robotic radical prostatectomy: Urinary continence and sexual function (part II). *Archivos Espanoles De Urologia, 60,* 767–776.

Rondorf-Klym, L.M., & Colling, J. (2003). Quality of life after radical prostatectomy [Online exclusive]. *Oncology Nursing Forum, 30,* E24–E32. doi:10.1188/03.ONF.E24-E32

Shelby, R.A., Taylor, K.L., Kerner, J.F., Coleman, E., & Blum, D. (2002). The role of community-based and philanthropic organizations in meeting cancer patient and caregiver needs. *CA: A Cancer Journal for Clinicians, 52,* 229–246. doi:10.3322/canjclin.52.4.229

Skjeldestad, F.E., & Hagen, B. (2008). Long-term consequences of gynecological cancer treatment on urinary incontinence: A population-based cross-sectional study. *Acta Obstetricia et Gynecologica Scandinavica, 87,* 469–475. doi:10.1080/00016340801948326

Smith, I.A., Shaw, E., & Rashid, P. (2009). Postprostatectomy stress urinary incontinence: Current and evolving therapies. *Australian Family Physician, 38,* 399–404.

Smither, A.R., Guralnick, M.L., Davis, N.B., & See, W.A. (2007). Quantifying the natural history of post-radical prostatectomy incontinence using objective pad test data. *BMC Urology, 7,* 2. doi:10.1186/1471-2490-7-2

Stafne, S.N., Salvesen, K.Å., Romundstad, P.R., Torjusen, I.H., & Mørkved, S. (2012). Does regular exercise including pelvic floor muscle training prevent urinary and anal incontinence during pregnancy? A randomised controlled trial. *BJOG: An International Journal of Obstetrics and Gynaecology, 119,* 1270–1280. doi:10.1111/j.1471-0528.2012.03426.x

Stothers, L., Thom, D., & Calhoun, E. (2005). Urologic diseases in America project: Urinary incontinence in males—demographics and economic burden. *Journal of Urology, 173,* 1302–1308. doi:10.1097/01.ju.0000155503.12545.4e

Talcott, J.A., Clark, J.A., Stark, P.C., & Mitchell, S.P. (2001). Long-term treatment related complications of brachytherapy for early prostate cancer: A survey of patients previously treated. *Journal of Urology, 166,* 494–499. doi:10.1016/S0022-5347(05)65970-8

Tang, D.H., Colayco, D.C., Khalaf, K.M., Piercy, J., Patel, V., Globe, D., & Ginsberg, D. (2014). Impact of urinary incontinence on healthcare resource utilization, health-related quality of life and productivity in patients with overactive bladder. *BJU International, 113,* 484–491. doi:10.1111/bju.12505

Tienforti, D., Sacco, E., Marangi, F., D'Addessi, A., Racioppi, M., Gulino, G., ... Bassi, P. (2012). Efficacy of an assisted low-intensity programme of perioperative pelvic floor muscle training in improving the recovery of continence after radical prostatectomy: A randomized controlled trial. *BJU International, 110,* 1004–1010. doi:10.1111/j.1464-410X.2012.10948.x

Urinary incontinence. (n.d.). In *The free dictionary.* Retrieved from http://medical-dictionary.thefreedictionary.com/urinary+incontinence

Van Kampen, M. (2006). In addition to usual care, pelvic floor exercises commenced preoperatively reduce incontinence after prostatectomy. *Australian Journal of Physiotherapy, 52,* 305. doi:10.1016/s0004-9514(06)70014-9

Van Kampen, M., de Weerdt, W., Van Poppel, H., de Ridder, D., Feys, H., & Baert, L. (2000). Effect of pelvic-floor re-education on duration and degree of incontinence after radical prostatectomy: A randomised controlled trial. *Lancet, 355,* 98–102. doi:10.1016/S0140-6736(99)03473-X

Varpe, P., Huhtinen, H., Rantala, A., Salminen, P., Rautava, P., Hurme, S., & Grönroos, J. (2011). Quality of life after surgery for rectal cancer with special reference to pelvic floor dysfunction. *Colorectal Disease, 13,* 399–405. doi:10.1111/j.1463-1318.2009.02165.x

Waller, J., & Pattison, N. (2013). Men's experiences of regaining urinary continence following robotic-assisted laparoscopic prostatectomy (RALP) for localised prostate cancer: A qualitative phenomenological study. *Journal of Clinical Nursing, 22,* 368–378. doi:10.1111/jocn.12082

Wallerstedt, A., Carlsson, S., Nilsson, A.E., Johansson, E., Nyberg, T., Steineck, G., & Wiklund, N.P. (2012). Pad use and patient reported bother from urinary leakage after radical prostatectomy. *Journal of Urology, 187,* 196–200. doi:10.1016/j.juro.2011.09.030

Walsh, E., & Hegarty, J. (2010). Men's experiences of radical prostatectomy as treatment for prostate cancer. *European Journal of Oncology Nursing, 14,* 125–133. doi:10.1016/j.ejon.2009.10.003

Wang, W., Huang, Q.M., Liu, F.P., & Mao, Q.Q. (2014). Effectiveness of preoperative pelvic floor muscle training for urinary incontinence after radical prostatectomy: A meta-analysis. *BMC Urology, 14,* 99. doi:10.1186/1471-2490-14-99

Weber, B.A., Roberts, B.L., Chumbler, N.R., Mills, T.L., & Algood, C.B. (2007). Urinary, sexual, and bowel dysfunction and bother after radical prostatectomy. *Urologic Nursing, 27,* 527–533.

Weber, B.A., Roberts, B.L., Mills, T.L., Chumbler, N.R., & Algood, C.B. (2008). Physical and emotional predictors of depression after radical prostatectomy. *American Journal of Men's Health, 2,* 165–171. doi:10.1177/1557988307312222

Yucel, S., & Baskin, L.S. (2004). An anatomical description of the male and female urethral sphincter complex. *Journal of Urology, 171,* 1890–1897. doi:10.1097/01.ju.0000124106.16505.df

Zhang, A.Y., Bodner, D.R., Fu, A.Z., Gunzler, D.D., Klein, E., Kresevic, D., ... Zhu, H. (2015). Effects of patient centered interventions on persistent urinary incontinence after prostate cancer treatment: A randomized, controlled trial. *Journal of Urology, 194,* 1675–1681. doi:10.1016/j.juro.2015.07.090

Zhang, A.Y., & Fu, A.Z. (2016). Cost-effectiveness of a behavioral intervention for persistent urinary incontinence in prostate cancer patients. *Psycho-Oncology, 25,* 421–427. doi:10.1002/pon.3849

Zullo, M.A., Plotti, F., Calcagno, M., Angioli, R., & Panici, P.B. (2008). Transurethral polydimethylsiloxane injection: A valid minimally invasive option for the treatment of postradical hysterectomy urinary incontinence. *Journal of Minimally Invasive Gynecology, 15,* 373–376. doi:10.1016/j.jmig.2007.12.005

Chapter 21 Study Questions

1. Which of the following cancers is NOT a genitourinary cancer?
   A. Bladder
   B. Lung
   C. Prostate
   D. Kidney

2. Which of the following is used to assess urinary incontinence in patients with prostate cancer in the United States?
   A. AUASS
   B. ICSmaleSF
   C. ICIQ-SF
   D. All of the above

3. Roughly how many men continued to leak at 12 months after prostate cancer treatment?
   A. 5%–10%
   B. 15%–20%
   C. 30%–40%
   D. 50%–60%

4. Pelvic floor muscle exercise (PFME) is believed to reduce prostatectomy urinary incontinence because it can strengthen muscles of the:
   A. Internal sphincter.
   B. External sphincter.
   C. Bladder.
   D. Abdomen.

5. Which of the following does NOT exacerbate urinary incontinence symptoms?
   A. Plenty of fluid intake
   B. Caffeinated drinks
   C. Obesity
   D. Diabetes

CHAPTER

22 Hematologic Issues

Patricia L. Adams, RN, MSN, AOCNS®

Introduction

Myelosuppression is the most common dose-limiting side effect and the most potentially life-threatening side effect related to systemic anticancer treatments (Gobel & O'Leary, 2007). It is crucial to understand the various manifestations of myelosuppression and the mechanisms by which they are induced in patients undergoing cancer therapy. It is then that proactive, effective nursing care can be delivered.

The manifestations of myelosuppression include neutropenia, thrombocytopenia, and anemia. Each may occur as the result of the suppressive effects on bone marrow function by cancer or cancer treatment. When suppression of bone marrow function occurs, adequate amounts of vital blood cells are reduced and the patient is at risk for experiencing complications that can be severe and life threatening. These include symptoms of infection related to neutropenia, bleeding as a consequence of thrombocytopenia, and symptoms of anemia. Each of these manifestations will be explored in detail.

Neutropenia

Overview

Neutropenia is a common toxicity of cancer chemotherapy. Neutrophils are the body's first line of defense against microbial invasion. Their main function is phagocytosis. The neutrophils constitute approximately 50%–60% of the total white blood cell count (Gobel & O'Leary, 2007). The neutrophil life span is six to eight hours once released from the bone marrow to the circulation (Camp-Sorrell, 2018). Neutropenia is defined as a reduction in circulating neutrophils. An absolute neutrophil count (ANC) of less than 1,500/mm^3 is generally the definition of neutropenia (Camp-Sorrell, 2018).

Risk Factors

Many risk factors exist for the development of neutropenia in patients with cancer. These factors may be categorized as patient specific, disease specific, or treatment related. Patient risk factors include the age and general health of the patient, history of prior cytotoxic therapy, and history of prior neutropenic fever. Individuals aged 65 years or older may experience age-related changes in their ability to metabolize, absorb, distribute, and excrete some chemotherapy agents (Lichtman, 2016). This may put them at greater risk for the development of neutropenic fevers. Studies demonstrated that older individuals with poor performance status had a significant risk for neutropenia (Gobel & O'Leary, 2007). Comorbid conditions such as cardiovascular disease, diabetes, liver disease, and chronic obstructive pulmonary disease increase the risk of neutropenia (Camp-Sorrell,

2018). The patient's current medications need to be reviewed. Medications such as ibuprofen, ranitidine, cimetidine, and phenytoin may cause neutropenia (Gobel & O'Leary, 2007).

Disease risk factors include the type and aggressiveness of the malignancy, whether it is a solid tumor or hematologic malignancy, the location of the disease, and whether it is an advanced stage. An elevated lactate dehydrogenase in individuals with lymphoma or leukemia increases risk for neutropenia (O'Leary, 2015).

Treatment risk factors include the type and dose of cytotoxic agents used, concurrent or prior radiation therapy, extensive prior chemotherapy, and absence of colony-stimulating factor therapy (Gobel & O'Leary, 2007). The treatment pattern also can be a risk factor for the development of neutropenia. *Dose intensity* is a term used to describe a cytotoxic treatment pattern achieved by increasing a single dose per cycle of cytotoxic agents (Venturini et al., 2005). The goal of dose-intense treatment is to administer the maximum tolerated dose of a cytotoxic agent to produce the most effective lethal impact on malignant cells, thereby achieving the best survival for the patient (Nirenberg et al., 2006a). Dose intensity is attained by administering cytotoxic drugs at the same dose per cycle with a shorter interval between treatment cycles (Venturini et al., 2005). The overall effect of dose-intensive treatment patterns is the delivery of a higher dose of cytotoxic agents over a shorter period of time. As a consequence, the incidence and severity of neutropenia are increased, and dose-intensive treatment plans must always include growth factor support (Nirenberg et al., 2006a).

High doses of specific immunosuppressive agents are used in the preparative regimens of hematopoietic stem cell transplantation, where the goal is to eradicate malignant hematopoietic stem cells and replace them with healthy progenitor cells. This process renders the patient profoundly neutropenic for a period of time (West & Mitchell, 2004).

Treatment with radiation to the large bones of the femur, pelvis, and mediastinum suppresses bone marrow function, potentially leading to an inability to produce adequate numbers of white blood cells. Patients at highest risk are those receiving chemotherapy and radiation concurrently, total body irradiation, splenic radiation, or wide field radiation encompassing more than 15% of active bone marrow in the field (Aistars, 2007).

Diagnosis

Neutrophils comprise the proportion of white blood cells that are immature (banded neutrophils) and mature (segmented neutrophils). Neutropenia exists when the ANC is below 1,500/mm^3 (National Cancer Institute Cancer Therapy Evaluation Program [NCI CTEP], 2010). This value is derived by multiplying the sum of the percent of banded and segmented neutrophils by the total white blood cell count divided by 100 (Marrs, 2006; Schwartzberg, 2006) (see Figure 22-1).

The severity of neutropenia is categorized as mild, moderate, or severe based on the ANC. The danger associated with abnormally low levels of neutrophils is that the risk of infection increases as the ANC decreases. A correlation exists between the severity and duration of neutropenia and the risk of infection in patients with cancer. The more severe and the longer the duration of neutropenia, more elevated the risk is for the development of severe, life-threatening infection (Schwartzberg, 2006) (see Table 22-1).

Chemotherapy-induced neutropenia can be a dose-limiting side effect, accounting for dose adjustments and dose delays that could potentially limit favorable outcomes for patients with cancer (Lyman, 2006). Complications resulting from chemotherapy-induced neutropenia, specifically febrile neutropenia, may lead to significant morbidity, mortality, and cost (Kuderer, Dale, Crawford, & Lyman, 2007; Nirenberg et al., 2006a). Febrile neutropenia can be a severe life-threatening complication of neutropenia.

Figure 22-1. Absolute Neutrophil Count Calculation

Formula

[segs (%) + bands (%)] × white blood cell count (cells/mm^3) = absolute value (cells/mm^3)

Example

[0.5% (segs) + 18% (bands)] = 0.185 × (1.0 × 10^3 cells/mm^3) = 185 absolute neutrophil count

Note. Based on information from Fischbach, 2000.

From "Evidence-Based Guidelines for the Management of Neutropenia Following Outpatient Hematopoietic Stem Cell Transplantation," by F. West and S.A. Mitchell, 2004, *Clinical Journal of Oncology Nursing, 8,* p. 602. Copyright 2004 by Oncology Nursing Society. Reprinted with permission.

In the absence of adequate numbers of circulating neutrophils, the classic signs of infection are muted or absent. Many times, the only symptom of life-threatening infection in a neutropenic patient may be a fever. Other symptoms that may be associated with infection include chills, myalgia (muscle pain), arthralgia (joint pain), mental status changes, anorexia, nausea and vomiting, cough, dyspnea, hypoxemia, hypotension, tachycardia, and pain or irritation at the site of the infection. However, many of the classic signs of infection, such as redness, purulence, and edema, may be absent in febrile patients who are neutropenic (Gobel & O'Leary, 2007). Neutrophil volume and function can be markedly suppressed by cancers such as hematologic malignancies and advanced stages of solid tumor malignancies that may have metastasized to bone marrow (Schwartzberg, 2006).

Treatment and Nursing Implications

Nurses should be aware of the significance of neutropenia in patients with cancer who are undergoing active therapy. Careful and proactive planning will result in successful cancer therapy outcomes for patients (O'Leary, 2015).

The Oncology Nursing Society has identified prevention of infection in patients with cancer as a nursing-sensitive patient outcome measure (Nirenberg et al., 2006b). Efficient and proactive assessment (see Figure 22-2), timely interventions, and expert patient education will facilitate successful outcomes in patients who are at risk. Although the occurrence of neutropenia may be an inevitable outcome of cytotoxic therapies, a number of strategies can reduce or prevent the complications and adverse sequelae (O'Leary, 2015).

Exogenous hematopoietic-stimulating factors are an effective pharmacologic strategy in preventing complications of neutropenia. Studies have demonstrated that the use of these agents has significantly reduced the length of hospital stay for the treatment of febrile neutropenia, reduced infection-related mortal-

Table 22-1. Absolute Neutrophil Count Grading and Risk for Infection

Grade	Absolute Neutrophil Count (/mm^3)	Risk for Infection
1	< LLN–1,500	No increased risk
2	1,500–1,000	Slightly increased risk
3	1,000–500	Moderately increased risk
4	< 500	High risk

LLN—lower limit of normal

Note. Based on information from National Cancer Institute Cancer Therapy Evaluation Program, 2010.

Figure 22-2. Risk Factors to Be Assessed for Neutropenia

Risk Factor	Yes	No
Comorbidities		
Chronic obstructive pulmonary disease		
Cardiovascular disease		
Liver disease		
Renal insufficiency		
Diabetes mellitus		
Baseline anemia		
Patient Related		
Increased age (> 65 years)		
Female sex		
Poor performance status (Eastern Cooperative Oncology Group ≥ 2)		
Poor nutritional status		
Decreased immune function		
Decreased body surface area		
Inpatient versus outpatient		
Cancer Related		
Bone marrow involvement of tumor		
Advanced cancer		
Type of malignancy: leukemia, lymphoma, lung cancer		
Elevated lactate dehydrogenase level (especially with non-Hodgkin lymphoma)		
Treatment Related		
Previous chemotherapy and type (specify) ________________		
Planned relative dose intensity		
Concurrent or prior irradiation to marrow		
Preexisting neutropenia (prolonged)		
History of severe neutropenia with chemotherapy		

(Continued on next page)

Figure 22-2. Risk Factors to Be Assessed for Neutropenia *(Continued)*

Risk Factor	Yes	No
Conditions With Increased Risk		
Open wounds		
Active infection		
Mucositis (Common Terminology Criteria for Adverse Events grades 3–4)		
Physical Examination		
Head-to-toe assessment, with high-risk areas for infection, perirectal area, oral mucosa, sinuses, lung, skin, and indwelling catheter sites		
Diagnostic Evaluation		
Complete blood count/differential, blood and other cultures, chemistry profile, chest x-ray		

Note. Based on information from Klastersky et al., 2000; Maxwell & Stein, 2006; Wujcik, 2004.

From "Prevention of Infection" (pp. 268–269), by J.M. Tipton in L.H. Eaton and J.M. Tipton (Eds.), *Putting Evidence Into Practice: Improving Oncology Patient Outcomes,* 2009, Pittsburgh, PA: Oncology Nursing Society.

ity, and shortened time to neutrophil recovery (Nirenberg et al., 2006a). The National Comprehensive Cancer Network® (NCCN®, 2016c) and the American Society of Clinical Oncology (Smith et al., 2015) have recognized the impact of growth factors and their use for primary prophylaxis of febrile neutropenia.

Patients who may be at risk for the development of neutropenia should be identified prior to treatment (see Figure 22-2). Risk assessments should include consideration of the disease to be treated and the treatment method. In addition, patient factors, such as comorbidities, age, and functional stability, should be assessed. A complete and thorough history and physical assessment should be completed with particular attention to potential sites of infection, such as the oral cavity and indwelling central vascular access devices. A plan of care or protocol should be established for specific preventive measures and steps to initiate in the event of fever in neutropenic patients (NCCN, 2017).

Patient education is paramount for nurses caring for patients with cancer and their families. Education should include teaching about the mechanism of action of chemotherapy, particularly its impact on neutrophils and their activity. Patients should understand the mechanism of action and importance of prophylactic agents, particularly exogenous hematopoietic-stimulating agents. Patients and families should be taught infection control measures, including avoiding environmental exposures, adhering to prophylactic measures, and incorporating personal hygiene practices into activities of daily living. Patients should be taught how to monitor themselves for symptoms of infections. Patients and families should be specifically instructed when and how to report symptoms of infections and any problems or concerns during active treatment (O'Leary, 2015).

Nurses should be aware of the significance of neutropenia in patients with cancer undergoing active therapy. Careful and proactive planning will contribute to successful patient outcomes (O'Leary, 2015).

Thrombocytopenia

Overview

Thrombocytopenia is defined as a platelet count of less than 150,000/mm^3 (George & Arnold, 2017). Platelets are produced in the bone marrow from megakaryocytes. Each megakaryocyte produces an estimated 1,000–5,000 platelets. The life span of the platelet is approximately 8–10 days in circulation, after which the monocyte–macrophage system removes them from circulation (George & Arnold, 2017).

A normal platelet count in adults is 150,000–450,000/mm^3 (George & Arnold, 2017). Under normal conditions, one-third of circulating platelets are sequestered in the spleen. Platelets play a vital role in the maintenance of hemostasis.

Risk Factors

Thrombocytopenia is a frequent consequence of myelosuppressive cancer therapy. The major mechanisms that cause thrombocytopenia in patients with cancer are decreased production, increased destruction, or platelet dysfunction. Platelet production by the bone marrow can be impaired when the marrow is suppressed or damaged. Causes associated with patients with cancer include active therapy with myelotoxic chemotherapy and radiation therapy to sites of platelet production. Chemotherapy agents with a greater potential to cause thrombocytopenia include gemcitabine, carboplatin, dacarbazine, fluorouracil, lomustine, mitomycin C, thiotepa, and trimetrexate (Camp-Sorrell, 2018). Bone marrow aplasia may be acquired via other means, such as hematologic disease, viral infections, vitamin B_{12} and folate deficiencies, and direct alcohol toxicity, which also may lead to thrombocytopenia (George & Arnold, 2017).

Disorders of increased platelet destruction include alloimmunization, disseminated intravascular coagulation, and thrombotic thrombocytopenic purpura–hemolytic uremic syndrome. Splenomegaly caused by sequestration of platelets can induce an apparent thrombocytopenia. Although total platelet volume remains normal, the number of functional platelets is decreased (George & Arnold, 2017).

A platelet count less than 50,000/mm^3 confers a moderate risk for bleeding. If the count decreases to less than 10,000/mm^3, a severe risk for a fatal hemorrhage may occur (Camp-Sorrell, 2018). The central nervous system, respiratory system, and gastrointestinal system are the major sites for hemorrhage.

Diagnosis

A platelet count less than 150,000/mm^3 on laboratory evaluation provides a diagnosis of thrombocytopenia. However, thrombocytopenia can have multiple causes, and obtaining a detailed history is important to identify the specific cause. Thrombocytopenia may initially exist without apparent symptoms. It is not unusual for thrombocytopenia to go undetected until signs and symptoms appear (George & Arnold, 2017).

Bleeding is the most common clinical presentation of thrombocytopenia and may be most apparent in mucosal surfaces and skin surfaces where it is manifested by petechiae and ecchymoses. Bleeding from superficial cuts and menorrhagia are common (George & Arnold, 2017). The most common cause of death from thrombocytopenia is bleeding into the central nervous system preceded by a traumatic event.

Treatment

Patients undergoing aggressive active therapy may receive several units of platelets over the course of active therapy. If the platelet count becomes less than 10,000–20,000/mm^3, a transfusion may be ordered; however, it may depend on whether the patient is bleeding (Camp-Sorrell, 2018). Platelet transfusions are a way of rapidly correcting dangerous levels of thrombocytopenia, but the process is not without risk (Yuan & Goldfinger, 2016). Platelet concentrates from random donors consist of platelets retrieved from several different human donors. A standard adult dose for prophylactic therapy is approximately one random donor unit per 10 kg of body weight, which is four to six units of pooled platelets or one apheresis unit. This dosing is expected to raise the platelet count as much as 30,000/mm^3 within 10 minutes of the infusion in an average-sized adult (Yuan & Goldfinger, 2016). However, the use of random donor platelets risks exposure of the patient to potential pathogens and antigens. Exposure to antigens may lead to the development of antibodies against future random donor platelets (alloimmunization).

Single-donor platelet products permit the collection of multiple units of platelets from a single donor with compatible antibodies for the patient. This method also has the advantages of reducing the patient's exposure to pathogenic organisms and minimizing the potential for alloimmunization. Restricting donor exposure will protect patients with cancer from potential pathogens (Yuan & Goldfinger, 2016).

It is important to obtain postinfusion platelet counts to evaluate the benefit of the transfusion. This is particularly important when thrombocytopenic patients are receiving transfusion specifically to safely undergo an invasive procedure.

Nursing Implications

Nursing care of patients who are at risk for the development of thrombocytopenia includes obtaining a detailed patient history (see Figure 22-3), reviewing laboratory assessments, and identifying risk factors. A detailed history of recent drug use is essential. Careful assessment of skin and mucous membranes, such as the oral cavity, is important. Patients who are undergoing active systemic therapy with aggressive chemotherapy regimens should be monitored and assessed on a regimented basis.

Proactive identification is important for patients who are at risk for developing thrombocytopenia as a sequela of either disease or treatment. Patient education is paramount in ensuring adherence to therapy and minimizing or preventing serious complications of thrombocytopenia. Patients should be taught what signs to look for that indicate bleeding (see Figure 22-4).

Anemia

Overview

Anemia is defined as a decrease in hemoglobin concentration and number of functional red blood cells or red blood cell volume to suboptimal levels (O'Leary, 2015). Anemia can have a detrimental impact on the performance status, quality of life, and therapeutic efficacy for patients with cancer (O'Leary, 2015).

The etiology of anemia can be categorized as (a) a decreased production of functional red blood cells, (b) an increased destruction of red blood cells, or (c) blood cell loss. Erythropoiesis is controlled by the growth factor erythropoietin. The kidneys produce erythropoietin in response to hypoxia. It is then transported to the bone marrow, where it stimulates the production of red blood cells in the bone marrow. Essential basic materials for this process include vitamin B_{12}, folic acid, and iron. Nutritional deficiencies or malabsorption syndromes can predispose patients to anemia in this manner (Coyer & Lash, 2008; O'Leary, 2015).

Anemia is the result of a reduction in circulating erythrocytes and thus a lowered hemoglobin level. With lowered hemoglobin levels, oxygen transport to tissues is diminished, causing tissue hypoxia (Coyer & Lash, 2008). Cancer-related anemia is frequently attributed to either direct tumor infiltration of the bone marrow, the effect of myelosuppres-

Figure 22-3. Assessment of Risk Factors for Bleeding

Assessment	Yes	No
Patient History		
Bleeding or clotting disorders		
Bleeding tendencies		
Petechiae		
Easy bruising		
Pain		
Headaches		
Nosebleeds		
Poor nutritional status		
Medication history (prescription, over the counter, vitamins/herbals)		
History of transfusions		
History of liver disease		
History of renal disease		
History of allergic reactions		
Known infections		
Type of malignancy		
Types of treatment		
Physical Assessment		
Body system review		
Performance status		
Diagnostic workup		
Laboratory data		

Note. Based on information from Friend & Pruett, 2004.

From "Prevention of Bleeding" (p. 254), by J.M. Tipton in L.H. Eaton and J.M. Tipton (Eds.), *Putting Evidence Into Practice: Improving Oncology Patient Outcomes*, 2009, Pittsburgh, PA: Oncology Nursing Society. Copyright 2009 by Oncology Nursing Society. Reprinted with permission.

sive antitumor therapy, or anemia of chronic disease (Coyer & Lash, 2008). Anemia of chronic disease is characterized by hypoplasia of bone marrow, decrease in red cell survival, decreased utilization of iron, and low serum erythropoietin level (Coyer & Lash, 2008).

Figure 22-4. Patient Education Regarding Thrombocytopenia

- Avoid use or overinflation of a blood pressure cuff or tourniquet use when platelet count is < 20,000/mm³.
- Avoid invasive procedures unless absolutely necessary; this includes rectal temperatures, enemas, suppositories, bladder catheterization, venipuncture, use of nasogastric tubes, finger sticks, or intramuscular or subcutaneous injections.
- Alter environment to avoid traumatic injuries, including padding side rails and clearing walkways.
- Avoid using sharp objects, such as straight-edge razors, in personal care.
- Wear shoes while ambulating to maintain skin integrity.
- Avoid activities that may lead to trauma.
- Use soft toothbrushes when brushing teeth to avoid gingival injury.
- Look for signs of new or uncontrolled bleeding, such as nosebleeds, dark tarry stools, easy bruising of the skin, and presence of petechiae.
- Notify healthcare provider for uncontrolled bleeding or signs of new bleeding.

Note. Based on information from Kurtin, 2016.

Risk Factors

Risk factors for anemia in patients with cancer may be multifactorial (O'Leary, 2015). Comorbidities, including hereditary disease, renal insufficiency, nutritional deficiencies, and anemia of chronic disease, may contribute to the anemia. Direct causes of anemia are the suppression of hematopoiesis by infiltration of the cancer cells into the bone marrow and the production of cytokines by cancer cells, which results in iron sequestration and a subsequent decrease in red blood cell production (NCCN, 2016a).

Higher rates of anemia have been observed with patients diagnosed with lung, ovarian, and head and neck cancers (NCCN, 2016a). This may be because of the use of platinum-containing chemotherapy agents commonly used for systemic therapy. The use of platinum-containing chemotherapy agents has been associated with increased incidence of anemia requiring transfusions (NCCN, 2016a). The myelosuppressive effects of chemotherapy agents may be cumulative over time with repeated cycles and increase the risk for anemia (NCCN, 2016a).

Diagnosis

The diagnosis of anemia is made by measuring the complete blood count, including a differential count. Other studies that should be included to characterize the etiology of anemia include reticulocyte count, iron studies, serum B_{12}, folate levels, stool for guaiac, lactate dehydrogenase, fractionated bilirubin, creatinine, bone marrow biopsy, hemoglobin electrophoresis, and direct Coombs test.

Anemia can be graded by severity based on hemoglobin concentration. NCI has established and published anemia toxicity scales (see Table 22-2). Severe anemia, also known as physiologic anemia, is associated with multiple adverse clinical symptoms, including headache, dyspnea, dizziness, poor mental status acuity, sleep disturbance, and sexual dysfunction. Severe anemia (grade 3) is defined as a hemoglobin level less than 8 g/dl (NCI CTEP, 2010). Severe anemia also can affect therapeutic outcomes and thus requires immediate intervention. Low hemoglobin levels can lead to treatment delays, delays in surgical intervention, or chemotherapy dose reductions, thereby decreasing the overall intensity required for successful outcomes. Tumor hypoxia particularly can limit effectiveness of radiation therapy. Cells that are not adequately oxygenated may be much less sensitive to the effects of ionizing radiation and may lead to treatment failure (Hurter & Bush, 2007).

In making the diagnosis and determining the treatment to correct anemia in patients with cancer, clinicians must consider other factors. It is important to evaluate the clinical manifestations and treatment context for each patient (NCCN, 2016a). Symptoms of acute-onset anemia include tachycardia, tachy-

Table 22-2. Anemia Grading

Grade	Description
1	Hgb < LLN–10.0 g/dl; < LLN–6.2 mmol/L; < LLN–100 g/L
2	Hgb < 10.0–8.0 g/dl; <6.2–4.9 mmol/L; < 100–80 g/L
3	Hgb < 8.0 g/dl; < 4.9 mmol/L; < 80 g/L; transfusion indicated
4	Life-threatening consequences; urgent intervention indicated
5	Death

Hgb—hemoglobin; LLN—lower limit of normal

Note. From *Common Terminology Criteria for Adverse Events* [v.4.03], by National Cancer Institute Cancer Therapy Evaluation Program, 2010. Retrieved from https://evs.nci.nih.gov/ftp1/CTCAE/CTCAE_4.03_2010-06-14_QuickReference_5x7.pdf.

pnea, and dyspnea on exertion; light-headedness; and fatigue. The physiologic compensation that occurs over time influences tissue demands for oxygen (Coyer & Lash, 2008). Subjective symptoms that should be evaluated include decreased activity tolerance and performance status.

Fatigue has been described as one of the most distressing side effects of cancer and cancer treatment and can have a serious impact on patients' quality of life (de Nijs, Ros, & Grijpdonck, 2008). It is defined as "a distressing, persistent subjective sense of physical, emotional, and/or cognitive tiredness or exhaustion related to cancer or cancer treatment that is not proportional to recent activity and interferes with usual functioning" (NCCN, 2016b, p. FT-1).

Fatigue is a prevalent symptom among patients with cancer and has been strongly attributed to anemia. Hypoxia-compromised organs and hemoglobin dysfunction have been proposed as mechanisms linking anemia to fatigue (Wang, 2008). Other theories have been proposed to explain the complex phenomenon of fatigue, including the effects of surgery; anesthesia; side effects of other antitumor therapies, such as hormone therapy, radiation therapy, or biotherapy; cachexia; other comorbidities; and abnormal production of inflammatory cytokines (Wang, 2008). Although the underlying etiology for fatigue continues to be explored (see Chapter 19), a known correlation exists between cancer-related fatigue and anemia (NCCN, 2016b).

Treatment

Treatment options for anemia are aimed at correcting the underlying cause of the anemia. The transfusion of packed red blood cells (PRBCs) or the administration of erythropoiesis-stimulating agents (ESAs) is indicated for select patients. The use of either of these treatment modalities carries potential risks as well as benefits (NCCN, 2016a).

Transfusion of PRBCs will rapidly increase hemoglobin and hematocrit levels. It is estimated that the transfusion of one unit of PRBCs will increase the hemoglobin by an increment of 1 g/dl or the hematocrit by 3% in an average-size adult. The amount of increase may be less if the patient is receiving concomitant fluid replacement (NCCN, 2016a).

Numerous safety processes have been incorporated over the past several years to ensure a safer blood supply in the United States. However, the potential risks associated with PRBC transfusion include bacterial contamination, viral infections, congestive heart failure, and iron overload (NCCN, 2016a).

The administration of ESAs has been shown to decrease the requirement of PRBC transfusion in patients with cancer who are actively undergoing chemotherapy. The risks associated with the use of these agents have become apparent in recent years when it was shown that a subset of patients with cancer tended to have a risk of shortened survival and tumor progression. Revised label warnings restrict the use of ESAs to the treatment of anemia in individuals undergoing myelosuppressive chemotherapy. The discontinuation of these agents once chemotherapy has been completed is strongly recommended. The warning for these agents further advises that physicians monitor hemoglobin levels and adjust dosing to maintain the lowest hemoglobin level necessary to avoid transfusions (NCCN, 2016a).

Other adverse events that have been associated with the use of ESAs include an increased risk of thromboembolic events, hypertension, and seizure activity (NCCN, 2016a).

In summary, the corrective measures for anemia in patients with cancer depend primarily on the underlying cause. The diagnosis of cancer and its various treatments should be considered primary risk factors for the development of anemia. Other risk factors include advanced age, nutritional deficiencies, chronic infections, and comorbidities such as congestive heart disease and renal insufficiencies (Hurter & Bush, 2007).

Corrective measures should be adopted and used based on the etiology of the anemia. They include (a) investigating for and correcting occult blood loss, such as gastrointestinal bleeding, (b) correcting nutritional deficiencies, (c) using ESAs when appropriate, (d) using PRBC transfusions when appropriate, and (e) discontinuing nephrotoxic agents when possible.

The risks and benefits of measures for correcting anemia are an important consideration that should be based on informed patient preferences, the treatment regimen, and the goals of the overall cancer therapy (NCCN, 2016a).

Nursing Implications

Care for patients with anemia begins with assessment of those potentially at risk for developing anemia, incorporating both subjective and objective data. Review of patients' history with attention to past use of cytotoxic agents, radiation therapy, surgical intervention, and current and recent nutritional deficits provides important baseline information. The identification of recent and past use of medications, including supplements, also should be included (Hurter & Bush, 2007).

Physical assessment parameters include the evaluation of skin and mucous membranes for paleness and pallor, petechiae and ecchymoses, poor skin turgor, and jaundice. Cardiopulmonary assessment should include evaluation for tachypnea and tachycardia. Patients should be assessed for symptoms of fatigue. Laboratory data should be obtained and regularly monitored to evaluate for response to interventions (Gobel & O'Leary, 2007; Hurter & Bush, 2007).

The safe administration of blood products and ESAs is recommended when indicated for correction of anemia in appropriate patients (NCCN, 2016a). Nurses should educate patients and family members on the mechanisms leading to anemia and the expected outcomes of interventions (O'Leary, 2015). Mitchell et al. (2014) suggested the following evidence-based interventions to combat fatigue during and following treatment:

- Work with the patient and family to improve assessment of fatigue and identify management strategies.
- Promote open communication between the patient, family, and caregiving team to facilitate discussions about fatigue's effects on daily life.
- Screen for the presence of treatable etiologic or contributing factors, including hypothyroidism, hypogonadism, adrenal insufficiency, cardiomyopathy, pulmonary dysfunction, concurrent distressing symptoms (pain, nausea, depression), emotional distress, sleep disturbances, anemia, nutritional compromise, fluid and electrolyte imbalances, and inactivity/physical deconditioning.
- Review current medications to identify any agent or medication interactions that may contribute to worsening fatigue.
- Consider attention-restoring activities, such as exposure to natural environments and pleasant distractions.

- Encourage a balanced diet with adequate intake of fluid, calories, protein, carbohydrates, fat, vitamins, and minerals.

Conclusion

Myelosuppression is a common, complex, and often serious consequence of cancer and cancer therapy. Nurses are in a unique position to appreciate the entire trajectory of the diagnosis and treatment for patients with cancer. Nurses can anticipate the need for potential interventions based on patients' likelihood for developing myelosuppression and proactively intervene through patient education and astute nursing assessment. It is an important nursing responsibility to provide education to patients and their families to help adhere to therapy and achieve optimal outcomes. Anticipating the potential outcomes of cancer diagnoses and treatments will position nurses to successfully meet the challenge of providing quality patient care.

The author would like to acknowledge Gail B. Johnson, RN, MSN, AOCN®, CNS, for her contribution to this chapter that remains unchanged from the first edition of this book.

References

Aistars, J. (2007). Radiation therapy. In M.E. Langhorne, J.S. Fulton, & S.E. Otto (Eds.), *Oncology nursing* (5th ed., pp. 346–359). St. Louis, MO: Elsevier Mosby.

Camp-Sorrell, D. (2018). Chemotherapy toxicities and management. In C.H. Yarbro, D. Wujcik, & B.H. Gobel (Eds.), *Cancer nursing: Principles and practice* (8th ed., pp. 497–554). Burlington, MA: Jones & Bartlett Learning.

Coyer, S.M., & Lash, A.A. (2008). Pathophysiology of anemia and nursing care implications. *Medsurg Nursing, 17,* 77–83, 91.

de Nijs, E.J.M., Ros, W., & Grijpdonck, M.H. (2008). Nursing intervention for fatigue during the treatment for cancer. *Cancer Nursing, 31,* 191–206. doi:10.1097/01.NCC.0000305721.98518.7c

Fischbach, F. (2000). *A manual of laboratory and diagnostic tests* (6th ed.). Philadelphia, PA: Lippincott.

Friend, P.H., & Pruett, J. (2004). Bleeding and thrombotic complications. In C.H. Yarbro, M.H. Frogge, & M. Goodman (Eds.), *Cancer symptom management* (3rd ed., pp. 233–251). Burlington, MA: Jones & Bartlett Learning.

George, J.N., & Arnold, D.M. (2017, January 9). Approach to the adult with unexplained thrombocytopenia [Literature review current through January 2017]. Retrieved from http://www.uptodate.com/contents/approach-to-the-adult-with-unexplained-thrombocytopenia

Gobel, B.H., & O'Leary, C. (2007). Bone marrow suppression. In M.E. Langhorne, J.S. Fulton, & S.E. Otto (Eds.), *Oncology nursing* (5th ed., pp. 488–504). St. Louis, MO: Elsevier Mosby.

Hurter, B., & Bush, N.J. (2007). Cancer-related anemia: Clinical review and management update. *Clinical Journal of Oncology Nursing, 11,* 349–359. doi:10.1188/07.CJON.349-359

Klastersky, J., Paesmans, M., Rubenstein, E.B., Boyer, M., Elting, L., Feld, R., ... Talcott, J. (2000). The Multinational Association for Supportive Care in Cancer risk index: A multinational scoring system for identifying low-risk febrile neutropenic cancer patients. *Journal of Clinical Oncology, 18,* 3038–3051.

Kuderer, N.M., Dale, D.C., Crawford, J., & Lyman, G.H. (2007). Impact of primary prophylaxis with granulocyte colony-stimulating factor on febrile neutropenia and mortality in adult cancer patients receiving chemotherapy: A systematic review. *Journal of Clinical Oncology, 25,* 3158–3167. doi:10.1200/JCO.2006.08.8823

Key Points

- Myelosuppression is the most common dose-limiting and most potentially life-threatening side effect related to systemic anticancer treatments.
- It is crucial to understand the various manifestations of myelosuppression and the mechanisms by which they are induced in patients receiving cancer therapy.
- By identifying the risk factors that contribute to neutropenia, thrombocytopenia, and anemia, the nurse can anticipate potential challenges successfully.

Kurtin, S. (2016). Alterations in hematologic and immune function. In J.K. Itano (Ed.), *Core curriculum for oncology nursing* (5th ed., pp. 322–339). St. Louis, MO: Elsevier.

Lichtman, S.M. (2016, June 23). Systemic chemotherapy for cancer in elderly persons [Literature review current through January 2017]. Retrieved from http://www.uptodate.com/contents/systemic-chemotherapy-for-cancer-in-elderly-persons

Lyman, G.H. (2006). Risks and consequences of chemotherapy-induced neutropenia. *Clinical Cornerstone, 8*(Suppl. 5), S12–S18. doi:10.1016/S1098-3597(06)80054-2

Marrs, J.A. (2006). Care of patients with neutropenia. *Clinical Journal of Oncology Nursing, 10,* 164–166. doi:10.1188/06.CJON.164-166

Maxwell, C., & Stein, A. (2006). Implementing evidence-based guidelines for preventing chemotherapy-induced neutropenia: From paper to clinical practice. *Community Oncology, 3,* 530–536. doi:10.1016/S1548-5315(11)70747-1

Mitchell, S.A., Hoffman, A.J., Clark, J.C., DeGennaro, R.M., Poirier, P., Robinson, C.B., & Weisbrod, B.L. (2014). Putting evidence into practice: An update of evidence-based interventions for cancer-related fatigue during and following treatment. *Clinical Journal of Oncology Nursing, 18,* 38–58. doi:10.1188/14.CJON.S3.38-58

National Cancer Institute Cancer Therapy Evaluation Program. (2010). *Common terminology criteria for adverse events* [v.4.03]. Retrieved from https://evs.nci.nih.gov/ftp1/CTCAE/CTCAE_4.03_2010-06-14_QuickReference_5x7.pdf

National Comprehensive Cancer Network. (2016a). *NCCN Clinical Practice Guidelines in Oncology (NCCN Guidelines®): Cancer- and chemotherapy-induced anemia* [v.1.2017]. Retrieved from http://www.nccn.org/professionals/physician_gls/pdf/anemia.pdf

National Comprehensive Cancer Network. (2016b). *NCCN Clinical Practice Guidelines in Oncology (NCCN Guidelines®): Cancer-related fatigue* [v.1.2017]. Retrieved from http://www.nccn.org/professionals/physician_gls/pdf/fatigue.pdf

National Comprehensive Cancer Network. (2016c). *NCCN Clinical Practice Guidelines in Oncology (NCCN Guidelines®): Myeloid growth factors* [v.2.2016]. Retrieved from http://www.nccn.org/professionals/physician_gls/pdf/myeloid_growth.pdf

National Comprehensive Cancer Network. (2017). *NCCN Clinical Practice Guidelines in Oncology (NCCN Guidelines®): Prevention and treatment of cancer-related infections* [v.2.2016]. Retrieved from http://www.nccn.org/professionals/physician_gls/pdf/infections.pdf

Nirenberg, A., Bush, A.P., Davis, A., Friese, C.R., Gillespie, T.W., & Rice, R.D. (2006a). Neutropenia: State of the knowledge part I. *Oncology Nursing Forum, 33,* 1193–1201. doi:10.1188/06.ONF.1193-1201

Nirenberg, A., Bush, A.P., Davis, A., Friese, C.R., Gillespie, T.W., & Rice, R.D. (2006b). Neutropenia: State of the knowledge part II. *Oncology Nursing Forum, 33,* 1202–1208. doi:10.1188/06.ONF.1202-1208

O'Leary, C. (2015). Neutropenia and infection. In C.G. Brown (Ed.), *A guide to oncology symptom management* (2nd ed., pp. 483–504). Pittsburgh, PA: Oncology Nursing Society.

Schwartzberg, L.S. (2006). Neutropenia: Etiology and pathogenesis. *Clinical Cornerstone, 8*(Suppl. 5), S5–S11. doi:10.1016/S1098-3597(06)80053-0

Smith, T.J., Bohlke, K., Lyman, G.H., Carson, K.R., Crawford, J., Cross, S.J., … Armitage, J.O. (2015). Recommendations for the use of WBC growth factors: American Society of Clinical Oncology clinical practice guideline update. *Journal of Clinical Oncology, 33,* 3199–3212. doi:10.1200/JCO.2015.62.3488

Venturini, M., Del Mastro, L., Aitini, E., Baldini, E., Caroti, C., Contu, A., … Bruzzi, P. (2005). Dose-dense adjuvant chemotherapy in early breast cancer patients: Results from a randomized trial. *Journal of the National Cancer Institute, 97,* 1724–1733. doi:10.1093/jnci/dji398

Wang, X.S. (2008). Pathophysiology of cancer-related fatigue. *Clinical Journal of Oncology Nursing, 12*(Suppl. 5), 11–20. doi:10.1188/08.CJON.S2.11-20

West, F., & Mitchell, S.A. (2004). Evidence-based guidelines for the management of neutropenia following outpatient hematopoietic stem cell transplantation. *Clinical Journal of Oncology Nursing, 8,* 601–613. doi:10.1188/04.CJON.601-613

Wujcik, D. (2004). Infection. In C.H. Yarbro, M.H. Frogge, & M. Goodman (Eds.), *Cancer symptom management* (3rd ed., pp. 252–275). Burlington, MA: Jones & Bartlett Learning.

Yuan, S., & Goldfinger, D. (2016, September 19). Clinical and laboratory aspects of platelet transfusion therapy [Literature review current through January 2017]. Retrieved from http://www.uptodate.com/contents/clinical-and-laboratory-aspects-of-platelet-transfusion-therapy

Chapter 22 Study Questions

1. The most common dose-limiting side effects for systemic anticancer treatments include:
   A. Neutropenia.
   B. Thrombocytopenia.
   C. Anemia.
   D. All of the above.

2. Which of the following statements related to neutrophils is correct?
   A. Their main function is phagocytosis.
   B. Their life span is one to three days after they have been released from the bone marrow to the circulation.
   C. Their role is second in the line of defense against microbial invasion.
   D. Both A and C are correct.

3. Patient education is essential for patients receiving chemotherapy. Education should include:
   A. The mechanism of action of the chemotherapy they will be receiving.
   B. Infection control measures.
   C. Symptoms that may represent an infection.
   D. All of the above.

4. Which chemotherapy agent has the greatest potential to cause thrombocytopenia?
   A. Doxorubicin
   B. Gemcitabine
   C. Methotrexate
   D. Paclitaxel

5. Which of the following is considered an evidence-based intervention to combat fatigue during and after chemotherapy?
   A. Promote open communication with the patient and family about how fatigue affects activities of daily living.
   B. Review current medications to identify any medication interactions that may contribute to worsening fatigue.
   C. Encourage a balanced diet with adequate intake of fluid, calories, protein, carbohydrates, fat, vitamins, and minerals.
   D. All of the above

CHAPTER

23 Hepatic Toxicities

Elizabeth Prechtel Dunphy, DNP, CRNP, BC, AOCN®

Introduction

To understand the management of hepatic symptoms related to cancer and cancer therapy, nurses need an understanding of the liver and its function. This chapter will review the basic anatomy, physiology, and pathology of the liver, along with liver function measurement. Physical findings and clinical symptoms will be summarized, followed by a review of clinical diagnoses related to liver dysfunction, such as ascites, encephalopathy, biliary obstruction, and veno-occlusive disease (sinusoidal obstruction syndrome), and their management. Lastly, processes related to hepatic symptom management as it relates to chemotherapy, surgery, radiation therapy, and liver-directed therapies will be addressed.

Liver Anatomy, Pathology, and Physiology

Anatomy

Anatomically, the liver is located in the right upper quadrant of the abdomen under the right rib cage against the diaphragm (see Figure 23-1). The liver is the largest gland/internal organ in the body. The liver is held in place by ligaments attached to the diaphragm, peritoneum, great vessels, and upper gastrointestinal (GI) organs. It is divided into the left and right lobes. The liver's right lobe is larger than the left. The lobes are further divided into eight segments (see Figure 23-2). The liver is unusual in that it has a dual blood supply: 20% of the liver blood flow is oxygen-rich from the hepatic

Figure 23-1. Location of the Liver in the Body

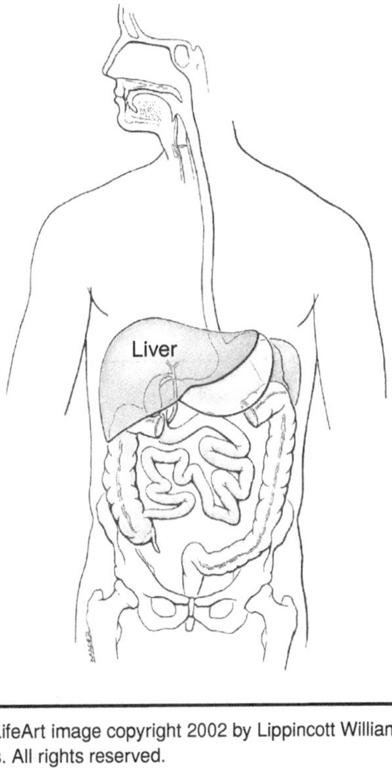

Note. LifeArt image copyright 2002 by Lippincott Williams & Wilkins. All rights reserved.

Figure 23-2. Liver Segments

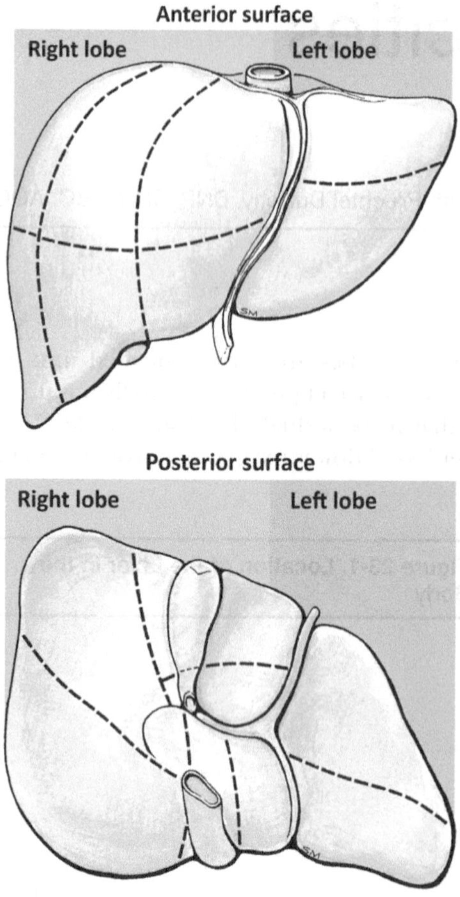

Note. LifeArt image copyright 2002 by Lippincott Williams & Wilkins.

artery, and 80% is nutrient-rich coming from the portal vein. The portal vein carries oxygenated, nutrient-rich blood from the spleen, intestine, and pancreas into the liver and to the hepatocytes (Ghany & Hoofnagle, 2012). Figure 23-3 shows the portal venous flow of the liver. The common hepatic artery enters the porta hepatis medial to the common bile duct and branches off the gastroduodenal artery to become the proper hepatic artery. It then bifurcates into the left and right hepatic arteries. Blood and waste products leave the liver via the hepatic veins and enter systemic circulation through the inferior vena cava (Groen, 1999). These are important concepts for nurses to keep in mind when evaluating patients with hepatic symptoms.

Pathology

Hepatocytes constitute two-thirds of the cells present in the liver. Other cell types include Kupffer cells, stellate cells, endothelial cells, and biliary epithelial cells. Kupffer cells are part of the reticuloendothelial system. Stellate cells store fat. Hepatocytes have many functions in maintaining homeostasis, including synthesis of essential serum proteins (albumin, carrier proteins, coagulation factors, hormonal and growth factors), production of bile and its carriers (bile acids, cholesterol, lecithin, phospholipids), regulation of nutrients (glucose, glycogen, lipids, cholesterol, amino acids), and metabolism and conjugation of lipophilic compounds (bilirubin, cations, drugs) for excretion in the bile or urine (Ghany & Hoofnagle, 2012).

Physiology

The liver has many functions, which are summarized in Figure 23-4. The liver maintains the processes of glycogenolysis and gluconeogenesis, supporting carbohydrate metabolism. Gluconeogenesis occurs when the liver metabolizes glucose into glycogen for storage; this usually occurs after meals. Glycogenolysis occurs when glucose is released from glycogen storage. Triglycerides are hydrolyzed by the liver into glycerol and free fatty acids, which are used to produce adenosine triphosphate. Fatty acids, necessary for the production of bile salts, steroid hormones, and components of plasma proteins, are then released into the bloodstream. The metabolism of amino acids in the liver occurs by the process of deamination (Groen, 1999).

Bilirubin is a by-product of the heme portion of red blood cells and is released when

Figure 23-3. Portal Venous Flow of the Liver

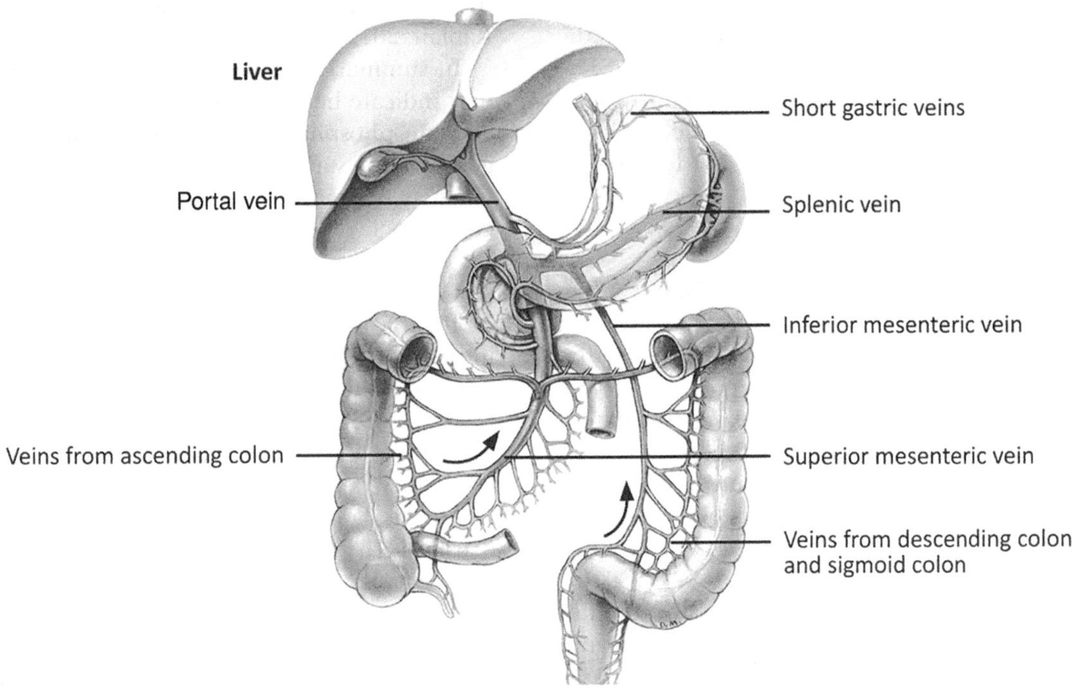

Note. LifeArt image copyright 2002 by Lippincott Williams & Wilkins. All rights reserved.

these cells are destroyed by the reticuloendothelial system. The released bilirubin binds to albumin in the blood as fat-soluble, unconjugated (indirect) bilirubin and then is conjugated by the liver to form water-soluble (direct) bilirubin, which is excreted via the bile into the GI tract. Vitamins A, D, E, K, and B_{12} are stored in the liver. Iron in the form of ferritin is stored in the liver, along with copper (Groen, 1999).

The liver synthesizes plasma proteins, albumin, and globulin. Albumin maintains the plasma oncotic pressure and the proper distribution of fluids between the vascular and interstitial compartments. The liver is the source of several clotting factors. It maintains homeostasis between thrombosis and hemorrhage by synthesizing fibrinogen, prothrombin, and factors I, II, IX, and X, all of which are necessary for clotting. The liver assists in the digestion and absorption of fats, cholesterol, and fat-soluble vitamins by secreting bile. Bile functions to emulsify and absorb fats (Groen, 1999).

Figure 23-4. Functions of the Liver

- Bilirubin formation
- Fat metabolism
- Drug metabolism
- Carbohydrate metabolism
- Protein synthesis
- Bile salt production
- Synthesis of clotting factors
- Vitamin and mineral storage
- Regeneration

Note. Based on information from Groen, 1999.

Lastly, the liver detoxifies endogenous and exogenous substances. Ammonia is a major toxic by-product excreted by the liver. Many chemotherapy agents are metabolized by the liver, as are alcohol and other medications. The liver also is able to inactivate steroid hormones. Although the liver is able to regenerate itself, 80% of it needs to be maintained for normal functioning (Groen, 1999).

Liver Laboratory Parameters

Liver function tests can be used to detect the presence of liver disease, distinguish among different types of liver disorders, gauge the extent of known liver disease, and follow the treatment response of tumors that involve the liver. Liver tests rarely indicate a specific diagnosis but may suggest a general category of liver disease (Pratt & Kaplan, 2012).

The most commonly used laboratory studies that aid in determining liver function are serum bilirubin, serum albumin, serum transaminases (aspartate aminotransferase [AST] and alanine aminotransferase [ALT]), and prothrombin time. Serum bilirubin measures hepatic conjugation and excretion, and serum albumin and prothrombin time measure protein synthesis. The transaminases or serum aminotransferases reflect hepatocellular injury (Ghany & Hoofnagle, 2012).

Enzymes that reflect damage to the hepatocytes are the serum aminotransferases or transaminases. The transaminases are sensitive indicators of liver cell injury and are most helpful in recognizing acute hepatocellular disease. They include AST and ALT. AST is found in the liver, cardiac muscle, skeletal muscle, kidneys, brain, pancreas, lungs, leukocytes, and erythrocytes. ALT is found primarily in the liver. These enzymes are released into the blood when damage to the liver cell membrane results in increased permeability (Pratt & Kaplan, 2012).

Ammonia is produced in the body during normal protein metabolism and by intestinal bacteria, primarily in the colon. The liver typically detoxifies ammonia by converting it to urea, which is excreted by the kidneys (Pratt & Kaplan, 2012).

In summary, abnormal AST and ALT levels may indicate hepatic injury, whereas abnormal alkaline phosphatase and bilirubin levels suggest a cholestatic pattern. These abnormalities may occur in overlapping patterns. These common liver tests have the following clinical implications: ALT and AST—hepatocellular damage; bilirubin—impaired cholestasis or biliary obstruction; alkaline phosphatase—impaired cholestasis or biliary obstruction; and prothrombin time and albumin—synthetic function (Green & Flamm, 2002). This is summarized in Table 23-1 along with the normal laboratory values.

Another way to grade the severity of liver disease is the Child-Pugh grading system. The system assigns 1–3 points based on the level of abnormality for five parameters: encephalopathy, ascites, albumin, prolongation of prothrombin time and international normalized ratio, and bilirubin. Class A is 5–6 points, good operative risk; class B is 7–9 points, moderate operative risk; and class C is 10–15 points, poor operative risk (National Comprehensive Cancer Network® [NCCN®], 2016; Pugh, Murray-Lyon, Dawson, Pietroni, & Williams, 1973). The Child-Pugh system was initially developed by hepatologists to stratify patients into risk groups. It is now used to assess prognosis in patients with cirrhosis and as criteria for evaluating patients prior to liver transplantation. The scoring system is a reliable predictor of survival in many liver diseases and predicts the likelihood of complications arising from cirrhosis. It also is used when evaluating patients for systemic therapy that may affect the liver.

Clinical Findings

Patients with liver disease related to cancer and its treatment may have myriad signs and

Table 23-1. Normal Values of Common Liver Function Tests and Implications of Abnormal Value

Test	Normal Range*	Implications
Alanine aminotransferase	5–35 U/L females 10–40 U/L males	Hepatocellular insult
Albumin	3.7–5.6 g/dl	Impaired synthetic liver function
Alkaline phosphatase	50–130 U/L females 65–260 U/L males	Cholestasis Biliary obstruction
Aspartate aminotransferase	5–30 U/L females 15–45 U/L males	Hepatocellular insult
Prothrombin time	11–16 seconds	Impaired synthetic liver function
Total bilirubin	Less than 1 mg/dl	Cholestasis Biliary obstruction

* Laboratory normal values from Wallach, 2000.

symptoms. Some may present with nonspecific symptoms, whereas others present with distinctive symptoms. Constitutional symptoms of liver disease include fatigue, weakness, and poor appetite, whereas liver-specific symptoms include jaundice, dark urine, light stools, itching, abdominal pain, and bloating (Kasper et al., 2016). Fatigue can be described as lethargy, weakness, listlessness, malaise, lack of stamina, or poor energy. It can be intermittent and variable. It may be related to other problems such as stress, anxiety, or concurrent illness. Nausea usually occurs with severe liver disease and may be provoked by food odors or eating fatty foods. Steatorrhea can occur in severe jaundice when there is a lack of bile acid reaching the intestine. Right upper quadrant pain occurs often in liver disease. Liver pain is often described as a constant dull ache that can radiate to the back or right shoulder (Grenon, 2018). Pruritus may occur as a result of obstructive jaundice and drug-induced cholestasis. Jaundice is a hallmark of liver disease and can be a marker of the severity of liver disease. Patients often report tea-colored urine and scleral icterus in conjunction with jaundice. Jaundice generally occurs when the bilirubin level is greater than 2.5 mg/dl (Ghany & Hoofnagle, 2012). Treatment of jaundice related to biliary obstruction, as well as ascites and encephalopathy, will be discussed in the next section.

Biliary Obstruction

Bilirubin is the end product of the degradation of hemoglobin—70%–90% of bilirubin is derived from the degradation of hemoglobin. This occurs primarily in the spleen, as well as in the Kupffer cells within the liver (Wolkoff, 2012). Malignant biliary obstruction often is caused by tumor in the biliary tree or extrinsic compression by pancreatic cancer, cholangiocarcinoma, metastatic disease, or lymphadenopathy in the portal or distal biliary area. Restoring biliary flow with relief of jaundice and pruritus is the primary goal in the palliation of biliary obstruction related to malignancy. It also can allow for the administration of chemotherapy in certain situations.

Three different types of mechanisms can be used for drainage: an external biliary drainage catheter, an internal-external biliary drainage catheter, or a stent. An external biliary drain enters a bile duct above the obstruction and drains bile into an external bag. An internal-external catheter enters the bile duct above the obstruction, crosses the obstruction, and enters the duodenum. An internal stent allows for internal drainage without the need for an external collection device. Patients should be monitored carefully for 48 hours after biliary drainage for signs and symptoms of bleeding or sepsis. Transient hemobilia (bleeding in or into the biliary ducts) may occur because the hepatic artery, portal vein, and bile ducts are next to each other within the portal triad. New or persistent hemobilia after catheter exchange often is the result of device malpositioning in an adjacent portal or hepatic vein branch. It usually can be corrected by catheter repositioning. If bleeding develops one to two weeks or more after the procedure, arterial injury should be suspected. An angiography should be done to identify the bleeding vessel, and vessel embolization should be considered. Sepsis usually manifests itself with rigors and fevers. IV antibiotics, hydration, and vasopressors are administered as indicated. Leakage around the catheter commonly is caused by catheter malpositioning (Boulay & Parepally, 2014; Covey & Brown, 2006b).

The mainstay of palliating jaundice is the placement of stents to relieve the obstruction. Biliary drainage by stent placement during endoscopic retrograde cholangiopancreatography (ERCP) has been shown to be safer and more successful than stent placement performed percutaneously. ERCP is associated with a lower incidence of bile leak, infection, and hemorrhage. During ERCP, the placement of the stent, as well as the ampulla and duodenum, can be directly visualized (Stern & Sturgess, 2008).

Stents can be either plastic or metal. The main problem with plastic stents is occlusion from a bacterial biofilm composed of protein, bilirubin, bacteria, and amorphous debris. Occlusion can lead to recurrent obstruction and subsequent jaundice or cholangitis. Plastic stents usually remain patent for approximately three months. Self-expanding metal biliary stents (SEMS) are made from either stainless steel or nickel. The benefit of a SEMS is its ability to expand from a relatively narrow delivery system to a diameter that allows for improved biliary flow and patency. Metal stents can remain patent for up to 12 months; however, they are not easily removed and cost significantly more than plastic stents. The primary causes of stent occlusion are tumor growth, epithelial hyperplasia, or obstruction caused by biliary sludge (Boulay & Parepally, 2014; Stern & Sturgess, 2008).

Ascites

Ascites is the excessive accumulation of extracellular fluid in the peritoneal cavity. The underlying pathophysiology of ascites is complicated. The most accepted theory is that arterial vasodilation occurs as a result of liver dysfunction. As liver disease progresses and arterial vasodilation increases, the renin–angiotensin–aldosterone system is activated. These mechanisms cause water and sodium absorption and vasoconstriction. This alters intestinal capillary permeability, which allows the fluid to move into the peritoneal cavity (Hansen, Sasaki, & Zucker, 2010; Sangisetty & Miner, 2012). In malignant ascites, water and sodium retention occurs in the abdominal cavity as a result of imbalance of peritoneal fluid production and drainage (Slusser, 2014). Risk factors for developing malignant ascites include the presence of an advanced neoplasm (lymphoma and colon, gastric, pancreatic, lung, ovarian, bladder, breast, and liver cancers) (Narayanan, Pezeshkmehr, Venkat, Guerrero, & Barbery, 2014). Cirrhosis, cardiac and renal disorders, radiation, hypoalbuminemia, and hypoproteinemia are often benign causes for ascites (Gordon, 2012).

Signs and symptoms of ascites include weight gain, abdominal distention, abdominal fullness or pressure, increased abdominal girth, peripheral edema, dyspnea, orthopnea, heartburn, distended abdominal wall veins, altered bowel habits, anorexia, and early satiety (Rogers, 2014). A thorough patient history and assessment by the nurse is important. It should include any history of liver damage, any contributing factors such as alcohol or drug use, history of bacterial peritonitis, the patient's current symptoms, and any amount of weight gain. Physical examination should include weight, vital signs, assessment for edema, and a thorough abdominal examination, including measurement of abdominal girth, eliciting a fluid wave, and evaluation for shifting dullness (Rogers, 2014; Slusser, 2014).

Diagnostic tests that should be considered are complete blood count (CBC), serum chemistries, liver function tests, and prothrombin time. An abdominal ultrasound can detect subtle ascites. Diagnosis of the cause of the ascites is made by paracentesis. Paracentesis is performed by needle aspiration of the ascitic fluid either at the bedside or under ultrasound guidance (Rogers, 2014).

Treatment of malignant ascites often initially includes paracentesis to relieve symptoms and obtain ascitic fluid for evaluation (Flaherty, 2015). Treatment also includes dietary sodium restriction, oral diuretic therapy, or a combination of the two. Free water intake should be limited to less than 1,500 ml a day with a maximum of 2,000 mg of sodium a day for nonmalignant ascites (Rogers, 2014). The data for diuretic use in malignant ascites are controversial and should be evaluated on an individual basis. The patient's breathing might be compromised, or the patient could be uncomfortable. The amount of fluid able to be removed safely is limited. Removing too much fluid can result in electrolyte disturbances, hypovolemia, hypotension, shock, or death. Frequently, the fluid reaccumulates rapidly.

Another method of relieving symptoms is through insertion of a peritoneovenous shunt. A peritoneovenous shunt is implanted in the abdomen and continuously shunts fluid from the abdomen into the venous system via a one-way valve. These shunts have been associated with complications such as shunt failure, pulmonary embolism, pulmonary edema, disseminated intravascular coagulation, and occlusion (Fleming, Alvarez-Secord, Von Gruenigen, Miller, & Abernethy, 2009).

Alternatively, PleurX™ and Aspira™ are two closed-drainage systems that are disposable and approved for use in management of malignant ascites. Both systems use vacuum-enhanced technology and have a maximum capacity of 1,000 ml. The catheter exit site dressing should be changed weekly, or sooner if it becomes wet (Flaherty, 2015; Narayanan et al., 2014). Additionally, a transjugular intrahepatic portosystemic shunt is a nonsurgical option used to decrease portal circulation pressure. Complications include occlusions that can lead to hepatic (i.e., portosystemic) encephalopathy (Rogers, 2014). If malignancy is causing the ascites, successful treatment of the malignancy with chemotherapy or radiation therapy may help reduce fluid accumulation (Collins, 2001).

No evidence-based standard guidelines exist for the management of malignant ascites. Treatment of malignant ascites is based on symptomatology and malignancy. Peritoneal catheters can improve quality of life and symptom control.

Encephalopathy

Hepatic encephalopathy is a complex neurologic state caused by hyperammonemia. It is believed that the causes of hepatic encephalopathy are multifactorial and can be attributed to neurotoxins, an increase in permeability of the blood-brain barrier, and changes in neurotransmitters. Encephalopathy is characterized by changes in mental state that can range from mild confusion to a coma. The first line of treatment is to identify and correct abnormalities, including electrolyte disturbances, dehydration, infections, bleeding, and effects from the use of sedatives (Fowler, 2013; Sharma & Sharma, 2015).

The mainstay of treatment for encephalopathy is the use of lactulose, a nonabsorbable disaccharide that lowers ammonia levels. Lactulose is metabolized in the colon, where bacteria break it down to lactic acid. The pH of the intestine decreases, thus affecting the absorption and production of ammonia. Lactulose is usually dosed at 10–30 ml two to four times a day. The goal is for the patient to have two to three soft stools a day. Nursing priorities include close monitoring of the patient's neurologic status, respiratory rate, and bowel activity (Fowler, 2015; Sargent, 2007; Sharma & Sharma, 2015).

Antimicrobials have also been used in the treatment of encephalopathy. Rifaximin is an antimicrobial with a broad spectrum of antibacterial activity. It is highly bioavailable and is minimally absorbed in the GI tract. When it was compared to other antibiotics in treatment of encephalopathy, rifaximin showed a greater reduction in blood ammonia levels (Di Piazza et al., 1991). Sharma et al. (2013) evaluated lactulose with rifaximin versus lactulose alone in overt hepatic encephalopathy. The study showed a significant decrease in mortality with the combination versus lactulose alone. Therefore, it is recommended that the two medications be used in combination for the treatment of hepatic encephalopathy.

Patients who undergo hematopoietic stem cell transplantation (HSCT) are at risk for developing encephalopathy, which can be caused by the conditioning regimen prior to transplantation, veno-occlusive disease, immunosuppressive drugs, infection, or cerebrovascular events. The clinical presentation may be as subtle as a change in mental status or as drastic as a seizure. Prophylactic treatment with phenytoin is given to patients who are treated with high-risk drugs such as busulfan. Close monitoring of drug levels and blood pressure management are paramount in patients undergoing HSCT (Saria & Gosselin-Acomb, 2007).

Sinusoidal Obstruction Syndrome

Hepatic sinusoidal obstruction syndrome (SOS), also called veno-occlusive disease, is a potential complication following HSCT. Clinical symptoms include weight gain, ascites, jaundice, and painful hepatomegaly (Senzolo, Germani, Cholongitas, Burra, & Burroughs, 2007; Wadleigh, Ho, Momtaz, & Richardson, 2003). DeLeve, Shulman, and McDonald (2002) suggested that the terminology *sinusoidal obstruction syndrome* was more appropriate than *veno-occlusive disease*; however, both terms are used interchangeably. The incidence of SOS after HSCT ranges from 0% to 70% (Senzolo et al., 2007). The diagnostic criteria for SOS include jaundice with a total bilirubin greater than 2 mg/dl with at least two of the following: hepatomegaly, ascites, or weight gain of more than 5% of the patient's total body weight (Jones et al., 1987).

The pathogenesis of SOS is thought to begin with injury of the hepatic venules. This vascular inflammatory process leads to the deposit of fibrin in the portal vessel, causing obstruction. The sinusoids become dilated, and hepatocytes become necrotic when collagen accumulates in the sinusoids and venules. Injury of the sinusoidal endothelial cells and the hepatocytes in zone three of the liver, located around the central veins, is an important initial event in hepatic SOS. The hepatocytes in zone three of the liver contain a high concentration of cytochrome P450 (CYP) enzymes, which metabolize many chemotherapy agents. Inability to metabolize those agents increases the risk of liver damage (Fan & Crawford, 2014; Krimmel & Williams, 2008), leading to liver dysfunction. Risk factors for developing SOS include a Karnofsky score of less than 90%, age older than 20 years, a history of liver disease, an intensive conditioning regimen, fungal infection (Pegram & Kennedy, 2001), an elevated AST prior to HSCT, previous abdominal irradiation, female gender, advanced malignancy, prior exposure to amphotericin B, increased number of days on broad-spectrum antibiotics, and increased number of days with fever before HSCT (Senzolo et al., 2007; Sosa, 2012; Wadleigh et al., 2003). SOS has been identified in patients who received alkylating agents such as oxaliplatin prior to surgical resection of metastatic tumors in the liver (Fan & Crawford, 2014).

The diagnosis of SOS is often a clinical diagnosis because of the danger of the patient bleeding during biopsy. The preferred method of pathologic diagnosis is transfemoral or transjugular liver biopsy and calculation of the hepatic venous pressure gradient. A percutaneous liver biopsy is not recommended. A Doppler ultrasound, magnetic resonance imaging (MRI), or computed tomography (CT) scan of the liver along with a hepatitis panel can help in making the clinical diagnosis (Krimmel & Williams, 2008). Findings on MRI, CT scan, or Doppler ultrasound would include splenomegaly, ascites, low portal venous flow, and high hepatic artery resistive index. If a liver biopsy is possible, it would reveal a hepatic venous pressure gradient of greater than 10 mm Hg. Liver biopsy is indicated in those with few diagnostic criteria, lack of thrombocytopenia, or coagulopathy (Levitsky & Sorrell, 2007).

The classic triad of SOS symptoms includes weight gain, tender hepatomegaly, and hyperbilirubinemia. Severe right upper quadrant pain often requires narcotic intervention. Often, elevation of bilirubin develops 6–10 days after HSCT followed by the development of edema and ascites. On physical examination, patients often have hepatomegaly and ascites. They also may have thrombocytopenia on laboratory studies. In this situation, the patient's weight gain is often refractory to diuretics, and the thrombocytopenia is refractory to platelet transfusion. Liver biopsy is considered the gold standard for diagnosis of hepatic SOS. This may be contraindicated in patients who are thrombocytopenic or neutropenic (Saria & Gosselin-Acomb, 2007; Sosa, 2012). Often, clinicians have to use clinical findings to establish the diagnosis. Because of this, clinical criteria to make the diagnosis of SOS have been formalized as stated previously (see also Chapter 14).

Effective treatment of hepatic SOS is elusive. Recognizing the risk factors is paramount. Prophylaxis with ursodeoxycholic acid, heparin, and defibrotide may be considered. Fifty percent of patients with severe SOS respond to defibrotide (Levitsky & Sorrell, 2007). Several studies have evaluated medications, including low-molecular-weight heparin and ursodeoxycholic acid, for the prevention of hepatic SOS, but results have varied (Essell et al., 1998; Giles et al., 2002; Ohashi et al., 2000; Park et al., 2002). Two studies with ursodeoxycholic acid showed a decrease in SOS incidence with its use (Essell et al., 1998; Ohashi et al., 2000); however, two other studies showed no benefit with the use of ursodeoxycholic acid (Giles et al., 2002; Park et al., 2000). In one of those studies, ursodeoxycholic acid was given with heparin (Park et al., 2000).

Treatment of SOS is primarily supportive. Prevention is a priority. The use of nonmyeloablative therapies in patients at risk for developing SOS has likely contributed to the decreasing incidence. Ascites associated with SOS is treated with sodium restriction, diuretics, and paracentesis. Correction of coagulopathies and prevention of infection are part of the supportive treatment (Sosa, 2012).

Mild hepatic SOS often resolves on its own without medical treatment. Moderate and severe SOS are treated with supportive care. Supportive care includes maintaining an adequate intake and output, adjusting medication doses if hepatic and renal impairment is present, and protecting kidney function. Nursing assessment should include the monitoring of laboratory studies (liver function tests, including liver enzymes and bilirubin levels), mental status, daily abdominal girth measurements, and daily weights. Supportive care should continue until SOS resolves or the liver cells regenerate (Krimmel & Williams, 2008; Sosa, 2012).

Liver Tumors

Both benign and malignant tumors can develop in the liver. Benign space-occupying lesions or abnormalities that arise in the liver include hemangiomas, adenomas, focal nodular hyperplasia, and hepatic cysts. Malignant liver tumors include hepatocellular cancer (HCC), angiosarcoma, hepatoblastoma, and cholangiocarcinoma. The most common cancers found in the liver are the result of metastatic disease from other primary cancer sites (Groen, 1999; NCCN, 2016). Primary liver cancers are most commonly adenocarcinomas that arise from epithelial cells. HCC, which accounts for the majority of liver cancer diagnoses, arises from hepatocytes (Grenon, 2018). Infection with hepatitis B and C viruses predisposes patients to the development of HCC. The majority of primary liver cancers are hepatocellular in origin. The remainder are cholangiocarcinomas, which arise from the bile duct epithelium. Occasionally, a mixed hepatocholangiocarcinoma histology may be present (Grenon, 2018).

In addition to tumors that originate in the liver, solid tumors have a propensity to spread to the liver. The true incidence of liver metastasis is unknown. The modality of spread to the liver is through the portal venous system. The most frequent causes of malignant hepatic disease are related to metastasis from GI tract tumors, breast and lung cancers, and melanoma. The increased frequency of the liver as a site of initial metastasis is thought to be caused by the liver's large blood supply from the portal and systemic circulation.

Management of primary liver malignancies and liver metastases often involves multiple treatment modalities, including surgical resection; liver-directed therapies, such as hepatic arterial infusion (HAI), transarterial chemoembolization, radioembolization, radiofrequency ablation (RFA), and radiation therapy; or systemic therapy (NCCN, 2016).

Therapies Used for Hepatic Toxicities

Surgery

Surgery offers patients with liver cancer the best chance for cure. Unfortunately, many patients are not eligible for liver resection (Groen, 1999; NCCN, 2016). Patients with lesions smaller than 5 cm and confined to the liver, with no evidence of vascular or lymph node involvement, are the best candidates for hepatic resection. The patient's Child-Pugh stage also is considered in the evaluation of surgical candidacy. The type of resection will depend on tumor location (Grenon, 2018).

Liver transplantation can be considered the best chance for long-term survival in patients with a localized HCC. The guidelines used to determine if a patient is eligible for liver transplantation include tumor size (one nodule less than 5 cm, one to three nodules less than 3 cm), the number of tumor nodules (less than three), the absence of vascular involvement, and a well-differentiated histology (Grenon, 2018). Because the waiting time for a liver transplant can be lengthy, localized treatments such as chemoembolization and RFA may be used in the interim to control disease growth.

Resection of hepatic metastasis is most appropriate in the setting of colorectal or breast cancer with a solitary metastatic lesion. It is not appropriate for patients with stomach and pancreatic cancer because of the aggressive nature of these cancers and the likelihood of the presence of other subclinical metastases. The guidelines for resection of liver metastasis include having no evidence of distant metastases or extrahepatic intra-abdominal metastases and no evidence of enlarged periportal lymph nodes. Liver lesions can be biopsied at the time of colorectal surgery with the intent to proceed with resection if it is a solitary lesion. An intraoperative ultrasound often is done to determine resectability and evaluate for the presence of smaller metastases (Grenon, 2018).

Postoperative care following a hepatic resection requires careful nursing monitoring. Patients typically are monitored in the intensive care unit immediately after the operation. Potential complications include hemorrhage, biloma, subphrenic abscess, ascites, liver failure, portal hypertension, and coagulopathy disturbances. Nurses should monitor the patient's vital signs, measure abdominal girth, monitor serial hemoglobin and hematocrit, obtain laboratory studies (including liver function tests and bilirubin), and observe for signs and symptoms of bleeding. Hepatic failure occurs as a result of portal vein thrombosis or insufficient hepatic parenchyma. Post-transplant care involves the same concepts as with a hepatic resection, in addition to the administration of immunosuppressive therapy to prevent organ rejection (Grenon, 2018).

Chemotherapy and Targeted Therapy

Liver injury can result following inhalation, ingestion, or parenteral administration of a number of pharmacologic and chemical agents. Hepatotoxic drugs and their metabolites can injure the hepatocyte directly by distorting cell membranes and other cellular molecules, causing the blockage of biochemical pathways and impairing cellular integrity. These injuries may lead to necrosis of hepatocytes, injury of bile ducts, cholestasis, blockage of pathways of lipid movement, and inhibition of protein synthesis or impairment of mitochondrial oxidation of fatty acids, resulting in fat accumulation or steatosis (Camp-Sorrell, 2018).

Drug toxicity can develop over weeks to months. Occasionally, reactions can occur weeks after a drug is discontinued. Hepatotoxicity related to chemotherapy can have a broad spectrum of clinical presentation from asymptomatic elevations in the serum enzymes to jaundice. Few guidelines are available to guide in the dosage of chemotherapy when hepatic dysfunction is present. Drugs that are hepatotoxic should be avoided when liver function tests are abnormal. Impaired liver function delays excretion and results in increased accumulation of chemotherapy in the plasma and tissues. Nurses should monitor liver function tests closely, as an elevation in the serum transaminases may be the first indication of hepatic toxicity (Camp-Sorrell, 2018).

Targeted therapies are biotherapy agents with specific molecular targets within and on cancer cells. Targeted therapies often block or interrupt pathways of cancer transformation and progression. Targeted therapies involve cell signaling or signal transduction. Cell signaling involves the communication of growth signals from outside the cell to the cell nucleus (Wujcik, 2018). See Chapter 10 for more detailed information on biotherapy and targeted therapies.

Liver metabolism of many chemotherapy and targeted agents occurs by the CYP enzyme system. Many cytotoxic drugs are either activated or inactivated by the CYP enzymes. The CYP enzymes play a key role in the metabolism of many of the targeted agents used to treat various cancers (Wujcik, 2018) (see Chapter 6). Tables 23-2 and 23-3 summarize chemotherapy and targeted therapy agents by class, listing their potential effects on the liver and management recommendations.

Liver-Directed Therapies

Hepatic tumors that are primarily supplied by the hepatic artery respond to liver-directed therapy better than tumors that are supplied by the portal vein. Liver-directed therapies include RFA, chemoembolization, radioembolization, and HAI. RFA is used in patients who choose not to undergo hepatic surgery or in patients who are not surgical candidates. Chemoembolization is used as a bridge in transplant candidates and in patients with advanced disease who are not surgical candidates. Embolization agents are injected into the hepatic arterial system, blocking blood flow to the small arterioles

Table 23-2. Chemotherapy Agents That Affect the Liver

Agent	Effect on Liver	Laboratory Abnormalities	Management Recommendations
Alkylating Agents Altretamine Busulfan Carboplatin Chlorambucil Cyclophosphamide Dacarbazine Estramustine Ifosfamide Lomustine Oxaliplatin Streptozocin Temozolomide Thiotepa	Metabolized in the liver	Elevated liver function tests (LFTs) and bilirubin	Monitor LFTs and bilirubin before and during treatment.
Antimetabolites Cladribine Clofarabine Cytarabine Decitabine 5-Azacytidine Floxuridine Gemcitabine hydrochloride Hydroxyurea (also classified as miscellaneous) Mercaptopurine Methotrexate Nelarabine Pentostatin Pralatrexate Thioguanine Trimetrexate	Metabolized in the liver	Elevated LFTs and bilirubin	Use with caution in patients with preexisting hepatic disease (5-azacytidine and cytarabine). Monitor LFTs at baseline and during and following treatment. Avoid concomitant hepatotoxic drugs (clofarabine and mercaptopurine). High doses increase risk of biliary sclerosis and fibrosis (floxuridine). Hemolytic uremic syndrome (gemcitabine)—decreased hemoglobin and platelets, and increased creatinine/blood urea nitrogen.
Anthracyclines Daunorubicin citrate Daunorubicin hydrochloride Doxorubicin hydrochloride Epirubicin hydrochloride	Metabolized and excreted in the liver	Elevated LFTs, bilirubin, and alkaline phosphatase	Dose adjust if hepatic dysfunction is present. Monitor LFTs at baseline and during and after treatment.
Antitumor Antibiotics Dactinomycin Idarubicin Mitomycin Mitoxantrone	Excreted in bile and urine unchanged	Elevated LFTs	Dose adjust in hepatic or renal dysfunction. Monitor LFTs before, during, and after treatment.

(Continued on next page)

Table 23-2. Chemotherapy Agents That Affect the Liver *(Continued)*

Agent	Effect on Liver	Laboratory Abnormalities	Management Recommendations
Fluoropyrimidines Capecitabine 5-Fluorouracil (5-FU)	Metabolized in the liver to 5-FU precursor (capecitabine) Metabolized in the liver (5-FU)	Elevated bilirubin	Monitor LFTs and bilirubin. Dose adjust with liver abnormalities.
Miscellaneous Arsenic trioxide Asparaginase Pegasparaginase Pemetrexed Procarbazine hydrochloride	Metabolized in the liver	Elevated LFTs	Arsenic is primarily stored in the liver. Asparaginase decreases hepatically derived clotting factors (excessive bleeding/clotting). Pegasparaginase is given intramuscularly to decrease hepatotoxicity. Procarbazine hydrochloride is metabolized by cytochrome P450 (CYP) enzymes. Monitor LFTs.
Nitrosoureas Carmustine	–	Elevated LFTs	Avoid concomitant use of hepatotoxic drugs.
Plant Alkaloids Etoposide Vinblastine Vincristine Vinorelbine tartrate	Excreted in the bile and metabolized in the liver	Elevated LFTs	Dose modify with hepatic dysfunction. CYP may affect enzymes' metabolism of the drug. Monitor LFTs at baseline and during treatment.
Taxanes Cabazitaxel Docetaxel Paclitaxel Paclitaxel protein-bound particles	Metabolized by CYP system	Elevated LFTs	Dose modify with hepatic dysfunction. Monitor LFTs at baseline and during treatment. Cabazitaxel should be avoided in hepatic insufficiency.
Topoisomerase Inhibitors Irinotecan Topotecan hydrochloride	Metabolized to active metabolite in the liver	Elevated LFTs	Use cautiously with CYP3A4 inhibitors. Monitor LFTs at baseline and during treatment.
Microtubule Inhibitors Ixabepilone Eribulin mesylate	Metabolized by CYP system	Elevated LFTs	Monitor LFTs at baseline and during treatment. Dose modify with hepatic dysfunction.

Note. Based on information from Wilkes & Barton-Burke, 2016.

Table 23-3. Targeted Therapies That Affect the Liver

Agent	Effect on Liver	Laboratory Abnormalities	Management Recommendations
Retinoids Bexarotene Tretinoin	Metabolized by cytochrome P450 (CYP) enzymes Excreted by hepatobiliary system	Elevated liver function tests (LFTs)	Monitor LFTs at baseline and during treatment.
Proteasome Inhibitors Bortezomib Carfilzomib	Oxidative metabolism through CYP enzymes	Elevated LFTs	Monitor LFTs at baseline and during treatment. Use with caution in patients with hepatic dysfunction. Hold for grade 3 or higher elevation in LFTs until resolved.
Tyrosine Kinase Inhibitors Afatinib Axitinib Bosutinib Cabozantinib Ceritinib Crizotinib Dasatinib Erlotinib Idelalisib Imatinib mesylate Lapatinib ditosylate Nilotinib Pazopanib Ponatinib Regorafenib Sorafenib Sunitinib	Extensively metabolized in the liver by CYP enzymes	Elevated LFTs Sorafenib can cause elevated lipase and amylase.	Monitor LFTs at baseline and during treatment. Use with caution in patients with hepatic dysfunction.
Fusion Protein Denileukin diftitox	Metabolized by proteolytic degradation and primarily excreted in the liver	Transient elevation of LFTs	Monitor laboratory values at baseline and during treatment.
Monoclonal Antibody Conjugated to a Cytotoxic Antibiotic Ado-trastuzumab Obinutuzumab	–	Elevated LFTs	Monitor LFTs and bilirubin at baseline and during treatment. Dose modify with hepatic dysfunction. Obinutuzumab can cause reactivation of hepatitis B. Patients should be screened before starting treatment.
Mammalian Target of Rapamycin Inhibitor Temsirolimus	Metabolized by CYP enzymes	Elevated LFTs	Monitor LFTs.

(Continued on next page)

Table 23-3. Targeted Therapies That Affect the Liver *(Continued)*

Agent	Effect on Liver	Laboratory Abnormalities	Management Recommendations
CYP17 Inhibitor Abiraterone acetate	–	Elevated LFTs	Monitor LFTs and bilirubin at baseline, every 2 weeks for first 3 months, then monthly thereafter. Dose adjust/discontinue for elevation in liver enzymes.
Angiogenesis Inhibitor Ziv-aflibercept	–	Elevated LFTs	Monitor LFTs.
Kinase Inhibitor (MEK Kinase) Trametinib	Metabolized by CYP enzymes	Elevated LFTs	Monitor LFTs. No dose adjustment for mild hepatic impairment. No data for dose with moderate or severe hepatic impairment.
Kinase Inhibitor (BRAF Kinase) Vemurafenib	Substrate of CYP enzymes		Monitor LFTs at baseline and then monthly during treatment.
Antiandrogen Bicalutamide Nilutamide		Elevated LFTs	Monitor LFTs at baseline and at regular intervals during treatment. Severe liver injury within first 3–4 months of therapy with bicalutamide. Nilutamide contraindicated in severe liver impairment.
Histone Deacetylase Inhibitor Belinostat Romidepsin	Metabolized by CYP enzymes	Elevated LFTs	Monitor LFTs before each treatment. Dose adjust/discontinue for elevation in liver enzymes.
Immune Checkpoint Inhibitor Ipilimumab		Elevated LFTs	Monitor LFTs before each treatment.
Immunomodulator Lenalidomide		Elevated LFTs	Monitor LFTs before each treatment. Stop medication if liver enzymes rise. Therapy can resume when liver enzymes return to normal. Dose adjustment should be considered.

Note. Based on information from Wilkes & Barton-Burke, 2016.

and capillaries leading to the tumor. Radioembolization is used for patients who are not candidates for surgery, in patients with metastatic cancer to the liver for certain malignancies, and for palliation. HAI is directed to the tumor.

Radiofrequency Ablation

RFA causes coagulative necrosis using a high-frequency alternating current that is delivered through an electrode placed in the center of the tumor. RFA involves the placement of a thin needle into the tumor under ultrasound, CT, and MRI guidance. Grounding pads are placed on the patient and connected to a generator to create a complete electrical circuit. The needle is used as an electrode to deliver alternating electrical current from the generator into the tumor and then to the dispersive electrodes or ground pads in a radiofrequency range of about 500 kilohertz. Temperatures in excess of 50°–60°C (122°–140°F) cause irreversible thermal damage to the cells and coagulation necrosis. This causes local ionic agitation and subsequent frictional heat. The by-products are reabsorbed by the body, excreted by the kidneys, and replaced by scar tissue in the liver (Locklin & Wood, 2005).

All tumors may be treated with RFA as long as the arterial supply to the tumor can be isolated. This type of ablation therapy works best on tumors 3 cm or smaller. Tumors larger than 3–5 cm may be treated with RFA in combination with chemoembolization (NCCN, 2016). RFA is indicated in nonsurgical candidates, those who choose not to undergo surgery, or those whose tumor is not resectable because of its location. Goals for RFA of neoplasms include cure, debulking, and palliation. The goal of palliative ablation may not include treatment of the entire tumor. Contraindications to RFA include coagulopathies that are not correctable and uncontrolled infection. RFA usually is performed in the outpatient setting with the patient under conscious sedation. RFA can be done percutaneously, laparoscopically, or intraoperatively (Locklin & Wood, 2005).

Before a liver RFA procedure, patients should have blood tests including a prothrombin time, partial thromboplastin time, CBC, blood urea nitrogen, serum creatinine, tumor markers, and liver function tests. Pretreatment scans may include CT scan, chest x-ray, or MRI to determine any contraindications to treatment. Patient education before and after the procedure is important. The frictional heat caused during the procedure may increase body temperature, and patients may experience diaphoresis. Skin burns are rare but can occur. To avoid skin burns, correct placement of the grounding pads is necessary. Nurses should check the grounding pads and patients' skin frequently. Once the needle is removed, an adhesive bandage is applied to the skin (Locklin & Wood, 2005).

After the liver is treated, patients may experience a postablation syndrome characterized by low-grade fever, aches, mild flu-like symptoms, and a general feeling of malaise. Patients should be made aware that these symptoms are normal, and they should continue oral hydration for five to seven days after the procedure (Locklin & Wood, 2005).

Chemoembolization

Hepatic artery chemoembolization is an alternative treatment for malignancies such as HCC and metastatic disease of the liver. It is used to suppress intrahepatic tumor growth, palliate symptoms, and improve survival.

Embolization may be done with or without chemotherapy. When chemotherapy is used, the procedure is termed *chemoembolization*. Doses of chemotherapy are based on hepatic function and not on body surface area, as chemotherapy is normally dosed. Therefore, higher chemotherapy drug concentrations can be given. This increased exposure enhances tumor necrosis (NCCN, 2016; Sangro, 2014).

The chemoembolization procedure requires the placement of a catheter in the femoral artery that is threaded into the hepatic artery. An angiogram is performed to verify the patency of the portal vein system before occlusion of the hepatic artery is performed. Once the catheter is in place, the interventional radiologist injects the chemotherapy and embolic agents until blood flow to the artery supplying the tumor stops. The use of embolization material minimizes the collateralization of blood flow by creating a vascular blockade. The chemotherapy agent undergoes degradation and resorption into the hepatic circulation, allowing vessels to reopen within 48–72 hours (Grenon, 2018).

Contraindications of embolization include advanced liver disease, active GI bleeding, encephalopathy, cirrhosis, portal vein occlusion, and Child-Pugh classification C. The most common adverse effects are nausea, vomiting, fever, and increased liver function tests. Increased liver function tests indicate the lysis of hepatocytes and the release of intracellular contents, signifying hepatic cellular death. Laboratory values that are monitored include CBC, electrolytes, and liver function tests (Grenon, 2018).

Patients may experience postembolization syndrome, which includes low-grade fever, abdominal pain, fatigue, nausea, and vomiting. These symptoms are often self-limiting. Management of postembolization syndrome includes symptom control. Patients may require IV hydration, prophylactic antibiotics, pain control, and antiemetics (Perez-Rojas, 2012).

Radioembolization

In radioembolization, microspheres containing yttrium-90 (^{90}Y), a beta-emitting isotope with a treatment range of 2 mm, are permanently implanted into hepatic tumors. This form of brachytherapy uses the liver's dual vascular anatomy to preferentially deliver radioactive particles to the tumor via the hepatic artery, avoiding injury to the normal liver parenchyma. Candidates include patients with solid tumors, adequate liver function, life expectancy of at least three months, and good performance status. Benefits have been seen in patients with low to moderate extrahepatic disease burden, prior liver radiation therapy, prior treatment with chemotherapy and biologic agents, and history of hepatic surgery or ablation. The majority of the clinical evidence has been reported in metastatic colorectal and neuroendocrine tumors and primary HCC. However, emerging data support the use of radioembolization in hepatic metastatic breast cancer, intrahepatic cholangiocarcinoma, and other metastatic tumor types (Kennedy, 2014).

Two commercial radioembolization products are available: resin microspheres (SIR-Spheres®) and glass microspheres (TheraSphere®), both of which use ^{90}Y as the therapeutic agent. Because the two types differ in composition, the amount of radiation carried per microsphere differs; however, the procedure itself is the same for both. The dose is calculated based on individual patients. Prior to treatment, the patient undergoes hepatic angiography to map the hepatic arterial system and protectively embolize any vessels that would permit microspheres to enter the GI tract. During the same procedure, a single photon emission computed tomography (known as SPECT) gamma camera scintigraphy is used to detect shunting into the pulmonary vasculature or GI tract (Kennedy, 2014).

The potential side effects of radioembolization are typically mild constitutional (fatigue) and GI issues limited to the first 7–14 days after treatment. Potentially serious or fatal radiation-induced liver disease (RILD) is extremely rare. The median time to treatment response is six months (Sangro, 2014). Future directions include using radioembolization combined with chemotherapy to maximize treatment response and improve patient outcomes. Transarterial chemoembolization and radioembolization often are used as complementary therapies.

Hepatic Arterial Infusion Chemotherapy

An alternative therapy for treatment of primary liver cancer or metastatic cancer to the liver is HAI of chemotherapy. Chemotherapy is delivered through the hepatic artery directly into the liver (Parks & Routt, 2015). HAI is appropriate for patients with primary liver cancer or if the liver is the only site of metastatic disease. The use of HAI is limited to a few specialized centers because of the high technical expertise required (Grenon, 2018).

HAI chemotherapy can be administered in several ways: via a percutaneously placed catheter, an arterial access port, or a surgically implanted port.

Implanted ports are placed during laparotomy or laparoscopy. The tip of the arterial port is placed in the common hepatic artery. The catheter is then connected to the port located in a surgically created subcutaneous pocket on either side of the rib cage, where it is sutured to the fascia. Dye is injected postoperatively to verify hepatic perfusion. A subcutaneous pump is placed in a similar manner to the port. During this procedure, the hepatic artery is cannulated by passing the catheter through the gastroduodenal artery into the hepatic artery. The catheter is then secured and connected to the pump, which is filled with chemotherapy or heparinized saline. The port and pump are accessed using a noncoring needle. The advantage of the port is that the flow rate can be controlled, whereas with the pump, flow rates and volumes can vary (Grenon, 2018).

Patients must meet certain criteria to be considered candidates for this treatment. The criteria include disease confined to the liver (single or multiple lesions not eligible for surgical resection), sufficient liver and kidney function, and vascular anatomy amenable to pump placement. Exclusion criteria include portal vein thrombosis because of the risk of hepatic ischemia (Parks & Routt, 2015).

Nurses who care for patients with HAI pumps need to know the mechanisms of action of the infusion pumps and how to care for patients with these pumps. Patients need to be educated regarding frequency of chemotherapy fills, implications if a scheduled fill is missed, and knowing when to report side effects to their healthcare providers. Nurses should become familiar with the protocol of their institution for administering and accessing the pump for chemotherapy fills (Parks & Routt, 2015).

Technical problems are associated with hepatic arterial ports, one of which is hepatic arterial thrombosis. There is no known way of avoiding this, so nurses must recognize the signs and symptoms, which include severe upper abdominal pain that radiates to the back during chemotherapy or at the time of flushing. Another problem is blockage of the catheter. Small amounts of urokinase pulsed into the port can open a blockage. To prevent this, nurses should maintain positive pressure at all times while the syringe is connected to the port, not allowing blood to pass back into the catheter. A third complication is the development of a duodenal fistula. This occurs after extravasation of HAI chemotherapy into the supraduodenal tissues and results in erosion of the duodenal walls that communicate with the gastroduodenal artery. As a result, upper GI bleeding occurs, which can be mild or severe depending on the location of the erosion and the amount of blood that passes into the duodenum (Barber & Fabugais-Nazario, 2003).

Radiation Therapy

Advances and highly conformal radiation therapy approaches used in cancer therapy, such as stereotactic body radiation therapy and proton therapy, have been found to be efficacious and safe as treatment modalities, but a risk for RILD still exists. RILD can occur from two weeks to four months following the completion of radiation therapy. Symptoms include elevated liver enzymes, tender hepatomegaly, and weight gain secondary to ascites. Laboratory findings include elevations of alkaline phosphatase, transaminases, and bilirubin (Kalogeridi et al., 2015). The clinical outcome ranges from mild, reversible damage to death. The pathology of RILD is veno-occlusive in nature, which is characterized by thrombosis within the central veins of the liver, producing hepatic congestion. The changes can occur in a lobe or a fraction of it; RILD rarely involves the entire liver. Analyses have demonstrated that increasing the mean liver dose correlates with the likelihood of developing RILD. Significant liver damage may not occur if a sufficient portion of the liver remains undamaged and can carry out normal liver function (Cao et al., 2007). Cao et al. (2007) demonstrated that the reduction in regional hepatic venous perfusion after radiation therapy is predicted by the accumulated liver dose and venous perfusion measured prior to the end of radiation therapy. This model has the potential to predict symptomatic radiation damage to the liver.

RILD most often is seen in patients receiving an allogeneic HSCT. This usually involves high-dose chemotherapy and total body irradiation. Patients who develop this complication can experience symptoms of jaundice, weight gain, right upper quadrant pain, hepatomegaly, ascites, and encephalopathy within one to four weeks after the transplant. The liver usually heals itself after subacute radiation injury, but chronic fibrosis may develop depending on the degree of radiation and chemotherapy injury. The damage resembles micronodular cirrhosis both pathologically and clinically. Irradiation to parts of the liver can cause localized fibrosis with no clinical sequelae of hepatic insufficiency if adequate compensation is present. No established therapies exist for RILD, but the use of steroids and anticoagulants has been suggested. The conventional dose of radiation to the liver is 30–35 centigray; doses greater than 50 centigray can cause radiation-induced hepatitis and liver failure (Grenon, 2018).

Conclusion

An understanding of the liver and its function is paramount to understanding the

Key Points

- Understanding liver function is essential to understanding the complications associated with liver toxicity in the treatment of patients with cancer.
- Biliary obstruction can be caused by cancer or cancer treatment. Restoring biliary flow with relief of jaundice and pruritus is the primary goal in the palliation of biliary obstruction related to malignancy.
- The most common risk factor for developing malignant ascites is the presence of an advanced neoplasm, particularly lymphoma and colon, gastric, pancreatic, lung, ovarian, bladder, breast, and liver cancers.
- In malignant ascites, successful treatment of the malignancy with chemotherapy or radiation therapy may help reduce fluid accumulation.
- Patients who undergo HSCT are at high risk for developing encephalopathy, which can be caused by the conditioning regimen prior to transplantation, veno-occlusive disease, immunosuppressive drugs, infection, or cerebrovascular events.
- Hepatic veno-occlusive disease, also called sinusoidal obstruction syndrome or SOS, is a potential complication following HSCT. Clinical symptoms include weight gain, ascites, jaundice, and painful hepatomegaly.
- The management of primary liver malignancies and liver metastases often involves multiple treatment modalities, including surgical resection; liver-directed therapies, such as HAI, transarterial chemoembolization, radioembolization, RFA, and radiation therapy; or systemic therapy.
- Many chemotherapy agents are metabolized by the liver, and monitoring liver function is essential.
- Advances in highly conformal radiation therapy approaches used in cancer therapy, such as stereotactic body radiation therapy and proton therapy, have been found to be efficacious and safe as treatment modalities, but risk for RILD still exists.

hepatic toxicities often associated with cancer and cancer therapies. It also helps to put complications arising from cancer and cancer therapies into perspective. Therefore, nurses need to have a basic knowledge and understanding of the assessment, diagnosis, and management of common hepatic toxicities related to cancer and cancer therapy.

References

Barber, F.D., & Fabugais-Nazario, L.E. (2003). What's old is new again: Patients receiving hepatic arterial infusion chemotherapy. *Clinical Journal of Oncology Nursing, 7,* 647–652. doi:10.1188/03.CJON.647-652

Boulay, B., & Parepally, M. (2014). Managing malignant biliary obstruction in pancreas cancer: Choosing the appropriate strategy. *World Journal of Gastroenterology, 20,* 9345–9353. Retrieved from http://www.wjgnet.com/1007-9327/full/v20/i28/9345.htm

Camp-Sorrell, D. (2018). Chemotherapy toxicities and management. In C.H. Yarbro, D. Wujcik, & B.H. Gobel (Eds.), *Cancer nursing: Principles and practice* (8th ed., 497–554). Burlington, MA: Jones & Bartlett Learning.

Cao, Y., Platt, J.F., Francis, I.R., Balter, J.M., Pan, C., Normolle, D., … Lawrence, T.S. (2007). The prediction of radiation-induced liver dysfunction using a local dose and regional venous perfusion model. *Medical Physics, 34,* 604–612. doi:10.1118/1.2431081

Collins, C.A. (2001). Ascites. *Clinical Journal of Oncology Nursing, 5,* 43–44.

Covey, A.M., & Brown, K.T. (2006). Palliative percutaneous drainage in malignant biliary obstruction. Part 2: Mechanisms and postprocedure management. *Journal of Supportive Oncology, 4,* 329–335.

DeLeve, L.D., Shulman, H.M., & McDonald, G.B. (2002). Toxic injury to hepatic sinusoids: Sinusoidal obstruction syndrome (veno-occlusive disease). *Seminars in Liver Disease, 22,* 27–42. doi:10.1055/s-2002-23204

Di Piazza, S., Filippazzo, M.G., Valenza, L.M., Morello, S., Pastore, L., Conti, A., … Pagliaro, L. (1991). Rifaximine versus neomycin in the treatment of portosystemic encephalopathy. *Italian Journal of Gastroenterology, 23,* 403–407.

Essell, J.H., Schroeder, M.T., Harman, G.S., Halvorson, R., Lew, V., Callander, N., … Thompson, J.M. (1998). Ursodiol prophylaxis against hepatic complications of allogeneic bone marrow transplantation: A randomized, double-blind, placebo-controlled trial. *Annals of Internal Medicine, 128,* 975–981. doi:10.7326/0003-4819-128-12_part_1-199806150-00002

Fan, C.Q., & Crawford, J.M. (2014). Sinusoidal obstruction syndrome (hepatic veno-occlusive disease). *Journal of Clinical and Experimental Hepatology, 4,* 332–346. doi:10.1016/j.jceh.2014.10.002

Flaherty, A. (2015). Management of malignancy-related ascites. *Oncology Nursing Forum, 42,* 96–99. doi:10.1188/15.ONF.96-99

Fleming, N.D., Alvarez-Secord, A., Von Gruenigen, V., Miller, M.J., & Abernethy, A.P. (2009). Indwelling catheters for the management of refractory malignant ascites: A systematic literature overview and retrospective chart review. *Journal of Pain and Symptom Management, 38,* 341–349. doi:10.1016/j.jpainsymman.2008.09.008

Fowler, C. (2013). Management of patients with complications of cirrhosis. *Nurse Practitioner, 38*(4), 14–22. doi:10.1097/01.NPR.0000427610.76270.45

Ghany, M., & Hoofnagle, J.H. (2012). Approach to the patient with liver disease. In D.L. Longo, A.S. Fauci, D.L. Kasper, S.L. Hauser, J.L. Jameson, & J. Loscalzo (Eds.), *Harrison's principles of internal medicine* (18th ed., pp. 2520–2527). Retrieved from http://accessmedicine.mhmedical.com

Giles, F., Garcia-Manero, G., Cortes, J., Thomas, D., Kantarjian, H., & Estey, E. (2002). Ursodiol does not prevent hepatic venoocclusive disease associated with Mylotarg therapy. *Haematologica, 87,* 1114–1116. Retrieved from http://www.haematologica.org/content/87/10/1114.long

Gordon, F.D. (2012). Ascites. *Clinics in Liver Disease, 16,* 285–299. doi:10.1016/j.cld.2012.03.004

Green, R.M., & Flamm, S. (2002). AGA technical review on the evaluation of liver chemistry test. *Gastroenterology, 123,* 1367–1384. doi:10.1053/gast.2002.36061

Grenon, N.N. (2018). Liver cancer. In C.H. Yarbro, D. Wujcik, & B.H. Gobel (Eds.), *Cancer nursing: Principles and practice* (8th ed., pp. 1651–1675). Burlington, MA: Jones & Bartlett Learning.

Groen, K.A. (1999). Primary and metastatic liver cancer. *Seminars in Oncology Nursing, 15,* 48–57. doi:10.1016/S0749-2081(99)80039-4

Hansen, L., Sasaki, A., & Zucker, B. (2010). End-stage liver disease: Challenges and practice implications. *Nursing Clinics of North America, 45,* 411–426. doi:10.1016/j.cnur.2010.03.005

Jones, R.J., Lee, K.S., Beschorner, W.E., Vogel, V.G., Grochow, L.B., Braine, H.G., … Rein, S. (1987). Venoocclusive disease of the liver following bone marrow transplantation. *Transplantation, 44,* 778–783. doi:10.1097/00007890-198712000-00011

Kalogeridi, M.-A., Zygogianni, A., Kyrgias, G., Kouvaris, J., Chatziioannou, S., Kelekis, N., & Kouloulias, V. (2015). Role of radiotherapy in management of hepatocellular carcinoma: A systematic review. *World Journal of Hepatology, 7,* 101–112. doi:10.4254/wjh.v7.i1.101

Kasper, D.L., Fauci, A.S., Hauser, S.L., Longo, D.L., Jameson, J., & Loscalzo, J. (Eds.). (2016). *Harrison's manual of medicine* (19th ed.). New York, NY: McGraw-Hill Education.

Kennedy, A. (2014). Radioembolization of hepatic tumors. *Journal of Gastrointestinal Oncology, 5,* 178–189. doi:10.3978/j.issn.2078-6891.2014.037

Krimmel, T., & Williams, L. (2008). Hepatic sinusoidal obstruction syndrome following hematopoietic stem cell transplantation. *Oncology Nursing Forum, 35,* 37–40. doi:10.1188/08.ONF.37-40

Levitsky, J., & Sorrell, M.F. (2007). Hepatic complications of hematopoietic cell transplantation. *Current Gastroenterology Reports, 9,* 60–65. doi:10.1007/s11894-008-0022-y

Locklin, J.K., & Wood, B.J. (2005). Radiofrequency ablation: A nursing perspective. *Clinical Journal of Oncology Nursing, 9,* 346–349. doi:10.1188/05.CJON.346-349

Narayanan, G., Pezeshkmehr, A., Venkat, S., Guerrero, G., & Barbery, K. (2014). Safety and efficacy of the PleurX catheter for the treatment of malignant ascites. *Journal of Palliative Medicine, 17,* 906–912. doi:10.1089/jpm.2013.0427

National Comprehensive Cancer Network. (2016). *NCCN Clinical Practice Guidelines in Oncology (NCCN Guidelines®): Hepatobiliary cancers* [v.2.2016]. Retrieved from http://www.nccn.org/professionals/physician_gls/pdf/hepatobiliary.pdf

Ohashi, K., Tanabe, J., Watanabe, R., Tanaka, T., Sakamaki, H., Maruta, A., … Yonekura, S. (2000). The Japanese multicenter open randomized trial of ursodeoxycholic acid prophylaxis for hepatic veno-occlusive disease after stem cell transplantation. *American Journal of Hematology, 64,* 32–38. doi:10.1002/(SICI)1096-8652(200005)64:1<32::AID-AJH6>3.0.CO;2-N

Park, S.H., Lee, M.H., Lee, H., Kim, H.S., Kim, K., Kim, W.S., … Kim, S.W. (2002). A randomized trial of heparin plus ursodiol vs heparin alone to prevent hepatic veno-occlusive disease after hematopoietic stem cell transplantation. *Bone Marrow Transplantation, 29,* 137–143. doi:10.1038/sj.bmt.1703342

Parks, L., & Routt, M. (2015). Hepatic artery infusion pump in the treatment of liver metastases. *Clinical Journal of Oncology Nursing, 19,* 316–320. doi:10.1188/15.CJON.316-320

Pegram, A.A., & Kennedy, L.D. (2001). Prevention and treatment of veno-occlusive disease. *Annals of Pharmacotherapy, 35,* 935–942. doi:10.1345/aph.10220

Perez-Rojas, E. (2012). Interventional radiology in oncology: Clinical management of patients undergoing transarterial chemoembolization for hepatic malignancies. *Clinical Journal of Oncology Nursing, 16,* 83–85. doi:10.1188/12.CJON.83-85

Pratt, D.S., & Kaplan, M.M. (2012). Evaluation of liver function. In D.L. Longo, A.S. Fauci, D.L. Kasper, S.L. Hauser, J.L. Jameson, & J. Loscalzo (Eds.), *Harrison's principles of internal medicine* (18th ed., pp. 2527–2531). Retrieved from http://accessmedicine.mhmedical.com

Pugh, R.N., Murray-Lyon, I.M., Dawson, J.L., Pietroni, M.C., & Williams, R. (1973). Transection of the oesophagus for bleeding oesophageal varices. *British Journal of Surgery, 60,* 646–649. doi:10.1002/bjs.1800600817

Rogers, M. (2014). Ascites. In D. Camp-Sorrell & R.A. Hawkins (Eds.), *Clinical manual for the oncology advanced practice nurse* (3rd ed., pp. 493–499). Pittsburgh, PA: Oncology Nursing Society.

Sangisetty, S.L., & Miner, T.J. (2012). Malignant ascites: A review of prognostic factors, pathophysiology and therapeutic measures. *World Journal of Gastrointestinal Surgery, 4,* 87–95. doi:10.4240/wjgs.v4.i4.87

Sangro, B. (2014). Chemoembolization and radioembolization. *Best Practice and Research Clinical Gastroenterology, 28,* 909–919. doi:10.1016/j.bpg.2014.08.009

Sargent, S. (2007). Pathophysiology and management of hepatic encephalopathy. *British Journal of Nursing, 16,* 335–339. doi:10.12968/bjon.2007.16.6.23003

Saria, M.G., & Gosselin-Acomb, T.K. (2007). Hematopoietic stem cell transplantation: Implications for critical care nurses. *Clinical Journal of Oncology Nursing, 11,* 53–63. doi:10.1188/07.CJON.53-63

Senzolo, M., Germani, G., Cholongitas, E., Burra, P., & Burroughs, A.K. (2007). Veno-occlusive disease: Update on clinical management. *World Journal of Gastroenterology, 13,* 3918–3924. doi:10.3748/wjg.v13.i29.3918

Sharma, B.C., Sharma, P., Lunia, M.K., Srivastava, G., Goyal, R., & Sarin, S.K. (2013). A randomized, double-blind, controlled trial comparing rifaximin plus lactulose with lactulose alone in treatment of overt hepatic encephalopathy. *American Journal of Gastroenterology, 108,* 1458–1463. doi:10.1038/ajg.2013.219

Sharma, P., & Sharma, B.C. (2015). Management of overt hepatic encephalopathy. *Journal of Clinical and Experimental Hepatology, 5*(Suppl. 1), S82–S87. doi:10.1016/j.jceh.2014.04.004

Slusser, K. (2014). Malignant ascites. In C.H. Yarbro, D. Wujcik, & B.H. Gobel (Eds.), *Cancer symptom management* (4th ed., pp. 241–262). Burlington, MA: Jones & Bartlett Learning.

Sosa, E.C. (2012). Veno-occlusive disease in hematopoietic stem cell transplantation recipients. *Clinical Journal of Oncology Nursing, 16,* 507–513. doi:10.1188/12.CJON.507-513

Stern, N., & Sturgess, R. (2008). Endoscopic therapy in the management of malignant biliary obstruction. *European Journal of Surgical Oncology, 34,* 313–317. doi:10.1016/j.ejso.2007.07.210

Wadleigh, M., Ho, V., Momtaz, P., & Richardson, P. (2003). Hepatic veno-occlusive disease: Pathogenesis, diagnosis and treatment. *Current Opinion in Hematology, 10,* 451–462. doi:10.1097/00062752-200311000-00010

Wallach, J. (2000). *Interpretation of diagnostic tests* (7th ed.). Philadelphia, PA: Lippincott Williams & Wilkins.

Wilkes, G.M., & Barton-Burke, M. (2016). *2016 oncology nursing drug handbook* (20th ed.). Burlington, MA: Jones & Bartlett Learning.

Wolkoff, A.W. (2012). The hyperbilirubinemias. In D.L. Longo, A.S. Fauci, D.L. Kasper, S.L. Hauser, J.L. Jameson, & J. Loscalzo (Eds.), *Harrison's principles of internal medicine* (18th ed., pp. 1999–2004). Retrieved from http://accessmedicine.mhmedical.com

Wujcik, D. (2018). Targeted therapy. In C.H. Yarbro, D. Wujcik, & B.H. Gobel (Eds.), *Cancer nursing: Principles and practice* (8th ed., pp. 653–680). Burlington, MA: Jones & Bartlett Learning.

Chapter 23 Study Questions

1. Malignant biliary obstruction often is caused by which of the following?
   A. Tumor in the biliary tree or extrinsic compression by metastatic disease
   B. Elevated liver enzymes
   C. Chemotherapy
   D. Tumor located in the stomach

2. Signs and symptoms of ascites include:
   A. Weight gain, nausea, and vomiting.
   B. Abdominal distention, nausea, and vomiting.
   C. Peripheral edema, cough, and right upper quadrant pain.
   D. Weight gain, abdominal distention, and early satiety.

3. The diagnostic criteria for sinusoidal obstruction syndrome include which of the following?
   A. Weight gain and ascites
   B. Right upper quadrant pain and ascites
   C. Jaundice, hepatomegaly, and ascites
   D. Hepatomegaly, right upper quadrant pain, and vomiting

4. The treatment of postembolization syndrome after chemoembolization often includes which of the following?
   A. No intervention
   B. IV hydration, prophylactic antibiotics, pain control, and antiemetics
   C. Watchful waiting
   D. Hospitalization

5. This form of brachytherapy uses the liver's unique dual vascular anatomy to preferentially deliver radioactive particles to the tumor via the hepatic artery, thus sparing the normal liver parenchyma.
   A. Chemoembolization
   B. Radiofrequency ablation
   C. Radioembolization
   D. Radiation therapy

CHAPTER

24 Hypersensitivity

Pamela Hallquist Viale, RN, MS, CS, ANP

Introduction

The increase in the number of oncologic treatments has offered patients more therapeutic options; consequently, hypersensitivity reactions (HSRs) have increased in number as well. Severe HSRs can result in the discontinuation of therapy or replacement by less effective agents (Mezzano, Giavina-Bianchi, Picard, Caiado, & Castells, 2014). Hypersensitivity reactions can result from exposure to any medication, but the incidence in the literature is variable. In general, HSRs occur in 5% of patients receiving oncology drugs, yet certain agents and drug classes carry a much higher risk (Lenz, 2007). HSRs can vary in intensity; patients may experience hives or wheals while others progress to anaphylaxis, which is often described as a serious, life-threatening reaction or a systemic HSR that is rapid in onset and capable of causing death (Simons et al., 2011). These reactions should be graded accordingly (see Table 24-1). Because of the serious nature of HSRs, oncology nurses must be able to anticipate, diagnose, and manage these reactions in patients receiving chemotherapy and monoclonal antibody therapy.

Pathophysiology

The mechanism of action for an HSR varies among agents (Lenz, 2007). An immune response can be innate, adaptive, or a combination of both (Joerger, 2012; Vogel, 2010). The innate response is nonspecific and rapid, presenting before drug exposure, versus the acquired adaptive response, which is specific in nature and capable of increasing the immune response with each successive exposure (Joerger, 2012). As cumulative exposure increases, the number of HSRs also can increase (Tham, Cheng, Tay, Alcasabas, & Shek, 2015). The pathophysiology for individual drug HSRs is not completely clear, but it appears that these reactions often produce immediate HSRs and seem to involve immunoglobulin (Ig) E (Boulanger et al., 2014). Four categories of HSRs exist: immediate IgE mediated (type 1), antibody mediated or cytotoxic (type II), immune complex mediated (type III), and delayed or cell mediated (type IV) (Gobel, 2007; Zanotti & Markham, 2001).

Types of Immune Reactions

Type I: Immunoglobulin E–Mediated Reactions

Type I HSRs are mediated by IgE (Makrilia, Syrigou, Kaklamanos, Manolopoulos, & Saif, 2010). This Ig is responsible for the degranulation of mast cells and basophils, progressing to the nonimmune-mediated histamine and cytokine release (Makrilia et al., 2010). His-

Table 24-1. National Cancer Institute Grading Criteria for Adverse Events: Hypersensitivity and Allergic Reactions

	Grade				
Event	**1**	**2**	**3**	**4**	**5**
Allergic reaction Defined as a disorder characterized by an adverse local or general response from allergen exposure.	Transient flushing or rash, drug fever < 38°C (< 100.4°F); intervention not indicated	Intervention or infusion interruption indicated; responds promptly to symptomatic treatment (e.g., antihistamines, NSAIDs, narcotics); prophylactic medications indicated for ≤ 24 hrs	Prolonged (e.g., not rapidly responsive to symptomatic treatment and/or brief interruption of infusion); recurrence of symptoms following initial improvement; hospitalization indicated for clinical sequelae (e.g., renal impairment, pulmonary infiltrates)	Life-threatening consequences; urgent intervention indicated	Death
Infusion-related reaction Defined as a disorder characterized by adverse reaction to the infusion of pharmacologic or biologic substances.	Mild transient reaction; infusion interruption not indicated; intervention not indicated	Therapy or infusion interruption indicated but responds promptly to symptomatic treatment (e.g., antihistamines, NSAIDs, narcotics, IV fluids); prophylactic medications indicated for ≤ 24 hrs	Prolonged (e.g., not rapidly responsive to symptomatic medication and/or brief interruption of infusion); recurrence of symptoms following initial improvement; hospitalization indicated for clinical sequelae	Life-threatening consequences; urgent intervention indicated	Death
Anaphylaxis Defined as a disorder characterized by an acute inflammatory reaction resulting from the release of histamine and histamine-like substances from mast cells, causing a hypersensitivity immune response. Clinically, it presents with breathing difficulty, dizziness, hypotension, cyanosis, and loss of consciousness and may lead to death.	–	–	Symptomatic bronchospasm, with or without urticaria; parenteral intervention indicated; allergy-related edema/angioedema; hypotension	Life-threatening consequences; urgent intervention indicated	Death

(Continued on next page)

Table 24-1. National Cancer Institute Grading Criteria for Adverse Events: Hypersensitivity and Allergic Reactions *(Continued)*

	Grade				
Adverse Event	**1**	**2**	**3**	**4**	**5**
Cytokine release syndrome A disorder characterized by nausea, headache, tachycardia, hypotension, rash, and shortness of breath; it is caused by the release of cytokines from the cells	Mild reaction; infusion interruption not indicated; intervention not indicated	Therapy or infusion interruption indicated but responds promptly to symptomatic treatment (e.g., antihistamines, NSAIDs, narcotics, IV fluids); prophylactic medications indicated for ≤ 24 hrs	Prolonged (e.g., not rapidly responsive to symptomatic medication and/or brief interruption of infusion); recurrence of symptoms following initial improvement; hospitalization indicated for clinical sequelae (e.g., renal impairment, pulmonary infiltrates)	Life-threatening consequences; pressor or ventilatory support indicated	Death
Serum sickness A disorder characterized by a delayed-type hypersensitivity reaction to foreign proteins derived from an animal serum. It occurs approximately 6–21 days after administration of the foreign antigen. Symptoms include fever, arthralgias, myalgias, skin eruptions, lymphadenopathy, chest marked discomfort, and dyspnea.	Asymptomatic; clinical or diagnostic observations only; intervention not indicated	Moderate arthralgia; fever, rash, urticaria, antihistamines indicated	Severe arthralgia or arthritis; extensive rash; steroids or IV fluids indicated	Life-threatening consequences; pressor or ventilatory support indicated	Death

NSAIDs—nonsteroidal anti-inflammatory drugs

Note. From *Common Terminology Criteria for Adverse Events* [v.4.03], by National Cancer Institute Cancer Therapy Evaluation Program, 2010. Retrieved from http://evs.nci.nih.gov/ftp1/CTCAE/CTCAE_4.03_2010-06-14_QuickReference_5x7.pdf.

tamine release occurs, the complement system is activated, and release of prostaglandins and inflammatory leukotrienes follows; these actions produce an antigen–antibody reaction (Kang & Saif, 2007). Although symptoms are often immediate, reactions can occur three to four hours after infusion of an agent (Kang & Saif, 2007). An important component of the reaction is the elevation of tryptase, a critical mast cell protease, which can be measured in the serum (Castells, 2015). Higher levels of tryptase correlate with the severity of the HSR (Castells, 2015).

Type II: Cytotoxic Reactions

Type II HSRs are referred to as *cytotoxic reactions.* The reaction takes place after the binding of cell surface antigens with IgG or IgM antibodies. The result of this interaction is the destruction or lysis of the target cell. Examples of a type II HSR are hemolytic anemia and hemolysis of red blood cells from a transfusion of incompatible blood (Gottlieb, Bordoni, Lawhead, & Feinberg, 2010).

Type III: Immune Complex–Mediated Reactions

Type III HSRs are also called *immune complex–mediated reactions.* In oncology, this type of reaction is seen with gamma globulin injections, commonly known as horse serum sickness. A network of immune complexes is formed by the interaction of antigens and antibodies within the tissues of the body. Another mechanism leading to type III reactions is the anaphylactoid reaction produced by complement activation through a classical immune system pathway. The resulting reaction may mimic a type I HSR (Gottlieb et al., 2010).

Type IV: Cell-Mediated Reactions

The final type of HSRs are type IV or *cell-mediated reactions,* also referred to as delayed HSRs. Delayed HSRs are inflammatory reactions that are initiated by mononuclear leukocytes. These "delayed" reactions occur 48–72 hours after exposure to an antigen as opposed to "immediate" HSRs (Viale & Yamamoto, 2010). This type of response occurs as a result of the interaction of sensitized T lymphocytes with antigens rather than by antigen–antibody binding. After interacting with antigens, the T cells release lymphokines, such as interleukins (Posadas & Pichler, 2007). Examples of type IV or delayed HSRs are tuberculosis, poison ivy, granulomas, and contact dermatitis caused by sensitivity to topical application of mechlorethamine for mycosis fungoides (Labovich, 1999).

Anaphylactoid Reactions

Another type of acute HSR to antineoplastic agents is referred to as *anaphylactoid* instead of anaphylactic. These anaphylactoid reactions present clinically as type I anaphylactic reactions but are not mediated by IgE. Mast cell degranulation and histamine release are components of anaphylactoid reactions, but the pathophysiology of the reaction appears to be subsequent to the release of cytokines and antibodies binding to antigen-expressing cells (Kang & Saif, 2007). These reactions are often seen after administration of monoclonal antibodies.

Reaction Symptoms

The European Network on Drug Allergy categorizes HSRs into two types based on the timing of symptoms after drug exposure: type 1, signifying an immediate reaction occurring within an hour of receiving drug, and type 2, a nonimmediate reaction occurring more than an hour after drug exposure (Joerger, 2012). Type 1 reactions exhibit urticaria, angioedema, rhinitis, conjunctivitis, bronchospasm, or anaphylaxis, whereas type 2 reactions display late urticaria, maculopapular rash, vasculitis, toxic epidermal necrolysis, Stevens-Johnson syndrome, or other systemic symptoms (Joerger, 2012). As discussed previously, immediate reactions are IgE mediated, while the nonimmediate reactions are T-cell mediated. Acute infusion reactions are described often as anaphylactic (IgE type 1 acute HSR) or anaphylactoid.

Reactions to Standard Chemotherapy

The chemotherapy drugs most frequently implicated in HSRs include taxanes, platinums, doxorubicin, asparaginase, and epipodophyllotoxins (Castells, 2015). Standard chemotherapy agent reactions appear to be related to type

1 hypersensitivity, resulting in the commonly seen symptoms of urticaria, rash, angioedema, bronchospasm, and alterations in blood pressure (Lenz, 2007). These commonly occurring symptoms result from the IgE-mediated release of histamines, leukotrienes, and prostaglandins from mast cells in the tissue and basophils in the peripheral blood (Lenz, 2007). Symptoms can rarely produce death from hypoxemia or shock (Joerger, 2012). The standard chemotherapy agents, their metabolites, or even the substance used to dissolve the agent (as in the case of Kolliphor® EL, formerly Cremophor® EL, which is used to render the drug soluble) also may be responsible for mast cell or basophil degranulation, resulting in similar IgE-mediated allergic reactions (Gradishar, 2006). Some patients experience atypical symptoms of HSR with administration of taxanes and oxaliplatin. These symptoms include hypertension, back and chest pain, and rigors (Castells, 2015).

Reactions to Monoclonal Antibodies

Monoclonal antibody treatment has resulted in varying degrees of infusion reaction, some severe enough to lead to patient death (Chung, 2008; Lenz, 2007). The mechanism of action for monoclonal antibody–associated infusion reaction is unclear (Chung, 2008). One theory suggests that the antibodies themselves interact with their molecular targets on specific target cells, tumor cells, or blood cells, thus promoting the release of inflammatory cytokines (Chung, 2008). The degree of humanization of the monoclonal antibody contributes to the potential for HSR; for example, mouse and chimeric antibodies can produce a rapid immune response and reaction, whereas humanized or fully human antibodies have a much lower potential for reaction because of their low immunogenicity (Pichler, 2006). Chimeric antibodies (frequently combined with mouse) contain greater than 50% human antibody compared to fully human antibodies (100%). Although fully human antibodies are considered less immunogenic, infusion reactions may still occur (Vogel, 2010). Acute infusion reactions occur generally in 3%–5% of patients treated with chimeric antibodies and can often be ameliorated by slowing the infusion rate and administering premedications. These reactions are usually not considered IgE mediated, but rather a result of a cytokine response (Wing, 2008). The infusion reactions occur most frequently with the first dose of the monoclonal antibody, and with some agents, such as trastuzumab or rituximab, subsequent doses may produce a lesser reaction (Baldo, 2013; Thompson et al., 2014). The incidence of infusion reactions varies with each agent, and risk factors can contribute to a higher incidence of HSR. In a retrospective analysis of trastuzumab-treated patients with breast cancer, the incidence of infusion reactions was 16.2% (32 out of 197 patients) and 1.8% of 1,788 doses (Thompson et al., 2014). In one report, rituximab reactions varied from 77% for the first infusion (with 10% grade 3–4), and by the fourth infusion, 30% of patients continued to react to the agent (Baldo, 2013). In another retrospective review of 222 cases of HSRs over a four-year period, 50% were found in patients receiving immunotherapeutic agents; most were grade 1 or 2 using the Common Terminology Criteria for Adverse Events criteria (DeMoor et al., 2011).

In rare cases, delayed reactions to monoclonal antibodies, such as trastuzumab, have occurred up to 24 hours after administration (Viale, 2009). Although rare, fatalities have occurred. It is believed T cells may mediate these delayed reactions (Posadas & Pichler, 2007).

Patients who experience an initial reaction that resolves after therapy and then develop recurrence of symptoms 1–72 hours after initial resolution of symptoms are considered to have biphasic reactions (Lieberman, 2005; Viale & Yamamoto, 2010). Biphasic reactions are seen with standard chemotherapy and monoclonal antibody treatment. Although the mechanism of action is not completely known, biphasic responses may occur because of inadequate initial treatment of the original reaction, allowing a resurgence of initial symptoms (Popa & Lerner, 1984). However, researchers have also proposed that this late response could be caused by a biphasic wave of histamine from mast cells or the activation of secondary inflammatory pathways following the initial HSR (Tole & Lieberman, 2007).

Risk Factors

Risk factors can increase the potential for a hypersensitivity event. These factors include the route of entry of the antigen, the amount of antigen introduced, the rate of antigen absorption, and the patient's degree of hypersensitivity to a particular agent (Labovich, 1999). The risk factors associated with an increased incidence of HSRs include age, gender, genetic makeup, nutritional status, stress level, hormonal factors, and environmental factors. Anaphylactic reactions occur more commonly if patients have a history of allergies, especially drug allergies. Previous exposure to a particular agent and failure to administer prophylactic medications are also considered risk factors for the development of HSRs (Polovich, Olsen, & LeFebvre, 2014).

Some drugs have specific risk factors which include the route of administration, duration of administration, and immunologic characteristics of the drug (Polovich et al., 2014). Without premedications prior to administration of protein drugs (such as L-asparaginase), the incidence of HSRs increases (Viale, 2009; Vogel, 2010).

Although any agent has the potential to cause an HSR, selected agents/classes have elevated risk. Platinum agents play a significant role in the armamentarium of oncology therapeutics for many different cancer types. Because of this, an increased incidence of HSRs has been documented. Although it is rare to see patients react to the initial course of therapy, allergic reactions can occur after a number of cycles. In particular, retreatment with carboplatin (usually administered over six cycles initially) often produces HSRs (in one series, 19%) (Boulanger et al., 2014). The overall incidence of HSR is calculated at 5%–20% with cisplatin and 1%–44% with carboplatin. Oxaliplatin, a mainstay of therapy for colorectal cancer, has an overall incidence of 10%–19%, although a recently published paper described reactions in up to 63% of patients after multiple exposures (Boulanger et al., 2014; Castells, 2015). Oxaliplatin-associated HSR can produce pruritus and erythema, as well as anaphylaxis in approximately 1% of cases (Joerger, 2012). In general, these reactions are seen with the seventh or eighth infusion. Skin testing may be appropriate to identify at-risk patients.

The risk factors for HSR to platinum therapy include an existing HSR to certain drugs and lifetime exposure to platinum drugs. The interval between the last cycle of the initial therapy and the first cycle of the second course is also considered a predictive variable; an increased incidence was seen in patients with carboplatin if the interval was more than 24 months (Schwartz et al., 2007). Once the patient is sensitized, a very small amount of medication can produce an HSR (Castells, 2015). Of note, recent data demonstrated that *BRCA* mutation carriers are at highest risk for HSR. In one study of 87 women with a *BRCA1* or *BRCA2* mutation, the participants had an increased susceptibility and a shorter time to carboplatin-associated HSR, suggesting that this group should receive additional counseling regarding risk for HSR (Moon et al., 2013).

Taxane reactions are associated with the Kolliphor EL diluent required to make the drug soluble; reactions to taxanes have been documented in up to 30% of all patients in published series (Joerger, 2012). Premedication (typically steroids and antihistamines) can reduce the incidence of reaction to approximately 4% or less and is critical to decrease HSRs (Castells, 2015; Joerger, 2012). Reactions typically occur with the first or second infusion. Premedication and rechallenge can be successful at reducing subsequent occurrences. A Kolliphor-free version of paclitaxel is approved in the treatment of several cancers. Patients with documented HSR to paclitaxel have been switched to docetaxel to reduce the incidence of HSR and still reacted; therefore, Kolliphor EL may not be the sole culprit in taxane reactions. More data are needed to fully identify the risk for taxane-induced HSRs (Castells, 2015).

Monoclonal antibodies, in general, can produce reactions as previously discussed, but specific agents have higher incidences of HSRs. Two agents, rituximab and trastuzumab, carry a higher risk—77% and 40% HSR with first infusion, respectively (Joerger, 2012). Cetuximab can produce HSRs in up to a quarter of patients treated with the antibody, usually at first exposure (Castells, 2015). As mentioned previously, the reactions generally occur with the first or second exposure to the antibody and are classic in their presentation, producing itching, flushing, respiratory symptoms, and gastrointestinal and cardiovascular involvement. In some cases, patients will experience fever and chills with body aches (Castells, 2015). Delayed reactions (type IV or cell mediated) can occur in patients receiving monoclonal antibodies, with symptoms seen within the first two weeks after treatment. Symptoms may include arthralgias and myalgias, rash, urticaria, and fever (Castells, 2015). Monoclonal antibodies also can cause a vast amount of cytokine release (cytokine release syndrome), producing effects anywhere from a flu-like syndrome to multiorgan failure along with classic infusion-related reactions (Castells, 2015).

Clinical Presentation

HSRs can occur with most chemotherapeutics and monoclonal antibody infusion, producing symptoms from IgE and non-IgE activation of mast cells and basophils (Castells, 2015). The subjective signs and symptoms of an HSR involve multiple systems and include generalized itching, chest tightness, agitation, uneasiness, dizziness, nausea, crampy abdominal pain, anxiety, sense of impending doom, desire to urinate or defecate, and chills. Objective signs include flushed appearance (edema of eyes, face, hands, or feet), localized or generalized urticaria, respiratory distress (with or without wheezing), hypotension, cyanosis, and difficulty speaking (Vogel, 2010).

Reactions usually occur within minutes of beginning an IV agent and peak within 15–30 minutes. Reactions to oral agents frequently occur within two hours but can be delayed up to several hours depending on the metabolism of the drug. HSR recurrence may be seen up to 24 hours after the initial appropriate premedications and precautions were followed (Viale & Yamamoto, 2010).

The most common causes of death from anaphylaxis are cardiovascular collapse and asphyxiation secondary to laryngeal edema and spasm. Cardiovascular collapse and shock can occur without any skin or respiratory symptoms (Labovich, 1999).

The main problems associated with a type II reaction are hemolytic anemia, cardiovascular collapse, and possibly death. Type III reactions result in the deposition of immune complexes in the tissues with varying degrees of tissue injury. Lastly, type IV or delayed HSRs are evidenced by mucositis, pneumonitis, contact dermatitis, granulomas, and homograft rejection as seen in graft-versus-host disease after a transplant (Posadas & Pichler, 2007).

Prevention of Hypersensitivity Reactions: Best Practices

Strategies to prevent HSRs involve multiple factors. A comprehensive allergy history is key, and patients with allergies to several other substances or drugs should be carefully assessed prior to therapy. Ascertaining an individual's degree of hypersensitivity to a particular drug is critical. The use of premedications, skin testing, and desensitization all play a vital role in reducing the number of HSRs in patients receiving chemotherapy and monoclonal antibody infusions. Infusion rates may need to be slowed or raised gradually to reduce risk. Certain geographic areas may place patients at higher risk; data suggest that patients receiving cetuximab in North Carolina and Tennessee have an increased incidence of HSRs (Viale, 2009; Vogel, 2010).

Premedication

The use of pharmacologic prophylaxis is recommended to reduce the frequency and severity of hypersensitivity reactions (Lenz, 2007). Pharmacologic strategies include the use of antihistamines, corticosteroids, or both. When administering paclitaxel, it is standard to administer dexamethasone, diphenhydramine, and an H_2 antagonist (Lenz, 2007; Viale, 2009; Vogel, 2010). Patients receiving monoclonal antibodies often require premedication; this strategy is not necessary with the administration of bevacizumab, panitumumab, or trastuzumab (Viale, 2010). Oral premedications are sometimes recommended; therefore, oncology nurses should ensure the premedication regimen has been followed appropriately. No standard regimen exists for all oncologic agents, and oncology nurses should monitor manufacturers' recommendations as well as their facility's protocol (Vogel, 2010).

Skin Testing and Desensitization

With the increase in HSRs, patient safety may be compromised (Castells, 2015). Additionally, patients may have to give up a potentially useful therapy because of an inability to tolerate infusion secondary to development of HSRs. Desensitization protocols have been used successfully, allowing patients to receive needed therapeutics. Evaluation of tryptase levels is an important marker during evaluation of hypersensitivity (Castells, 2015). Skin testing is used to determine IgE sensitization and select appropriate patients to undergo desensitization protocols (Castells, 2015). Although no standardized approaches to skin testing exist, it is generally recommended to wait two to four weeks after the initial anaphylactic reaction. Both skin pricks and intradermal concentrations have been used to determine sensitivity. Vesicant agents cannot be used for skin testing because of skin toxicity (Castells, 2015).

Currently, no standardized protocol exists for drug desensitization. Castells has published extensively on desensitization protocol experiences, yielding a 12-step protocol to administer doubling doses of antigen at fixed time intervals. This approach has been used successfully in several hundred patients (Castells, 2015). Wong, Ling, Patil, Banerji, and Long (2014) studied 48 patients with oxaliplatin-induced HSR. Immediate HSR skin testing was performed to stratify risk, and the drug desensitization protocols were administered based on clinical history, skin test results, and the patient's experience with the protocol previously. Although HSRs occurred during the study, all patients were ultimately desensitized successfully. In another trial, Madrigal-Burgaleta et al. (2013) reported that desensitization was successful in 188 of 189 oxaliplatin administrations. No breakthrough reactions occurred in 94% of the desensitizations, with most noted to be mild. Desensitization protocols have helped patients receive monoclonal antibody therapy as well (Gottlieb et al., 2010).

Nursing Implications

Before administering the initial dose of a drug to a patient who has a strong likelihood of experiencing an HSR, nurses should perform either an intradermal skin test or scratch test or administer a test dose of the drug in question. For patients who have received prior doses of carboplatin, a skin test is suggested after the seventh dose of the drug, as the risk of HSR can increase after multiple doses (Polovich et al., 2014).

Nurses need to be familiar with the potential side effects of the drugs to be administered so that they can take the necessary precautions. Knowledge of appropriate premedication regimens is absolutely essential to decrease the risk of an HSR. Before administering the drug, nurses should ensure that emergency equipment and medications are readily available. Required emergency equipment and medications include oxygen supplies, cardiac monitor, defibrillator, intubation supplies, epinephrine 1:1,000 or 1:10,000, diphenhydramine 50 mg, corticosteroids such as methylprednisolone sodium succinate 125 mg, and other drugs, such as aminophylline and dopamine sulfate. Isotonic IV fluids including normal saline or lactated Ringer solution must be available to maintain blood pressure should the need arise (Viale, 2009). Strategies may include the use of resuscitation protocols or algorithms readily available at the bedside or the appropriate medication (Viale, 2009).

Vital signs, including blood pressure, pulse, and respiratory rate, need to be assessed before, during, and after administration of the drug. Nurses need to prioritize their duties so they are able to remain with the patient for 15–30 minutes after administering the agent. A free-flowing IV infusion should be maintained at all times during the drug administration (Polovich et al., 2014).

If the patient begins to experience signs and symptoms of an HSR, administration of the offending agent must be stopped immediately, the IV infusion maintained, and a call for help be made, as the nurse must remain with the patient. The patency of the patient's airway must be assessed, as well as the blood pressure, pulse, and respiratory rate. Oxygen should be administered at a high flow rate. The patient should be lowered to a supine position to perfuse the organs with blood (Viale, 2009). Documentation of events should include appropriate grading of the reaction (see Figure 24-1).

Nurses must be prepared to administer medications as prescribed by the institution's protocol. These medications may include epinephrine, diphenhydramine, albuterol, and methylprednisolone (see Figure 24-1). Someone must remain with the patient and be prepared to administer CPR, as well as provide emotional support to the patient and family (Polovich et al., 2014). Careful documentation is critical. Studies have documented that caring for a patient who experiences an HSR or event can be stressful for both the nurse and the patient (Colwell et al., 2007). Patients who experience a severe HSR may have a biphasic reaction or recurrence of symptoms within 24 hours of the first reaction. It is advisable, therefore, to hospitalize and closely monitor patients who have severe HSRs for a 24-hour period (Viale & Yamamoto, 2010).

It is not clear whether an offending antineoplastic agent should be used again if the patient experienced a serious HSR. As premedications will often prevent a reaction to an antineoplastic agent, healthcare professionals may choose to rechallenge the patient with this same regimen. Desensitization may offer patients an additional option.

Conclusion

Oncology nurses administering therapeutic treatments should be aware of the risk for HSRs with standard chemotherapy and monoclonal antibody treatments. Although severe HSRs are not common, these reactions can be disruptive and distressing for both patients and nurses. Rare, fatal reactions have occurred. Prompt recognition, evaluation, and treatment of HSRs is imperative for optimal outcomes.

Figure 24-1. Management of Hypersensitivity and Anaphylactic Reactions

1. Review the patient's allergy history.
2. Consider prophylactic medications with hydrocortisone or an antihistamine in atopic/allergic individuals. (This requires a physician's order.)
3. Patient and family education: Assess the patient's readiness to learn. Inform the patient of the potential for an allergic reaction and instruct to report any unusual symptoms, such as the following:
   - Uneasiness or agitation
   - Abdominal cramping
   - Itching
   - Chest tightness
   - Light-headedness or dizziness
   - Chills
4. Ensure that emergency equipment and medications are readily available.
5. Obtain baseline vital signs and note the patient's mental status.
6. As appropriate, perform a scratch test, intradermal skin test, or test dose before administering the full dosage (this requires a physician's order). If there is no reaction, the remaining dose can be administered. If an allergic response is suspected, discontinue the test dose (unless it has been completed), maintain the IV line, and notify the physician.
7. For a localized allergic response:
   - Evaluate symptoms; observe for urticaria, wheals, and localized erythema.
   - Administer diphenhydramine or hydrocortisone as per the physician's order.
   - Monitor vital signs every 15 minutes for 1 hour.
   - Continue subsequent dosing or desensitization program according to the physician's order.
   - If a "flare" reaction appears along the vein with doxorubicin or daunorubicin, flush the line with saline.
     - Ensure that extravasation has not occurred.
     - Administer hydrocortisone 25–50 mg IV with a physician's order, followed by a 0.9% normal saline flush. This may be adequate to resolve the flare reaction.
     - Once the flare reaction has resolved, continue slow infusion of the drug.
     - Monitor for repeated flare episodes. It is preferable to change the IV site if possible.
8. For a generalized allergic response, either anaphylactoid (patient has never been exposed to the drug before) or anaphylaxis (patient has severe hypersensitivity reaction after having received the drug before), assess for the following signs or symptoms (these usually occur within the first 15 minutes of the start of the infusion or injection):
   - Generalized itching
   - Chest tightness
   - Agitation
   - Uneasiness
   - Dizziness
   - Nausea
   - Crampy abdominal pain
   - Anxiety
   - Sense of impending doom
   - Desire to urinate or defecate
   - Chills
   - Objective signs
   - Flushed appearance (edema of face, hands, or feet)
   - Localized or generalized urticaria
   - Respiratory distress with or without wheezing
   - Hypotension
   - Cyanosis
   - Difficulty speaking

(Continued on next page)

Figure 24-1. Management of Hypersensitivity and Anaphylactic Reactions *(Continued)*

9. For a generalized allergic response:
   - Stop the infusion immediately and notify the physician.
   - Maintain the IV line with the appropriate solution to expand the vascular space (e.g., normal saline).
   - If not contraindicated, ensure maximum rate of infusion if the patient is hypotensive.
   - Position the patient to promote perfusion of the vital organs; the supine position is preferred.
   - Monitor vital signs every 2 minutes until stable, then every 5 minutes for 30 minutes, then every 15 minutes as ordered.
   - Reassure the patient and the family.
   - Maintain the airway and anticipate the need for CPR.
   - All medications must be administered with a physician's order.
   - Anticipate administering the following medications for the following effects:
     – Vasoconstriction to increase cardiac output and blood pressure
   - Epinephrine 1:1,000, 0.3–0.5 ml IVP (peds), or 0.3–0.5 mg IM or SC every 10–15 min; or, if hypotensive, 1:10,000, 0.5–1.0 ml (0.1 mg) IVP in adults (peds 1:1,000, 0.01 ml/kg [up to 0.3 ml] IV)
   - Dopamine 2–20 mcg/kg/min IV (adults)
     – Antihistamines to stop allergic release of histamines
   - Diphenhydramine 25–50 mg IVP (adults), 1 mg/kg IV or IM with 50 mg max (peds)
   - Ranitidine 50 mg IV or famotidine 20 mg IV (adults)
     – Bronchodilation: aminophylline 5 mg/kg IV over 30 min (adults)
     – Anti-inflammation/bronchodilation: steroids. Hydrocortisone 100–500 mg IV (peds 1–2 mg/kg); or methylprednisolone 30–50 mg IV (peds 0.3–0.5 mg/kg); or dexamethasone 10–20 mg IVP (peds 1–2 mg/kg); or hydrocortisone 100–500 mg IV (peds 1–2 mg/kg)
10. Document the incident in the medical record according to institution policy and procedures.
11. Physician-guided desensitization may be necessary for subsequent dosing.

IM—intramuscular; IVP—intravenous push; peds—pediatric patients; SC—subcutaneous

Note. Based on information from Polovich et al., 2014; Viale, 2009; Vogel, 2010.

Key Points

- With a larger arsenal of chemotherapy agents, HSRs have increased in number as well.
- The mechanism of action for hypersensitivity varies among agents.
- The four categories of hypersensitivity agents are immediate IgE mediated (type I), antibody mediated (type II), immune complex mediated (type III), and delayed or cell mediated (type IV).
- Reactions seen with standard chemotherapy agents most commonly appear to be related to type I hypersensitivity.
- Type I reactions may include urticaria, rash, angioedema, bronchospasm, and alterations in blood pressure.
- Monoclonal antibody infusions may produce varying degrees of infusion reaction, and some can be severe enough to lead to patient death.
- The use of premedication is recommended to reduce the frequency and severity of HSRs and may include antihistamines, corticosteroids, or both.
- Oncology nurses need to be familiar with the potential side effects of chemotherapy agents and be prepared to manage HSRs.

The author would like to acknowledge Susan P. Epting, RN, MSN, AOCNS®, for her contribution to this chapter that remains unchanged from the first edition of this book.

References

Baldo, B.A. (2013). Adverse events to monoclonal antibodies used for cancer therapy: Focus on hypersensitivity responses. *OncoImmunology, 2,* e26333. doi:10.4161/onci.26333

Boulanger, J., Boursiquot, J.N., Cournoyer, G., Lemieux, J., Masse, M.S., Almanric, K., & Guay, M.P. (2014). Management of hypersensitivity to platinum and taxane-based chemotherapy: CEPO review and clinical recommendations. *Current Oncology, 21,* e630–e641. doi:10.3747/co.21.1966

Castells, M.C. (2015). Anaphylaxis to chemotherapy and monoclonal antibodies. *Immunology and Allergy Clinics of North America, 35,* 335–348. doi:10.1016/j.iac.2015.01.011

Chung, C.H. (2008). Managing premedications and the risk for reactions to infusional monoclonal antibody therapy. *Oncologist, 13,* 725–732. doi:10.1634/theoncologist.2008-0012

Colwell, H.H., Mathias, S.D., Ngo, N.H., Gitlin, M., Lu, Z.J., & Knoop, T. (2007). The impact of infusion reactions on oncology patients and clinicians in the inpatient and outpatient practice settings: Oncology nurses' perspectives. *Journal of Infusion Nursing, 30,* 153–160. doi:10.1097/01.NAN.0000270674.13439.5b

DeMoor, P.A., Matusov, Y., Kelly, C., Kolan, S., Barnachea, L., & Bazhenova, L.A. (2011). A retrospective review of the frequency and nature of acute hypersensitivity reactions at a medium-sized infusion center: Comparison to reported values and inconsistencies found in literature. *Journal of Cancer, 2,* 153–164. doi:10.7150/jca.2.153

Gobel, B.H. (2007). Hypersensitivity reactions to biological drugs. *Seminars in Oncology Nursing, 23,* 191–200. doi:10.1016/j.soncn.2007.05.009

Gottlieb, G.R., Bordoni, R.E., Lawhead, R.A., & Feinberg, B.A. (2010). Successful outpatient desensitization of cancer patients with hypersensitivity reactions to chemotherapy. *Community Oncology, 7,* 452–457. doi:10.1016/S1548-5315(11)70425-9

Gradishar, W.J. (2006). Albumin-bound paclitaxel: A next-generation taxane. *Expert Opinion on Pharmacotherapy, 7,* 1041–1053. doi:10.1517/14656566.7.8.1041

Joerger, M. (2012). Prevention and handling of acute allergic and infusion reactions in oncology. *Annals of Oncology, 23*(Suppl. 10), x313–x319. doi:10.1093/annonc/mds314

Kang, S.P., & Saif, M.W. (2007). Infusion-related and hypersensitivity reactions of monoclonal antibodies used to treat colorectal cancer—Identification, prevention, and management. *Journal of Supportive Care in Oncology, 5,* 451–457.

Labovich, T.M. (1999). Acute hypersensitivity reactions to chemotherapy. *Seminars in Oncology Nursing, 15,* 222–231. doi:10.1016/S0749-2081(99)80010-2

Lenz, H.-J. (2007). Management and preparedness for infusion and hypersensitivity reactions. *Oncologist, 12,* 601–609. doi:10.1634/theoncologist.12-5-601

Lieberman, P. (2005). Biphasic anaphylactic reactions. *Annals of Allergy, Asthma and Immunology, 95,* 217–226. doi:10.1016/S1081-1206(10)61217-3

Madrigal-Burgaleta, R., Berges-Gimeno, M.P., Angel-Pereira, D., Ferreiro-Monteagudo, R., Guillen-Ponce, C., Pueyo, C., ... Alvarez-Cuesta, E. (2013). Hypersensitivity and desensitization to antineoplastic agents: Outcomes of 189 procedures with a new short protocol and novel diagnostic tools assessment. *Allergy, 68,* 853–861. doi:10.1111/all.12105

Makrilia, N., Syrigou, E., Kaklamanos, I., Manolopoulos, L., & Saif, M.W. (2010). Hypersensitivity reactions associated with platinum antineoplastic agents: A systematic review. *Metal-Based Drugs, 2010,* Article 207084. doi:10.1155/2010/207084

Mezzano, V., Giavina-Bianchi, P., Picard, M., Caiado, J., & Castells, M. (2014). Drug desensitization in the management of hypersensitivity reactions to monoclonal antibodies and chemotherapy. *BioDrugs, 28,* 133–144. doi:10.1007/s40259-013-0066-x

Moon, D.H., Lee, J.-M., Noonan, A.M., Annunziata, C.M., Minasian, L., Houston, N., ... Kohn, E.C. (2013). Deleterious BRCA1/2 mutation is an independent risk factor for carboplatin hypersensitivity reactions. *British Journal of Cancer, 109,* 1072–1078. doi:10.1038/bjc.2013.389

Pichler, W.J. (2006). Adverse side-effects to biologic agents. *Allergy, 61,* 912–920. doi:10.1111/j.1398-9995.2006.01058.x

Polovich, M., Olsen, M., & LeFebvre, K.B. (Eds.). (2014). *Chemotherapy and biotherapy guidelines and recommendations for practice* (4th ed.). Pittsburgh, PA: Oncology Nursing Society.

Popa, V.T., & Lerner, S.A. (1984). Biphasic systemic anaphylactic reaction: Three illustrative cases. *Annals of Allergy, 53,* 151–155.

Posadas, S.J., & Pichler, W.J. (2007). Delayed drug hypersensitivity reactions—New concepts. *Clinical and Experimental Allergy, 37,* 989–999. doi:10.1111/j.1365-2222.2007.02742.x

Schwartz, J.R., Bandera, C., Bradley, A., Brard, L., Legare, R., Granai, C.O., & Dizon, D.S. (2007). Does the platinum-free interval predict the incidence or severity of hypersensitivity reactions to carboplatin? The experience from Women and Infants' Hospital. *Gynecologic Oncology, 105,* 81–83. doi:10.1016/j.ygyno.2006.10.047

Simons, F.E.R., Ardusso, L.R.F., Biló, M.B., El-Gamal, Y.M., Ledford, D.K., Ring, J., ... Thong, B.Y. (2011). World Allergy Organization guidelines for the assessment and management of anaphylaxis. *World Allergy Organization Journal, 4,* 13–37. doi:10.1097/WOX.0b013e318211496c

Tham, E.H., Cheng, Y.K., Tay, M.H., Alcasabas, A.P., & Shek, L.P.-C. (2015). Evaluation and management of hypersensitivity reactions to chemotherapy agents. *Journal of Postgraduate Medicine, 91,* 145–150. doi:10.1136/postgradmedj-2014-132686

Thompson, L.M., Eckmann, K., Boster, B.L., Hess, K.R., Michaud, L.B., Esteva, F.J., ... Barnett, C.M. (2014). Incidence, risk factors, and management of infusion-related reactions in breast cancer patients receiving trastuzumab. *Oncologist, 19,* 228–234. doi:10.1634/theoncologist.2013-0286

Tole, J.W., & Lieberman, P. (2007). Biphasic anaphylaxis: Review of incidence, clinical predictors, and observation recommendations. *Immunology and Allergy Clinics of North America, 27,* 309–326. doi:10.1016/j.iac.2007.03.011

Viale, P.H. (2009). Management of hypersensitivity reactions: A nursing perspective. *Oncology, 23*(2, Suppl. 1), 26–30. Retrieved from http://www.cancernetwork.com/oncology-journal/management-hypersensitivity-reactions-nursing-perspective

Viale, P.H., & Yamamoto, D.S. (2010). Biphasic and delayed hypersensitivity reactions: Implications for oncology nursing. *Clinical Journal of Oncology Nursing, 14,* 347–356. doi:10.1188/10.CJON.347-356

Vogel, W.H. (2010). Infusion reactions: Diagnosis, assessment, and management [Online exclusive]. *Clinical Journal of Oncology Nursing, 14,* E10–E21. doi:10.1188/10.CJON.E10-E21

Wing, M. (2008). Monoclonal antibody first dose cytokine release syndromes—Mechanisms and prediction. *Journal of Immunotoxicology, 5,* 11–15. doi:10.1080/15476910801897433

Wong, J.T., Ling, M., Patil, S., Banerji, A., & Long, A. (2014). Oxaliplatin hypersensitivity: Evaluation, implications of skin testing, and desensitization. *Journal of Allergy and Clinical Immunology: In Practice, 2,* 40–45. doi:10.1016/j.jaip.2013.08.011

Zanotti, K.M., & Markman, M. (2001). Prevention and management of antineoplastic-induced hypersensitivity reactions. *Drug Safety, 24,* 767–779. doi:10.2165/00002018-200124100-00005

Chapter 24 Study Questions

1. Which of the following statements is NOT true?
   A. As cumulative exposure to a drug increases, the number of hypersensitivity reactions (HSRs) also can increase.
   B. Drug reactions often produce immediate HSRs and most often involve immunoglobulin E (IgE).
   C. Five categories of HSRs exist.
   D. IgE is responsible for degranulation of mast cells and basophils, leading to histamine and cytokine release.

2. Which of the following chemotherapy agents frequently is linked to HSRs?
   A. Platinum
   B. Methotrexate
   C. 5-Fluorouracil
   D. Vincristine

3. The subjective signs and symptoms of an HSR involve multiple symptoms. The patient may complain of:
   A. Generalized itching and chest tightness.
   B. Nausea or crampy abdominal pain.
   C. Anxiety and/or an impending sense of doom.
   D. Desire to urinate or defecate.
   E. All of the above.

4. HSRs can be immediate or delayed. Delayed reactions can be biphasic and have been observed up to 24 hours or more after the initial presentation of HSR. Which of the following is the most likely cause of a biphasic reaction?
   A. The type of agent administered
   B. Inadequate initial treatment of the original reaction
   C. Administration of the agent too quickly
   D. Administration of the agent in a normal saline solution

5. Pharmacologic prophylaxis is recommended to reduce the frequency and severity of HSR. Which of the following strategies often is recommended prior to administration of specific agents?
   A. Dexamethasone
   B. Diphenhydramine
   C. H_2 antagonist
   D. Opioids
   E. All except D

CHAPTER

25 Oncologic Emergencies

Colleen M. O'Leary, MSN, RN, AOCNS®, and Diana McMahon, MSN, RN, OCN®

Introduction

Cancer remains the second leading cause of death in the United States, with an estimated 1,685,210 new cases in 2016 and accounting for almost 600,000 annual deaths (American Cancer Society, 2016). Cancer-related emergencies can occur any time during the disease trajectory and often are the initial indication of cancer. These emergent conditions can occur because of the cancer itself or as a result of cancer treatment. Timely recognition of oncologic emergencies with swift interventions can prolong survival and improve quality of life for patients with cancer. Different resources list a variety of conditions that can be considered oncologic emergencies that are beyond the scope of this text. This chapter will focus on six common emergent conditions seen in patients with cancer. These include sepsis, tumor lysis syndrome, hypercalcemia of malignancy, metastatic spinal cord compression, cardiac tamponade, and superior vena cava syndrome.

Sepsis

Definition

Roger Bone, along with associates of the American College of Chest Physicians and the Society of Critical Care Medicine, defined sepsis as a cluster of symptoms that represent a systemic response to infection (Bone, 1996). Sepsis occurs along a continuum of infection, bacteremia, systemic inflammatory response syndrome (SIRS), septic shock, and multiple organ dysfunction syndrome. It is the leading cause of death among patients with cancer who are receiving chemotherapy (Bos, Smeets, Dumay, & de Jonge, 2013). Prompt recognition and management is critical in the care of patients with cancer.

Incidence

Febrile neutropenia (FN) is the most common cause of sepsis in patients with cancer (O'Leary, 2018). FN occurs in 10%–40% of patients with solid tumors, and the incidence rises to more than 80% in patients with hematologic cancers (Aarts et al., 2013; Flowers et al., 2013). It is widely accepted that more than 50% of patients with FN or bacteremia will develop sepsis. Severe sepsis occurs in 20%–30% of these patients, and septic shock is seen in 5%–10% of patients (Ahn, Lee, Lim, & Lee, 2013; Legrand et al., 2012).

Risk Factors

Granulocytopenia with resulting FN is the most common risk factor for the development of sepsis in patients with cancer (O'Leary, 2018). Other factors that put patients at risk for septic shock are patient-, disease-, or treatment-related (Apostolopoulou, Raftopoulos, Terzis, & Elefsiniotis, 2010; O'Leary, 2018) (see Figure 25-1).

Pathophysiology

The entire pathophysiology of sepsis is not clearly understood. However, what is known is that some type of inflammatory stimulus, usually gram-negative bacteria, triggers a systemic inflammatory response. With this inflammatory response, proinflammatory cytokines are released. A negative feedback system in the immune system causes additional anti-inflammatory cytokines to release in response to the others. In initial stages, the release of all of the cytokines causes arterial dilation, decreasing peripheral artery resistance, which, in turn, increases cardiac output. As the systemic response continues, cardiac output decreases, blood pressure falls, and the typical symptoms of septic shock appear (O'Leary, 2018).

Figure 25-1. Risk Factors for Sepsis

Patient Related
- Age > 65 years
- Age < 1 year

Disease Related
- Febrile neutropenia
- Malignancy (especially lymphoma, leukemia, and multiple myeloma)
- Splenectomy
- Malnutrition
- Hospitalization
- Skin or mucous membrane breakdown

Treatment Related
- Corticosteroids
- Immunosuppressive therapies
- Chemotherapy
- Radiation therapy
- Antibiotic use
- Invasive procedure
- Devices in place

Note. Based on information from Apostolopoulou et al., 2010; O'Leary, 2018.

Clinical Manifestations

The continuum of sepsis has distinct clinical manifestations with each stage (Bone, 1996). The first stage is infection with an inflammatory response of normally sterile environments to the presence of a pathogen. However, in patients who are neutropenic, the only sign of infection may be fever because the number of neutrophils is inadequate to mount a normal inflammatory response. When the pathogen enters the bloodstream, bacteremia occurs, which is determined by positive blood cultures. The next stage SIRS exists when two or more of the following occur: temperature greater than 100.4°F (38°C) or less than 96.8°F (36°C), heart rate greater than 90 beats per minute, respiratory rate greater than 20 breaths per minute or partial pressure of carbon dioxide in arterial blood ($PaCO_2$) less than 32 mm Hg, and white blood cell count greater than 12,000/mm^3 or less than 4,000/mm^3 or more than 10% bands. When the patient meets SIRS criteria and a documented infection is present, the patient is diagnosed with sepsis. With severe sepsis, organ dysfunction, hypoperfusion, or hypertension occurs and is manifested by lactic acidosis, oliguria, or acute mental status changes. Septic shock occurs when hemodynamic stability cannot occur, despite aggressive fluid challenges. The final stage of the sepsis continuum is multiple organ dysfunction syndrome, where the function of one or more organs is altered, resulting in the immediate need for intervention for homeostasis to occur (see Table 25-1).

Assessment

Nurses must include a thorough patient history when assessing for sepsis to help determine possible contributing factors. History should include burns, trauma, infec-

Table 25-1. Clinical Manifestations of Sepsis

Stage	Manifestations
Infection	Inflammatory response (Fever may be the only sign in patients with neutropenia.)
Bacteremia	Inflammatory response and positive blood culture
Systemic inflammatory response syndrome	Two or more of the following: • Temperature > 100.4°F (38°C) or < 96.8°F (36°C) • Heart rate > 90 beats/min • Respiratory rate > 20 breaths/min or partial pressure of carbon dioxide in arterial blood ($PaCO_2$) < 32 mm Hg • White blood cells > 12,000/mm^3 or < 4,000/mm^3 or > 10% bands
Sepsis	Systemic inflammatory response syndrome criteria met Documented infection
Severe sepsis	Organ dysfunction, hypoperfusion, or hypertension with the following: • Lactic acidosis • Oliguria • Acute mental status changes
Septic shock	Hemodynamic instability despite aggressive fluid challenges
Multiple organ dysfunction syndrome	Alteration in function of one or more organs

Note. Based on information from Bone, 1996.

tion, nutritional status, recent blood product administration, surgery (placement of port/central venous catheter), malignancy, immunosuppression, mucositis grades 3–4, HIV, and diabetes. Recent medication history of steroids, antipyretics, chemotherapy, herbals, and antibiotics should be obtained. Medical history also should include any chronic diseases, use of indwelling medical devices, recent surgeries, and cancer treatments, including radiation therapy (Widmeier & Wesley, 2014).

Two tools are commonly used to assess for and detect sepsis: the Acute Physiology and Chronic Health Evaluation (APACHE) and the Modified Early Warning Score (MEWS). The APACHE is most commonly used in intensive care units and is based on 17 physiologic variables with additional points added for age and comorbidities (O'Leary, 2015). The higher the score, the greater the chance of death. This tool often is used to determine the course and aggressiveness of treatment.

The MEWS was first developed as a tool to improve communication between nurses and the medical team when the nurse first detected signs of deterioration in the patient. This tool is used to help determine if a higher level of care is needed and to facilitate that move if necessary. It details specific physical parameters, including blood pressure, pulse, respiratory rate, temperature, and level of consciousness. Each parameter is given a score based on the results of the measure. A MEWS score greater than 4 is associated with an increased risk of death and indicates the need for an immediate move to a higher level of care (O'Leary, 2015).

Management

Because the sepsis continuum is rapidly moving and potentially fatal, it is imperative to manage the clinical manifestations in an organized fashion to have the best outcomes. The Surviving Sepsis Campaign and the Institute for Healthcare Improvement have worked together since 2008 to develop management strategies for sepsis, which were updated in 2015 (Dellinger, 2015). They describe care bundles that indicate what interventions should be put into place within specific time frames. According to these management bundles, within the first three hours of determination of sepsis, the healthcare team should determine lactate level, obtain blood cultures prior to antibiotic administration, administer broad-spectrum antibiotics, and administer 30 ml/kg of crystalloid for hypotension or increased lactate (Dellinger, 2015). It is important to accomplish all of the interventions because they each may indicate or affect different outcomes. Lactate is measured because a lactate level greater than 4 mmol/L indicates organ hypoperfusion even in patients with a normal blood pressure and may be the first indication of impending sepsis with organ dysfunction (O'Leary, 2018).

Additional interventions also should be accomplished within six hours of a sepsis diagnosis. These include administering vasopressors if hypotension does not respond to initial fluid resuscitation, reassessing volume status and tissue perfusion with documentation of results, and remeasuring the lactate level (Dellinger, 2015). Vasopressors are used with continued hypotension to maintain a mean arterial pressure greater than 65 mm Hg. A central venous catheter is needed if arterial hypotension continues or the lactate is greater than 4 mmol/L in order to measure a central venous pressure (CVP) of greater than 8 mm Hg and central venous oxygen saturation ($ScvO_2$) greater than 70% (Dellinger, 2015). Reassessment of volume status can be accomplished by either a repeat focused examination after initial fluid resuscitation to include vital signs, cardiopulmonary status, capillary refill, pulse, and skin findings or two of the following: measurement of CVP, measurement of $ScvO_2$, bedside cardiovascular ultrasound, or dynamic assessment of fluid responsiveness with passive leg raise or fluid challenge (Dellinger, 2015).

Finally, in addition to these more urgent bundles, the Surviving Sepsis Campaign and the Institute for Healthcare Improvement describe a management bundle that can be started at the onset of sepsis and should be completed within 24 hours. These interventions include administering a low-dose corticosteroid when the addition of vasopressors does not maintain blood pressure, maintaining a blood glucose between the lower limit of normal and 180 mg/dl, and, for mechanically ventilated patients, maintaining an inspiratory plateau pressure of 30 cm H_2O or less (Dellinger et al., 2013).

Nursing Interventions

Hand hygiene remains the most effective tool for prevention of infections. Nurses should be the model of good hand hygiene with their patients. Oral care with gentle brushing, flossing, and bland oral rinses can help to prevent oral mucosal breakdown. It is important to avoid placement of catheters when possible and to remove Foley catheters as soon as possible. Injection ports on IV tubing or vascular catheters should be scrubbed with an appropriate antiseptic before access. Sterile dressings should be applied to vascular access devices. Catheter sites should be inspected and palpated for tenderness regularly. Implanted port needles should be changed every seven days. IV administration sets should be changed every 96 hours or when compromised or soiled. Encouraging yearly influenza vaccine for patients, as well as receiving the influenza vaccine, is important (Wilson et al., 2007). Employing evidence-based preventive strategies, along with thorough assessment and rapid identification of infection and sepsis, is critical for positive patient outcomes (see Figure 25-2).

Figure 25-2. Nursing Interventions for Prevention of Sepsis

- Practice proper hand hygiene.
- Perform oral care.
- Avoid indwelling catheters when possible.
- Remove Foley catheters as soon as possible.
- Scrub the hub of injection ports with antiseptic prior to accessing.
- Place sterile dressings on vascular access devices.
- Inspect and palpate catheter sites for tenderness regularly.
- Change implanted port needles every 7 days.
- Change IV administration sets every 96 hours or when compromised or soiled.
- Encourage yearly influenza vaccine for patients.
- Receive yearly influenza vaccine.
- Ensure rapid recognition of sepsis.

Note. Based on information from Wilson et al., 2017; Zitella et al., 2014.

Patient Education

The first step in preventing sepsis is rigorous attention to prevention of infections in patients with cancer. It is important to teach patients, families, and caregivers interventions to prevent infection, especially during neutropenic periods. Education should include the potential for neutropenia, as well as the potential for sepsis if left unchecked. If sepsis occurs, patients and families should be educated regarding the treatments and potential outcomes, including the risk of death if not managed appropriately.

Tumor Lysis Syndrome

Definition

Tumor lysis syndrome (TLS) is an oncologic emergency associated with the breakdown of tumors following chemotherapy. When tumor cells are destroyed, they release massive amounts of potassium, phosphorus, and uric acid into the circulation, resulting in hyperkalemia, hyperphosphatemia, secondary hypocalcemia, and hyperuricemia and their associated metabolic changes. When these metabolic changes occur in the setting of cancer chemotherapy, it generally is accepted to be TLS (Mirrakhimov, Voore, Khan, & Ali, 2015).

Incidence

The incidence of TLS varies depending on the type of cancer. The most common malignancies associated with TLS include the hematologic malignancies with a large number of rapidly growing tumor cells that are sensitive to chemotherapy. High-grade acute lymphoblastic leukemia (ALL) carries the greatest risk (Wilson & Berns, 2014). In addition to ALL, other malignancies associated with TLS include acute myeloid leukemia (AML) and Burkitt lymphoma (Abu-Alfa & Younes, 2010; Howard, Jones, & Pui, 2011). Although much less common, cases have been reported of TLS associated with radiation therapy, dexamethasone treatment, thalidomide therapy, and newer biologic therapies, including bortezomib and rituximab (Bose & Qubaiah, 2011).

Risk Factors

TLS risk is determined by a number of factors, including the patient's age, type and stage of the cancer, lactate dehydrogenase (LDH) level, white blood cell count, baseline renal function, and comorbidities (Cairo, Coiffier, Reiter, & Younes, 2010). TLS is most frequently associated with aggressive hematologic malignancies but has been seen in highly proliferative solid tumors as well. Hematologic cancers that put patients at the highest risk include ALL, AML, and Burkitt lymphoma. Solid tumors that have been associated with TLS include small cell lung cancer, germ cell tumors, inflammatory breast cancer, melanoma, and testicular cancer (Lewis, Hendrickson, & Moynihan, 2011). Elevated LDH and impaired renal function also place patients at higher risk for TLS (Cairo et al., 2010) (see Figure 25-3).

Figure 25-3. Risk Factors for Tumor Lysis Syndrome

- Advanced age
- Lactate dehydrogenase > 2 × upper limit of normal
- White blood cell count ≥ 100,000/mm³
- Renal insufficiency
- Renal failure
- Dehydration
- Preexisting uremia or hyperuricemia
- Decreased urine flow
- Acidic urine
- Highly proliferative solid tumors
  - Small cell lung cancer
  - Germ cell tumors
  - Inflammatory breast cancer
  - Melanoma
  - Testicular cancer
- Acute lymphoblastic leukemia
- Acute myeloid leukemia
- Burkitt lymphoma

Note. Based on information from Cairo et al., 2010; Lewis et al., 2011.

Pathophysiology

TLS occurs most commonly after antineoplastic therapy but can occur spontaneously in very large tumors. When tumor cells are broken down, intracellular materials are released into the extracellular areas. These materials include potassium, phosphorus, and uric acid. The kidneys usually are able to compensate for the release of these agents, but with the rapid degradation of cells, the kidneys can become overwhelmed and unable to remove these electrolytes. When this happens, hyperkalemia with ensuing hypocalcemia, hyperuricemia, and hyperphosphatemia occurs. In addition, calcium and uric acid can precipitate in the renal tubules, causing crystals to form, which can lead to acute kidney injury, thus worsening the clearance of toxins (Ñamendys-Silva et al., 2015).

Clinical Manifestations

As stated, the clinical manifestations of TLS occur as a result of electrolyte abnormalities, including hyperkalemia, hyperphosphatemia, hyperuricemia, and hypocalcemia.

Hyperkalemia

Defined as serum potassium greater than 6 mEq/L or an increase of 25% from baseline, hyperkalemia occurs 6–72 hours following cytotoxic therapy (McCurdy & Shanholtz, 2012). Hyperkalemia can manifest as muscle cramps, fatigue, anorexia, paresthesias, and cardiac dysfunction. It can potentially be the deadliest of TLS consequences, depending on the degree of imbalance. Several electrocardiographic changes can occur, ranging from mild changes to complete heart block, ventricular tachycardia, ventricular fibrillation, and asystole.

Hyperphosphatemia

The amount of phosphorus in tumor cells is four times that in normal cells (Wagner & Arora, 2014). Because of this, when tumor cells are broken down, hyperphosphatemia may occur. Hyperphosphatemia is defined as serum phosphate of 4.5 mg/dl or greater or a 25% increase from baseline and occurs 24–48 hours after initiation of therapy. Increasing rates of serum phosphorus can lead to renal failure and secondary hypocalcemia (Sarno, 2013). When the phosphorus level rises significantly, patients may experience nausea, vomiting, lethargy, and seizures. Severely elevated levels can lead to a greater risk of calcium deposits in the renal tubules and heart, which can lead to renal failure and cardiac arrhythmias. Symptoms include tetany, muscle spasm, paresthesias, and seizures, which occur because of increased neuromuscular and cardiac excitability.

Hypocalcemia

Hypocalcemia can occur secondary to hyperphosphatemia because of the precipitation of phosphate with calcium into tissue. Hypocalcemia is defined as a calcium level below 2.1 mmol/L. The patient can be asymptomatic. However, when symptoms occur, they are classified as muscular, cardiovascular, and neurologic. Muscular symptoms include muscle cramps and spasms, paresthesias, and tetany. Cardiovascular symptoms include ventricular arrhythmia, heart block, and hypotension. Confusion, delirium, hallucinations, and seizures are neurologic symptoms that can occur. Rarely, more severe symptoms may occur, which include bradycardia, cardiac failure, coma, and death (Pi et al., 2016).

Hyperuricemia

Hyperuricemia is defined as serum uric acid of 8 mg/dl or greater or a 25% increase from baseline three days before or seven days after initiation of therapy (Cairo et al., 2010). Uric acid is normally cleared by the kidneys, but with the rapid rise in uric acid following tumor cell lysis, the kidneys are overwhelmed and uric acid crystals begin to form. Symptoms of hyperuricemia include nausea, vomiting, diarrhea, anorexia, and acute kidney failure (McCurdy & Shanholtz, 2012). If uric acid stones form, patients also can experience severe flank pain.

Assessment

Assessment for TLS should begin with a complete history and physical. Baseline laboratory values include complete blood count with platelets, renal functions, electrolytes, uric acid, and LDH. Assessment is divided into laboratory TLS and clinical TLS (Cairo et al., 2010). Currently, TLS is defined as a 25% increase in uric acid, potassium, or phosphorus and/or a 25% decrease in calcium within three days prior to or seven days after initiation of treatment (Cairo et al., 2010). Absolute values for these electrolytes are also critical. These include uric acid of 8 mg/dl or greater, potassium of 6 mg/dl or greater, phosphorus of 4.5 mg/dl or greater, or calcium of 7 mg/dl or less (Cairo et al., 2010).

Clinical assessment for TLS includes monitoring for symptoms of electrolyte imbalances together with the laboratory values. In addition, a creatinine of 1.5 times or more the upper limit of normal, seizure, cardiac arrhythmia, or sudden death are defined as clinical TLS (Cairo et al., 2010).

Management

Prevention is the key to management of TLS. Prevention strategies should always be implemented in patients at high risk for TLS. Hydration is the hallmark preventive strategy. IV fluids should be initiated 24–48 hours prior to start of therapy and continue for as long as 72 hours after therapy with a goal of maintaining urine output greater than 100 ml/hr (Pession et al., 2011). Pharmacologic therapy should include the hypouricemic agents such as allopurinol and rasburicase. Allopurinol works by blocking the transformation of hypoxanthine and xanthine to uric acid. Administration of allopurinol should begin up to three days before therapy (Kennedy, Koontz, & Rao, 2011). Rasburicase is an enzyme that causes rapid reduction in uric acid by converting uric acid to a more water-soluble state (Bose & Qubaiah, 2011). Whereas allopurinol only reduces uric acid levels after treatment is initiated, rasburicase can also lower preexisting hyperuricemia.

Regardless of vigorous preventive measures, some patients will still develop TLS. It is important to routinely monitor serum electrolyte level. Management of electrolyte imbalances is required. Electrolyte replacements should be given to bring levels back to normal. If correcting electrolyte levels is not possible, dialysis may be warranted. Dialysis is started for potassium levels greater than 7 mEq/L, uric acid levels greater than 10 mg/dl, or phosphorus levels greater than 10 mg/dl along with increasing blood urea nitrogen and creatinine levels (Lewis et al., 2011).

Nursing Interventions

Nursing management of TLS can be categorized into three main areas: prevention, early detection, and symptom management. Prevention of TLS is a key nursing role. Interventions that fall into this category include identifying patients at high risk for TLS, reviewing current medications, and removing additional sources of potassium and phosphorus (Mackiewicz, 2012). Vigilant monitoring of vital signs, intake and output, and weight is critical for early detection. Additionally, reviewing and noting any changes in electrolytes or urinalysis is warranted. Symptom management activities include monitoring electrocardiogram changes, providing vigorous hydration and diuresis, managing medications, and implementing possible seizure precautions (Mackiewicz, 2012) (see Figure 25-4).

Patient Education

Nurses play a crucial role in monitoring and recognizing signs of TLS. Nurses should provide information to patients and families about the possibility of TLS, including associated signs and symptoms of fluid and electrolyte imbalances. It is important to educate patients and families about taking allopurinol or rasburicase as ordered.

Hypercalcemia of Malignancy

Definition

Hypercalcemia is a complex metabolic disorder and defined as serum calcium level greater than 11 mg/dl or ionized serum calcium level greater than 1.29 mmol/L (Evenepoel et al., 2010; Rosner & Dalkin, 2012). Hypercalcemia can present as a life-threatening metabolic emergency.

Incidence

Hypercalcemia is a significant and common oncologic complication, occurring in up to 30% of patients with cancer (Rosner & Dalkin, 2012). It is the most common metabolic disorder associated with cancer. In early stages of cancer, the incidence is less than 5%, but it is identified most often in advanced stages of disease and recognized as a sign of poor prognosis (Rosner & Dalkin, 2012).

Risk Factors

Hypercalcemia can occur in patients with hematologic cancers and solid tumors. The most common malignancies associated with hypercalcemia include lung, breast, and renal cell cancer, multiple myeloma, and T-cell lymphoma and leukemia. Hypercalcemia also occurs in patients with head and neck, gynecologic, and prostate cancer. Bisphosphonate treatment in patients with metastatic bone disease may decrease the incidence of hypercalcemia (see Figure 25-5).

Pathophysiology

Calcium is the most plentiful mineral in the body and vital in maintaining cell mem-

Figure 25-4. Nursing Interventions for Tumor Lysis Syndrome

Prevention	Early Detection	Symptom Management
• Identify patients at risk. • Review current medications. • Remove additional sources of potassium and phosphorus.	• Monitor vital signs. • Monitor intake and output. • Monitor weight. • Review changes in electrolytes and urinalysis.	• Monitor electrocardiogram changes. • Institute vigorous hydration. • Promote diuresis. • Manage medications. • Implement seizure precautions.

Note. Based on information from Mackiewicz, 2012.

Figure 25-5. Risk Factors for Hypercalcemia of Malignancy

- Secondary to secretion of parathyroid hormone-related protein due to the following cancers:
  - Squamous cell (e.g., lung)
  - Renal
  - Ovarian
  - Endometrial
  - Lymphoma
  - Breast
- Bone metastasis with osteolytic lesions due to the following:
  - Breast cancer
  - Multiple myeloma
  - Lymphoma
- Leukemia
- Ectopic hyperparathyroidism
- Vitamin D–secreting lymphomas

Note. Based on information from Rosner & Dalkin, 2012; Wagner & Arora, 2014.

brane permeability (muscle contraction, nerve and brain function), bone formation, and blood coagulation. Serum calcium levels indicate both ionized and bound forms of the mineral. While 99% of the body's calcium is stored in bones and teeth, 1% circulates in the bloodstream and is regulated by hormones, the kidneys, and bones. Approximately half of the total serum calcium is bound to proteins, mainly albumin, and is inactive, whereas the other 50% is found in the form of free ions and is biologically active (Perrone & Monteiro, 2016). The kidneys play an important role in calcium homeostasis. When disease such as cancer causes destruction of bone, the kidneys will attempt to compensate by increasing calcium exertion significantly before the increased calcium overwhelms renal compensatory mechanisms, resulting in hypercalcemia (Rosner & Dalkin, 2012). Bone is always in the process of remodeling. Osteoblast cells are responsible for bone formation, and osteoclasts are responsible for bone resorption or breakdown. Hypercalcemia results when osteoclasts increase the bone resorption, resulting in excess blood calcium that the kidneys cannot excrete (Rosner & Dalkin, 2012).

Hypercalcemia in patients with cancer can be related to different mechanisms but most commonly is caused by the release of parathyroid hormone-related peptide (PTHrP) from tumor cells and less often by the release of substances from tumor cells that activate vitamin D. This release results in increased blood calcium levels, production of proteins that stimulate osteoclasts and inhibit osteoblasts (most common with metastatic cancer or multiple myeloma), dehydration and kidney insufficiency or failure, and decreased physical activity (Rosner & Dalkin, 2012). Less frequently, tumor cells produce cytokines that can lead to calcium reabsorption, causing osteoclasts to be active at the site of tumor cells, resulting in the breakdown of bones and an increased calcium level (Rosner & Dalkin, 2012).

Clinical Manifestations

The symptoms of hypercalcemia can develop slowly and may be unrelated to the actual calcium level. Older patients often experience more symptoms than younger patients. Prompt treatment of hypercalcemia is important not only to relieve symptoms but also to improve the patient's quality of life and ensure continuation of the cancer treatment. Hypercalcemia can be fatal if untreated (Rosner & Dalkin, 2012).

Symptoms of hypercalcemia can be nonspecific and attributed to the primary disease or treatment. Signs and symptoms of hypercalcemia involve many different systems, including the following (Pi et al., 2016):

- Neurologic: headache, restlessness, lethargy, changes in mental status including confusion and disorientation, seizures, coma
- Musculoskeletal: fatigue, bone pain, pathologic fractures, myopathy
- Cardiac: irregular heartbeat, heart attack, electrocardiogram changes

- Gastrointestinal: anorexia, nausea, vomiting, constipation, abdominal pain
- Renal: polyuria, polydipsia, renal failure

Assessment

Assessment for hypercalcemia includes a thorough history. Specific information related to hypercalcemia of malignancy includes the patient's symptoms, disease status, and treatment and medication regimens. Symptoms that have a rapid onset are more commonly associated with hypercalcemia of malignancy. Disease status may be indicative as more advanced disease and metastatic bone disease can contribute to hypercalcemia.

Laboratory tests for hypercalcemia may include serum calcium, ionized (total) calcium, serum albumin, and parathyroid hormone level (PTHrP). Ionized calcium is the most dependable test for hypercalcemia, with results greater than 1.29 mmol/L considered elevated (Evenepoel et al., 2010). However, if this test is not available, the serum calcium may be estimated using a formula that adjusts for decreases in serum albumin. It is important to review the patient's albumin results when using the total serum calcium level, as a decreased level can give a false-normal result. A corrected calcium level can be calculated using the total serum calcium and albumin levels.

No absolute calcium level exists at which all patients become symptomatic; rather, the rate of rise appears to be more significant. Patients tolerate fairly high calcium levels if the increase is gradual (Behl, Hendrickson, & Moynihan, 2010). The PTHrP level should not be used to direct the initial management of hypercalcemia; however, it may be helpful along the treatment trajectory (Behl et al., 2010).

Management

Treatment of the underlying disease is critical in patients with hypercalcemia. Patients presenting with hypercalcemia may be approaching the last weeks of life if effective treatment for the underlying cancer diagnosis is not available. The management of hypercalcemia is dependent on symptoms, the underlying disease, and laboratory results. The degree of symptoms helps to guide interventions (see Table 25-2). Initially, fluid replacement will begin rehydration and diuresis to promote excretion of calcium from the kidneys and dilute the serum (Lewis et al., 2011). Hydration alone may not be able to correct hypercalcemia.

Bisphosphonates may inhibit bone loss and decrease the risk of skeletal-related events. In addition to being the first-line treatment for cancer-related hypercalcemia, IV bisphosphonates may be administered routinely in the management of patients with metastatic bone disease to decrease osteoclastic activity (Dietzek, Connelly, Cotugno, Bartel, & McDonnell, 2015). Calcitonin may be administered intramuscularly or subcutaneously to decrease serum calcium levels by inhibiting osteoclasts in the bone and increasing urinary excretion of the mineral. Corticosteroids may be given in conjunction to allow for a longer effect of the calcitonin (Mirrakhimov, 2015). Because of its rapid onset of action, calcitonin may serve as a safety net while other treatment modalities are reaching their therapeutic effect (Mirrakhimov, 2015). Finally, denosumab, a fully humanized monoclonal antibody, has been effective in inhibiting osteoclast production and survival (Mirrakhimov, 2015). This subcutaneous injection is administered every four weeks and has the potential to cause severe hypocalcemia, usually seen within two to four days after administration (Mirrakhimov, 2015).

Nursing Interventions

Nursing care for patients with hypercalcemia is directed at prevention and early detection. Preventive measures for high-risk patients include hydration and mobilization with emphasis on safety (see Figure 25-6).

Table 25-2. Nursing Interventions for Hypercalcemia of Malignancy

Category	Interventions
Mild, asymptomatic hypercalcemia	Administer additional fluids, usually intravenously. Establish effective bowel plan. Promote ambulation and other weight-bearing activities. Eliminate medications that elevate calcium, including thiazide diuretics, nonsteroidal anti-inflammatory drugs, and over-the-counter medications containing calcium.
Moderate to severe hypercalcemia	Treat underlying cancer. Initiate fluid replacement. Administer bisphosphonate medications to decrease or stop the breakdown of bone; consider denosumab if hypercalcemia is refractory to bisphosphonates. Administration of calcitonin with or without steroid medication may decrease the breakdown of bone and the uptake of calcium from food (in some types of cancer, such as lymphoma); however, steroid side effects must be considered. Consider dialysis to treat patients with renal failure related to severe hypercalcemia.

Note. Based on information from Lewis et al., 2011; Rosner & Dalkin, 2012; Wagner & Arora, 2012.

Figure 25-6. Safety Measures for Patients With Hypercalcemia of Malignancy

- Assistance with ambulation as needed
- Bed position/side rails for patients with mental status changes
- Transfer devices for immobile patients to decrease risk of fractures
- Seizure precautions for severely elevated calcium levels

Identifying patients at risk, monitoring vital signs and laboratory values, reviewing medications, performing a physical assessment, and looking for signs of dehydration, weight loss, loss of muscle strength, and mental status changes are key. Hypercalcemia therapy may include fluid and electrolyte replacement. Patients are at risk for electrolyte imbalance, fatigue, acute confusion, falls, and nausea, thus suggesting the need for careful assessment of renal, neurologic, gastrointestinal, cardiac, and musculoskeletal changes. Patient and caregiver education is crucial, as well as providing emotional support during a complicated treatment regimen, usually with an advanced disease process.

Patient Education

Patients and caregivers must be familiar with the symptoms of hypercalcemia and the need to promptly report them to their healthcare provider. Cancer-related hypercalcemia is not caused by having too much calcium in the diet, so patients must be instructed that decreasing dietary calcium intake is not helpful.

In addition to adhering to the medical management of hypercalcemia, patients should be advised to maintain good fluid intake, control nausea and vomiting, maintain physical activity (including weight-bearing activity), check with a healthcare provider before taking over-the-counter medications (some can increase calcium levels), and follow up for laboratory testing to monitor calcium levels and renal function (Lewis et al., 2011).

Metastatic Spinal Cord Compression

Definition

Metastatic spinal cord compression (MSCC) is a relatively common emergent condition associated with advanced cancer. It is defined as a compression to the cord itself or the spinal nerves and nerve roots by either metastatic lesions or direct invasion into the cord, which can cause neurologic impairment (Farrell, 2013).

Incidence

An estimated 20,000 patients develop MSCC each year in the United States (Becker & Baehring, 2015). Patients with solid tumors have a higher incidence of metastasis to the spine, with cancers of the breast, lung, and prostate having the highest incidence, each accounting for approximately 15%–20% of cases (Lewis et al., 2011). Because people are living longer with cancer, the incidence of MSCC is likely to increase (Harel & Angelov, 2010).

Risk Factors

Several factors are considered when determining risk of developing MSCC. The two most common risk factors are tumor type and patient age. Patients with tumors that have a high risk of spreading to the bones, such as breast, lung, and prostate, are at a higher risk for MSCC. The timing of MSCC development differs by type of cancer. In patients with breast cancer, MSCC generally develops later in the course of the disease—on average, 43 months after diagnosis (Becker & Baehring, 2015). However, in other diseases, such as lung cancer, especially non-small cell lung cancer, multiple myeloma, and non-Hodgkin lymphoma, MSCC may be the first indication of disease (Becker & Baehring, 2015). Generally, patients in their 40s through 60s are at a greater risk for development of MSCC (Becker & Baehring, 2015).

Pathophysiology

MSCC can occur via three different processes. The most common way is when a metastatic tumor mass presses against and compresses the spinal cord by expanding into the vertebral body and epidural space. A second process is when the tumor erodes the vertebral body, causing it to collapse and send bone fragments into the epidural space. The third and least common process occurs when the tumor directly invades the vertebral space without destruction of bone (Kaplan, 2013).

Clinical Manifestations

Back pain for a prolonged period of time often is the first symptom in 90%–98% of patients with MSCC (Bowers, 2015). Because back pain can precede other symptoms by up to four months, misdiagnosis is a risk. Therefore, MSCC should be considered in anyone who has known spinal metastasis or cancer and develops new back pain (National Institute for Health and Care Excellence [NICE], n.d.). Symptoms of MSCC are dependent on the area of the spine where the compression occurs. Pain in the thoracic and cervical spine is uncommon in other conditions and thus should be considered a red flag in people with a history of cancer (Bowers, 2015). Patients with lower spinal pain often present with localized spinal tenderness, spinal pain aggravated by straining, or nighttime spinal pain preventing sleep (Bowers, 2015; NICE, n.d.). A hallmark sign of MSCC is pain that intensifies when raising legs in a supine position and often is rated at a high number. When left untreated, pain from MSCC can quickly develop into neurologic symptoms. The next most common symptom is limb weakness to the point where the patient is unable to ambulate unassisted (Bowers, 2015). Motor deficits are more common than sensory deficits. However, when a lesion is within two nerve root levels, sensory deficits often occur. Once neurologic symptoms start, they can quickly develop into paralysis from which patients rarely recover even with treatment (Bowers, 2015). Some patients experience other neurologic symptoms without ever experiencing spinal pain. These include increased difficulty walking, altered sensation in the limbs, or new, unexplained bladder or bowel problems (Bowers, 2015; NICE, n.d.).

Assessment

Assessment for MSCC should include both physical and diagnostic evaluations. A thorough history should also be obtained as part of the physical assessment. A comprehensive pain assessment as part of the history should include onset, location, intensity, quality, exacerbating and relieving factors, prior interventions for relief of pain, and use of any pain-relieving medications (Ferrell, 2010). Prior and current cancer history should be obtained, as well as a comprehensive medication list including over-the-counter medications, herbal remedies, and nutritional supplements. Additionally, exploration of preexisting and comorbid conditions is warranted.

Physical examination should include assessment of back pain, as well as musculoskeletal, sensory, and autonomic function. The musculoskeletal assessment encompasses observation of posture, spinal curvature, gait, and coordination. Evaluation of the patient's ability to sense pain, temperature, light touch, vibration, and position (proprioception) is included in the sensory assessment. Any changes in bowel and bladder function are important aspects in assessing autonomic function.

Historically, plain radiographic studies, myelography, bone scans, and positron-emission tomography have all been used to diagnose MSCC. However, magnetic resonance imaging (MRI) has been determined to be the gold standard for diagnosis (Bowers, 2015).

Management

In 2014, NICE reviewed its guidelines for the care of patients with MSCC (Bowers, 2015). According to NICE, MSCC should be considered a medical emergency and necessitates admission to the hospital. Additional recommendations include use of bed rest with log-rolling, administration of dexamethasone 16 mg daily while awaiting treatment swelling along with a protein pump inhibitor, provision of adequate pain control, and, most importantly, an MRI of the total spine within 24 hours (Bowers, 2015). The steroids are given to help reduce pressure caused by spinal cord edema, thus relieving pain and improving neurologic symptoms.

Treatment modalities include surgery, radiation therapy, and symptom management. Surgery should only be used in patients with a good prognosis and life expectancy of more than three months. Indicators that surgery could be beneficial are a histologic finding of multiple myeloma, lymphoma, or breast, prostate, or renal cancers; good motor function at presentation; good performance status; limited comorbidity; single-level spinal disease; absence of visceral metastasis; and a long interval from primary diagnosis (Bowers, 2015). However, a majority of patients diagnosed with MSCC do not meet these criteria and therefore would be unsuitable for surgery. Radiation therapy is the most common treatment and should begin within 24 hours of MSCC diagnosis. Radiation therapy is given to relieve compression of the spine and nerve roots. It is very effective at providing pain relief and improving or stabilizing neurologic deficits.

Nursing Interventions

Nursing care should begin with emotional support for patients and families. Pain management is vital and can include nonsteroidal anti-inflammatory drugs, steroids, and nonopioid and opioid analgesia. Nurses can help to protect the spinal cord by maintaining patients in a flat position with neutral spine alignment and gradually assisting them to sitting. Other supportive interventions would include thromboprophylaxis, meticulous skin care to prevent pressure ulcers, and management of bladder and bowel function, as well as managing circulatory and respiratory function (Agency for Healthcare Research and Quality, 2012) (see Figure 25-7).

Figure 25-7. Nursing Interventions for Metastatic Spinal Cord Compression

- Emotional support for patients and families
- Pain management
  - Nonsteroidal anti-inflammatory drugs
  - Steroids
  - Nonopioid analgesia
  - Opioid analgesia
- Protection of spinal cord
  - Flat position with neutral spine alignment
  - Gradual assistance to sitting position
- Supportive interventions
  - Thromboprophylaxis
  - Pressure ulcer prevention
  - Management of bowel and bladder function
  - Management of circulatory function
  - Management of respiratory function

Note. Based on information from Agency for Healthcare Research and Quality, 2012.

Patient Education

Patient education should include risks for MSCC and the signs and symptoms to report to healthcare providers. Once a diagnosis is confirmed, teaching should include pain management and safety and mobility issues. Upon discharge to home, patients and families need to be educated about bowel and bladder regimens, patient safety, rehabilitation, and medications.

Cardiac Tamponade

Definition

Cardiac tamponade is a compression of the heart that occurs when blood or fluids accumulate in the pericardial sac. The excess pressure from the fluid prevents the heart from functioning properly, resulting in increased intrapericardial pressure and decreased cardiac output. Cardiac tamponade in patients with cancer is rarely an initial presenting symptom; however, it is life threatening and requires immediate care.

Incidence

Pericardial disease is present in 7%–12% of patients with cancer (Lestuzzi, 2010). Pericardial effusion is the most common manifestation of malignant pericardial disease, but cardiac tamponade is the most serious complication. As cancer screening and treatment have improved, more patients with cancer are living longer, increasing the prevalence of pericardial neoplastic disease (Scheinin & Sosa-Herrera, 2014).

Risk Factors

Primary tumors of the pericardium are rare but include mesothelioma and sarcomas (Patel & Sheppard, 2011). Cancers that most frequently metastasize to the pericardium by direct local extension include lung, breast, and esophageal cancers, whereas melanoma, leukemia, and lymphoma more commonly spread via the blood or lymphatic system. Additionally, patients may develop pericardial disease related to chemotherapy toxicity, radiation greater than 4,000 cGy to the chest, and opportunistic infections (Refaat & Katz, 2011).

Pathophysiology

The heart is enclosed in a two-layer protective sac called the pericardium. The pericardial space lies between the parietal and visceral layers. This space holds up to 50 ml of fluid that acts as a lubricant. A pericardial effusion results as fluids accumulate, causing a decrease in left ventricular filling, increased pressure, and compression of the heart muscle and decreased cardiac output. The rate and volume of fluid accumulation, as well as the health of the pericardium, affect the hemodynamic impact of the increase in pressure.

Fluid accumulation in the pericardial space can develop slowly or rapidly. The pericardial sac may stretch to accommodate up to 2 L of fluid if the accumulation occurs slowly over a period of time, whereas a rapid accumulation of fluid can make a patient symptomatic at 100 ml (Kaplan, 2018). Toxicities related to pericardial effusion are scored on a 1–5 scale, with cardiac tamponade considered a grade 4 (Story, 2013).

Clinical Manifestations

Neoplastic cardiac tamponade can go undetected until a substantial decrease occurs in cardiac output. It can have a variety of clinical presentations depending on the fluid volume and rate of accumulation. Tamponade classically presents with the Beck triad: hypotension, elevated jugular venous pressure, and diminished heart sounds. However, many patients will not present with all three symptoms. Patient complaints may be nonspecific, but exertional dyspnea, tachycardia, and chest discomfort are most frequently noted. Other signs of tamponade include pulsus paradoxus (greater than 10 mm Hg variation in systolic pressure with inspiration), a classic "water bottle" silhouette of the heart, electrocardiogram changes, peripheral edema, pericardial rub, and hepatomegaly (Lewis et al., 2011).

Assessment

A complete patient history is an important component of the assessment. A patient with a known primary tumor of the heart, a tumor that extends into the pericardium, or an obstruction of mediastinal lymph nodes may warrant closer evaluation. In addition, patients who have had chemotherapy (especially anthracyclines, interferon, interleukin, and granulocyte macrophage–colony-stimulating factor), radiation to the mediastinum, or comorbidities such as heart disease, connective tissue disorders, tuberculosis, and history of cardiac surgery may have additional indicators that necessitate a thorough cardiac evaluation (Story, 2013).

Physical assessment coupled with the appropriate diagnostic studies is key to diagnosing neoplastic cardiac tamponade, as it can mimic other diseases, including congestive heart failure. Cardiac tamponade is most commonly and accurately diagnosed with echocardiography. Other diagnostic tests include chest x-ray, electrocardiogram, computed tomography, and MRI. A percutaneous pericardiocentesis may be performed with a large effusion or tamponade so that the source of the fluid can be assessed for transudate versus exudate. This also may decrease symptoms temporarily. Figure 25-8 lists components of the cardiopulmonary assessment in cardiac tamponade (Kaplan, 2018; Story, 2013).

Management

The immediate goals of treatment are to remove the accumulated fluid and reverse the hemodynamic effects of tamponade. Medical management will be determined by the patient's current status, tumor type, responsiveness to cancer treatments, and comorbid conditions. Fluid resuscitation may be appropriate for hypovolemic patients who present hemodynamically unstable. However, fluids also could increase an already elevated intrapericardial pressure and further compromise coronary perfusion. Treatment modalities for neoplastic cardiac tamponade include pericardiocentesis to provide immediate relief of symptoms and the mechanical constriction of

Figure 25-8. Cardiopulmonary Assessment in Cardiac Tamponade

- Blood pressure
- Pulse
- Heart rhythm and sounds
- Pulse pressures
- Jugular vein distention
- Respiratory status and lung sounds
- Perfusion
- Hemodynamic pressures
- Electrolyte abnormalities

Note. Based on information from Story, 2013.

tamponade; however, reaccumulation of fluid within as soon as 48 hours has been noted (Scheinin & Sosa-Herrera, 2014). Pericardial instillation of sclerosing or chemotherapy agents can be used to mechanically prevent the reaccumulation of fluids by promoting adhesion of the pericardial layers. Radiation therapy or chemotherapy is used for disease control if the tumor is sensitive to the treatment modality. Surgical treatments such as a pericardiotomy are used to create a "pericardial window," or a pericardioperitoneal shunt to drain fluid from the pericardial sac to the pleural or peritoneal space.

Nursing Interventions

Nurses play an important role in recognizing the signs and symptoms of cardiac tamponade so that patients can receive prompt diagnostic evaluation and appropriate treatment for this life-threatening event. Nursing assessment should focus on the patient's cardiac and respiratory status, altered tissue perfusion, pain, and anxiety. Monitoring and reporting subtle changes in heart sounds and vital signs along with assessment of pulsus paradoxus and jugular venous pressure are crucial for the recognition of tamponade progression.

Physical features and symptoms often are confused with other conditions, so knowledge of the patient's history is essential. Frequent assessment of cardiopulmonary status is crucial to early identification and intervention in cardiac tamponade (see Figure 25-8). Without intervention, late signs and symptoms of cardiac tamponade (see Figure 25-9) will eventually lead to heart failure and cardiac arrest.

Nurses should carefully maintain optimal pulmonary status, including administering oxygen as ordered, elevating the head of the bed, encouraging energy-conserving activities, and promoting respiratory hygiene. Supporting cardiac status may include IV fluids, vasopressors, comfort measures, and medications for pain and anxiety. Preparing patients for invasive procedures and encouraging relaxation techniques may further reduce psychosocial distress and the workload of the heart.

Figure 25-9. Late Signs and Symptoms of Cardiac Tamponade

- Dyspnea at rest
- Orthopnea
- Increased retrosternal chest pain or heaviness may disappear
- Mental status changes
- Cyanosis
- Hoarseness, dysphagia
- Coughing
- Hiccups
- Anxiety and sense of impending doom
- Apprehension
- Tachycardia (greater than 100 beats/min)
- Increased jugular vein distention
- Muffled/absent heart sounds
- Friction rub
- Narrowed pulse pressure
- Pulsus paradoxus > 10 mm Hg
- Oliguria
- Peripheral edema
- Beck triad (increased central venous pressure, hypotension, and distant heart sounds)

Note. Based on information from Kaplan, 2018; Story, 2013.

Patient Education

Patients at risk for cardiac tamponade should be able to identify the early signs and symptoms of malignant pericardial disease and report changes to their healthcare provider immediately. Education to help patients and families minimize the severity of the symptoms and maximize safety includes assistance with activities of daily living, paced ambulation/activities to decrease energy expenditure, oxygen therapy as needed, elevation of the head of the bed while resting, and medication management of pain and dyspnea. A serious condition such as cardiac tamponade can increase patient and family anxiety; thus, emotional support and a calm environment are crucial.

Superior Vena Cava Syndrome

Definition

Superior vena cava syndrome (SVCS) is a composite of signs and symptoms resulting from an internal or external obstruction of the superior vena cava due to tumor or thrombus. The obstruction results in decreased blood return to the heart, decreased cardiac output, and increased venous congestion and edema.

Incidence

Although benign diseases can cause SVCS, malignant disease accounts for more than two-thirds of adult cases (Wilson, Detterbeck, & Yahalom, 2007). Almost 75% of all cancer-related SVCS diagnoses are attributed to bronchogenic cancer, most frequently small cell lung cancer (Rice, Rodriguez, & Light, 2006). Lymphomas (15%) and metastatic disease (7%), especially breast tumors, are significant contributors to the development of SVCS (Rice et al., 2006).

Risk Factors

Oncologic risk factors for SVCS include disease- and treatment-related complications. Malignant diseases related to this syndrome include breast, lung, and esophageal cancers, in addition to lymphoma and metastatic disease. Central vascular access devices commonly used in the treatment of cancer put patients at risk for line thrombosis, which can result in an internal superior vena cava vessel obstruction. Prior radiation therapy to the mediastinum also contributes to the risk for SVCS (McNally, 2018).

Pathophysiology

The superior vena cava is a thin-walled, low-pressure major blood vessel that carries venous drainage from the head and upper extremities to the heart. This vessel is surrounded by relatively rigid structures in the mediastinum, including multiple lymph nodes. SVCS results when an obstruction blocks the superior vena cava vessel, interfering with venous return to the heart. Tumors or enlarged lymph nodes may externally obstruct the vessel, whereas a thrombus or clot may occlude the vessel internally. SVCS results in increased venous pressure and decreased cardiac output (McNally, 2018).

Clinical Manifestations

SVCS usually has a slow onset, and although clinical presentation may be alarming, early symptoms are usually not life threatening. Collateral circulation may develop and divert blood around the obstruction, delaying the onset of symptoms. Symptoms of SVCS can be divided into common early signs and late signs and symptoms (see Figure 25-10).

Figure 25-10. Signs and Symptoms of Superior Vena Cava Syndrome

Common
- Cough (productive or nonproductive)
- Dyspnea
- Hoarseness
- Dysphagia
- Difficulty buttoning shirt collar
- Neck and thoracic vein distention
- Discoloration of thoracic area
- Facial erythema
- Edema of head, neck, and upper extremities

Late
- Cyanosis of the face and upper torso
- Decreased or absent peripheral pulses
- Congestive heart failure
- Decreased blood pressure
- Chest pain
- Mental status changes, including irritability and lethargy
- Tachypnea, tachycardia, or orthopnea
- Orbital edema
- Visual disturbances
- Syncope
- Stridor
- Severe headache

Note. Based on information from Koetters, 2012; McNally, 2018.

Assessment

SVCS may be the presenting symptom of malignancy or may develop in a patient with a cancer diagnosis. A thorough patient history is key to revealing the cause and severity of symptoms (McNally, 2018). Because SVCS is most commonly associated with lung cancer, patients without a cancer diagnosis should be questioned regarding smoking habits, environmental exposures, and previous radiation to the mediastinum to identify risk factors for cancer. Additionally, patients with a recent vascular access device insertion, history of preexisting coronary disease, hypertension, or heart failure may be at increased risk for SVCS (McNally, 2018).

Patients with cancer most frequently present with upper body edema and shortness of breath. Blood pressure may be high in the arms and low in the legs. The identification of patients at risk for SVCS should focus on the presence of symptoms that require timely intervention to prevent airway compromise or cerebral edema (Lepper et al., 2011). Blockage of the superior vena cava may be seen on chest radiography, computed tomography of the chest, MRI of the chest, coronary angiography, Doppler ultrasound, and radionuclide ventriculography (Colen, 2008). IV contrast dye study is used to identify central line thrombosis (Colen, 2008).

Management

Management of SVCS includes treatment of the underlying cause and presenting symptoms. Treatment and prognosis are dependent on the cause of the obstruction. SVCS may require radiation or chemotherapy to decrease the size of a tumor mass. Radiation is frequently considered the standard treatment for obstructive SVCS and may provide symptom relief within three to four days (Koetters, 2012). However, chemotherapy is the most common treatment for SVCS caused by small cell lung cancer (Koetters, 2012). A stent may need to be placed to decompress an occluded vessel. Steroids and diuretics can be used to temporarily relieve edema and respiratory distress. Thrombolytic treatment is administered for central line complications.

Nursing Interventions

The goals of nursing care include identification and careful assessment of high-risk patients. Respiratory, cardiac, and neurologic examinations can provide a baseline for disease management and complications. Patients may have increased anxiety because of respiratory symptoms requiring supportive management, including oxygen therapy, a calm environment, and assistance with activities of daily living to decrease energy expenditure. In addition, a 45° elevation of the head of the bed, monitoring of input and output, daily laboratory studies and weight, and assessment of skin integrity may be indicated. If the SVCS is life threatening, patients may be intubated.

Patient Education

Patients and caregivers should be taught to recognize and report symptoms to their healthcare provider immediately. Nurses should advise patients on basic symptom management techniques to decrease respiratory distress, including elevation of the head of the bed, use of oxygen as ordered, paced activities, antianxiety medications if needed, and ensuring environmental safety, including the use of a walker and removal of floor rugs. Additionally, removing rings, avoiding restrictive clothing, and elevating upper extremities to promote venous return may help to reduce symptoms related to circulatory compromise.

Conclusion

The most common oncologic emergencies include sepsis, TLS, hypercalcemia, MSCC, cardiac tamponade, and SVCS. These syndromes are seen throughout the cancer trajectory. Nurses need to be keenly aware of the signs and symptoms of oncologic emergencies for early identification and intervention to obtain the best outcomes for patients.

References

Aarts, M.J., Peters, F.P., Mandigers, C.M., Derksen, M.W., Stouthard, J.M., Nortier, H.J., … Tjan-Heijnen, V.C.G. (2013). Primary granulocyte colony-stimulating factor prophylaxis during the first two cycles only or throughout all chemotherapy cycles in patients with breast cancer at risk for febrile neutropenia. *Journal of Clinical Oncology, 31,* 4290–4296. doi:10.1200/JCO.2012.44.6229

Abu-Alfa, A.K., & Younes, A. (2010). Tumor lysis syndrome and acute kidney injury: Evaluation, prevention, and management. *American Journal of Kidney Diseases, 55*(5, Suppl. 3), S1–S13. doi:10.1053/j.ajkd.2009.10.056

Agency for Healthcare Research and Quality. (2012). *Guideline summary: Metastatic spinal cord compression. Diagnosis and management of adults at risk of and with metastatic spinal cord compression.* Retrieved from https://www.guideline.gov/content.aspx?id=14326

Ahn, S., Lee, Y.-S., Lim, K.S., & Lee, J.-L. (2013). Adding procalcitonin to the MASCC risk-index score could improve risk stratification of patients with febrile neutropenia. *Supportive Care in Cancer, 21,* 2303–2308. doi:10.1007/s00520-013-1787-6

American Cancer Society. (2016). *Cancer facts and figures 2016.* Retrieved from http://www.cancer.org/acs/groups/content/@research/documents/document/acspc-047079.pdf

Apostolopoulou, E., Raftopoulos, V., Terzis, K., & Elefsiniotis, I. (2010). Infection probability score, APACHE II and Karnofsky scoring systems as predictors of bloodstream infec-

Key Points

- Sepsis is seen on a continuum from infection to multiple organ dysfunction syndrome.
- Rapid identification of sepsis is critical in reducing mortality.
- Three-hour and six-hour intervention bundles should guide management decisions.
- TLS is more common in hematologic malignancies and solid tumors with high tumor burden.
- TLS occurs most often after treatment begins as a result of tumor destruction and the release of tumor by-products into the circulation.
- TLS is characterized by hyperkalemia, hyperphosphatemia, hypocalcemia, and hyperuricemia.
- Hypercalcemia is the most common metabolic disorder associated with cancer and occurs in up to 30% of patients with cancer.
- Bisphosphonate and denosumab treatment in patients with metastatic bone disease may decrease the incidence of hypercalcemia.
- MSCC most often occurs later in the disease trajectory.
- Prompt recognition and treatment of MSCC is imperative to avoid potentially irreversible paralysis and increased mortality.
- Cardiac tamponade is a potentially life-threatening condition that can result from the malignant process, the metastatic process, or the cancer treatment itself.
- Tamponade classically presents with the Beck triad: hypotension, elevated jugular venous pressure, and diminished heart sounds.
- Oncologic risk factors for SVCS include malignant disease, as well as treatment-related complications, such as central vascular access devices and prior radiation therapy to the mediastinum.
- SVCS usually has a slow onset, and early symptoms are usually not life threatening; however, advanced symptoms may include life-threatening respiratory distress, cyanosis of the face, tachypnea, syncope, orthopnea, and stridor.

tion onset in hematology-oncology patients. *BMC Infectious Diseases, 10,* 135. doi:10.1186/1471-2334-10-135

Becker, K.P., & Baehring, J.M. (2015). Spinal cord compression. In V.T. DeVita Jr., T.S. Lawrence, & S.A. Rosenberg (Eds.), *Cancer: Principles and practice of oncology* (10th ed., pp. 1816–1821). Philadelphia, PA: Wolters Kluwer Health/Lippincott Williams & Wilkins.

Behl, D., Hendrickson, A.W., & Moynihan, T.J. (2010). Oncologic emergencies. *Critical Care Clinics, 26,* 181–205. doi:10.1016/j.ccc.2009.09.004

Bone, R.C. (1996). The sepsis syndrome: Definition and general approach to management. *Clinics in Chest Medicine, 17,* 175–181. doi:10.1016/S0272-5231(05)70307-5

Bos, M.M.E.M., Smeets, L.S., Dumay, I., & de Jonge, E. (2013). Bloodstream infections in patients with or without cancer in a large community hospital. *Infection, 41,* 949–958. doi:10.1007/s15010-013-0468-1

Bose, P., & Qubaiah, O. (2011). A review of tumour lysis syndrome with targeted therapies and the role of rasburicase. *Journal of Clinical Pharmacy and Therapeutics, 36,* 299–326. doi:10.1111/j.1365-2710.2011.01260.x

Bowers, B. (2015). Recognizing metastatic spinal cord compression. *British Journal of Community Nursing, 20,* 162–165. doi:10.12968/bjcn.2015.20.4.162

Cairo, M.S., Coiffier, B., Reiter, A., & Younes, A. (2010). Recommendations for the evaluation of risk and prophylaxis of tumour lysis syndrome (TLS) in adults and children with malignant diseases: An expert TLS panel consensus. *British Journal of Haematology, 149,* 578–586. doi:10.1111/j.1365-2141.2010.08143.x

Colen, F.N. (2008). Oncologic emergencies: Superior vena cava syndrome, tumor lysis syndrome and spinal cord compression. *Journal of Emergency Nursing, 34,* 535–537. doi:10.1016/j.jen.2007.09.012

Dellinger, R.P. (2015). The Surviving Sepsis Campaign: Where have we been and where are we going? *Cleveland Clinic Journal of Medicine, 82,* 237–244. doi:10.3949/ccjm.82gr.15001

Dellinger, R.P., Levy, M.M., Rhodes, A., Annane, D., Gerlach, H., Opal, S.M., ... Moreno, R. (2013). Surviving Sepsis Campaign: International guidelines for management of severe sepsis and septic shock, 2012. *Intensive Care Medicine, 39,* 165–228. doi:10.1007/s00134-012-2769-8

Dietzek, A., Connelly, K., Cotugno, M., Bartel, S., & McDonnell, A.M. (2015). Denosumab in hypercalcemia of malignancy: A case series. *Journal of Oncology Pharmacy Practice, 21,* 143–147. doi:10.1177/1078155213518361

Evenepoel, P., Bammens, B., Claes, K., Kuypers, D., Meijers, B.K.I., & Vanrenterghem, Y. (2010). Measuring total blood calcium displays a low sensitivity for the diagnosis of hypercalcemia in incident renal transplant recipients. *Clinical Journal of the American Society of Nephrology, 5,* 2085–2092. doi:10.2215/CJN.02460310

Farrell, C. (2013). Bone metastases: Assessment, management and treatment options. *British Journal of Nursing, 22*(Suppl. 7), S4–S11. doi:10.12968/bjon.2013.22.Sup7.S4

Ferrell, B. (2010, November 4). Pain management at the end of life. Retrieved from http://www.medscape.com/viewarticle/731405

Flowers, C.R., Seidenfeld, J., Bow, E.J., Karten, C., Gleason, C., Hawley, D.K., ... Ramsey, S.D. (2013). Antimicrobial prophylaxis and outpatient management of fever and neutropenia in adults treated for malignancy: American Society of Clinical Oncology clinical practice guideline. *Journal of Clinical Oncology, 31,* 794–810. doi:10.1200/JCO.2012.45.8661

Harel, R., & Angelov, L. (2010). Spine metastasis: Current treatments and future directions. *European Journal of Cancer, 46,* 2696–2707. doi:10.1016/j.ejca.2010.04.025

Howard, S.C., Jones, D.P., & Pui, C.-H. (2011). The tumor lysis syndrome. *New England Journal of Medicine, 364,* 1844–1854. doi:10.1056/NEJMra0904569

Kaplan, M. (2013). Spinal cord compression. In M. Kaplan (Ed.), *Understanding and managing oncologic emergencies: A resource for nurses* (2nd ed., pp. 337–383). Pittsburgh, PA: Oncology Nursing Society.

Kaplan, M. (2018). Cardiac tamponade. In C.H. Yarbro, D. Wujcik, & B.H. Gobel (Eds.), *Cancer nursing: Principles and practice* (8th ed., pp. 1075–1094). Burlington, MA: Jones & Bartlett Learning.

Kennedy, L.D., Koontz, S., & Rao, K. (2011). Emerging role of rasburicase in the management of increased plasma uric acid levels in patients with hematologic malignancies. *Journal of Blood Medicine, 2011*(2), 1–6. doi:10.2147/JBM.S9648

Koetters, K.T. (2012). Superior vena cava syndrome. *Journal of Emergency Nursing, 38,* 135–138. doi:10.1016/j.jen.2010.08.019

Legrand, M., Max, A., Peigne, V., Mariotte, E., Canet, E., Azowlay, E., ... Debrumetl, A. (2012). Survival in neutropenic patients with severe sepsis or septic shock. *Critical Care Medicine, 40,* 43–49. doi:10.1097/CCM.0b013e31822b50c2

Lepper, P.M., Ott, S.R., Hoppe, H., Schumann, C., Stammberger, U., Bugalho, A., ... Hamacher, J. (2011). Superior vena cava syndrome in thoracic malignancies. *Respiratory Care, 56,* 653–666. doi:10.4187/respcare.00947

Lestuzzi, C. (2010). Neoplastic pericardial disease: Old and current strategies for diagnosis and management. *World Journal of Cardiology, 2,* 270–279. doi:10.4330/wjc.v2.i9.270

Lewis, M.A., Hendrickson, A.W., & Moynihan, T.J. (2011). Oncologic emergencies: Pathophysiology, presentation, diagnosis, and treatment. *CA: A Cancer Journal for Clinicians, 61,* 287–314. doi:10.3322/caac.20124

Mackiewicz, T. (2012). Prevention of tumor lysis syndrome in an outpatient setting. *Clinical Journal of Oncology Nursing, 16,* 189–193. doi:10.1188/12.CJON.189-193

McCurdy, M.T., & Shanholtz, C.B. (2012). Oncologic emergencies. *Critical Care Medicine, 40,* 2212–2222. doi:10.1097/CCM.0b013e31824e1865

McNally, G.A. (2018). Superior vena cava syndrome. In C.H. Yarbro, D. Wujcik, & B.H. Gobel (Eds.), *Cancer nursing: Principles and practice* (8th ed., pp. 1187–1195). Burlington, MA: Jones & Bartlett Learning.

Mirrakhimov, A.E. (2015). Hypercalcemia of malignancy: An update of pathogenesis and management. *North American Journal of Medical Sciences, 7,* 483–493. doi:10.4103/1947-2714.170600

Mirrakhimov, A.E., Voore, P., Khan, M., & Ali, A.M. (2015). Tumor lysis syndrome: A clinical review. *World Journal of Critical Care Medicine, 4*(2), 130–138. doi:10.5492/wjccm.v4.i2.130

Ñamendys-Silva, S.A., Arredondo-Armenta, J.M., Plata-Menchaca, E.P., Guevara-García, H., García-Guillén, F.J., Rivero-Sigarroa, E., & Herrera-Gómez, A. (2015). Tumor lysis syndrome in the emergency department: Challenges and solutions. *Open Access Emergency Medicine, 7,* 39–44. doi:10.2147/OAEM.S73684

National Institute for Health and Care Excellence. (n.d.). Metastatic spinal cord compression overview. Retrieved from https://pathways.nice.org.uk/pathways/metastatic-spinal-cord-compression

O'Leary, C. (2015). Neutropenia and infection. In C.G. Brown (Ed.), *A guide to oncology symptom management* (2nd ed., pp. 483–504). Pittsburgh, PA: Oncology Nursing Society.

O'Leary, C. (2018). Septic shock. In C.H. Yarbro, D. Wujcik, & B.H. Gobel (Eds.), *Cancer nursing: Principles and practice* (8th ed., pp. 1135–1151). Burlington, MA: Jones & Bartlett Learning.

Patel, J., & Sheppard, M.N. (2011). Primary malignant mesothelioma of the pericardium. *Cardiovascular Pathology, 20,* 107–109. doi:10.1016/j.carpath.2010.01.005

Perrone, D., & Monteiro, M. (2016). The chemistry of calcium. In V.R. Preedy (Ed.), *Calcium: Chemistry, analysis, function and effects* (pp. 67–74). Washington, DC: Royal Society of Chemistry.

Pession, A., Masetti, R., Gaidano, G., Tosi, P., Rosti, G., Aglietta, M., … Pane, F. (2011). Risk evaluation, prophylaxis, and treatment of tumor lysis syndrome: Consensus of an Italian expert panel. *Advances in Therapy, 28,* 684–697. doi:10.1007/s12325-011-0041-1

Pi, J., Kang, Y., Smith, M., Earl, M., Norigian, Z., & McBride, A. (2016). A review in the treatment of oncologic emergencies. *Journal of Oncology Pharmacy Practice, 22,* 625–638. doi:10.1177/1078155215605661

Refaat, M.M., & Katz, W.E. (2011). Neoplastic pericardial effusion. *Clinical Cardiology, 34,* 593–598. doi:10.1002/clc.20936

Rice, T.W., Rodriguez, R.M., & Light, R.W. (2006). The superior vena cava syndrome: Clinical characteristics and evolving etiology. *Medicine, 85,* 37–42. doi:10.1097/01.md.0000198474.99876.f0

Rosner, M.H., & Dalkin, A.C. (2012). Onco-nephrology: The pathophysiology and treatment of malignancy-associated hypercalcemia. *Clinical Journal of the American Society of Nephrology, 7,* 1722–1729. doi:10.2215/CJN.02470312

Sarno, J. (2013). Prevention and management of tumor lysis syndrome in adults with malignancy. *Journal of the Advanced Practitioner in Oncology, 4,* 101–106.

Scheinin, S.A., & Sosa-Herrera, J. (2014). Cardiac tamponade resembling an acute myocardial infarction as the initial manifestation of metastatic pericardial adenocarcinoma. *Methodist DeBakey Cardiovascular Journal, 10,* 124–128. doi:10.14797/mdcj-10-2-124

Story, K.T. (2013). Cardiac tamponade. In M. Kaplan (Ed.), *Understanding and managing oncologic emergencies: A resource for nurses* (2nd ed., pp. 43–68). Pittsburgh, PA: Oncology Nursing Society.

Wagner, J., & Arora, S. (2014). Oncologic metabolic emergencies. *Emergency Medicine Clinics of North America, 32,* 509–525. doi:10.1016/j.emc.2014.04.003

Widmeier, K., & Wesley, K. (2014). Infection detection: Identifying and understanding sepsis in the prehospital setting. *Journal of Emergency Medical Services, 39,* 34–37.

Wilson, B.J., Ahmed, F., Crannell, C.E., Crego, W., Dixon, K., Erb, C.H., … Zitella, L. (2017, January 25). Putting evidence into practice: Prevention of infection. Retrieved from https://www.ons.org/practice-resources/pep/prevention-infection

Wilson, F.P., & Berns, J.S. (2014). Tumor lysis syndrome: New challenges and recent advances. *Advances in Chronic Kidney Disease, 21,* 18–26. doi:10.1053/j.ackd.2013.07.001

Wilson, L.D., Detterbeck, F.C., & Yahalom, J. (2007). Superior vena cava syndrome with malignant causes. *New England Journal of Medicine, 356,* 1862–1869. doi:10.1056/NEJMcp067190

Zitella, L.J., Erb, C.H., Hammer, M.J., Peterson, M.E., & Wilson, B.J. (2014). Prevention of infection. In M. Irwin & L.A. Johnson (Eds.), *Putting evidence into practice: A pocket guide to cancer symptom management* (pp. 211–232). Pittsburgh, PA: Oncology Nursing Society.

Chapter 25 Study Questions

1. What is the most common cause of sepsis in patients with cancer?
   A. Poor performance status
   B. Advanced age
   C. Neutropenia
   D. Thrombocytopenia

2. What is NOT a hallmark sign of tumor lysis syndrome?
   A. Hypokalemia
   B. Hyperphosphatemia
   C. Hypocalcemia
   D. Hyperuricemia

3. The symptoms of hypercalcemia can develop slowly and may be unrelated to the actual calcium level.
   A. True
   B. False

4. An *early* sign of metastatic spinal cord compression is:
   A. Limb weakness.
   B. Gait disturbances.
   C. Severe constipation.
   D. Back pain.

5. Malignant cardiac tamponade symptoms may be nonspecific, but the most frequent patient complaints include:
   A. Exertional dyspnea.
   B. Tachycardia.
   C. Chest discomfort.
   D. All of the above.

6. Superior vena cava syndrome is most frequently associated with:
   A. Breast cancer.
   B. Bronchogenic cancer.
   C. Lymphoma.
   D. Metastatic disease.

CHAPTER

26 Pain

Suzanne Walker, CRNP, MSN, AOCN®, BC

Introduction

Pain is one of the most feared symptoms of the cancer experience. More than half of patients with cancer report experiencing pain throughout the disease trajectory. The highest rates occur among patients with advanced cancer. However, up to one-third of patients who have completed curative therapy experience chronic pain as well (National Cancer Institute, 2016; van den Beuken-van Everdingen et al., 2007). Of these patients, more than one-third describe their pain as moderate or severe. Chronic pain may result in sleep disorders, changes in personal relationships, decreases in functional capacity, and loss of work days (Kroenke et al., 2010; McCarberg, Nicholson, Todd, Palmer, & Penles, 2008). Chronic pain has also been linked to higher rates of anxiety and depression, diminished quality of life, and shortened survival (Annagür, Uguz, Apiliogullari, Kara, & Gunduz, 2014; Oliveira et al., 2014; Rayment et al., 2013). Despite these facts, up to one-third of all patients with cancer continue to have inadequately managed pain (Greco et al., 2014).

Numerous barriers exist to adequate pain management in patients with cancer. Patient-related barriers include fear of addiction, association with disease progression, and concerns about side effects (Kwon, 2014). Provider-related barriers to pain management include poor assessment and lack of knowledge over side effect concerns, as well as fear of addiction (Kwon, 2014). System-related barriers include inhibitory regulatory policies and formulary issues (Cherny, Baselga, de Conno, & Radbruch, 2010) and gaps or deficiencies in prescription drug coverage (Wieder, DeLaRosa, Bryan, Hill, & Amadio, 2014). Cultural barriers may exist as well. A recent meta-analysis of cultural differences between Asian and Western patients with cancer pain revealed that Asian patients may perceive more barriers to cancer pain management than their Western counterparts (Chen, Tang, & Chen, 2012). Meghani, Byun, and Gallagher (2012) noted that African American and Hispanic patients have been identified as more likely to experience pain management disparities than non-minority patients. Nurses are in a key position to assess pain in patients with cancer and to intervene to improve pain control in these vulnerable populations.

Definition

The International Association for the Study of Pain (2012) defines pain as "an unpleasant sensory and emotional experience associated with actual or potential tissue damage, or described in terms of such damage." McCaffery and Pasero further defined pain as "whatever the experiencing person says it is, existing whenever he says it does" (McCaffery & Pasero, 1999, p. 17).

Etiology

Pain may be classified as either acute or chronic. Acute pain typically is construed as pain that has a well-defined source and resolves within six weeks (von Gunten, 2011). Acute pain is usually associated with tissue injury and manifested through an autonomic nervous system response (Brant, 2018). Chronic pain may be defined as pain persisting for more than three months (LeBlanc & Abernethy, 2015). Breakthrough pain implies a temporary flare in otherwise stable pain. The etiology of pain in patients with cancer may be related to the underlying illness or secondary to diagnostic- or treatment-related sequelae. Direct tumor invasion may occur from a primary tumor or metastasis. Treatment-related pain may occur as a result of surgery or other invasive procedures, radiation, or systemic therapies, such as chemotherapy. Procedural pain from surgery may be acute, such as incisional pain, or chronic, as in the case of postmastectomy or post-thoracotomy pain syndromes. Radiation therapy also may cause both acute (e.g., esophagitis, mucositis) and chronic (e.g., brachial plexopathy) types of pain. Examples of pain secondary to systemic therapy include chemotherapy-induced peripheral neuropathy and bone pain from colony-stimulating factors. Chemotherapy agents may induce peripheral neuropathy, a painful condition caused by irritation of the peripheral nerves.

Pathophysiology

Pain is a complex and multidimensional process involving not only physiologic components but also emotional and psychological components (Renn & Dorsey, 2005). The fact that pain pathways in the patient with cancer may be dependent on the type of pain that the individual is experiencing adds to the complexity of this common yet difficult to treat symptom. Adding to the complexity, many patients with cancer experience a combination of pain types, leading to challenges in assessment and management of cancer pain.

Pain may be classified as either nociceptive (somatic or visceral) or neuropathic. Somatic pain is described as pain originating from an identifiable, easily localized source, such as a bone metastasis. This type of pain may be characterized as aching, stabbing, throbbing, or sharp. Visceral pain is not well localized and may be referred to various sites. It may be described as deep or squeezing (Foley, 2005). Pleural involvement secondary to an underlying lung carcinoma is an example of visceral pain. Neuropathic pain results from a lesion or disease of the somatosensory system (International Association for the Study of Pain, 2012) and may be described as burning, electric shock–like, or numbness and tingling (Brunelli et al., 2014). Examples of neuropathic pain include peripheral neuropathy and postmastectomy pain syndrome.

Nociceptive pain occurs when a noxious stimulus activates nociceptors (afferent, or ascending, neurons that sense pain) located on nerve endings on skin, bones, organs, and connective tissue (von Gunten, 2011). The activating pain stimulus may be either exogenous, such as hot objects, or endogenous, such as inflammatory mediators. Two types of nociceptors exist: myelinated A fibers and demyelinated C fibers. The A fibers transmit signals quickly, and the C fibers process signals more slowly (von Gunten, 2011). The signal is then transmitted along these nerve fibers to the dorsal horn of the spinal cord, where f neurotransmitters are released to signal higher-level neurons that communicate via the thalamus with the cerebral cortex and limbic system in the brain. Some of these neurotransmitters include substance P, serotonin, prostaglandins, and endorphins (von Gunten, 2011). The cerebral cortex is where pain interpretation occurs, while the limbic system is responsible for the emotional and affective components of pain (Katz & Rothenberg, 2005). The descending pathways are modulatory pathways in the central nervous system, which may inhibit release of neurotransmitters or impair the function of neurotransmitter receptors. This pathway may alter pain with either inhibition or exacerbation (Renn & Dorsey, 2005). Opioid receptors are located in both ascending and descending pathways (Foley, 2005).

Neuropathic pain involves a dysfunction in the processing of information by either the peripheral or central nervous system (Brant, 2018). The exact mechanism is not well understood and may be multifactorial, including an increase in sodium and calcium channels (Raphael et al., 2010) and stimulation of N-methyl-D-aspartate receptor by glutamate, which can regulate pain transmission (von Gunten, 2011). These changes can result in the phenomena of allodynia (pain elicited by what is normally a nonpainful stimulus) or hyperalgesia (an increased response to a painful stimulus) that may be associated with neuropathic pain.

Assessment

Nurses are in a key position to assess pain in patients with cancer. Assessment tools range from rudimentary linear scales to complex multidimensional questionnaires. The American Pain Society recommends that all patients be routinely screened for pain in addition to undergoing a comprehensive pain assessment and frequent reassessment following interventions (Gordon et al., 2005). Basic pain scales such as visual analog scales, numeric pain intensity scales, and simple descriptive pain intensity scales (see Figure 26-1) are easily administered, one-dimensional measurements of pain. These scales require little investment of time, yet they may fail to capture the multidimensional nature of pain.

Commonly used multidimensional pain assessment tools include the McGill Pain Questionnaire (MPQ) and the Brief Pain Inventory (BPI). The MPQ is an extensive questionnaire that assesses evaluative, sensory, and affective aspects of pain (Melzack, 1975). Drawings of the human body are included for documenting specific locations of pain. The BPI, originally developed as the Wisconsin Brief Pain Questionnaire (Daut, Cleeland, & Flanery, 1983), is a multidimensional assessment tool commonly used for cancer-specific pain (see Figure 26-2). Short versions of both pain scales are available.

Pain may be associated with other symptoms in patients with cancer. McCorkle and Young (1978) developed a symptom distress scale, which assesses multiple symptoms commonly experienced by patients with cancer. In 2001, Dodd et al., coined the term *symptom clusters* to represent the concurrent presentation of multiple symptoms. Other results suggested these clusters could affect functional status and patient outcomes (Dodd et al., 2001). A systematic review of studies on advanced cancers identified pain as part of a cluster along with dyspnea, drowsiness, and fatigue (Dong, Butow, Costa, Lovell, & Agar, 2014). Therefore, assessment of pain in the context of other symptoms is essential, as the symptom of pain may not exist as a sole entity.

Assessment of pain in older adults or cognitively impaired individuals presents distinct challenges to nurses. Traditional pain measurement scales may not be appropriate for use with these patients. Of concern, many of the tools developed for pain assessment in cognitively impaired patients were developed for older adult patients with dementia. Because dementia has varying degrees of symptoms, not all tools will be appropriate for all patients. Other tools have only been tested in the pediatric population or not thoroughly validated. Researchers have found that older adult patients without significant cognitive impairment may find the verbal descriptor scale the most preferable (Peters, Patijn,

Figure 26-1. Visual Pain Rating Scales

Visual Analog Scale

No Pain ____ Worst Imaginable Pain

Numeric Scale

No Pain 0 1 2 3 4 5 6 7 8 9 10 Worst Imaginable Pain

& Lamé, 2007), although Closs, Barr, Briggs, Cash, and Seers (2004) suggested this tool may be beneficial for use in patients with cognitive impairment as well. The Iowa Pain Thermometer is an adapted form of the verbal descriptor scale, also with use in the older adult population (Herr, Spratt, Garand, & Li, 2007). In patients with significant dementia, scales incorporating assessments of behavioral cues, such as the Pain Assessment in Advanced Dementia Scale, the Non-communicative Patient's Pain Assessment Instrument, and the Abbey Pain Scale, have been used (Lukas, Barber, Johnson, & Gibson, 2013).

Management

The World Health Organization (WHO) developed the WHO Pain Ladder, a three-step approach to pain management with recommendations for management of all levels of pain (see Figure 26-3). The ladder begins with the use of non-narcotic opioid analgesics, such as nonsteroidal anti-inflammatory drugs (NSAIDs), and progresses to mild and eventually strong opioid analgesics, with or without an adjuvant medication (WHO, n.d.). Because cancer pain may have different mechanisms of action, a tailored approach to pain management is important.

The Oncology Nursing Society (ONS) Putting Evidence Into Practice (PEP) resources for symptom management have a topic that covers acute, chronic, breakthrough, and intractable types of pain. This resource is periodically updated and revised to provide authoritative direction and guidelines for care of patients with pain due to cancer and its treatment (www.ons.org/practice-resources/pep/pain). Each topic has designated classification schema based on the supporting evidence (or lack thereof) to assist nurses in choosing the best and most effective interventions to treat patients' pain or educate families about different medications and their routes for treatment. Types of approaches and analgesics are provided for subtopics of pain with a list of articles reviewed to categorize the intervention, organized according to the type of article: research evidence, systematic review/meta-analysis, and guideline/expert opinion (Miaskowski et al., 2017).

This section of the chapter will describe various categories of analgesics used for pain management, as well as their mechanism of action and toxicities.

Non-Narcotic Analgesics

According to the WHO ladder, nonopioid analgesics should be considered for mild pain. This includes agents such as NSAIDs and acetaminophen.

Aspirin, or acetylsalicylic acid, was first developed at the end of the 19th century (Botting, 2010). Although aspirin is considered an NSAID, it differs from other NSAIDs through irreversible inhibition of platelet aggregation. It is associated with aspirin-exacerbated respiratory disease, a condition characterized by adult-onset asthma, nasal polyps,

Figure 26-2. Brief Pain Inventory

STUDY ID #:__________ DO NOT WRITE ABOVE THIS LINE HOSPITAL #:__________

Brief Pain Inventory (Short Form)

Date: ____/____/____ Time: _______

Name: __________________ __________________ ______________

Last First Middle Initial

1. Throughout our lives, most of us have had pain from time to time (such as minor headaches, sprains, and toothaches). Have you had pain other than these every-day kinds of pain today?

   1. Yes 2. No

2. On the diagram, shade in the areas where you feel pain. Put an X on the area that hurts the most.

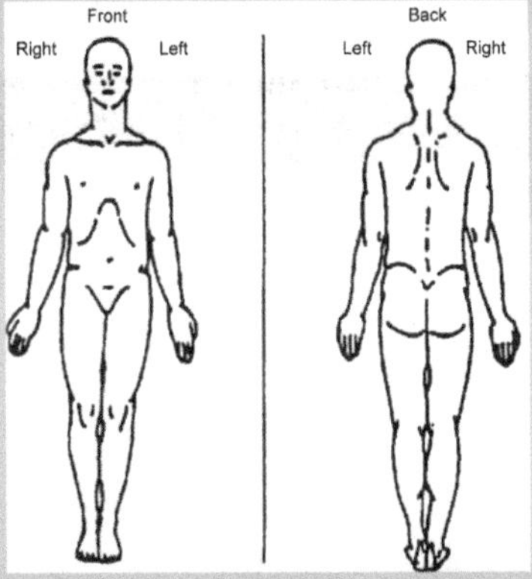

3. Please rate your pain by circling the one number that best describes your pain at its worst in the last 24 hours.

0	1	2	3	4	5	6	7	8	9	10
No Pain										Pain as bad as you can imagine

4. Please rate your pain by circling the one number that best describes your pain at its least in the last 24 hours.

0	1	2	3	4	5	6	7	8	9	10
No Pain										Pain as bad as you can imagine

5. Please rate your pain by circling the one number that best describes your pain on the average.

0	1	2	3	4	5	6	7	8	9	10
No Pain										Pain as bad as you can imagine

6. Please rate your pain by circling the one number that tells how much pain you have right now.

0	1	2	3	4	5	6	7	8	9	10
No Pain										Pain as bad as you can imagine

(Continued on next page)

Figure 26-2. Brief Pain Inventory *(Continued)*

STUDY ID #:__________ DO NOT WRITE ABOVE THIS LINE HOSPITAL #:__________

Date: ____/____/____ Time: ________

Name: ________________ ________________ ________________

Last First Middle Initial

7. What treatments or medications are you receiving for your pain?

8. In the last 24 hours, how much relief have pain treatments or medications provided? Please circle the one percentage that most shows how much relief you have received.

0%	10%	20%	30%	40%	50%	60%	70%	80%	90%	100%
No Relief										Complete Relief

9. Circle the one number that describes how, during the past 24 hours, pain has interfered with your:

A. General Activity

0	1	2	3	4	5	6	7	8	9	10
Does not Interfere										Completely Interferes

B. Mood

0	1	2	3	4	5	6	7	8	9	10
Does not Interfere										Completely Interferes

C. Walking Ability

0	1	2	3	4	5	6	7	8	9	10
Does not Interfere										Completely Interferes

D. Normal Work (includes both work outside the home and housework)

0	1	2	3	4	5	6	7	8	9	10
Does not Interfere										Completely Interferes

E. Relations with other people

0	1	2	3	4	5	6	7	8	9	10
Does not Interfere										Completely Interferes

F. Sleep

0	1	2	3	4	5	6	7	8	9	10
Does not Interfere										Completely Interferes

G. Enjoyment of life

0	1	2	3	4	5	6	7	8	9	10
Does not Interfere										Completely Interferes

Note. Copyright 1991 by Charles S. Cleeland, PhD, Pain Research Group. Used with permission.

rhinosinusitis, and hypersensitivity to aspirin or NSAIDs (Rajan, Wineinger, Stevenson, & White, 2015).

Traditional NSAIDs, or nonselective cyclooxygenase (COX)-1 and COX-2 inhibitors such as ibuprofen and naproxen, inhibit COX-1 and COX-2 enzymes, leading to a reduction in the production of prostanoids, the key regulators of inflammatory pain (Chen, Yang, & Grosser, 2013). Prostaglandins, along with thromboxane A2, are collectively identified as prostanoids. The desired effects of agents that inhibit these compounds include analgesia and anti-inflammation (Gargiulo, Capodanno, Longo, Capranzano, & Tamburino, 2014). Unwanted side effects/toxicities occur in the gastrointestinal, hepatic, cardiovascular, and renal systems, plus effects on blood pressure and platelet aggregation (Ong, Lirk, Tan, & Seymour, 2007). Inhibition of thromboxane A2 produces a temporary impairment of platelet aggregation (Gargiulo et al., 2014). A recent meta-analysis demonstrated an increased risk of venous thromboembolism in NSAID users (Ungprasert, Srivali, Wijarnpreecha, Charoenpong, & Knight, 2015). These results could have significant implications for patients with cancer who, because of their underlying malignancy, may already be at risk for development of venous thromboembolism.

Gastrointestinal adverse effects of NSAIDs include ulcer development and associated sequelae such as nausea, vomiting, heartburn, dyspepsia, strictures, and colitis (Gupta & Eisen, 2009; Lane & Kim, 2006). These untoward effects are a result both of COX-1 inhibition and direct mucosal irritation, although COX-1 inhibition appears to be the most important factor (Sostres, Gargallo, Arroyo, & Lanas, 2010). COX-1 is present in many normal tissues, including the gastrointestinal tract, where it protects the gastric mucosa via prostacyclin.

Toxicity risk factors include advanced age, history of a prior ulcer, concomitant use of corticosteroids or anticoagulants, high doses or combinations of NSAIDs, *Helicobacter pylori* infection, and a serious systemic illness (Sostres et al., 2010; Wolfe, Lichtenstein, & Singh, 1999). Agents shown to reduce the risk of gastroduodenal ulcers in patients receiving

Figure 26-3. World Health Organization Pain Ladder

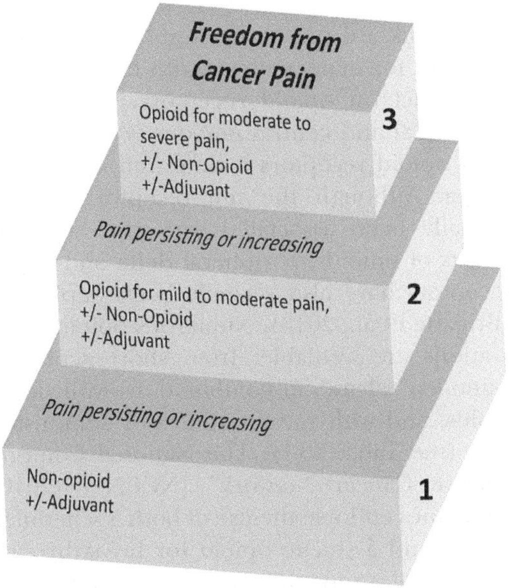

The World Health Organization has developed a three-step "ladder" for cancer pain relief. If pain occurs, there should be prompt oral administration of drugs in the following order: nonopioids (aspirin and paracetamol); then, as necessary, mild opioids (codeine); then strong opioids such as morphine, until the patient is free of pain. To calm fears and anxiety, additional drugs—"adjuvants"—should be used. To maintain freedom from pain, drugs should be given "by the clock"—that is, every 3–6 hours—rather than "on demand." This three-step approach of administering the right drug in the right dose at the right time is inexpensive and 80%–90% effective. Surgical intervention on appropriate nerves may provide further pain relief if drugs are not wholly effective.

Note. From *WHO's Cancer Pain Ladder for Adults*, by World Health Organization. Retrieved from http://www.who.int/cancer/palliative/painladder/en. Copyright 2016 by World Health Organization. Reprinted with permission.

chronic NSAID therapy include misoprostol, double-dose histamine-2 receptor antagonists, and proton pump inhibitors. Of note, dose histamine-2 receptor antagonists have not been proven to prevent complications from ulcers (Lanza, Chan, & Quigley, 2009; Rostom et al., 2002).

Prostaglandins are involved in renal function through the regulation of vascular tone, sodium and water homeostasis, and the release of renin enzyme that controls fluid volume and arterial vasoconstriction. Inhibition of prostaglandins through the use of NSAIDs may cause edema, hypertension, and even acute renal failure in less than 1% of users (Curiel & Katz, 2013; Weir, 2002). Prior to recommending this class of drugs, it is necessary to recognize patients who might be at risk for developing renal toxicity from NSAIDs, such as older adults and those with cirrhosis, congestive heart failure, hypertension, or underlying renal disease, or patients taking concomitant medications such as diuretics or angiotensin-converting enzyme inhibitors (Curiel & Katz, 2013; Weir, 2002). Importantly, a more recent systematic review of regular-dose NSAID use among patients with chronic kidney disease demonstrated no significant progression of chronic kidney disease in this population (Nderitu, Doos, Jones, Davies, & Kadam, 2013).

COX-2 inhibitors are selective inhibitors of the COX-2 enzyme. COX-2, not COX-1, is required for relief of inflammatory pain (Cannon & Cannon, 2012). COX-2 inhibitors have been shown to exhibit less gastrointestinal toxicity than traditional NSAIDs (Jarupongprapa, Ussavasodhi, & Katchamart, 2013). Some studies have demonstrated an increased risk of cardiovascular complications, including myocardial infarction (Coxib and Traditional NSAID Trialists' Collaboration, 2013). Celecoxib is the only COX-2 inhibitor currently available in the United States.

Acetaminophen is a weak analgesic with an unknown mechanism of action (Bandschapp, Filitz, Urwyler, Koppert, & Ruppen, 2011). It is safe and well tolerated as long as dosing follows established guidelines. The most serious adverse effect is hepatotoxicity if dosed improperly. Many combination products for pain management include acetaminophen. Patients should be educated regarding the concomitant use of these products to avoid acetaminophen overdose.

Opioids

Opioids are the cornerstone of pain management for many patients with cancer. These agents act on opioid receptors in both the peripheral and central nervous systems. Common opioid receptors include mu, delta, and kappa. Although the mu receptor has historically been associated with the analgesic effects of opioids, peripheral delta and kappa receptors have also recently been implicated (Brigatte et al., 2013). Numerous opioid preparations are available, from short acting to extended release, in combinations with nonopioids, and with various routes of administration (see Table 26-1). The National Comprehensive Cancer Network® (NCCN®) (2016) guidelines endorse the use of both a scheduled opioid and a rescue opioid for breakthrough pain. Oral preparations are the most common, but other routes may be considered when appropriate (NCCN, 2016).

Morphine is the prototypical opioid because of its familiarity and wide range of available routes of administration, including oral, rectal, and parenteral. The rectal route of morphine has been shown to be an effective route of administration and may be considered for patients at the end of life when alternative routes are inappropriate or unavailable (De Conno et al., 1995; Maloney, Kesner, Klein, & Bockenstette, 1989). Sublingual absorption of morphine has not been shown to be an effective route of administration, and this practice is not recommended (Reisfield & Wilson, 2007). Other commonly used opioids include oxycodone, hydrocodone, fentanyl, oxymorphone, and hydromorphone. Metha-

Table 26-1. Commonly Used Opioids

Name	Route	Strength	Dosing Interval
Fentanyl*	Transdermal	In mcg/hour: 12, 25, 50, 75, 100	72 hrs
	Transmucosal (buccal)	In mcg: 100, 200, 400, 600, 800	4 hrs; may repeat × 1 within 30 min of initial dose
	Transmucosal (buccal)	In mcg: 200, 400, 600, 800, 1,200, 1,600	4 hrs; may repeat × 1 within 30 min of start of initial dose
	Transmucosal (buccal)	In mcg: 200, 400, 600, 800, 1,200	2 hrs; no more than 4 doses/day
	Transmucosal (sublingual)	In mcg: 100, 200, 300, 400, 600, 800	2 hrs; may repeat × 1 after 30 min
	Transmucosal (nasal spray)	In mcg: 100, 400	2 hrs
	Transmucosal (sublingual spray)	In mcg: 100, 200, 400, 600, 800	4 hrs; may repeat × 1 after 30 min
Hydrocodone	Oral	In mg: 20, 30, 40, 60, 80, 100, 120	24 hrs
	Oral	In mg: 10, 15, 20, 30, 40, 50	12 hrs
Hydromorphone	Oral, rectal, parenteral	Oral in mg: 2, 4, 8; also available as oral solution 5 mg/5 ml; Rectal: 3 mg Injection in mg/ml: 1, 2, 4, 10 (Dilaudid HP®)	Oral: 4–6 hrs Rectal: 6–8 hrs Injection: 4–6 hrs
	Oral extended-release	In mg: 8, 12, 16, 32	24 hrs
Morphine sulfate	Oral extended-release	In mg: 30, 45, 60, 75, 90, 120	24 hrs
	Oral sustained-release	In mg: 10, 20, 30, 40, 50, 60, 80, 100, 200	12–24 hrs
	Oral sustained-release	In mg: 15, 30, 60, 100, 200	8–12 hrs
Morphine sulfate immediate-release	Oral immediate-release; solution Parenteral	In mg: 15, 30 Solution: 10 mg/5 ml, 20 mg/5 ml Concentrate: 20 mg/ml Various doses	4 hrs
Oxycodone	Oral controlled-release	In mg: 10, 15, 20, 30, 40, 60, 80	12 hrs
Oxycodone HCl	Oral immediate-release Solution	5 mg 5 mg/ml; 20 mg/ml	4–6 hrs

(Continued on next page)

Table 26-1. Commonly Used Opioids *(Continued)*

Name	Route	Strength	Dosing Interval
Oxymorphone HCl	Oral, parenteral	Oral: In mg: 5, 10 Parenteral: 1 mg/ml	4–6 hrs
	Oral extended-release	In mg: 5, 7.5, 10, 15, 20, 30, 40	12 hrs
Hydrocodone + acetaminophen	Oral	Various strengths/combinations	4–6 hrs
Oxycodone + acetaminophen	Oral	Various strengths/combinations	4–6 hrs

* Fentanyl preparations should be used in opioid-tolerant patients only.

Note. Based on information from Actavis Pharma, Inc., 2014; Cephalon, Inc., 2011, 2013; Depomed, Inc., 2015; Endo Pharmaceuticals Inc., 2014a, 2014b; INSYS Therapeutics, Inc., 2014; Janssen Pharmaceuticals, Inc., 2014; Mallinckrodt Brand Pharmaceuticals, Inc., 2015; *Monthly Prescribing Reference Nurse Practitioners' Edition*, 2015; National Comprehensive Cancer Network, 2016; Pernix Therapeutics, LLC, 2015; Pfizer Inc., 2014; Purdue Pharma L.P., 2014b, 2014c, 2014d; Sentynl Therapeutics, Inc., 2015.

done also may be useful for some patients. The selection of opioid may be based on many factors, including pain level, cost, tolerability, concomitant medications, desired preparation (i.e., immediate or sustained release), or comorbidities. For example, the NCCN (2016) guidelines endorse a cautious approach to the use of morphine, hydromorphone, oxymorphone, hydrocodone, and codeine in patients with unstable renal function because of possible accumulation of toxic metabolites resulting in increased neurotoxicity.

Fentanyl

Fentanyl is available in both transdermal and transmucosal preparations. Transdermal fentanyl is an appropriate alternative opioid when oral opioids are contraindicated. Because transdermal fentanyl takes 20–72 hours to reach peak concentrations after initial application, it is not indicated for acute pain or for opioid-naïve patients (Janssen Pharmaceuticals, Inc., 2014). Transdermal fentanyl has been shown to produce less constipation (Hadley, Derry, Moore, & Wiffen, 2013), as well as less sedation and nausea, than oral morphine (Yang et al., 2010). Impaired absorption could be an issue, especially in patients with cancer cachexia (Heiskanen et al., 2009).

Six transmucosal formulations of fentanyl are also available with indications for treatment of breakthrough cancer pain in patients who are opioid tolerant. Formulations include a sublingual spray, nasal spray, lozenge, buccal tablet, buccal film, and sublingual tablet. Some evidence supports that the transmucosal fentanyl preparations may have superior efficacy compared with morphine sulfate immediate-release preparations (Jandhyala & Fullarton, 2012), as well as a quicker onset of action and improved patient satisfaction (Davies et al., 2013). The nasal spray formulation can have a faster onset of action but shorter duration than the buccal and sublingual transmucosal versions (Twycross, Prommer, Myhalyo, & Wilcock, 2012). Clinicians must be aware that all transmucosal fentanyl preparations are part of a risk evaluation and mitigation strategy (REMS) program (discussed later in chapter).

Methadone

Methadone is a cost-effective oral opioid that has analgesic properties similar to morphine (Nicholson, Watson, Derry, & Wiffen, 2017).

Methadone is uniquely different from morphine because it has variable pharmacokinetics with the potential for cumulative toxicity. Titration and switching from other opioids to methadone can be challenging, and NCCN (2016) recommends consulting a pain or palliative care specialist unless the practitioner has experience with methadone. Additionally, methadone has been found to prolong the QT interval of the electrocardiogram (ECG) for some patients (van den Beuken-van Everdingen, Geurts, & Patijn, 2013). The American Pain Society, in conjunction with the Heart Rhythm Society, has issued recommendations for ECG monitoring in patients prescribed methadone (Chou et al., 2014). Methadone prescriptions should therefore be initiated and managed by healthcare professionals experienced with its use.

Miscellaneous Medications

Tramadol is an analgesic with both opioid and nonopioid (inhibition of serotonin and norepinephrine) properties (Raffa et al., 1992). Even at maximum doses, it is less potent than other opioids (NCCN, 2016). Additionally, a systematic review by Tassinari et al. (2011) found inconclusive data to support the use of tramadol over acetaminophen with codeine for mild to moderate cancer pain.

Transdermal buprenorphine is a partial mu agonist that is approved for severe chronic pain when alternative options are unacceptable. This analgesic can be useful in patients with neuropathic pain or renal impairment, especially with low rates of respiratory depression (Pergolizzi et al., 2009). Transdermal buprenorphine is most appropriate for opioid-naïve patients or those on low-dose opioids because of the risk of withdrawal in patients who have developed opioid dependence (Portenoy & Ahmed, 2014). This group of patients may require referral to a pain specialist (NCCN, 2016). Because QTc prolongation of the ECG can be observed at higher doses, a maximum recommended dose of 20 mcg/hr should not be exceeded (Purdue Pharma L.P., 2014a).

Opioids Not Recommended for Practice

Certain opioids are not useful for the treatment of cancer pain. These include meperidine, propoxyphene, and codeine. Meperidine is converted into its metabolite, normeperidine, which can produce significant neurotoxicity, including seizure activity, with chronic use and in patients with renal insufficiency (Seifert & Kennedy, 2004). A meta-analysis conducted in chronic noncancer pain found no benefit of either codeine or propoxyphene (often administered in conjunction with acetaminophen) compared to NSAIDs or tricyclic antidepressants (Furlan, Sandoval, Mailis-Gagnon, & Tunks, 2006). A more recent Cochrane review of codeine for cancer pain demonstrated that although codeine may offer some efficacy over placebo, unacceptable toxicities could limit its use in this population. More rigorously conducted studies are required (Straube et al., 2014).

Risk Evaluation and Mitigation Strategy Programs

REMS programs were developed by the U.S. Food and Drug Administration (FDA) in 2007 to ensure that the benefits of certain high-risk drugs outweighed the risk. In 2012, opioid agents were included to address prescription drug abuse across the United States. The opioid REMS programs include requirements for manufacturers to provide training to opioid prescribers and also written educational materials on safe use to both patients and providers. Opioid analgesics included as part of REMS programs are the long-acting and extended-release opioids, transmucosal immediate-release fentanyl preparations, transdermal fentanyl, and buprenorphine, plus analgesic forms of methadone (U.S. FDA, 2013).

Opioid Dosing and Conversion

The initial starting dose of opioids is dependent on the specific opioid selected, the severity of the pain, and the route of administration. Oral morphine is the prototypical agent, but alternative opioids or routes of administration could be considered based on patient-specific needs. Nurses caring for patients with cancer must be aware there is no ceiling to opioid dosing. Patients started on a controlled-release formulation of opioid should also receive a concomitant prescription for breakthrough pain using an immediate-release opioid at a dose that is 10%–20% of the total daily dose of the sustained-release opioid (NCCN, 2016). Similarly, for patients receiving a continuous IV opioid infusion, consideration may be given to bolus doses equivalent to 50% of the hourly rate at an interval of every 8–10 minutes (Prommer, 2015). Upward dose titrations for uncontrolled pain should increase the total daily dose (combination of long-acting and breakthrough) by 50%–100% for moderate to severe pain (NCCN, 2016). These titrations should occur regularly until adequate pain control is achieved. The frequency of dose titration should be based on the pain severity and the opioid analgesic formulation. For example, oral morphine has a more rapid onset of action and shorter duration than transdermal fentanyl, so it can be titrated more frequently than transdermal fentanyl. Conversely, when opioid analgesics are no longer needed, the dose should be tapered by 20%–25% every one to two days until the dose reaches an equivalent of 30 mg of morphine per day, and it can then be discontinued after two days (Gordon & Dahl, 2015). Patients who require opioid rotation should be switched to an equianalgesic dose of the comparable opioid (see Table 26-2). If the pain is controlled at the time of conversion, a dose reduction of 25%–50% should be considered to prevent incomplete cross-tolerance between opioids. If the pain is uncontrolled, then a rate of 100%–125% may be used (NCCN, 2016).

Opioid Adverse Effects

Constipation is a common toxicity of opioids, affecting up to 85% of individuals who use these agents, and can cause reductions in quality of life (Abramowitz et al., 2013). Unlike most other adverse effects from opioids, patients do not usually experience tolerance to constipation. Opioids interfere with bowel function by inhibiting normal peristalsis and secretion (Thomas et al., 2008). The NCCN (2016) guidelines recommend prevention of opioid constipation with the use of a stimulant laxative, such as senna, with or without a stool softener, or polyethylene glycol. A randomized trial comparing senna plus placebo to senna plus docusate showed no benefit with the addition of docusate (Tarumi, Wilson, Szafran, & Spooner, 2013). For more information on constipation, see Chapter 20.

Nurses should increase the laxative dose when the opioid dose is increased (NCCN, 2016). Treatment of persistent constipation should include the use of additional laxatives, such as bisacodyl, lactulose, magnesium citrate, magnesium hydroxide, or polyethylene glycol (NCCN, 2016). Opioid rotation to a less-constipating opioid, such as fentanyl or methadone, also may be an option (NCCN, 2016). Methylnaltrexone, a mu-opioid receptor antagonist, has demonstrated efficacy in treating opioid-induced constipation (Thomas et al., 2008) and should be considered when laxative therapy has been unsuccessful (NCCN, 2016). Both lubiprostone and naloxegol have demonstrated efficacy in the treatment of opioid-induced constipation but are not approved for use in the cancer population. The use of fiber-bulking agents is not recommended in patients with advanced illness who are taking opioids, as they can worsen constipation if adequate fluid intake is not maintained (Thomas et al., 2008).

Opioid-induced nausea, typically temporary, can be caused by stimulation of the chemoreceptor trigger zone, gastric stasis, or enhanced vestibular sensitivity (Smith & Laufer, 2014). NCCN (2016) guidelines recommend treating opioid-induced nausea with antiemetics and using an antiemetic prior to the opioid dose as prophylaxis treatment in patients with a prior history of opioid-induced nausea. Antiemetics may include agents such as prochlorpera-

Table 26-2. Equianalgesic Doses of Opioid Analgesics

Analgesic	Oral Dose (mg)	Intravenous Dose (mg)
Codeine	200	–
Hydrocodone	30	–
Morphine	30	10
Oxycodone	20	–
Methadone*	–	–
Hydromorphone	7.5	1.5
Fentanyl†	–	–
Oxymorphone‡	–	–

*Dose is variable. Consult with a pain or palliative care specialist if unfamiliar with methadone dosing.

†When converting from oral morphine to transdermal fentanyl, consider a 2:1 ratio (2 mg/day oral morphine to 1 mcg/hr of transdermal fentanyl).

‡For conversion from oral morphine to oxymorphone, use a conversion factor of 0.333:1.

Note. Based on information from Berdine & Nesbit, 2006; Endo Pharmaceuticals Inc., 2014a; National Comprehensive Cancer Network, 2016.

zine, haloperidol, metoclopramide, corticosteroids, or serotonin antagonists (NCCN, 2016). No evidence has shown that one agent is more effective than another, but the NCCN guidelines recommend initially considering the use of prochlorperazine, haloperidol, or metoclopramide. Opioid rotation should be considered if nausea persists for more than one week (NCCN, 2016).

Pruritus is an adverse effect of opioids and is more commonly seen with the neuraxial route of administration (de la Cruz & Bruera, 2010). Possible causes involve stimulation of receptors such as mu-opioid, dopamine, serotonin, gamma-aminobutyric acid, and glycine, as well as prostaglandins (Ganesh & Maxwell, 2007). Clinicians should note that pruritus is an adverse effect and not necessarily an allergic reaction. Management strategies include the use of antihistamines, opioid rotation, low-dose nalbuphine PRN, ondansetron, and continuous-infusion naloxone (NCCN, 2016). Opioid rotation also should be considered if rash or hives indicative of a true allergy are present.

Approximately 20%–60% of patients receiving opioids will experience some degree of sedation (Cherny et al., 2001). Patients should be informed that sedation is usually transient, persisting for only a few days, and most commonly occurs with the initiation of opioids or substantial dose increases (McNicol et al., 2003). The concomitant use of other sedating medications used by patients with cancer may exacerbate the sedating effects of opioids. Strategies for managing sedation that persists for more than a few days include dose reduction; addition of a nonopioid analgesic to allow for dose reduction; opioid rotation; or central nervous system stimulants, such as caffeine, methylphenidate, dextroamphetamine, or modafinil (NCCN, 2016).

Respiratory depression may be a potentially life-threatening adverse effect of opioids. Opioids interfere with normal functioning of the respiratory center in the brain stem, producing respiratory depression and, ultimately, apnea (McNicol et al., 2003). However, this toxicity is rare in individuals on chronic doses of opioids (McNicol et al., 2003). Respiratory depression is also uncommon in opioid-naïve patients (Clemens, Quednau, & Klaschik, 2008). Additionally, use of opioids seems to be safe in patients with underlying respiratory disease (Walsh, Rivera, & Kaiko, 2003). The fear of respiratory depression should not be a reason for failing to utilize opioids. The use of an opioid antagonist, such as naloxone, may be considered for impending or serious respiratory depression when respirations are below 8 breaths/min (McNicol et al., 2003). If respiratory depression occurs, the NCCN (2016) guidelines recommend administering a dose of naloxone every 30–60 seconds until improvement occurs, with consideration of continuous-infusion naloxone for patients on opioids with a long half-life. The American Society for Pain Management Nursing has also published guidelines on monitoring for opioid-induced respiratory depression (Jarzyna et al., 2011).

Adjuvant Analgesics

Adjuvant analgesics are recommended as possible additions to the pain armamentarium at all three steps of the WHO pain ladder (WHO, n.d.), as well as by the NCCN (2016) guidelines and the ONS PEP resource for chronic pain (Miaskowski et al., 2017). Many of these agents have been studied in conditions unrelated to cancer, such as non–cancer-related neuropathy, seizures, and depression. Most recommendations for patients with cancer are based on data extrapolated from these studies or on expert opinion. Although adjuvant analgesics can be administered as single agents, they often are combined with opioids (McDonald & Portenoy, 2006). The following section will focus on adjuvant analgesics that are commonly used in patients with cancer, including anticonvulsants, antidepressants, corticosteroids, and topical agents (see Table 26-3). Many of these agents are used to treat neuropathic pain. Anticonvulsants and antidepressants are the categories of choice for the management of cancer-related neuropathic pain (McDonald & Portenoy, 2006; NCCN, 2016).

Anticonvulsants

The mechanism of action of anticonvulsants for neuropathic pain is poorly understood. This class is divided into first-generation agents (e.g., phenytoin, carbamazepine) and second-generation agents (e.g., gabapentin, pregabalin, lamotrigine). Most first-generation anticonvulsants have demonstrated inconsistent results in treating neuropathic pain (Dworkin et al., 2007). They also have significant adverse effects and drug interactions resulting in decreased frequency of use, particularly with the availability of less toxic alternatives (Lussier, Huskey, & Portenoy, 2004). Therefore, it is suggested they be reserved for third-line therapy for the treatment of neuropathic cancer pain (Dworkin et al., 2007).

Gabapentin, a second-generation anticonvulsant, is recommended as first-line therapy in the treatment of neuropathic pain (Dworkin et al., 2007). Gabapentin works by inhibiting calcium flow into a neuron, reducing hyperactivity (McDonald & Portenoy, 2006). Gabapentin has shown some efficacy in both general chronic neuropathic pain (Moore, Wiffen, Derry, Toelle, & Rice, 2014) and neuropathic cancer pain (Caraceni et al., 2004; Keskinbora, Pekel, & Aydinli, 2007; Mishra, Bhatnagar, Goyal, Rana, & Upadhya, 2012). Gabapentin is well tolerated, with dizziness and somnolence as the most common dose-limiting toxicities (Dworkin et al., 2007). No significant drug interactions exist (Dworkin et al., 2007). Slow titration is recommended to limit adverse effects. The typical starting dose is 100–300 mg daily with titration every three to five days to achieve a usual maximum dose of 3,600 mg daily in divided doses. Dose adjustments for renal impairment are recommended (NCCN, 2016).

Table 26-3. Adjuvant Analgesics

Agent	Usual Starting Dose	Usual Daily Dose
Anticonvulsants		
Gabapentin	100–300 mg/day	900–3,600 mg/day in 2–3 divided doses
Pregabalin	150 mg/day	150–300 mg BID
Antidepressants		
Tricyclics		
• Amitriptyline	10–25 mg every night	50–150 mg every night
• Desipramine	10–25 mg every night	50–150 mg every night
• Imipramine	10–25 mg every night	50–200 mg every night
• Nortriptyline	10–25 mg every night	50–150 mg every night
Selective serotonin and norepinephrine reuptake inhibitors		
• Venlafaxine*	37.5–75 mg/day	75–225 mg/day
• Duloxetine	20–30 mg/day	60–120 mg/day
Corticosteroids		
Dexamethasone	Variable†	Variable†
Local Anesthetics		
Lidocaine (topical)	Up to 3 patches at once for 12 hours in a 24-hour period	Depends on surface area of pain; up to 3 patches for up to 12 hours in a 24-hour period

*In divided doses if immediate-release formulation used

†The lowest dose for the shortest duration should be considered. A moderate dose of 8 mg is appropriate but should be discontinued after 1 week if there is no improvement in pain.

Note. Based on information from Endo Pharmaceuticals Inc., 2015; McDonald & Portenoy, 2006; *Monthly Prescribing Reference Nurse Practitioners' Edition*, 2015; National Comprehensive Cancer Network, 2016; Paulsen et al., 2013.

The NCCN (2016) guidelines include pregabalin as a recommended coanalgesic. Pregabalin has a mechanism of action similar to gabapentin. It has shown efficacy in a variety of non–cancer-related neuropathic pain conditions (Moore, Straube, Wiffen, Derry, & McQuay, 2010). In a randomized trial in chronic neuropathic cancer pain, pregabalin was found to be more effective than opioids and with fewer toxicities (Raptis et al., 2014). The toxicity profile is similar to gabapentin, but a more rapid titration may be possible (McDonald & Portenoy, 2006). Like gabapentin, dose reductions for renal impairment are indicated (NCCN, 2016).

Lamotrigine is approved for seizures as well as bipolar disorder, but it has not shown significant activity in neuropathic pain (Wiffen, Derry, & Moore, 2013). Additionally, it has the potential for drug interactions and may cause severe cutaneous hypersensitivity reactions, including Stevens-Johnson syndrome (McDonald & Portenoy, 2006). Because many other adjuvant analgesics with proven efficacy are available, lamotrigine does not appear to have a role in the cancer patient population.

Antidepressants

Antidepressants have been primarily utilized for neuropathic pain, but most of the research has occurred in patients without cancer. The classes of drugs that have been studied include tricyclic antidepressants, selective serotonin reuptake inhibitors, and selective serotonin and norepinephrine reuptake inhibitors. In general, the data for the use of selective serotonin reuptake inhibitors in cancer-related pain have been inconclusive, and they are not typically recommended (Miaskowski et al., 2017). The dose necessary to achieve pain relief is often lower than the antidepressant dose with these agents. One benefit of using antidepressants for pain is that they may be helpful in patients with underlying depression or insomnia.

Tricyclic antidepressants have been available for many years. They consist of both secondary (nortriptyline and desipramine) and tertiary (amitriptyline and imipramine) amines. Side effects are common, with up to 20% of individuals discontinuing use secondary to toxicity (Saarto & Wiffen, 2007). Common adverse effects include sedation, orthostatic hypotension, dry mouth, constipation, and urinary retention. Tricyclic antidepressants should be avoided in patients with underlying cardiac disease or in patients at risk for suicide (Dworkin et al., 2007). Secondary amines are better tolerated than tertiary amines and should be the initial choice of tricyclic antidepressants. Dosing should start low and be titrated slowly to the minimally effective dose. Because of numerous side effects and availability of more effective alternatives, tricyclic antidepressants should not be considered as initial therapy (Derry, Wiffen, Aldington, & Moore, 2015; Hearn, Moore, Derry, Wiffen, & Phillips, 2014; Moore, Derry, Aldington, Cole, & Wiffen, 2015).

More evidence exists for the use of selective serotonin and norepinephrine reuptake inhibitors for pain relief than for the use of selective serotonin reuptake inhibitors. Two such agents, venlafaxine and duloxetine, have demonstrated efficacy in studies of general neuropathic pain (Kadiroglu et al., 2008; Lunn, Hughes, & Wiffen, 2014; Razazian et al., 2014), as well as cancer-related neuropathic pain. Duloxetine has exhibited effectiveness for chemotherapy-induced peripheral neuropathy (Otake et al., 2015; Yang et al., 2012), and venlafaxine has been helpful in both the prevention and treatment of postmastectomy pain syndrome (Reuben, Makari-Judson, & Lurie, 2004; Tasmuth, Härtel, & Kalso, 2002). Selective serotonin and norepinephrine reuptake inhibitors are tolerated with fewer adverse effects than the tricyclic antidepressants (Lussier et al., 2004). Many experts recommend inclusion of these agents in the first-line treatment of neuropathic pain (Dworkin et al., 2007; Miaskowski et al., 2017; NCCN, 2016).

Bone Resorptive Agents

Bone resorptive agents may be useful adjunctive therapies for chronic cancer pain (Miaskowski et al., 2017; NCCN, 2016). Bisphosphonates are compounds that inhibit the activity of osteoclasts on bone resorption. They can decrease the incidence of pain and skeletal complications in patients with a variety of malignancies (Mhaskar et al., 2012; Wong, Stockler, & Pavlakis, 2012; Yuen, Shelley, Sze, Wilt, & Mason, 2006). Bisphosphonates are available both orally and intravenously. Those commonly used in clinical practice include IV pamidronate and zoledronic acid. Both agents appear to be equivalent with respect to efficacy (Mhaskar et al., 2012); however, the infusion time for zoledronic acid is shorter. The most worrisome side effects of bisphosphonates are renal toxicity and osteonecrosis of the jaw. Nurses should assess patients' serum creatinine level prior to each infusion. The dose may need to be reduced or withheld if baseline creatinine clearance is low (Novartis Pharmaceuticals Corp., 2015).

Denosumab is a monoclonal antibody against receptor-activated nuclear factor kappa-B ligand (known as RANKL), involved with osteoclast formation (Kostenuik et al., 2009). Several large studies have shown it can reduce skeletal-related events, as well as pain across a variety of solid tumors (Henry et al., 2014; Peddi, Lopez-Olivo, Pratt, & Suarez-Almazor, 2013; Wong et al., 2012). Denosumab has been compared with zoledronic acid and has evidence of superiority with regard to both skeletal events and pain (Henry et al., 2014; Peddi et al., 2013). Both agents have similar rates of osteonecrosis of the jaw, but denosumab has less nephrotoxicity (Peddi et al., 2013). However, denosumab is responsible for higher rates of hypocalcemia (Henry et al., 2014; Peddi et al., 2013). Regular monitoring of serum calcium is warranted.

Corticosteroids

Corticosteroids have been used for many years in patients with cancer. They are inexpensive and widely available. Corticosteroids act by decreasing inflammation, which may contribute to cancer-related pain. Although a paucity of data exists to support the use of steroids in the oncology population, NCCN recommends the use of steroids for malignant pain (NCCN, 2016). Typical scenarios where corticosteroids may be useful include in spinal cord compression, liver capsule pain, and bone involvement. Corticosteroids have significant long-term complications that include osteoporosis, proximal myopathy, hyperglycemia, Cushing syndrome, and gastrointestinal bleeding. In patients with a limited life expectancy, these side effects may not be relevant. To avoid precipitating an adrenal crisis, healthcare providers must exercise caution when discontinuing high-dose corticosteroids or prescribing them for long periods of time. A slow taper is recommended.

Topical Anesthetics

Topical lidocaine is indicated for treatment of postherpetic neuralgia, but it also can be effective in other pain syndromes, such as postmastectomy and post-thoracotomy pain (Devers & Galer, 2000). Although a recent Cochrane Review failed to identify quality evidence from randomized trials to support its general use for neuropathic pain, the authors acknowledged smaller studies and anecdotal reports demonstrating efficacy (Derry, Wiffen, Moore, & Quinlan, 2014). Additionally, the low toxicity profile of lidocaine makes it an attractive adjuvant option for some patients. Topical lidocaine is available in a patch form, applied locally to the painful area. It works peripherally by blocking sodium channels necessary for the initiation and conduction of nerve impulses (Cleary, 2007). Lidocaine patches are well tolerated with only mild skin irritation noted in one study (Devers & Galer, 2000).

Interventional Strategies for Pain Management

Interventional techniques for pain management in patients with cancer include the employment of nerve blocks, administration of spinal or regional analgesics, radiofrequency ablation, and vertebroplasty or kyphoplasty. Interventional strategies may be considered when nerve blocks may be effective for pain relief or when less invasive techniques have been ineffective or too toxic (NCCN, 2016).

Neurolytic Blocks

Neurolytic (nerve) blocks involve instillation of either alcohol or phenol into a nerve, nerve root, or plexus, causing destruction of the nerve (Sloan, 2004). Examples of commonly employed nerve blocks in patients with cancer include celiac plexus and superior hypogastric blocks. The celiac plexus is a collection of nerves located in the retroperitoneum extending from the T12 to L1 levels (Adolph &

Benedetti, 2006). Celiac plexus blocks can be employed for a variety of gastrointestinal cancers that can invade this structure. Possible primary cancer sites include esophageal, pancreatic, gastric, or hepatic malignancies (Sloan, 2004). A meta-analysis showed that approximately 90% of patients experienced pain relief with celiac nerve blocks (Eisenberg, Carr, & Chalmers, 1995). A systematic review performed in 2011 confirmed the effectiveness of this procedure for upper abdominal cancers (Nagels, Pease, Bekkering, Cools, & Dobbels, 2013). Contemporary minimally invasive approaches through the use of ultrasound-guided techniques are currently being studied. The most common adverse effects associated with celiac plexus blocks are local discomfort, diarrhea, and hypotension (Eisenberg et al., 1995; Nagels et al., 2013).

Superior hypogastric blocks are used for pain secondary to pelvic malignancies. The superior hypogastric plexus is a ganglionic nerve bundle that combines with the pelvic splanchnic nerves to form the inferior hypogastric plexus to supply various pelvic organs (Adolph & Benedetti, 2006). Data are limited on the efficacy of this procedure; however, one study of 227 patients with malignant pelvic pain reported that 72% of patients who underwent superior hypogastric plexus block experienced satisfactory pain control without the development of complications (Plancarte, de Leon-Casasola, El-Helaly, Allende, & Lema, 1997). More recently, Mishra, Bhatnagar, Rana, Khurana, and Thulkar (2013) demonstrated that ultrasound-guided superior hypogastric plexus block reduced morphine consumption and improved patient satisfaction over oral morphine alone. The combination of celiac and superior hypogastric plexus blocks for upper abdominal cancers is gaining interest as well, with some evidence that the combination is superior to celiac plexus block alone (Huang et al., 2014).

Additional sites to utilize blocks include the brachial plexus, intercostal nerve, dorsal root ganglion, or ganglion impar. These measures may be temporary, as some nerves have the ability to regenerate. For example, the duration of improvement in pain and quality of life was less than three months in research studies by Huang et al. (2014). Neurolytic blocks therefore are typically reserved for individuals with a limited life expectancy (Adolph & Benedetti, 2006).

Spinal Analgesia

Spinal analgesia involves administration of analgesics directly into the spinal region, where they work centrally to inhibit nociception. Either epidural or intrathecal (subarachnoid) routes are used. Both routes have been shown to be effective for the relief of cancer pain (Ballantyne et al., 2005; Hayek, Deer, Pope, Panchal, & Patel, 2011; Jeon et al., 2012). The selection of one site over another has not been clearly defined. Epidural catheters are easily placed but require an external catheter or pump, so their use is limited to days to weeks because of concerns about catheter dislodgment. The intrathecal route can be preferable for chronic use because conversion to an implantable pump provides a programmable system that is self-contained below the skin with no exposed wires or equipment. Fewer adverse effects arise with spinal analgesia; the most common include skin site or catheter infections (Adolph & Benedetti, 2006). Patients who receive intraspinal opioid analgesia have reported high rates of pruritus, which may be a dose-dependent phenomenon (Slappendel, Weber, Benraad, van Limbeek, & Dirksen, 2000). Spinal analgesia is indicated in patients whose pain is not controlled with systemic analgesics or when the toxicity is unacceptable (NCCN, 2016). Various delivery systems, either external or implantable, are available. The decision regarding which system to use depends on a variety of issues, including cost, life expectancy of the patient, and patient/caregiver ability to manage the device (Burton et al., 2004). The most commonly used intraspinal agent is morphine (Hassenbusch &

Portenoy, 2000), but a variety of other opioids or anesthetics may be employed.

Radiofrequency Ablation

Radiofrequency ablation (RFA) involves the heating of tissues to high temperatures, thereby precipitating coagulation necrosis and subsequent tissue death (Patti, Neeman, & Wood, 2002). This procedure involves placing a small catheter to deliver an electrical current into the tumor, leading to thermal injury (Locklin & Wood, 2005). RFA has been used for a variety of malignant conditions and is approved for thermal ablation of soft tissues (U.S. FDA, 2008). The procedure has demonstrated efficacy in small studies with respect to cancer pain in both soft tissue pain (Locklin, Mannes, Berger, & Wood, 2004) and pain related to bone metastases (Aono et al., 2008; Belfiore et al., 2008; Gevargez & Groenemeyer, 2008). RFA has even demonstrated usefulness in patients with cancer who have body or face pain requiring partial cordotomies (Raslan, 2008). Complications are variable depending on the target site. Postablation syndrome consisting of mild flu-like symptoms may occur. Patients should be well hydrated following the procedure to limit complications from postablation syndrome (Locklin & Wood, 2005).

Vertebroplasty and Kyphoplasty

Vertebroplasty and kyphoplasty have been extensively studied in patients with osteoporotic vertebral fractures. Both procedures have demonstrated ability to provide effective pain control in patients with metastatic vertebral cancers (Berenson et al., 2011; Burton et al., 2011). Vertebroplasty entails the injection of a cement compound into the involved vertebra to provide stability and reduce pain. The most common complication is cement leakage, which is estimated to occur in 9%–38% of patients undergoing the procedure (Fourney et al., 2003; Weill et al., 1996). The majority of these leakages are asymptomatic and not clinically significant. Kyphoplasty differs from vertebroplasty in that an inflatable balloon is used to heighten the vertebral body before cement is injected (Berenson et al., 2011). Kyphoplasty has been found to be a very safe procedure, with similar adverse events noted in the kyphoplasty and control groups in one large randomized trial (Berenson et al., 2011).

Radiation Therapy

External beam radiation therapy has been used for many years for palliation of cancer-related symptoms such as pain. It is particularly useful in patients with painful bone metastases for which other effective treatments do not exist. The efficacy of radiation therapy has been established in patients with painful bone metastases, with nearly 25% experiencing complete pain control (Chow, Harris, Fan, Tsao, & Sze, 2007). Schedules with various fractions of external beam radiation have been employed, but it appears that single-fraction therapy may be just as effective as multifraction therapy for palliation of bone pain (Chow et al., 2007; Lutz et al., 2011). Although the single-fraction schedule offers more convenience to patients, the risk of retreatment to the same site is higher. Newer modalities such as stereotactic body radiation therapy may be considered for some patients under specific circumstances (Lutz et al., 2011).

Radioisotopes and Radionuclides

Radioisotopes, referred to as *systemic radiation therapy* by Hillegonds, Franklin, Shelton, Vijayakumar, and Vijayakumar (2007), have been used to target multiple sites of bone metastases. These compounds, which are administered in a single outpatient IV injection, have been shown to reduce pain related to bone metastases (Roqué i Figuls, Martinez-Zapata, Scott-Brown, & Alonso-Coello, 2011). Examples of radioisotopes currently in use include samarium-153 and strontium-89, with no apparent differences in efficacy between the two (Roqué i Figuls et al., 2011). Radioisotopes have traditionally been used in the late stages of disease in individuals with advanced bone metastases (Hillegonds et al., 2007). The most concerning toxicity of these agents is myelosuppression, particularly leukopenia and thrombocytopenia (Roqué i Figuls et al., 2011). Appropriate patient selection for radioisotopes should include assessment of prior myelosuppressive therapy and current marrow function, as well as patient life expectancy and candidacy for other palliative pain measures (Mercadante & Fulfaro, 2007). Detailed instructions regarding radiation precautions must be provided to the patients because radioactivity will be present in urine for approximately 12 hours after administration. Blood counts should be monitored weekly for at least eight weeks (Lantheus Medical Imaging, Inc., 2014).

More recently, a novel bone-seeking calcium mimetic radionuclide has emerged for the management of bone metastases in patients with castration-resistant prostate cancer. Radium-223 is an alpha particle–emitting agent that delivers targeted radiation to osteoblastic bone metastases while sparing the bone marrow (Vengalil, O'Sullivan, & Parker, 2012). It has been shown to reduce the risk of symptomatic skeletal-related events, as well as improve survival (Parker et al., 2013; Sartor et al., 2014). The myelosuppression common with other radionuclides has not been evident with radium-223. In one study, researchers noted fewer adverse events in the study drug group compared to the placebo group (Parker et al., 2013).

Surgery

Literature to support the use of surgery for palliation of cancer pain is limited. Studies have generally been small or looked at outcomes such as survival rather than symptom palliation. Despite this fact, surgeons in one survey estimated that palliative surgical procedures accounted for more than 20% of cancer operations (McCahill et al., 2002). The most prominent literature appears to be related to the treatment of spinal cord compression or spine metastases. Quan et al. (2011) prospectively followed 118 patients who underwent spinal surgery for vertebral metastases and noted improvements in pain, function, and quality of life. The improvements persisted until death or at the completion of the 12-month follow-up period. Wu et al. (2010) also discovered improvements in quality of life in patients with spinal metastases who were treated surgically compared to those who were managed without surgery. Historically, surgery for pain palliation in patients with cancer has been indicated when less invasive interventions are unsuccessful or toxicity of those interventions is unacceptable (McCahill & Ferrell, 2002). Other factors to consider prior to palliative surgery in patients with cancer include the likelihood of improvement in pain control and quality of life, the patient's prognosis, and cost-effectiveness (Miner, 2005).

Chemotherapy

Chemotherapy offers effective pain palliation for a variety of tumor types (Andreopoulou et al., 2004; Bang et al., 2005; Shelley et al., 2006). Because chemotherapy has the potential for serious toxicities, however, selection of candidates for palliative chemotherapy should include a risk-benefit analysis. In addition to potential toxicity, other factors to be considered include patient prognosis and the likelihood of the treatment's ability to improve quality of life or decrease symptoms (Browner & Carducci, 2005). See Chapter 9 for a more detailed review of chemotherapy.

Integrative Therapies

The use of integrative therapies is commonplace, with 95% of patients with cancer reporting their use of integrative therapies. Perhaps even more importantly, 20%–77% of patients do not inform their physicians of their use

(Davis, Oh, Butow, Mullan, & Clarke, 2012). Patients with cancer who experience pain may be even more likely than other patients to utilize certain integrative therapy treatments (Bardia, Greeno, & Bauer, 2007). Oncology nurses are likely to recommend integrative therapy practices to their patients (Kwekkeboom, Bumpus, Wanta, & Serlin, 2008). A systematic review of nonpharmacologic therapies for cancer-related pain revealed a lack of good evidence for many of these recommendations (Hökkä, Kaakinen, & Pölkki, 2014). NCCN (2016) guidelines, however, recommend the use of certain integrative therapies for pain that may be alleviated by these measures, particularly in frail older adult patients. The National Center for Complementary and Integrative Health, a division of the National Institutes of Health, is dedicated to the scientific research of complementary and integrative therapies for health care and is a good resource for both consumers and healthcare providers. According to NCCN, examples of integrative therapies that may have the potential for temporarily alleviating pain in patients with cancer include massage, acupuncture, and select mind–body interventions (NCCN, 2016).

Cannabinoids

Cannabinoids are a group of compounds found in the cannabis plant (Miaskowski et al., 2017). The most common of these are delta-9-tetrahydrocannabinol and cannabidiol (Pertwee, 2006). They interact with certain endogenous cannabinoid receptors involved in analgesia (Portenoy et al., 2012). The ONS PEP resource (Miaskowski et al., 2017) recommends cannabis/cannabinoids as likely to be effective for chronic cancer pain. Various routes of administration have been studied, including oral, oromucosal, and inhalation (Miaskowski et al., 2017). Side effects may include nausea, vomiting, dizziness, somnolence, and disorientation (Portenoy et al., 2012).

Mind–Body Interventions

Mind–body interventions include techniques such as hypnosis, relaxation, guided imagery, and distraction. Hypnosis and guided imagery have both been recognized as potential integrative therapies for pain in patients with cancer (NCCN, 2016), and music therapy may be beneficial as well (Miaskowski et al., 2017). Hypnosis has been practiced for many years and was initially shown to reduce oral pain in patients with cancer who had received a bone marrow transplant (Syrjala, Cummings, & Donaldson, 1992). More recently, Cramer et al. (2015) conducted a systematic review of hypnosis in patients with breast cancer and found promising evidence that it can be helpful with a variety of symptoms, including pain. Hypnosis appears to be a well-tolerated intervention, with no differences in adverse events noted between the hypnosis and control arms (Cramer et al., 2015).

Guided imagery involves the use of visualization or imagination to induce relaxation (Gatlin & Schulmeister, 2007). It may be combined with other techniques, such as relaxation. These interventions may be beneficial adjuncts for reducing pain in patients with cancer (Kwekkeboom, Cherwin, Lee, & Wanta, 2010). The positive effects may be transient, however, as one study on relaxation produced short-term but not chronic pain control (Anderson et al., 2006). According to Cassileth and Keefe (2010), the low cost and absence of significant adverse effects may make mind–body interventions such as guided imagery an attractive option for clinicians and patients.

Music interventions that have been studied range from listening to prerecorded music provided by medical staff to participation in programs administered by trained music therapists (Archie, Bruera, & Cohen, 2013; Bradt, Dileo, Magill, & Teague, 2016). Music therapy may include activities such as listening, singing, and composition (Tsai et al., 2014). Both a systematic review (Tsai et al., 2014) and a Cochrane review (Bradt et al., 2016) provide evidence for the use of music interventions to relieve cancer pain. This low-risk intervention may be a useful complement to other pain relief measures.

Acupuncture

Acupuncture involves the use of thin needles that either manually or electronically stimulate various anatomic points on the body. Its mechanism of action is purported to involve the regulation of energy. Conclusions have been conflicting regarding the efficacy of acupuncture for cancer pain. Both a Cochrane review (Paley, Johnson, Tashani, & Bagnall, 2015) and a systematic review (Garcia et al., 2013) failed to demonstrate sufficient evidence to endorse the use of acupuncture for cancer-related pain. A more recent systematic review of acupuncture in the oncology palliative care setting identified this modality as a potentially useful option for cancer pain relief (Lian, Pan, Zhou, & Zhang, 2014). In an integrative overview, Towler, Molassiotis, and Brearley (2013) concluded that the use of acupuncture may have some benefit for cancer pain and that consideration should be given to incorporation of acupuncture into a holistic patient care approach. The side effects of acupuncture are mild, with minimal bruising or bleeding at the site (Lian et al., 2014).

Massage Therapy and Reflexology

Massage therapy involves the manual manipulation of soft tissue, whereas reflexology involves the application of pressure to the feet, hands, or ears. A recent meta-analysis demonstrated the effectiveness of pain relief with massage therapy in patients with diverse cancer diagnoses. Foot reflexology appeared even more successful at cancer pain reduction than other forms of massage (Lee, Kim, Yeo, Kim, & Lim, 2015). Massage therapy is a well-tolerated technique without significant adverse effects (Kutner et al., 2008). Importantly, massage therapists should be adequately trained in the care of patients with cancer, as techniques may require modification for this population.

Although additional larger randomized studies are required to draw conclusions about the efficacy of many integrative therapies, there appears to be little downside for patients with cancer who are in pain. In a systematic review of multiple types of integrative therapy interventions, no adverse effects were reported (Bardia et al., 2007). Patients should be provided the necessary tools to make informed decisions regarding the use of such therapies. They also should be instructed not to forgo evidence-based, conventional therapies in their quest for integrative therapy treatments.

Psychoeducational Interventions

The area where nursing may have the greatest impact on cancer-related pain is with the use of psychoeducational interventions. Psychoeducational interventions often are divided into skills-based and educational strategies and may encompass techniques such as providing written or audiovisual materials, coaching, cognitive behavioral therapy, hypnosis, and relaxation with imagery. A combination of approaches can be useful for some patients. Numerous studies have demonstrated the effectiveness of these interventions (Lee, Hyun, et al., 2015; Ling, Lui, & So, 2012; Marie, Luckett, Davidson, Lovell, & Lal, 2013; Syrjala et al., 2014). The most promising of these interventions include patient-centered or individualized approaches that focus on patient self-efficacy/empowerment and are incorporated into routine cancer care (Lovell et al., 2014; Marie et al., 2013). The nursing profession is critical for implementing these psychoeducational programs, with one meta-analysis identifying nearly two-thirds of interventions provided by nurses (Gorin et al., 2012).

Conclusion

Many patients with cancer will experience some degree of pain throughout the disease trajectory. Numerous causes of pain exist in patients with cancer, including treatment-related or disease-related causes. Nurses should conduct thorough and frequent pain assessments in these patients. Available treatment options are dependent on the type or cause of pain. Nurses who care for patients with cancer must be aware of the various etiologies of cancer pain, as well as treatment strategies. Many organizations such as the American Pain Society, NCCN, and ONS offer pain guidelines that oncology nurses can refer to for current recommendations. Nurses can and should continue to play a major role in advocating for adequate pain management for all patients with cancer.

References

Abramowitz, L., Béziaud, N., Labreze, L., Giardina, V., Caussé, C., Chuberre, B., ... Perrot, S. (2013). Prevalence and impact of constipation and bowel dysfunction induced by strong opioids: A cross-sectional survey of 520 patients with cancer pain: DYONISOS study. *Journal of Medical Economics, 16,* 1423–1433. doi:10.3111/13696998.2013.851082

Actavis Pharma, Inc. (2014). *Kadian® (morphine sulfate)* [Package insert]. Parsippany, NJ: Author.

Adolph, M.D., & Benedetti, C. (2006). Percutaneous-guided pain control: Exploiting the neural basis of pain sensation. *Gastroenterology Clinics of North America, 35,* 167–188. doi:10.1016/j.gtc.2005.12.009

Anderson, K.O., Cohen, M.Z., Mendoza, T.R., Guo, H., Harle, M.T., & Cleeland, C.S. (2006). Brief cognitive-behavioral audiotape interventions for cancer-related pain: Immediate but not long-term effectiveness. *Cancer, 107,* 207–214. doi:10.1002/cncr.21964

Andreopoulou, E., Ross, P.J., O'Brien, M.E.R., Ford, H.E.R., Priest, K., Eisen, T., ... Smith, I.E. (2004). The palliative benefits of MVP (mitomycin C, vinblastine and cisplatin) chemotherapy in patients with malignant mesothelioma. *Annals of Oncology, 15,* 1406–1412. doi:10.1093/annonc/mdh356

Annagür, B.B., Uguz, F., Apiliogullari, S., Kara, I., & Gunduz, S. (2014). Psychiatric disorders and association with quality of sleep and quality of life in patients with chronic pain: A SCID-based study. *Pain Medicine, 15,* 772–781. doi:10.1111/pme.12390

Aono, M., Nakamura, H., Ieguchi, M., Hoshi, M., Taguchi, S., & Takami, M. (2008). Radiofrequency ablation for metastatic bone tumors [Abstract 20720]. *Journal of Clinical Oncology, 26*(Suppl.). Retrieved from http://meeting.ascopubs.org/cgi/content/short/26/15_suppl/20720

Archie, P., Bruera, E., & Cohen, L. (2013). Music-based interventions in palliative cancer care: A review of quantitative studies and neurobiological literature. *Supportive Care in Cancer, 21,* 2609–2624. doi:10.1007/s00520-013-1841-4

Key Points

- Pain is one of the most feared symptoms of the cancer experience, with more than half of patients experiencing pain at some point throughout the cancer trajectory.
- Numerous barriers to appropriate cancer pain management have been identified from the patient, provider, and systems perspective.
- Cancer pain may be classified as acute or chronic, and further classified as either nociceptive (somatic or visceral) or neuropathic.
- The etiology of cancer pain may be multifactorial and consequential to the underlying disease or diagnostic- or treatment-related sequelae.
- Routine screening for pain is essential, and numerous pain assessment tools have been validated for this purpose.
- Pain management strategies may include a variety of pharmacologic, interventional, and nonpharmacologic options.
- Pharmacologic options may include classes of medications such as non-narcotic analgesics, opioid analgesics, or adjuvant medications.
- Opioids often are the cornerstone of cancer pain management and are available in a variety of formulations. Side effects often are predictable and manageable through a variety of pharmacologic and nonpharmacologic strategies.

Ballantyne, J.C., Carwood, C.M., Gupta, A., Bennett, M.I., Simpson, K.H., Dhandapani, K., ... Baraniddharan, G. (2005). Comparative efficacy of epidural, subarachnoid, and intracerebroventricular opioids in patients with pain due to cancer. *Cochrane Database of Systematic Reviews, 2005*(2). doi:10.1002/14651858.CD005178

Bandschapp, O., Filitz, J., Urwyler, A., Koppert, W., & Ruppen, W. (2011). Tropisetron blocks analgesic action of acetaminophen: A human pain model study. *Pain, 152,* 1304–1310. doi:10.1016/j.pain.2011.02.003

Bang, S.-M., Park, S.H., Kang, H.G., Jue, J.I., Cho, I.H., Yun, Y.H., ... Lee, J.H. (2005). Changes in quality of life during palliative chemotherapy for solid cancer. *Supportive Care in Cancer, 13,* 515–521. doi:10.1007/s00520-004-0708-0

Bardia, A., Greeno, E., & Bauer, B.A. (2007). Dietary supplement usage by patients with cancer undergoing chemotherapy: Does prognosis or cancer symptoms predict usage? *Journal of Supportive Oncology, 5,* 195–198.

Belfiore, G., Tedeschi, E., Ronza, F.M., Belfiore, M.P., Della Volpe, T., Zeppetella, G., & Rotondo, A. (2008). Radiofrequency ablation of bone metastases induces long-lasting palliation in patients with untreatable cancer. *Singapore Medical Journal, 49*(7), 565–570.

Berdine, H.J., & Nesbit, S.A. (2006). Equianalgesic dosing of opioids. *Journal of Pain and Palliative Care Pharmacotherapy, 20,* 79–84.

Berenson, J., Pflugmacher, R., Jarzem, P., Zonder, J., Schechtman, K., Tillman, J.B., ... Vrionis, F. (2011). Balloon kyphoplasty versus non-surgical fracture management for treatment of painful vertebral body compression fractures in patients with cancer: A multicentre, randomised controlled trial. *Lancet Oncology, 12,* 225–235. doi:10.1016/S1470-2045(11)70008-0

Botting, R.M. (2010). Vane's discovery of the mechanism of action of aspirin changed our understanding of its clinical pharmacology. *Pharmacological Reports, 62,* 518–525. doi:10.1016/S1734-1140(10)70308-X

Bradt, J., Dileo, C., Magill, L., & Teague, A. (2016). Music interventions for improving psychological and physical outcomes in cancer patients. *Cochrane Database of Systematic Reviews, 2016*(8). doi:10.1002/14651858.CD006911.pub3

Brant, J.M. (2018). Cancer pain. In C.H. Yarbro, D. Wujcik, & B.H. Gobel (Eds.), *Cancer nursing: Principles and practice* (8th ed., pp. 781–816). Burlington, MA: Jones & Bartlett Learning.

Brigatte, P., Konno, K., Gutierrez, V.P., Sampaio, S.C., Zambelli, V.O., Picolo, G., ... Cury, Y. (2013). Peripheral *kappa* and *delta* opioid receptors are involved in the antinociceptive effect of crotalphine in a rat model of cancer pain. *Pharmacology Biochemistry and Behavior, 109,* 1–7. doi:10.1016/j.pbb.2013.04.012

Browner, I., & Carducci, M.A. (2005). Palliative chemotherapy: Historical perspective, applications, and controversies. *Seminars in Oncology, 32,* 145–155. doi:10.1053/j.seminoncol.2004.11.014

Brunelli, C., Bennett, M.I., Kaasa, S., Fainsinger, R., Sjøgren, P., Mercadante, S., ... Caraceni, A. (2014). Classification of neuropathic pain in cancer patients: A Delphi expert survey report and EAPC/IASP proposal of an algorithm for diagnostic criteria. *Pain, 155,* 2707–2713. doi:10.1016/j.pain.2014.09.038

Burton, A.W., Mendoza, T., Gebhardt, R., Hamid, B., Nouri, K., Perez-Toro, M., ... Koyyalagunta, D. (2011). Vertebral compression fracture treatment with vertebroplasty and kyphoplasty: Experience in 407 patients with 1,156 fractures in a tertiary cancer center. *Pain Medicine, 12,* 1750–1757. doi:10.1111/j.1526-4637.2011.01278.x

Burton, A.W., Rajagopal, A., Shah, H.N., Mendoza, T., Cleeland, C., Hassenbusch, S.J., III, & Arens, J.F. (2004). Epidural and intrathecal analgesia is effective in treating refractory cancer pain. *Pain Medicine, 5,* 239–247. doi:10.1111/j.1526-4637.2004.04037.x

Cannon, C.P., & Cannon, P.J. (2012). Physiology. COX-2 inhibitors and cardiovascular risk. *Science, 336,* 1386–1387. doi:10.1126/science.1224398

Caraceni, A., Zecca, E., Bonezzi, C., Arcuri, E., Tur, R.Y., Maltoni, M., ... De Conno, F. (2004). Gabapentin for neuropathic cancer pain: A randomized controlled trial from the Gabapentin Cancer Pain Study Group. *Journal of Clinical Oncology, 22,* 2909–2917. doi:10.1200/JCO.2004.08.141

Cassileth, B.R., & Keefe, F.J. (2010). Integrative and behavioral approaches to the treatment of cancer-related neuropathic pain. *Oncologist, 15*(Suppl. 2), 19–23. doi:10.1634/theoncologist.2009-S504

Cephalon, Inc. (2011). *Actiq® (fentanyl citrate)* [Package insert]. Frazer, PA: Author.

Cephalon, Inc. (2013). *Fentora® (fentanyl buccal tablet)* [Package insert]. Frazer, PA: Author.

Chen, C.H., Tang, S.T., & Chen, C.H. (2012). Meta-analysis of cultural differences in Western and Asian patient-perceived barriers to managing cancer pain. *Palliative Medicine, 26,* 206–221. doi:10.1177/0269216311402711

Chen, L., Yang, G., & Grosser, T. (2013). Prostanoids and inflammatory pain. *Prostaglandins and Other Lipid Mediators, 104–105,* 58–66. doi:10.1016/j.prostaglandins.2012.08.006

Cherny, N.I., Baselga, J., de Conno, F., & Radbruch, L. (2010). Formulary availability and regulatory barriers to accessibility of opioids for cancer pain in Europe: A report from the ESMO/EAPC Opioid Policy Initiative. *Annals of Oncology, 21,* 615–626. doi:10.1093/annonc/mdp581

Cherny, N.I., Ripamonti, C., Pereira, J., Davis, C., Fallon, M., McQuay, H., ... Ventafridda, V. (2001). Strategies to manage the adverse effects of oral morphine: An evidence-based report. *Journal of Clinical Oncology, 19,* 2542–2554. doi:10.1200/JCO.2001.19.9.2542

Chou, R., Cruciani, R.A., Fiellin, D.A., Compton, P., Farrar, J.T., Haigney, M.C., … Zeltzer, L. (2014). Methadone safety: A clinical practice guideline from the American Pain Society and College on Problems of Drug Dependence, in collaboration with the Heart Rhythm Society. *Journal of Pain, 15,* 321–337. doi:10.1016/j.jpain.2014.01.494

Chow, E., Harris, K., Fan, G., Tsao, M., & Sze, W.M. (2007). Palliative radiotherapy trials for bone metastases: A systematic review. *Journal of Clinical Oncology, 25,* 1423–1436. doi:10.1200/JCO.2006.09.5281

Cleary, J.F. (2007). The pharmacologic management of cancer pain. *Journal of Palliative Medicine, 10,* 1369–1394. doi:10.1089/jpm.2007.9842

Clemens, K.E., Quednau, I., & Klaschik, E. (2008). Is there a higher risk of respiratory depression in opioid-naïve palliative care patients during symptomatic therapy of dyspnea with strong opioids? *Journal of Palliative Medicine, 11,* 204–216. doi:10.1089/jpm.2007.0131

Closs, S.J., Barr, B., Briggs, M., Cash, K., & Seers, K. (2004). A comparison of five pain assessment scales for nursing home residents with varying degrees of cognitive impairment. *Journal of Pain and Symptom Management, 27,* 196–205. doi:10.1016/j.jpainsymman.2003.12.010

Coxib and Traditional NSAID Trialists' Collaboration. (2013). Vascular and upper gastrointestinal effects of non-steroidal anti-inflammatory drugs: Meta-analyses of individual participant data from randomised trials. *Lancet, 382,* 769–779. doi:10.1016/S0140-6736(13)60900-9

Cramer, H., Lauche, R., Paul, A., Langhorst, J., Kümmel, S., & Dobos, G.J. (2015). Hypnosis in breast cancer care: A systematic review of randomized controlled trials. *Integrative Cancer Therapies, 14,* 5–15. doi:10.1177/1534735414550035

Curiel, R.V., & Katz, J.D. (2013). Mitigating the cardiovascular and renal effects of NSAIDs. *Pain Medicine, 14*(Suppl. 1), S23–S28. doi:10.1111/pme.12275

Daut, R.L., Cleeland, C.S., & Flanery, R.C. (1983). Development of the Wisconsin Brief Pain Questionnaire to assess pain in cancer and other diseases. *Pain, 17,* 197–210. doi:10.1016/0304-3959(83)90143-4

Davies, A., Buchanan, A., Zeppetella, G., Porta-Sales, J., Likar, R., Weismayr, W., … Stenberg, M. (2013). Breakthrough cancer pain: An observational study of 1000 European oncology patients. *Journal of Pain and Symptom Management, 46,* 619–628. doi:10.1016/j.jpainsymman.2012.12.009

Davis, E.L., Oh, B., Butow, P.N., Mullan, B.A., & Clarke, S. (2012). Cancer patient disclosure and patient-doctor communication of complementary and alternative medicine use: A systematic review. *Oncologist, 17,* 1475–1481. doi:10.1634/theoncologist.2012-0223

De Conno, F., Ripamonti, C., Saita, L., MacEachern, T., Hanson, J., & Bruera, E. (1995). Role of rectal route in treating cancer pain: A randomized crossover clinical trial of oral versus rectal morphine administration in opioid-naïve cancer patients with pain. *Journal of Clinical Oncology, 13,* 1004–1008. doi:10.1200/JCO.1995.13.4.1004

de la Cruz, M., & Bruera, E.D. (2010). Opioid side effects and management. In E.D. Bruera & R.K. Portenoy (Eds.), *Cancer pain: Assessment and management* (2nd ed., pp. 230–254). New York, NY: Cambridge University Press.

Depomed, Inc. (2015). *Lazanda® (fentanyl)* [Package insert]. Newark, CA: Author.

Derry, S., Wiffen, P.J., Aldington, D., & Moore, R.A. (2015). Nortriptyline for neuropathic pain in adults. *Cochrane Database of Systematic Reviews, 2015*(1). doi:10.1002/14651858.CD011209.pub2

Derry, S., Wiffen, P.J., Moore, R.A., & Quinlan, J. (2014). Topical lidocaine for neuropathic pain in adults. *Cochrane Database of Systematic Reviews, 2014*(7). doi:10.1002/14651858.CD010958.pub2

Devers, A., & Galer, B.S. (2000). Topical lidocaine patch relieves a variety of neuropathic pain conditions: An open-label study. *Clinical Journal of Pain, 16,* 205–208. doi:10.1097/00002508-200009000-00005

Dodd, M., Janson, S., Facione, N., Faucett, J., Froelicher, E.S., Humphreys, J., … Taylor, D. (2001). Advancing the science of symptom management. *Journal of Advanced Nursing, 33,* 668–676.

Dong, S.T., Butow, P.N., Costa, D.S.J., Lovell, M.R., & Agar, M. (2014). Symptom clusters in patients with advanced cancer: A systematic review of observational studies. *Journal of Pain and Symptom Management, 48,* 411–450. doi:10.1016/j.jpainsymman.2013.10.027

Dworkin, R.H., O'Connor, A.B., Backonja, M., Farrar, J.T., Jensen, T.S., Kalso, E.A., … Wallace, M.S. (2007). Pharmacologic management of neuropathic pain: Evidence-based recommendations. *Pain, 132,* 237–251. doi:10.1016/j.pain.2007.08.033

Eisenberg, E., Carr, D.B., & Chalmers, T.C. (1995). Neurolytic celiac plexus block for treatment of cancer pain: A meta-analysis. *Survey of Anesthesiology, 39,* 382.

Endo Pharmaceuticals Inc. (2014a). *Opana® ER (oxymorphone hydrochloride)* [Package insert]. Malvern, PA: Author.

Endo Pharmaceuticals Inc. (2014b). *Opana® injection (oxymorphone hydrochloride)* [Package insert]. Malvern, PA: Author.

Endo Pharmaceuticals Inc. (2015). *Lidoderm® (lidocaine patch 5%)* [Package insert]. Malvern, PA: Author.

Foley, K.M. (2005). Management of cancer pain. In V.T. DeVita, S. Hellman, & S.A. Rosenberg (Eds.), *Can-*

cer: Principles and practice of oncology (7th ed., pp. 2615–2649). Philadelphia, PA: Lippincott Williams & Wilkins.

Fourney, D.R., Schomer, D.F., Nader, R., Chlan-Fourney, J., Suki, D., Ahrar, K., ... Gokaslan, Z.L. (2003). Percutaneous vertebroplasty and kyphoplasty for painful vertebral body fractures in cancer patients. *Journal of Neurosurgery, 98*(Suppl. 1), 21–30. doi:10.3171/spi.2003.98.1.0021

Furlan, A.D., Sandoval, J.A., Mailis-Gagnon, A., & Tunks, E. (2006). Opioids for chronic noncancer pain: A meta-analysis of effectiveness and side effects. *Canadian Medical Association Journal, 174,* 1589–1594. doi:10.1503/cmaj.051528

Ganesh, A., & Maxwell, L.G. (2007). Pathophysiology and management of opioid-induced pruritus. *Drugs, 67,* 2323–2333. doi:10.2165/00003495-200767160-00003

Garcia, M.K., McQuade, J., Haddad, R., Patel, S., Lee, R. Yang, P., ... Cohen, L. (2013). Systematic review of acupuncture in cancer care: A synthesis of the evidence. *Journal of Clinical Oncology, 31,* 952–960. doi:10.1200/JCO.2012.43.5818

Gargiulo, G., Capodanno, D., Longo, G., Capranzano, P., & Tamburino, C. (2014). Updates on NSAIDs in patients with and without coronary artery disease: Pitfalls, interactions and cardiovascular outcomes. *Expert Review of Cardiovascular Therapy, 12,* 1185–1203. doi:10.1586/14779072.2014.964687

Gatlin, C.G., & Schulmeister, L. (2007). When medication is not enough: Nonpharmacologic management of pain. *Clinical Journal of Oncology Nursing, 11,* 699–704. doi:10.1188/07.CJON.699-704

Gevargez, A., & Groenemeyer, D.H.W. (2008). Image-guided radiofrequency ablation (RFA) of spinal tumors. *European Journal of Radiology, 65,* 246–252. doi:10.1016/j.ejrad.2007.03.026

Gordon, D.B., & Dahl, J.L. (2015). Fast Facts and Concepts #95: Opioid withdrawal. Retrieved from http://www.mypcnow.org/blank-nonh6

Gordon, D.B., Dahl, J.L., Miaskowski, C., McCarberg, B., Todd, K.H., Paice, J.A., ... Carr, D.B. (2005). American Pain Society recommendations for improving the quality of acute and cancer pain management: American Pain Society Quality of Care Task Force. *Archives of Internal Medicine, 165,* 1574–1580. doi:10.1001/archinte.165.14.1574

Gorin, S.S., Krebs, P., Badr, H., Janke, E.A., Jim, H.S.L., Spring, B., ... Jacobsen, P.B. (2012). Meta-analysis of psychosocial interventions to reduce pain in patients with cancer. *Journal of Clinical Oncology, 30,* 539–547. doi:10.1200/JCO.2011.37.0437

Greco, M.T., Roberto, A., Corli, O., Deandrea, S., Bandieri, E., Cavuto, S., & Apolone, G. (2014). Quality of cancer pain management: An update of a systematic review of undertreatment of patients with cancer. *Journal of Clinical Oncology, 32,* 4149–4154. doi:10.1200/JCO.2014.56.0383

Gupta, M., & Eisen, G.M. (2009). NSAIDs and the gastrointestinal tract. *Current Gastroenterology Reports, 11,* 345–353. doi:10.1007/s11894-009-0053-z

Hadley, G., Derry, S., Moore, R.A., & Wiffen, P.J. (2013). Transdermal fentanyl for cancer pain. *Cochrane Database of Systematic Reviews, 2013*(10). doi:10.1002/14651858.CD010270.pub2

Hassenbusch, S.J., & Portenoy, R.K. (2000). Current practices in intraspinal therapy—A survey of clinical trends and decision making. *Journal of Pain and Symptom Management, 20*(2), S4–S11. doi:10.1016/S0885-3924(00)00203-7

Hayek, S.M., Deer, T.R., Pope, J.E., Panchal, S.J., & Patel, V.B. (2011). Intrathecal therapy for cancer and non-cancer pain. *Pain Physician, 14,* 219–248.

Hearn, L., Moore, R.A., Derry, S., Wiffen, P.J., & Phillips, T. (2014). Desipramine for neuropathic pain in adults. *Cochrane Database of Systematic Reviews, 2014*(9). doi:10.1002/14651858.CD011003.pub2

Heiskanen, T., Mätzke, S., Haakana, S., Gergov, M., Vuori, E., & Kalso, E. (2009). Transdermal fentanyl in cachectic cancer patients. *Pain, 144,* 218–222. doi:10.1016/j.pain.2009.04.012

Henry, D., Vadhan-Raj, S., Hirsh, V., von Moos, R., Hungria, V., Costa, L., ... Yeh, H. (2014). Delaying skeletal-related events in a randomized phase 3 study of denosumab versus zoledronic acid in patients with advanced cancer: An analysis of data from patients with solid tumors. *Supportive Care in Cancer, 22,* 679–687. doi:10.1007/s00520-013-2022-1

Herr, K., Spratt, K.F., Garand, L., & Li, L. (2007). Evaluation of the Iowa Pain Thermometer and other selected pain intensity scales in younger and older adult cohorts using controlled clinical pain: A preliminary study. *Pain Medicine, 8,* 585–600. doi:10.1111/j.1526-4637.2007.00316.x

Hillegonds, D.J., Franklin, S., Shelton, D.K., Vijayakumar, S., & Vijayakumar, V. (2007). The management of painful bone metastases with an emphasis on radionuclide therapy. *Journal of the National Medical Association, 99,* 785–794.

Hökkä, M., Kaakinen, P., & Pölkki, T. (2014). A systematic review: Non-pharmacological interventions in treating pain in patients with advanced cancer. *Journal of Advanced Nursing, 70,* 1954–1969. doi:10.1111/jan.12424

Huang, L., Tao, F., Wang, Z., Wan, H., Qu, P., & Zheng, H. (2014). Combined neurolytic block of celiac and superior hypogastric plexuses for incapacitating upper abdominal cancer pain. *Journal of the Balkan Union of Oncology, 19,* 826–830.

INSYS Therapeutics, Inc. (2014). *Subsys® (fentanyl sublingual spray)* [Package insert]. Phoenix, AZ: Author.

International Association for the Study of Pain. (2012, May 22). IASP taxonomy. Retrieved from http://www.iasp-pain.org/Education/Content.aspx?ItemNumber=1698#Pain

Jandhyala, R., & Fullarton, J. (2012). Various formulations of oral transmucosal fentanyl for breakthrough cancer pain: An indirect mixed treatment comparison meta-analysis. *BMJ Supportive and Palliative Care, 2,* 156–162. doi:10.1136/bmjspcare-2011-000139

Janssen Pharmaceuticals, Inc. (2014). *Duragesic® (fentanyl transdermal system)* [Package insert]. Titusville, NJ: Author.

Jarupongprapa, S., Ussavasodhi, P., & Katchamart, W. (2013). Comparison of gastrointestinal adverse effects between cyclooxygenase-2 inhibitors and non-selective, non-steroidal anti-inflammatory drugs plus proton pump inhibitors: A systematic review and meta-analysis. *Journal of Gastroenterology, 48,* 830–838. doi:10.1007/s00535-012-0717-6

Jarzyna, D., Jungquist, C.R., Pasero, C., Willens, J.S., Nisbet, A., Oakes, L., ... Polomano, R.C. (2011). American Society for Pain Management Nursing guidelines on monitoring for opioid-induced sedation and respiratory depression. *Pain Management Nursing, 12,* 118–145. doi:10.1016/j.pmn.2011.06.008

Jeon, Y.S., Lee, J.A., Choi, J.W., Kang, E.G., Jung, H.S., Kim, H.K., ... Joo, J.D. (2012). Efficacy of epidural analgesia in patients with cancer pain: A retrospective observational study. *Yonsei Medical Journal, 53,* 649–653. doi:10.3349/ymj.2012.53.3.649

Kadiroglu, A.K., Sita, D., Kayabasi, H., Tuzcu, A.K., Tasdemir, N., & Yilmaz, M.E. (2008). The effect of venlafaxine HCl on painful peripheral diabetic neuropathy in patients with type 2 diabetes mellitus. *Journal of Diabetes and Its Complications, 22,* 241–245. doi:10.1016/j.jdiacomp.2007.03.010

Katz, W.A., & Rothenberg, R. (2005). Section 3: The nature of pain: Pathophysiology. *Journal of Clinical Rheumatology, 11*(Suppl. 2), S11–S15. doi:10.1097/01.rhu.0000158686.43637.af

Keskinbora, K., Pekel, A.F., & Aydinli, I. (2007). Gabapentin and an opioid combination versus opioid alone for the management of neuropathic cancer pain: A randomized open trial. *Journal of Pain and Symptom Management, 34,* 183–189. doi:10.1016/j.jpainsymman.2006.11.013

Kostenuik, P.J., Nguyen, H.Q., McCabe, J., Warmington, K.S., Kurahara, C., Sun, N., ... Sullivan, J.K. (2009). Denosumab, a fully human monoclonal antibody to RANKL, inhibits bone resorption and increases BMD in knock-in mice that express chimeric (murine/human) RANKL. *Journal of Bone and Mineral Research, 24,* 182–195. doi:10.1359/jbmr.081112

Kroenke, K., Theobald, D., Wu, J., Loza, J.K., Carpenter, J.S., & Tu, W. (2010). The association of depression and pain with health-related quality of life, disability, and health care use in cancer patients. *Journal of Pain and Symptom Management, 40,* 327–341. doi:10.1016/j.jpainsymman.2009.12.023

Kutner, J.S., Smith, M.C., Corbin, L., Hemphill, L., Benton, K., Mellis, B.K., ... Fairclough, D.L. (2008). Massage therapy versus simple touch to improve pain and mood in patients with advanced cancer: A randomized trial. *Annals of Internal Medicine, 149,* 369–379. doi:10.7326/0003-4819-149-6-200809160-00003

Kwekkeboom, K.L., Bumpus, M., Wanta, B., & Serlin, R.C. (2008). Oncology nurses' use of nondrug pain interventions in practice. *Journal of Pain and Symptom Management, 35,* 83–94. doi:10.1016/j.jpainsymman.2007.02.037

Kwekkeboom, K.L., Cherwin, C.H., Lee, J.W., & Wanta, B. (2010). Mind-body treatments for the pain-fatigue-sleep disturbance symptom cluster in persons with cancer. *Journal of Pain and Symptom Management, 39,* 126–138.

Kwon, J.H. (2014). Overcoming barriers in cancer pain management. *Journal of Clinical Oncology, 32,* 1727–1733. doi:10.1016/j.jpainsymman.2006.12.011

Lane, M.E., & Kim, M.-J. (2006). Assessment and prevention of gastrointestinal toxicity of non-steroidal anti-inflammatory drugs. *Journal of Pharmacy and Pharmacology, 58,* 1295–1304. doi:10.1111/j.2042-7158.2006.tb01645.x

Lantheus Medical Imaging, Inc. (2014). *Quadramet® (samarium Sm 153 lexidronam)* [Package insert]. N. Billerica, MA: Author.

Lanza, F.L., Chan, F.K.L., & Quigley, E.M.M. (2009). Guidelines for prevention of NSAID-related ulcer complications. *American Journal of Gastroenterology, 104,* 728–738. doi:10.1038/ajg.2009.115

LeBlanc, T.W., & Abernethy, A.P. (2015). Management of cancer pain. In V.T. DeVita Jr., T.S. Lawrence, & S.A. Rosenberg (Eds.), *Cancer: Principles and practice of oncology* (10th ed., pp 2084–2104). Philadelphia, PA: Wolters Kluwer Health/Lippincott Williams & Wilkins.

Lee, S.-H., Kim, J.-Y., Yeo, S., Kim, S.-H., & Lim, S. (2015). Meta-analysis of massage therapy on cancer pain. *Integrative Cancer Therapies, 14,* 297–304. doi:10.1177/1534735415572885

Lee, Y.J., Hyun, M.K., Jung, Y.J., Kang, M.J., Keam, B., & Go, S.J. (2015). Effectiveness of education interventions for the management of cancer pain: A systematic review. *Asian Pacific Journal of Cancer Prevention, 15,* 4787–4793. doi:10.7314/APJCP.2014.15.12.4787

Lian, W.-L., Pan, M.-Q., Zhou, D.-H., & Zhang, Z.-J. (2014). Effectiveness of acupuncture for palliative care in cancer patients: A systematic review. *Chinese Journal of Integrative Medicine, 20,* 136–147. doi:10.1007/s11655-013-1439-1

Ling, C.-C., Lui, L.Y.Y., & So, W.K.W. (2012). Do educational interventions improve cancer patients' quality of life and reduce pain intensity? Quantitative systematic review. *Journal of Advanced Nursing, 68,* 511–520. doi:10.1111/j.1365-2648.2011.05841.x

Locklin, J.K., Mannes, A., Berger, A., & Wood, B.J. (2004). Palliation of soft tissue cancer pain with radiofrequency ablation. *Journal of Supportive Oncology, 2,* 439–445.

Locklin, J.K., & Wood, B.J. (2005). Radiofrequency ablation: A nursing perspective. *Clinical Journal of Oncology Nursing, 9,* 346–349. doi:10.1188/05.CJON.346-349

Lovell, M.R., Luckett, T., Boyle, F.M., Phillips, J., Agar, M., & Davidson, P.M. (2014). Patient education, coaching, and self-management for cancer pain. *Journal of Clinical Oncology, 32,* 1712–1720. doi:10.1200/JCO.2013.52.4850

Lukas, A., Barber, J.B., Johnson, P., & Gibson, S.J. (2013). Observer-rated pain assessment instruments improve both the detection of pain and the evaluation of pain intensity in people with dementia. *European Journal of Pain, 17,* 1558–1568. doi:10.1002/j.1532-2149.2013.00336.x

Lunn, M.P.T., Hughes, R.A.C., & Wiffen, P.J. (2014). Duloxetine for treating painful neuropathy, chronic pain or fibromyalgia. *Cochrane Database of Systematic Reviews, 2014*(1). doi:10.1002/14651858.CD007115.pub3

Lussier, D., Huskey, A.G., & Portenoy, R.K. (2004). Adjuvant analgesics in cancer pain management. *Oncologist, 9,* 571–591. doi:10.1634/theoncologist.9-5-571

Lutz, S., Berk, L., Chang, E., Chow, E., Hahn, C., Hoskin, P., … Hartsell, W. (2011). Palliative radiotherapy for bone metastases: An ASTRO evidence-based guideline. *International Journal of Radiation Oncology, Biology, Physics, 79,* 965–976. doi:10.1016/j.ijrobp.2010.11.026

Mallinckrodt Brand Pharmaceuticals, Inc. (2015). *Exalgo® (hydromorphone HCl)* [Package insert]. Hazelwood, MO: Author.

Maloney, C.M., Kesner, R.K., Klein, G., & Bockenstette, J. (1989). The rectal administration of MS Contin: Clinical implications of use in end stage cancer. *American Journal of Hospice and Palliative Medicine, 6,* 34–35. doi:10.1177/104990918900600409

Marie, N., Luckett, T., Davidson, P.M., Lovell, M., & Lal, S. (2013). Optimal patient education for cancer pain: A systematic review and theory-based meta-analysis. *Supportive Care in Cancer, 21,* 3529–3537. doi:10.1007/s00520-013-1995-0

McCaffery, M., & Pasero, C. (1999). *Pain: Clinical manual* (2nd ed.). St. Louis, MO: Mosby.

McCahill, L.E., & Ferrell, B. (2002). Palliative surgery for cancer pain. *Western Journal of Medicine, 176,* 107–110.

McCahill, L.E., Krouse, R., Chu, D., Juarez, G., Uman, G.C., Ferrell, B., & Wagman, L.D. (2002). Indications and use of palliative surgery—Results of Society of Surgical Oncology survey. *Annals of Surgical Oncology, 9,* 104–112. doi:10.1245/aso.2002.9.1.104

McCarberg, B.H., Nicholson, B.D., Todd, K.H., Palmer, T., & Penles, L. (2008). The impact of pain on quality of life and the unmet needs of pain management: Results from pain sufferers and physicians participating in an internet survey. *American Journal of Therapeutics, 15,* 312–320. doi:10.1097/MJT.0b013e31818164f2

McCorkle, R., & Young, K. (1978). Development of a symptom distress scale. *Cancer Nursing, 1,* 373–378. doi:10.1097/00002820-197810000-00003

McDonald, A.A., & Portenoy, R.K. (2006). How to use antidepressants and anticonvulsants as adjuvant analgesics in the treatment of neuropathic cancer pain. *Journal of Supportive Oncology, 4,* 43–52.

McNicol, E., Horowicz-Mehler, N., Fisk, R.A., Bennett, K., Gialeli-Goudas, M., Chew, P.W., … Carr, D. (2003). Management of opioid side effects in cancer-related and chronic noncancer pain: A systematic review. *Journal of Pain, 4,* 231–256. doi:10.1016/S1526-5900(03)00556-X

Meghani, S.H., Byun, E., & Gallagher, R.M. (2012). Time to take stock: A meta-analysis and systematic review of analgesic treatment disparities for pain in the United States. *Pain Medicine, 13,* 150–174. doi:10.1111/j.1526-4637.2011.01310.x

Melzack, R. (1975). The McGill pain questionnaire: Major properties and scoring methods. *Pain, 1,* 277–299. doi:10.1016/0304-3959(75)90044-5

Mercadante, S., & Fulfaro, F. (2007). Management of painful bone metastases. *Current Opinion in Oncology, 19,* 308–314. doi:10.1097/CCO.0b013e3281214400

Mhaskar, R., Redzepovic, J., Wheatley, K., Clark, O.A.C., Miladinovic, B., Glasmacher, A., … Djulbegovic, B. (2012). Bisphosphonates in multiple myeloma: A network meta-analysis. *Cochrane Database of Systematic Reviews, 2012*(5). doi:10.1002/14651858.CD003188.pub3

Miaskowski, C.A., Brant, J.M., Caldwell, P., Eaton, L., Gallagher, E., Gallagher, N., … Yeh, C.-H. (2017). Putting evidence into practice: Pain. Retrieved from https://www.ons.org/practice-resources/pep/pain

Miner, T.J. (2005). Palliative surgery for advanced cancer: Lessons learned in patient selection and outcome assessment. *American Journal of Clinical Oncology, 28,* 411–414. doi:10.1097/01.coc.0000158489.82482.2b

Mishra, S., Bhatnagar, S., Goyal, G.N., Rana, S.P.S., & Upadhya, S.P. (2012). A comparative efficacy of amitriptyline, gabapentin, and pregabalin in neuropathic cancer pain: A prospective randomized double-blind placebo-controlled study. *American Journal of Hospice and Palliative Medicine, 29,* 177–182. doi:10.1177/1049909111412539

Mishra, S., Bhatnagar, S., Rana, S.P.S., Khurana, D., & Thulkar, S. (2013). Efficacy of the anterior ultrasound-guided superior hypogastric plexus neurolysis in pelvic cancer pain in advanced gynecological cancer patients. *Pain Medicine, 14,* 837–842. doi:10.1111/pme.12106

Monthly prescribing reference nurse practitioners' edition. (2015). New York, NY: Haymarket Media.

Moore, R.A., Derry, S., Aldington, D., Cole, P., & Wiffen, P.J. (2015). Amitriptyline for neuropathic pain in adults. *Cochrane Database of Systematic Reviews, 2015*(7). doi:10.1002/14651858.CD008242.pub3

Moore, R.A., Straube, S., Wiffen, P.J., Derry, S., & McQuay, H.J. (2010). Pregabalin for acute and chronic pain in adults. *Cochrane Database of Systematic Reviews, 2010*(3). doi:10.1002/14651858.CD007076.pub2

Moore, R.A., Wiffen, P.J., Derry, S., Toelle, T., & Rice, A.S.C. (2014). Gabapentin for chronic neuropathic pain and fibromyalgia in adults. *Cochrane Database of Systematic Reviews, 2014*(4). doi:10.1002/14651858.CD007938.pub3

Nagels, W., Pease, N., Bekkering, G., Cools, F., & Dobbels, P. (2013). Celiac plexus neurolysis for abdominal cancer pain: A systematic review. *Pain Medicine, 14,* 1140–1163. doi:10.1111/pme.12176

National Cancer Institute. (2016). Cancer pain (PDQ®) [Health professional version]. Retrieved from https://www.cancer.gov/about-cancer/treatment/side-effects/pain/pain-hp-pdq

National Comprehensive Cancer Network. (2016). *NCCN Clinical Practice Guidelines in Oncology (NCCN Guidelines®): Adult cancer pain* [v.2.2016]. Retrieved from http://www.nccn.org/professionals/physician_gls/pdf/pain.pdf

Nderitu, P., Doos, L., Jones, P.W., Davies, S.J., & Kadam, U.T. (2013). Non-steroidal anti-inflammatory drugs and chronic kidney disease progression: A systematic review. *Family Practice, 30,* 247–255. doi:10.1093/fampra/cms086

Nicholson, A.B., Watson, G.R., Derry, S., & Wiffen, P.J. (2017). Methadone for cancer pain. *Cochrane Database of Systematic Reviews, 2007*(4). doi:10.1002/14651858.CD003971.pub3

Novartis Pharmaceuticals Corp. (2015). *Zometa® (zoledronic acid)* [Package insert]. East Hanover, NJ: Author.

Oliveira, K.G., von Zeidler, S.V., Podestá, J.R.V., Sena, A., Souza, E.D., Lenzi, J., ... Gouvea, S.A. (2014). Influence of pain severity on the quality of life in patients with head and neck cancer before antineoplastic therapy. *BMC Cancer, 14,* 39. doi:10.1186/1471-2407-14-39

Ong, C.K.S., Lirk, P., Tan, C.H., & Seymour, R.A. (2007). An evidence-based update on nonsteroidal anti-inflammatory drugs. *Clinical Medicine and Research, 5,* 19–34. doi:10.3121/cmr.2007.698

Otake, A., Yoshino, K., Ueda, Y., Sawada, K., Mabuchi, S., Kimura, T., ... Kimura, T. (2015). Usefulness of duloxetine for paclitaxel-induced peripheral neuropathy treatment in gynecological cancer patients. *Anticancer Research, 35,* 359–364. Retrieved from http://ar.iiarjournals.org/content/35/1/359.long

Paley, C.A., Johnson, M.I., Tashani, O.A., & Bagnall, A.-M. (2015). Acupuncture for cancer pain in adults. *Cochrane Database of Systematic Reviews, 2015*(10). doi:10.1002/14651858.CD007753.pub3

Parker, C., Nilsson, S., Heinrich, D., Helle, S.I., O'Sullivan, J.M., Fosså, S.D., ... Sartor, O. (2013). Alpha emitter radium-223 and survival in metastatic prostate cancer. *New England Journal of Medicine, 369,* 213–223. doi:10.1056/NEJMoa1213755

Patti, J.W., Neeman, Z., & Wood, B.J. (2002). Radiofrequency ablation for cancer-associated pain. *Journal of Pain, 3,* 471–473. doi:10.1054/jpai.2002.126785

Paulsen, Ø., Aass, N., Kaasa, S., & Dale, O. (2013). Do corticosteroids provide analgesic effects in cancer patients? A systematic literature review. *Journal of Pain and Symptom Management, 46,* 96–105. doi:10.1016/j.jpainsymman.2012.06.019

Peddi, P., Lopez-Olivo, M.A., Pratt, G.F., & Suarez-Almazor, M.E. (2013). Denosumab in patients with cancer and skeletal metastases: A systematic review and meta-analysis. *Cancer Treatment Reviews, 39,* 97–104. doi:10.1016/j.ctrv.2012.07.002

Pergolizzi, J.V., Jr., Mercadante, S., Echaburu, A.V., Van den Eynden, B., de Faría Fragoso, R.M., Mordarski, S., ... Slama, O. (2009). The role of transdermal buprenorphine in the treatment of cancer pain: An expert panel consensus. *Current Medical Research and Opinion, 25,* 1517–1528. doi:10.1185/03007990902920731

Pernix Therapeutics, LLC. (2015). *Zohydro® ER (hydrocodone bitartrate)* [Package insert]. Morristown, NJ: Author.

Pertwee, R.G. (2006). Cannabinoid pharmacology: The first 66 years. *British Journal of Pharmacology, 147,* S163–S171. doi:10.1038/sj.bjp.0706406

Peters, M.L., Patijn, J., & Lamé, I. (2007). Pain assessment in younger and older pain patients: Psychometric properties and patient preference of five commonly used measures of pain intensity. *Pain Medicine, 8,* 601–610. doi:10.1111/j.1526-4637.2007.00311.x

Pfizer Inc. (2014). *Avinza® (morphine sulfate capsule, extended release)* [Package insert]. New York, NY: Author.

Plancarte, R., de Leon-Casasola, O.A., El-Helaly, M., Allende, S., & Lema, M.J. (1997). Neurolytic superior hypogastric plexus block for chronic pelvic pain associated with cancer. *Regional Anesthesia, 22,* 562–568.

Portenoy, R.K., & Ahmed, E. (2014). Principles of opioid use in cancer pain. *Journal of Clinical Oncology, 32,* 1662–1670. doi:10.1200/JCO.2013.52.5188

Portenoy, R.K., Ganae-Motan, E.D., Allende, S., Yanagihara, R., Shaiova, L., Weinstein, S., ... Fallon, M.T. (2012). Nabiximols for opioid-treated cancer patients with poorly-controlled chronic pain: A randomized, placebo-controlled, graded-dose trial. *Journal of Pain, 13,* 438–449. doi:10.1016/j.jpain.2012.01.003

Prommer, E. (2015). Fast Facts and Concepts #92: Patient controlled analgesia in palliative care. Retrieved from http://www.mypcnow.org/blank-ypz41

Purdue Pharma L.P. (2014a). *Butrans® (buprenorphine patch, extended release)* [Package insert]. Stamford, CT: Author.

Purdue Pharma L.P. (2014b). *Hysingla™ ER (hydrocodone bitartrate tablet, extended release)* [Package insert]. Stamford, CT: Author.

Purdue Pharma L.P. (2014c). *MS Contin® (morphine sulfate tablet, film coated, extended release)* [Package insert]. Stamford, CT: Author.

Purdue Pharma L.P. (2014d). *Oxycontin® (oxycodone hydrochloride tablet, film coated, extended release)* [Package insert]. Stamford, CT: Author.

Quan, G.M.Y., Vital, J.-M., Aurouer, N., Obeid, I., Palussiére, J., Diallo, A., & Pointillart, V. (2011). Surgery improves pain, function and quality of life in patients with spinal metastases: A prospective study on 118 patients. *European Spine Journal, 20,* 1970–1978. doi:10.1007/s00586-011-1867-6

Raffa, R.B., Friderichs, E., Reimann, W., Shank, R.P., Codd, E.E., & Vaught, J.L. (1992). Opioid and nonopioid components independently contribute to the mechanism of action of tramadol, an "atypical" opioid analgesic. *Journal of Pharmacology and Experimental Therapeutics, 260,* 275–285.

Rajan, J.P., Wineinger, N.E., Stevenson, D.D., & White, A.A. (2015). Prevalence of aspirin-exacerbated respiratory disease among asthmatic patients: A meta-analysis of the literature. *Journal of Allergy and Clinical Immunology, 135,* 676–681. doi:10.1016/j.jaci.2014.08.020

Raphael, J., Ahmedzai, S., Hester, J., Urch, C., Barrie, J., Williams, J., ... Sparkes, E. (2010). Cancer pain: Part 1: Pathophysiology, oncological, pharmacological, and psychological treatments: A perspective from the British Pain Society endorsed by the UK Association of Palliative Medicine and the Royal College of General Practitioners. *Pain Medicine, 11,* 742–764. doi:10.1111/j.1526-4637.2010.00840.x

Raptis, E., Vadalouca, A., Stavropoulou, E., Argyra, E., Melemeni, A., & Siafaka, I. (2014). Pregabalin vs. opioids for the treatment of neuropathic cancer pain: A prospective, head-to-head, randomized, open-label study. *Pain Practice, 14,* 32–42. doi:10.1111/papr.12045

Raslan, A.M. (2008). Percutaneous computed tomography-guided radiofrequency ablation of upper spinal cord pain pathways for cancer-related pain. *Operative Neurosurgery, 62*(Suppl. 1), S226–S234. doi:10.1227/01.neu.0000317397.16089.f5

Rayment, C., Hjermstad, M.J., Aass, N., Kaasa, S., Caraceni, A., Strasser, F., ... Bennett, M.I. (2013). Neuropathic cancer pain: Prevalence, severity, analgesics and impact from the European Palliative Care Research Collaborative–Computerised Symptom Assessment study. *Palliative Medicine, 27,* 714–721. doi:10.1177/0269216312464408

Razazian, N., Baziyar, M., Moradian, N., Afshari, D., Bostani, A., & Mahmoodi, M. (2014). Evaluation of the efficacy and safety of pregabalin, venlafaxine, and carbamazepine in patients with painful diabetic peripheral neuropathy: A randomized, double-blind trial. *Neurosciences, 19,* 192–198. Retrieved from https://www.ncbi.nlm.nih.gov/pmc/articles/PMC4727652/pdf/Neurosciences-19-192.pdf

Reisfield, G.M., & Wilson, G.R. (2007). Rational use of sublingual opioids in palliative medicine. *Journal of Palliative Medicine, 10,* 465–475. doi:10.1089/jpm.2006.0150

Renn, C.L., & Dorsey, S.G. (2005). The physiology and processing of pain: A review. *AACN Clinical Issues, 16,* 277–290. doi:10.1097/00044067-200507000-00002

Reuben, S.S., Makari-Judson, G., & Lurie, S.D. (2004). Evaluation of efficacy of the perioperative administration of venlafaxine XR in the prevention of postmastectomy pain syndrome. *Journal of Pain and Symptom Management, 27,* 133–139. doi:10.1016/j.jpainsymman.2003.06.004

Roqué i Figuls, M., Martinez-Zapata, M.J., Scott-Brown, M., & Alonso-Coello, P. (2011). Radioisotopes for metastatic bone pain. *Cochrane Database of Systematic Reviews, 2011*(7). doi:10.1002/14651858.CD003347.pub2

Rostom, A., Dube, C., Wells, G.A., Tugwell, P., Welch, V., Jolicoeur, E., ... Lanas, A. (2002). Prevention of NSAID-induced gastroduodenal ulcers. *Cochrane Database of Systematic Reviews, 2002*(4). doi:10.1002/14651858.CD002296

Saarto, T., & Wiffen, P.J. (2007). Antidepressants for neuropathic pain. *Cochrane Database of Systematic Reviews, 2007*(4). doi:10.1002/14651858.CD005454.pub2

Sartor, O., Coleman, R., Nilsson, S., Heinrich, D., Helle, S.I., O'Sullivan, J.M., ... Parker, C. (2014). Effect of radium-223 dichloride on symptomatic skeletal events in patients with castration-resistant prostate cancer and bone metastases: Results from a phase 3, double-blind, randomised trial. *Lancet Oncology, 15,* 738–746. doi:10.1016/S1470-2045(14)70183-4

Seifert, C.F., & Kennedy, S. (2004). Meperidine is alive and well in the new millennium: Evaluation of meperidine usage and patterns and frequency of adverse drug reactions. *Pharmacotherapy, 24,* 776–783. doi:10.1592/phco.24.8.776.36066

Sentynl Therapeutics, Inc. (2015). *Abstral® (fentanyl sublingual tablets)* [Package insert]. Solana Beach, CA: Author.

Shelley, M., Harrison, C., Coles, B., Stafforth, J., Wilt, T.J., & Mason, M. (2006). Chemotherapy for hormone-refractory prostate cancer. *Cochrane Database of Systematic Reviews, 2006*(4). doi:10.1002/14651858.CD005247.pub2

Slappendel, R., Weber, E.W.G., Benraad, B., van Limbeek, J., & Dirksen, R. (2000). Itching after intrathecal morphine: Incidence and treatment. *European Journal of Anaesthesiology, 17,* 616–621. doi:10.1097/00003643-200010000-00004

Sloan, P.A. (2004). The evolving role of interventional pain management in oncology. *Journal of Supportive Oncology, 2,* 491–506.

Smith, H.S., & Laufer, A. (2014). Opioid induced nausea and vomiting. *European Journal of Pharmacology, 722,* 67–78. doi:10.1016/j.ejphar.2013.09.074

Sostres, C., Gargallo, C.J., Arroyo, M.T., & Lanas, A. (2010). Adverse effects of non-steroidal anti-inflammatory drugs (NSAIDs, aspirin and coxibs) on upper gastrointestinal tract. *Best Practice and Research Clinical Gastroenterology, 24,* 121–132. doi:10.1016/j.bpg.2009.11.005

Straube, C., Derry, S., Jackson, K.C., Wiffen, P.J., Bell, R.F., Strassels, S., & Straube, S. (2014). Codeine, alone and with paracetamol (acetaminophen), for cancer pain. *Cochrane Database of Systematic Reviews, 2014*(9). doi:10.1002/14651858.CD006601.pub4

Syrjala, K.L., Cummings, C., & Donaldson, G.W. (1992). Hypnosis or cognitive behavioral training for the reduction of pain and nausea during cancer treatment: A controlled clinical trial. *Pain, 48,* 137–146. doi:10.1016/0304-3959(92)90049-H

Syrjala, K.L., Jensen, M.P., Mendoza, M.E., Yi, J.C., Fisher, H.M., & Keefe, F.J. (2014). Psychological and behavioral approaches to cancer pain management. *Journal of Clinical Oncology, 32,* 1703–1711. doi:10.1200/JCO.2013.54.4825

Tarumi, Y., Wilson, M.P., Szafran, O., & Spooner, G.R. (2013). Randomized, double-blind, placebo-controlled trial of oral docusate in the management of constipation in hospice patients. *Journal of Pain and Symptom Management, 35,* 2–13. doi:10.1016/j.jpainsymman.2012.02.008

Tasmuth, T., Härtel, B., & Kalso, E. (2002). Venlafaxine in neuropathic pain following treatment of breast cancer. *European Journal of Pain, 6,* 17–24. doi:10.1053/eujp.2001.0266

Tassinari, D., Drudi, F., Rosati, M., Tombesi, P., Sartori, S., & Maltoni, M. (2011). The second step of the analgesic ladder and oral tramadol in the treatment of mild to moderate cancer pain: A systematic review. *Palliative Medicine, 25,* 410–423. doi:10.1177/0269216311405090

Thomas, J., Karver, S., Cooney, G.A., Chamberlain, B.H., Watt, C.K., Slatkin, N.E., ... Israel, R.J. (2008). Methylnaltrexone for opioid-induced constipation in advanced illness. *New England Journal of Medicine, 358,* 2332–2343. doi:10.1056/NEJMoa0707377

Towler, P., Molassiotis, A., & Brearley, S.G. (2013). What is the evidence for the use of acupuncture as an intervention for symptom management in cancer supportive and palliative care: An integrative overview of reviews. *Supportive Care in Cancer, 21,* 2913–2923. doi:10.1007/s00520-013-1882-8

Tsai, H.F., Chen, Y.R., Chung, M.H., Liao, Y.M., Chi, M.J., Chang, C.C., & Chou, K.R. (2014). Effectiveness of music intervention in ameliorating cancer patients' anxiety, depression, pain, and fatigue: A meta-analysis. *Cancer Nursing, 37,* E35–E50. doi:10.1097/NCC.0000000000000116

Twycross, R., Prommer, E.E., Myhalyo, M., & Wilcock, A. (2012). Fentanyl (transmucosal). *Journal of Pain and Symptom Management, 44,* 131–149. doi:10.1016/j.jpainsymman.2012.05.001

Ungprasert, P., Srivali, N., Wijarnpreecha, K., Charoenpong, P., & Knight, E.L. (2015). Non-steroidal anti-inflammatory drugs and risk of venous thromboembolism: A systematic review and meta-analysis. *Rheumatology, 54,* 736–742. doi:10.1093/rheumatology/keu408

U.S. Food and Drug Administration. (2008, September 26). Radiofrequency ablation devices. Retrieved from http://www.fda.gov/safety/medwatch/safetyinformation/safetyalertsforhumanmedicalproducts/ucm152662.htm

U.S. Food and Drug Administration. (2013, March 1). Questions and answers: FDA approves a risk evaluation and mitigation strategy (REMS) for extended-release and long-acting (ER/LA) opioid analgesics. Retrieved from http://www.fda.gov/Drugs/DrugSafety/InformationbyDrugClass/ucm309742.htm

van den Beuken-van Everdingen, M.H., de Rijke, J.M., Kessels, A.G., Schouten, H.C., van Kleef, M., & Patijn, J. (2007). Prevalence of pain in patients with cancer: A systematic review of the past 40 years. *Annals of Oncology, 18,* 1437–1449. doi:10.1093/annonc/mdm056

van den Beuken-van Everdingen, M.H., Geurts, J.W., & Patijn, J. (2013). Prolonged QT interval by methadone: Relevance for daily practice? A prospective study in patients with cancer and noncancer pain. *Journal of Opioid Management, 9,* 263–267. doi:101097/SPC.0bo13e328355eo82

Vengalil, S., O'Sullivan, J.M., & Parker, C.C. (2012). Use of radionuclides in metastatic prostate cancer: Pain relief and beyond. Current Opinion in *Supportive and Palliative Care, 6,* 310–315. doi:10.1097/SPC.0b013e328355e082

von Gunten, C.F. (2011). Pathophysiology of pain in cancer. *Journal of Pediatric Hematology/Oncology, 33*(Suppl.), S12–S18. doi:10.1097/MPH.0b013e31821218a7

Walsh, T.D., Rivera, N.I., & Kaiko, R. (2003). Oral morphine and respiratory function amongst hospice inpatients with advanced cancer. *Supportive Care in Cancer, 11,* 780–784. doi:10.1007/s00520-003-0530-0

Weill, A., Chiras, J., Simon, J.M., Rose, M., Sola-Martinez, T., & Enkaoua, E. (1996). Spinal metastases: Indications for and results of percutaneous injection of acrylic surgical cement. *Radiology, 199,* 241–247. doi:10.1148/radiology.199.1.8633152

Weir, M.R. (2002). Renal effects of nonselective NSAIDs and coxibs. *Cleveland Clinic Journal of Medicine, 69*(Suppl. 1), SI53–SI58. doi:10.3949/ccjm.69.Suppl_1.SI53

Wieder, R., DeLaRosa, N., Bryan, M., Hill, A.M., & Amadio, W.J (2014). Prescription coverage in indigent patients affects the use of long-acting opioids in the management of cancer pain. *Pain Medicine, 15,* 42–51. doi:10.1111/pme.12238

Wiffen, P.J., Derry, S., & Moore, R.A. (2013). Lamotrigine for chronic neuropathic pain and fibromyalgia in adults. *Cochrane Database of Systematic Reviews, 2013*(12). doi:10.1002/14651858.CD006044.pub4

Wolfe, M.M., Lichtenstein, D.R., & Singh, G. (1999). Gastrointestinal toxicity of nonsteroidal antiinflammatory drugs. *New England Journal of Medicine, 340,* 1888–1899. doi:10.1056/NEJM199906173402407

Wong, M.H.F., Stockler, M.R., & Pavlakis, N. (2012). Bisphosphonates and other bone agents for breast cancer. *Cochrane Database of Systematic Reviews, 2012*(2). doi:10.1002/14651858.CD003474.pub3

World Health Organization. (n.d.). WHO's cancer pain ladder for adults. Retrieved from http://www.who.int/cancer/palliative/painladder/en

Wu, J., Zheng, W., Xiao, J.R., Sun, X., Liu, W.Z., & Guo, Q. (2010). Health-related quality of life in patients with spinal metastases treated with or without spinal surgery: A prospective, longitudinal study. *Cancer, 116,* 3875–3882. doi:10.1002/cncr.25126

Yang, Q., Xie, D.-R., Jiang, Z.-M., Ma, W., Zhang, Y.-D., Bi, Z.-F., & Chen, D.-L. (2010). Efficacy and adverse effects of transdermal fentanyl and sustained-release oral morphine in treating moderate-severe cancer pain in Chinese population: A systematic review and meta-analysis. *Journal of Experimental and Clinical Cancer Research, 29,* 67. doi:10.1186/1756-9966-29-67

Yang, Y.H., Lin, J.K., Chen, W.S., Lin, T.Z., Yang, S.H., Jiang, J.K., ... Teng, H.W. (2012). Duloxetine improves oxaliplatin-induced neuropathy in patients with colorectal cancer: An open-label pilot study. *Supportive Care in Cancer, 20,* 1491–1497. doi:10.1007/s00520-011-1237-2

Yuen, K.K., Shelley, M., Sze, W.M., Wilt, T.J., & Mason, M. (2006). Bisphosphonates for advanced prostate cancer. *Cochrane Database of Systematic Reviews, 2006*(4). doi:10.1002/14651858.CD006250

Chapter 26 Study Questions

1. Pain may be classified as neuropathic or:
   A. Serotonergic.
   B. Receptive.
   C. Dopaminergic.
   D. Nociceptive.

2. When administering nonsteroidal anti-inflammatory drugs, it is important to monitor:
   A. Renal function.
   B. Calcium levels.
   C. Endocrine function.
   D. Potassium levels.

3. Which of the following opioids is NOT recommended for management for cancer pain?
   A. Morphine
   B. Hydromorphone
   C. Meperidine
   D. Fentanyl

4. A patient was initiated on morphine two days ago. She informs her nurse that she has been feeling somewhat sedated since then. The nurse should:
   A. Inform the patient that this is a normal side effect that will likely persist for just a few days.
   B. Administer naloxone 1 mg now and every 30–60 seconds until sedation resolves.
   C. Recommend opioid rotation to oxycodone.
   D. Hold the next dose of morphine and administer ibuprofen instead.

5. Examples of interventional strategies for pain management include all of the following EXCEPT:
   A. Kyphoplasty.
   B. Hypnosis.
   C. Radiofrequency ablation.
   D. Nerve blocks.

CHAPTER

27 Peripheral Neuropathy

Melissa F. Saxon, RN, MSN, FNP, AOCNP®

Introduction

Peripheral neuropathy (PN) is defined as "a condition in which there is alteration in function and structure of the motor, sensory, or autonomic components of a peripheral nerve" (Grisdale & Armstrong, 2014, p. 1137). This dysfunction occurs outside of the central nervous system and results in peripheral neuropathic signs and symptoms including numbness, pain, burning, tingling, and paresthesias (Polovich, Olsen, & LeFebvre, 2014; Postma & Heimans, 2000).

Although the exact incidence of PN is currently unknown, the subjective nature of PN, unstandardized approaches to measurement and grading, the lack of current methods to detect PN during its early stages, and the difficulties in clinical assessment and diagnosis all affect the actual incidence rates reported in the oncology setting (Ocean & Vahdat, 2004). Therefore, oncology nurses need to be knowledgeable regarding the impact of PN and its consequences on patients with cancer and to maintain that knowledge by keeping up with current information in the literature. According to Holden and Felde (1987), "Much of the difficulty educating individuals about peripheral neuropathy secondary to treatment arises as a result of lack of knowledge on the part of physicians and nurses" (p. 13).

Risk Factors

PN has multiple causes and is a common feature of many disease states. Patients diagnosed with PN may have risk factors, such as metabolic disorders, nutritional deficiencies, inherited neurologic disorders, and ischemic diseases, which may increase the severity of the neuropathy after treatment with chemotherapy or radiation therapy. PN can be classified as either acquired or hereditary and commonly is associated with other systemic disorders, such as alcohol abuse, atherosclerotic heart disease, Charcot-Marie-Tooth disease, diabetes, HIV, herpes zoster, thyroid disorders, cachexia, and vitamin B deficiencies, especially B_{12} and B_9 (folic acid) (Armstrong & Gilbert, 2002; Polovich et al., 2014). Risk factors for the development of PN include age greater than 60 years, any preexisting PN from another comorbid condition, neurologic damage resulting from previous administration of radiation therapy to the spinal area, concurrent use of neurotoxic chemotherapies, and a history of cumulative doses of specific chemotherapy agents (i.e., cisplatin, vincristine, and taxanes) (Polovich et al., 2014).

Drug-induced neuropathies are frequent, and many common medications are known to cause PN. These include amiodarone, colchicine, hydralazine, isoniazid, metronidazole, nitrofurantoin, phenytoin, and the statins (Slade, 2005).

Neurotoxic chemotherapy and biologic agents appear to target the sensory component of the nervous system because, like most drugs, they are unable to cross the blood-brain barrier, where motor nerves are located (Wampler & Rosenbaum, 2008). Several chemotherapy and biologic drugs are classified as neurotoxic and must be dose-limited because of the development of chemotherapy-induced PN, including cisplatin, oxaliplatin, and bortezomib (Polovich et al., 2014) (see Figure 27-1).

Pathophysiology

Although the exact mechanism of the development of PN is unknown, numerous causes exist, and damage to the nerves can be cumulative and irreversible (Grisdale & Armstrong, 2014). The nervous system consists of three distinct systems responsible for different activities in the human body. The autonomic system maintains homeostasis, which includes regulation of blood pressure and intestinal motility. The motor (efferent) system is composed of the nerve fibers, also known as axons, which control reflexes and muscle strength. The sensory (afferent) portion of the nervous system includes both large and small axons. The large axons are used to detect vibration and proprioception, and the small axons detect temperature and pain (Farabee, 2001). Both large and small fibers carry sensation for light touch. Damage from known risk factors causes degeneration of both the axon and the myelin sheath, a protective coating that surrounds the axon, and because the injury is at the cellular level, recovery often is not possible (Poncelet, 1998). The velocity of electrical conduction through a nerve is reduced when the axon is no longer protected by the myelin sheath. This results in signs of PN such as the loss of deep tendon reflexes (Hickey, 2014).

Although PN most commonly is associated with chemotherapy, radiation therapy also may cause PN, albeit less frequently. PN symptoms caused by radiation may not occur for months or years (Belka, Budach, Kortmann, & Bamberg, 2001).

Figure 27-1. Chemotherapy and Biotherapy Drugs That Cause Peripheral Neuropathy

- Bortezomib
- Cisplatin
- Docetaxel
- Gemcitabine
- Oxaliplatin
- Paclitaxel
- Thalidomide
- Vinblastine
- Vincristine
- Vinorelbine

Note. Based on information from Polovich et al., 2014.

Assessment

Patient report of PN is subjective in nature. Currently, few reliable and valid instruments are available to assist patients in their quality-of-life (QOL) assessment or to determine how PN is affecting their physical and role function.

Patients with neuropathy may present with reports of pain, tingling, or numbness in the fingers or toes. Sensory peripheral neuropathies are commonly distinctive and distally progressive and usually manifest as sensory-type symmetrically distributed symptoms, such as tingling, numbness, burning, or increased sensitivity in a stocking-glove distribution (Almadrones, McGuire, Walczak, Florio, & Tian, 2004). Large fiber neuropathies may cause electric shock–like sensations, especially in the lower extremities (Grisdale & Armstrong, 2014). Damage in any of these areas can cause significant impairment in routine activities. For example, numbness of the fingers and toes may create safety issues such as an exaggerated tolerance of hot and cold temperatures (Visovsky,

Collins, Abbott, Aschenbrenner, & Hart, 2007), the inability to grasp and hold on to the handle of a pot of hot food, or tripping over throw rugs.

Current PN measurement systems involve subjective self-reports, objective clinical assessments, and grading based on numerous scales, which lack the standardization and reliability that is imperative when attempting to determine the degree and severity of PN. Varying scales are available for subjective assessment of PN and its impact on QOL issues for patients, including physical and role function. These scales must be adapted to correspond to the particular disease and the neurotoxic agent being used. Ocean and Vahdat (2004) reported that QOL scales may be more important than quantitative scales in assessing the impact of PN on patients with cancer.

Several toxicity grading systems are currently in use to assist in the accuracy and reliability of PN documentation. These include the following:

- Ajani Motor Neuropathy Scale (Ajani, Welch, Raber, Fields, & Krakoff, 1990) (see Table 27-1)
- Common Terminology Criteria for Adverse Events (National Cancer Institute Cancer Therapy Evaluation Program, 2010) (see Table 27-2)
- Total Neuropathy Scale (Cavaletti et al., 2003) (see Table 27-3)
- Eastern Cooperative Oncology Group Toxicity Scale for Peripheral Neuropathy (Oken et al., 1982) (see Table 27-4)

Most clinicians are unable to agree on one particular scale to use in practice settings. The unstandardized approach to grading and measurement has led to PN being underreported, and these inconsistencies may not reveal the true impact of PN on patients with cancer. Research that determines the efficacy, reliability, and validity of the current scales and compares them to each other needs to be completed. Until a "gold standard" scale for assessing PN is determined, institutions and healthcare entities need to agree on one particular grading system and use it in all oncology clinical settings to follow and report the incidence of PN in patients with cancer.

The primary duties related to PN of nurses caring for patients with cancer are assessment, determination, and documentation of the presence and severity of the symptoms of PN and their effect on patients' activities of daily living and QOL (Barker, 2008; Hausheer, Schilsky, Bain, Berghorn, & Lieberman, 2006). Assessment of these changes as part of the clinical examination at every treatment and follow-up visit can guide the oncology team in implement-

Table 27-1. Ajani Motor Neuropathy Scale

	Grade				
Type of Neuropathy	**0**	**1**	**2**	**3**	**4**
Motor neuropathy	None	Mild intermittent muscle weakness	Persistent weakness but able to ambulate	Unable to ambulate	Complete paralysis
Sensory neuropathy	None	Paresthesia and decreased deep tendon reflexes	Absence of deep tendon reflexes, mild to moderate functional abnormality	Severe paresthesias, severe functional abnormality	Complete loss of function and sensory loss

Note. Based on information from Ajani et al., 1990.

Table 27-2. Common Terminology Criteria for Adverse Events Grading for Neuropathic Conditions

Adverse Event	Grade 1	Grade 2	Grade 3	Grade 4	Grade 5
Paresthesia A disorder characterized by functional disturbances of sensory neurons resulting in abnormal cutaneous sensations of tingling, numbness, pressure, cold, and warmth that are experienced in the absence of a stimulus	Mild symptoms	Moderate symptoms; limiting instrumental ADL	Severe symptoms; limiting self-care ADL	–	–
Dysesthesia A disorder characterized by distortion of sensory perception, resulting in an abnormal and unpleasant sensation	Mild sensory alteration	Moderate sensory alteration; limiting instrumental ADL	Severe sensory alteration; limiting self-care ADL	–	–
Peripheral motor neuropathy A disorder characterized by inflammation or degeneration of the peripheral motor nerves	Asymptomatic; clinical or diagnostic observations only; intervention not indicated	Moderate symptoms; limiting instrumental ADL	Severe symptoms; limiting self-care ADL; assistive device indicated	Life-threatening consequences; urgent intervention indicated	Death
Peripheral sensory neuropathy A disorder characterized by inflammation or degeneration of the peripheral sensory nerves	Asymptomatic; loss of deep tendon reflexes or paresthesia	Moderate symptoms; limiting instrumental ADL	Severe symptoms; limiting self-care ADL	Life-threatening consequences; urgent intervention indicated	Death

ADL—activities of daily living

Note. From *Common Terminology Criteria for Adverse Events* [v.4.03], by National Cancer Institute Cancer Therapy Evaluation Program, 2010. Retrieved from http://evs.nci.nih.gov/ftp1/CTCAE/CTCAE_4.03_2010-06-14_QuickReference_5x7.pdf.

ing interventions such as discontinuing the drug or altering its dose to prevent further damage from developing (Almadrones et al., 2004).

During the initial and ongoing assessment of patients with cancer, oncology nurses should be aware of signs and symptoms that could be related to noncancerous systemic disorders or medications. Further evaluation may be warranted prior to the initiation or continuation of a neurotoxic agent to prevent further damage to the peripheral nervous system. It is essential that a thorough past and current medical history be obtained and documented (Barker, 2008), as well as a three-generational family history, because hereditary neuropathies are common. A comprehensive patient history is important to include a review of current medications, as well as vitamins and over-the-counter products, to minimize potential neurologic adverse events (Bromberg, 2005).

Table 27-3. Total Neuropathy Scale

	Grade				
Item Measured	**0**	**1**	**2**	**3**	**4**
Autonomic symptoms	None	1	2	3	4 or 5
Motor symptoms	None	Slight difficulty	Moderate difficulty	Requires assistance	Functionally disabling
Peroneal amplitude	Normal or reduced < 5%	76%–96%	51%–75%	26%–50%	0%–25%
Pin sensibility	None	Reduced in fingers and toes	Reduced to ankle	Reduced to elbow or knee	Reduced above elbow or knee
Reflexes	None	Reduced ankle reflex	Absent ankle reflex	All reflexes reduced	All reflexes absent
Sensory symptoms	None	Limited to fingers and toes	Extension to ankle or wrist	Extension to knee or elbow	Extension to above the knee or below the elbow, functionally disabling
Sural amplitude	Normal or reduced < 5%	76%–96%	51%–75%	26%–50%	0%–25%
Vibration sensation	Normal–125	126–150	151–200	201–300	> 300
Vibration sensibility	None	Reduced in fingers and toes	Moderate difficulty, reduced up to wrist or ankle	Reduced to elbow or knee	Reduced to above elbow or knee

Note. Based on information from Cavaletti et al., 2003.

Table 27-4. Eastern Cooperative Oncology Group Toxicity Scale for Peripheral Neuropathy

Grade	Description
0	None
1	Decreased deep tendon reflexes, mild constipation, mild paresthesias
2	Absent deep tendon reflexes, severe constipation, mild weakness
3	Severe neuropathic pain, obstipation, bladder dysfunction, severe weakness
4	Respiratory dysfunction, surgical intervention for obstipation, paralysis with confinement to bed/wheelchair

Note. Based on information from Oken et al., 1982.

Prevention and Treatment

Currently, no measures exist that can be implemented to prevent the development of PN in patients receiving neurotoxic drugs. While no treatments are available to reverse PN, oncology nurses can take a proactive approach in minimizing its devastating effects (Armstrong, Almadrones, & Gilbert, 2005). This includes recognizing and treating any preexisting conditions; obtaining a full medical history to establish if PN exists prior to therapy, and if so, determining whether a neurotoxic drug will be used in the treatment regimen; carefully assessing and monitoring for PN to determine if the agent must be discontinued based on the severity of the neuropathy (Armstrong et al., 2005); and educating patients with PN about measures to maintain or improve personal safety (Visovsky, Collins, Hart, Abbott, & Aschenbrenner, 2009).

The occurrence of PN can lead to delays in treatment, modification of doses, and possible discontinuation of therapy if the neuropathy becomes severe. If PN has developed, the continuation of the neurotoxic drug or drugs may lead to a permanent loss of function and irreversible nerve damage that can severely affect patients' QOL (Armstrong et al., 2005; Hausheer et al., 2006; Polovich et al., 2014).

No current method used in practice is able to detect and evaluate PN in its early stages. The Oncology Nursing Society's Putting Evidence Into Practice (PEP) resource for PN suggests options for treatment of PN with evidence-based results for the best approaches plus those that are not likely to be effective (Tofthagen et al., 2017). Duloxetine has been categorized as likely to be effective to reduce PN, and suggested dosing and timing are included in the PEP resource at www.ons.org/intervention/duloxetine-0 (Tofthagen et al., 2017). Gabapentin is an anticonvulsant that has also been found to be effective against PN when combined with low-dose opioids (Tofthagen et al., 2017). Neuropathy cannot be reversed, but oncology nurses can take a proactive approach in minimizing its devastating effects, including informing patients that PN may occur and educating them about the signs and symptoms of PN to report (Visovsky et al., 2009).

Visovsky et al. (2009) reported that patients may benefit from the use of assistive devices, such as a cane or orthotic, although this will not directly improve the effects of PN. Other interventions for PN that have been studied in small or noncancer populations include acupuncture, exercise (progressive resistance, aerobics, and stretching), pulsed infrared light therapy, and transcutaneous electrical nerve stimulation and high-frequency external muscle stimulation (Tofthagen et al., 2017). All have shown some benefit, but none have been studied in large, randomized clinical trials of patients with cancer or have established evidence of benefit (Tofthagen et al., 2017). It is important for clinicians and patients to determine together whether an assistive device or intervention would be appropriate for an individual patient.

PN is not a new phenomenon, but with the development of newer agents known to cause neurotoxicity, as well as combination chemotherapies with larger doses being administered, PN is becoming a much more common side effect in the oncology setting (Trivedi, Hershman, & Crew, 2015). Gaps in current evidence about PN include the need for clinical examination to include focused monitoring of subjective PN symptoms and standardized guidelines for grading, as well as inconsistencies in grading interpretation by the examiner and the introduction of potential prophylactic measures. Oncology nurses should address these gaps when evaluating the holistic needs of patients with PN and forming a protocol that addresses the areas that can be managed by the oncology team. The subjective assessment, measurement, and minimization of PN remain relatively unexplored, and further studies are needed to develop a reliable, standardized approach to this common toxicity.

Nursing Implications

The promotion of thorough and competent care is essential in caring for individuals at risk for or diagnosed with PN. Oncology nurses are in an ideal situation to assist in identifying patient risk factors, clinically assessing patients for PN, using current tools for grading PN, recognizing potential prophylactic measures to prevent or minimize PN, and educating patients about safety measures. Conducting and documenting a baseline neurologic assessment is imperative and allows oncology professionals to determine if underlying conditions exist that may affect the treatment regimen (Armstrong et al., 2005; Barker, 2008). Ongoing assessment for PN should be done at each chemotherapy or biotherapy treatment and indefinitely at follow-up visits thereafter. To assess for PN, nurses should evaluate pertinent findings from the patient examination (see Figure 27-2). They also should assess patients with PN for pain.

Patients should have a baseline audiogram prior to receiving treatment with cisplatin and carboplatin, and periodically thereafter, to assess their hearing (Polovich et al., 2014). Multidisciplinary management of these patients is often necessary, including referrals to neurologists, physical therapists, speech therapists, occupational therapists, and audiologists to properly guide the care of patients experiencing PN (Polovich et al., 2014). The addition of these members of the healthcare team should occur at the onset of symptoms and continue throughout the entire treatment process, as well as after the regimen has been completed.

Patient Education

Nurses can make a major impact on the QOL of patients with PN by teaching both patients and families about measures to maintain or improve patient safety (Visovsky et al., 2009). Specific teaching points (Visovsky et al., 2009) include the following:

- Inform patients and families that PN is an adverse effect from one or more of the drugs the patients will receive. Instruct patients receiving oxaliplatin that cold temperatures may induce PN symptoms, and encourage them to avoid temperature extremes (Tipton, 2009).
- Educate patients about the signs and symptoms of PN, whom to notify immediately if the signs or symptoms develop, and contact phone numbers.
- Teach patients to visually inspect their hands and feet daily for signs of PN, and encourage patients to use footwear that is not restrictive or tight.
- Teach patients and families to critically evaluate their home for possible dangers, such as throw rugs, hallway clutter, or furniture.
- Teach patients and families preventive measures for safety, including turning the temperature down on the hot water heater to prevent scalding, checking bath water with a thermometer to make sure it is less than 48.9°C (120°F), keeping extremities warm in cold weather, placing a nonskid mat in the bathtub or shower, and asking for assistance with specific cooking chores such as draining hot water from food or removing food from an oven.
- Instruct patients not to use alcohol or recreational drugs that might affect their cognition and potentially create unsafe situations (Sandstrom, 1996).
- Refer patients to support groups, rehabilitation services, or faith-based community organizations for additional emotional support, as well as support in the home.

The oncology nurse's role is unique in educating patients and their families about PN and holistically managing those patients who develop or are at risk for developing PN. Follow-up care should be active and continuous, as the needs of patients with PN change rapidly.

Figure 27-2. Sample Baseline Assessment for Chemotherapy-Induced Peripheral Neuropathy

Assessment	Yes	No
History of diabetes		
Arthritis or other connective tissue disease		
Peripheral vascular disease		
Chronic alcohol use		
History of HIV/AIDS		
History of chemical exposures		
History of previous neurotoxic chemotherapy		
• Taxanes (paclitaxel, docetaxel, nanoparticle albumin paclitaxel)		
• Epothilones (ixabepilone)		
• Vinca alkaloids (vincristine, vinblastine, vinorelbine)		
• Platinum compounds (cisplatin, carboplatin, oxaliplatin)		
• Angiogenesis agents (thalidomide)		
• Proteasome inhibitors (bortezomib)		
Current symptoms of neuropathy: Sensory (numbness and tingling, burning or stabbing pain in hands or feet, diminished reflexes)		
Review medication list (prescription, over-the-counter, and vitamins/herbals)		
Pertinent physical examination findings		
• Vibration sense with tuning fork		
• Proprioception		
• Deep tendon reflexes		
• Cutaneous sensation		
• Muscle strength		
• Gait/balance		

Note. Based on information from Visovsky & Daly, 2004; Wickham, 2007; Wilkes, 2004.

From "Peripheral Neuropathy" (p. 236), by J.M. Tipton in L.H. Eaton and J.M. Tipton (Eds.), *Putting Evidence Into Practice: Improving Oncology Patient Outcomes*, 2009, Pittsburgh, PA: Oncology Nursing Society. Copyright 2009 by Oncology Nursing Society. Reprinted with permission.

Conclusion

PN is a dysfunction in the peripheral nerve system and can cause pain, numbness, burning, tingling, and paresthesias in patients with cancer. The inability to detect PN in the early stages, clinician difficulties in assessment and diagnosis, and unstandardized approaches to its measurement can affect the QOL of patients who may already be devastated by a cancer diagnosis. It is imperative that oncology nurses be well informed of the risk factors, pathophysiology, assessment, prevention, and treatment of PN, as well as the nursing implications for patients receiving therapy that may potentiate or cause PN, to prevent further neurologic complications of the cancer treatment.

Key Points

- Chemotherapy and radiation therapy can cause PN.
- Drug-induced neuropathies are frequent, and many common medications are known to cause PN. These include aminoglycosides, amiodarone, colchicine, hydralazine, isoniazid, metronidazole, nitrofurantoin, phenytoin, and the statins.
- PN is a dysfunction in the peripheral nerve system and can cause pain, numbness, burning, tingling, and paresthesias in patients with cancer.
- Neuropathy cannot be reversed.
- Nursing assessment for PN should include hearing tests.
- A comprehensive patient history is important and should include a review of current medications, as well as vitamins and over-the-counter products, to minimize potential neurologic adverse events.
- Varying PN assessment scales are available for the subjective assessment of PN and its impact on QOL issues for patients, including physical and role function.
- The Oncology Nursing Society PEP resource on PN includes interventions likely to be effective for PN, as well as those that are not as effective, which could be important for patient education.
- The oncology nurse's role is unique in educating patients and their families about PN and holistically managing those patients who develop or are at risk for developing PN.

References

Ajani, J.A., Welch, S.R., Raber, M.N., Fields, W.S., & Krakoff, I.H. (1990). Comprehensive criteria for assessing therapy-induced toxicity. *Cancer Investigation, 8,* 147–159. doi:10.3109/07357909009017560

Almadrones, L., McGuire, D.B., Walczak, J.R., Florio, C.M., & Tian, C. (2004). Psychometric evaluation of two scales assessing functional status and peripheral neuropathy associated with chemotherapy for ovarian cancer: A Gynecologic Oncology Group study. *Oncology Nursing Forum, 31,* 615–623. doi:10.1188/04.ONF.615-623

Armstrong, T., Almadrones, L., & Gilbert, M.R. (2005). Chemotherapy-induced peripheral neuropathy. *Oncology Nursing Forum, 32,* 305–311. doi:10.1188/05.ONF.305-311

Armstrong, T., & Gilbert, M.R. (2002). Chemotherapy-induced peripheral neuropathy. In W.T. Fetner (Ed.), *The female patient* (pp. 27–30). Chatham, NJ: Quadrant HealthCom.

Barker, E. (2008). *Neuroscience nursing: A spectrum of care* (3rd ed.). St. Louis, MO: Elsevier Mosby.

Belka, C., Budach, W., Kortmann, R.D., & Bamberg, M. (2001). Radiation induced CNS toxicity—Molecular and cellular mechanisms. *British Journal of Cancer, 85,* 1233–1239. doi:10.1054/bjoc.2001.2100

Bromberg, M.B. (2005). An approach to the evaluation of peripheral neuropathies. *Seminars in Neurology, 25,* 153–159. doi:10.1055/s-2005-871323

Cavaletti, G., Bogliun, G., Marzorati, L., Zincone, A., Piatti, M., Colombo, N., … Zanna, C. (2003). Grading of chemotherapy-induced peripheral neurotoxicity using the Total Neuropathy Scale. *Neurology, 61,* 1297–1300. doi:10.1212/01.WNL.0000092015.03923.19

Farabee, M.J. (2001). *Online biology book.* Retrieved from http://www2.estrellamountain.edu/faculty/farabee/biobk/biobooktoc.html

Grisdale, K.A., & Armstrong, T.S. (2014). Peripheral neuropathy. In D. Camp-Sorrell & R.A. Hawkins (Eds.), *Clinical manual for the oncology advanced practice nurse* (3rd ed., pp. 1137–1149). Pittsburgh, PA: Oncology Nursing Society.

Hausheer, F.H., Schilsky, R.L., Bain, S., Berghorn, E.J., & Lieberman, F. (2006). Diagnosis, management, and evaluation of chemotherapy-induced peripheral neuropathy. *Seminars in Oncology, 33,* 15–49. doi:10.1053/j.seminoncol.2005.12.010

Hickey, J.V. (2014). *The clinical practice of neurological and neurosurgical nursing* (7th ed.). Philadelphia, PA: Wolters Kluwer Health/Lippincott Williams & Wilkins.

Holden, S., & Felde, G. (1987). Nursing care of patients experiencing cisplatin-related peripheral neuropathy. *Oncology Nursing Forum, 14,* 13–17.

National Cancer Institute Cancer Therapy Evaluation Program. (2010). *Common terminology criteria for adverse events* [v.4.03]. Retrieved from https://evs.nci.nih.gov/ftp1/CTCAE/CTCAE_4.03_2010-06-14_QuickReference_5x7.pdf

Ocean, A.J., & Vahdat, L.T. (2004). Chemotherapy-induced peripheral neuropathy: Pathogenesis and emerging therapies. *Supportive Care in Cancer, 12,* 619–625. doi:10.1007/s00520-004-0657-7

Oken, M.M., Creech, R.H., Tormey, D.C., Horton, J., Davis, T.E., McFadden, E.T., & Carbone, P.P. (1982). Toxicity and response criteria of the Eastern Cooperative Oncology Group. *American Journal of Clinical Oncology, 5,* 649–655. doi:10.1097/00000421-198212000-00014

Polovich, M., Olsen, M., & LeFebvre, K.B. (Eds.). (2014). *Chemotherapy and biotherapy guidelines and recommendations for practice* (4th ed.). Pittsburgh, PA: Oncology Nursing Society.

Poncelet, A.N. (1998). An algorithm for the evaluation of peripheral neuropathy. *American Family Physician, 57,* 755–764. Retrieved from http://www.aafp.org/afp/980215ap/poncelet.html

Postma, T.J., & Heimans, J.J. (2000). Grading of chemotherapy-induced peripheral neuropathy. *Annals of Oncology, 11,* 509–513. doi:10.1023/A:1008345613594

Sandstrom, S.K. (1996). Nursing management of patients receiving biological therapy. *Seminars in Oncology Nursing, 12,* 152–162. doi:10.1016/S0749-2081(96)80009-X

Slade, J. (2005). Neurological toxicities associated with cancer chemotherapeutic agents. *U.S. Pharmacist, 4*(Onc. Suppl.), 3–18.

Tipton, J.M. (2009). Peripheral neuropathy. In L.H. Eaton & J.M. Tipton (Eds.), *Putting evidence into practice: Improving oncology patient outcomes* (pp. 235–241). Pittsburgh, PA: Oncology Nursing Society.

Tofthagen, C.S., Visovsky, C., Camp-Sorrell, D., Collins, M.L., Erb, C.H., Olson, E.K., & Wood, S.K. (2017, February 20). ONS PEP resource: Peripheral neuropathy. Retrieved from https://www.ons.org/practice-resources/pep/peripheral-neuropathy

Trivedi, M.S., Hershman, D.L., & Crew, K.D. (2015). Management of chemotherapy-induced peripheral neuropathy. *American Journal of Hematology/Oncology, 11*(1), 4–10. Retrieved from http://www.gotoper.com/publications/ajho/2015/2015jan/management-of-chemotherapy-induced-peripheral-neuropathy

Visovsky, C., Collins, M., Abbott, L.I., Aschenbrenner, J., & Hart, C. (2007). Putting Evidence Into Practice®: Evidence-based interventions for chemotherapy-induced peripheral neuropathy. *Clinical Journal of Oncology Nursing, 11,* 901–913. doi:10.1188/07.CJON.901-913

Visovsky, C., Collins, M., Hart, C., Abbott, L.I., & Aschenbrenner, J.A. (2009). ONS PEP resource: Peripheral neuropathy. In L.H. Eaton & J.M. Tipton (Eds.), *Putting evidence into practice: Improving oncology patient outcomes* (pp. 243–252). Pittsburgh, PA: Oncology Nursing Society.

Visovsky, C., & Daly, B.J. (2004). Clinical evaluation and patterns of chemotherapy-induced peripheral neuropathy. *Journal of the American Academy of Nurse Practitioners, 16,* 353–359. doi:10.1111/j.1745-7599.2004.tb00458.x

Wampler, M.A., & Rosenbaum, E.H. (2008, April 2). Chemotherapy-induced peripheral neuropathy fact sheet. Retrieved from http://www.cancersupportivecare.com/nervepain.php

Wickham, R. (2007). Chemotherapy-induced peripheral neuropathy: A review and implications for oncology nursing practice. *Clinical Journal of Oncology Nursing, 11,* 361–376. doi:10.1188/07.CJON.361-376

Wilkes, G.M. (2004). Peripheral neuropathy. In C.H. Yarbro, M.H., Frogge, & M. Goodman (Eds.), *Cancer symptom management* (3rd ed., pp. 333–358). Burlington, MA: Jones & Bartlett Learning.

Chapter 27 Study Questions

1. Which of the following chemotherapy agents is NOT often associated with chemotherapy-induced peripheral neuropathy?
   A. Taxanes
   B. Vinca alkaloids
   C. Platinum-based drugs
   D. Doxorubicin

2. Which of the following risk factors is NOT associated with the increased development of chemotherapy-induced peripheral neuropathy?
   A. Age younger than 60 years
   B. Previous radiation therapy to the spinal area resulting in neurologic damage
   C. Preexisting peripheral neuropathy from Charcot-Marie-Tooth disease
   D. Concurrent or later use of aminoglycoside antibiotics

3. Symptoms of sensory peripheral neuropathies include all of the following EXCEPT:
   A. Tingling.
   B. Numbness.
   C. Shock-like sensations.
   D. Burning.

4. The primary role of the oncology nurse in managing patients with chemotherapy-induced peripheral neuropathy includes all of the following EXCEPT:
   A. Diagnosis of chemotherapy-induced peripheral neuropathy.
   B. Careful assessment and monitoring for chemotherapy-induced peripheral neuropathy.
   C. Educating the patient about measures to maintain or improve personal safety.
   D. Notifying the physician if chemotherapy-induced peripheral neuropathy exists prior to initiation of a neurotoxic drug.

5. Medications for peripheral neuropathy that have evidence showing effectiveness include which of the following?
   A. Duloxetine and gabapentin
   B. Cyclobenzaprine
   C. Low-dose opioids with lidocaine
   D. Pregabalin

CHAPTER

28 Pulmonary Toxicities

Vickie Connelly Murphy, PA-C, and Vickie Shannon, MD

Introduction

Significant advancements in cancer treatment strategies over the past 20 years have included the development of new therapeutic agents within the class of conventional chemotherapies, as well as a rapidly growing class of novel immunomodulating and molecular-targeted therapies. In addition, new radiation techniques and delivery systems have led to improvements in the management of radiation-sensitive tumors. Each of these treatment modalities has the potential to produce clinically significant lung injury. Drug-induced lung injury (DILI) patterns have increased as new anticancer agents, and new classes of these agents, have expanded. Lung injury is a common sequela of radiation therapy to the thorax for chest wall or intrathoracic malignancies. In addition to lung toxicities, airway disease associated with infusion reactions is a common problem during the administration of monoclonal antibody therapies. In many centers, the administration of cancer drugs is a primary responsibility of the oncology nursing staff. Thus, oncology nurses should be able to identify patients at risk, recognize the clinical signs of lung toxicity, and provide optimal prophylactic measures and symptom management.

This chapter will review clinically important lung injury patterns associated with conventional chemotherapy agents, targeted therapies, and radiation therapy. The discussion will include risk factors for lung injury, the pathologic mechanisms of treatment-related lung damage, where known, and treatment advances that have emerged in this field.

Lung Injury Caused by Conventional and Targeted Anticancer Agents

Toxicity to the lungs results in stereotypical lung injury patterns that may differ both in frequency and intensity, depending on the therapeutic class of the drug (see Table 28-1). While all patterns of pulmonary injury may be seen following exposure to both classes of drugs, vasculopathies, infusion reactions, and pleural effusions are more common following targeted therapies (Barber & Ganti, 2011). Severe myelosuppression and mucositis leading to increased risks for opportunistic pneumonias and aspiration pneumonitis are more often sequelae of conventional chemotherapy (Guntur & Dhand, 2012; Quinn, Alam, Aminazad, Marshall, & Choong, 2013). Approximately 10%–20% of all patients treated with antineoplastic therapies may develop some form of DILI. Estimates may reach 30%–40% (Shannon & Price, 1998; Snyder & Hertz, 1988) following exposure to some agents but was as low

Table 28-1. Patterns of Lung Injury and Suspected Antineoplastic Agents

Lung Injury Patterns	Conventional Chemotherapy	Monoclonal Antibodies	Small Molecule Inhibitors	Immunotherapies
Airway disease with bronchospasm or anaphylaxis Hypersensitivity pneumonitis	Gemcitabine Taxanes: paclitaxel/docetaxel Cyclophosphamide Ifosfamide L-Asparaginase Cisplatin, carboplatin Oxaliplatin Nitrosoureas [carmustine (BCNU), lomustine (CCNU)] Melphalan Methotrexate Pemetrexed Procarbazine Topotecan Liposomal doxorubicin/daunorubicin Etoposide/teniposide Mitomycin C/vinca alkaloid regimens Ixabepilone	Most monoclonal antibodies	Imatinib Carfilzomib Temsirolimus Everolimus Sunitinib	–
Bronchiolitis obliterans	Topotecan	Cetuximab Panitumumab Trastuzumab	Bortezomib	Thalidomide Tumor necrosis factor-7
Nonspecific interstitial pneumonitis Usual interstitial pneumonitis Pulmonary fibrosis	Methotrexate Gemcitabine Fludarabine Cyclophosphamide Ifosfamide Temozolomide Nitrosoureas (BCNU, CCNU) Melphalan Taxanes: paclitaxel/docetaxel Mitomycin C/vinca alkaloid regimens	Rituximab Cetuximab Panitumumab Alemtuzumab Trastuzumab Ado-trastuzumab emtansine	Everolimus Temsirolimus Gefitinib Erlotinib Sorafenib Imatinib Dasatinib Nilotinib Bosutinib Bortezomib Carfilzomib Crizotinib Vandetanib Idelalisib Trametinib Vemurafenib Ruxolitinib	Thalidomide Lenalidomide Pomalidomide Nivolumab Ipilimumab Pembrolizumab

(Continued on next page)

Table 28-1. Patterns of Lung Injury and Suspected Antineoplastic Agents *(Continued)*

Lung Injury Patterns	Conventional Chemotherapy	Monoclonal Antibodies	Small Molecule Inhibitors	Immunotherapies
Eosinophilic pneumonia	Cyclophosphamide Oxaliplatin Cytarabine Fludarabine Bleomycin Etoposide Teniposide Taxanes: paclitaxel/docetaxel Nitrosoureas (BCNU, CCNU) Methotrexate Procarbazine	–	–	Thalidomide Interleukin-2
Capillary leak/noncardiogenic pulmonary edema	Busulfan Bleomycin Cyclophosphamide Ifosfamide	Cetuximab Rituximab Alemtuzumab Ofatumumab All-trans-retinoic acid Arsenic trioxide	Gefitinib Erlotinib Everolimus Ruxolitinib	Interleukin therapies Interferon-7
Diffuse alveolar damage and/or acute respiratory distress syndrome with or without diffuse alveolar hemorrhage	Cyclophosphamide Ifosfamide Busulfan Temozolomide Oxaliplatin Bleomycin Mitomycin C/vinca alkaloid regimens Methotrexate Azathioprine Cytarabine Fludarabine Gemcitabine Pemetrexed Zinostatin Topotecan Etoposide Taxanes: paclitaxel/docetaxel All-trans-retinoic acid Arsenic trioxide	Cetuximab Panitumumab Bevacizumab Alemtuzumab Rituximab Obinutuzumab Ofatumumab Ibritumomab Trastuzumab Pertuzumab Gemtuzumab Ipilimumab	Gefitinib Erlotinib Imatinib Sorafenib Vandetanib Idelalisib Crizotinib Ruxolitinib Everolimus Temsirolimus Bortezomib Ruxolitinib	Thalidomide Interleukin-2

(Continued on next page)

Table 28-1. Patterns of Lung Injury and Suspected Antineoplastic Agents *(Continued)*

Lung Injury Patterns	Conventional Chemotherapy	Monoclonal Antibodies	Small Molecule Inhibitors	Immunotherapies
Hemoptysis unrelated to diffuse alveolar hemorrhage/acute respiratory distress syndrome	–	Bevacizumab Alemtuzumab Rituximab Pazopanib	–	Interleukin-2 Tumor necrosis factor Interferon-7
Pleural effusion	Gemcitabine Fludarabine Docetaxel Cyclophosphamide Methotrexate Mitomycin C/vinca alkaloid regimens All-trans-retinoic acid Arsenic trioxide Procarbazine	Panitumumab	Imatinib Dasatinib > bosutinib > nilotinib Ponatinib	Thalidomide Interleukin-2 Interferon-7
Pulmonary hypertension	Bleomycin Mitomycin C/vinca alkaloid regimens Gemcitabine Nitrosoureas (BCNU, CCNU)	–	Dasatinib	–
Thromboembolism	Tamoxifen	Bevacizumab Ponatinib Pazopanib Crizotinib	Sunitinib	Thalidomide

Note. Based on information from Camus, Bonniaud, et al., 2004; Camus, Fanton, et al., 2004; Camus, Kudoh, et al., 2004; Dabydeen et al., 2012; Dy & Adjei, 2013; Ryu, 2010; Shannon & Price, 1998; Sleijfer, 2001.

as 9.5% in a recent study of drug-induced acute lung injury (Dhokarh et al., 2012). This susceptibility to drug-induced injury relates, in part, to the fact that the lungs receive the entire blood supply and thus have greater exposure to potentially toxic agents than other organ systems. The pathogenesis of DILI is poorly understood. Cytokine release, recruitment of inflammatory cells, and oxidative injury due to the release of oxygen free radicals have been implicated in direct injury to the type II pneumocytes and the alveolar capillary endothelium. In addition, drug-induced activation of lymphocytes and alveolar macrophages results in cell-mediated lung injury. Finally, impairment of alveolar wall repair caused by epidermal growth factor receptor (EGFR) inhibition on type II pneumocytes is a more recently implicated cause of lung injury (Sleijfer, 2001; Vahid & Marik, 2008).

Risk factors for DILI vary with the different drug classes and include older age, cumulative dose, concomitant or sequential radiation therapy, high oxygen administration, prior lung injury, and the use of multidrug regimens (see Figure 28-1). These factors significantly influ-

Figure 28-1. Risk Factors for Drug-Induced Lung Injury

- Older age (> 65 years)
- Cumulative dosage of drug
- Concomitant or sequential radiation therapy
- High inspired oxygen administration
- Prior lung disease
- Multidrug regimens

Note. Based on information from Merrill, 2016; Rovirosa & Valduvieco, 2010.

ence disease occurrence, severity of the injury, and latency periods between drug exposure and clinical symptoms (Barber & Ganti, 2011; Guntur & Dhand, 2012; Ryu, 2010).

The clinical manifestations of DILI are nonspecific. Nonproductive cough, low-grade fevers, hypoxemia, and dyspnea are common presenting symptoms, which may progress insidiously over several weeks to two months after drug exposure. Late-onset manifestations, occurring two months to years after completion of the drug, have been described following exposure to bleomycin, busulfan, cyclophosphamide, gemcitabine, mitomycin C, and the nitrosoureas (Bacakoğlu et al., 2003; Barber & Ganti, 2011; Cooper, White, & Matthay, 1986a, 1986b; Sostman, Matthay, & Putman, 1977; White & Stover, 1984). Wheezing, with or without a concomitant rash, may signal a hypersensitivity reaction. The lung examination often is clear, although bibasilar rales may be auscultated, particularly in the setting of pulmonary fibrosis. Clinical manifestations vary with the individual agents. Symptoms may develop following the first or subsequent treatment cycles (Guntur & Dhand, 2012; Ryu, 2010; Sostman et al., 1977; Vahid & Marik, 2008).

Other than drug rechallenge, no specific diagnostic tests or pathognomonic histopathologic findings exist to establish the diagnosis of DILI. Recrudescence of clinical signs and symptoms following challenge testing, which involves the administration of small doses of the implicated agent after a period of drug withdrawal, establishes the diagnosis. This approach to diagnosis, however, is not recommended, particularly when a conventional chemotherapy agent is the suspected culprit, because of unpredictable and sometimes severe adverse reactions. The diagnosis of DILI thus relies on the temporal association between drug exposure and the development of lung injury, the presence of a recognized clinical pattern following exposure to a drug that is a known or suspected culprit, and the exclusion of competing diagnoses that may mimic DILI, such as infection, aspiration pneumonitis, radiation injury, acute lung injury/acute respiratory distress syndrome (ARDS), pulmonary edema, and cancer relapse (see Figure 28-2) (Camus, 2004; Camus, Bonniaud, et al., 2004; Camus, Fanton, Bonniaud, Camus, & Foucher, 2004; Camus, Kudoh, & Ebina, 2004).

Radiographic patterns of DILI are variable. Infiltrates are most often bibasilar or peripheral and may be alveolar, interstitial, or mixed. Pleural effusions and focal nodular consolidations that mimic tumor involvement have also been described. A decrease in diffusing capacity for carbon monoxide (DLCO) may represent the initial and only derangement upon pulmonary function testing. In advanced cases, a restric-

Figure 28-2. Clinical Clues to Drug-Induced Lung Injury

- Temporal association between drug exposure and development of lung injury
- Recognition of clinical pattern of lung injury typically associated with individual agent
- Exclusion of competing diagnosis (i.e., infection, aspiration, pneumonitis, radiation injury, acute lung injury, acute respiratory distress syndrome, pulmonary edema, and cancer relapse)
- Improvement of lung injury with drug withdrawal
- Provocative testing with drug rechallenge (not recommended with most agents)

Note. Based on information from Merrill, 2016; Rovirosa & Valduvieco, 2010.

tive lung defect may be seen. Airflow obstruction has also been described, particularly following taxane and monoclonal antibody therapies (Akoun, Milleron, Cadranel, & Mayaud, 1992; Hirsch et al., 1996; Quinn et al., 2013).

Withdrawal of the drug is required in most cases. Corticosteroids may decrease symptoms of DILI in steroid-responsive lung injury patterns, such as hypersensitivity pneumonitis, eosinophilic pneumonia, and bronchiolitis obliterans with organizing pneumonia (BOOP). In patients with glucocorticoid-responsive lung disorders and signs of severe acute, subacute, or progressive pulmonary toxicity (dyspnea at rest, decrease in oxygen saturation below 90% or more than 4% below baseline), systemic corticosteroid therapy should be considered. Prednisone or its equivalent, dosed at 40–60 mg daily, is generally used, although no evidence-based guidelines for corticosteroid therapy in this setting exist. Intravenous methylprednisolone is preferred for patients on mechanical ventilation or those with impending respiratory failure. Steroids are typically tapered over one to three months, depending on the response to therapy. Any decision to reintroduce the offending agent must be based on the individual drug, the severity of the toxicity reaction, and the availability of alternative therapies (Guntur & Dhand, 2012).

Specific Clinicopathologic Syndromes

The clinical and histopathologic presentation of DILI is highly variable from one therapeutic class of drugs to the next. In addition, individual agents within a certain therapeutic class may induce similar patterns of lung injury with widely varying frequencies. Individual drug toxicities may be confined to the pulmonary interstitium, alveoli, pleura, pulmonary circulation, or airways, or, alternatively, may involve multiple intrathoracic structures. Organization of potentially toxic drugs by clinical syndromes may facilitate association of these drugs with their clinical presentations. These clinical syndromes are discussed in the following sections.

Interstitial Lung Disease

Interstitial lung disease (ILD) consists of widely varied histopathologic patterns of interstitial pneumonitis, which have varying clinical presentations and response to steroids. Interstitial pneumonitis may progress to pulmonary fibrosis. Nonspecific interstitial pneumonitis is the most common form of drug-induced ILD. Symptoms of dry cough, pleuritic chest pain, low-grade fever, and progressive dyspnea may develop insidiously over weeks to several months following drug exposure (Matsuno, 2012). Pleural based, lower lobe predominant, ground glass attenuations, reticular lines, mosaic patterns, and small nodules are common radiographic findings, which may develop well after clinical symptoms. Several forms of drug-induced ILD, including nonspecific interstitial pneumonitis, hypersensitivity pneumonitis, and eosinophilic pneumonia, tend to be steroid responsive. However, progression to end-stage, potentially fatal fibrotic lung disease, despite drug withdrawal and corticosteroid therapy, has been described following all histologic forms of interstitial lung disease.

Interstitial Pneumonitis

Bleomycin-induced interstitial pneumonitis (BIP) occurs in up to 20% of treated patients, typically 4–10 weeks after bleomycin administration (Jules-Elysee & White, 1990; Schwaiblmair et al., 2012; Yousem, Lifson, & Colby, 1985). Risk factors for BIP include advanced age (older than 70 years), uremia, and multiagent therapy. Increased risk of toxicity has been described with a cumulative dose greater than 400 U. BIP may progress to respiratory failure associated with diffuse alveolar damage and ARDS. Concomitant or sequential radiation therapy also may potentiate BIP. Importantly, the use of high inspired oxygen administration even months or years after bleomycin exposure has been associated with BIP (Donat & Levy, 1998; Schwaiblmair et al., 2012; Sleijfer, 2001). This association has been largely anecdotal, and questions remain regarding the threshold dose of oxygen, the duration of oxygen therapy, and the latency period between bleomycin and high oxygen exposure that confer an increased risk. General recommendations for supplemental oxygen in bleomycin-exposed patients include close monitoring with titration to achieve oxygen saturations at or above 89%–92% (Schwaiblmair et al., 2012). Monitoring the DLCO with pulmonary function testing is generally recommended for patients with known lung disease or abnormal lung function at baseline and as the cumulative dose of bleomycin approaches 400 U. Although reductions in DLCO are considered early markers of BIP, threshold cutoffs for drug withdrawal based on declining DLCO have not been established. Drug withdrawal is recommended for symptomatic patients and patients with changes suggestive of BIP on imaging studies (see Figure 28-3). Withdrawal of bleomycin also should be considered among patients with declining DLCO values of 30%–60% below baseline (Donat & Levy, 1998; Schwaiblmair et al., 2012; Sleijfer, 2001). Steroid therapy may be helpful early in BIP but is of no proven benefit during the fibrotic stages of the disease.

Other conventional chemotherapy agents that have been commonly associated with interstitial pneumonitis include 1,3-bis(2-chloroethyl)-1-nitrosourea (BCNU), busulfan, gemcitabine, methotrexate, procarbazine, cyclophosphamide, and the taxanes (paclitaxel, docetaxel). Busulfan and methotrexate are unique in their predilection for upper lobe–predominant interstitial pneumonitis and fibrosis. Late presentations of interstitial pneumonitis, occurring two months to years after drug exposure, have been described following cyclophosphamide, busulfan, bleomycin, mitomycin C, and BCNU and gentamycin therapies. Pulmonary fibrosis is a common sequela of late lung injury, which may progress to progressive respiratory failure and death. BCNU-related lung injury is dose related, with higher rates of toxicity seen when cumulative doses

Figure 28-3. Bleomycin-Induced Lung Injury

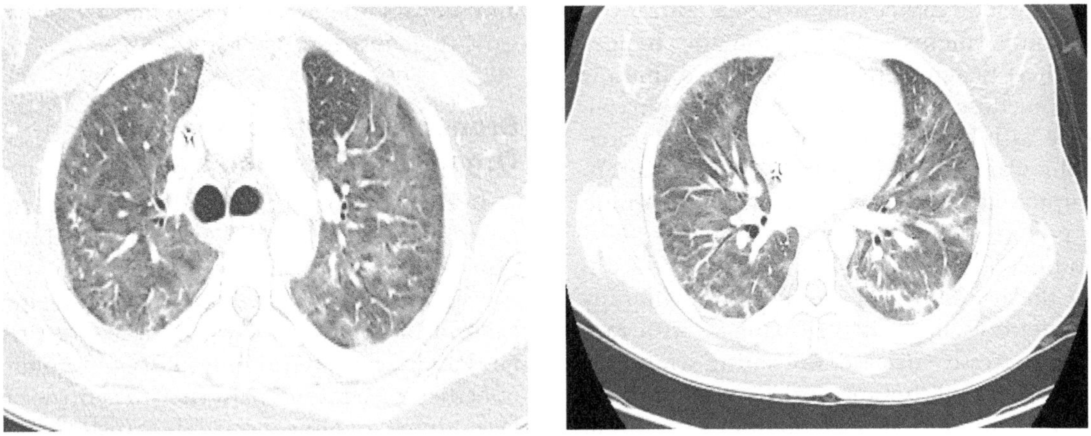

Fatal bleomycin-induced lung injury in a 25-year-old woman who underwent surgery for a fractured femur under general anesthesia. Bleomycin-based chemotherapy for Hodgkin lymphoma was completed 4 months prior. Autopsy showed diffuse alveolar damage and fibrotic lung disease.

of the drug exceed 1,500 mg/m^2. Pneumothorax and pulmonary fibrosis involving predominantly the middle and upper lobes have been reported years after BCNU exposure (Matsuno, 2012; Shannon & Price, 1998).

Interstitial pneumonitis has also been described following molecular-targeted therapies, including mammalian target of rapamycin (mTOR) inhibitors (everolimus, temsirolimus); EGFR inhibitors (gefitinib, erlotinib, cetuximab, panitumumab); multikinase angiogenesis inhibitors (sorafenib); the HER2 inhibitor trastuzumab; Bcr-Abl inhibitors (imatinib, dasatinib, nilotinib, bosutinib); proteasome inhibitors (bortezomib, carfilzomib); the ALK inhibitor crizotinib; the c-Met inhibitor tivantinib; and immunomodulatory agents (thalidomide, lenalidomide, pomalidomide, nivolumab, ipilimumab). Asymptomatic changes on chest imaging studies following targeted therapies are common, although fulminant respiratory failure, particularly following rituximab, EGFR inhibitors, and mTOR inhibitors, has been well described (Dabydeen et al., 2012; Duran et al., 2014; Gartrell et al., 2014; Maroto et al., 2011). Symptoms, when they do occur, typically develop within two to six months following therapy. Common symptoms include dry cough, dyspnea, and fever. For some patients with asymptomatic changes on chest imaging studies, continued therapy without dose interruption and close surveillance with high-resolution computed tomography scans are reasonable. The approach to symptomatic patients is guided by the grade of pneumotoxicity, which may include dose modification or interruption, with or without the institution of corticosteroid therapy (Montani et al., 2012). In patients with rapidly progressive disease, worsening symptoms despite steroid therapy or dose reduction, or severe symptoms at presentation, withdrawal of the culprit agent is indicated. Hospitalization and high-dose steroids (at least 2 mg/kg/day of prednisone or its equivalent) is recommended for these patients, with a gradual taper after symptoms improve (Dy & Adjei, 2013).

Hypersensitivity Pneumonitis

The syndrome of hypersensitivity pneumonitis comprises dyspnea, dry cough, and rash occurring three to four weeks following repeated drug exposure. Symptoms may wax and wane without adjustments in therapy. Unlike nonspecific interstitial pneumonitis, patients with hypersensitivity pneumonitis commonly present with upper lobe–predominant disease. Poorly formed granulomas and bronchoalveolar lavage lymphocytosis are common histopathologic findings. Among the drugs associated with hypersensitivity pneumonitis, methotrexate is the most well studied. Hypersensitivity pneumonitis has been reported following oral, IV, intrathecal, and intramuscular routes of methotrexate administration, sometimes associated with hilar adenopathy and pleural effusions. These findings, coupled with histologic evidence of ill-defined granulomas, should raise suspicion for methotrexate-related lung disease. Favorable outcomes with complete resolution of clinical signs and symptoms following drug withdrawal and steroid therapy occur in most cases of early-stage disease.

Bronchiolitis Obliterans With Organizing Pneumonia

BOOP has been attributed to certain antineoplastic agents, as well as a rare complication of allogeneic hematopoietic stem cell transplantation. In both settings, the clinical and radiographic presentations are similar. Patchy, peripheral, migratory pulmonary opacities, tree-in-bud pattern with centrilobular nodules, and linear opacities are described in both settings, rendering determination of exact causal associations difficult (see Figure 28-4). Agents including bleomycin, busul-

Figure 28-4. Bronchiolitis Obliterans With Organizing Pneumonia

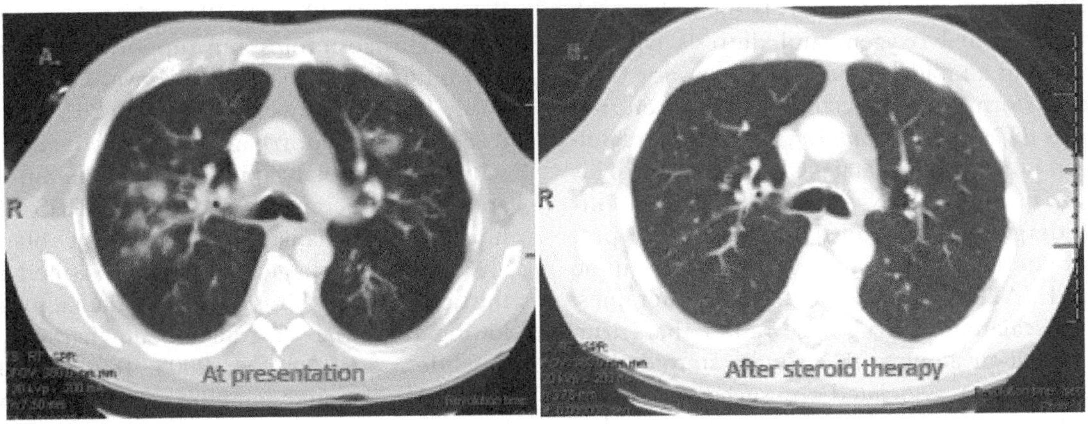

Biopsy-proven bronchiolitis obliterans with organizing pneumonia in a 63-year-old man treated with cyclophosphamide-based chemotherapy for non-Hodgkin lymphoma (A). A repeat computed tomography scan of the chest (B) performed 3 weeks later showed marked improvement in the lung lesions after a 3-week course of steroid therapy.

fan, BCNU, cyclophosphamide, methotrexate, thalidomide, bortezomib, cetuximab, panitumumab, and interferon gamma have been implicated as potential causes of drug-induced BOOP (Shannon & Price, 1998). Patients typically respond well to corticosteroid therapy along with withdrawal of the offending agent.

Eosinophilic Pneumonia

Fludarabine, interleukin-2, infliximab, methotrexate, and bleomycin are the most frequent offending agents in the setting of acute eosinophilic pneumonia. Elevated eosinophils in peripheral blood and on bronchoscopic lavage fluid, along with radiographic findings of homogeneous opacities with a predilection for the peripheral lungs and upper lobes, suggest the diagnosis. A reverse pulmonary edema pattern is highly suggestive of eosinophilic pneumonia. Other agents that have been implicated in the development of eosinophilic pneumonia include cyclophosphamide, busulfan, oxaliplatin, gemcitabine, etoposide, thalidomide, interleukin-2, the nitrosoureas (BCNU, lomustine [CCNU]), and the taxanes (paclitaxel, docetaxel). Symptom resolution with drug withdrawal and corticosteroid therapy has been reported; however, progression to ARDS and respiratory failure may occur, despite therapy.

Noncardiogenic Pulmonary Edema

Drug-induced noncardiogenic pulmonary edema (NCPE) is characterized by a bland pulmonary capillary leak syndrome, which is typically unrelated to drug dosage or duration of therapy. Common radiographic findings include a central bat-wing pattern or bilateral peripheral airspace disease with air bronchograms. Unlike cardiogenic pulmonary edema, Kerley B lines, cardiomegaly, and vascular redistribution are rare. Anticancer agents most often implicated in the development of NCPE include bleomycin, busulfan, cyclophosphamide, the molecular-targeted agents (cetuximab, erlotinib, gefitinib), the antilymphocyte monoclonal antibodies (alemtuzumab, ofatumumab, rituximab), the mTOR inhibitors (everolimus, temsirolimus), and interleukin therapies (see Figure 28-5). Symptoms are typically self-limited, although NCPE leading to ARDS has been described. Drug withdrawal, supplemental oxygen, and diuresis typically result in a rapid response and recovery. Cytokine storm with associated NCPE is referred to as *differentiation syndrome*, which is characterized by potentially fatal NCPE and ARDS. This can be particularly associated with patients undergoing induction therapy for acute promyelocytic leukemia with all-trans-retinoic acid (ATRA) or arsenic trioxide therapies. De-escalation of drug dose rather than drug withdrawal along with systemic steroid therapy has been associated with successful resolution of toxicity in patients with mild to moderate forms of this syndrome (Luesink & Jansen, 2010; Rogers & Yang, 2012). Ruxolitinib, a novel JAK1 and JAK2 inhibitor, causes a cytokine rebound reaction that may lead to life-threatening NCPE and ARDS. The preemptive use of corticosteroids and supportive therapy may mitigate this reaction (Beauverd & Samii, 2014; Tefferi, Litzow, & Pardanani, 2011). Diffuse alveolar hemorrhage is typically seen as a sequela of alveolar-capillary membrane injury and thus is a common sequela of ARDS/diffuse alveolar damage. Occasionally, bland alveolar hemorrhage has been described in the absence of diffuse alveolar damage following rituximab and alemtuzumab therapy (Sachdeva & Matuschak, 2008; Tefferi et al., 2011). Massive and sometimes fatal bleeding has been reported during bevacizumab therapy for treatment of central airway tumors (Sandler, 2007).

Figure 28-5. Interleukin-2–Induced Noncardiogenic Pulmonary Edema

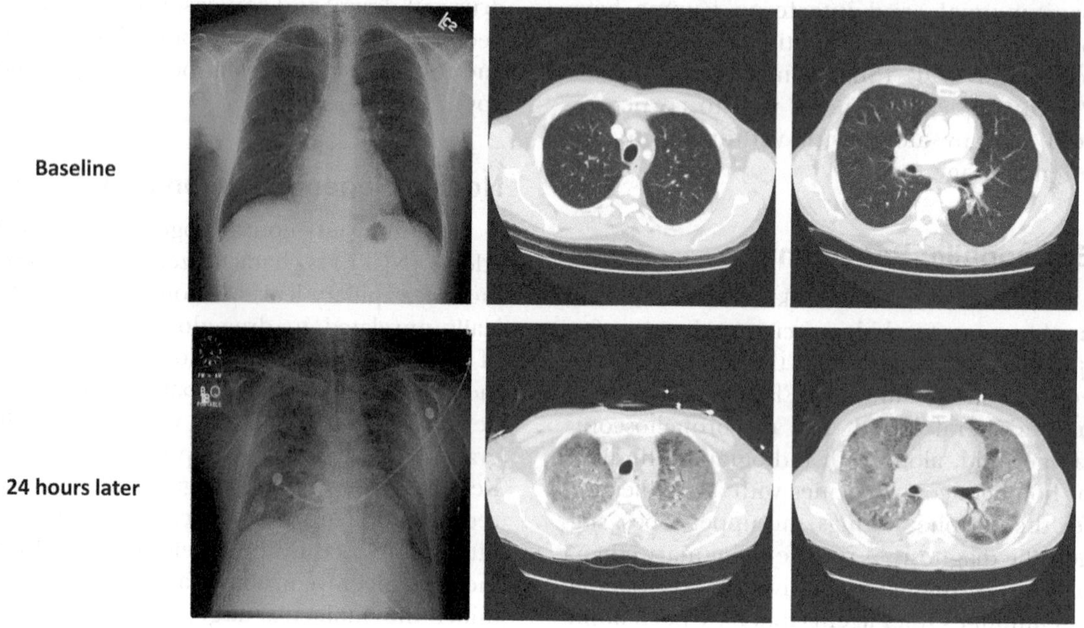

A 57-year-old man developed severe dyspnea 24 hours following cycle 1 of interleukin-2 (IL-2) therapy for malignant melanoma. Chest radiograph and computed tomography scans of the chest 24 hours later demonstrated diffuse alveolar infiltrates with small bilateral pleural effusions. These findings, along with the absence of Kerley B lines and normal cardiac silhouette, are consistent with noncardiogenic pulmonary edema, which was thought to be IL-2 induced.

Pleural Disease

Drug-induced pleural disease is most frequently seen after treatment with methotrexate, docetaxel, gemcitabine, azathioprine, interleukin-2, ATRA, and interferon gamma chemotherapies. The reaction presents as pleural effusions with or without pulmonary infiltrates and may resolve spontaneously following drug withdrawal. The benefit of steroid therapy in drug-induced pleural disease has not been established (Shannon & Price, 1998). Pleural fibrosis has been described as a late manifestation of cyclophosphamide, BCNU, and bleomycin toxicity.

Pulmonary Vascular Disease

Drug-induced vasculopathies, including thromboembolism and pulmonary hypertension, have been described following the use of conventional and targeted cancer therapies. Increased rates of thromboembolism have been reported following tamoxifen therapy. Thromboembolic events with rates ranging from 14%–43% have been reported among recipients of thalidomide-based chemotherapy given in combination with steroids, doxorubicin, or BCNU (Procopio et al., 2014; Sandler, 2007; see Figure 28-6). The vascular endothelial growth factor inhibitors, bevacizumab, sunitinib, and sorafenib, also are associated with thromboembolic events (Procopio et al., 2014; Sandler, 2007).

Thromboembolism causing significant clot burden within the pulmonary vasculature may lead to pulmonary hypertension, which is typically transient. Persistent pulmonary hypertension may occur as a result of drug-induced pulmonary arterial hypertension (PAH) and drug-related pulmonary veno-occlusive disease. Severe PAH has been reported following treatment with dasatinib, a Bcr-Abl tyrosine kinase inhibitor. Dasatinib-induced PAH may be only partially reversible in most cases after drug withdrawal. Immediate drug withdrawal without rechallenge is recommended once PAH is suspected (Abratt & Morgan, 2002; Godinas et al., 2013; Montani et al., 2012). Other chemotherapy drugs with potential PAH risk include interferon and zinostatin. Zinostatin is a novel antitumor antibiotic that may cause hypertrophy of the pulmonary vasculature wall, leading to PAH. Bleomycin and BCNU have been implicated in the development of fibrous obliteration of pulmonary venules and small pulmonary veins, leading to pulmonary veno-occlusive disease and persistent pulmonary hypertension.

Figure 28-6. Massive Pulmonary (Saddle) Embolus

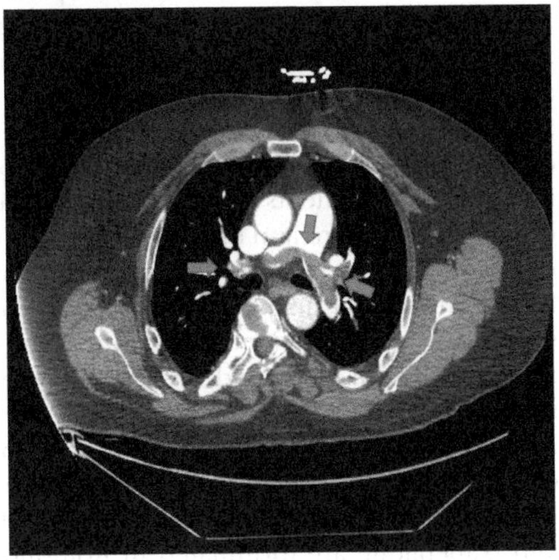

Massive pulmonary (saddle) embolism (arrows) in a patient treated with thalidomide and steroids for malignant melanoma.

Drug-Induced Airway Disease and Infusion Reactions

Severe bronchospasm following concurrent or sequential administration of a vinca alkaloid and mitomycin therapy has been reported (Dyke, 1984; Rivera, Kris, Gralla, & White, 1995). Drug-induced bronchospasm more often occurs as a consequence of infusion reactions. Intravenous infusion of many of the conventional antineoplastic therapies and virtually all monoclonal antibody therapy may trigger infusion reactions. Infusion reactions may represent allergic, immunoglobulin E–mediated, type I anaphylaxis reactions (carboplatin, oxaliplatin, and L-asparaginase) or, alternatively, may occur as nonallergic anaphylactoid reactions due to cytokine release (most monoclonal antibodies). Individual patients may have a higher rate of infusion reactions and more severe reactions depending on certain risk factors (see Figure 28-7). The clinical manifestations range from simple dry cough, dyspnea, and wheezing to anaphylaxis with associated hypoxia, hypotension, and death. Both the drug and the vehicle in which the drug is formulated may be implicated in the development of some infusion reactions. For example, paclitaxel, teniposide, and ixabepilone are formulated in Kolliphor® EL, formerly Cremophor® EL, which is highly allergenic and thought to be responsible for inducing the infusion reaction. Docetaxel and etoposide are both formulated in polysorbate 80 and may trigger similar allergic responses. Standard prophylaxis with histamine receptor antagonists and steroids prior to taxane administration has reduced the incidence of taxane-induced bronchospasm from 30% to 2% (Markman, 2003). However, breakthrough infusion reactions may occur despite prophylaxis.

Figure 28-7. Factors That May Increase the Risk of Infusion Reactions

- History of asthma or atopy
- Iodine or seafood allergies
- Concomitant use of beta-adrenergic blockers
- Concurrent autoimmune disease
- Higher than standard drug doses
- Newly diagnosed, chemotherapy-naïve patients
- Patients with hematologic malignancies (e.g., mantle cell lymphoma, chronic lymphocytic leukemia, small lymphocytic leukemia)
- Previous exposure to the inciting drug

Note. Based on information from Vogel, 2010.

The National Cancer Institute proposed grading criteria for cytokine release infusion reactions in 2006 (Camus, 2004: Camus, Bonniaud, et al., 2004; Camus, Fanton, et al., 2004; Camus, Kudoh, et al., 2004; see Table 28-2). Most, but not all, of the infusion reactions caused by monoclonal antibody infusions tend to be nonallergic and are associated with milder (grade 1–2) symptoms. Anaphylactic reactions following infusion with this group of drugs do occur, particularly during rituximab, trastuzumab, alemtuzumab, cetuximab, and gemtuzumab administration, but are less frequent than those following some conventional chemotherapy infusions. Allergic infusion reactions tend to occur early, within the first few minutes of the infusion, whereas nonallergic infusion reactions may occur later, typically within 30–120 minutes after starting the infusion. Cytokine release tends to diminish and symptoms subside as the tumor burden shrinks with additional cycles of therapy. Therefore, in contrast to type I allergic reactions, after some monoclonal antibody infusions, a brief cessation of therapy followed by initiation of antihistamines and resumption of therapy with adjustments in the monoclonal antibody infusion rate may be an acceptable approach in the management of mild cytokine release reactions. Immediate withdrawal of the offending agent is generally recommended following a type I anaphylactic reaction. Reintroduction of the offending agent following an anaphylactic reaction is discouraged.

The initial severity of an anaphylactic reaction does not predict its outcome. Mild reactions may progress rapidly to life-threatening cardiovascular or respiratory failure. Intravenous infusion of many of the cancer agents is the responsibility of most oncology nurses. Thus, the ability to identify the signs and symptoms of infusion reactions and a working knowledge of preventive measures and the acute management of these events by the oncology nursing team are mandatory. Infusion centers and facilities that administer oncology agents should always be prepared with mandatory

Table 28-2. Grading Criteria and Suggested Interventions for Infusion Reactions and Hypersensitivity Reactions

Grade	Signs/Symptoms	Treatments/Interventions	Outcome
1	Mild dry cough, transient flushing, mild rash, low-grade fever (< 38°C [100.4°F])	Drug interruption not indicated; no intervention indicated	Usually good
2	Sustained flushing, urticaria, dyspnea, fever > 38°C (100.4°F)	Interrupt infusion, promptly institute medical interventions including administration of antihistamines, nonsteroidal anti-inflammatory drugs (NSAIDs), narcotics, IV fluids, and steroids; continue medications for 24–72 hours.	Usually prompt response to medical interventions
3	Symptomatic bronchospasm with or without urticaria, parenteral medication(s) indicated, allergy-related edema/angioedema or hypotension	Initiate antihistamines, NSAIDs, narcotics, IV fluid resuscitation, vasopressors, steroids, glucagon, and bronchodilators if indicated; continue medications for 24–72 hours.	Poor response to treatment; symptom recurrence with resumption of therapy; hospitalization usually indicated for clinical sequelae such as renal impairment, hypotension, or pulmonary infiltrates
4	Anaphylaxis; life-threatening symptoms	Hospitalize the patient with intensive care; implement ventilator or vasopressor support as indicated; administer antihistamines, NSAIDs, narcotics, IV fluid resuscitation, vasopressors, steroids, glucagon, or bronchodilators as indicated.	Early withdrawal of agent and initiation of supportive care may improve outcome.

Note. Based on information from Camus, 2004: Camus, Bonniaud, et al., 2004; Camus, Fanton, et al., 2004; Camus, Kudoh, et al., 2004; Vogel, 2010.

supplies, equipment, medications, and a thoroughly trained staff. All of the nursing staff should be familiar with written emergency protocols. Standing orders for emergent treatment of infusion reactions are prudent and may reduce critical delays in treatment while waiting for the clinician's order. Delays in recognition of the signs and symptoms of anaphylaxis may result in increased morbidity and mortality. Because infusion reactions may be delayed by several hours after infusion, close monitoring during and for several hours following drug infusion is critical.

Supportive therapy for infusion reactions may include epinephrine, fluid resuscitation, dopamine, glucagon, histamine agents, and bronchodilators. Systemic corticosteroids have been shown to improve symptoms, decrease the duration of a reaction, and prevent biphasic (recurrent) reactions, but they are of no benefit in the acute management of anaphylaxis (Brown, Mullins, & Gold, 2006). Close surveillance with monitoring of vital signs every 15 minutes is recommended. Patients should be observed for at least four hours after resolution of symptoms. Lengthier observations are advised for some patients, depending on the risk factors for interstitial pneumonitis and the severity of the reaction. Up to 20% of patients may develop a recrudescence of bronchospasm (biphasic episode) within 8–72 hours of successful treatment. Rates of biphasic reactions tend to be highest among patients with initial severe reactions. Recurrent symptoms may be as severe as or worse than the initial event. No specific protocols for the length of inpatient observation have been established, but having longer observation periods for individuals with severe initial reactions seems reasonable. Recurrence of symptoms also may occur if the half-life of the rescue medication is shorter than that of the offending agent. Oncology nurses must be familiar with these factors and incorporate them into their treatment strategies. Figure 28-8 lists other observations that are important in nursing documentation of infusion events. At discharge, patients and families should be educated regarding the need for close observation and immediate reporting of any suspicious delayed symptoms to the medical team.

Figure 28-8. Recommended Components of Nursing Documentation for Drugs With Potential Infusion Reactions

1. Preassessment
   a. Exact times of drug administration
   b. Drug dosage
   c. Prior exposures to each agent, if any
   d. Cycle number
   e. Infusion rates
2. During infusion
   a. Initial symptoms and course of progression
   b. Symptom onset relative to drug administration
   c. Symptom duration and severity
   d. Need for therapeutic intervention response to therapy, including specific intervention and timing of response to therapy
3. After infusion
   a. Close observation with documentation of the duration of the observation period following drug exposure
   b. Need for extended periods of observation or escalation of care
   c. Follow-up instructions to the patient and family for continued careful observation and timing of delayed reactions

Note. Based on information from Vogel, 2010.

Other Clinicopathologic Syndromes

The development of noncaseating granulomas is a rare manifestation of DILI that may be indistinguishable from sarcoidosis. Conventional antineoplastic agents that have been implicated in the development of this disorder include methotrexate, procarbazine, sirolimus, and interferon (Marzouk, Saleh, Kannass, & Sharma, 2004; Sybert & Butler, 1978). Recent reports of sarcoid-like reactions following exposure to the immunomodulating agents, ipilimumab and nivolumab, have been described (Ortega & Drabkin, 2015). Drug withdrawal may result in disease regression.

Radiation-Induced Lung Injury

Radiation-induced lung injury (RILI) is the most common dose-limiting complication following thoracic radiation and chemoradiation regimens. The precise incidence of clinically significant lung toxicity is unknown. Radiation pneumonitis and radiation fibrosis represent the acute and late phases, respectively, of RILI and are the most frequent forms of radiation toxicity.

Classic radiation pneumonitis is predictable and dose dependent, with the injury confined to the irradiated lung field. Factors that influence the appearance and severity of RILI may be divided into those associated with radiation delivery, such as total radiation dose, dose per fraction, volume of irradiated lung, and beam characteristics and arrangements, and clinical factors, including preexisting lung disease, underlying poor pulmonary reserve, prior radiation therapy, multimodality regimens, and rapid steroid withdrawal. Radiation injury is rarely seen following radiation doses less than 20 Gy but occurs at increased rates once the dose exceeds 40 Gy (see Figure 28-9) (Marks et al., 2003; Movsas, Raffin, Epstein, & Link, 1997; Rovirosa & Valduvieco, 2010).

Symptoms of fever, dry cough, dyspnea, and pleuritic chest pain typically develop insidiously within one to three months and peak at three to four months after initial radiation therapy. Certain radiation-sensitizing drugs, such as mitomycin, cyclophosphamide, vincristine, doxorubicin, bleomycin, gemcitabine, the taxanes, and actinomycin D, may potentiate the severity of radiation injury or shorten the latency period between radiation exposure and the development of RILI (Phillips, 1992).

Depending on the degree of lung injury, generalized malaise and weight loss may develop with disease progression. Early radiographic changes include diffuse haze with indistinct vascular margins within the irradiated field. As the injury evolves, patchy areas of consolidation with air bronchograms may coalesce and lead to well-demarcated areas of volume loss, linear densities, and bronchiectasis within the treatment portals (see Figure 28-10). Spontaneous pneumothoraces may occur as sequelae of RILI. Ipsilateral pleural effusions also occur, typically within six months of completion of radiation therapy. Late effusions, occurring one to five years after completion of thoracic radiation, have also been reported. On examination, these effusions are cytologically negative and frequently demonstrate only reactive mesothelial cells. The effusions are typically small and asymptomatic, although dyspnea and pleuritic chest pain have been described. Radiation injury to the pulmonary vasculature has rarely been implicated in the development of pulmonary veno-occlusive disease. Pulmonary hypertension resulting from this form of radiation injury tends to be recalcitrant and irreversible. Other rare complications of thoracic radiation include BOOP and eosinophilic pneumonia. Both entities have been described following breast irradiation and are characterized by migratory pulmonary opacities occurring one to three months after completion of radiation therapy. A prior history of asthma or atopy and the presence of blood or tissue eosinophilia help to support the diagnosis. The opacities may occur outside of the irradiated field and tend to be steroid responsive (Cornelissen et al., 2007; Cottin et al., 2004). The physical examination may be normal or, alternatively, may reveal nonspecific rales, a pleural rub, or dullness to percussion. An erythematous rash that outlines the radiation port may be seen; however, this does not correlate with the occurrence or severity of radiation pneumonitis. Pulmonary function testing also may be normal. With significant lung injury, a restrictive defect with reductions in the DLCO is seen. These findings, when they occur, typically develop two to three months after completing radiation therapy and may progress over time with the development of pulmonary fibrosis.

Figure 28-9. Factors Associated With Radiation-Induced Lung Injury

- Total dose of radiation
- Dose per fraction
- Time-dose factor
- Type of radiation (conventional, intensity modulated, stereotactic body)
- Volume of lung irradiated
- Radiation portals and beam arrangements and characteristics
- Preexisting fibrotic lung disease
- Underlying pulmonary reserve
- Prior radiation therapy
- Rapid steroid withdrawal
- Multimodality regimens
- Radiation-sensitizing chemotherapy agents
- Possible genetic susceptibility

Note. Based on information from Merrill, 2016; Rovirosa & Valduvieco, 2010.

Figure 28-10. Radiation Fibrosis

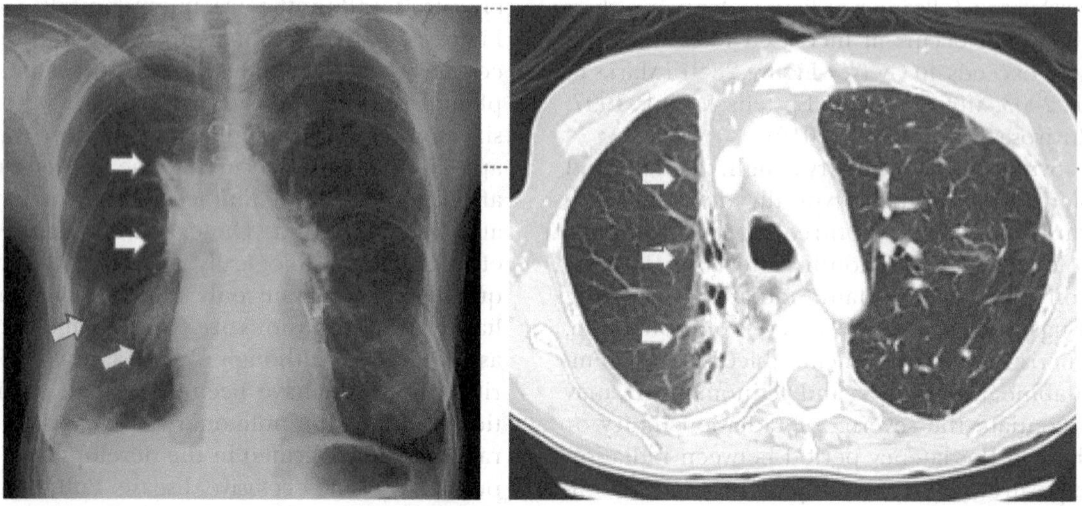

Radiation fibrosis 1 year following radiation to the right hilar area for treatment of metastatic sarcoma. Notice the right-sided volume loss with well-demarcated linear densities (white arrows) that outline the radiation treatment portal. Traction bronchiectasis also is seen. Multiple metastatic lesions are noted, with the largest one overlying the right lower lobe (gray arrows).

The diagnosis of radiation pneumonitis is based on the onset of symptoms and signs relative to completion of thoracic radiation, the presence of compatible radiographic changes, and the exclusion of competing diagnoses. Mimickers of RILI include infection, drug-induced pneumonitis, and tumor progression. Computed tomography is more sensitive than conventional chest radiographs in detecting the subtle lung changes following radiation treatment and correlate with the phase of lung injury. Bronchoscopy may be helpful in excluding competing diagnoses such as infection or tumor. In cases that are clinically atypical for RILI, transbronchial biopsies may be useful; however, no histopathologic changes are pathognomonic for RILI.

Radiation fibrosis develops in virtually all patients with radiation exposures of 40 Gy or greater regardless of clinical manifestations of pneumonitis. This late phase of RILI usually is radiographically apparent by six months and stabilizes over the ensuing one to two years after thoracic irradiation (Quinn et al., 2013; Rovirosa & Valduvieco, 2010).

Newer strategies for radiation therapy, including conformal therapy and intensity-modulated radiation therapy, have been developed to deliver adequate doses to the tumor while limiting exposure to normal lung. However, these newer radiation modalities and delivery systems can cause lung injury. The typical well-demarcated area of consolidation that conforms to the radiation treatment field associated with conventional radiation therapy may not be as obvious with the newer modalities, which renders diagnosis more difficult (Liao, Travis, & Tucker, 1995; Quinn et al., 2013; Rovirosa & Valduvieco, 2010).

Radiation recall pneumonitis describes a rare inflammatory reaction that is confined to a previously irradiated field and is triggered by the administration of certain chemotherapy and targeted agents. The inflammatory response may occur within several weeks of exposure to the inflammatory trigger, which may be months to years following completion of radiation therapy. The clinical presentation of radiation recall pneumonitis includes dry cough, fever, and dyspnea, accompanied by ground-glass opacities and areas of consolidation that conform to the prior radiation treatment portal. Taxane- and anthracycline-based therapies are the most frequent inciting agents. Other drugs, including gemcitabine, etoposide, vinorelbine, trastuzumab, and erlotinib, also have been implicated in the development of this disease (Ding, Ji, Li, Zhang, & Wang, 2011; Lee et al., 2014; Onal, Abali, Koc, & Kara, 2012; Schwarte, Wagner, Karstens, & Bremer, 2007). This type of pneumonitis occurs shortly after administration of the inciting antineoplastic agent, which can be weeks to months following completion of radiation therapy. Standard treatment includes withdrawal of the precipitating agent. Systemic corticosteroid therapy has been tried with varied success. Successful reintroduction of the inciting agent has been described (Ding et al., 2011; Schwarte et al., 2007).

Conclusion

Careful assessment of potential respiratory toxicities in patients receiving radiation therapy, chemotherapy, or biologic therapy is important for early detection and intervention. A variety of symptoms associated with pulmonary toxicities can occur early or years after therapy. Radiographic changes due to chemotherapy can occur in a classic diffuse reticular pattern as ground-glass opacities and are usually bilateral. Early radiographic changes due to radiation therapy appear as diffuse haziness and ground-glass opacification, whereas later changes occur as infiltrate or dense consolidation that corresponds to the region of radiation exposure. With targeted therapies, the radiographic changes range from diffuse bilateral lung infiltrates to normal findings. Physical examination results can include dyspnea

Key Points

- Oncology nurses should be able to identify patients at risk, recognize the clinical signs of lung toxicity, and provide optimal prophylactic measures and symptom management.
- The most common toxicities following targeted therapies are vasculopathies, infusion reactions, and pleural effusions.
- The pulmonary clinical manifestations of cancer treatment–associated infusion reactions range from simple dry cough, dyspnea, and wheezing to anaphylaxis with associated hypoxia, hypotension, and death. Both the drug and the vehicle in which the drug is formulated may be implicated in the development of some infusion reactions.
- Patients who received methotrexate, docetaxel, gemcitabine, azathioprine, interleukin-2, ATRA, and interferon gamma chemotherapies should be monitored for drug-induced pleural disease.
- Cytokine release associated with monoclonal antibody infusion tends to diminish and symptoms subside as the tumor burden shrinks with additional cycles of therapy.
- RILI is the most common dose-limiting complication following thoracic radiation and chemoradiation regimens.
- A variety of chemotherapy (bleomycin, busulfan, chlorambucil, cyclophosphamide, doxorubicin, ifosfamide, methotrexate, mitomycin, vinblastine, and vincristine) and targeted therapies (alemtuzumab, bevacizumab, cetuximab, rituximab, and trastuzumab) are predisposed to radiation pneumonitis.
- Radiation recall pneumonitis describes a rare inflammatory reaction that is confined to a previously irradiated field and is triggered by the administration of certain chemotherapy and targeted agents.

and nonproductive cough to moist rales, pleural friction rub, and tachypnea with cyanosis.

The authors would like to acknowledge Dawn Camp-Sorrell, RN, MSN, FNP, AOCN®, for her contribution to this chapter that remains unchanged from the first edition of this book.

References

Abratt, R.P., & Morgan, G.W. (2002). Lung toxicity following chest irradiation in patients with lung cancer. *Lung Cancer, 35,* 103–109. doi:10.1016/S0169-5002(01)00334-8

Akoun, G.M., Milleron, B.J., Cadranel, J.L., & Mayaud, C.M. (1992). Pulmonary pathology of drug origin. *Revue du Praticien, 42,* 2593–2599.

Bacakoğlu, F., Atasever, A., Ozhan, M.H., Gurgun, C., Ozkilic, H., & Guzelant, A. (2003). Plasma and bronchoalveolar lavage fluid levels of endothelin-1 in patients with chronic obstructive pulmonary disease and pulmonary hypertension. *Respiration, 70,* 594–599. doi:10.1159/000075204

Barber, N.A., & Ganti, A.K. (2011). Pulmonary toxicities from targeted therapies: A review. *Targeted Oncology, 6,* 235–243. doi:10.1007/s11523-011-0199-0

Beauverd, Y., & Samii, K. (2014). Acute respiratory distress syndrome in a patient with primary myelofibrosis after ruxolitinib treatment discontinuation. *International Journal of Hematology, 100,* 498–501. doi:10.1007/s12185-014-1628-5

Brown, S.G., Mullins, R.J., & Gold, M.S. (2006). Anaphylaxis: Diagnosis and management. *Medical Journal of Australia, 185,* 283–289.

Camus, P. (2004). Interstitial lung disease in patients with non-small-cell lung cancer: Causes, mechanisms and management. *British Journal of Cancer, 91*(Suppl. 2), S1–S2. doi:10.1038/sj.bjc.6602060

Camus, P., Bonniaud, P., Fanton, A., Camus, C., Baudaun, N., & Foucher, P. (2004). Drug-induced and iatrogenic infiltrative lung disease. *Clinics in Chest Medicine, 25,* 479–519. doi:10.1016/j.ccm.2004.05.006

Camus, P., Fanton, A., Bonniaud, P., Camus, C., & Foucher, P. (2004). Interstitial lung disease induced by drugs and radiation. *Respiration, 71,* 301–326. doi:10.1159/000079633

Camus, P., Kudoh, S., & Ebina, M. (2004). Interstitial lung disease associated with drug therapy. *British Journal of Cancer, 91*(Suppl. 2), S18–S23. doi:10.1038/sj.bjc.6602063

Cooper, J.A., Jr., White, D.A., & Matthay, R.A. (1986a). Drug-induced pulmonary disease. Part 1: Cytotoxic drugs. *American Review of Respiratory Disease, 133,* 321–340.

Cooper, J.A., Jr., White, D.A., & Matthay, R.A. (1986b). Drug-induced pulmonary disease. Part 2: Noncytotoxic drugs. *American Review of Respiratory Disease, 133,* 488–505.

Cornelissen, R., Senan, S., Antonisse, I.E., Liem, H., Tan, Y.K., Rudolphus, A., & Aerts, J.G. (2007). Bronchiolitis obliterans organizing pneumonia (BOOP) after thoracic radiotherapy for breast carcinoma. *Radiation Oncology, 2*(2), 1–5. doi:10.1186/1748-717X-2-2

Cottin, V., Frognier, R., Monnot, H., Levy, A., DeVuyst, P., Cordler, J.-F., & Groupe d'Etudes et de Recherche sur les Maladies "Orphelines" Pulmonaires. (2004). Chronic eosinophilic pneumonia after radiation therapy for breast cancer. *European Respiratory Journal, 23,* 9–13. doi:10.1183/09031936.03.00071303

Dabydeen, D.A., Jagannathan, J.P., Ramaiya, N., Krajewski, K., Schutz, F.A., Cho, D.C., ... Choueiri, T.K. (2012). Pneumonitis associated with mTOR inhibitors therapy in patients with metastatic renal cell carcinoma: Incidence, radiographic findings and correlation with clinical outcome. *European Journal of Cancer, 48,* 1519–1524. doi:10.1016/j.ejca.2012.03.012

Dhokarh, R., Li, G., Schmickl, C.N., Kashyap, R., Assudani, J., Limper, A.H., & Gajic, O. (2012). Drug-associated acute lung injury: A population-based cohort study. *Chest, 142,* 845–850. doi:10.1378/chest.11-2103

Ding, X., Ji, W., Li, J., Zhang, X., & Wang, L. (2011). Radiation recall pneumonitis induced by chemotherapy after thoracic radiotherapy for lung cancer. *Radiation Oncology, 6*(24), 1–6. doi:10.1186/1748-717x-6-24

Donat, S.M., & Levy, D.A. (1998). Bleomycin associated pulmonary toxicity: Is perioperative oxygen restriction necessary? *Journal of Urology, 160,* 1347–1352. doi:10.1016/S0022-5347(01)62533-3

Duran, I., Goebell, P.J., Papazisis, K., Ravaud, A., Weichhart, T., Rodriguez-Portal, J.A., & Budde, K. (2014). Drug-induced pneumonitis in cancer patients treated with mTOR inhibitors: Management and insights into possible mechanisms. *Expert Opinion on Drug Safety, 13,* 361–372. doi:10.1517/14740338.2014.888056

Dy, G.K., & Adjei, A.A. (2013). Understanding, recognizing, and managing toxicities of targeted anticancer therapies. *CA: A Cancer Journal for Clinicians, 63,* 249–279. doi:10.3322/caac.21184

Dyke, R. (1984). Acute bronchospasm after a vinca alkaloid in patients previously treated with mitomycin. *New England Journal of Medicine, 310,* 389. doi:10.1056/NEJM198402093100611

Gartrell, B.A., Ying, J., Sivendran, S., Boucher, K.M., Choueiri, T.K., Sonpavde, G., ... Galsky, M.D. (2014). Pulmonary complications with the use of mTOR inhibitors in targeted cancer therapy: A systematic review and meta-analysis. *Targeted Oncology, 9,* 195–204. doi:10.1007/s11523-013-0289-2

Godinas, L., Guignabert, C., Seferian, A., Perros, F., Bergot, E., Sibille, Y., ... Montani, D. (2013). Tyrosine kinase inhibitors in pulmonary arterial hypertension: A double-edge sword? *Seminars in Respiratory and Critical Care Medicine, 34,* 714–724. doi:10.1055/s-0033-1356494

Guntur, V.P., & Dhand, R. (2012). Pulmonary toxicity of chemotherapeutic agents. In M.C. Perry (Ed.), *Perry's the chemotherapy source book* (5th ed., pp. 206–213). Philadelphia, PA: Wolters Kluwer Health/Lippincott Williams & Wilkins.

Hirsch, A., Vander Els, N., Straus, D.J., Gomez, E.G., Leung, D., Portlock, C.S., & Yahalom, J. (1996). Effect of ABVD chemotherapy with and without mantle or mediastinal irradiation on pulmonary function and symptoms in early-stage Hodgkin's disease. *Journal of Clinical Oncology, 14,* 1297–1305.

Jules-Elysee, K., & White, D.A. (1990). Bleomycin-induced pulmonary toxicity. *Clinics in Chest Medicine, 11,* 1–20.

Lee, H.E., Jeong, N.J., Lee, Y., Seo, Y.J., Kim, C.D., Lee, J.H., & Im, I. (2014). Radiation recall dermatitis and pneumonitis induced by trastuzumab (Herceptin®). *International Journal of Dermatology, 53,* e159–e160. doi:10.1111/j.1365-4632.2012.05788.x

Liao, Z.X., Travis, E.L., & Tucker, S.L. (1995). Damage and morbidity from pneumonitis after irradiation of partial volumes of mouse lung. *International Journal of Radiation Oncology, Biology, Physics, 32,* 1359–1370. doi:10.1016/0360-3016(94)00660-D

Luesink, M., & Jansen, J.H. (2010). Advances in understanding the pulmonary infiltration in acute promyelocytic leukaemia. *British Journal of Haematology, 151,* 209–220. doi:10.1111/j.1365-2141.2010.08325.x

Markman, M. (2003). Management of toxicities associated with the administration of taxanes. *Expert Opinion on Drug Safety, 2,* 141–146. doi:10.1517/14740338.2.2.141

Marks, L.B., Yu, X., Vujaskovic, Z., Small, W., Jr., Folz, R., & Anscher, M.S. (2003). Radiation-induced lung injury. *Seminars in Radiation Oncology, 13,* 333–345. doi:10.1016/S1053-4296(03)00034-1

Maroto, J.P., Hudes, G., Dutcher, J.P., Logan, T.F., White, C.S., Krygowski, M., ... Berkenblit, A. (2011). Drug-related pneumonitis in patients with advanced renal cell carcinoma treated with temsirolimus. *Journal of Clinical Oncology, 29,* 1750–1756. doi:10.1200/JCO.2010.29.2235

Marzouk, K., Saleh, S., Kannass, M., & Sharma, O.P. (2004). Interferon-induced granulomatous lung disease. *Current Opinion in Pulmonary Medicine, 10,* 435–440. doi:10.1097/01.mcp.0000134400.88832.9c

Matsuno, O. (2012). Drug-induced interstitial lung disease: Mechanisms and best diagnostic approaches. *Respiratory Research, 13,* 39. doi:10.1186/1465-9921-13-39

Merrill, W.W. (2016, July 19). Radiation-induced lung injury [Literature review current through February 2017]. Retrieved from http://www.uptodate.com/contents/radiation-induced-lung-injury

Montani, D., Bergot, E., Günther, S., Savale, L., Bergeron, A., Bourdin, A., ... Humbert, M. (2012). Pulmonary arterial hypertension in patients treated by dasatinib. *Circulation, 125,* 2128–2137. doi:10.1161/CIRCULATIONAHA.111.079921

Movsas, B., Raffin, T.A., Epstein, A.H., & Link, C.J., Jr. (1997). Pulmonary radiation injury. *Chest, 111,* 1061–1076. doi:10.1378/chest.111.4.1061

Onal, C., Abali, H., Koc, Z., & Kara, S. (2012). Radiation recall pneumonitis caused by erlotinib after palliative definitive radiotherapy. *Onkologie, 35,* 191–194. doi:10.1159/000337616

Ortega, R.M.M., & Drabkin, H.A. (2015). Nivolumab in renal cell carcinoma. *Expert Opinion on Biological Therapy, 15,* 1049–1060. doi:10.1517/14712598.2015.1049596

Phillips, T.L. (1992). Effects of chemotherapy and irradiation on normal tissues. *Frontiers in Radiation Therapy and Oncology, 26,* 45–54. doi:10.1159/000421054

Procopio, G., Verzoni, E., Biondani, P., Grassi, P., Testa, I., Garanzini, E., & de Braud, F. (2014). Rationale and protocol of RESORT, a randomized, open-label, multicenter phase II study to evaluate the efficacy of sorafenib in patients with advanced renal cell carcinoma after radical resection of the metastases. *Tumori, 100,* e28–e30. doi:10.1700/1430.15834

Quinn, T., Alam, N., Aminazad, A., Marshall, M.B., & Choong, C.K.C. (2013). Decision making and algorithm for the management of pleural effusions. *Thoracic Surgery Clinics, 23,* 11–16. doi:10.1016/j.thorsurg.2012.10.009

Rivera, M.P., Kris, M.G., Gralla, R.J., & White, D.A. (1995). Syndrome of acute dyspnea related to combined mitomycin plus vinca alkaloid chemotherapy. *American Journal of Clinical Oncology, 18,* 245–250. doi:10.1097/00000421-199506000-00012

Rogers, J.E., & Yang, D. (2012). Differentiation syndrome in patients with acute promyelocytic leukemia. *Journal of Oncology Pharmacy Practice, 18,* 109–114. doi:10.1177/1078155211399163

Rovirosa, A., & Valduvieco, I. (2010). Radiation pneumonitis. *Clinical Pulmonary Medicine, 17,* 218–222. doi:10.1097/CPM.0b013e3181efac67

Ryu, J.H. (2010). Chemotherapy-induced pulmonary toxicity in lung cancer patients. *Journal of Thoracic Oncology, 5,* 1313–1314. doi:10.1097/JTO.0b013e3181e9dbb9

Sachdeva, A., & Matuschak, G.M. (2008). Diffuse alveolar hemorrhage following alemtuzumab. *Chest, 133,* 1476–1478. doi:10.1378/chest.07-2354

Sandler, A. (2007). Bevacizumab in non–small cell lung cancer. *Clinical Cancer Research, 13,* s4613–s4616. doi:10.1158/1078-0432.CCR-07-0647

Schwaiblmair, M., Behr, W., Haeckel, T., Märkl, B., Foerg, W., & Berghaus, T. (2012). Drug induced interstitial lung disease. *Open Respiratory Medicine Journal, 6,* 63–74. doi:10.2174/1874306401206010063

Schwarte, S., Wagner, K., Karstens, J.H., & Bremer, M. (2007). Radiation recall pneumonitis induced by gemcitabine. *Strahlentherapie und Onkologie, 183,* 215–217. doi:10.1007/s00066-007-1688-z

Shannon, V., & Price, K. (1998). Pulmonary complications of cancer therapy. *Anesthesiology Clinics of North America, 16,* 563–585. doi:10.1016/S0889-8537(05)70043-2

Sleijfer, S. (2001). Bleomycin-induced pneumonitis. *Chest, 120,* 617–624. doi:10.1378/chest.120.2.617

Snyder, L.S., & Hertz, M.I. (1988). Cytotoxic drug-induced lung injury. *Seminars in Respiratory Infection, 3,* 217–228.

Sostman, H.D., Matthay, R.A., & Putman, C.E. (1977). Cytotoxic drug-induced lung disease. *American Journal of Medicine, 62,* 608–615. doi:10.1016/0002-9343(77)90424-7

Sybert, A., & Butler, T.P. (1978). Sarcoidosis following adjuvant high-dose methotrexate therapy for osteosarcoma. *Archives of Internal Medicine, 138,* 488–489. doi:10.1001/archinte.1978.03630270094033

Tefferi, A., Litzow, M.R., & Pardanani, A. (2011). Long-term outcome of treatment with ruxolitinib in myelofibrosis. *New England Journal of Medicine, 365,* 1455–1457. doi:10.1056/NEJMc1109555

Vahid, B., & Marik, P.E. (2008). Infiltrative lung diseases: Complications of novel antineoplastic agents in patients with hematological malignancies. *Canadian Respiratory Journal, 15,* 211–216. doi:10.1155/2008/305234

Vogel, W.H. (2010). Infusion reactions: Diagnosis, assessment and management. *Clinical Journal of Oncology Nursing, 14,* E10–E21. doi:10.1188/10.CJON.E10-E21

White, D.A., & Stover, D.E. (1984). Severe bleomycin-induced pneumonitis: Clinical features and response to corticosteroids. *Chest, 86,* 723–728. doi:10.1378/chest.86.5.723

Yousem, S.A., Lifson, J.D., & Colby, T.V. (1985). Chemotherapy-induced eosinophilic pneumonia: Relation to bleomycin. *Chest, 88,* 103–106. doi:10.1378/chest.88.1.103

Chapter 28 Study Questions

1. Which of the following patient characteristics increases the likelihood of the patient being diagnosed with a pulmonary toxicity related to cancer therapy?
   A. Cumulative dose of chemotherapy to date is less than the lifetime dose
   B. History of secondhand smoke
   C. 71 years of age
   D. Male gender

2. A person receiving radiation to the chest is most likely to experience which of the following with the development of a pulmonary toxicity?
   A. Onset of symptoms within 10–15 minutes after completing the treatment
   B. Development of symptoms six weeks after completing radiation therapy
   C. High-grade fever since treatment seven days ago with nasal congestion
   D. Asymptomatic with dry cough

3. Match the following pulmonary toxicity risk factors with their treatment type or types:

A. Preexisting pulmonary disease	1. Chemotherapy
B. Age	2. Radiation
C. High concentration of oxygen (> 35%)	3. Targeted therapies

SECTION IV

Issues for Cancer Survivors and Their Families

CHAPTER 29

Developmental Life Stage Issues

Janet Harden, PhD, RN

Introduction

As people age, they experience physical, intellectual, and psychosocial changes associated with their developmental life stage. A life-span perspective suggests that adults experience a series of gains and losses across the life span (Baltes, 1987, 1997). Gains are more pronounced in young adulthood and tend to be balanced in middle adulthood; in later adulthood, the losses exceed the gains (Orth, Maes, & Schmitt, 2015). Efforts to balance gains and losses in different life domains are essential to personal development over the life span. When a person's own resources are insufficient to solve a problem, strategies such as seeking information or acquiring new skills are used. If these strategies are insufficient to improve the situation, emotional responses such as hopelessness, resignation, or depression can follow as a result of blocked goals (Brandtstädter & Renner, 1990). As adults age, they also use accommodation as a way to neutralize problems.

Accommodation includes a psychological reorientation, which consists of people adjusting their aspiration levels, revising goals to be consistent with abilities, realigning priorities, and performing a cognitive reappraisal of their life (Schmutte & Ryff, 1997). Middle-aged and older adults tend to shift their goal orientation toward maintenance and loss prevention, while younger adults tend to focus on growth goals (Ebner, Freund, & Baltes, 2006). All of these adaptive strategies can lead to a personal paradigm shift changing individuals' beliefs about themselves and their world. The strategies are used to minimize physical, psychological, and social changes that develop in mid-life and older age. Accommodation of preferences, most common at a later age, may account for high life satisfaction reported by older adults even in the face of circumstances generally regarded as highly aversive, such as a cancer diagnosis (Friedman & Ryff, 2012; Rothermund & Brandstädter, 2003; Rustoen, Moum, Wiklund, & Hanestad, 1999).

Cancer is a major life stressor that can disrupt the lifestyles and routines of all involved. Preexisting factors within the family unit related to life cycle changes influence the struggle that families face in adjusting to a cancer diagnosis. Most family members have some ongoing life stressors that relate to their role in the family. For the patient, physical symptoms, changes in responsibilities, financial issues, and diminished social interactions are factors that contribute to stress within the couple. Families often need to deal with many disease-related stressors in addition to other stressors that are part of the developmental life cycle. These age-related stressors exist concurrently and can affect the family's ability to adjust to illness. Researchers have found that older age was related to fewer daily stressors, which, in turn, was related to less negative affect, which may influence the way patients and families respond to a cancer diagnosis (Charles et al., 2010).

Couples face developmental changes related to their stage in life, including a redistribution of role and power between the partners that can affect the balance in their relationship (Rowland, 1990). Families actively work to develop new patterns of functioning as they age and thus adapt to their new circumstances. Most family members have unresolved concurrent stress related to their role within the family. With the addition of new stressors related to illness, prior strains may become more pronounced. Because people's needs and stressors change across the life span, information about the time at which cancer occurs and the treatment consequences that interfere with or threaten developmental tasks provides insight for nurses into the psychological issues that may develop during the diagnosis, treatment, and recovery periods.

Early Adulthood (Ages 20–39)

Early adulthood is a life stage in which the individual explores the adult world and seeks a comfortable fit between self and society. A key developmental task of this stage is achievement of intimacy and closeness to others, particularly sexually. During this stage, youthful plans are pursued, jobs and careers are begun, and future advancement plans are mapped out. This is a period filled with much satisfaction in terms of sexuality, family life, creativity, and occupational advancements (Levinson, 1986). This same time period is also filled with much stress as young adults enter marriage, begin parenthood, and assume financial obligations. Erikson (1963) has referred to this stage as *intimacy versus isolation*. A mature sexual relationship is an important part of this stage, and the inability to achieve this relationship results in isolation and threatens goal attainment (Erikson, 1963). A cancer illness at this time can dramatically affect the young adult's ability to form and sustain close relationships, to achieve career goals, and to maintain independence (Rowland, 1990). Feelings of vulnerability and a lack of a secure, healthy future can interfere with the establishment of relationships. Family development related to forming and maintaining close relationships, commitment to each other, and achievement of work goals can be affected, all of which can have a deleterious effect on self-esteem. Cancer treatment can affect physical appearance and compromise fertility (Smith et al., 2013). Because cancer treatment often necessitates dependence on others, the young adult's self-esteem can be further threatened. This increased dependence can result in anger and frustration (Rowland, 1990).

In a large study (N = 398) of cancer survivors, younger survivors were at greater risk for mood disturbance and reported higher levels of anxiety and depression than an age-matched comparison group (Costanzo, Ryff, & Singer, 2009). Similarly, in another study of individuals with chronic illness, disruption in lifestyle was greater in the younger participants, contributing to higher depressive symptoms (Devins, 1993). Healthcare providers need to be vigilant for symptoms of depression in young patients and survivors.

Research in young cancer survivors (mean age of 32 years) has shown that they believed that their experience with cancer made their family relationship closer, which enhanced their potential parenting skills (Schover, Rybicki, Martin, & Bringelsen, 1999). Sixty percent of study participants wanted to be a parent, yet 58% did not want to leave a spouse with young children to raise alone, thus creating a dilemma. Interestingly, in this study, although men were chosen because their cancer treatment was likely to impair fertility, only 60%

had any memory of a healthcare provider discussing fertility before cancer treatment. Fewer recalled being given the option of banking sperm (51%), and still fewer had a discussion about health risks to children conceived after treatment (26%). Only 43% of the men in this study were given information about the risk of cancer for their children.

Infertility was a source of distress for all survivors but was greater in those who were childless at the time of treatment (Schover, Brey, Lichtin, Lipshultz, & Jeha, 2002; Williams, 2013). Patients often noted that the topic of infertility was not discussed with them prior to treatment (Morrow et al., 2014). Some participants worried about the potential risk to their children of inherited cancer or birth defects. Women worried that pregnancy would increase the chance of cancer recurrence. A small number of women were concerned that cancer treatment effects would result in a high-risk pregnancy (Schover et al., 1999). In a large study (N = 523) of young adults, results showed that more than 50% reported that cancer had a negative impact on plans for having children (Bellizzi et al., 2012). Young female survivors of breast cancer have indicated a desire for more information on coping with the psychosocial distress following treatment and for recommendations to rehabilitative care to address this need (Takahashi, 2014). Healthcare providers need to make a concerted effort to disseminate information and support resources for these young survivors who experience a variety of issues related to interpersonal relationships, sexuality, fertility, and even employment.

Research has shown that young adult patients with cancer have a need to meet with other young people with cancer (Kurtz, Given, Given, & Kurtz, 1994). Developmentally, the need for social connection is strong during this stage. Some research has shown that social activity in one's 20s affects socialization such as emotional closeness in later life (Carmichael, Reis, & Duberstein, 2015). Younger adults have reported that their quality of life is somewhat compromised as a result of cancer and its treatment (Monteiro, Torres, Morgadinho, & Pereira, 2013). They often miss experiences common in this age group, such as dating, leaving home, and establishing independence (D'Agostino, Penney, & Zebrack, 2011). Identity development is a key component of health development in young adults. To minimize the disruption caused by cancer, it is important for young adults to stay connected with their peers. Same-age peers may help young adult patients with cancer to develop coping skills that lead to positive health behaviors. In addition, seeing others who have had similar experiences survive treatment and form meaningful friendships may promote social and psychological well-being.

In a large longitudinal study (N = 148) of caregivers of patients with cancer, young female caregivers (younger than age 50) reported higher levels of negative impact on their schedule secondary to role strain (work outside the home, household chores, and child rearing) (Nijboer et al., 2000). Other studies have shown that younger caregivers are more vulnerable in terms of mental health and psychological well-being (Mor, Allen, & Malin, 1994; Vinokur, Threatt, Vinokur-Kaplan, & Satariano, 1990). Younger caregivers face multiple responsibilities inherent with younger families and, consequently, may experience a greater impact on their schedule. The social and economic consequences related to lost wages coupled with increasing expenses can be devastating, resulting in depression and anxiety. Some research has shown that the burden experienced by younger caregivers was somewhat mitigated by support from their network of friends (Kurtz et al., 1994).

In summary, a cancer illness during young adulthood threatens young adults' ability to form close relationships, achieve career goals, and maintain independence. Young caregivers have more role strain and are at risk for developing psychological distress. Social and economic consequences of a cancer illness during young adulthood can lead to increased anxiety, depression, anger, and frustration (Rowland, 1990) (see Table 29-1).

Middle Adulthood (Ages 40–59)

Middle adulthood is characterized by the achievement of personal goals. During middle age, the adult serves an important role in the family and workplace, sharing knowledge and wisdom with young people by drawing on previous life experiences (Erikson, 1963). While some aspects of physical functioning decline, such as physical strength, many cognitive functions peak (Ryff, 1995). In addition, psychological variables such as self-confidence and self-mastery also peak during this stage. Fewer financial responsibilities and a higher earning capacity result in more economic stability for some couples, whereas others experience an increased financial strain related to educational expenses of college-bound children. In addition, many couples worry that they do not have enough money saved in preparation for retirement.

Personal accomplishments are frequently recognized and rewarded in middle adulthood. Baltrusch, Seidel, Stangel, and Waltz (1988) referred to this age as the first phase of aging, which begins around age 50. During this phase, a transition from biologic tasks (such as fathering or birthing and rearing children) and social tasks (such as marriage and finding

Table 29-1. Developmental Tasks and the Effects of a Cancer Illness

Developmental Stage	Developmental Tasks	Threats Created by a Cancer Diagnosis
Early adulthood (ages 20–39)	Intimacy versus isolation Achievement of intimacy Formation of mature sexual relationships Pursuance of careers Occupational achievement Stress related to marriage and parenthood Increased financial obligations	Ability to form close relationships Ability to maintain career goals Ability to maintain independence
Middle adulthood (ages 40–59)	Achievement of personal goals Peaking of cognitive and psychological variables Launching of adult children Responsibilities to aging parents	Ability to continue work Forced early retirement Financial insecurity Disruption of sexual relationship
Young-old (ages 60–74)	Establishment of new life goals after retirement Increased marital satisfaction Development of comorbid conditions Fulfillment of retirement dreams	Interruption of life plans Decreased sense of security for future Emotional distress in spousal caregiver
Old-old (age 75 and older)	Physical, social, psychological, and economic changes Demands on individuals' ability to respond to changes in health Tendency to minimize degree of threat from illness	Decreased mobility Increased loneliness Physically more compromised by treatment

Note. Based on information from Arber & Evandrou, 1993; Baltrusch et al., 1988; Erikson, 1963; Harden et al., 2002, 2006; Keller, Leventhal, & Larson, 1989; Keller, Leventhal, Prohaska, et al., 1989; Kurtz et al., 1994; Kutner et al., 1992; Levinson, 1986; Mellon, 2002; Mor et al., 1994; Newman & Newman, 1999; Northouse et al., 2000; Rowland, 1990; Ryff, 1995; Woods & Lewis, 1995.

a job) is beginning. For many couples, children are maturing and leaving home, leading to fewer responsibilities around the house, an increased desire for companionship, and possibly new levels of intimacy and sexual desire. Some couples find the increased time together stressful as they work to renew their relationship.

A significant challenge of middle age is effectively responding to the additional responsibilities related to caring for aging parents while still being involved with teenaged or young adult children. People in this stage are characterized by taking care of things and managing the negative and positive occurrences they face (Levinson, 1986). While they are the senior members in the workforce, concurrently they are beginning to prepare for the next phase of life.

The occurrence of an illness during ages 50–64 may force early retirement and produce financial hardships, as well as feelings of anger, frustration, and loss of professional identity related to being cheated of a full career and a healthy retirement (Harden, Northouse, & Mood, 2006; Kelly, 2004; Nishigaki et al., 2007). Despite the fact that some people are retiring earlier than in previous generations, work continues to be a major source of social status, self-esteem, and social contact, as well as financial well-being. Some people find it necessary to return to work following retirement to supplement their retirement income. People who are forced to leave their employment before they are ready may experience a variety of reactions, such as happiness, sadness, anger, or depression (Arber & Evandrou, 1993). Psychological issues and physical changes associated with aging can threaten self-image, and self-image can be further threatened by a diagnosis of cancer. Downing et al. (2015) found that adults aged 55–65 years reported poorer quality of life than adults older than 65 years diagnosed with cancer, possibly related to prior expectations of relatively good health during this time period. Middle-aged adults also were more likely to report unmet needs related to emotional and family problems (Parry, Lomax, Morningstar, & Fairclough, 2012).

In a longitudinal study (N = 48) of women (mean age of 43 years) with chronic illness, including breast cancer, researchers found that the illness affected marital adjustment, which, in turn, affected family life, parent–child relationships, and family functioning (Woods & Lewis, 1995). Further, they found that in a breast cancer population (mean age of 54 years), an interrelationship existed between the women's level of adjustment and their husband's adjustment; if women experienced emotional distress, so did the husband. A cancer illness frequently brought changes in sexual relationships, which were sometimes related to physical dysfunction and sometimes to clinical depression. Working through the effects of these changes within couples and restoring some level of intimacy is an added challenge in the survival phase for couples.

In a large study (N = 112) looking at the effect of symptom burden on patients, the researchers found that many in the sample experienced a loss of dignity ("feeling like I am no longer who I was") related to the number of symptoms they were experiencing (Vehling & Mehnert, 2014). Feelings of loss of dignity were associated with hopelessness and the desire to hasten death (Monforte-Royo, Villavicencio-Chávez, Tomás-Sábado, & Balaguer, 2011). Dignity-conserving care and interventions may help preserve patients' integrity and counter feelings of worthlessness in this age group.

Kent et al. (2012) found that health information needs varied by age, with the greatest need in the younger group of survivors (participants ranged from younger than age 50 to older than age 80). This study was a survey of 1,197 survivors more than five years from the original diagnosis. More than half of the survivors expressed a desire for more information about side effects and symptoms, tests and treatments, health promotion, and interpersonal/emotional needs. Findings indicated that needs were similar across cancer sites. Greater information need was associated with poorer mental well-being. Further, findings suggested that despite the number of years since diagnosis, survivors had lingering questions related to their cancer and its treatment. Healthcare providers need to provide survivors with the information and tools needed to maintain good long-term health.

In a mixed design study of caregivers of autologous bone marrow transplant recipients, caregivers reported continued caretaking responsibilities one to six years following transplantation, which included physical, emotional, and monitoring care of the survivor in addition to the caregiver's work and childcare responsibilities (Boyle et al., 2000). These caregivers reported a continued need for support for themselves but found that the availability of support decreased over time. In this same study, when caregivers' expectations of the survivor's "return to normal" were not met, frustration and emotional distress increased. Caregivers found that the end of treatment brought anxiety as well as relief. The survivors were physically and emotionally weakened, and the caregivers often were not prepared for the continued need for assistance, which left the caregivers overwhelmed and stressed. Research shows that spouses of cancer survivors continued to experience intrusive thoughts 18 months after treatment (Baider, Koch, Esacson, & De-Nour, 1998). Distress in this group was higher for the spouses than for the survivors.

Some caregivers have expressed concern about being the sole provider for the family. Researchers have reported that disability among cancer survivors is common, with nearly 16.8% of working-age cancer survivors reporting an inability to work (Hewitt, Rowland, & Yancik, 2003). This created added strain on the caregiver. Some caregivers felt trapped in their current job because of the need for continued insurance benefits. Others purposefully took different jobs to get better or supplemental insurance coverage (Hewitt et al., 2003; National Cancer Institute, 2003).

In summary, a cancer illness during middle adulthood threatens the middle adult's sexual relationships and self-esteem, as well as the ability to achieve personal goals and financial security. Caregivers continue to care for patients' physical and emotional needs into survivorship. Intrusive thoughts about cancer often continue following the completion of treatment, leading to higher stress levels in caregivers. The inability to reach personal goals and establish financial stability was a source of personal disappointment to couples in this age group. Research has found that the social and economic consequences related to lost wages coupled with increasing expenses of treatment can result in depression and anxiety (Mor et al., 1994). A cancer illness during this developmental phase can have significant financial consequences and threats to self-esteem. Anger, frustration, and depression can result from forced early retirement (see Table 29-1).

Young-Old (Ages 60–74)

The second phase of aging begins with retirement and includes establishing new life goals for the remainder of life (Baltrusch et al., 1988). Adults in this stage face mortality issues, and they must come to terms with their life as it was, as it is, and with what remains. Reminiscing takes place as people review their life to make sense of it, to enable them to accept their current life, and to prepare them to focus on the present and future. While purpose and personal growth may decrease with age, environmental mastery and positive relations tend to increase with age (Ryff, 1995). Some aspects of perceived control decline, such as control over children or physical functioning, whereas others, such as marital satisfaction, increase in later adulthood. A perceived lack of control has been associated with increased stress and poor immune system functioning (Lachman, 2001). Although fewer critical events occur in late adulthood, those that do are associated with greater stress (Baltrusch et al., 1988).

In their mid-60s and early 70s, most adults have entered retirement and a transitional status. They may review the past successes and failures of their life as they adjust to new roles. Many view retirement as a welcome relief from the day-to-day stress of the work environment. However, for others, retirement is a stressor that challenges self-esteem and causes feelings of uselessness and depression because of the lack of a job, a lack of a defined role, and decreased income (Newman & Newman, 1999). Changes in social interactions can lead to loneliness. While many adults in this stage of life continue to experience good health, concurrently they are beginning to experience the physical changes related to aging and the development of comorbid conditions. Couples in this life stage often look forward to fulfilling their dreams for retirement and quality time together. A cancer diagnosis disrupts plans for the idyllic retirement. Fears about becoming dependent and having to ask for help further threaten self-esteem. Fear of being left alone can create anxiety for the spouse.

In a large study of cancer survivors (N = 123) and their families (N = 246) (mean age of 65 years), families continued up to six years after treatment to express concern about the survivor dealing with long-term effects of treatment (Mellon, 2002). Families found that the treatment severely debilitated the survivor. Treatment was harsh, and the survivor had no internal resources left to manage the long lasting side effects. Recovery was a slow process that many survivors had not anticipated. Adult children were a source of support for survivors in this age group (Mellon, 2002). Research in couples living with prostate cancer found that treatment and side effects caused interruptions in their life (Harden et al., 2002). Plans for travel during retirement were disrupted or put on hold. Worry about recurrence was constant for many; others expressed a decreased sense of future security (Harden et al., 2006). Cancer survivors who were women were more likely than men to have unmet needs related to financial issues, whereas prostate cancer survivors were more likely to express concerns related to physical problems and personal control, especially related to inability to control urine and lack of sexual function (Burg et al., 2015).

Nijboer et al. (2000) found that older caregivers (older than 65 years) experienced caregiving as less negative over time because it caused less disruption to their schedule. However, a study by Northouse, Mood, Templin, Mellon, and George (2000) of a colon cancer population (mean age of 61 years) found that spouses reported more emotional distress than their partners. Furthermore, spousal caregivers experiencing negative role adjustments directly affected patient role adjustment.

Some research indicates that couples in the young-old group felt this life stage was a "good age" to be able to manage a cancer illness (Harden et al., 2006). Retirement meant they could come and go as needed for treatment and could rest if they wanted. Additionally, couples felt satisfied with the things they had accomplished in life. Accommodation of preferences most common in middle and late adulthood may account for high life satisfaction reported by older adults in the face of adverse living circumstances (Schmutte & Ryff, 1997). Furthermore, research showed that patients in this age group had better mental quality of life, higher self-efficacy, and less negative appraisal of illness than patients who were younger or older (Harden et al., 2008).

In summary, a cancer illness during the young-old developmental phase may have less psychological impact related to feelings of accomplishment for the completion of life tasks and less disruption of schedules. Debilitating treatment effects may result in changes in socialization and feelings of loneliness for patients and caregivers. Fear of being left alone may increase caregiver anxiety, resulting in disrupted rest patterns. A cancer illness during this developmental phase may have less negative psychological effect on the patient but cause higher levels of caregiver distress (see Table 29-1).

Old-Old (Age 75 and Older)

Recognizing that the span of years in late adulthood is varied, researchers have begun to explore differences within this older age group, proposing that old age is not one but several phases (Smith, 2001). Biogenetic, health, and personal life factors create differences within this age span. Baltes (1998) referred to a "fourth age" and defined it as beginning at the chronologic age where 50% of the person's birth cohort has died. At this point, biologic factors are predominant in the aging process. Within the life span, the fourth age is a phase that creates a great demand on individuals' ability to respond to changes in their health. As a person ages, the time needed for adaptation or recovery increases. Baltrusch et al. (1988) also referred to the age beginning at about 75 years and lasting until death as a separate phase of aging. During this period, the adult loses a certain amount of independence and autonomy. Individuals in this phase often experience many physical, social, psychological, and economic changes.

Studies of aging and illness report that older individuals are increasingly vulnerable to illness and are correspondingly less able to recover (Keller, Leventhal, Prohaska, & Leventhal, 1989). These beliefs may result in tendencies by older adults to minimize the degree of threat and avoid seeking information about disease either because they are fearful of the outcome or because they believe these conditions are inevitable and must be accepted as part of life. Studies have shown that older survivors report fewer unmet needs, which may be related to the tendency to minimize the effects of illness or the tendency to focus on non–cancer-related problems (Burg et al., 2015). Confusing symptoms of aging with symptoms of illness can cause older adults to view their symptoms as a natural consequence of aging and, therefore, to discount symptoms. Many older adults accept physical decline as part of the aging process and actually expect to feel some degree of ill health as normal (Keller, Leventhal, & Larson, 1989; Luggen, 1998; Rowland & Bellizzi, 2014). This often leads to a delay in seeking treatment.

As couples move into the mid-70s and beyond, they begin to experience a greater decline in physical abilities, resulting in increased susceptibility to illness, greater difficulty in managing complex medical regimens or medication schedules, and less adaptability to unfamiliar environments and treatment (Rowland, 1990). Challenges related to dealing with chronic illness and impairments in physical, sensory, and cognitive function have a pervasive impact on managing daily routines. As people age, their ability to adapt to declining health may reach a critical limit. How a person manages an illness may depend on his or her ability to compensate for changes related to both cancer and old age (Esbensen, Swane, Hallberg, & Thomé, 2008). A recent study showed a strong reciprocal relationship between functional limitations and quality of life in patients with cancer aged 75 years and older (Hamama-Raz, Shrira, Ben-Ezra, & Palgi, 2015). The main finding was that the oldest patients with low quality of life were at the highest risk of a decline in functional status. Functional status represents the ability to accomplish essential functions of daily life. Healthcare providers need to be especially vigilant with older patients because of this relationship and the ramifications it can have on tolerance to cancer therapy. Furthermore, receiving help from their adult children has been associated with lower quality of life (Esbensen, Thomé, & Thomsen, 2012). Although the help is appreciated, this reversal in roles from providing help to the adult children to receiving help often is associated with functional decline, which has a negative effect on quality of life (Esbensen et al., 2012; Harden et al., 2006).

In addition, social contact often is decreased in the old-old group because of decreased mobility and the death of family and friends, which can lead to loneliness. The strain of dealing with the effects of chronic illness, age-related frailty, functional impairment, and social losses can stress older adults. The mobility patterns common in American society increase the likelihood that adult children live a distance from the aging person and therefore are unable to provide support on an ongoing basis (Boyle & Engelking, 1993).

Researchers have demonstrated that age affects a person's perception of illness (Keller, Leventhal, Prohaska, et al., 1989; Steverink, Westerhof, Bode, & Dittman-Kohli, 2001). Older adults are less likely than middle-aged adults to express emotion related to illness. Longevity appears to prepare older adults for loss and disappointment in later life. Deimling, Kahana, Bowman, and Schaefer (2002) found that increasing age had a protective effect on psychological distress related to a cancer diagnosis. They postulated that people at age 80 were less concerned with the likelihood of recurrence and consequently less distressed. Research has demonstrated that older people tend to be health optimists, having more favorable health perceptions than objective physical data can support (Berg & Upchurch, 2007; Kutner et al., 1992). Because of these perceptions, older people tend to use different reference points to rate their overall feelings of health and health-related satisfaction. These attitudes by older adults have affected researchers' ability to detect the effects of illness on the quality of life in the older population.

Quality-of-life studies in patients with newly diagnosed cancer found that older adults reported better quality of life in all scales tested (Kutner et al., 1992). They viewed their health as good in the presence of overt pathology. Earlier research by Mor et al. (1994) found that older patients with cancer exhibited fewer and less severe psychosocial problems than younger patients with cancer. Older patients were more physically compromised than younger patients, perhaps related to comorbid conditions; however, social disruption related to needing assistance and adhering to intensive treatment protocols and burden on caregivers was less prevalent and less intense in older patients. The passage of time may mitigate the negative effect of cancer on patients and their families. As people age, the fear of recurrence may represent less of a threat than it does for a younger family.

When the patient experiences a reduction in energy level and difficulty in bending, lifting, and walking that restricts activities of daily living and instrumental activities of daily living related to treatment, the partner is the first to take an active part in compensating for the shortcomings in an effort to maintain life as it was before treatment (Jakobsson, Hallberg, & Lovén, 1997). Couples in a long-standing relationship rely on each other to meet daily challenges and maintain independence. Care of an ill or disabled spouse is a role frequently taken on in old age. Some spouses find this role fulfilling, whereas others find it stressful. Spouses report a sense of responsibility by virtue of marriage to fulfill this role.

Cancer prevalence increases with age, with people older than age 65 accounting for 60% of newly diagnosed cases and 70% of cancer deaths (Berger et al., 2006), yet research in older adults is limited and often excludes patients older than age 70 (Johnson, 2011). Effects of cancer treatment in older adults can vary widely, yet it would be erroneous to assume that a cancer diagnosis in older adults will not evoke a range of feelings similar to those experienced by a younger person (Kane, 1991). Healthcare providers need to consider the health literacy of older patients in communications and printed materials, as older patients tend to have lower health literacy, which may have an effect on their interactions with providers (Johnson, 2011). Much research is still needed to understand how age is related to psychological health and recovery in this age group.

In summary, a cancer illness during the old-old developmental phase may have fewer negative effects on patients. As people age, they often use different reference points related to overall feelings of health and expect the development of comorbidities as part of the aging process. Consequently, they are less concerned about recurrence, resulting in less psychological distress. However, the treatment for cancer is more difficult to manage, recovery is slower as a result of weakened physical and psychological reserves, and fatigue is a factor that affects both social relationships and engagement in pleasurable activities. Because of their advanced age and the responsibilities of caregiving, old-old spousal caregivers are at risk for immediate and long-term negative effects on their physical and psychological health (see Table 29-1).

Conclusion

Patients with cancer and their families face many disease-related stressors in addition to other stressors that are part of the developmental life cycle. These age-related stressors exist concurrently and can affect a family's ability to adjust to illness. Information about the time at which cancer occurs and the treatment consequences that interfere with or threaten developmental tasks enables understanding of the psychological and quality-of-life issues that may develop during the diagnosis, treatment, recovery, and survivorship periods. Understanding the developmental life stage at which cancer occurs can help healthcare providers identify needs specific to the patient and the family at the time of care.

Key Points

- A life-span perspective suggests that adults experience changes across their life span that requires them to adjust their individual beliefs about themselves and their world.
- Adults use adaptive strategies to minimize physical, psychological, and social changes that develop in mid-life and older age.
- Cancer is a major life stressor that can disrupt the lifestyles and routines of all involved.
- A cancer illness during young adulthood can dramatically affect individuals' ability to form and sustain close relationships, achieve career goals, and maintain independence, resulting in feelings of vulnerability and insecurity about their future that can interfere with the establishment of relationships.
- Young adults who are childless at the time of a cancer diagnosis need to discuss the topic of infertility with their healthcare providers to diminish their distress.
- Middle-aged adults aged 55–65 years report poorer quality of life than older adults and are more likely to report unmet needs related to emotional and family problems.
- Symptom burden in middle-aged adults can lead to feelings of loss of dignity associated with feelings of hopelessness and even a desire to hasten death, making interventions designed to counter these feelings of worthlessness important.
- A cancer illness during the young-old developmental phase (ages 60–74) may have less psychological impact related to feelings of accomplishment for completion of life tasks, but debilitating treatment effects may result in changes in socialization and feelings of loneliness for patients and caregivers.
- The oldest patients (age 75 years and older) who have low quality of life are at the highest risk for decline in functional status related to weakened physical and psychological reserves and fatigue.
- Because cancer affects people in various developmental life stages, understanding the life stage at which cancer occurs can help healthcare providers identify needs specific to the patient and the family at the time of care.

References

Arber, S., & Evandrou, M. (1993). Mapping the territory. In S. Arber & M. Evandrou (Eds.), *Ageing, independence and the life course* (pp. 9–26). Bristol, PA: Jessica Kingsley Publishers.

Baider, L., Koch, U., Esacson, R., & De-Nour, A.K. (1998). Prospective study of cancer patients and their spouses: The weakness of marital strength. *Psycho-Oncology, 7,* 49–56. doi:10.1002/(SICI)1099-1611(199801/02)7:1<49::AID-PON312>3.0.CO;2-Z

Baltes, M.M. (1998). The psychology of the oldest-old: The fourth age. *Current Opinion in Psychiatry, 11,* 411–415. doi:10.1097/00001504-199807000-00009

Baltes, P.B. (1987). Theoretical propositions of life-span developmental psychology: On the dynamics between growth and decline. *Developmental Psychology, 23,* 611–626. doi:10.1037/0012-1649.23.5.611

Baltes, P.B. (1997). On incomplete architecture of human ontogeny: Selection, optimization, and compensation as foundation of developmental theory. *American Psychologist, 54,* 366–380. doi:10.1037/0003-066X.52.4.366

Baltrusch, H.F., Seidel, J., Stangel, W., & Waltz, M.E. (1988). Psychosocial stress, aging, and cancer. *Annals of the New York Academy of Sciences, 521,* 1–15. doi:10.1111/j.1749-6632.1988.tb35261.x

Bellizzi, K.M., Smith, A.S., Schmidt, S., Keegan, T.H.M., Zebrack, B., Lynch, C.F., ... Simon, M. (2012). Positive and negative psychosocial impact of being diagnosed with cancer as an adolescent or young adult. *Cancer, 118,* 5155–5162. doi:10.1002/cncr.27512

Berg, C.A., & Upchurch, R. (2007). A developmental-contextual model of couples coping with chronic illness across the adult life span. *Psychological Bulletin, 133,* 920–954. doi:10.1037/0033-2909.133.6.920

Berger, N.A., Savvides, P., Koroukian, S.M., Kahana, E.F., Deimling, G.T., Rose, J.H. ... Miller, R.H. (2006). Cancer in the elderly. *Transactions of the American Clinical and Climatological Association, 117,* 147–156.

Boyle, D.M., Blodgett, L., Gnesdiloff, S., White, J., Bamford, A.M., Sheridan, M., & Beveridge, R. (2000). Caregiver quality of life after autologous bone marrow transplantation. *Cancer Nursing, 23,* 193–203. doi:10.1097/00002820-200006000-00006

Boyle, D.M., & Engelking, C. (1993). Cancer in the elderly: The forgotten priority. *European Journal of Cancer Care, 2,* 101–107. doi:10.1111/j.1365-2354.1993.tb00176.x

Brandtstädter, J., & Renner, G. (1990). Tenacious goal pursuit and flexible goal adjustment: Explication and age-related analysis of assimilative and accommodative strategies of coping. *Psychology and Aging, 5,* 58–67. doi:10.1037/0882-7974.5.1.58

Burg, M.A., Adorno, G., Lopez, E.D.S., Loerzel, V., Stein, K., Wallace, C., & Sharma, D.K.B. (2015). Current unmet needs of cancer survivors: Analysis of open-ended responses to the American Cancer Society Study of Cancer Survivors II. *Cancer, 121,* 623–630. doi:10.1002/cncr.28951

Carmichael, C.L., Reis, H.T., & Duberstein, P.R. (2015). In your 20s it's quantity, in your 30s it's quality: The prognostic value of social activity across 30 years of adulthood. *Psychology and Aging, 30,* 95–105. doi:10.1037/pag0000014

Charles, S.T., Luong, G., Almeida, D.M., Ryff, C., Sturm, M., & Love, G. (2010). Fewer ups and downs: Daily stressors mediate age differences in negative affect. *Journal of Gerontology: Psychological Sciences, 65B,* 279–286. doi:10.1093/geronb/gbq002

Costanzo, E.S., Ryff, C.D., & Singer, B.H. (2009). Psychosocial adjustment among cancer survivors: Findings from a national survey of health and well-being. *Health Psychology, 28,* 147–156. doi:10.1037/a0013221

D'Agostino, N.M., Penney, A., & Zebrack, B. (2011). Providing developmentally appropriate psychosocial care to adolescent and young adult cancer survivors. *Cancer, 117,* 2329–2334. doi:10.1002/cncr.26043

Deimling, G.T., Kahana, B., Bowman, K.F., & Schaefer, M.L. (2002). Cancer survivorship and psychological distress in later life. *Psycho-Oncology, 11,* 479–494. doi:10.1002/pon.614

Devins, G.M. (1993). Psychosocial impact of illness from a developmental-systems perspective: New directions for health psychology. *Canadian Journal of Behavioural Science, 25,* 329–331. doi:10.1037/h0084918

Downing, A., Morris, E.J.A., Richards, M., Corner, J., Wright, P., Sebag-Montefiore, D., ... Glasser, A.W. (2015). Health-related quality of life after colorectal cancer in England: A patient-reported outcomes study of individuals 12 to 36 months after diagnosis. *Journal of Clinical Oncology, 33,* 616–624. doi:10.1200/JCO.2014.56.6539

Ebner, N.C., Freund, A.M., & Baltes, P.B. (2006). Developmental changes in personal goal orientation from young to late adulthood: From striving for gains to maintenance and prevention of losses. *Psychology and Aging, 21,* 664–678. doi:10.1037/0882-7974.21.4.664

Erikson, E.H. (1963). *Childhood and society.* New York, NY: W.W. Norton.

Esbensen, B.A., Swane, C.E., Hallberg, I., & Thomé, B. (2008). Being given a cancer diagnosis in old age: A phenomenological study. *International Journal of Nursing Studies, 45,* 393–405. doi:10.1016/j.ijnurstu.2006.09.004

Esbensen, B.A., Thomé, B., & Thomsen, T. (2012). Dependency in elderly people newly diagnosed with cancer – A mixed method study. *European Journal of Oncology Nursing, 16,* 137–144. doi:10.1016/j.ejon.2011.04.011

Friedman, E.M., & Ryff, C.D. (2012). Living well with medical comorbidities: A biopsychosocial perspective. *Journals of Gerontology, Series B: Psychological Sciences and Social Science, 67,* 535–544. doi:10.1093/geronb/gbr152

Hamama-Raz, Y., Shrira, A., Ben-Ezra, M., & Palgi, Y. (2015). The recursive effects of quality of life and functional limitation among older adult cancer patients: Evidence from the Survey of Health, Ageing and Retirement in Europe. *European Journal of Cancer Care, 24,* 205–212. doi:10.1111/ecc.12300

Harden, J.K., Northouse, L.L., Cimprich, B., Pohl, J.M., Liang, J., & Kershaw, T. (2008). The influence of developmental life stage on quality of life in survivors of prostate cancer and their partners. *Journal of Cancer Survivorship, 2,* 84–94. doi:10.1007/s11764-008-0048-z

Harden, J.K., Northouse, L.L., & Mood, D.W. (2006). Qualitative analysis of couples' experience with prostate cancer by age cohort. *Cancer Nursing, 29,* 367–377. doi:10.1097/00002820-200609000-00004

Harden, J.K., Schafenacker, A., Northouse, L.L., Mood, D., Smith, D., Pienta, K., ... Baranowski, K. (2002). Couples' experiences with prostate cancer: Focus group research. *Oncology Nursing Forum, 29,* 701–709. doi:10.1188/02.ONF.701-709

Hewitt, M., Rowland, J.H., & Yancik, R. (2003). Cancer survivors in the United States: Age, health, and disability. *Journal of Gerontology: Series A: Biological Sciences and Medical Sciences, 58,* 82–91. doi:10.1093/gerona/58.1.m82

Jakobsson, L., Hallberg, I.R., & Lovén, L. (1997). Experiences of daily life and life quality in men with prostate cancer: An explorative study. Part I. *European Journal of Cancer Care, 6,* 108–116. doi:10.1046/j.1365-2354.1997.00019.x

Johnson, M. (2011). Chemotherapy treatment decision making by professionals and older patients with cancer: A narrative review of the literature. *European Journal of Cancer Care, 21,* 3–9. doi:10.1111/j.1365-2354.2011.01294.x

Kane, R.A. (1991). Psychosocial issues: Psychological and social issues for older people with cancer. *Cancer, 68*(Suppl. 11), 2514–2518. doi:10.1002/1097-0142(19911201)68:11+<2514::AID-CNCR2820681506>3.0.CO;2-D

Keller, M.L., Leventhal, E.A., & Larson, B.A. (1989). Aging: The lived experience. *International Journal of Aging and Human Development, 29*(1), 67–82. doi:10.2190/DEQQ-AAUV-NBU0-3RMY

Keller, M.L., Leventhal, H., Prohaska, T.R., & Leventhal, E.A. (1989). Beliefs about aging and illness in a community sample. *Research in Nursing and Health, 12,* 247–255. doi:10.1002/nur.4770120407

Kelly, D. (2004). Patients with colorectal cancer expressed a loss of adulthood related to a loss of professional and sexual identity, dignity, privacy, independence, and ability to socialise. *Evidence-Based Nursing, 7,* 126.

Kent, E., Arora, N.K., Rowland, J.H., Bellizzi, K.M., Forsythe, L.P., Hamilton, A.S., ...Aziz, N.M. (2012). Health information needs and health-related quality of life in a diverse population of long-term cancer survivors. *Patient Education and Counseling, 89,* 345–352. doi:10.1016/j.pec.2012.08.014

Kurtz, M., Given, G.W., Given, B.A., & Kurtz, J.C. (1994). The interaction of age, symptoms, and survival status on physical and mental health of patients with cancer and their families. *Cancer, 74*(Suppl. 7), 2071–2078. doi:10.1002/1097-0142(19941001)74:7+<2071::AID-CNCR2820741715>3.0.CO;2-R

Kutner, N., Ory, M., Baker, D., Schechtman, K., Hornbrook, M., & Mulrow, C. (1992). Measuring the quality of life of the elderly in health promotion interventions clinical trials. *Public Health Reports, 107,* 530–538.

Lachman, M.E. (2001). Psychology of adult development. In N.J. Smelser & P.B. Baltes (Eds.), *International encyclopedia of the social and behavioral sciences* (pp. 135–139). doi:10.1016/b0-08-043076-7/01650-8

Levinson, D.J. (1986). A conception of adult development. *American Psychologist, 41,* 3–13. doi:10.1037/0003-066X.41.1.3

Luggen, A.S. (1998). Chronic pain in older adults: A quality of life issue. *Journal of Gerontological Nursing, 24*(2), 48–54. doi:10.3928/0098-9134-19980201-13

Mellon, S. (2002). Comparisons between cancer survivors and family members on meaning of the illness and family quality of life. *Oncology Nursing Forum, 29,* 1117–1125. doi:10.1188/02.ONF.1117-1125

Monforte-Royo, C., Villavicencio-Chávez, C., Tomás-Sábado, J., & Balaguer, A. (2011). The wish to hasten death: A review of clinical studies. *Psycho-Oncology, 20,* 795–804. doi:10.1002/pon.1839

Monteiro, S., Torres, A., Morgadinho, R., & Pereira, A. (2013). Psychosocial outcomes in young adults with cancer: Emotional distress, quality of life and personal growth. *Archives of Psychiatric Nursing, 27,* 299–305. doi:10.1016/j.apnu.2013.08.003

Mor, V., Allen, S., & Malin, M. (1994). The psychosocial impact of cancer on older versus younger patients and their families. *Cancer, 74*(Suppl. 7), 2118–2127. doi:10.1002/1097-0142(19941001)74:7+<2118::AID-CNCR2820741720>3.0.CO;2-N

Morrow, P.K., Broxson, A.C., Munsell, M.F., Basen-Enquist, K., Rosenblum, C.K., Schover, L.R., ... Hortobagyi, G.N. (2014). Effect of age and race on quality of life in young breast cancer survivors. *Clinical Breast Cancer, 14,* e21–e31. doi:10.1016/j.clbc.2013.10.003

National Cancer Institute. (2003). *After cancer treatment ends—The impact on caregivers and families.* Bethesda, MD: Author.

Newman, B., & Newman, P. (1999). *Development through life: A psychosocial approach* (7th ed.). Belmont, CA: Wadsworth.

Nijboer, C., Triemstra, M., Tempelaar, R., Mulder, M., Sanderman, R., & van den Bos, G.A.M. (2000). Patterns of caregiving experiences among partners of cancer patients. *Gerontologist, 40,* 738–746. doi:10.1093/geront/40.6.738

Nishigaki, M., Oya, M., Ueno, M., Arai, M., Yamaguchi, T., Muto, T., & Kazuma, K. (2007). The influence of life stage on psychosocial adjustment in colorectal cancer patients. *Journal of Psychosocial Oncology, 25,* 71–87. doi:10.1300/J077v25n04_05

Northouse, L.L., Mood, D., Templin, T., Mellon, S., & George, T. (2000). Couples' patterns of adjustment to colon cancer. *Social Science and Medicine, 50,* 271–284. doi:10.1016/S0277-9536(99)00281-6

Orth, U., Maes, J., & Schmitt, M. (2015). Self-esteem development across the life span: A longitudinal study with a large sample from Germany. *Developmental Psychology, 51,* 248–259. doi:10.1037/a0038481

Parry, C., Lomax, J.B., Morningstar, E.A., & Fairclough, D.L. (2012). Identification and correlates of unmet service needs in adult leukemia and lymphoma survivors after treatment. *Journal of Oncology Practice, 8,* e135–e141. doi:10.1200/JOP.2011.000464

Rothermund, K., & Brandstädter, J. (2003). Coping with deficits and losses in later life: From compensatory action to accommodation. *Psychology and Aging, 18,* 896–905. doi:10.1037/0882-7974.18.4.896

Rowland, J. (1990). Developmental states and adaptation: Adult model. In J.C. Holland & J.H. Rowland (Eds.), *Handbook of psychooncology: Psychological care of the patient with cancer* (pp. 25–43). New York, NY: Oxford University Press.

Rowland, J.H., & Bellizzi, K.M. (2014). Cancer survivorship issues: Life after treatment and implications for an aging population. *Journal of Clinical Oncology, 32,* 2662–2668. doi:10.1200/JCO.2014.55.8361

Rustoen, T., Moum, T., Wiklund, I., & Hanestad, B.R. (1999). Quality of life in newly diagnosed cancer patients. *Journal of Advanced Nursing, 29,* 490–498. doi:10.1046/j.1365-2648.1999.00912.x

Ryff, C.D. (1995). Psychological well-being in adult life. *Current Directions in Psychological Science, 4,* 99–104. doi:10.1111/1467-8721.ep10772395

Schmutte, P.S., & Ryff, C.D. (1997). Personality and well-being: Reexamining methods and meanings. *Journal of Personality and Social Psychology, 73,* 549–559. doi:10.1037/0022-3514.73.3.549

Schover, L.R., Brey, K., Lichtin, A., Lipshultz, L.I., & Jeha, S. (2002). Knowledge and experience regarding cancer, infertility, and sperm banking in younger male survivors. *Journal of Clinical Oncology, 20,* 1880–1889. doi:10.1200/JCO.2002.07.175

Schover, L.R., Rybicki, L.A., Martin, B.A., & Bringelsen, K.A. (1999). Having children after cancer: A pilot survey of survivors' attitudes and experiences. *Cancer, 86,* 697–709. doi:10.1002/(SICI)1097-0142(19990815)86:4<697::AID-CNCR20>3.0.CO;2-J

Smith, A.W., Bellizzi, K.M., Keegan, T.H.M., Zebrack, B., Chen, V.W., Neale, A.V., ... Lynch, C.F. (2013). Health-related quality of life of adolescent and young adult patients with cancer in the United States: The adolescent and young adult health outcomes and patient experience study. *Journal of Clinical Oncology, 31,* 2136–2145. doi:10.1200/JCO.2012.47.3173

Smith, J. (2001). Old age and centenarians. In N.J. Smelser & P.B. Baltes (Eds.), *International encyclopedia of the social and behavioral sciences* (pp. 10843–10847). doi:10.1016/b0-08-043076-7/01705-8

Steverink, N., Westerhof, G., Bode, C., & Dittmann-Kohli, F. (2001). The personal experience of aging, individual resources, and subjective well-being. *Journal of Gerontology: Series B: Psychological Sciences and Social Sciences. 56,* P364–P373. doi:10.1093/geronb/56.6.P364

Takahashi, M. (2014). Psychosocial distress among young breast cancer survivors: Implications for healthcare providers. *Breast Cancer, 21,* 664–669. doi:10.1007/s12282-013-0508-9

Vehling, S., & Mehnert, A. (2014). Symptom burden, loss of dignity, and demoralization in patients with cancer: A mediation model. *Psycho-Oncology, 23,* 283–290. doi:10.1002/pon.3417

Vinokur, A.D., Threatt, B.A., Vinokur-Kaplan, D., & Satariano, W.A. (1990). The process of recovery from breast cancer for younger and older patients: Changes during the first year. *Cancer, 65,* 1242–1254. doi:10.1002/1097-0142(19900301)65:5<1242::AID-CNCR2820650535>3.0.CO;2-1

Williams, K.A. (2013). Adolescent and young adult oncology: An emerging subspecialty. *Clinical Journal of Oncology Nursing, 17,* 292–296. doi:10.1188/13.CJON.292-296

Woods, N.F., & Lewis, F.M. (1995). Women with chronic illness: Their views of their families' adaptations. *Health Care for Women International, 16,* 135–148. doi:10.1080/07399339509516165

Chapter 29 Study Questions

1. Having few daily stressors and less negative effect resulting from a cancer diagnosis is most common in which of the following age groups?
   A. Early adulthood
   B. Middle adulthood
   C. Young-old
   D. Old-old

2. Healthcare providers need to be vigilant for symptoms of depression in all patients with cancer, but in which of the following age groups is it more likely?
   A. Early adulthood
   B. Middle adulthood
   C. Young-old
   D. Old-old

3. Young adults who have a cancer diagnosis have expressed which of the following? *(choose all that apply)*
   A. Closer relationships with family as a result of the cancer diagnosis and treatment
   B. Fear of being left alone
   C. Decline in physical abilities
   D. Concerns about infertility and future childbearing

4. Adapting to the challenges of a cancer diagnosis is most difficult for which of the following age groups?
   A. Early adulthood
   B. Middle adulthood
   C. Young-old
   D. Old-old

5. A cancer illness during middle adulthood primarily has which of the following effects?
   A. Threats to ability to form close relationships, achieve career goals, and maintain independence
   B. Few negative effects such as psychosocial distress related to cancer treatment and recurence
   C. Threats to achievement of personal goals, financial security, and self-esteem
   D. Changes in socialization and unfulfilled dreams

CHAPTER

30 Ethical Issues

Teresa A. Savage, PhD, RN, and Lisa Anderson-Shaw, DrPH, MA, MSN

Introduction

Ethics, bioethics, clinical ethics, medical ethics, nursing ethics, morality—numerous terms are used to describe the foundation of decision making in the healthcare arena. Although all the terms listed can be used to describe the same process, this chapter will use the term *bioethics*. Bioethics is defined as "the ethical issues in health and the delivery of health care" (Bosek & Savage, 2007, p. 446). Nursing has always had at its very core the desire to help maintain health, improve health, or alleviate the suffering of human beings. This obligation to help also may be seen as the obligation to do good (i.e., beneficence).

However, in nurses' attempts to do good, advances in technology and pharmacology also make it possible for them to do harm to their patients. How, then, do clinicians make decisions or help their patients make informed choices about their own health care that take into account the benefits and burdens of treatment options to arrive at the "right" decision?

Many theories and models of decision making in bioethics can assist providers and patients when faced with difficult decisions with no clear-cut answer. One frequently used approach is the application of specific principles to the specific situation. These principles include **autonomy**—the ability of an individual to make decisions consistent with his or her values; **beneficence**—the idea that treatments and providers should act in ways that are of benefit; **nonmaleficence**—to act in a way to minimize or avoid harm; and **justice**—which can take many forms but usually means that the just allocation of healthcare resources is based on need and the expected outcome (Beauchamp & Childress, 2013). For example, based on the just allocation of resources, aggressive lifesaving care might not be justified for a patient with end-stage cancer who is already in the dying process.

Another decision-making approach is looking at the overall utility of a treatment for a patient. If the outcome of a specific treatment is thought to be of benefit to the patient, the treatment has utility; if it is not thought to be of help or benefit, it does not have utility and therefore should not be applied. Patients or family members sometimes insist on treatment that may not offer any benefit and may be causing significant morbidity, but they do not want to "give up" on the quest for a cure.

A third bioethics analytical approach that often is used is called the *four topics analysis*. This method sorts key elements of a specific case into four topics: medical indications, patient preferences, quality of life, and contextual features. The medical indications and patient preferences are the most important factors, but considerations of quality of life from the patient's perspective and other contextual features enter into the process as well (Jonsen, Siegler, & Winslade, 2015). Many other theories, tools, and approaches are available to help healthcare providers with difficult situations, and these come from various disciplines, such as philosophy, theology, literature, and psychology (see Table 30-1). It is important to remember that whatever tools or processes are used, the task is "to foster a range of ethical skills and sensitivities, and . . . to deepen understanding of the context of ethical decision making" in the clinical context (McCarthy, 2006, p. 164).

Table 30-1. Approaches to Decision Making

Approach	Primary Elements
Principles of biomedical ethics (principlism) (Beauchamp & Childress, 2013)	Autonomy, beneficence, nonmaleficence, and justice
Utilitarian/consequence-based	Greatest good for the greatest number Balance of good and bad outcomes
Four-box/four topics (Jonsen et al., 2015)	Medical indications, patient preferences, quality of life, and contextual features
Kantian theory/obligation-based (deontology)	Rule-based Actions are more important than outcomes
Liberal individualism/rights-based	The legitimate role of government involvement or noninvolvement based on individual rights
Communitarian/community-based	Fundamental ethics come from the community members—common good, communal values, traditions, and social goods
Care ethics	Preservation of relationships; relief of burden; self-sacrifice

Nurses' Role

Nurses, in general, take care of and are with people often at their most vulnerable times, when they are sick, healing, disrupted, and dying. They interact not only with patients but also with their family, friends, and loved ones. In doing so, nurses learn much about patients' lives, problems, treatments, healthcare decisions, and maybe even how they wish to live and die.

In oncology, nurses provide care in a variety of settings, including acute care hospitals, clinics and outpatient areas, homes, emergency departments, and palliative care and hospice settings. Nurses practice at various levels of care, including advanced practice nursing. Because nurses are positioned in a role with patients and their families that often allows more time to get to know them more personally, nurses at all practice levels and settings have a unique ethical role in the care of patients with cancer. One very important role for oncology nurses at all levels is to educate patients and families and facilitate the use of advance directives for health care for all patients. This will be discussed in more depth later in the chapter, and the authors highly encourage using advance directives as a communication tool for difficult conversations. Patients often wait for the provider to raise the issue of advance care planning, yet in many cases, providers wait for patients to ask (Lum, Sudore, & Bekelman, 2015).

Oncology nurses have a great understanding of chemotherapy agents and various procedures and can be very helpful in educating patients and families about these treatments, including side effects, specific precautions, and follow-up needs. In addition, patients often feel comfortable with their nurses and may ask specific questions or seek additional information from them. In acute settings, it may be that the patient is trying to make a decision among treatment options and the nurse is able to identify the patient's educational needs. Or, the nurse may see a possible disconnect between what the patient and family are expecting from a specific treatment and what the treatment team believes will be the ultimate outcome. At some level, past experience with a specific cancer and treatment may lead nurses to recognize ideas of unrealistic expectations by patients or families. At that time, it might be helpful to ask for a meeting with the family and treatment team to review expectations. Perhaps a conflict exists between the patient's goals and treatment team's goals for the patient. In such cases, the nurse may feel caught in the middle. It often is helpful to deal with these issues early, as soon as they are identified. Discussions between the patient and treatment team are the first place to start. In any discussions, include key consultants, such as other medical specialties, psychology, social work, or ethics consultation.

Palliative care focuses on improving the quality of life of patients who have serious illnesses. Hospice is a type of palliative care that is provided at the end of life. In a hospice nursing role, the goal of treatment has changed from the eradication of disease to the alleviation of suffering. The nursing role may be very influential in planning and delivering end-of-life care. At times, the medical team, family, or patients may not be willing to forgo curative treatments for patients who are clearly in the dying process. This is a difficult situation, and the oncology nurse may be in the best position to advocate for changing the treatment goal from a more aggressive curative goal to an aggressive palliative care goal. Medicare and Medicaid now provide coverage for Medicare "beneficiaries with advanced cancers, chronic obstructive pulmonary disease, congestive heart failure and human immunodeficiency virus/acquired immunodeficiency syndrome (HIV/AIDS)" who may receive hospice and curative services at the same time (Centers for Medicare and Medicaid Services, 2016). For example, radiation treatments to shrink a mass had been considered strictly curative and were unavailable to someone in hospice. The change permits the patient and hospice team to consider a wider range of options for palliation. A family team meeting in these situations can be very valuable for patients, family members, and loved ones, as well as all levels of the oncology team (see Table 30-2).

Diagnosis—Truth-Telling, Prognosis, Treatment Options, and Hope

Is it ever permissible to lie to a patient? What happens if a patient asks a question that the nurse is not comfortable answering? What if the truth is very bad news, and the nurse does not want to tell the patient? Does telling the truth about a terminal diagnosis take away hope for the patient?

Table 30-2. The Nurse's Role in Advocating for Patients and Families

Patient and Family Needs	Nurse's Role
Lack of knowledge about cancer treatment	Educate about chemotherapy, radiation therapy, other treatments and procedures, possible side effects, precautions, and follow-up needs.
Lack of knowledge about advance directives	Provide information about the types of advance directives; facilitate communication to complete advance directives.
"Disconnect" between patient's expressed goals and treatment team's goals	Facilitate communication between key people (e.g., physician, patient, family member); coordinate team meeting; seek ethics consultation when needed.
Lack of knowledge about end-of-life care	Provide information on end-of-life care, palliative care, and hospice care; assist in planning and delivering end-of-life care.

Oncology nurses often face these questions in clinical practice. One of the most frequently reported ethical issues for oncology nurses is "uncertainties and barriers to truth telling" (McLennon, Uhrich, Lasiter, Chamness, & Helft, 2013, p. 114). Provision 1 of the American Nurses Association's Code of Ethics for Nurses states that "the nurse practices with compassion and respect for the inherent dignity, worth, and unique attributes of every person" (American Nurses Association, 2015, p. v). To fully respect a person's dignity and worth, nurses should never lie to their patients or their family members and loved ones. Individuals have a right to the truth about their health, their care, and their treatment options if they are to make truly autonomous and informed decisions. Patients may feel ambivalent about hearing the prognosis, so it is helpful to begin by asking patients what they know and what they want to know. This follows the principle of autonomy, which is based on a person's right to self-determination. The importance of care has to do with the cultivation of the relationship between the nurse and patient and, in doing so, respecting the patient's right to be told the diagnosis and prognosis.

Physicians often have difficulty in estimating survival in patients with cancer. Calling it the "surprise" question, Moss et al. (2010) offered this question as a way to focus on prognosis: "Would I be surprised if this patient died in the next year?" (p. 837). The answer is helpful in deciding when to discuss end-of-life care rather than aggressive curative treatment. Instruments such as the POLST (Physicians [or Practitioners] Orders for Life-Sustaining Treatment) are intended for use with people with life-limiting or chronic conditions or fragile health who are not expected to live another year and can be useful in broaching difficult conversations. POLST will be discussed in more detail later in the chapter.

Nurses report that they often feel "in the dark" about what patients have been told and what their prognosis is (McLennon et al., 2013, p. 119). Patients are referred for hospice in their last days of life, when, as nurses in this study believe, patients might have made different choices had they been told their prognosis sooner. When prognostic information is withheld, inaccurate, or incomprehensible to the patient, nurses want to intervene to ensure that patients get timely, accurate, understandable information. However, they feel constrained by the power differential in the hospital or cancer center hierarchy, in which it is the physician's responsibility to share the prognosis. Frequent team conferences would provide a forum for nurses to raise questions and support their physician colleagues in having the difficult conversations. Nurses and other members of the team could then move forward in helping patients and their families with advance care planning (McLennon et al., 2013).

Some cultural norms exist that view nondisclosure of a terminal illness as a way of protecting a person. Lying or not disclosing the truth is an infraction on the rights of the person or the person's surrogate decision maker, and the truth should always be disclosed. However, being culturally sensitive does not have to compromise this stand. When true cultural norms dictate that the treatment team withhold the truth of a clinical situation from a patient, the team and family should hold a thoughtful meeting to discuss and develop an action plan that is culturally sensitive but that does not infringe on the rights of the individual patient or the provider who feels ethically obligated to disclose specific information. The patient may refuse to hear the diagnosis, prognosis, and treatment options and designate someone else to make the decision.

Caregiver Burden, Moral Distress, and Impact on Treatment Decisions

Caring for patients with cancer can be very emotional for nurses, especially if the nurses have been caring for a patient over a long time and have built a relationship with the patient and family. Therefore, an ethical dilemma can arise when nurses are unable to provide the type of care that they believe is needed. For example, a patient is in the dying process and not able to make medical decisions, but the family wants to continue aggressive curative therapy. The nurse, in honoring the patient's stated wishes, may believe that forgoing curative treatment is the right thing to do, but the nurse feels powerless to change the situation. The stress of such situations can sometime be profound and may even progress into moral distress. Moral distress is defined as "the pain or anguish in response to a situation in which a nurse (a) recognizes an ethical problem, (b) realizes the professional obligation to take action to address that problem, and (c) considers the ethically correct action to take" but feels constrained to act (Rushton & Kurtz, 2015, p. 4). They go on to say that "moral courage . . . compels nurses to speak up and speak out about ethically problematic situations. Moral courage requires that nurses discern the boundaries of acceptable norms of practice that arise from their Code of Ethics and possess the ability to articulate alignments with and infractions of those norms" (Rushton & Kurtz, 2015, p. 17). Situations such as providing aggressive treatment for patients with terminal disease or inadequate pain and symptom control at the end of life significantly contribute to feelings of frustration and moral distress in nurses. Epstein and Hamric (2009) described a moral residue and a crescendo effect from repeated and inadequately resolved moral distress experiences. *Moral residue* is the uncomfortable feeling that lingers after a morally distressing situation has passed. It leads the nurse to feel distress earlier and more intensely in future situations. The growing moral residue has a *crescendo effect*, where the mounting moral distress and residue reach a critical point for the nurse. The University of Virginia instituted a Moral Distress Consult Service within their Ethics Consultation Service. In 2013, they averaged one consult per month (Boyle, 2013). Rushton and Kurtz (2015) described other strategies to identify and manage moral distress. They cited two tools to identify moral distress: the 4 A's to Rise Above Moral Distress, developed by the American Association of Critical-Care Nurses (n.d.), and the Moral Distress Thermometer, developed by Wocial and Weaver (2013). Rushton and Kurtz (2015) also provided individual and institutional building capacities to reduce moral distress. It is important for providers who work in oncology to take time to discuss stressful situations and events in a safe environment. Figure 30-1 lists some effects of and interventions for moral distress. Regular sessions with colleagues to discuss feelings and experiences might be helpful. Inviting a mental health professional or bioethics consultant to a session might help provide insight into the sources of stress and the identification of effective coping techniques. One tactic to avoid escalation of stressful situations is to conduct a case conference when a nurse is feeling moral distress. Case conferences should be multidisciplinary, including nurses, physicians, ethicists, clergy, social workers, and others involved in the care of a particular patient. It may be appropriate for the patient or the patient's surrogate decision maker to be involved in these meetings so that the treatment plan can be discussed and then implemented in such a way that gives true benefit to the patient and alleviates staff members' feelings of powerlessness or frustration.

Advance Care Planning

Advance Directives

The right to make one's healthcare decisions is based on the principle of respect for autonomy and is taken very seriously in Western healthcare settings. The principle of autonomy is exercised by the use of advance directives, which are devised in advance of illness and must be written when a person has the capacity to make informed decisions. Examples of written advance directives include living wills, durable power of attorney for health care, and uniform (i.e., portable from one setting to another) do-not-resuscitate orders. Both federal legislation, such as the Patient Self-Determination Act (PSDA) of 1990, and state statutes articulate the ways in which each state authorizes advance directives. The federal PSDA law applies to all healthcare institutions receiving Medicare and Medicaid funds and requires that all adults receiving medical care be given written information about their rights under the law to make decisions about their medical care, which includes the right to accept or refuse such care. In addition to state and federal laws, the Joint Commission has specific standards related to advance directives.

Figure 30-1. Effects of Moral Distress and Interventions to Reduce Moral Distress

Potential Provider Effects of Moral Distress

1. Feelings of lack of support from colleagues
2. Feelings of lack of support from administrators
3. Feelings of lack of support from the institution
4. Job dissatisfaction
5. Physical symptoms of stress

Interventions to Reduce Moral Distress

1. Recognize clinical situations that may cause provider moral distress.
2. Recognize in self and others when symptoms of moral distress are evident.
3. Hold multidisciplinary case conferences to discuss cases or situations that might be causing provider moral distress.
4. Provide opportunities for staff to interact with mental health counselors when stressful situations occur in the clinical areas.
5. Provide a safe clinical environment for providers to feel comfortable to discuss stressful situations.
6. Develop institutional policies that support providers with moral distress.

Key Points of Family/Team Meeting to Minimize Provider Moral Distress

1. Keep the patient and family informed of current health status and prognosis.
2. Ask the patient and family to discuss possible health outcomes and their goals.
3. Seek information about advance directives early in the treatment phase.
4. Offer emotional and spiritual support services, such as social work and pastoral care, to the patient and family throughout the treatment phase.
5. Be honest with the patient and family when they ask direct questions related to death and dying.

Note. Based on information from Cohen & Erickson, 2006; Ferrell, 2006; Sundin-Huard & Fahy, 1999; Zuzelo, 2007.

The most common forms of advance directives are living wills and healthcare power of attorney (see Table 30-3). The *living will* is a document that goes into effect when the person, in the opinion of the attending physician, has a terminal illness with a life expectancy of six months or less. The document allows the person to give specific written instructions about future medical treatments, such as mechanical ventilation, surgeries, or CPR. It can be limited in its effect by state law; for example, Illinois does not allow the withdrawal of nutrition and hydration if it would be the primary cause of death (Illinois Living Will Act, 2007). With the *healthcare power of attorney,* also called *durable power of attorney for health care,* the patient names a person (a proxy or agent) to make healthcare decisions for the patient if he or she loses decisional capacity. This document also allows the patient to describe preferences regarding specific treatment options, as well as to name successive agents should the first person be unavailable to take the role of proxy or agent. For example, the current version of the Illinois Health Care Surrogate Act was updated in 2014 to include the POLST (Illinois Health Care Surrogate Act, 2014). POLST is an order form, portable from one setting to another, in which the patient's physician, or in some states, the advanced practice nurse or physician's assistant, writes an order for the specific level of resuscitation the patient desires (National POLST Paradigm Office, n.d.). The form has categories to indicate if the patient

Table 30-3. Advance Directives

Type	Description	Advantages	Disadvantages
Living will	The patient must have a terminal condition; this document specifies treatment that the patient does not want if dying (e.g., CPR, blood transfusion, ventilator support, dialysis, surgery). In some states, the patient may not forgo nutrition and hydration.	Patient can list specific conditions and specific treatments to be withheld or withdrawn.	Variations between states exist regarding interpretation, so nurses should check with their institution's legal department regarding a patient forgoing nutrition and hydration.
Durable power of attorney for health care; power of attorney for health care	Document designates a surrogate decision maker if the patient is no longer able to participate in decision making. Surrogate can make all the decisions that the patient would have made if capable, including decision to forgo nutrition and hydration.	Surrogate may authorize treatment as well as the withdrawal of treatment, including nutrition and hydration.	It may not be clear if the surrogate is following the patient's wishes or making decisions based on what the surrogate would choose, not what the patient would choose.
Do-not-resuscitate (DNR) order	Physician order entered into a patient's medical record specifying what measures are to be withheld if there is cardiac or respiratory arrest that will result in death if not treated	Clarifies for the rest of the healthcare team what should be done if there is a cardiac or respiratory arrest	A DNR order can be written by the physician without consent of the patient or family, which can create conflict and tension between the patient, family, and healthcare team.

Note. Advance directives are written when the patient is capable of participating in decision making and only apply when the patient lacks capacity to participate in decision making.

wants full CPR or no resuscitation, comfort measures only, limited medical interventions, intubation and medical ventilation, and three options for artificially administered nutrition (none, defined period of time, or long term). Prior to a form like the POLST, patients who did not want to be resuscitated needed to have separate do-not-resuscitate (DNR) orders written for inpatient, outpatient, and home. The POLST form differs from DNR orders in that patients can also explicitly indicate which treatments they wish to have, such as antibiotics or a blood transfusion.

Advance directives are important for patients, their family members and loved ones, and healthcare institutions because they provide insight into the patients' wishes when the patients can no longer participate in decision making. It is important for all patients and their families to receive information on advance directives and be allowed to discuss these options with their healthcare providers. However, with the nature of many cancer diagnoses and prognoses, it is especially important in oncology. Although discussions about advance directives can be difficult, they should be viewed in a positive way as helping patients to have some control over their situation and future health care. Advance directives also allow people to have conversations about illness, death, and dying with their family and loved ones that often are avoided in society. Research shows that patients and healthcare providers avoid discussing end-of-life issues—both wait for the other to broach the topic, but neither does so (Spoelhof & Elliott, 2012). However, advance directives may allow people to have hope that their pain will be controlled and may relieve some of the fear and suffering that accompany a terminal cancer diagnosis and the expectation that they will be provided with the care that they choose.

Only about 26% of Americans have prepared an advance directive document (Rao, Anderson, Lin, & Laux, 2014). The major reasons people reported for not having an advance directive were lack of knowledge about what an advance directive was and the belief that their family knew their wishes, so the advance directive would be unnecessary. Rao et al.'s (2014) findings showed that women with college or graduate education, higher income, and a chronic condition were more likely to have an advance directive. Non-Whites were less likely to have an advance directive. Morhaim and Pollack (2013) found a slightly higher percentage, 30%, of American adults have an advance directive. They too found that few non-Whites had completed an advance directive, owing to cultural differences in decision making, mistrust of the healthcare system, and lack of communication with their healthcare providers. Great opportunity exists for oncology nurses to assist patients with preparing advance directives and communicating their wishes to their family. Although advance directives were designed to represent a patient's wishes when the patient cannot communicate, they also can save patients from the pain, suffering, and financial burden when unwanted medical interventions are withheld per the patient's wishes.

Aid in Dying

End-of-life care can be very challenging for oncology nurses. However, nurses can positively affect many aspects of end-of-life care. Pain is among the most common and most feared symptoms in individuals at the end of life (Paice, 2015). Although aggressive palliative care can help make pain and other symptoms tolerable, some patients may fear that at some point the pain and suffering will not be controllable, and they may consider requesting assistance in dying. Many patients, 62%–86% of those with advanced cancer and 24%–60% of those actively being treated, experience pain, and often are undertreated for the pain (Paice & Von Roenn, 2014). However, in both Washington and Oregon, states that have legalized physician-assisted suicide (PAS), most patients seek PAS not because of uncontrollable pain, but because of a loss of autonomy (87%–91%), inability to engage in enjoyable activities (88%–89%), loss of dignity (65%–75%), loss of bodily functions (28%–53%), being a burden on family, friends, or caregivers (22%–36%), inadequate pain control or concern about it (22%–35%), and financial implications of treatment (0%–4%) (Loggers et al., 2013). These data also reveal that 81%–100% of the patients who sought PAS have terminal cancer. Aid in dying is a very controversial topic throughout the world, as physicians and nurses struggle with their duty to care for and maintain life and yet desire to end the pain and suffering of their patients.

In 1994, the voters of Oregon approved the Oregon Death With Dignity Act (1995). This act "delineates the limited circumstances under which a physician may prescribe, but not actually administer, a lethal prescription for a patient" (Rich, 2002, p. 354). As such, because the provider is not administering the lethal dose, this action would be considered passive, rather than active, euthanasia. *Euthanasia* literally means "good death" and often has been associated with the term *mercy killing*, which is "deliberately and directly killing a sufferer to relieve pain" (Jonsen et al., 2015). Active euthanasia is illegal in the United States; physician-assisted death is legal in California, Colorado, Montana, New Mexico, Oregon, Vermont, and Washington at this time. Data from Oregon show that less than one-half of 1% of deaths in Oregon are from PAS (Orentlicher, Pope, & Rich, 2014).

The proponents of PAS garnered much publicity in 2014 when a young woman, Brittany Maynard, who was diagnosed with a terminal glioblastoma, declared her intent to move to Oregon from California so that she could legally seek PAS. Compassion and Choices, an organization advocating legalization of PAS, promoted her story and established a fund in her name. Although she said she was not ready to die on the date she had identified, two days later, she died from ingesting the prescribed medication (Shoichet, 2014). She was dubbed the "new face of the assisted-dying movement" because she was atypical of older patients seeking PAS (Angell, 2014). Despite her compelling story, opposition to PAS remains.

The Catholic Church is the largest constituency opposing PAS on religious grounds (Purvis, 2012). Disability groups such as Not Dead Yet were created solely to oppose PAS. Opposition rests on concern that the rules are not stringent enough to prevent non-terminally ill or clinically depressed patients from accessing PAS. Some patients who are uninsured or underinsured may view PAS as an option if they cannot get treatment. Prognostication is difficult, and thus some patients may prematurely end their lives out of fear of the future; at least one patient in Oregon lived three years after obtaining a prescription for PAS (Finlay & George, 2011).

The American Nurses Association (2013), the American Medical Association (2016b), the Oncology Nursing Society (2011), and the Hospice and Palliative Nurses Association (2011) all prohibit nurses and physicians from participating in assisted suicide. For nurses working in states where PAS is legal, nurses are encouraged to follow their state nurses' association guidelines on PAS. Nurses who have a moral objection to participation may declare a conscientious objection and provide for a safe, timely transfer of the patient's care to another nurse without the objection.

Palliative Sedation

When patients experience unremitting, intractable pain and suffering, they may choose to have enough nonopioid medication to keep them sedated or in a comatose state. When sedation is an issue in relieving uncontrolled physical symptoms, providers often feel a conflict with the balance of controlling symptoms and possible respiratory depression. It is feared that too much sedation (which might be needed to control pain and suffering) can actually cause patient death. However, the ethical principle of beneficence, as well as the doctrine of double effect, would allow for control of pain and suffering even if death is the result. The doctrine of double effect "affirms that the risk for an unintended consequence of treatment is justified when the purpose and intention of the treatment is to benefit the patient; the situation is sufficiently grave to merit the risk; and the desired benefit is not achieved via the adverse effect" (Eisenchlas, 2007, p. 211). That is to say that the intent for palliative sedation (formerly called terminal sedation) is to relieve the physical symptoms and not to cause the death of the patient; however, accepting death as a possible consequence of relieving symptoms is ethically permissible.

It should be noted that "the use of sedation in end-of-life care is not controversial" (Gallagher & Wainwright, 2007, p. 42). In fact, sedation often is used in healthcare settings to assist patients for a number of reasons, such as pain and symptom management, aid in sleeping, reduction of agitation, and conscious sedation for diagnostic procedures such as magnetic resonance imaging scans or colonoscopies. However, in palliative care situations, the care requested by patients or their decision maker, as well as the actions taken by the providers, should be carefully examined to ensure that proper standards of care are followed for each situation. The Hospice and Palliative Nurses Association (2016) affirmed the use of palliative sedation at the end of life. In all cases, however, pain and symptom assessment and management in patients with cancer should be a high priority for healthcare providers.

The use of palliative sedation in patients who are experiencing existential angst is controversial. Even in some European countries that have had physician-assisted dying for years, controversy still exists over palliative sedation for existential pain (Anquinet et al., 2014; Varelius, 2014). The American Medical Association (2016a) specifically addresses the issue: "Physicians may offer palliative sedation to unconsciousness to address refractory clinical symptoms, not to respond to existential suffering arising from such issues as death anxiety, isolation, or loss of control. Existential suffering should be addressed through appropriate social, psychological or spiritual support" (p. 60).

Role of Ethics Consultants and Ethics Committees

Most hospitals in the United States have some mechanism in place to deal with ethical issues and questions in clinical practice. Many institutions have ethics committees to serve this purpose. Although ethics committees have been in use since the 1950s, the use has increased since the boom of medical technology in the 1970s. In 1992, the Joint Commission required hospitals to have mechanisms for the consideration of ethical issues "in the care of patients and to educate caregivers and patients on bioethical issues" (Fry-Revere, 1992, p. 15). As a result of Joint Commission standards supporting institutional ethics committees, constantly advancing medical technology, and issues of medical futility and end of life, ethics committees are now an important part of the healthcare landscape.

Most ethics committees encourage interdisciplinary membership in which nurses, physicians, social workers, clergy, and other providers can participate in discussions on clinical cases, patient rights, and ethics policies, as well as provide education to members and the entire institution on relevant clinical ethics topics. Ethical issues that frequently arise in clinical oncology services include end-of-life decisions, questions of medical futility, decisional capacity, patient autonomy, and advance directives, to name a few. Ethics committees are available to discuss difficult issues with providers in a safe and confidential environment. In addition, ethics committees can assist with questions related to institutional policy.

Many healthcare institutions have clinical ethics consultation services as well as an ethics committee. Clinical ethics consultants provide consultation to patients, providers, and family members. The ethics consultant may be able to provide timely and efficient assistance to staff or family when waiting to convene the ethics committee. Often, the ethics consultant is also a member of the ethics committee and brings cases back to the committee meetings for discussion. With complicated clinical ethics situations, the consultant may call on members of the ethics committee for emergency meetings to obtain interdisciplinary input. With the use of secure online discussion boards, consultants also may post consultation notes for the ethics committee members to review and provide input for added advice and support.

Although educational training for clinical ethics consultants varies, they usually have formal training and education in the field of bioethics. The American Society for Bioethics and Humanities (2011) developed the core competencies for healthcare ethics consultants, and there has been movement toward development of certifying examinations (Fox, 2014) or quality attestation portfolios. It is important that oncology clinicians use all of the institutional resources available to them to provide the optimum care to their patients. These resources include but are not limited to social services, clergy, and ethics consultants or committees.

Informed Consent

After the diagnosis of cancer, the patient and healthcare team explore treatment options. Treatment regimens usually fall into one of three categories: standard treatment—treatment whose efficacy is known through rigorous clinical trials; experimental treatment—treatment whose efficacy is under investigation; and "compassionate care"—treatment whose efficacy for a particular condition is unproven, but the patient does not meet inclusion criteria for a clinical study. (See Chapter 13 for additional information on clinical trials.) Before the patient agrees to treatment, he or she needs to understand whether the treatment is standard or experimental, the possible risks and benefits, any alternatives, and the likely consequences if treatment is declined. For many cancers, clinical trials are conducted to find better treatments with fewer side effects.

For patients to make an informed decision, they must receive information in a way that is understandable to them, free of jargon, and in the language they speak and understand. The healthcare team should share information with patients in such a way that patients do not feel coerced to accept or reject the choices. Patients should give their consent or refusal voluntarily. Patients should receive enough detail to gain a full understanding of the treatment, including the procedures, possible risks, expected benefits, and alternatives. Patients may ask about costs and what their insurance will cover. Because the diagnosis of cancer can be frightening to patients and their families, it is difficult for patients to listen and retain information the first time it is given. Repeating discussions, explanations, and conversations with patients and families is helpful. Patients should be told if treatment is time sensitive and whether they need to make a decision within a specific time period. If the treating physician, usually an oncologist, thinks the patient may be eligible for inclusion in a clinical trial, the patient must receive this additional information.

For inclusion in a randomized controlled clinical trial, patients must meet certain eligibility criteria and agree to be randomly assigned to a group—either a control group, which receives standard treatment, or the experimental group (National Cancer Institute, 2016b). Some studies may have more than one experimental group. Both the treatment team and the patients are blind to the group assignment. As with standard treatment, patients who are considering experimental treatment need additional information. They need to understand random assignment and that although the treatment team hopes that patients will benefit from inclusion in the study, the primary purpose of the study is to determine which treatment is more effective or has fewer adverse side effects (if it is a phase III clinical trial). Oncologists are often part of regional or national study groups that are funded to investigate cancer therapies. The treating oncologist may also be an investigator in the study. This dual role can pose an ethical challenge for the physician. The primary obligation of a treating physician is to the patient and working for the best interests of the patient. The primary obligation of the researcher is to conduct the study with rigor and in adherence with the Nuremberg Code (see Figure 30-2) so that results of the study are valid and reliable.

Each institution has one or more institutional review boards (IRBs) that may comprise faculty from medical centers and affiliated universities and nonaffiliated, nonscientist community members. The charge of the IRB is to ensure that the study will be conducted in an ethical way to minimize harm to human subjects/participants (U.S. Department of Health and Human Services, 2009a).

Patients who agree to be in a clinical trial are referred to as *human subjects* or *research participants.* This label is an important distinction from the label of *patients,* as subjects/participants are owed different ethical obligations than patients. Patients who agree to be in a clinical trial but who experience a change that makes them ineligible to continue in the study may be withdrawn from the study. The investigator/treating physician may withdraw them because inclusion of their data may confound the results or because the patients are experi-

Figure 30-2. Nuremberg Code Directives for Human Experimentation

1. The voluntary consent of the human subject is absolutely essential.
   This means that the person involved should have legal capacity to give consent; should be so situated as to be able to exercise free power of choice, without the intervention of any element of force, fraud, deceit, duress, over-reaching, or other ulterior form of constraint or coercion; and should have sufficient knowledge and comprehension of the elements of the subject matter involved, as to enable him to make an understanding and enlightened decision. This latter element requires that, before the acceptance of an affirmative decision by the experimental subject, there should be made known to him the nature, duration, and purpose of the experiment; the method and means by which it is to be conducted; all inconveniences and hazards reasonably to be expected; and the effects upon his health or person, which may possibly come from his participation in the experiment.
   The duty and responsibility for ascertaining the quality of the consent rests upon each individual who initiates, directs or engages in the experiment. It is a personal duty and responsibility which may not be delegated to another with impunity.
2. The experiment should be such as to yield fruitful results for the good of society, unprocurable by other methods or means of study, and not random and unnecessary in nature.
3. The experiment should be so designed and based on the results of animal experimentation and a knowledge of the natural history of the disease or other problem under study that the anticipated results will justify the performance of the experiment.
4. The experiment should be so conducted as to avoid all unnecessary physical and mental suffering and injury.
5. No experiment should be conducted where there is an a priori reason to believe that death or disabling injury will occur; except, perhaps, in those experiments where the experimental physicians also serve as subjects.
6. The degree of risk to be taken should never exceed that determined by the humanitarian importance of the problem to be solved by the experiment.
7. Proper preparations should be made and adequate facilities provided to protect the experimental subject against even remote possibilities of injury, disability, or death.
8. The experiment should be conducted only by scientifically qualified persons. The highest degree of skill and care should be required through all stages of the experiment of those who conduct or engage in the experiment.
9. During the course of the experiment, the human subject should be at liberty to bring the experiment to an end if he has reached the physical or mental state where continuation of the experiment seems to him to be impossible.
10. During the course of the experiment, the scientist in charge must be prepared to terminate the experiment at any stage, if he has probable cause to believe, in the exercise of the good faith, superior skill and careful judgment required of him, that a continuation of the experiment is likely to result in injury, disability, or death to the experimental subject.

Note. From *Trials of War Criminals Before the Nuremberg Military Tribunals Under Control Council Law No. 10*, Vol. 2, pp. 181–182, 1949, Washington, DC: U.S. Government Printing Office. Retrieved from https://history.nih.gov/research/downloads/nuremberg.pdf.

encing unacceptable side effects, toxicity, or risks. The investigator/treating physician must balance the potential benefit/risk to the patient while upholding the highest rigor in research; rigor in research will benefit patients in the future. If the patient appears to be responding to the experimental treatment but is no longer eligible to continue in the study, the physician can apply for a compassionate drug use, which permits the physician to use the experimental treatment with this specific patient (American Cancer Society, 2016).

Patients may mistakenly believe that the experimental treatment will definitely benefit them, because otherwise their physicians would not tell them about the study. Appelbaum, Lidz, and Grisso (2004) first coined the phrase *therapeutic misconception*, which occurs when study participants erroneously assume that the study protocol will be altered to meet their specific needs or they incorrectly estimate the likelihood of medical benefit from inclusion in the study. A number of studies have demonstrated that patients decide to enroll in clinical trials based on trust in their physicians, so a physician's mere suggestion that the patient consider enrolling in a clinical trial can be a powerful influence in the patient's decision of whether to participate (Appelbaum et al., 2004; Dresser, 2002). Lidz et al. (2015) suggested three steps to reduce therapeutic misconception when recruiting participants for clinical trials: (a) describe the scientific reasoning underpinning the study (i.e., why randomization and blinding are critical), (b) admit that if the best approach were known, the study would not be necessary, and (c) avoid having anyone on the treatment team involved in recruitment. The recruiter should avoid the usual appearance of a clinician, such as wearing a lab coat and stethoscope.

Some cynicism exists about participation in medical research, such as in the African American community, where past atrocities occurred, such as the Tuskegee Syphilis Study (Jones, 1993). In a study to increase participation in cancer clinical trials among the African American community, researchers found that despite an increase in knowledge about cancer clinical trials, participation and retention of African Americans remains low (Green et al., 2015).

Nurses who care for patients undergoing treatment, whether standard, experimental, or compassionate, participate in the informed consent process by telling patients what they are doing, responding to their questions, and referring them to the physician, research coordinator, or another appropriate person to ensure their questions are answered (see Figure 30-3). If a patient is in a clinical trial, it is very important for nurses to follow the protocol and to alert the research team if a deviation from the protocol occurs.

Figure 30-3. The Nurse's Role in Informed Consent for Treatment

- Observe and document the informed consent process between the patient (and family, if present) and the treating physician or researcher.
- Provide the patient with the informed consent document.
- Provide time for the patient to read and consider participation (or acceptance of a treatment).
- Assess the patient's understanding with interactive questioning, a written questionnaire, or by having the patient explain specific parts of the informed consent document in his or her own words.
- Clarify the information for the patient. Provide resources (e.g., videotapes, audiotapes, interactive computer programs, refer the patient to www.cancer.gov website, discussions with qualified professional and lay individuals). Answer the patient's questions until the patient states that he or she has enough information to make a decision.
- Obtain verbal assent prior to each administration of therapy.
- Notify the physician or researcher if further discussion is needed because the patient or family has questions that the nurse is unable to answer.
- Explain any procedures and provide any instructions related to the treatment; for example, the physician obtains consent from the patient for placement of a central venous catheter, and the nurse explains the daily care of a central line, ways to secure it, how to shower with it, and so on.

Note. Based on information from Klimaszewski, 2015; National Cancer Institute, 2016a.

Futility

The concept of medical futility has become a hotbed of ethical conflict and yet there is no consensus on a definition. Medical technology has improved to the point that people may continue biological life (assisted by technology) long after they have lost the ability to respond or interact with their environment. Providers are asked to prolong life-sustaining treatments or to add further aggressive curative treatments or procedures even when the clinical outcome is not expected to improve the overall clinical situation.

A general definition of futility is "serving no useful purpose: completely ineffective" ("Futile," n.d.). The definition of futility is important and useful in clinical situations; however, it does not take into account values, beliefs, or goals that a patient or loved one may have regarding a "useful purpose." Clinical goals are very important and often guide the overall treatment plan. If the clinical goals are not shared by the patient and family, though, consensus on futility will not be reached. Rather than focus on futility, the team should shift the focus to immediate goals of patient comfort and family support. The clinically indicated treatments, such as mechanical ventilation, opioids, oxygen, and blood transfusions, would be evaluated in light of their likelihood of producing comfort for the patient.

In the qualitative aspect of futility, though, the value of the treatment is assessed. For example, a patient with lung cancer is severely hypoxic. His family is coming in from another state to see him. He asks to receive any treatment that will keep him alive and lucid until he has said his good-byes to his family. The treatment team thinks they can buy him some time by intubating him and putting him on a ventilator. The team expects that even on the ventilator, he will eventually die from his lung cancer, but they may be able to keep him alive for a few more days. Treatment in this case is not physiologically futile; it will keep him alive for a few days. But the treatment will not cure him or keep him alive indefinitely. Should it be offered?

Suppose that same patient with lung cancer has lapsed into a coma. His family members arrive and are extremely distraught that they were unable to see him while he was still conscious. They beg the treatment team to do whatever they can to keep him alive and help him to regain consciousness. The team explains to the family that they may be able to keep him alive a little longer with a ventilator, but he most likely will not regain consciousness. He is dying, and the ventilator will only prolong his dying. The family, however, believes there is value in extending his life; they want the team to try. Knowing that the patient also wanted to try further treatment to stay alive to see his family, the treatment team agrees to try the ventilator and titration of medication to see if he regains consciousness. Not everyone on the treatment team believes this is an ethical course of action; hence, some members of the team experience moral distress.

Futility as a Power Struggle

Rubin (1998) viewed futility as a power struggle between patients and providers. Patients "demand" treatment that the treatment team believes would be futile. However, the decision to treat is the physician's decision. If futility is seen as a unilateral judgment made by the physician, then patients have no say in the decision and their autonomy is denied. However, if futility is viewed as Rubin proposes, as a "negotiated reality," then the healthcare providers and patients engage in conversation to determine each other's goals (see Figure 30-4). A patient's (or surrogate's) autonomy, however, should not be threatened by a discussion in which goals are clarified and all treatment

Figure 30-4. Questions for Patients and Families to Ask Their Healthcare Providers

- Can you describe the treatment options for this condition?
- What is involved in each of these treatments?
- Which treatment or combination of treatments offers the best chance of cure?
- What are the possible side effects of each treatment option?
- What can be done to minimize the side effects?
- How will these treatments affect my daily living?
- If cure is unlikely, how much longer can these treatments extend my life?

Note. Patients also may want to review websites such as the National Cancer Institute's site (www.cancer.gov), especially sections on questions to ask when considering participation in a clinical trial (www.cancer.gov/about-cancer/treatment/clinical-trials/questions).

options and rationales are reviewed. As Caplan (2012) stated,

> Autonomy is not threatened by hearing the thoughtful opinion of experts about what they deem the best course of action. Autonomy is also not so fragile that it cannot withstand challenging, through questioning, or probing to make sure that choices are truly informed, authentic, and sincere. In seeking consent to stop [treatment], physicians ought not fear introducing their experience and evidence-based point of view in framing patients' and surrogates' choices. Physicians should be open to dissent, pushback, and disagreement, but making an expert view known is part of patient advocacy. (p. 1041)

Patients and family members may have high, unrealistic expectations of medicine and believe that medicine can produce miracles. Schneiderman, Faber-Langendoen, and Jecker (1994) suggested that patients fear abandonment when there is no curative treatment to offer. Patients may benefit from aggressive palliative care to manage their symptoms, relieve their pain and distress, and provide emotional and spiritual support. Twenty percent of patients with cancer in the United States have chemotherapy in the last 14 days before they die (Smith & Hillner, 2010). For patients who want treatment for metastatic disease with a poor prognosis and the team believes treatment offers marginal benefits, Smith and Hillner (2010) offered a decision aid to facilitate the discussion. The aid focuses on survival data with or without the requested treatment and shifts attention to other end-of-life issues.

Roeland et al. (2014) offered another perspective on facilitating medical decisions using *palliative paternalism*. They defined this as

> an approach to communication with limited open-ended questions that utilizes well-informed, discrete, concrete options during medical discussions, in order to reduce confusion and suffering by avoiding nonbeneficial care. Palliative paternalism provides a communication approach that determines the appropriate level of patient autonomy . . . [and] must always be grounded in compassion for patients, as well [as] humility, recognizing the limitations to understanding many aspects of each individual's illness experience. (p. 416)

The authors praise nursing's long-standing attention to the needs of patients when cure is elusive. However, it is not uncommon that patients, especially those in intensive care units, receive treatment that nurses believe are futile. Providing care to those patients takes a toll on the nursing staff in terms of moral distress.

Moral Distress and Futility

Moral distress, discussed earlier in this chapter, was originally defined as when "one knows the right thing to do, but institutional constraints make it nearly impossible to pursue the right course of action" (Jameton, 1984, p. 6). Oncology nurses have identified the question of futility as one of the greatest sources of moral distress for them (Ferrell, 2006). When nurses view the treatment they are providing as causing more harm than good, they feel as though they are physically abusing dying patients. As advocates for patients, nurses wish to give compassionate end-of-life care. Yet when there are disagreements about care or poor communication between the healthcare team and the patient and family, moral distress can result. There may be no greater challenge than to frankly discuss dying with a patient. These discussions require skill, a depth of knowledge and experience, and courage. Most oncologists and palliative care physicians have these skills, but some do not and may avoid having these discussions or may conduct them in a less-than-optimal way. Even after the most skillful delivery, patients and families may reject what they hear and demand treatment that the healthcare team believes would be ineffective in reaching the patient's stated goals. Schofield, Carey, Love, Nehill, and Wein (2006) recommended, based on currently available evidence, steps to facilitate the conversation to move from curative to palliative treatment.

Oncology nursing, whether one enters the specialty immediately upon becoming a nurse or after practicing in another area of nursing, requires nurses who can work with patients who are suffering and dying (Ferrell & Coyle, 2008). Even when no ethical conflict exists in a patient's care, being present and authentic with each patient can take a toll on the nurse. Ethical conflict and moral distress can exacerbate an already stressful work environment. Novice nurses experiencing moral distress may find support and guidance from more seasoned oncology nurses. Forums such as nursing ethics rounds may help in providing a vehicle for discussing ethical issues in a constructive, structured format. Interestingly, in an institutionwide study of moral distress, Whitehead, Herbertson, Hamric, Epstein, and Fisher (2015) found that moral distress was higher than average in clinicians who had end-of-life and pain management training. These authors observed that this may occur when clinicians know the best practices in end-of-life care but are unable to enact them in their practice setting. They concluded that education alone is not sufficient to minimize moral distress. Informal consultation and ethics education seminars may present other avenues to reduce moral distress, as nurses may be unaware that they can ask for an ethics consultation, are prohibited by hospital policy to initiate an ethics consultation, or are reluctant to do so for fear of reprisal from other members of the team (Gordon & Hamric, 2006).

Pediatric Issues

Decision Making for Children

Upon reaching the age of majority (18 in most states, 19 or 21 in others), an individual is considered an adult and can make decisions, enter into contracts, and get married. Before that day, parents or legal guardians must give consent for medical treatment, except in states that have specific statutes regarding instances of emergencies, substance abuse treatment, mental health treatment, and pregnancy and birth control. The same informed consent process as discussed previously is followed to obtain consent from the parents for medical treatment of their child (see also Chapter 12). Cancer treatment for children is available through clinical trials to find more efficacious, less toxic treatments. The treating physician and treatment team often are part of a consortium of hospitals and oncology providers, such as the Children's Oncology Group (COG). COG is a collaboration of more than 200 children's hospitals and 9,000 members involved in clinical research (COG, n.d.). Oncology programs that are part of COG follow precise protocols for including children in clinical trials. The research must adhere to the specific federal regulations for including children that are published in part 46, subpart D of the *Code of Federal Regulations* (U.S. Department of Health and Human Services, 2009c). For multisite studies, each hospital's IRB also must approve each study, although proposed changes to the Common Rule would provide for a central IRB to be used for multisite studies (Hudson & Collins, 2015). Regulations also require that permission be obtained from parents to include the child in the clinical trial, and, depending on the age of the child, assent is obtained from the child. *Assent* is the affirmative agreement to participate in the clinical trial. Absence of objection is not considered giving assent. The investigator or a designee explains the study to the parents, and after they have considered all the options and had their questions answered, they decide if they want their child to be included in the study. If parents decide not to include their child in the study, they have the option of seeking standard treatment, which is the best available treatment known for the child's particular type of cancer.

Assent

Once parents give permission for the child to be enrolled in the study, assent is sought from the child. The investigator usually has prepared descriptions of the study for different ages, so that the person obtaining assent (often the investigator, research nurse, resident physician, or clinical research coordinator) can explain the study to the child in language geared toward the child's developmental level. Children as young as 14 years old use the same decision-making strategies as adults (Weithorn, 1983; Weithorn & Campbell, 1982). Typically, children younger than 7 years old may not be asked to assent to be in the study; for children 7–14 years of age, verbal assent is sought; and for children older than 14, verbal and written assent is sought. The UCLA Office of the Human Research Protection Program (2012) identified the ages of 7 through 12 when important developmental milestones are reached that influence the child's ability to give assent. They proposed that children at age 13 may be capable of independent decision making but that this should be verified by a capacity assessment. The act of seeking assent demonstrates respect for the child's developing autonomy. If, however, the child has the prospect of direct benefit by participating in the study, federal regulations at 45 CFR 46 subpart D (§ 46.408) specify that parental permission is required but assent is not. It logically follows that if a child's refusal will not be honored, then assent should not be sought. In a study to examine how well children aged 7–18 years of age understand clinical trials, Unguru, Sill, and Kamani (2010) found that most children did not understand the research, although they had repeated explanations, and they did not feel involved in the decision to participate in research. The researchers concluded that tools to facilitate a child's understanding would be helpful.

The regulations concerning parental consent and child assent were adopted in 1979. In 2011, the Office for Human Research Protections sought public comment and recommendations for updating and improving regulations. A table comparing existing issues, recommendations, and rationale for change is available at www.hhs.gov/ohrp/humansubjects/anprmchangetable.html.

Disagreement Regarding Treatment

Regardless of whether the child receives standard or experimental treatment, when there is disagreement between the parents and older child, ethical conflict exists. It is expected that a younger child who does not understand the illness or treatment may object and even physically resist injections, blood draws, chemotherapy infusions, and bad-tasting oral medications. Older children who understand their situation may grow weary of feeling ill and being away from friends and school. Nurses experience distress when they must continue the treatment despite the child's objections, especially when the prognosis is poor and the child is at the end stage of the illness. Although advance directives are not legally recognized in minors, they can be used to discuss treatment goals and end-of-life preferences with adolescents (Rushton & Lynch, 1992). Parents regret the pain and discomfort the child must bear during treatment, but they hope that the treatment will result in cure. If the child's condition deteriorates and is not responding to treatment, nurses may advocate for discontinuing noxious treatment and interventions, especially if the child is refusing treatments and invasive procedures. The parents may be approached to discuss limiting treatment in terms of stopping invasive interventions and withholding CPR if the child has a respiratory or cardiac arrest. It is hard to imagine something more difficult for parents to decide. In the author's (TAS) experience, some parents have said they cannot agree to a DNR order because it signifies that they are "giving up" on their child.

Discussions with parents should focus on the goals of the care the child receives. The child may continue to receive treatment that serves a palliative purpose, such as radiation to shrink a tumor that is causing pain or loss of function, but is not likely to cure the child. The healthcare team should provide aggressive pain and symptom management, as well as psychological, emotional, and spiritual support for the child and parents. If disagreement remains between the child and parents, or between the parents and treatment team, an ethics consultation may be helpful. Some oncology programs have regular ethics rounds with an ethics consultant to preemptively address potential conflicts. In extreme cases, the child may go to court to be declared a mature minor for the purposes of making healthcare decisions.

One major ethical issue in pediatric cancer is the undertreatment of pain. Seventy-six percent of children with cancer report pain, and nearly 92% experience pain in the last month of life (Anghelescu et al., 2015). For social and cultural reasons, some parents do not want their children to receive opioids, so the pain may be undertreated. Children who get treatments on an outpatient basis may rely on parents to manage pain relief at home. Nurses should educate parents about best practices in assessing and managing cancer pain in children (Herr, Coyne, McCaffery, Manworren, & Merkel, 2011).

Treatment of Vulnerable Populations

Anyone with cancer may feel vulnerable—feeling at risk for dying, experiencing side effects or complications from treatment, or feeling powerless and susceptible. For the purposes of this chapter, a vulnerable person is one who has additional threats to his or her autonomy. Three groups will be discussed: prisoners, homeless individuals, and people with disabilities.

Prisoners

By virtue of their confinement, whether in a facility or on home arrest, prisoners lack autonomy. This is important in oncology, when treatment may be provided within clinical trials. When ethical guidelines for human subjects research were being developed, prisoners were identified as a group requiring special protection (U.S. Department of Health and Human Services, 2009b). If a prisoner may potentially be enrolled in a study, the IRB that reviews the study must have a member who has knowledge or experience with prisons, such as a former prisoner, family member of a prisoner, prison employee or consultant, or someone working on a parole board. Hayes (2006) offered suggestions for enhancing informed consent for research with vulnerable populations, such as prisoners, and those suggestions can be useful for the informed consent process for treatment. End-of-life care also poses a challenge for the prisoner population. Progress has been made, though, with the formation of the National Prison Hospice Association (www.npha.org).

Homeless People

Another vulnerable group is homeless people. Cancer treatment often requires support from family and friends. That support can be in the form of physical care, as well as emotional and financial support. People who are homeless lack the resources that would give them options in care. They require hospitalization because they do not have running water, refrigeration, or a secure place to store medicines and practice good hygiene. Although they are destitute, they may be eligible for public funding for health care through the Patient Protection and Affordable Care Act. They may be transient as they search for a place to stay and their next meal. Lacking funds for transportation, they may not be able to return to the facility where they received cancer treatment. End-of-life care for the homeless is also a challenge, and some hospices may provide unreimbursed care. Once hospitalized, if patients who are homeless lose their decision-making capacity, a surrogate must be found. People who are homeless often are unbefriended; they are unable to identify a family member or friend who can act as a surrogate decision maker (Pope & Sellers, 2012). This can result in overtreatment, with the default decision being to treat, as the patient's wishes are not known. No family members or friends are available to assume surrogacy, and the guardianship process can be expensive and protracted. Pope and Sellers (2012) identified strategies that some institutions have adopted to address these situations, such as creation of surrogate decision-making committees. These committees are composed of volunteers, many with a clinical, legal, or social service background, or consumers. They review the evidence as to whether the person lacks capacity and then determine what is in the person's best interests based on what information is known about the person. Pope and Sellers also called for states to amend their unwieldy guardianship procedures or for institutions to adopt policies for decision making for the unbefriended.

People With Disabilities

People with disabilities have difficulty accessing healthcare services (National Council on Disability, 2009). Hospital and clinic facilities are designed for the mainstream population. Facilities may have ramps, electric doors, and "handicapped accessible" toilet stalls, but many do not have the equipment or properly trained personnel to assist people with disabilities. For example, a 60-year-old man with post-polio syndrome requires assistance in moving onto a gurney for a computed tomography scan. Because he will be in a supine position for a prolonged period of time, he also needs a ventilator during the scan. Or, as another example, someone who is deaf may require assistance in the informed consent process or when being taught about the care of a central line. The Americans With Disabilities Act, passed in 1991, mandated that physicians' offices and healthcare facilities accommodate people with disabilities, but the law has been weakened by challenges from businesses fearing excessive costs for accommodation. Some hospitals have created a position for an ombudsman to facilitate the care of patients with disabilities. Oncology nurses should avail themselves of the services of this person. For hospitals or clinics without this resource, nurses should start by finding out from the people with disabilities what they need, where special services or equipment can be obtained, and how to make their clinic visit or hospitalization safe and productive. This shows respect for individuals with disabilities, honors their autonomy, and reduces their vulnerability.

Another situation that places a person with a disability in a vulnerable position is when healthcare providers make treatment decisions based on the person's disability. Assumptions may be made that the quality of life for a person with extensive physical disability is so poor that lifesaving cancer treatment should not be offered (Gill, 2006). Quality-of-life determinations are subjective and cannot be made by another person. Albrecht and Devlieger (1999) described the "disability paradox" in which people with disabilities report their quality of life as the same or higher than people without disabilities. Assumptions and biases should be suspended, and treatment decisions should be based on the informed decision making of the person with a disability or the parents of a child with a disability.

Another possible situation of vulnerability is when a person with a disability has altered functioning so that critical signs of complications are undetected. Communication with the person with the disability and family members is extremely important to deliver safe care. Consultation with the person's primary care providers, or with other healthcare providers with expertise in caring for people with disabilities, may be very helpful.

Rehabilitation for Patients With a Cancer Diagnosis

People are surviving and living longer with cancer than ever before. The effects of the disease, and often of the treatment, can be debilitating. The continuum of oncology treatment, though, may not extend beyond periodic monitoring for recurrence or managing sequelae of the disease and treatment. As cancer is reconceptualized from a terminal disease to a chronic disease, the field of cancer rehabilitation is growing (Franklin, 2007). Deconditioning from inactivity or disuse, fatigue, or pain is addressed through a multidisciplinary approach. Even with metastatic disease, when the prognosis is uncertain or known to be terminal, rehabilitation to improve function and quality of life should be offered as tolerated. Palliative care and hospice also should be available to patients in cancer rehabilitation.

Conclusion

Oncology nursing is a challenging specialty. Ethical issues abound, and nurses need to use resources to facilitate decision making, resolve conflicts, and cope with the daily witnessing of suffering and dying. The emotional highs of successful treatment and grateful patients contrast the lows of loss, moral distress, and organizational problems. Hamric (1999) found that nurses who had ethics education, had a sense of their influence in their work setting, had reached a level of clinical expertise, and had ethical concern were more likely to take steps to resolve ethical issues. Oncology units would benefit by having nurses who embrace advocacy and have the support of their peers, physician colleagues, administrators, and the nursing community.

References

Albrecht, G.L., & Devlieger, P.J. (1999). The disability paradox: High quality of life against all odds. *Social Science and Medicine, 48,* 977–988. doi:10.1016/S0277-9536(98)00411-0

American Association of Critical-Care Nurses. (n.d.). The 4 A's to rise above moral distress. Retrieved from http://www.nursingworld.org/MainMenuCategories/EthicsStandards/Courage-and-Distress/AACN-Framework-and-Moral-Distress.html

American Cancer Society. (2016). Compassionate drug use. Retrieved from http://www.cancer.org/treatment/treatmentsandsideeffects/clinicaltrials/compassionate-drug-use

American Medical Association. (2016a). Opinions on caring for patients at the end of life, subsection 5.6: Sedation to unconsciousness in end-of-life care. Retrieved from https://www.ama-assn.org/sites/default/files/media-browser/code-2016-ch5.pdf

American Medical Association. (2016b). Opinions on caring for patients at the end of life, subsection 5.7: Phy-

Key Points

- Ethical issues faced by patients and families and by nurses in oncology settings are pervasive, and the bioethical principles of autonomy, beneficence, nonmaleficence, and justice are useful in analyzing situations.
- Moral distress among nurses and other professionals caring for patients with cancer often occurs; it is very important that when nurses experience such distress that processes are in place to minimize and manage moral distress.
- Institutional ethics committees can assist patients, families, and staff with conflicts regarding end-of-life care, informed consent, advance directives, and issues related to futility of treatment, for example.

sician-assisted suicide. Retrieved from https://www.ama-assn.org/sites/default/files/media-browser/code-2016-ch5.pdf

American Nurses Association. (2013). Position statement: Euthanasia, assisted suicide, and aid in dying. Retrieved from http://www.nursingworld.org/euthanasiaanddying

American Nurses Association. (2015). *Code of ethics for nurses with interpretive statements.* Silver Spring, MD: Author.

American Society for Bioethics and Humanities. (2011). *Core competencies for health care ethics consultation* (2nd ed.). Glenview, IL: Author.

Angell, M. (2014). The Brittany Maynard effect: How she is changing the debate on assisted dying. *Washington Post.* Retrieved from http://www.washingtonpost.com/opinions/the-brittany-maynard-effect-how-she-is-changing-the-debate-on-assisted-dying/2014/10/31/efc75078-5df0-11e4-8b9e-2ccdac31a031_story.html

Anghelescu, D.L., Snaman, J.M., Trujillo, L., Sykes, A.D., Yuan, Y., & Baker, J.N. (2015). Patient-controlled analgesia at the end of life at a pediatric oncology institution. *Pediatric Blood and Cancer, 62,* 1237–1244. doi:10.1002/pbc.25493

Anquinet, L., Rietjens, J., van der Heide, A., Bruinsma, S., Janssens, R., Deliens, L., ... Seymour, J. (2014). Physicians' experience and perspectives regarding the use of continuous sedation until death for cancer patients in the context of psychological and existential suffering at the end of life. *Psycho-Oncology, 23,* 539–546. doi:10.1002/pon.3450

Appelbaum, P.S., Lidz, C.W., & Grisso, T. (2004). Therapeutic misconception in clinical research: Frequency and risk factors. *IRB: Ethics and Human Research, 26*(2), 1–8. doi:10.2307/3564231

Beauchamp, T.L., & Childress, J.F. (2013). *Principles of biomedical ethics* (7th ed.). New York, NY: Oxford University Press.

Bosek, M.S.D., & Savage, T.A. (2007). *The ethical component of nursing education: Integrating ethics into clinical experience.* Philadelphia, PA: Lippincott Williams & Wilkins.

Boyle, R. (2013). Ethics committee annual report—2012–2013. Retrieved from www.uvagomagnet.com/pdfs/ep/ep17exhibits/exhibit-ep17b-ethicscommitteereport2012-2013.pdf

Caplan, A.L. (2012). Little hope for medical futility. *Mayo Clinic Proceedings, 87,* 1040–1041. doi:10.1016/j.mayocp.2012.09.003

Centers for Medicare and Medicaid Services. (2016). Medicare care choices model [Fact sheet]. Retrieved from https://innovation.cms.gov/initiatives/Medicare-careChoices

Children's Oncology Group. (n.d.). About us. Retrieved from https://www.childrensoncologygroup.org/index.php/aboutus

Cohen, J.S., & Erickson, J.M. (2006). Ethical dilemmas and moral distress in oncology nursing practice. *Clinical Journal of Oncology Nursing, 10,* 775–780. doi:10.1188/06.CJON.775-780

Dresser, R. (2002). The ubiquity and utility of the therapeutic misconception. *Social Philosophy and Policy, 19,* 271–294. doi:10.1017/S0265052502192119

Eisenchlas, J.H. (2007). Palliative sedation. *Current Opinion in Supportive and Palliative Care, 1,* 207–212. doi:10.1097/SPC.0b013e3282f19f87

Epstein, E.G., & Hamric, A.B. (2009). Moral distress, moral residue, and the crescendo effect. *Journal of Clinical Ethics, 20,* 330–342.

Ferrell, B.R. (2006). Understanding the moral distress of nurses witnessing medically futile care. *Oncology Nursing Forum, 33,* 922–930. doi:10.1188/06.ONF.922-930

Ferrell, B.R., & Coyle, N. (2008). The nature of suffering and the goals of nursing. *Oncology Nursing Forum, 35,* 241–247. doi:10.1188/08.ONF.241-247

Finlay, I.G., & George, R. (2011). Legal physician-assisted suicide in Oregon and The Netherlands: Evidence concerning the impact on patients in vulnerable groups—Another perspective on Oregon's data. *Journal of Medical Ethics, 37,* 171–174. doi:10.1136/jme.2010.037044

Fox, E. (2014). Developing a certifying examination for health care ethics consultants: Bioethicists need help. *American Journal of Bioethics, 14*(1), 1–4. doi:10.1080/15265161.2014.873243

Franklin, D.J. (2007). Cancer rehabilitation: Challenges, approaches, and new directions. *Physical Medicine and Rehabilitation Clinics of North America, 18,* 899–924. doi:10.1016/j.pmr.2007.07.007

Fry-Revere, S. (1992). *The accountability of bioethics committees and consultants.* Hagerstown, MD: University Publishing Group.

Futile. (n.d.). In *Merriam-Webster's online dictionary* (11th ed.). Retrieved from http://www.merriam-webster.com/dictionary/futile

Gallagher, A., & Wainwright, P. (2007). Terminal sedation: Promoting ethical nursing practice. *Nursing Standard, 21*(34), 42–46. doi:10.7748/ns2007.05.21.34.42.c4551

Gill, C.J. (2006). Disability, constructed vulnerability, and socially conscious palliative care. *Journal of Palliative Care, 22,* 183–189.

Gordon, E.J., & Hamric, A.B. (2006). The courage to stand up: The cultural politics of nurses' access to ethics consultation. *Journal of Clinical Ethics, 17,* 231–254.

Green, M.A., Michaels, M., Blakeney, N., Odulana, A.A., Isler, M.R., Richmond, A., ... Corbie-Smith, G. (2015). Evaluating a community-partnered cancer clinical trials pilot intervention with African American communities. *Journal of Cancer Education, 30,* 158–166. doi:10.1007/s13187-014-0764-1

Hamric, A.B. (1999). The nurse as a moral agent in modern health care. *Nursing Outlook, 47*(3), 106. doi:10.1016/S0029-6554(99)90001-5

Hayes, M.O. (2006). Prisoners and autonomy: Implications for the informed consent process with vulnerable populations. *Journal of Forensic Nursing, 2,* 84–89. doi:10.1097/01263942-200606000-00006

Herr, K., Coyne, P.J., McCaffery, M., Manworren, R., & Merkel, S. (2011). Pain assessment in the patient unable to self-report: Position statement with clinical practice recommendations. *Pain Management Nursing, 12,* 230–250. doi:10.1016/j.pmn.2011.10.002

Hospice and Palliative Nurses Association. (2011). HPNA position statement: Role of the nurse when hastened death is requested. Retrieved from http://hpna.advancingexpertcare.org/wp-content/uploads/2015/08/Role-of-the-Nurse-When-Hastened-Death-is-Requested.pdf

Hospice and Palliative Nurses Association. (2016). HPNA position statement: Palliative sedation. Retrieved from http://advancingexpertcare.org/wp-content/uploads/2016/01/Palliative-Sedation.pdf

Hudson, K.L., & Collins, F.S. (2015). Bringing the Common Rule into the 21st century. *New England Journal of Medicine, 373,* 2293–2296. doi:10.1056/NEJMp1512205

Illinois Health Care Surrogate Act, 755 Ill. Comp. Stat. 40/1 Ch. 110 1/2 para. 851–1. (2014). Retrieved from http://www.ilga.gov/legislation/ilcs/ilcs3.asp?ActID=2111&ChapterID=60

Illinois Living Will Act, 755 Ill. Comp. Stat. 35/2 Ch. 110 1/2 para. 702 § 2(d). (2007). Retrieved from http://www.ilga.gov/legislation/ilcs/ilcs3.asp?ActID=2110&ChapAct=755%26nbsp%3BILCS%26nbsp%3B35%2F&ChapterID=60&ChapterName=ESTATES&ActName=Illinois+Living+Will+Act

Jameton, A. (1984). *Nursing practice: The ethical issues.* Englewood Cliffs, NJ: Prentice-Hall.

Jones, J.H. (1993). *Bad blood: The Tuskegee syphilis experiment* (New and expanded ed.). New York, NY: Free Press.

Jonsen, A.R., Siegler, M., & Winslade, W.J. (2015). *Clinical ethics: A practical approach to ethical decisions in clinical medicine* (8th ed.). New York, NY: McGraw-Hill Education.

Klimaszewski, A.D. (2015). Informed consent. In A.D. Klimaszewski, M. Bacon, J.A. Eggert, E. Ness, J.G. Westendorp, & K. Willenberg (Eds.), *Manual for clinical trials nursing* (3rd ed., pp. 113–125). Pittsburgh, PA: Oncology Nursing Society.

Lidz, C.W., Albert, K., Appelbaum, P., Dunn, L.B., Overton, E., & Pivovarova, E. (2015). Why is therapeutic misconception so prevalent? *Cambridge Quarterly of Healthcare Ethics, 24,* 231–241. doi:10.1017/S096318011400053X

Loggers, E.T., Starks, H., Shannon-Dudley, M., Back, A.L., Appelbaum, F.R., & Stewart, F.M. (2013). Implementing a Death with Dignity program at a comprehensive cancer center. *New England Journal of Medicine, 368,* 1417–1424. doi:10.1056/NEJMsa1213398

Lum, H.D., Sudore, R.L., & Bekelman, D.B. (2015). Advance care planning in the elderly. *Medical Clinics of North America, 99,* 391–403. doi:10.1016/j.mcna.2014.11.010

McCarthy, J. (2006). A pluralist view of nursing ethics. *Nursing Philosophy, 7,* 157–164. doi:10.1111/j.1466-769X.2006.00272.x

McLennon, S.M., Uhrich, M., Lasiter, S., Chamness, A.R., & Helft, P.R. (2013). Oncology nurses' narratives about ethical dilemmas and prognosis-related communication in advanced cancer patients. *Cancer Nursing, 36,* 114–121. doi:10.1097/NCC.0b013e31825f4dc8

Morhaim, D.K., & Pollack, K.M. (2013). A personal, economic, public policy, and public health crisis. *American Journal of Public Health, 103*(6), e8–e10. doi:10.2105/AJPH.2013.301316

Moss, A.H., Lunney, J.R., Culp, S., Auber, M., Kurian, S., Rogers, J., ... Abraham, J. (2010). Prognostic significance of the "surprise" question in cancer patients. *Journal of Palliative Medicine, 13,* 837–840. doi:10.1089/jpm.2010.0018

National Cancer Institute. (2016a). Informed consent. Retrieved from https://www.cancer.gov/about-cancer/treatment/clinical-trials/patient-safety/informed-consent

National Cancer Institute. (2016b). Phases of clinical trials. Retrieved from https://www.cancer.gov/about-cancer/treatment/clinical-trials/what-are-trials/phases

National Council on Disability. (2009). *Current state of health care for people with disabilities.* Retrieved from http://www.ncd.gov/publications/2009/Sept302009

National POLST Paradigm Office. (n.d.). POLST and advance directives. Retrieved from http://polst.org/advance-care-planning/polst-and-advance-directives

Oncology Nursing Society. (2011). Role of the nurse when hastened death is requested (endorsed position statement, Hospice and Palliative Nurses Association). Retrieved from https://www.ons.org/advocacy-policy/positions/ethics/hastened-death

Oregon Death With Dignity Act, Or. Rev. Stat. §§ 127.800–.897 (1995).

Orentlicher, D., Pope, T.M., & Rich, B.A. (2014). The changing legal climate for physician aid in dying. *JAMA, 311,* 1961–1962. doi:10.1001/jama.2014.4117

Paice, J.A. (2015). Pain at the end of life. In B.R. Ferrell, N. Coyle, & J. Paice (Eds.), *Textbook of palliative nursing* (4th ed., pp. 135–153). New York, NY: Oxford University Press.

Paice, J.A., & Von Roenn, J.H. (2014). Under- or overtreatment of pain in the patient with cancer: How to achieve proper balance. *Journal of Clinical Oncology, 32,* 1721–1726. doi:10.1200/JCO.2013.52.5196

Pope, T.M., & Sellers, T. (2012). Legal briefing: The unbefriended: Making healthcare decisions for patients without surrogates (Part 1). *Journal of Clinical Ethics, 23,* 84–96.

Purvis, T.E. (2012). Debating death: Religion, politics, and the Oregon Death With Dignity Act. *Yale Journal of Biology and Medicine, 85,* 271–284.

Rao, J.K., Anderson, L.A., Lin, F.-C., & Laux, J.P. (2014). Completion of advance directives among U.S. consumers. *American Journal of Preventive Medicine, 46,* 65–70. doi:10.1016/j.amepre.2013.09.008

Rich, B. (2002). Oregon versus Ashcroft: Pain relief, physician-assisted suicide, and the controlled substances act. *Pain Medicine, 3,* 353–360. doi:10.1046/j.1526-4637.2002.02056.x

Roeland, E., Cain, J., Onderdonk, C., Kerr, K., Mitchell, W., & Thornberry, K. (2014). When open-ended questions don't work: The role of palliative paternalism in difficult medical decisions. *Journal of Palliative Medicine, 17,* 415–420. doi:10.1089/jpm.2013.0408

Rubin, S.B. (1998). *When doctors say no: The battleground of medical futility.* Bloomington, IN: Indiana University Press.

Rushton, C.H., & Kurtz, M.J. (2015). *Moral distress and you: Supporting ethical practice and moral resilience in nursing.* Silver Spring, MD: American Nurses Association.

Rushton, C.H., & Lynch, M.E. (1992). Dealing with advance directives for critically ill adolescents. *Critical Care Nurse, 12*(5), 31–37.

Schneiderman, L.J., Faber-Langendoen, K., & Jecker, N.S. (1994). Beyond futility to an ethic of care. *American Journal of Medicine, 96,* 110–114. doi:10.1016/0002-9343(94)90130-9

Schofield, P., Carey, M., Love, A., Nehill, C., & Wein, S. (2006). Would you like to talk about your future treatment options? Discussing the transition from curative cancer treatment to palliative care. *Palliative Medicine, 20,* 397–406. doi:10.1191/0269216306pm1156oa

Shoichet, C.E. (2014). Brittany Maynard, advocate for 'death with dignity,' dies. Retrieved from http://www.cnn.com/2014/11/02/health/oregon-brittany-maynard/index.html

Smith, T.J., & Hillner, B.E. (2010). Explaining marginal benefits to patients, when "marginal" means additional but not necessarily small. *Clinical Cancer Research, 16,* 5981–5986. doi:10.1158/1078-0432.CCR-10-1278

Spoelhof, G.D., & Elliott, B. (2012). Implementing advance directives in office practice. *American Family Physician, 85,* 461–466.

Sundin-Huard, D., & Fahy, K. (1999). Moral distress, advocacy and burnout: Theorising the relationships. *International Journal of Nursing Practice, 5,* 8–13. doi:10.1046/j.1440-172x.1999.00143.x

UCLA Office of the Human Research Protection Program. (2016, June 9). *Guidance and procedures: Child assent and permission by parents or guardians.* Retrieved from http://ora.research.ucla.edu/OHRPP/Documents/Policy/9/ChildAssent_ParentPerm.pdf

Unguru, Y., Sill, A.M., & Kamani, N. (2010). The experiences of children enrolled in pediatric oncology research: Implications for assent. *Pediatrics, 125,* e876–e883. doi:10.1542/peds.2008-3429

U.S. Department of Health and Human Services. (2009a). Code of Federal Regulations: Title 45, Vol. 1, Part 46, Subpart A: Basic HHS policy for protection of human research subjects. Retrieved from http://ohsr.od.nih.gov/guidelines/45cfr46.html#46.108

U.S. Department of Health and Human Services. (2009b). Code of Federal Regulations: Title 45, Vol. 1, Part 46, Subpart C: Additional protections pertaining to biomedical and behavioral research involving prisoners as subjects. Retrieved from http://www.hhs.gov/ohrp/sites/default/files/ohrp/policy/ohrpregulations.pdf

U.S. Department of Health and Human Services. (2009c). Code of Federal Regulations: Title 45, Vol. 1, Part 46, Subpart D: Additional protections for children involved as subjects in research. Retrieved from http://www.hhs.gov/ohrp/sites/default/files/ohrp/policy/ohrpregulations.pdf

Varelius, J. (2014). On the relevance of an argument as regards the role of existential suffering in the end-of-life context. *Journal of Medical Ethics, 40,* 114–116. doi:10.1136/medethics-2013-101803

Weithorn, L.A. (1983). Children's capacities to decide about participation in research. *IRB: Ethics and Human Research, 5*(2), 1–5. doi:10.2307/3563792

Weithorn, L.A., & Campbell, S.B. (1982). The competency of children and adolescents to make informed treatment decisions. *Child Development, 53,* 1589–1598. doi:10.2307/1130087

Whitehead, P.B., Herbertson, R.K., Hamric, A.B., Epstein, E.G., & Fisher, J.M. (2015). Moral distress among healthcare professionals: Report of an institution-wide survey. *Journal of Nursing Scholarship, 47,* 117–125. doi:10.1111/jnu.12115

Wocial, L.D., & Weaver, M.T. (2013). Development and psychometric testing of a new tool for detecting moral distress: The Moral Distress Thermometer. *Journal of Advanced Nursing, 69,* 167–174. doi:10.1111/j.1365-2648.2012.06036.x

Zuzelo, P.R. (2007). Exploring the moral distress of registered nurses. *Nursing Ethics, 14,* 344–359. doi:10.1177/0969733007075870

Chapter 30 Study Questions

1. Why is the POLST (Physicians [or Practitioners] Orders for Life-Sustaining Treatment) form so important for patients with life-limiting conditions?
   A. It only goes into effect if the patient is in the terminal phase of disease.
   B. Like other advance directives, it does not need a physician/provider signature.
   C. Providers are not legally bound to follow the directives of the form.
   D. It is a legal order, signed by a physician, and must be honored in all care settings, including the home.

2. One of the most frequently reported ethical issues for oncology nurses is related to truth telling. What is the best response if a patient asks the nurse, "What is my diagnosis?" but the family asked that the patient not be told?
   A. Because the patient has a right to know, the nurse should tell the patient the diagnosis.
   B. Discuss with the family the reasons for the request to withhold this information; explain that for the patient to make informed decisions regarding treatment, the patient needs this information, and then develop a plan with the family to respond to the patient's question.
   C. Meet with the family and insist that they tell the patient his or her diagnosis.
   D. Tell the patient to ask the doctor.

3. Therapeutic misconception is:
   A. A patient's belief that a research protocol will be altered to provide the patient maximum benefit.
   B. The patient's belief that research subjects will be randomly assigned to the control or experimental group.
   C. The patient's belief that eligibility criteria for inclusion will be waived for the sickest patients.
   D. The patient's belief that research is conducted to benefit future patients.

4. Futility is an elusive concept, as its meaning may differ among patients, families, and the healthcare team. Which view of futility might facilitate a constructive discussion among all the stakeholders?
   A. Physiologic futility: the desired treatment will not work
   B. Qualitative futility: the desired treatment will not produce the desired outcome
   C. Negotiated reality: a mutual discussion to arrive at goals and ways to reach the goals
   D. Futility: an inappropriate use of resources

5. Under what conditions is it ethically permissible to provide palliative sedation?
   A. Unrelenting, unmanageable suffering of the patient
   B. Existential angst
   C. Unrelieved intense pain
   D. A and C

CHAPTER

31 Palliative Care

Ruth R. Zalonis, RN, MSN, OCN®, CHPN, GC-C

Introduction

Many people and clinicians think palliative care is hospice, but it's not. Moreover, they think that patients give up curative or life-sustaining care, but they don't.

—C. Dahlin in Sherner, 2015, p. 17

Palliative care (PC) is a concept whose time has come. As the healthcare system shifts from an acute disease model to a chronic disease model of health care (Meier & Sieger, 2004), PC will demonstrate its eminent usefulness. This chapter will explore its fitness for the new model of care and the ways it accomplishes its goals. PC is "patient and family centered care that optimizes quality of life by anticipating, preventing and treating suffering" (Hospice and Palliative Nurses Association [HPNA], 2013a). In today's evolving practice, a simultaneous care model calls for life-prolonging treatment and comfort care given *concurrently* for those diagnosed with a serious, life-limiting illness (Wittenberg-Lyles, Goldsmith, & Ragan, 2011) rather than waiting until the end of life (EOL). Instead, PC should be offered throughout the illness trajectory (HPNA, 2013a), that is, from the time of diagnosis until EOL.

Many disease states that proved fatal in past generations are now controlled or cured. Despite the benefits to individuals of this trend, the consequences are the accumulation of chronic disease states (comorbidities). Multiple chronic diseases present in the individual influence what medical treatment is feasible and useful in the context of life-limiting disease. PC providers take into account all comorbidities when formulating a treatment plan.

PC pays particular attention to the suffering experienced by individuals during their illness journey. In his seminal work of 1982, Dr. Eric Cassel, professor emeritus of public health at Cornell University, decried the lack of regard by his colleagues for the suffering of patients in their care, not only related to the disease state but also to the treatment of the disease (Cassel, 1982). "The relief of suffering . . . is considered one of the primary goals of medicine by patients and lay persons, but not by the medical profession" (Cassel, 1982, p. 640). Cassel wrote of the historical mind–body dichotomy proposed by the French philosopher René Descartes, which he contended was useful for scientific advancement but was injurious to individuals when used medically. It does not help us understand suffering. Instead, he contended, although individuals have "many facets" (p. 640), they exist as unified wholes. People cannot be reduced to their respective parts (Cassel, 1982).

This leads us to consider the ways in which individuals experience suffering. Dame Cicely Saunders, founder of the hospice movement (a movement related to PC, but not the same), pioneered the concept of "total pain" (Mehta & Chan, 2008). Saunders proposed that "pain should be understood as having physical, psychological, social, emotional, and spiritual components" (Mehta & Chan, 2008, p. 27). Assaults to the person by serious disease act on all aspects: body, mind, and spirit. PC chooses to address all aspects of suffering, unlike standard medicine, which tends to focus on the specialty of the clinician.

Pivotal to any discussion of PC is the recognition of the individual's illness journey—a person's values, preferences, and goals of treatment. A whole-person orientation provides patient-centered, not disease-centered, care. The structure and process that PC uses to accomplish patient-centered care will be discussed throughout the chapter.

Historical Development of Palliative Care

Historically, PC is a new subspecialty, beginning in the 1970s through the efforts of Dr. Balfour Mount, a Canadian physician (Duffy, 2005). Dr. Mount spent time with Dame Cicely Saunders in London, where she had begun her work with the terminally ill in 1948 (National Hospice and Palliative Care Organization [NHPCO], 2016a). When Mount returned to Canada, he chose the term *palliative,* which means to improve the quality of something, to describe his new concept of care (Duffy, 2005). This revolutionary type of care "focused on maximizing quality of life" (Lynch, Dahlin, Hultman, & Coakley, 2011, p. 106), not on EOL alone, as hospice does.

Palliative Care: What It Is, What It Is Not

How, then, does PC relate to hospice? First and foremost, the two terms are not synonymous. While all hospice is palliative in the general sense of amelioration, not all PC is hospice. The practice of PC is broad, whereas hospice is narrow. The two terms relate to one another as indicated in Figure 31-1. PC can be inclusive of hospice.

PC is provided "regardless of the state of disease" (Lynch et al., 2011, p. 106), is not restricted by settings, and thus can be provided in inpatient, outpatient, or home settings (NHPCO, n.d.-b). Although hospice care is generally restricted to the expected last six months of life, PC has no such restrictions. Acceptance of PC does not preclude curative treatment, unlike hospice, which focuses on comfort alone.

Despite the focus on comfort in the last six months of life with hospice, the use of hospice services does not amount to "giving up" but instead "giving over" to a different kind of care. Hospice care is not the stage where "nothing more can be done." This is not only erroneous but cruel. What this phrase actually means is that no more *curative options* are available. Instead, skillfully administered hospice aggressively treats suffering in all its forms: body, mind, and spirit. There is much that can be done in the treatment of physical pain, shortness of breath, nausea, and constipation, as

Figure 31-1. Relationship of Hospice and Palliative Care

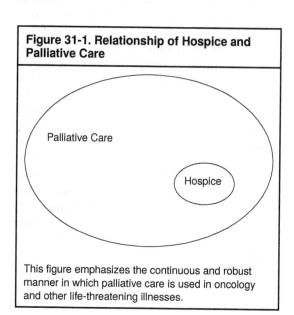

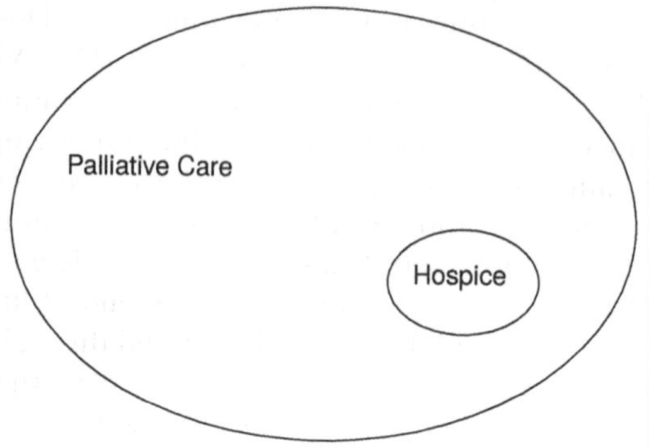

This figure emphasizes the continuous and robust manner in which palliative care is used in oncology and other life-threatening illnesses.

well as spiritual and emotional pain and other forms of suffering. Hospice is considered the model for compassionate EOL care (NHPCO, 2016b). Medicare pays for bereavement counseling services for a period up to one year following the patient's death (Centers for Medicare and Medicaid Services, 2015).

Furthermore, hospice is not limited to only those who are actively dying, but rather is available to those whose life expectancy is approximately six months or less. However, hospice is frequently underused until death is imminent. The Centers for Medicare and Medicaid Services (2014) Center for Medicare reported that the percentage of Medicare decedents who died while receiving the hospice benefit increased from 35% in 2007 to 44% in 2012. However, NHPCO reported that approximately 35.5% of those receiving hospice services in 2014 died or were discharged within seven days of admission (NHPCO, 2015). Author and healthcare chaplain Hank Dunn (n.d.) has written of the tragedy of late hospice referrals. Hospice professionals may not have time to adequately control pain and meet all the emotional and spiritual needs of the patient and family before death occurs (Dunn, 2012). Despite the frequent late referrals, a recent study by the NHPCO revealed that 94% of those who received hospice services rated them as very good to excellent (NHPCO, n.d.-a).

Need for Palliative Care Guidelines and Evaluation

As the concept of PC gained ground in health care, the need for standardization and evaluation became evident. In 2004, a coalition of PC organizations formed the National Consensus Project for Quality Palliative Care (NCP) and developed the *Clinical Practice Guidelines for Quality Palliative Care* (HPNA, 2013a). The objective was to provide a means for a structured, consistent evaluation of PC programs (HPNA, 2013a). The guidelines were revised in 2009 and 2013. Likewise, in 2006, the National Quality Forum, an organization that promotes improving the health care of Americans, used the guidelines as a basis for its national strategy for PC (HPNA, 2013a).

NCP addresses eight domains of PC: (a) structure and processes of care, (b) physical aspects of care, (c) psychological and psychiatric aspects of care, (d) social aspects of care, (e) spiritual, religious, and existential aspects of care, (f) cultural aspects of care, (g) care at the EOL, and (h) ethical and legal aspects of care (NCP, n.d.-a). These domains enable quality assessment and improvement initiatives by PC practitioners. Together, NCP and the National Quality Forum are foundational in ensuring and evaluating the consistency and effectiveness of PC. In addition, the Center to Advance Palliative Care provides outreach and technical assistance to U.S. hospitals about what data to collect and analyze for "strategic planning, quality improvement and demonstration of palliative care program impact" (Weissman, Morrison, & Meier, 2010, p. 179).

Structure of Palliative Care Services

PC uses a team approach to provision of services (World Health Organization, n.d.-b). The use of an interdisciplinary team allows access to multiple skill sets for the benefit of patients and their families. The philosophy of team culture, a "mutual appreciation of goals" (Jünger, Pestinger, Elsner, Krumm, & Radbruch, 2007, p. 348), allows for "higher levels of autonomy, flat hierarchy, more realistic workloads, and higher levels of personal feedback by colleagues, patients and relatives" (Jünger et al., 2007, p. 347). Teams allow flexibility in addressing the needs of the whole person: physical, emotional, psychosocial, and spiritual. The team treats the patient and family as the *unit of care*. In this approach, the patient defines what the family is (Lynch et al., 2011). Teams may include some or all of the following (NCP, n.d.-b): physician, advanced practice nurse, nurse, case manager, social worker, chaplain, pharmacist, and volunteers. Assistance from ancillary departments such as respiratory therapy, physical and occupational therapy, music therapy, and dietary services may occur. The exact membership of the team will depend on the setting and organization. Settings for the provision of PC include acute care hospitals, outpatient clinics, and community settings, such as assisted living, a personal care facility, or the home.

Process of Palliative Care: Communication, Collaboration, and Continuity

Communication

Multidirectional communication is foundational to the process of providing PC services. In PC, communication is not simply the transmission of information but the "mutual creation of meaning by both communicators" (Wittenberg-Lyles, Goldsmith, Ferrell, & Ragan, 2013, p. 1). As Wittenberg-Lyles et al. (2013) so aptly stated, "Both communicators are speaking and listening, sending and receiving" (p. 1). This is a fundamentally reciprocal process. In this give-and-take pattern of communication, information flows in all directions among the team, patient, and family, as well as the primary physician, consulting physicians, and those in ancillary departments. A web of communication is created.

Communication within the team itself will be ongoing during the acute phase, bringing to bear each discipline's expertise. Communication will continue temporally throughout the disease trajectory as care needs change and additional discussions about goals and services are needed (Zalonis & Slota, 2014).

The collegial atmosphere of the team promotes the free flow of information. When effective communication occurs, it empowers patients and families, reduces uncertainty, and creates an environment of safety and trust (Wittenberg-Lyles et al., 2013). This atmosphere encourages the patient and family to share their stories, and thus, the team shifts the focus from the team to the patient (Wittenberg-Lyles et al., 2013), thereby providing patient-centered care.

Communication in PC frequently occurs in an emotionally charged environment. Patients and families are trying to sort out their lives after receiving bad news about a life-limiting diagnosis. Wittenberg-Lyles et al. (2013) delineated two levels of meaning that occur in any communication with the team: the content level and the relationship level. Speaking the words of a message, the "task" (p. 4), provides the *content* of communication, but the *relationship* is usually conveyed by nonverbal cues. Nonverbal cues become preeminent because researchers note that as much as 80% of communication is nonverbal (Wittenberg-Lyles et al., 2013). Examples are maintaining eye contact, positioning, and showing focused attentiveness without distraction (Wittenberg-Lyles et al., 2013). Effective, expert communicators are needed for these sensitive situations, as the relationship of trust rests upon the words and nonverbal cues being consistent.

Collaboration

PC teams operate in challenging environments. In decision making, "because certainty cannot be obtained, the right answer to problems [in PC] has to be created or produced through moral reflection" (Hermsen & Ten Have, 2005, p. 564). Multiple solutions present themselves. A cooperative dialogue ensues in an atmosphere of mutual respect, as no one discipline has a corner on "absolute moral truth" (Hermsen & Ten Have, 2005, p. 565). A joint decision by the team can produce a balanced and prudent decision, although this decision by nature retains an element of uncertainty (Hermsen & Ten Have, 2005).

During ongoing discussions, the team members answer questions about patient autonomy, caregiver differences of opinion, safety, resource requirements, and feasibility. Openness and flexibility are important attributes if collaboration is to succeed (Jünger et al., 2007). A participant in Jünger et al.'s (2007) study stated that having a common vision of what is desired to be achieved is essential.

Continuity

According to *Growth of Palliative Care in U.S. Hospitals: 2015 Snapshot* (Center to Advance Palliative Care, 2015), achieving well-coordinated care across healthcare settings is a prime goal of PC programs. Families frequently have little experience in access to, or knowledge of, helpful services and resources to transition from the hospital. The PC team matches resources and services with patient and family needs after the patient has left an acute care setting. Supportive services are available in a variety of settings, such as outpatient clinics, the home, personal care homes, or long-term care facilities. The PC team's expertise in understanding the rules governing services and the routes of access remains an important function. Recommendations by the team also reflect the changes in care needs due to progressive illness. For example, a PC team might refer to a palliative home care agency initially that also offers hospice care in preparation for future need. Or, the patient might begin with a referral to home care, then transition to palliative home care, and later to hospice. Or, alternatively, a patient might use an outpatient PC clinic as long as feasible and then transition to hospice.

In summary, the patient's prognosis and illness trajectory will provide direction about care needs. PC teams are experienced in eliciting goals and needs, working in a collegial manner, and facilitating access to services. These activities of the PC process exemplify the 3 C's of PC: communication, collaboration, and continuity.

The Family Meeting

A primary vehicle used by the PC team is the family meeting. Wittenberg-Lyles et al. (2011) described the family meeting as enabling "the family to take an active role in the physician-patient consultation" (p. 308). The meeting can occur in a variety of settings, either inpatient or outpatient. It serves to establish the preferences and wishes of patients in relation to their diagnosis and prognosis and to clarify goals in light of information provided. Ideally, the patient is a full participant in these discussions. If the individual is unable to participate, then a surrogate decision maker acts in the patient's stead. In advanced illness, it may be problematic for the surrogate to determine preferences if prior conversations did not occur when the patient was lucid. This highlights the need to begin conversations at the time of diagnosis, or at least early after diagnosis. A series of meetings may better serve the patient and family, but depending on the state of illness and the setting, this may not be feasible.

The physical environment of the family meeting is important. Usually, the team chooses a quiet, comfortable place for the discussions. A designated leader initiates the discussion (Weissman, Quill, & Arnold, 2015), but who occupies this role depends on the makeup of the team. Frequently the leader is a physician or advanced practice nurse. The leader begins by introducing himself or herself and the team members. Family members are introduced. The leader initiates the conversation by determining what understanding the patient and family have about status and prognosis. Any misconceptions must be dealt with at this stage (Weissman et al., 2015). Next, the leader summarizes the patient and family's understanding to confirm that everyone is on common ground (Weissman et al., 2015). These foundational steps are necessary prior to moving to discussions about wishes, preferences, and goals. (Advance directives also may be addressed in family meetings.) Once preferences and goals are established, the team proposes a plan of care. A reciprocal discussion ensues; the plan is amended, if needed, and then implemented. The team will make referrals for services and help to transition the patient to another setting with services agreed upon during the meetings. Patient-centered discussions in a compassionate atmosphere promote trust and adherence to the plan.

Symptom Management

PC seeks to address the multifactorial nature of suffering that often accompanies serious illness. *Suffering* is defined as a state of severe distress induced by loss of intactness of person (HPNA, 2012). Diagnosis with a serious, life-limiting illness frequently catalyzes a break in personhood. Causes of suffering may be physical, such as breathlessness, nausea and vomiting, constipation, diarrhea, pain, or delirium, but other causes often may be emotional, social, or spiritual.

Causes of pain in serious illness are often complex and may complicate a patient's expression of pain (Mehta & Chan, 2008). In PC, the concept of total pain may serve to inform understanding and treatment of distress (Mehta & Chan, 2008). Total pain encompasses not only physical pain due to tissue damage, but also the emotional, psychosocial, spiritual, and cultural aspects of pain. PC treats pain of the body, mind, and spirit. Dame Cicely Saunders pioneered this concept in her hospice work (Mehta & Chan, 2008). The whole-person perspective can also be traced to Florence Nightingale. In her foundational work, *Notes on Nursing: What It Is and What It Is Not*, Nightingale observed that suffering extended beyond bodily expression (Lynch et al., 2011, p. 107).

The experience of physical pain is a common symptom in serious illness, as well as being one of the most feared symptoms (HPNA, 2012). Nurses should not fear to adequately relieve pain; a large body of research has demonstrated that pain medication does not hasten death. Rather, unrelieved pain hastens death by consuming physical energy and decreasing mobility (HPNA, 2012).

Descriptions of pain are subjective and individual. Nursing pioneer Margo McCaffery revolutionized pain management in 1968 by her stance that "pain is what the person says it is and exists whenever he or she says it does" (as cited in Ferrell, 2005, p. 88). By this definition, pain is viewed from the perspective of the one who has it: the sufferer. This perspective meshes perfectly with the holistic principles of PC.

In the population that receives PC, the person assessing pain needs to be able to separate acute and chronic pain. Although both types need to be addressed, their manifestations may be quite different. For those with chronic pain, for example, facial expression may not correlate with the expectations of the assessor. Nurses can avoid this pitfall if they recall McCaffery's dictum.

Chronic pain can be defined as pain that lasts more than six weeks and affects a person's sense of well-being and quality of life (Lambert, 2010). It usually falls into two categories: nociceptive or neuropathic (Medtronic, n.d.). Nociceptive pain is usually due to tissue damage and can encompass pain from benign causes, as well as tumors or metastatic disease. Its quality is sharp or throbbing, whereas neuropathic pain is usually burning or shooting and results from damage to nerves (Medtronic, n.d.). Both types of chronic pain often exist simultaneously in patients with cancer and require skillful handling by the PC team. The PC physician or nurse practitioner on the team will take into account "biopsychosocial factors in addition to spiritual and cultural issues" (Lambert, 2010, p. 436) when addressing pain.

Nociceptive pain may respond well to nonsteroidal anti-inflammatory drugs (NSAIDs) or opioids, whereas neuropathic pain may respond better to agents such as gabapentin, pregabalin, amitriptyline, or duloxetine hydrochloride (Lambert, 2010). People who have received certain chemotherapy agents, such as platinum-based compounds, vinca alkaloids, or taxanes, frequently have neuropathic pain (Polovich, Olsen, & LeFebvre, 2014).

When nonopioid analgesia alone is insufficient for effective pain management, opioids are then warranted. When mild opioids such as codeine are ineffective, strong opioids such as morphine and hydromorphone should be added (World Health Organization, n.d.-a). Additional medications, adjuvants, which address fear and anxiety, are recommended in conjunction with analgesics (World Health Organization, n.d.-a). Opioid doses may be lowered by simultaneous use of nonopioids such as NSAIDs (Coyne, 2015). Because cancer pain is frequently multifactorial in nature, combination pharmacology is more effective than opioids alone. An effective pain regimen may include NSAIDs, agents such as gabapentin, and opioids.

As presented by the World Health Organization pain ladder, adjuvants for the relief of other symptoms are necessary to obtain quality of life. Symptoms such as nausea may respond to antiemetics, for example, ondansetron or prochlorperazine, but agents such as dexamethasone, metoclopramide, or lorazepam may also be needed for refractory nausea, depending on the exact cause (Polovich et al., 2014).

Breathlessness may respond to morphine. For those with renal compromise, hydromorphone may be used instead because of its lower levels of active metabolites (Coyne, 2015). Morphine is very flexible because it comes in long- and short-acting oral forms as well as rectal, subcutaneous, and IV preparations. The intramuscular route is not recommended because it has unreliable absorption and a rapid drop in action and is painful (Wells, Pasero, & McCaffery, 2008). Tablets or oral solutions of morphine also are available. Because breathlessness has both sensory and affective components, techniques such as a handheld fan, pursed-lip breathing, and anxiety relief also may be used (Booth, Chin, & Spathis, 2015).

Bone pain, common in metastatic disease of breast, lung, and prostate cancers, is challenging to treat. Opioids alone may be insufficient, and additional classes of medications may be helpful. Bone pain may be amenable to use of bisphosphonates, which inhibit osteolysis (Coyne, 2015). Massage therapy, hydrotherapy, and daily stretching and exercise have demonstrated benefits to those with bone pain (Coyne, 2015).

Constipation frequently accompanies opioid use, or may be a feature of the disease process. As-needed (PRN) administration of opioids is not recommended; instead, a daily regimen is prescribed. Docusate sodium, polyethylene glycol, and/or senna used daily in conjunction with PRN suppositories, sodium phosphate enemas, or milk of magnesia (*Nursing2017 Drug Handbook*, 2017) often is necessary to provide regular evacuation.

Other symptoms may include anxiety and depression. Anxiety may respond well to anxiolytics (Cope et al., 2016). Depression, a common accompaniment to a cancer diagnosis, may respond well to agents such as citalopram, duloxetine, or fluoxetine (Cope et al., 2017). Excess secretions also may occur in advanced disease. Excess secretions at EOL respond to treatment with glycopyrrolate, given IV; atropine sulfate ophthalmic drops, given sublingually; or scopolamine, administered via transdermal patch (Bailey & Harman, 2017).

Concerns about the use of opioids and associated respiratory depression for those needing PC or hospice are generally unfounded. The PC physician or nurse practitioner will generally perform a trial of analgesics initially at a low dose, and then titrate the dose upward according to the estimated pain intensity based on pathology and analgesic history (Herr, Coyne, McCaffery, Manworren, & Merkel, 2011). Alert patients do not suddenly experience respiratory depression; it typically develops only as sedation is increased (Wells et al., 2008). Therefore, the nurse needs to monitor sedation levels and administer doses accordingly. Relying on pulse oximetry levels alone is not recommended because a decreased oxygen saturation is a later indication of respiratory depression (Wells et al., 2008).

In a landmark study, Marks and Sachar (1973) reported that physicians' misconceptions regarding use of narcotic analgesics led to undertreatment of pain and therefore needless suffering in patients. Since then, research has consistently demonstrated that pain is undertreated (Wells et al., 2008). Changes in level of consciousness in a state of advanced illness may be due to the disease process, not medication. The benefit of having the PC team on board is that altered levels of consciousness can be investigated and appropriately treated.

The concern about overtreatment with opioids causes the harmful effects of unrelieved pain to be ignored. Negative effects occur in the endocrine, metabolic, cardiovascular, gastrointestinal, and immune systems (Wells et al., 2008). The endocrine system releases excess hormones, producing fat catabolism, weight loss, and inflammation (Wells et al., 2008). For those with cancer, stress and pain can suppress natural killer cells that act to prevent tumor growth and the process of metastasis (Wells et al., 2008).

Spiritual distress can have a significant effect on suffering and generally complicate the treatment of physical pain. In a recent study of patients with advanced cancer receiving PC, 40 of 91 patients (44%) reported spiritual pain (Delgado-Guay et al., 2011). All humans are intrinsically spiritual because all individuals have relationships "with themselves, others, nature, and the significant or sacred" (HPNA, 2010). The team chaplain and other team members understand that each person has unique beliefs, values, and practices (HPNA, 2010). As the team uncovers the causes of spiritual distress, it will address brokenness and create space for healing (HPNA, 2010).

Barriers to Use of Palliative Care

As noted previously, PC as a new subspecialty emerged in the 1970s (Duffy, 2005). The prime barrier to obtaining PC services is a lack of knowledge by both the public and clinicians. Many believe that PC is equivalent to hospice, which they wrongly impute as "giving up." Further needs for the nurse's role of educator in this area are described in the Nursing Implications section later in this chapter.

Avoidance of the subject of death and dying is also a barrier. Even after the passage of the Patient Self-Determination Act in 1991, the majority of people have not completed a living will. Research by the Agency for Healthcare Research and Quality showed that when the records of the terminally ill were retrieved, less than 50% had an advance directive (Kass-Bartelmes & Hughes, 2003). Some clinicians and families have concerns that engaging PC will "take away hope." In fact, this fear is unfounded.

Value of Palliative Care

A randomized controlled trial performed by Temel et al. (2010) showed that the difficulties of providing data about the value of early PC were unfounded. This landmark study demonstrated the benefit of providing PC services at the time of diagnosis of a serious, life-limiting illness. The researchers found that those in the intervention arm of the study (those who received PC at the time of diagnosis) had a longer median survival, as well as marked improvement in quality of life and mood. Longer survival was accomplished even when compared to those who received aggressive treatment up to EOL (Temel et al., 2010). The authors hypothesized that earlier referral may have resulted in better symptom management, which, in turn, translated into longer survival. Rates of depression differed between the two arms of the study, with half as many patients suffering from depression in the intervention arm (Temel et al., 2010). This study also demonstrated that more patients in the intervention arm had addressed advance directives by EOL.

In the ENABLE III randomized controlled trial, researchers found that early PC improved survival, reduced depression, and relieved family caregiver depression and stress (Bakitas et al., 2015; Dionne-Odom et al., 2015). Analysis compared patients who were referred to PC within 30–60 days of diagnosis with those whose initiation of PC was delayed for three months. One-year survival rates were 63% in the early referral group and 48% in the delayed referral group (Bakitas et al., 2015). Hospitals' use of the intensive care unit and emergency department was lower in the early PC group (Bakitas et al., 2015). Median survival in the early intervention group was 18.3 months compared with 11.8 months in the delayed group (Bakitas et al., 2015). Furthermore, the early intervention group was more likely to have a home death (Bakitas et al., 2015), consistent with other studies of those receiving early PC. A common theme in the general population is the wish to die at home.

Jack, Hillier, Williams, and Oldham (2004) investigated a different advantage to receiving early PC. The aim of the study was to determine whether those who received early PC had more "insight into their disease and prognosis" (p. 47). The intervention did demonstrate an improvement in insight, confirming the previous results in other studies (Jack et al., 2004). Healthcare providers in the study thought that PC involvement allowed patients to explore their understanding from a patient perspective and allowed more open communication (Jack et al., 2004).

In a follow-up study to Temel et al. (2010), Yoong et al. (2013) demonstrated the difference between PC visits and oncology visits by patients. While oncology visits focused on cancer treatment and medical complications, PC visits emphasized "managing symptoms, strengthening coping, and cultivating illness understanding and prognosis awareness" (p. 283). The authors also learned that early PC visits were related to building relationships, while final visits were where EOL discussions occurred (Yoong et al., 2013). This should help to allay fears of clinicians who have concerns about PC referral "taking away hope."

In summary, evidence supports that early initiation of PC has multiple benefits to both patients and families. Yoong et al. (2013) noted that because cancer treatment is now very complex, requiring considerable time and attention from the oncologist directing the regimen and managing medical complications of the treatment, collaboration with the PC team allows the oncologist to focus on cancer therapy. The PC team can manage the "psychological, social, and emotional aspects of illness" (Yoong et al., 2013, p. 288). Early initiation of PC is recommended by a number of organizations, including HPNA (2013b), the American Academy of Hospice and Palliative Medicine (2008), the Center to Advance Palliative Care (n.d.), and the American Society of Clinical Oncology (Ferrell et al., 2017). The National Comprehensive Cancer Network® (2017) guidelines state that all patients should be screened for PC needs during their initial visit, as well as at appropriate intervals and as clinically indicated. NHPCO and the Center to Advance Palliative Care (n.d.) state that PC should be offered along with curative and restorative treatment. Initiation of PC should begin before occurrence of a healthcare crisis (HPNA, 2013b). The primary objective should be to provide maximum benefit to patients and their families.

Nursing Implications

The constant presence of nurses among patients receiving PC emphasizes that nurses are critical to the provision of high-quality PC. They find themselves in a unique position to have conversations about healthcare interventions and patients' preferences, values, and goals related to these interventions (HPNA, 2013b). Patients facing a serious diagnosis tend to feel very vulnerable and benefit from the skill, experience, and compassion of nurses. Patients rely on nurses to be their advocates, that is, to ensure that their wishes and preferences are honored (HPNA, 2013b).

Nurses need to be proactive in their pursuit of PC education as the healthcare system moves from an acute care model of disease to a chronic care model. The End-of-Life Nursing Education Consortium (ELNEC) is an excellent resource and supports the report on improving care in serious illness issued by the Health and Medicine Division of the National Academies of Sciences, Engineering, and Medicine (formerly the Institute of Medicine) (Field & Cassel, 1997; Malloy, Virani, Kelly, Harrington-Jacobs, & Ferrell, 2008). ELNEC is available at many sites in the United States and worldwide. Participating in ELNEC training enables nurses to communicate more effectively with the PC team about patients' needs, gain expertise in symptom management, provide needed care to families, and advocate for the relief of suffering (see www.aacn.nche.edu/ELNEC). HPNA and the Oncology Nursing Society also provide high-quality information and opportunities related to PC, such as print and online journals, workshops and conferences, and online courses (see http://hpna.advancingexpertcare.org and www.ons.org).

Nurses should endeavor to become expert in symptom management. Becoming knowledgeable about safe pain management will help to prevent the undertreatment of pain and its subsequent harmful effects (Wells et al., 2008). Adequate monitoring by nurses is the best prevention of untoward sedation (Wells et al., 2008).

Nurses' role in making information understandable to patients and their families is paramount. Promoting understanding is one of the abilities needed by healthcare professionals involved with shared decision making (Kawasaki, 2014; Légaré et al., 2011). In the face of receiving bad news, anxiety and shock often require the nurse to reinforce information presented, correct misconceptions, and interpret "medicalese." Without adequate understanding, informed decision making cannot occur.

Because nurses spend more time with patients than other providers, they may have many opportunities to develop a good understanding of patient and family wishes and preferences. The nurse's role in advance care planning is recognized in the HPNA (2013a) position statement, "The Nurse's Role in Advance Care Planning," and is considered a core element of palliative nursing practice. Assisting families to formulate and then verbalize these wishes to their healthcare providers is a valuable service nurses provide. In doing so, nurses promote patient autonomy, one of the prevailing bioethical principles of today's health care (Zalonis & Slota, 2014).

When nurses communicate with providers about the appropriateness of initiating involvement of the PC team, patients and their families have the opportunity to explore at length their wishes and goals. Participation of the PC team and the nurse when surrogates must make decisions for the patient adds another measure of support. However, it may also enable families to feel that their substituted judgment is in line with patient wishes and that autonomy has been protected. Preferences and values are explored and addressed at length in family meetings.

Another valuable service provided by nurses is that of presence. This is simply *being there* and "that quality that makes patients and their families feel that their nurses are there for them" (Wittenberg-Lyles et al., 2013, p. 10). Tellingly, the term *healing presence* is often used in nursing literature, which confers the aura of nonverbal attentiveness and compassionate witness. There is power in the nurse's *being* alone. Empathy flows from presence and is one of the core attributes of healing presence (Wittenberg-Lyles et al., 2013). From healing presence, a therapeutic relationship is created. Ferrell and Coyle (2008) stated that in the midst of fears and anxieties, the nurse's presence speaks through "the chaos and depersonalization of the healthcare environment" (p. 109). Providing presence is a priceless gift.

In the milieu of a therapeutic relationship, patients and families feel free to share their feelings: uncertainty, fear, depression, and pent-up emotions. Kawasaki (2014) cited the sharing of feelings and emotions as a beneficial nursing technique in shared decision-making situations. Patients may fear that asking questions will make them appear foolish (Jack et al., 2004), but nurses can ameliorate fear in the context of a therapeutic relationship.

Conclusion

The commitment to prevent suffering and treat total pain, see the person instead of the disease, and treat the patient and family as the unit of care are hallmarks of PC. Furthermore, the commitment to inform and facilitate self-determination and uphold autonomy is another hallmark of PC. The simultaneous care model is recommended in current practice, that is, providing PC concurrently with life-sustaining treatment. PC should be initiated at the time of a serious, life-limiting diagnosis. In addition, the reality of the need to emphasize that PC is not hospice remains.

The American Academy of Hospice and Palliative Medicine's (2008) position statement on access to palliative care and hospice states that PC should be a "fundamental component of excellent medical care, not an alternative after other approaches have been pursued." HPNA supports the stance that "all patients with a serious or life-threatening illness should have access to high-quality palliative care" (HPNA, 2013a, p. 3).

Advancing the use of PC is within the purview of nurses. Facilitating access to a team of experts who can deal with the complex problems experienced by people with serious disease is a valuable service nurses can provide. Research demonstrates that provision of PC enables patients to be more satisfied with their overall care, feel that they have improved communication with their providers, and avoid intensive care units and emergency department visits (National Quality Forum, n.d.). Furthermore, a body of evidence has now emerged demonstrating the value of PC through randomized controlled trials: increased median survival, increased mood, and decreased caregiver stress.

A great deal of literature on PC communication focuses on physician–patient communication and breaking bad news. Instead, Button, Gavin, and Keogh (2015) focused on the continual presence of nurses. Nurses help to interpret bad news and provide the gift of presence by listening to family concerns (Button et al., 2015). Communication is foundational to all nursing practice, but particularly in PC, where patients and families must confront life-limiting diagnoses.

Estimates show that by 2030 there will be twice as many older adults in the United States than in 2000 (National Quality Forum, n.d.); therefore, the need for PC services will only become more pressing. As nurse scientist Betty Ferrell (2012) stated, through PC, "we offer what the nation needs—quality, patient-centered, cost-effective, compassionate care for patients and families" (p. 447). In an environment today where Americans tend to deny death and view death as a failure of the healthcare system (Malloy et al., 2008), PC can provide a sensible and comprehensive alternative. Nurse scientist Barbara Gomes (2015), in analyzing the ENABLE III trial results, asked as the title of her editorial, "palliative care: if it makes a difference, why wait?" (p. 1420).

Many healthcare professionals provide valuable aspects of PC. Yet, throughout the present and future of PC, nurses will be an abiding presence, combining the science of expert skills with the art of caring.

Key Points

- PC and hospice are not synonymous.
- All hospice care is palliative, but not all PC is hospice.
- A team of healthcare professionals provides PC services.
- The patient and family is the *unit of care* in PC.
- PC should be offered from the time of diagnosis of a serious, life-limiting illness throughout the illness to EOL.
- Patients can receive PC while also receiving curative treatment.
- Nurses are an abiding presence in the provision of PC services.

References

American Academy of Hospice and Palliative Medicine. (2008, March 11). Position statements: Statement on access to palliative care and hospice. Retrieved from http://aahpm.org/positions/access

Bailey, F.A., & Harman, S.M. (2017, February 27). Palliative care: The last hours and days of life [Literature review current through February 2017]. Retrieved from https://www.uptodate.com/contents/palliative-care-the-last-hours-and-days-of-life

Bakitas, M.A., Tosteson, T.D., Li, Z., Lyons, K.D., Hull, J.G., Li, Z., … Ahles, T.A. (2015). Early versus delayed initiation of concurrent palliative oncology care: Patient outcomes in the ENABLE III randomized controlled trial. *Journal of Clinical Oncology, 33,* 1438–1445. doi:10.1200/JCO.2014.58.6362

Booth, S., Chin, C., & Spathis, A. (2015). The brain and breathlessness: Understanding and disseminating a palliative care approach. *Palliative Medicine, 29,* 396–398. doi:10.1177/0269216315579836

Button, E.B., Gavin, N.C., & Keogh, S.J. (2015). Exploring palliative care provision for recipients of allogeneic hematopoietic stem cell transplantation who relapsed. *Oncology Nursing Forum, 41,* 370–381. doi:10.1188/14.ONF.370-381

Cassel, E.J. (1982). The nature of suffering and the goals of medicine. *New England Journal of Medicine, 306,* 639–645. doi:10.1056/NEJM198203183061104

Center to Advance Palliative Care. (n.d.). About palliative care. Retrieved from http://www.capc.org/about/palliative-care

Center to Advance Palliative Care. (2015). Growth of palliative care in U.S. hospitals: 2015 snapshot (2000–2013). Retrieved from https://media.capc.org/filer_public/92/40/92407399-0cef-4754-8eb7-01dbeaed6946/capc_growth_snapshot_2015_final.pdf

Centers for Medicare and Medicaid Services. (2014). Center for Medicare. Retrieved from https://www.cms.gov/Medicare/Medicare-Fee-for-Service-Payment/Hospice/Downloads/March-2014-NHPCO-Slides.pdf

Centers for Medicare and Medicaid Services. (2015). *Medicare benefit policy manual.* Retrieved from https://www.cms.gov/Regulations-and-Guidance/Guidance/Manuals/downloads/bp102c09.pdf

Cope, D.G., Fulcher, C.D., Berkowitz, A., Coignet, H., Conley, S., Doherty, A., … Walker, D.K. (2016, September 1). ONS PEP resource: Anxiety. Retrieved from https://www.ons.org/practice-resources/pep/anxiety

Cope, D.G., Fulcher, C.D., Berkowitz, A., Coignet, H., Conley, S., Doherty, A., … Walker, D.K. (2017, February 27). ONS PEP resource: Depression. Retrieved from https://www.ons.org/practice-resources/pep/depression

Coyne, P.E. (2015). Symptom management of bone metastasis at end of life. *Journal of Hospice and Palliative Nursing, 17,* 183–188. doi:10.1097/NJH.0000000000000152

Delgado-Guay, M.O., Hui, D., Parsons, H.A., Govan, K., De la Cruz, M., Thorney, S., & Bruera, E. (2011). Spirituality, religiosity, and spiritual pain in advanced cancer patients. *Journal of Pain and Symptom Management, 41,* 986–994. doi:10.1016/j.jpainsymman.2010.09.017

Dionne-Odom, J.N., Azuero, A., Lyons, K.D., Hull, J.G., Tosteson, T., Li, Z., … Bakitas, M.A. (2015). Benefits of early versus delayed palliative care to informal family caregivers of patients with advanced cancer: Outcomes from the ENABLE III randomized controlled trial. *Journal of Clinical Oncology, 33,* 1446–1452. doi:10.1200/JCO.2014.58.7824

Duffy, A. (2005, April 25). A moral force: The story of Dr. Balfour Mount. *The Ottawa Citizen,* p. E8. Retrieved from http://www.virtualhospice.ca/Assets/Bal%20Mount%20article_20090310154705.pdf

Dunn, H. (n.d.). Bio. Retrieved from http://www.hankdunn.com/about/bio

Dunn, H. (2012, July 11). Hospice care too long? Retrieved from http://hankdunn.com/hospice-care-too-long

Ferrell, B. (2005). Ethical perspectives on pain and suffering. *Pain Management Nursing, 6,* 83–90. doi:10.1016/j.pmn.2005.06.001

Ferrell, B. (2012). From the editor. *Journal of Hospice and Palliative Nursing, 14,* 447. doi:10.1097/NJH.0b013e3182693387

Ferrell, B., & Coyle, N. (2008). *The nature of suffering and the goals of nursing.* New York, NY: Oxford University Press.

Ferrell, B.R., Temel, J.S., Temin, S., Alesi, E.R., Balboni, T.A., Basch, E.M., ... Smith, T.J. (2017). Integration of palliative care into standard oncology care: American Society of Clinical Oncology clinical practice guideline update. *Journal of Clinical Oncology, 35,* 96–112. doi:10.1200/JCO.2016.70.1474

Field, M.J., & Cassel, C.K. (Eds.). (1997). *Approaching death: Improving care at the end-of-life* [Report of the Institute of Medicine Task Force]. Washington, DC: National Academies Press.

Gomes, B. (2015). Palliative care: If it makes a difference, why wait? [Editorial]. *Journal of Clinical Oncology, 33,* 1420–1421. doi:10.1200/JCO.2014.60.5386

Hermsen, M.A., & Ten Have, H.A.M.J. (2005). Palliative care teams: Effective through moral reflection. *Journal of Interprofessional Care, 19,* 561–568. doi:10.1080/13561820500404871

Herr, K., Coyne, P.J., McCaffery, M., Manworren, R., & Merkel, S. (2011). Pain assessment in the patient unable to self-report: Position statement with clinical practice recommendations. *Pain Management Nursing, 12,* 230–250. doi:10.1016/j.pmn.2011.10.002

Hospice and Palliative Nurses Association. (2010). HPNA position statement: Spiritual care. Retrieved from http://hpna.advancingexpertcare.org/wp-content/uploads/2014/09/Spiritual-Care-Position-Statement-FINAL-1010.pdf

Hospice and Palliative Nurses Association. (2012). HPNA position statement: Pain management. Retrieved from http://hpna.advancingexpertcare.org/wp-content/uploads/2015/08/Pain-Management.pdf

Hospice and Palliative Nurses Association. (2013a). HPNA position statement: Assuring high quality in palliative nursing. Retrieved from http://hpna.advancingexpertcare.org/wp-content/uploads/2015/08/Assuring-High-Quality-in-Palliative-Care.pdf

Hospice and Palliative Nurses Association. (2013b). HPNA position statement: The nurse's role in advance care planning. Retrieved from http://hpna.advancingexpertcare.org/wp-content/uploads/2014/09/The_Nurses_Role_in_ACP_Position_Statement_111513.pdf

Jack, B., Hillier, V., Williams, A., & Oldham, J. (2004). Hospital-based palliative care teams improve the insight of cancer patients into their disease. *Palliative Medicine, 18,* 46–52. doi:10.1191/0268216304pm846oa

Jünger, S., Pestinger, M., Elsner, F., Krumm, N., & Radbruch, L. (2007). Criteria for successful multiprofessional cooperation in palliative care teams. *Palliative Medicine, 21,* 347–354. doi:10.1177/0269216307078505

Kass-Bartelmes, B.L., & Hughes, R. (2003). Advance care planning: Preferences for care at the end of life. *Research in Action, 12.* Retrieved from https://archive.ahrq.gov/research/findings/factsheets/aging/endliferia/endria.html

Kawasaki, Y. (2014). Consultation techniques using shared decision making for patients with cancer and their families. *Clinical Journal of Oncology Nursing, 18,* 701–706. doi:10.1188/14.CJON.701-706

Lambert, M. (2010). ICSI releases guideline on chronic pain assessment and management. *American Family Physician, 82,* 434–439. Retrieved from http://www.aafp.org/afp/2010/0815/p434.html

Légaré, F., Stacey, D., Pouliot, S., Gauvin, F.-P., Desroches, S., Kryworuchko, J., ... Graham, I.D. (2011). Interprofessionalism and shared decision-making in primary care: A stepwise approach towards a new model. *Journal of Interprofessional Care, 25,* 18–25. doi:10.3109/13561820.2010.490502

Lynch, M., Dahlin, C., Hultman, T., & Coakley, E.E. (2011). Palliative care nursing: Defining the discipline? *Journal of Hospice and Palliative Nursing, 13,* 106–111. doi:10.1097/NJH.0b013e3182075b6e

Malloy, P., Virani, R., Kelly, K., Harrington-Jacobs, H., & Ferrell, B. (2008). Seven years and 50 courses later: End-of-Life Nursing Education Consortium continues commitment to provide excellent palliative care education. *Journal of Hospice and Palliative Nursing, 10,* 233–239. doi:10.1097/01.NJH.0000319163.35596.59

Marks, R.M., & Sachar, E.J. (1973). Undertreatment of medical inpatients with narcotic analgesics. *Annals of Internal Medicine, 78,* 173–181. doi:10.7326/0003-4819-78-2-173

Medtronic. (n.d.). Improving life by easing chronic pain: Common types of chronic pain. Retrieved from http://www.medtronicneuro.com.au/chronic_pain_commontypes.html

Mehta, A., & Chan, L.S. (2008). Understanding the concept of "total pain": A prerequisite for pain control. *Journal of Hospice and Palliative Nursing, 10,* 26–32. doi:10.1097/01.NJH.0000306714.50539.1a

Meier, D.E., & Sieger, C.E. (2004). *A guide to building a hospital-based palliative care program.* New York, NY: Center to Advance Palliative Care.

National Comprehensive Cancer Network. (2017). *NCCN Clinical Practice Guidelines in Oncology (NCCN Guidelines®):*

Palliative care [v.1.2017]. Retrieved from www.nccn.org/professionals/physician_gls/pdf/palliative.pdf

National Consensus Project for Quality Palliative Care. (n.d.-a). References. Retrieved from http://www.nationalconsensusproject.org/DisplayPage.aspx?Title=References

National Consensus Project for Quality Palliative Care. (n.d.-b). Welcome. Retrieved from http://www.nationalconsensusproject.org/Default.aspx

National Hospice and Palliative Care Organization. (n.d.-a). Key hospice messages: Hospice: It's about how you live. Retrieved from http://www.nhpco.org/press-room/key-hospice-messages

National Hospice and Palliative Care Organization. (n.d.-b). Palliative care: An explanation of palliative care. Retrieved from http://www.nhpco.org/palliative-care-4

National Hospice and Palliative Care Organization. (2015). *NHPCO's facts and figures: Hospice care in America.* Retrieved from http://www.nhpco.org/sites/default/files/public/Statistics_Research/2015_Facts_Figures.pdf

National Hospice and Palliative Care Organization. (2016a, March 28). History of hospice care. Retrieved from http://www.nhpco.org/history-hospice-care

National Hospice and Palliative Care Organization. (2016b, December 16). Hospice care. Retrieved from http://www.nhpco.org/about/hospice-care

National Quality Forum. (n.d.). Palliative care and end-of-life care. Retrieved from http://www.qualityforum.org/topics/palliative_care_and_end-of-life_care.aspx

Nursing2017 drug handbook (37th ed.). (2017). Philadelphia, PA: Wolters Kluwer.

Polovich, M., Olsen, M., & LeFebvre, K.B. (Eds.). (2014). *Chemotherapy and biotherapy guidelines and recommendations for practice* (4th ed.). Pittsburgh, PA: Oncology Nursing Society.

Sherner, T. (2015). Palliative care provides support throughout treatment, not just at end of life. *ONS Connect, 30*(2), 16–20. Retrieved from http://connect.ons.org/issue/june-2015/up-front/palliative-care-provides-support-throughout-treatment-not-just-at-end-of-life

Temel, J.S., Greer, J.A., Muzikansky, A., Gallagher, E.R., Admane, S., Jackson, V.A., … Lynch, T.J. (2010). Early palliative care for patients with metastatic non–small-cell lung cancer. *New England Journal of Medicine, 363,* 733–742. doi:10.1056/NEJMoa1000678

Weissman, D.E., Morrison, R.S., & Meier, D.E. (2010). Center to Advance Palliative Care palliative care clinical care and customer satisfaction metrics consensus recommendations. *Journal of Palliative Medicine, 13,* 179–184. doi:10.1089/jpm.2009.0270

Weissman, D.E., Quill, T., & Arnold, R.M. (2015). Fast Facts and Concepts #223: The family meeting: Starting the conversation. Retrieved from http://www.mypcnow.org/blank-u77fm

Wells, N., Pasero, C., & McCaffery, M. (2008). Improving the quality of care through pain assessment and management. In R.G. Hughes (Ed.), *Patient safety and quality: An evidence-based handbook for nurses.* Retrieved from http://www.ncbi.nlm.nih.gov/books/NBK2658/#ch17.sl

Wittenberg-Lyles, E., Goldsmith, J., Ferrell, B., & Ragan, S.L. (2013). *Communication in palliative nursing.* New York, NY: Oxford University Press.

Wittenberg-Lyles, E., Goldsmith, J., & Ragan, S. (2011). The shift to early palliative care: A typology of illness journeys and the role of nursing. *Clinical Journal of Oncology Nursing, 15,* 304–310. doi:10.1188/11.CJON.304-310

World Health Organization. (n.d.-a). WHO's cancer pain ladder for adults. Retrieved from http://www.who.int/cancer/palliative/painladder/en

World Health Organization. (n.d.-b). WHO definition of palliative care. Retrieved from http://www.who.int/cancer/palliative/definition/en

Yoong, J., Park, E.R., Greer, J.A., Jackson, V.A., Gallagher, E.R., Pirl, W.F., … Temel, J.S. (2013). Early palliative care in advanced lung cancer: A qualitative study. *JAMA Internal Medicine, 173,* 283–290. doi:10.1001/jamainternmed.2013.1874

Zalonis, R., & Slota, M. (2014). The use of palliative care to promote autonomy in decision making. *Clinical Journal of Oncology Nursing, 18,* 707–711. doi:10.1188/14.CJON.707-711

Chapter 31 Study Questions

1. The concept of "total pain" is used in palliative care because:
   A. Patients with serious illness have a great deal of pain.
   B. Patients receiving palliative care find pain crippling.
   C. Families have difficulty in dealing with the pain of serious illness.
   D. This concept encompasses pain in body, mind, and spirit.

2. The simultaneous care model in palliative care enables:
   A. A number of different treatments.
   B. Life-sustaining treatment concurrently with comfort care.
   C. Comfort care to overwhelm life-sustaining treatment.
   D. Provision of palliative care after all curative interventions have been exhausted.

3. Which of the following is a primary vehicle used by the palliative care team to promote patient preferences and goals?
   A. Teamwork
   B. Family meeting
   C. Medication regimen
   D. Chaplain's services

4. The 3 C's of palliative care are:
   A. Consensus, continuity, and communication.
   B. Communication, creativity, and consensus.
   C. Communication, collaboration, and continuity.
   D. Congruence, collaboration, and consensus.

5. Temel et al. (2010) demonstrated that early initiation of palliative care:
   A. Took away hope.
   B. Freed the patient from pain.
   C. Increased median survival.
   D. Made family members depressed.

CHAPTER

32 Psychosocial Issues

Ellen Giarelli, EdD, RN, CRNP

Introduction

Cancer is a whole-body disease affecting the body, mind, and spirit. Patients will experience the burdens imposed by this disease differently and can take acute or chronic paths. Family members and formal caregivers may share the emotional consequences as patients traverse the cancer trajectory from symptom identification to the end of life (Holland, 1982). In 2005, Kazak proposed a general model of prevention informed by work with children with a cancer diagnosis and their families. The model proposed that all illnesses and trauma have psychosocial consequences. Applying this model to cancer care in general, all individuals affected with any cancer, and members of their families, are at risk to suffer from psychosocial consequences and must deal with the issues surrounding end-of-life care (Douglas & Daly, 2014; Dy et al., 2011).

The term *psychosocial* refers to one's psychological state or development in interactions with a social environment. *Psychology* is the study of mental processes and behavior. The *social environment*, or *context*, is the influence of social position, roles, culture, and relationships that as a whole may influence the psychology.

Contrasted with social psychology, which attempts to explain social patterns of behavior in a general sense, the concept of *psychosocial* is used to describe the unique internal processes that occur within the individual. It often is discussed in the context of psychosocial interventions, which may be behavioral, educational, or pharmacologic (Baltrusch & Waltz, 1985) and employ technology (Kaltenbaugh et al., 2015).

A growing body of research supports the integration of body and mind such that they are now considered inseparable. Nummenmaa, Glerean, Hari, and Hietanen (2014) demonstrated that emotions are felt in the body, and somatosensory feedback may trigger conscious emotional experiences by mapping bodily sensations associated with different emotions after stimulating an emotion. They further illustrated that this somatosensory system is culturally universal. While their study demonstrated that emotions affect the physical body, corresponding studies have linked emotional consequences to disease, and emotional pathologies to specific brain regions (Carlson et al., 2015; Denollet et al., 2006). Conversations about the mind–body phenomenon are at the heart of medicine and the soul of cancer care.

Both patients and family members may be affected and have feelings of anger, fear, uncertainty, sadness, hopelessness, distress, loneliness, grief, and relief. Mental health may be compromised by anxiety and depression, while social problems are largely interpersonal and economic. The family that faces a cancer diagnosis may experience interpersonal discord, loss of emotional support and partnership, and economic burdens from the loss of employment and the high costs of care. Bultz and Carlson (2005), among others (e.g., Salmon, Clark, McGrath, & Fisher, 2015), have labeled emotional distress as the sixth vital sign in cancer care. Every kind of cancer, mode of therapy, or cluster of symptoms carries with it psychosocial issues. For example, individuals treated with targeted therapy to inhibit epithelial growth factors will likely develop acne-like facial rashes that may generate extreme embarrassment and lead to social isolation. The facial disfigurement caused by head and neck cancer causes profound psychological trauma and has a significant impact on self-esteem (Callahan, 2004; Coffman, 2015). In another example, a person with lung cancer may feel guilty for having smoked cigarettes despite warnings from family and friends. This person's caregivers may be angry and blame the patient for "causing" his own suffering (Lobchuk, McClement, McPherson, & Cheang, 2008; MacNeil et al., 2010).

With the advent of cancer predisposition genetic testing came a new set of psychological problems. For the patient with breast and ovarian cancer syndrome, familial adenomatous polyposis, or multiple endocrine neoplasia, the cancer trajectory may begin with presymptomatic risk assessment and determination of genetic mutation carrier status. Knowledge of such risk may generate fear, worry, and other psychosocial consequences perhaps decades before the onset of disease, or even when the development of cancer is not absolute. People who are offered predisposition testing must struggle with the choice to know their risk. If one chooses to know, he or she may face a different kind of fear of the future and potential loss of a loved one.

A new area of research examines the motivations of individuals who seek genetic testing, as well as its impact on risk perception and self-concept. Motivators appear to influence a person's adherence to and decision making about preventive strategies and lifestyle changes. This domain of psychosocial research promises to offer insights that may be applied to improve risk prevention (Bleiker, Esplen, Meiser, Petersen, & Patenaude, 2013).

Every aspect of cancer care will have psychological and social correlates that are inseparable and, to varying degrees, may closely follow the clinical course.

Conceptualizing Psychosocial Aspects

A number of methods exist to conceptualize psychosocial issues in cancer care and guide the management of psychosocial problems. One way is to use a systems approach, which considers the individual in the context of social systems, such as the family, the healthcare community, and the larger social network. A systems approach allows for the selective study and treatment of psychosocial problems at the interface of patients with their immediate and extended family members, friends, employers, and associates in larger cultural and social networks.

A robust body of literature supports a family-centered approach to psychosocial issues and a careful consideration of the role of culture, race, and ethnicity (Lillie et al., 2014). Over the decades, studies of family responses to cancer have shown strong evidence of family distress (Bachner, O'Rourke, & Carmel, 2011; Baider & De-Nour, 1988; Germino et al., 1998; Haase & Phillips, 2004; Lewis & Deal, 1995; Pellegrino et al., 2010) along with shared decision making (Obeidat, Homish, & Lally, 2013). Multiple factors influence couple and family adjustment (Hilton, 1993; Hilton, Crawford, & Tarko, 2000; Lewis, 1993), and distress among family members influences psychosocial issues for patients (Given & Given, 1992; Heiniger, Butow, Price, & Charles, 2013) and especially parents (Long & Marsland, 2011; Miedema, Hamilton, Fortin, Easley, & Matthews, 2010).

When using a systems approach, a nurse may identify a recipient of psychosocial interventions within concentric circles of care, and at any time treatment may be directed to a patient or a combination of the patient and his or her relations. This approach acknowledges that individuals who know, love, and care for the person with cancer will attempt to apprehend that person's reality and empathize with the person who is suffering. Figure 32-1 is an illustration of how concentric circles of care can be used to identify and plan nursing care.

Another model, the Human Response to Illness Model (Mitchell, Gallucci, & Fought, 1991; Nesbitt & Sawatzky, 2009), provides a comprehensive framework to explain how psychosocial factors interact with physiologic processes. In this model, psychosocial variables are depicted as interacting with psychological, pathophysiologic, behavioral, and experiential perspectives. Psychosocial processes that may generate stress or distress, such as coping and finding meaning in illness, and the availability of social support may have a direct or indirect influence on health and illness (McCance, Forshee, & Shelby, 2006; Milberg, Wåhlberg, & Krevers, 2014; Miller & Schnoll, 2000; Rolland & Williams, 2005). Hansen and Sawatzky (2008) proposed that a sufficiently intense and unresolved stress response may lead to pathology and exacerbate existing illness. Referring to this model allows oncology nurses to expand their focus to include the following (Cohen, Jenkins, Holston, & Carlson, 2013):

- Impact of psychological distress on symptoms and disease progression in the patient
- Impact of psychological distress among family members at risk for cancer
- Role of culture, spirituality or religion, and other support networks and social relationships on cancer-related psychological distress
- Health literacy as a complex of understanding and proactive decision making for optimal patient-centered outcomes

Figure 32-1. Concentric Circles of Psychosocial Care in Oncology Nursing

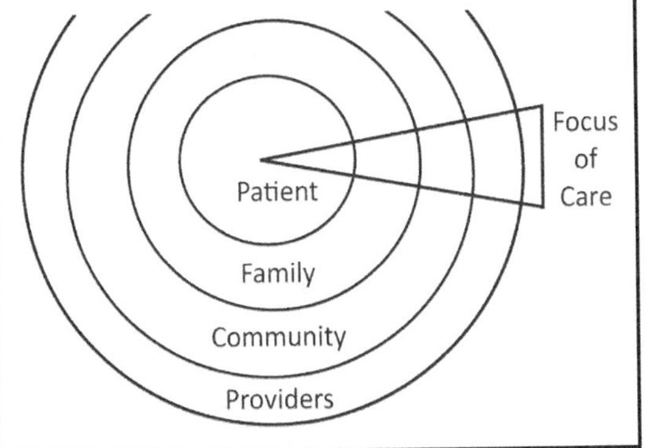

Another approach is to conceptualize and manage psychosocial aspects of cancer as occurring over time. The natural path of any long-lasting disease or health condition can be thought of as proceeding in phases. This concept of time provides nurses with a way to think longitudinally about the course of the illness for patients and families. With this approach, nurses may examine the evolution of psychological pathology and illness in affected and unaffected family members as a consequence of a loved one's cancer diagnosis.

The most common progression is from crisis (or onset) to chronic to terminal. For example, with the advent of presymptomatic genetic testing, the natural trajectory of illness has shifted. A patient and family may experience additional psychosocial crises at the points of genetic testing, post-testing counseling, and prior to any symptomatology (Kinney et al., 2014; Rolland, 1999). Patients and families may experience long stretches of chronic psychological distress as they presumptively wait for symptoms to begin and the genotype to be expressed. Living day to day with the burdens of disease may be exhausting physically, emotionally, and socially.

This chapter takes a temporal and noncategorical approach to psychosocial issues. The temporal appraisal follows psychosocial factors from prediagnosis to disease recurrence or metastasis. The noncategorical appraisal considers that the diagnosis of cancer, in general, is followed by certain emotions and behavioral responses.

Psychosocial issues are continually studied by clinicians and researchers who adjust the variables to examine experiences based on age, sex, diagnosis, treatment setting, treatment approaches, and contextual factors, and tailor research designs to selected populations. However, the fundamental underlying psychosocial issues are universal and enduring. The most important habit of mind for oncology nurses to develop is to expect that patients and families will experience some version of psychosocial distress as a result of the diagnosis. Nurses must understand basic concepts, search the most contemporary evidence, and prepare to intervene based on patients' and families' specific and individual set of circumstances. The nurse has a significant role in all aspects of cancer care, and psychosocial care in particular (Sheldon, Harris, & Arcieri, 2012).

Traumatic Events in the Cancer Trajectory

Psychological trauma is a type of damage to one's mental state that occurs as a result of a traumatic event. Such an event may be a brief experience, a series of experiences, or chronic negative experiences that overwhelm a person's ability to cope or integrate the events with one's life. Many aspects of cancer care, from diagnosis to treatment, can be traumatic. Along the cancer continuum, certain events are more likely to be experienced as traumatic: learning one's risk for cancer; finding a sign of cancer; waiting for test results; learning the diagnosis; treatment aspects (awaiting, changing, and ending treatment; dealing with side effects; and treatment failure); recurrence, progression, or metastasis; and facing death.

Cancer and Post-Traumatic Stress Disorder

People who experience a trauma have four traits in common: the event was unexpected; the event was psychologically overwhelming; the person was unprepared or unable to cope with it; and the person felt he or she could do nothing to prevent or mitigate the event (Feldman, Sorocco, & Bratkovich, 2014; Kangas, Henry, & Bryant, 2002; Smith, Redd, Peyser, & Vogl, 1999). The event does not determine whether an experience is traumatic; rather, it is the subjective interpretation by that person. Based on this definition, the number of reports of post-traumatic stress disorder (PTSD) among cancer survivors and their relatives is growing (Kangas et al., 2002; Mehnert & Koch, 2007; Smith et al., 1999; Yi & Kim, 2014). The risk of PTSD for parental caregivers of children with cancer is especially high. In general, parents do adjust and cope with their child's cancer, but a significant majority experience post-traumatic stress symptoms (Jones, 2012). In addition, cultural factors may influence how an individual manifests distress.

Shim and Park (2012) found that having no religion, impaired levels of overall functioning, and "multiple psychological morbidities," including PTSD, were associated with suicidality in Korean patients with cancer. Survivorship issues have become and will remain an important area of research as treatments improve (Badger et al., 2011; Haj Mohammad et al., 2015; Santin, Treanor, Mills, & Donnelly, 2014). The cancer experience is highly complex, and labeling it as a trauma is still under scrutiny.

Psychosocial Impact Along the Cancer Trajectory

Most patients undergoing cancer treatment and their families experience periods of distress that correspond with the clinical course of cancer. For a small portion of patients, psychomorbidity or severe psychiatric problems may occur that require referral for psychiatric intervention. According to the National Comprehensive Cancer Network® (NCCN®), "Distress is a multifactorial unpleasant emotional experience of a psychological (i.e., cognitive, behavioral, emotional), social, and/or spiritual nature that may interfere with the ability to cope effectively with cancer, its physical symptoms, and its treatment" (NCCN, 2016, p. DIS-2). Distress ranges from common and normal feelings, such as distraction, difficulty concentrating, and loss of appetite, to problems that are disabling, such as despair and cognitive dysfunction. An individual's response to distress can be "normal" and anticipated, or extreme and disabling (see Figure 32-2). In the practical sense, by observing patients and families across the life span and by position on the cancer trajectory, oncology nurses can identify times when their interventions may have the greatest therapeutic effect. In the theoretical sense, it allows researchers and clinicians to observe changes over time in response to disease and treatment. Varied aspects of normal living are affected, such as sexuality, the experience of pain, cognitive function, and development in children, because many cancers are being redefined as chronic rather than acute, life-threatening conditions (Morse & Fife, 1996).

Psychosocial Response to Learning One's Risk

It is estimated that 5%–10% of all cancers are due to a genetic predisposition (National Cancer Institute [NCI], 2015). Many studies have been conducted to evaluate a person's risk for cancer syndromes, such as hereditary breast and ovarian cancer (HBOC) syndrome, Lynch syndrome and colorectal cancers, multiple endocrine neoplasia, and melanoma. The principles of risk assessment and reporting of findings are shared across patient populations. Findings from one set of studies (i.e., assess-

Figure 32-2. Parameters of Psychosocial Distress in Cancer Care

Normal and Common Feelings
- Vulnerability
- Uncertainty
- Sadness
- Nervousness
- Worry
- Anger
- Fear
- Guilt
- Grief

Common Psychosocial Consequences
- Impaired sleep
- Impaired appetite, temporary loss of appetite
- Mental distraction
- Difficulty concentrating
- Impaired body image
- Loss of interest in usual activities (temporary)
- Loss of interest in sexual relations (temporary)
- Questioning and asking "why"
- Limiting social contact
- Family discord/disruption

Disabling Feelings
- Clinical depression
- Severe anxiety
- Panic
- Extreme anger, outbursts
- Existential and spiritual crisis
- Hopelessness, despair

Disabling Responses
- Sleep disorder (long-standing)
- Eating disorders
- Sexual dysfunction (without physiologic or anatomic etiology)
- Loss of faith
- Social isolation and withdrawal from family and friends
- Anhedonia
- Rejection of help
- Abuse or neglect
- Preoccupation with loss and death
- Suicidal ideation

ment of women at risk for HBOC) apply to other cohorts of patients.

Women who participate in cancer risk assessment experience unexpected feelings and the need for help in navigating their healthcare future and finding social support (Crotser & Dickerson, 2010). Some women at risk for HBOC are at increased risk for elevated levels of psychological distress that includes intrusive thoughts, compromised well-being, and avoidance (Schwartz et al., 2002); the study authors predicted that such women would benefit from additional, tailored support. Den Heijer et al. (2013) implemented a tailored support system for a cohort of women undergoing breast cancer risk assessment and reported a significant reduction in the participants' feelings of intrusion and avoidance. They further identified that predictors of long-term distress were passive and palliative coping styles, excessive breast self-examination, and overestimation of breast cancer risk (den Heijer et al., 2013).

Despite concerns about the likelihood of negative psychological responses to genetic testing for disease risk (Lerman et al., 1998), no systematic negative long-term psychological outcomes have been demonstrated (Hamilton, Lobel, & Moyer, 2009; Heshka, Palleschi, Howley, Wilson, & Wells, 2008). Reports in the literature have attributed this to (a) the success of genetic counseling in facilitating adaptation, (b) receiving genetic results as the benefits of reducing uncertainty regarding risk, and (c) provision of information to guide screening and prevention decisions (Heiniger et al., 2013; Lammens et al., 2010; van Asperen et al., 2002). These optimistic reports emphasize the role that healthcare providers, including nurses, play in the pre- and post-testing counseling process.

Nurses have important roles in assessing support networks of individuals seeking cancer risk assessment, providing anticipatory guidance on risk communication, and remaining sensitive to the impact of cancer screening and risk analysis on a patient's self-concept, hope, and psychological well-being. Crotser and Dickerson (2010) called for more research to examine cancer risk communication among diverse groups of women.

Family Cluster Effect

The participation of family members is a desired outcome in cancer care because of the role of social support in well-being. Lapointe et al. (2012) examined this effect on psychosocial variables in families undergoing *BRCA1* and *BRCA2* genetic testing for cancer susceptibility. They reported that family cluster effects reached significance for the majority of behavioral and psychosocial variables associated with predisposition testing, including perceived health status, general distress, psychological adjustment, risk perception, and motivation for genetic testing, regardless of family size. They concluded that this effect should be routinely accounted for when studying psychosocial aspects of genetic testing. By extension, one may presume that the family cluster effect should also be routinely accounted for when evaluating the psychosocial consequences along the patient's cancer trajectory and the content and process of psychosocial interventions.

Spirituality and Religion

NCI (2016) defined *religion* as a set of beliefs and practices associated with an organized group, and *spirituality* as the search for ultimate meaning through religion or other paths. Spiritual distress is unresolved religious or spiritual conflict and doubt that may arise from the diagnosis of cancer.

Approximately 50%–90% of patients with cancer view religion and spirituality as personally important, and association has been demonstrated between spirituality and improved coping and quality of life (Balboni et al., 2007). For example, high spirituality may reduce anxiety, mitigate sadness and the sense of isolation, help a person cope with effects of treatment, and allow a person to feel personal growth as a consequence of living with cancer (Lillis, 2014). Stephenson and Berry (2014) conducted an extensive review of the literature to conclude that substantive evidence supports that uncertainty and spirituality may coexist and blend to influence a patient's experiences, especially at the end of life. Spirituality and religion recur in the literature as key determinants of enhanced coping and improved resilience and mitigators of distress among patients with cancer and their families.

Responses to Diagnosis

The diagnosis of a life-threatening illness causes emotional distress for patients and their family members. The threat to life and security is real, and fear is an appropriate response. The patient will fear physical, emotional, and social harm. Weisman and Worden (1977) described the first 100 days after the initial diagnosis as a period of existential crisis. The crisis is a state of panic or feeling of intense emotional discomfort. It comes from a sense of being alone and isolated and the realization of one's own mortality. During this time, patients may be deeply concerned or preoccupied with issues of life, death, and purpose. Parents experience similar feelings (Sulkers et al., 2015).

Family members face similar fears. Fear becomes irrational when the depth and strength of the emotion does not match the probable consequences of the illness. Among members of families with hereditary cancers, those who were ineligible for genetic testing experienced more cancer-related distress than tested individuals, and cancer-related emotional distress was lower, in general, among those who declined testing (Heiniger et al., 2013).

Responses to Treatment

Patients treated with surgery, chemotherapy, and radiation therapy will experience some, or many, long-term side effects that can impair quality of life. Caregivers of patients similarly experience stress and distress as they observe the daily and sometimes unrelenting physical effects on their loved ones. For example, in studies of patients with testicular cancer and their partners, authors have reported that patients (and couples) experienced the start of chemotherapy as the most psychologically stressful point in the cancer continuum, causing problems in social and physical functioning and mental health (Tuinman et al., 2007; Vidrine et al., 2010). Adjustment patterns differed between patients and their partners, with patients reporting a low quality of life after the completion of chemotherapy. For most couples, the quality of life returned to normal levels one year after diagnosis, but a minority needed clinical attention for severe stress response. After a traumatic experience with treatment, a person may reexperience the mental and physical anguish and avoid reminders, or triggers, of the experience.

Hospitalization and beginning treatment contributes to depressive symptoms. In a study of patients beginning chemotherapy, Wedding et al. (2007) observed that female patients, patients with solid tumors, and those with functional limitations had significantly higher scores for somatic and affective depressive symptoms on the Beck Depression Inventory. Depression has been studied extensively among patients diagnosed with cancer (Robinson, Kissane, Brooker, & Burney, 2015; Walker & Sharpe, 2014) and remains one of the most significant psychosocial consequences of a cancer diagnosis.

Among children with cancer, the psychosocial impact of treatment can be stressful for patients, parents, and siblings (Sulkers et al., 2015). According to McCaffrey (2006), major stressors for children with cancer were treatment procedures, especially chemotherapy; loss of control; the hospital environment; relapses; and fear of dying. Parents and siblings (depending on their age) will variably apprehend the child's distressing experiences and may agonize about anticipated psychosocial issues, such as dealing with altered body image, assault to the child's self-esteem, and transition back into "ordinary" life.

Nurses are in the best position to screen for distress during treatments and provide early intervention to improve health outcomes and quality of life. Mahendran et al. (2014) found that nurses who received training in managing psychosocial issues during cancer care obtained positive gains in applied knowledge and practice behaviors that were sustained over three months. The authors predicted that these gains would eventually lead to staff empowerment and care improvement.

Response to Recurrence and Metastasis

Of all the phases of cancer, recurrence or metastasis may induce the most disturbing feelings. These events can bring the loss of hope for recovery, intense fears of death, and difficulty continuing to manage the emotional consequences and deteriorating functional ability (Andersen, Shapiro, Farrar, Crespin, & Wells-Digregorio, 2005; Given & Given, 1992; Mahon & Casperson, 1995; Mahon, Cella, & Donovan, 1990; Paiva, Souza, & Paiva, 2015).

Not all people experience recurrence the same way. Yang, Thornton, Shapiro, and Andersen (2008) found that in patients with breast cancer, in the year after recurrence, physical health and functioning showed no improvement, whereas quality of life and mood generally improved and stress declined. Compared to a first diagnosis, recurrence caused significantly lower anxiety and confusion. The authors concluded that despite physical burden, patients with recurrent breast cancer exhibited resilience, and some showed steady improvement in psychological adjustment. Over time, the management of physical symptoms becomes especially important to facilitate coping.

With many cancers now being considered chronic diseases, the terms *recurrence* and *metastasis* are perceived differently, as well. Instead of approaching cancer as a finite phenomenon, nurses may help patients with the psychosocial experience of "living with cancer." Lang, France, Williams, Humphris, and Wells (2013) conceptualized core psychosocial experiences that occur when patients must adapt to cancer as a chronic condition. These are uncertainty and waiting for the future, disruption of daily life, diminished self, making sense of the experience, sharing the burden, and finding a path. The issue that dominated the experiences of this group of patients was the day-to-day challenges compounded by social and existential change. Patients' sense of self and perceptions of the future were affected by whether they saw life as diminished, merely changed, or enhanced by the experience of cancer.

Caregiver-Specific Responses

Several factors are associated with caregivers' responses to a patient's cancer. The multiple roles held by caregivers, such as employee, parent, spouse, or child, influence their psychological adjustment over the patient's cancer trajectory. Kim, Baker, Spillers, and Wellisch (2006) studied the relationship among caregiver roles and adjustment and reported that the more social roles a caregiver carries out, the more likely that the caregiver will experience stress and negative effects. Caregivers may experience sleep disorders, reduced employment and income, social withdrawal, and physical problems.

Among family caregivers, those with more limited social networks, those with more restriction in their daily activities, and those who were younger reported the highest burden (Goldstein et al., 2004; Jones, Whitford, & Bond, 2015; Utne, Miaskowski, Paul, & Rustøen, 2013). Young caregivers with low income and limited education are at greater risk for psychosocial stress when their dependent member (e.g., spouse, child, parent) is diagnosed (Lewis & Deal, 1995; Northouse, Katapodi, Song, Zhang, & Mood, 2010; Palos et al., 2011). Nurses can be instrumental in helping family members deal with the burdens of caregiving (see Figure 32-3).

Nursing Management of Psychosocial Aspects

Assessment

To be effective in a therapeutic relationship, oncology nurses must learn how to assess a patient's ability to adjust to the new diagnosis, treatment, recurrence, or prognosis. Nurses may help patients and family members to recognize, accept, and work through their negative feelings. Healthcare professionals are responsible for identifying those who need additional help to deal with psychological distress.

Some psychosocial responses to cancer may be present at any time and affect quality of life; therefore, they should be evaluated as a matter of routine. NCCN advocates that distress, like pain, "should be recognized, monitored, documented, and treated promptly at all stages of disease and in all settings" (NCCN, 2016, p. DIS-3). NCCN created a Distress Thermometer that quickly and easily measures distress on a 0–10 scale. An accompanying problem checklist aids in identifying etiologies, such as practical, spiritual, physical, emotional, and familial problems. NCCN recommends that patients complete these screening tools at each visit and that clinicians review the outcome. The Distress Thermometer and problem checklist screening tools are available online (see NCCN, 2016). Clinical pathways are available for treating the etiologies or distress using a multidisciplinary approach (Vitek, Rosenzweig, & Stollings, 2007). Instruments are available for research and clinical practice to assess anxiety (Spielberger, 1983), mood (McNair, Lorr, & Droppleman, 1971), impact of an event (Horowitz, Wilner, & Alvarez, 1979), perceived stress (Cohen, Kamarck, & Mermelstein, 1983), coping (Folkman & Lazarus, 1985), quality of life (Ferrans, 1990), and depression (Sellick & Edwardson, 2007). Tools also are available to evaluate the psychosocial impact on informal (family) caregivers, including the Caregiver Burden Scale (Stetz, 1987) and the Caregiver Quality of Life Index (Weitzner & McMillan, 1999). Another useful instrument for screening is the Brief Symptom Inventory (Derogatis, 2008). This tool is used to collect patient-reported data and to help support clinical decision making at intake and during the treatment course in multiple settings. The Brief Symptom Inventory assesses psychological problems and progress over time.

Figure 32-3. Family Caregiver Responses and Goals

Responses
- Sleep problems
- Marital problems
- Reduced employment
- Social isolation
- Depression
- Guilt
- Anxiety
- Physical symptoms
- Fatigue

Goals
- Set realistic expectations for self as caregiver.
- Set realistic expectations for loved one with cancer.
- Plan time for self.
- Make time for family.
- Talk about feelings.
- Seek out and use community resources.
- Manage emotions.

Depression Versus Fatigue

Differentiation between fatigue and depression is needed, as patients may feel both. Fatigue is one of the most common symptoms in the cancer experience and is more prevalent than clinical depression (Jacobs & Piper, 1995). People who are fatigued may experience low energy, low motivation, anhedonia (the "total loss of feeling pleasure in normally pleasurable acts" [*Dorland's Illustrated Medical Dictionary*, 2007, p. 92]), decreased sex drive, and decreased concentration. A person who is depressed may express feelings of worthlessness, self-loathing, shame, guilt, suicidal ideation, and a wish to hasten death.

Quality of Life

Quality of life is a broad concept that reflects a subjective evaluation of well-being. Quality of life is a critical construct in psychosocial oncology. Health-related quality of life is a multidimensional experience that incorporates psychological and social adjustment and well-being. One's health-related quality of life is a function of the extent of the perceived gap between expectations and experiences surrounding the four dimensions of well-being (psychological, physical, social, and spiritual) (Padilla, Mishel, & Grant, 1992). As Ferrell and Coyle (2008) attested, "Suffering is common across phases of cancer. It is thoroughly individual and intensely personal" (p. 241), and witnessing suffering is the everyday work of nurses. Wise oncology nurses anticipate the probability that a patient is suffering and are ever-vigilant for signs of psychological suffering that may affect quality of life. Nurses should ask as they observe: what is the patient saying and not saying, and how is the patient acting? The answers to these questions will uncover the impact of an event.

Psychosocial Interventions

Interventions have been developed for distress during different phases of the cancer trajectory, from diagnosis through active treatment to end of life (Carlson & Bultz, 2003; Grov & Valeberg, 2012; Watson, 1995). The types of treatment available are listed in Figure 32-4. Lewis (2004) recommended that psychosocial research, and thereafter, interventions, should focus on the family system because interventions targeted to individuals have the potential to benefit the family as a whole and vice versa. The overall aim of family-centered interventions is to maintain family function and integrity as best as possible. This can be accomplished using psychoeducational approaches. Teaching problem-solving skills may prevent psychosocial morbidity (Bultz, Speca, Brasher, Geggie, & Page, 2000; Sahler et al., 2013).

Figure 32-4. Treatment for Psychosocial Distress

Types of Psychosocial Interventions	Means to Deliver
• Professional counseling • Peer counseling, with professional assistance • Peer and/or professional support • Cognitive behavioral therapy – Short-term, situational – Long-term, coping and adaptation	• Print materials • Peer-modeling videos • One-on-one, telephone • In person, one-on-one • In person, family based • In person, support group

Psychosocial interventions lower anxiety, improve perceived social support, and improve immune function among patients with cancer (Andersen et al., 2004). Interventions may include strategies to reduce stress, improve mood, alter health behaviors, and maintain adherence to cancer treatment and care.

Psychoeducation

Psychoeducation is also called *reeducation* and sometimes is referred to as *cognitive reframing.* It refers to the education offered to people who suffer from a psychological disturbance. The principle behind psychoeducation is that the more knowledge patients have of their illness, the better they will be able to live with their condition. Most often, psychoeducational training involves patients with emotional or psychiatric disorders such as schizophrenia, clinical depression, anxiety, eating disorders, and personality disorders (Bäuml, Froböse, Kraemer, Rentrop, & Pitschel-Walz, 2006; Hogarty et al., 1991). However, psychoeducation has been used with patients with physical illnesses. Patients' own strengths, resources, and coping skills are identified and reinforced to avoid relapse and contribute to their own health and wellness on a long-term basis. It may be difficult for patients and some family members to accept the diagnosis; therefore, one specific use of psychoeducation is to destigmatize the psychological and social responses to a diagnosis of cancer and thereby diminish some barriers to treatment. Through an improved view of the causes and effects of the illness and treatment and short- and long-term expectations, patients and families gain a broader view of the overall illness. Figure 32-5 lists some elements of psychoeducation.

Cognitive Behavioral Stress Management

Cognitive behavioral therapy (CBT) emphasizes the relationship among thinking, feeling, and doing. CBT deals with the way people manipulate their thoughts and feelings, which they attach to their past, present, or future, and explores the maladaptive connections between these thoughts and feelings, which the person may not notice independently. CBT helps people to realize and identify negative, destructive thoughts and feelings and work on changing them into healthy and productive ones, along with changing their behavior patterns from maladaptive to adaptive ones (Epstein, 2006; Ledley, 2005; León-Pizarro et al., 2007).

CBT targets problem areas and helps individuals to develop effective problem-solving techniques. The therapist and client work collaboratively on problem identification, treatment planning, and outcome evaluation. The client is taught how to use different kinds of relaxation techniques, such as deep diaphragmatic breathing, progressive muscle relaxation, and the tension-and-release approach (Epstein, 2006; Ledley, 2005; León-Pizarro et al., 2007).

Research is ongoing and has produced mixed results. In a systematic review of seven CBT studies, short-term improvement was found in depressive symptoms in patients with

Figure 32-5. Elements of Psychoeducation

Information Transfer
- Symptoms of the disease
  - Physical signs
  - Emotional consequences
  - Social impact, including effect on family system
- Etiologic factors contributing to cancer development
  - Behavior
  - Exposure
  - Genetics
  - Epigenetics
- Treatment concepts
  - Options available
  - Advantages and disadvantages
  - Risks and benefits
  - Expected responses
  - Short- and long-term expectations
  - Follow-up care
  - Inheritance/childbearing issues
  - Lifelong quality of life

Emotional Issues
- Identifying/understanding feelings in self
- Identifying/understanding the feelings expressed by others
- Managing personal emotional responses
- Dealing with the emotional reactions of others
- Exchange of experiences with others

Supportive Care
- Medication with psychotherapeutics
  - Antidepressants
  - Anxiolytics
  - Mood stabilizers
  - Other
- Medication to mitigate contributing factors
  - Analgesics for pain
  - Antipyretics for fever
  - Antibiotics for infections
- Medication interaction effects
- Cooperation approach to problem solving, and adherence to treatment recommendations
- Assistance in self-help
  - Training in self-monitoring
  - Training of family members in patient monitoring

prostate cancer (Chien, Liu, Chien, & Liu, 2014). However, findings are equivocal: some reported favorable outcomes (Brothers, Yang, Strunk, & Andersen, 2011; Guo et al., 2013), while others reported no effect (Boesen et al., 2011; Groarke, Curtis, & Kerin, 2013; Korstjens et al., 2011; Serfaty, Wilkinson, Freeman, Mannix, & King, 2012). The format, frequency, and timing of the intervention program varied across studies. Content also can be diverse and often includes education or relaxation-training activities. These varied methodological approaches may have contributed to inconsistent results across studies.

A psychotherapist determines whether a particular client may benefit from this approach. CBT can be used with many patients with cancer and their family members across age ranges and presenting problems. CBT has been favored among clinicians, and intervention protocols often include stress management treatments to reduce social disruption, increase emotional well-being, generate positive mental states and benefit finding, foster positive lifestyle changes, and reinforce positive affect (Epstein, 2006; Ledley, 2005; León-Pizarro et al., 2007). Antoni et al. (2006) reported beneficial effects on stress management after 199 women newly treated for breast cancer received an intervention comprising these aspects. Furthermore, CBT can be self-administered (Krischer, Xu, Meade, & Jacobsen, 2007). Specific techniques include guided imagery and relaxation (Nunes et al., 2007) and positive self-talk (Schnur & Montgomery, 2008). CBT is useful for pain management, self-image, hot flashes, and insomnia, among other symptoms (Epstein & Dirksen, 2007). The two approaches, individual and group therapy, are best applied based on the specific and individual needs of the patients or the social group (i.e., family and family dynamics).

Psychotherapy and Disclosure

Disclosure is the release of previously unshared or unexpressed thoughts and feelings resulting in reduced psychological work to repress unpleasant thoughts or emotions. According to Pennebaker and Seagal (1999), translating distress into language helps people to move through and beyond a negative experience such as cancer. It also may occur through expressive writing. Laccetti (2007) found that using positive-affect words was related to emotional well-being for patients with cancer attempting to reintegrate the experience with life.

Benefit Finding and Finding Meaning

One of the most significant acts of supportive care for patients and families is to help them clarify "meaning" in the context of cancer. Kim, Schulz, and Carver (2007) identified six domains of benefit finding in caregiving: acceptance, empathy, appreciation, family, positive self-view, and reprioritization. The researchers reported that actively accepting what happened and appreciating new relationships with others improved caregivers' adaptation.

Dignity Therapy

Some work has been done in examining a novel intervention called *dignity therapy*, which is designed to address psychosocial and existential distress among terminally ill patients. Dignity therapy invites a patient to discuss issues that matter most or that he or she would most want to be remembered by others. Dignity therapy redirects the patient's thoughts to the individual's self-worth, self-respect, and desired esteem (Chochinov et al., 2005).

Improving Quality of Life

Cella (1991) suggested four ways to improve quality of life for a patient: treat the disease, treat the symptoms and side effects, enhance communications, and reframe attitudes. In the context of psychosocial oncology, enhancing communication and reframing attitudes will have the greatest impact on psychosocial well-being. Oncology nurses may intervene by continually exploring how the experience of cancer is evolving over time and help patients to align their expectations (for cure, for health, for relief, for social relationships) with the actual experience (prognosis, availability of palliation, functional changes). This realigning helps patients to adjust their attitudes and modify expectations.

Spiritual Care

Oncology nurses should respectfully support patients' use of spiritual coping during the illness and encourage them to speak with their clergy or spiritual leader, if relevant, or refer them to the hospital chaplain or a support group that addresses spiritual issues during illness (Balboni et al., 2007; Lin & Bauer-Wu, 2003). Culture and spirituality may be included in the assessment and provide fundamental information on a system of support that is not well understood but known to be important. Nurses may consider the family cluster effect at the onset of assessment and conduct a comprehensive family evaluation. The family's coping style, experiences of distress, and overall perceptions of cancer and cancer care will inevitably influence the patient's psychosocial response.

A spiritual assessment will contribute to best-practice nursing care. It may include questions related to the following: religious affiliation, if any; beliefs or philosophy of life, spirituality, or religion as a source of strength; participation in a religious community; the use of prayer or meditation; loss of faith; and concerns about death, the afterlife, and end-of-life planning (Lewis, 2008; NCI, 2016).

Supportive Psychotherapy and Supportive Social Networks

Personal support has been associated with reducing symptom distress, decreasing hopelessness, and improving quality of life. Families also have important roles in providing supportive care to patients with cancer. Manning-Walsh (2005) reported that social support from family members and friends helped to decrease the negative effects of symptoms. Hopelessness is negatively correlated with social support, such that the more family members and friends can be involved in a supportive way, the less likely a patient is to experience hopelessness (Tan & Karabulutlu, 2005). Steginga, Pinnock, Gardner, Gardiner, and Dunn (2005) reported that among men with prostate cancer, peer support was rated positively by most men, and a high satisfaction with support groups was linked to better quality of life, lower pain, and higher perceived clinician support for group participation. Eton, Lepore, and Helgeson (2005) studied psychological distress in the spouses of men treated for early-stage prostate carcinoma. They found that the spouses reported more cancer distress than patients, and the degree of distress was inversely associated with social support.

Because of the major role of family and friends in mitigating the psychosocial effects of cancer on patients, healthcare providers should educate family members in techniques that encourage, offer assistance, and convey a sense that someone is available to listen, learn, and lend a hand.

Psychotherapy occurs within a structured encounter between a trained therapist and patient, alone or with significant others. The problems associated with a cancer diagnosis and treatment may be clinically diagnosable, as well as everyday problems. Most forms of psychotherapy use only spoken conversation, but some use other forms of communication, such as the written word, artwork, drama, narrative story, music, or therapeutic touch.

Psychotherapeutic interventions treat patients using the medical model of illness and cure, but not all psychotherapeutic approaches follow the model. Some practitioners, such as those from the humanistic schools, see themselves in an educator or helper role. Because sensitive topics often are discussed during psychotherapy, therapists are expected, and usually legally bound, to respect client or patient confidentiality.

Mitigating and Compounding Distress

Several situational and personal factors mitigate or compound a person's psychosocial response to cancer. These include personal and social history, developmental issues, patients with special needs, practical problems, and culture and attitude.

Personal and Social History

Personal and social variables may increase a person's risk of experiencing disabling distress. A patient or family member may have a history of psychiatric disorders, substance abuse, or suicide attempts. Nurses should evaluate patients' cognitive function and ascertain a history of developmental delay, intellectual disability, or learning exceptionality. Healthcare providers must adjust all instructional materials and person-to-person discussion for individuals with these exceptionalities.

During psychosocial interventions, oncology nurses must consider the possible impact of social problems, such as inability of the family caregiver to provide support, solitary living, or lack of a support network, or financial problems. Situational factors may potentiate feelings of anger, hopelessness, and fear and play a role in the patient's rejection of treatments judged to be too costly. In addition to psychiatric history and limited social support, other factors may predict poor coping and increase the likelihood of psychosocial distress. These include alcohol or drug abuse or addiction history; recent significant losses (e.g., loss of spouse or job); a pessimistic outlook on life in general; and an inflexible way of coping (Rowland & Baker, 2005; Stanton et al., 2005).

Developmental Issues

The experience of childhood cancer, for some, may produce chronic psychological and cognitive impairments that hinder adjustment and quality of life even after cancer is cured. The risk is greater for those who are female, with a low educational level, and with low household incomes (Hudson et al., 2003). It is not known how developmental stage at the time of diagnosis influences the experience of cancer. However, it is well documented that the younger the age, the less there is insight, and therefore less ability to master developmental tasks and manage the stress and consequences of illness (Nelson, Haase, Kupst, Clarke-Steffen, & Brace-O'Neill, 2004; Ritchie, 1992). It is certainly possible that the younger the age at diagnosis, the greater the likelihood of developmental and cognitive delay, and these two factors affect potential educational achievement and adjustment in later life.

At any point in the cancer trajectory, patients have developmental needs. This is especially true for children with cancer, as well as for young adolescent and adult survivors of childhood cancers. The best psychosocial nursing care aims to facilitate the young person's development of a positive view of the impact of the cancer experience (Servitzoglou, Papadatou, Tsiantis, & Vasilatou-Kosmidis, 2008).

For young patients with cancer and survivors of childhood cancer, issues of self-esteem are especially important and may predict later psychosocial adjustment (Overbaugh & Sawin, 1992). An enhanced self-image has been associated with positive adjustment to stressors among children (Stern, Norman, & Zevon, 1993). The aims of psychosocial interventions are to promote normalcy throughout the cancer experience (Cantrell, 2007; Ritchie, 2001). See Chapter 29 for additional information.

Patients With Special Needs

Very little is known regarding the risk of neoplasms among people with developmental and other disabilities and their psychosocial issues and needs. Patja, Eero, and Livanainen (2001) reported that people with intellectual disability had an increased risk of cancer of the gallbladder, thyroid, and brain. Liu and Clark (2010) reported that women with disabilities faced significant barriers in accessing health care and routine preventive services and were less likely to report having had a mammogram or Pap test. Similar findings were reported in 2010 (Mehta, Fung, Kistler, Chang, & Walter, 2010). A description of the care of patients with autism spectrum disorder undergoing cancer surgery did not specifically address psychosocial issues and how they should be managed (Dell et al., 2008). Furthermore, the psychosocial experiences of patients with cancer with comorbid disorders, such as multiple sclerosis, deafness, spinal cord injuries, and other disabilities, are not well understood or sufficiently addressed in the literature. Nurses working in cancer care must be mindful of the additional psychological and social burdens associated with these comorbid disorders when planning care.

Practical Problems

Practical concerns for patients and their families are numerous and are related to the integrity of social support systems and financial security. Nurses may not be able to help directly but may be able to offer guidance to patients and family members who require public assistance. Nurses may provide a plan of care that includes a list of community resources and examples of strategies that have worked for other patients. The first step in addressing practical problems is to assess their existence and discuss possible resources.

One practical concern that affects all other issues is finances. The cost of cancer care continually increases. If a patient has insufficient financial resources, he or she may not be able to adhere to basic medical recommendations or receive curative or palliative care, medications, physical therapy, and other supportive or medical services. Even the simple expectation of attending a follow-up visit may not be possible if the patient does not have access to, or cannot pay for, transportation (see Figure 32-6).

Cultural and Attitudinal Barriers to Psychosocial Care

Around the world, for centuries, families withheld diagnoses of cancer from loved ones whom they perceived as vulnerable or not capable of dealing with the stigma and fear (Holland, 2004). An old custom of "never telling" was applied to spare the patient from emotional agony because death was presumed to be inevitable. Although many cancers are now thought to be chronic conditions, the stigma remains. Different cultures deal differently with the fear and stigma. According to Holland (2004), in the past 50 years, increased openness in the dialogue between healthcare providers and patients and families led to the first psychosocial studies of patients with cancer. Prejudice and stigma remain attached to mental illness, and emotional breakdowns are associated with weakness. Prejudices are barriers to the identification and comprehensive treatment of psychosocial distress. The veneer of culture imposes additional nuances to the cancer experience. Within the context of the therapeutic relationship, oncology nurses must consider the effect of culture when assessing psychosocial health.

Figure 32-6. Practical Problems Associated With Cancer

- Illiteracy or language barriers
- Barriers to access to medical care; lack of medical insurance
- Costs of cancer treatments
- Financial implications for the family
- Comorbidities that impair food preparation, medication taking, treatment adherence, and activities of daily living
- Limitations in access to transportation
- Job-related difficulties (work increase, decrease, or change in responsibilities)
- School-related difficulty

Conclusion

Many excellent sources of information and guidance are available on psychosocial oncology, including journals such as *Psycho-Oncology*, *Journal of Psychosocial Oncology*, and *Oncology Nursing Forum*, as well as non–oncology-specific journals such as *Psychosomatic Medicine*, *Health Education and Behavior*, and *Journal of Genetic Counseling*. Diverse perspectives on the best approach to care are continually evolving as more data are collected and more principles hold up when applied to practice. Responsible oncology nurses keep abreast of the state of the science and the endeavor to keep their practice holistic, contemporary, and evidence based.

References

Andersen, B.L., Farrar, W.B., Golden-Kreutz, D.M., Glaser, R., Emery, C.F., Crespin, T., … Carson, W.E. (2004). Psychological, behavioral, and immune changes after a psychological intervention: A clinical trial. *Journal of Clinical Oncology, 22,* 3570–3580. doi:10.1200/JCO.2004.06.030

Andersen, B.L., Shapiro, C.L., Farrar, W.B., Crespin, T., & Wells-Digregorio, S. (2005). Psychological responses to cancer recurrence. *Cancer, 104,* 1540–1547. doi:10.1002/cncr.21309

Key Points

- Cancer is a whole-body disease, affecting the body, mind, and spirit.
- The patient experience of cancer is personal, and the burdens imposed by this disease may differ by the course of the trajectory (acute or chronic).
- The term *psychosocial* refers to one's psychological state or development in interactions with a social environment. *Psychology* is the study of mental processes and behavior. The *social environment*, or *context*, is the influence of social position, roles, culture, and relationships that as a whole may influence the psychology.
- Both patients and family members may be affected and have feelings of anger, fear, uncertainty, sadness, hopelessness, distress, loneliness, grief, and relief, and a patient's mental health may be compromised by anxiety and depression.
- The family of a patient with cancer may experience interpersonal discord, loss of emotional support and partnership, and economic burdens from the loss of employment and the high costs of care. The threat to life and security is real, and fear is an appropriate response.
- Major stressors for children with cancer are treatment procedures, especially chemotherapy; loss of control; the hospital environment; relapses; and fear of dying.
- Parents and siblings (depending on their age) will variably apprehend the child's distressing experiences and may agonize about anticipated psychosocial issues, such as dealing with altered body image, assault to the child's self-esteem, and transition back into "ordinary" life.
- With the advent of cancer predisposition genetic testing came new psychological problems associated with presymptomatic risk assessment and determination of genetic mutation carrier status, which may generate fear, worry, and other psychosocial consequences perhaps decades before the onset of disease or even when the development of cancer is not absolute.
- A systems approach considers the individual in the context of social systems, such as the family, the healthcare community, and the larger social network, and allows for the selective study and treatment of psychosocial problems at the interface of patients with their immediate and extended family members, friends, employers, and associates in larger cultural and social networks.
- Approximately 50%–90% of patients with cancer view religion and spirituality as personally important, and association has been demonstrated between spirituality and improved coping and quality of life.

Antoni, M.H., Lechner, S.C., Kazi, A., Wimberly, S.R., Sifre, T., Urcuyo, K.R., ... Carver, C.S. (2006). How stress management improves quality of life after treatment for breast cancer. *Journal of Consulting and Clinical Psychology, 74,* 1143–1152. doi:10.1037/0022-006X.74.6.1143

Bachner, Y.G., O'Rourke, N., & Carmel, S. (2011). Fear of death, mortality communication, and psychological distress among secular and religiously observant family caregivers of terminal cancer patients. *Death Studies, 35,* 163–187. doi:10.1080/07481187.2010.535390

Badger, T.A., Segrin, C., Figueredo, A.J., Harrington, J., Sheppard, K., Passalacqua, S., ... Bishop, M. (2011). Psychosocial interventions to improve quality of life in prostate cancer survivors and their intimate or family partners. *Quality of Life Research, 20,* 833–844. doi:10.1007/s11136-010-9822-2

Baider, L., & De-Nour, A.K. (1988). Adjustment to cancer: Who is the patient—the husband or the wife? *Israel Journal of Medical Sciences, 24,* 631–636.

Balboni, T.A., Vanderwerker, L.C., Block, S.D., Paulk, M.E., Lathan, C.S., Peteet, J.R., & Prigerson, H.G. (2007). Religious and spiritual support among advanced cancer patients and associations with end-of-life treatment preferences and quality of life. *Journal of Clinical Oncology, 25,* 555–560. doi:10.1200/JCO.2006.07.9046

Baltrusch, H.J.F., & Waltz, M. (1985). Cancer from a biobehavioral and social epidemiological perspective. *Social Science and Medicine, 20,* 789–794. doi:10.1016/0277-9536(85)90332-6

Bäuml, J., Froböse, T., Kraemer, S., Rentrop, M., & Pitschel-Walz, G. (2006). Psychoeducation: A basic psychotherapeutic intervention for patients with schizophrenia and their families. *Schizophrenia Bulletin, 32*(Suppl. 1), S1–S9. doi:10.1093/schbul/sbl017

Bleiker, E.M.A., Esplen, M.J., Meiser, B., Petersen, H.V., & Patenaude, A.F. (2013). 100 years Lynch syndrome: What have we learned about psychosocial issues? *Familial Cancer, 12,* 325–339. doi:10.1007/s10689-013-9653-8

Boesen, E.H., Karlsen, R., Christensen, J., Paaschburg, B., Nielsen, D., Bloch, I.S., ... Johansen, C. (2011). Psychosocial group intervention for patients with primary breast cancer: A randomised trial. *European Journal of Cancer, 47,* 1363–1372. doi:10.1016/j.ejca.2011.01.002

Brothers, B.M., Yang, H.C., Strunk, D.R., & Andersen, B.L. (2011). Cancer patients with major depressive disorder: Testing a biobehavioral/cognitive behavior intervention. *Journal of Consulting and Clinical Psychology, 79,* 253–260. doi:10.1037/a0022566

Bultz, B.D., & Carlson, L.E. (2005). Emotional distress: The sixth vital sign in cancer care. *Journal of Clinical Oncology, 23,* 6440–6441. doi:10.1200/JCO.2005.02.3259

Bultz, B.D., Speca, M., Brasher, M., Geggie, P.H., & Page, S.A. (2000). A randomized controlled trial of a brief psychoeducational support group for partners of early stage breast cancer patients. *Psycho-Oncology, 9,* 303–313. doi:10.1002/1099-1611(200007/08)9:4<303::AID-PON462>3.0.CO;2-M

Callahan, C. (2004). Facial disfigurement and sense of self in head and neck cancer. *Social Work in Health Care, 40,* 73–87. doi:10.1300/J010v40n02_05

Cantrell, M.A. (2007). Health-related quality of life in childhood cancer: State of the science. *Oncology Nursing Forum, 34,* 103–111. doi:10.1188/07.ONF.103-111

Carlson, L.E., Beattie, T.L., Giese-Davis, J., Faris, P., Tamagawa, R., Fick, L.J., ... Speca, M. (2015). Mindfulness-based cancer recovery and supportive-expressive therapy maintain telomere length relative to controls in distressed breast cancer survivors. *Cancer, 121,* 476–484. doi:10.1002/cncr.29063

Carlson, L.E., & Bultz, B.D. (2003). Cancer distress screening: Needs, models, and methods. *Journal of Psychosomatic Research, 55,* 403–409. doi:10.1016/S0022-3999(03)00514-2

Cella, D.F. (1991). Functional status and quality of life: Current views on measurement and intervention. In *Functional status and quality of life in persons with cancer: Selected papers from First National Conference on Cancer Nursing Research* (pp. 1–12). Atlanta, GA: American Cancer Society.

Chien, C.H., Liu, K.L., Chien, H.T., & Liu, H.E. (2014). The effects of psychosocial strategies on anxiety and depression of patients diagnosed with prostate cancer. *International Journal of Nursing Studies, 51,* 28–38. doi:10.1016/j.ijnur stu.2012.12.019

Chochinov, H.M., Hack, T., Hassard, T., Kristjanson, L.J., McClement, S.E., & Harlos, M. (2005). Dignity therapy: A novel psychotherapeutic intervention for patients near the end of life. *Journal of Clinical Oncology, 23,* 5520–5525. doi:10.1200/JCO.2005.08.391

Coffman, K.L. (2015). Psychiatric evaluation of the face transplant candidate. *Current Opinion in Organ Transplantation, 20,* 222–228. doi:10.1097/MOT.0000000000000168

Cohen, M.Z., Jenkins, D., Holston, E.C., & Carlson, E.D. (2013). Understanding health literacy in patients receiving hematopoietic stem cell transplantation. *Oncology Nursing Forum, 40,* 508–515. doi:10.1188/13.ONF.508-515

Cohen, S., Kamarck, T., & Mermelstein, R. (1983). A global measure of perceived stress. *Journal of Health and Social Behavior, 24,* 385–396. doi:10.2307/2136404

Crotser, C.B., & Dickerson, S.S. (2010). Learning about a twist in the road: Perspectives of at-risk relatives learning of potential for cancer. *Oncology Nursing Forum, 37,* 723–733. doi:10.1188/10.ONF.723-733

Dell, D.D., Feleccia, M., Hicks, L., Longstreth-Papsun, E., Politsky, S., & Trommer, C. (2008). Care of patients with autism spectrum disorder undergoing surgery for cancer. *Oncology Nursing Forum, 35,* 177–182. doi:10.1188/08.ONF.177-182

den Heijer, M., Seynaeve, C., Vanheusden, K., Timman, R., Duivenvoorden, H.J., Tilanus-Linthorst, M., ... Tibben, A. (2013). Long-term psychological distress in women at risk for hereditary breast cancer adhering to regular surveillance: A risk profile. *Psycho-Oncology, 22,* 598–604. doi:10.1002/pon.3039

Denollet, J., Pedersen, S.S., Ong, A.T., Erdman, R.A., Serruys, P.W., & van Domburg, R.T. (2006). Social inhibition modulates the effect of negative emotions on cardiac prognosis following percutaneous coronary intention in the drug-eluting stent era. *European Heart Journal, 27,* 171–177. doi:10.1093/eurheartj/ehi616

Derogatis, L.R. (2008). *BSI—Brief Symptom Inventory: Assessments for educational, clinical, and psychological use.* San Antonio, TX: Pearson Education.

Dorland's illustrated medical dictionary (31st ed.). (2007). Philadelphia, PA: Elsevier Saunders.

Douglas, S.L., & Daly, B.J. (2014). Effect of an integrated cancer support team on caregiver satisfaction with end-of-life care [Online exclusive]. *Oncology Nursing Forum, 41,* E248–E255. doi:10.1188/14.ONF.E248-E255

Dy, S.M., Asch, S.M., Lorenz, K.A., Weeks, K., Sharma, R.K., Wolff, A.C., & Malin, J.L. (2011). Quality of end-of-life care for patients with advanced cancer in an academic medical center. *Journal of Palliative Medicine, 14,* 451–457. doi:10.1089/jpm.2010.0434

Epstein, D.R., & Dirksen, S.R. (2007). Randomized trial of a cognitive-behavioral intervention for insomnia in breast cancer survivors [Online exclusive]. *Oncology Nursing Forum, 34,* E51–E59. doi:10.1188/07.ONF.E51-E59

Epstein, N. (2006). *Enhancing cognitive-behavioral therapy for couples: A contextual approach.* Washington, DC: American Psychological Association.

Eton, D.T., Lepore, S.J., & Helgeson, V.S. (2005). Psychological distress in spouses of men treated for early-stage prostate carcinoma. *Cancer, 103,* 2411–2418. doi:10.1002/cncr.21092

Feldman, D.B., Sorocco, K.H., & Bratkovich, K.L. (2014). Treatment of posttraumatic stress disorder at the end-of-life: Application of the Stepwise Psychosocial Palliative Care model. *Palliative and Supportive Care, 12,* 233–243. doi:10.1017/S1478951513000370

Ferrans, C.E. (1990). Development of a quality-of-life index for patients with cancer. *Oncology Nursing Forum, 17*(Suppl. 3), 15–21.

Ferrell, B.R., & Coyle, N. (2008). The nature of suffering and the goals of nursing. *Oncology Nursing Forum, 35,* 241–247. doi:10.1188/08.ONF.241-247

Folkman, S., & Lazarus, R.S. (1985). *Ways of coping questionnaire.* Redwood City, CA: Mind Garden.

Germino, B.B., Mishel, M.H., Belyea, M., Harris, L., Ware, A., & Mohler, J. (1998). Uncertainty in prostate cancer: Ethnic and family patterns. *Cancer Practice, 6,* 107–113. doi:10.1046/j.1523-5394.1998.1998006107.x

Given, B., & Given, C.W. (1992). Patient and family caregiver reaction to new and recurrent breast cancer. *Journal of the American Medical Women's Association, 47,* 201–206, 212.

Goldstein, N.E., Concato, J., Fried, T.R., Kasl, S.V., Johnson-Hurzeler, R., & Bradley, E.H. (2004). Factors associated with caregiver burden among caregivers of terminally ill patients with cancer. *Journal of Palliative Care, 20,* 38–43.

Groarke, A., Curtis, R., & Kerin, M. (2013). Cognitive-behavioural stress management enhances adjustment in women with breast cancer. *British Journal of Health Psychology, 18,* 623–641. doi:10.1111/bjhp.12009

Grov, E.K., & Valeberg, B.T. (2012). Does the cancer patient's disease stage matter? A comparative study of caregivers' mental health and health related quality of life. *Palliative and Supportive Care, 10,* 189–196. doi:10.1017/S1478951511000873

Guo, Z., Tang, H.-Y., Li, H., Tan, S.-K., Feng, K.-H., Huang, Y.-C., ... Jiang, W. (2013). The benefits of psychosocial interventions for cancer patients undergoing radiotherapy. *Health and Quality of Life Outcomes, 11,* 121. doi:10.1186/1477-7525-11-121

Haase, J., & Phillips, C.R. (2004). The adolescent/young adult experience. *Journal of Pediatric Oncology Nursing, 21,* 145–149. doi:10.1177/1043454204264385

Haj Mohammad, N., Walter, A.W., van Oijen, M.G., Hulshof, M.C., Bergman, J.J., Anderegg, M.C., ... van Laarhoven, H.W. (2015). Burden of spousal caregivers of stage II and III esophageal cancer survivors 3 years after treatment with curative intent. *Supportive Care in Cancer, 23,* 3589–3598. doi:10.1007/s00520-015-2727-4

Hamilton, J.G., Lobel, M., & Moyer, A. (2009). Emotional distress following genetic testing for hereditary breast and ovarian cancer: A meta-analytic review. *Health Psychology, 28,* 510–518. doi:10.1037/a0014778

Hansen, F., & Sawatzky, J.V. (2008). Stress in patients with lung cancer: A human response to illness. *Oncology Nursing Forum, 35,* 217–223. doi:10.1188/08.ONF.217-223

Heiniger, L., Butow, P.N., Price, M.A., & Charles, M. (2013). Distress in unaffected individuals who decline, delay, or remain ineligible for genetic testing for hereditary diseases: A systematic review. *Psycho-Oncology, 22,* 1930–1945. doi:10.1002/pon.3235

Heshka, J.T., Palleschi, C., Howley, H., Wilson, B., & Wells, P.S. (2008). A systematic review of perceived risks, psychological and behavioral impacts of genetic testing. *Genetics in Medicine, 10,* 19–32. doi:10.1097/GIM.0b013e31815f524f

Hilton, B.A. (1993). A study of couple communication patterns when coping with early stage breast cancer. *Canadian Oncology Nursing Journal, 3,* 159–166. doi:10.5737/1181912x34159166

Hilton, B.A., Crawford, J.A., & Tarko, M.A. (2000). Men's perspectives on individual and family coping with their wives' breast cancer and chemotherapy. *Western Journal of Nursing Research, 22,* 438–459. doi:10.1177/01939450022044511

Hogarty, G.E., Anderson, C.M., Reiss, D.J., Kornblith, S.J., Greenwald, D.P., Ulrich, R.F., & Carter, M. (1991). Family psychoeducation, social skills training and maintenance chemotherapy in the aftercare treatment of schizophrenia: II. Two-year effects of a controlled study on relapse and adjustment. *Archives of General Psychiatry, 48,* 340–347. doi:10.1001/archpsyc.1991.01810280056008

Holland, J.C. (Ed.). (1982). *Psychological aspects of cancer.* Philadelphia, PA: Lea & Febiger.

Holland, J.C. (2004). IPOS Sutherland Memorial Lecture: An international perspective on the development of psychosocial oncology: Overcoming cultural and attitudinal barriers to improve psychosocial care. *Psycho-Oncology, 13,* 445–459. doi:10.1002/pon.812

Horowitz, M., Wilner, N., & Alvarez, W. (1979). Impact of Event Scale: A measure of subjective stress. *Psychosomatic Medicine, 41,* 209–218. doi:10.1097/00006842-197905000-00004

Hudson, M.M., Mertens, A.C., Yasui, Y., Hobbie, W., Chen, H., Gurney, J.G., ... Oeffinger, K.C. (2003). Health status of adult long-term survivors of childhood cancer: A report from the Childhood Cancer Survivor Study. *JAMA, 290,* 1583–1592. doi:10.1001/jama.290.12.1583

Jacobs, L.A., & Piper, B.F. (1995). The phenomenon of fatigue and the cancer patient. In R. McCorkle, M. Grant, M. Frank-Stromborg, & S.B. Baird (Eds.), *Cancer nursing: A comprehensive textbook* (pp. 1193–1210). Philadelphia, PA: Saunders.

Jones, B.L. (2012). The challenge of quality care for family caregivers in pediatric cancer care. *Seminars in Oncology Nursing, 28,* 213–220, doi:10.1016/j.soncn.2012.09.003

Jones, S.B., Whitford, H.S., & Bond, M.J. (2015). Burden on informal caregivers of elderly cancer survivors: Risk versus resilience. *Journal of Psychosocial Oncology, 33,* 178–198. doi:10.1080/07347332.2014.1002657

Kaltenbaugh, D.J., Klem, M.L., Hu, L., Turi, E., Haines, A.J., & Lingler, J.H. (2015). Using web-based interventions to support caregivers of patients with cancer: A systematic review. *Oncology Nursing Forum, 42,* 156–164. doi:10.1188/15.ONF.156-164

Kangas, M., Henry, J.L., & Bryant, R.A. (2002). Posttraumatic stress disorder following cancer: A conceptual and empirical review. *Clinical Psychology Review, 22,* 499–524. doi:10.1016/S0272-7358(01)00118-0

Kazak, A.E. (2005). Evidence-based interventions for survivors of childhood cancer and their families. *Journal of Pediatric Psychology, 30,* 29–39. doi:10.1093/jpepsy/jsi013

Kim, Y., Schulz, R., & Carver, C.S. (2007). Benefit finding in the cancer caregiving experience. *Psychosomatic Medicine, 69,* 283–291. doi:10.1097/PSY.0b013e3180417cf4

Kim, Y.F.B., Baker, F., Spillers, R.L., & Wellisch, D.K. (2006). Psychological adjustment of cancer caregivers with multiple roles. *Psycho-Oncology, 15,* 795–804. doi:10.1002/pon.1013

Kinney, A.Y., Butler, K.M., Schwartz, M.D., Mandelblatt, J.S., Boucher, K.M., Pappas, L.M., ... Campo, R.A. (2014). Expanding access to *BRCA1/2* genetic counseling with telephone delivery: A cluster randomized trial. *Journal of the National Cancer Institute, 106*(12), dju328. doi:10.1093/jnci/dju328

Korstjens, I., Mesters, I., May, A.M., van Weert, E., van den Hout, J.H., Ros, W., ... van den Borne, B. (2011). Effects of cancer rehabilitation on problem-solving, anxiety and depression: A RCT comparing physical and cognitive-behavioural training versus physical training. *Psychology and Health, 26*(Suppl. 1), 63–82. doi:10.1080/08870441003611569

Krischer, M.M., Xu, P., Meade, C.D., & Jacobsen, P.B. (2007). Self-administered stress management training in patients undergoing radiotherapy. *Journal of Clinical Oncology, 25,* 4657–4662. doi:10.1200/JCO.2006.09.0126

Laccetti, M. (2007). Expressive writing in women with advanced breast cancer. *Oncology Nursing Forum, 34,* 1019–1024. doi:10.1188/07.ONF.1019-1024

Lammens, C.R., Aaronson, N.K., Wagner, A., Sijmons, R.H., Ausems, M.G., Vriends, A.H., ... Bleiker, E.M. (2010). Genetic testing in Li-Fraumeni syndrome: Uptake and psychosocial consequences. *Journal of Clinical Oncology, 28,* 3008–3014. doi:10.1200/JCO.2009.27.2112

Lang, H.R., France, E., Williams, G., Humphris, G., & Wells, M. (2013). The psychological experience of living with head and neck cancer: A systematic review and meta-synthesis. *Psycho-Oncology, 22,* 2648–2663. doi:10.1002/pon.3343

Lapointe, J., Abdous, B., Camden, S., Bouchard, K., Goldgar, D., Simard, J., & Dorval, M. (2012). Influence of the family cluster effect on psychosocial variables in families undergoing *BRCA1/2* genetic testing for cancer susceptibility. *Psycho-Oncology, 21,* 515–523. doi:10.1002/pon.1936

Ledley, D.R. (2005). *Making cognitive-behavioral therapy work: Clinical process for new practitioners.* New York, NY: Guilford Press.

León-Pizarro, C., Gich, I., Barthe, E., Rovirosa, A., Farrús, B., Casas, F., ... Arcusa, A. (2007). A randomized trial of the effect of training in relaxation and guided imagery techniques in improving psychological and quality-of-life indices for gynecologic and breast brachytherapy patients. *Psycho-Oncology, 16,* 971–979. doi:10.1002/pon.1171

Lerman, C., Hughes, C., Lemon, S.J., Main, D., Snyder, C., Durham, C., ... Lynch, H.T. (1998). What you don't know can hurt you: Adverse psychologic effects in members of *BRCA1*-linked and *BRCA2*-linked families who decline genetic testing. *Journal of Clinical Oncology, 16,* 1650–1654.

Lewis, F.M. (1993). Psychosocial transitions and the family's work in adjusting to cancer. *Seminars in Oncology Nursing, 9,* 127–129. doi:10.1016/S0749-2081(05)80109-3

Lewis, F.M. (2004). Family-focused oncology nursing research. *Oncology Nursing Forum, 31,* 288–292. doi:10.1188/04.ONF.288-292

Lewis, F.M., & Deal, L.W. (1995). Balancing our lives: A study of the married couple's experience with breast cancer recurrence. *Oncology Nursing Forum, 22,* 943–953.

Lewis, L.M. (2008). Spiritual assessment in African-Americans: A review of measures of spirituality used in health research. *Journal of Religion and Health, 47,* 458–475. doi:10.1007/s10943-007-9151-0

Lillie, S.E., Janz, N.K., Friese, C.R., Graff, J.J., Schwartz, K., Hamilton, A.S., ... Hawley, S.T. (2014). Racial and ethnic variation in partner perspectives about the breast cancer treatment decision-making experience. *Oncology Nursing Forum, 41,* 13–20. doi:10.1188/14.ONF.13-20

Lillis, B.S. (2014). Understanding the complex role of a hospice spiritual counselor. *American Journal of Hospice and Palliative Medicine, 31,* 353–355. doi:10.1177/1049909113494746

Lin, H.R., & Bauer-Wu, S.M. (2003). Psycho-spiritual well-being in patients with advanced cancer: An integrative review of the literature. *Journal of Advanced Nursing, 44,* 69–80. doi:10.1046/j.1365-2648.2003.02768.x

Liu, S.Y., & Clark, M.A. (2010). Breast and cervical cancer screening practices among disabled women aged 40–75: Does quality of the experience matter? *Journal of Women's Health, 17,* 1321–1329. doi:10.1089/jwh.2007.0591

Lobchuk, M., McClement, S.E., McPherson, C., & Cheang, M. (2008). Does blaming the patient with lung cancer affect the helping behavior of primary caregivers? *Oncology Nursing Forum, 35,* 681–689. doi:10.1188/08.ONF.681-689

Long, K.A., & Marsland, A.L. (2011). Family adjustment to childhood cancer: A systematic review. *Clinical Child and Family Psychology Review, 14,* 57–88. doi:10.1007/s10567-010-0082-z

MacNeil, G., Kosberg, J.I., Durkin, D.W., Dooley, W.K., DeCoster, J., & Williamson, G.M. (2010). Caregiver mental health and potentially harmful caregiving behavior: The central role of caregiver anger. *Gerontologist, 50,* 76–86. doi:10.1093/geront/gnp099

Mahendran, R., Chua, J., Peh, C.X., Lim, H.A., Ang, E.N., Lim, S.E., & Kua, E.H. (2014). Knowledge, attitudes, and practice behaviors (KaPb)of nurses and the effectiveness of a training program in psychosocial cancer care. *Supportive Care in Cancer, 22,* 2049–2056. doi:10.1007/s00520-014-2172-9

Mahon, S.M., & Casperson, D.S. (1995). Psychosocial concerns associated with recurrent cancer. *Cancer Practice, 3,* 372–380.

Mahon, S.M., Cella, D.F., & Donovan, M.I. (1990). Psychosocial adjustment to recurrent cancer. *Oncology Nursing Forum, 17*(Suppl. 3), 47–52.

Manning-Walsh, J. (2005). Social support as a mediator between symptom distress and quality of life in women with breast cancer. *Journal of Obstetric, Gynecologic and Neonatal Nursing, 34,* 482–493. doi:10.1177/0884217505278310

McCaffrey, C.N. (2006). Major stressors and their effects on the well-being of children with cancer. *Journal of Pediatric Nursing, 21,* 59–66. doi:10.1016/j.pedn.2005.07.003

McCance, K.L., Forshee, B.A., & Shelby, K.L. (2006). Stress and disease. In K.L. McCance & S.E. Huether (Eds.), *Pathophysiology: The biologic basis for disease in adults and children* (pp. 311–332). St. Louis, MO: Elsevier Mosby.

McNair, D., Lorr, M., & Droppleman, L. (1971). *Psychiatric outpatient mood scale.* Boston, MA: Boston University Medical Center.

Mehnert, A., & Koch, U. (2007). Prevalence of acute and post-traumatic stress disorder and comorbid mental disorders in breast cancer patients during primary cancer care: A prospective study. *Psycho-Oncology, 16,* 181–188. doi:10.1002/pon.1057

Mehta, K.M., Fung, K.Z., Kistler, C.E., Chang, A., & Walter, L.C. (2010). Impact of cognitive impairment on screening mammography use in older US women. *American Journal of Public Health, 100,* 1917–1923. doi:10.2105/AJPH.2008.158485

Miedema, B., Hamilton, R., Fortin, P., Easley, J., & Matthews, M. (2010). "You can only take so much, and it took everything out of me": Coping strategies used by parents of children with cancer. *Palliative and Supportive Care, 8,* 197–206. doi:10.1017/S1478951510000015

Milberg, A., Wåhlberg, R., & Krevers, B. (2014). Patients' sense of support within the family in the palliative care context: What are the influencing factors? *Psycho-Oncology, 23,* 1340–1349. doi:10.1002/pon.3564

Miller, S.M., & Schnoll, R.A. (2000). When seeing is feeling: A cognitive-emotional approach to coping with health stress. In M. Lewis & J. Haviland-Jones (Eds.), *Handbook of emotions* (2nd ed., pp. 538–557). New York, NY: Guilford Press.

Mitchell, P.H., Gallucci, B., & Fought, S.G. (1991). Perspectives on human response to health and illness. *Nursing Outlook, 39,* 154–157.

Morse, J.M., & Fife, B. (1996). Coping with a partner's cancer: Adjustment at four stages of the illness trajectory. *Oncology Nursing Forum, 25,* 751–760.

National Cancer Institute. (2015). The genetics of cancer. Retrieved from https://www.cancer.gov/about-cancer/causes-prevention/genetics

National Cancer Institute. (2016). Spirituality in cancer care (PDQ®) [Health professional version]. Retrieved from http://www.cancer.gov/about-cancer/coping/day-to-day/faith-and-spirituality/spirituality-hp-pdq

National Comprehensive Cancer Network. (2016). *NCCN Clinical Practice Guidelines in Oncology (NCCN Guidelines®): Distress management* [v.2.2016]. Retrieved from http://www.nccn.org/professionals/physician_gls/PDF/distress.pdf

Nelson, A.E., Haase, J., Kupst, M.J., Clarke-Steffen, L., & Brace-O'Neill, J. (2004). Consensus statements: Interventions to enhance resilience and quality of life in adolescents with cancer. *Journal of Pediatric Oncology Nursing, 21,* 305–307. doi:10.1177/1043454204267925

Nesbitt, J., & Sawatzky, J.A. (2009). Using the Human Response to Illness Model to assess altered level of consciousness in patients with subdural hematomas. *Canadian Journal of Neuroscience Nursing, 31*(2), 6–12.

Northouse, L.L., Katapodi, M.C., Song, L., Zhang, L., & Mood, D.W. (2010). Interventions with family caregivers of cancer patients: Meta-analysis of randomized trials. *CA: A Cancer Journal for Clinicians, 60,* 317–339. doi:10.3322/caac.20081

Nummenmaa, L., Glerean, E., Hari, R., & Hietanen, J.K. (2014). Bodily maps of emotions. *Proceedings of the National Academy of Sciences of the United States of America, 111,* 646–651. doi:10.1073/pnas.1321664111

Nunes, D.F.T., Rodriguez, A.L., Hoffmann, F.d.S., Luz, C., Filho, A.P.F.B., Paira, A., ... Bauer, M.E. (2007). Relaxation and guided imagery program in patients with breast cancer undergoing radiotherapy is not associated with neuroimmunomodulatory effects. *Journal of Psychosomatic Research, 63,* 647–655. doi:10.1016/j.jpsychores.2007.07.004

Obeidat, R.F., Homish, G.G., & Lally, R.M. (2013). Shared decision making among individuals with cancer in non-Western cultures: A literature review. *Oncology Nursing Forum, 40,* 454–463. doi:10.1188/13.ONF.454-463

Overbaugh, K.A., & Sawin, K. (1992). Future life expectations and self-esteem of the adolescent survivor of childhood cancer. *Journal of Pediatric Oncology Nursing, 9,* 8–16. doi:10.1177/104345429200900103

Padilla, G.V., Mishel, M.H., & Grant, M.M. (1992). Uncertainty, appraisal and quality of life. *Quality of Life Research, 1,* 155–165. doi:10.1007/BF00635615

Paiva, C.E., Souza, P.H., & Paiva, B.S.R. (2015). Discussion about the prevalence of mental disorders depending on the different phases of cancer care within the cancer continuum [Letter to the editor]. *Journal of Clinical Oncology, 33,* 1516. doi:10.1200/jco.2014.60.0023

Palos, G.R., Mendoza, T.R., Liao, K.P., Anderson, K.O., Garcia-Gonzalez, A., Hahn, K., ... Cleeland, C.S. (2011). Caregiver symptom burden: The risk of caring for an underserved patient with advanced cancer. *Cancer, 117,* 1070–1079. doi:10.1002/cncr.25695

Patja, K., Eero, P., & Livanainen, M. (2001). Cancer incidence among people with intellectual disability. *Journal of Intellectual Disability Research, 45,* 300–307. doi:10.1046/j.1365-2788.2001.00322.x

Pellegrino, R., Formica, V., Portarena, I., Mariotti, S., Grenga, I., Del Monte, G., & Roselli, M. (2010). Caregiver distress in the early phases of cancer. *Anticancer Research, 30,* 4657–4663. Retrieved from http://ar.iiarjournals.org/content/30/11/4657.long

Pennebaker, J.W., & Seagal, J.D. (1999). Forming a story: The health benefits of narrative. *Journal of Clinical Psychology, 55,* 1243–1254. doi:10.1002/(SICI)1097-4679(199910)55:10<1243::AID-JCLP6>3.0.CO;2-N

Ritchie, M.A. (1992). Psychosocial functioning of adolescents with cancer: A developmental perspective. *Oncology Nursing Forum, 19,* 1497–1501.

Ritchie, M.A. (2001). Self-esteem and hopefulness in adolescents with cancer. *Journal of Pediatric Nursing, 16,* 35–42. doi:10.1053/jpdn.2001.20551

Robinson, S., Kissane, D.W., Brooker, J., & Burney, S. (2015). A systematic review of the demoralization syndrome in individuals with progressive disease and cancer: A decade of research. *Journal of Pain and Symptom Management, 49,* 595–610. doi:10.1016/j.jpainsymman.2014.07.008

Rolland, J.S. (1999). Families and genetic fate: A millennial challenge. *Families, Systems, and Health, 17,* 123–133. doi:10.1037/h0089890

Rolland, J.S., & Williams, J.K. (2005). Toward a biopsychosocial model for 21st-century genetics. *Family Process, 44,* 3–24. doi:10.1111/j.1545-5300.2005.00039.x

Rowland, J.H., & Baker, F. (2005). Introduction: Resilience of cancer survivors across the lifespan. *Cancer, 104*(Suppl. 11), 2543–2548. doi:10.1002/cncr.21487

Sahler, O.J., Dolgin, M.J., Phipps, S., Fairclough, D.L., Askins, M.A., Katz, E.R., ... Butler, R.W. (2013). Specificity of problem-solving skills training in mothers of children newly diagnosed with cancer: Results of a multisite randomized clinical trial. *Journal of Clinical Oncology, 31,* 1329–1335. doi:10.1200/jco.2011.39.1870

Salmon, P., Clark, L., McGrath, E., & Fisher, P. (2015). Screening for psychological distress in cancer: Renewing the research agenda. *Psycho-Oncology, 24,* 262–268. doi:10.1002/pon.3640

Santin, O., Treanor, C., Mills, M., & Donnelly, M. (2014). The health status and health service needs of primary caregivers of cancer survivors: A mixed methods approach. *European Journal of Cancer Care, 23,* 333–339. doi:10.1111/ecc.12157

Schnur, J.B., & Montgomery, G.H. (2008). Hypnosis and cognitive-behavioral therapy during breast cancer radiotherapy: A case report. *American Journal of Clinical Hypnosis, 50,* 209–215. doi:10.1080/00029157.2008.10401624

Schwartz, M.D., Peshkin, B.N., Hughes, C., Main, D., Isaacs, C., & Lerman, C. (2002). Impact of *BRCA1/BRCA2* mutation testing on psychologic distress in a clinic-based sample. *Journal of Clinical Oncology, 20,* 514–520. doi:10.1200/JCO.20.2.514

Sellick, S.M., & Edwardson, A.D. (2007). Screening new cancer patients for psychologic distress using the hospital anxiety and depression scale. *Psycho-Oncology, 16,* 534–542. doi:10.1002/pon.1085

Serfaty, M., Wilkinson, S., Freeman, C., Mannix, K., & King, M. (2012). *The ToT Study: Helping With Touch or Talk (ToT)*: A pilot randomised controlled trial to examine the clinical effectiveness of aromatherapy massage versus cognitive behaviour therapy for emotional distress in patients in cancer/palliative care. *Psycho-Oncology, 21,* 563–569. doi:10.1002/pon.1921

Servitzoglou, M., Papadatou, D., Tsiantis, I., & Vasilatou-Kosmidis, H. (2008). Psychosocial functioning of young adolescent and adult survivors of childhood cancer. *Supportive Care in Cancer, 16,* 29–36. doi:10.1007/s00520-007-0278-z

Sheldon, L., Harris, D., & Arcieri, C. (2012). Psychosocial concerns in cancer care: The role of the oncology nurse. *Clinical Journal of Oncology Nursing, 16,* 316–319. doi:10.1188/12.CJON.316-319

Shim, E.-J., & Park, J.-H. (2012). Suicidality and its associated factors in cancer patients: Results of a multi-center study in Korea. *International Journal of Psychiatry in Medicine, 43,* 381–403. doi:10.2190/PM.43.4.g

Smith, M.Y., Redd, W.H., Peyser, C., & Vogl, D. (1999). Post-traumatic stress disorder in cancer: A review. *Psycho-Oncology, 8,* 521–537. doi:10.1002/(SICI)1099-1611(199911/12)8:6<521::AID-PON423>3.0.CO;2-X

Spielberger, C.D. (1983). *State-trait anxiety inventory.* Redwood City, CA: Mind Garden.

Stanton, A.L., Ganz, P.A., Rowland, J.H., Meyerowitz, B.E., Krupnick, J.L., & Sears, S.R. (2005). Promoting adjustment after treatment for cancer. *Cancer, 104*(Suppl. 11), 2608–2613. doi:10.1002/cncr.21246

Steginga, S.K., Pinnock, C., Gardner, M., Gardiner, R.A., & Dunn, J. (2005). Evaluating peer support for prostate cancer: The Prostate Cancer Peer Support Inventory. *BJU International, 95,* 46–50. doi:10.1111/j.1464-410X.2005.05247.x

Stephenson, P.S., & Berry, D.M. (2014). Spirituality and uncertainty at the end of life. *Oncology Nursing Forum, 41,* 33–39. doi:10.1188/14.ONF.33-39

Stern, M., Norman, S.L., & Zevon, M.A. (1993). Adolescents with cancer: Self-image and perceived social support as indexes of adaptation. *Journal of Adolescent Research, 8,* 124–142. doi:10.1177/074355489381009

Stetz, K.M. (1987). Caregiving demands during advanced cancer: The spouse's needs. *Cancer Nursing, 10,* 260–268. doi:10.1097/00002820-198710000-00004

Sulkers, E., Tissing, W.J., Brinksma, A., Roodbol, P.F., Kamps, W.A., Stewart, R.E., ... Fleer, J. (2015). Providing care to a child with cancer: A longitudinal study on the course, predictors, and impact of caregiving stress during the first year after diagnosis. *Psycho-Oncology, 24,* 318–324. doi:10.1002/pon.3652

Tan, M., & Karabulutlu, E. (2005). Social support and hopelessness in Turkish patients with cancer. *Cancer Nursing, 28,* 236–240. doi:10.1097/00002820-200505000-00013

Tuinman, M.A., Hoekstra, H.J., Sleijfer, D.T., Fleer, J., Vidrine, D.J., Gritz, E.R., & Hoekstra-Weebers, J.E.H.M. (2007). Testicular cancer: A longitudinal pilot study on stress response symptoms and quality of life in couples before and after chemotherapy. *Supportive Care in Cancer, 15,* 279–286. doi:10.1007/s00520-006-0119-5

Utne, I., Miaskowski, C., Paul, S.M., & Rustøen, T. (2013). Association between hope and burden reported by family caregivers of patients with advanced cancer. *Supportive Care in Cancer, 21,* 2527–2535. doi:10.1007/s00520-013-1824-5

van Asperen, C.J., van Dijk, S., Zoeteweij, M.W., Timmermans, D.R.M., de Bock, G.H., Meijers-Heijboer, E.J., ... Otten, W. (2002). What do women really want to know? Motives for attending familial breast cancer clinics. *Journal of Medical Genetics, 39,* 410–414. doi:10.1136/jmg.39.6.410

Vidrine, D.J., Hoekstra-Weebers, J.E., Hoekstra, H.J., Tuinman, M.A., Marani, S., & Gritz, E.R. (2010). The effects of testicular cancer treatment on health-related quality of life. *Urology, 75,* 636–641. doi:10.1016/j.urology.2009.09.053

Vitek, L., Rosenzweig, M., & Stollings, S. (2007). Distress in patients with cancer: Definition, assessment, and suggested interventions. *Clinical Journal of Oncology Nursing, 11,* 413–418. doi:10.1188/07.CJON.413-418

Walker, J., & Sharpe, M. (2014). Integrated management of major depression for people with cancer. *International Review of Psychiatry, 26,* 657–668. doi:10.3109/09540261.2014.981512

Watson, A. (1995). Psychosocial oncology clinical nurse specialist enhances staff and patient well-being. Interview by Mary Beth Tombes. *ONS News, 10*(8), 5.

Wedding, U., Koch, A., Röhrig, B., Pientka, L., Sauer, H., Höffken, K., & Maurer, I. (2007). Requestioning depression in patients with cancer: Contribution of somatic and affective symptoms to Beck's Depression Inventory. *Annals of Oncology, 18,* 1875–1881. doi:10.1093/annonc/mdm353

Weisman, A.D., & Worden, J.W. (1977). The existential plight in cancer: Significance of the first 100 days. *International Journal of Psychiatry in Medicine, 7*, 1–15. doi:10.2190/UQ2G-UGV1-3PPC-6387

Weitzner, M.A., & McMillan, S.C. (1999). The Caregiver Quality of Life Index-Cancer (CQOLC) Scale: Revalidation in a home hospice setting. *Journal of Palliative Care, 15*(2), 13–20.

Yang, H.C., Thornton, L.M., Shapiro, C.L., & Andersen, B.L. (2008). Surviving recurrence: Psychological and quality-of-life recovery. *Cancer Nursing, 112*, 1178–1187. doi:10.1002/cncr.23272

Yi, J., & Kim, M.A. (2014). Postcancer experiences of childhood cancer survivors: How is posttraumatic stress related to posttraumatic growth? *Journal of Traumatic Stress, 27*, 461–467. doi:10.1002/jts.21941

Chapter 32 Study Questions

1. A patient has been diagnosed with a stage I basal cell carcinoma with no lymph node involvement, no metastasis, and limited risk of recurrence, yet the patient's fear is overwhelming and all-consuming and, in effect, paralyzes the patient's ability to move past the crisis stage of diagnosis. Which statement is true?
   A. The patient's fear is reasonable and expected.
   B. This level of fear is not rational and may suggest comorbid psychopathology.
   C. The diagnosis is probably not accurate and a second opinion is needed.
   D. Paralysis may be a side effect of basal cell carcinoma.

2. Certain characteristics can alert nurses to the risk for depression after a diagnosis. A female patient has been diagnosed with a solid tumor in her abdomen. Which of the following characteristics is NOT a risk factor?
   A. Young age
   B. Female gender
   C. Solid tumor
   D. Reduced functional status

3. Major stressors for children with cancer include:
   A. Treatment procedures.
   B. The hospital environment.
   C. Fear of dying.
   D. All of the above.

4. Which of the following are types of psychosocial interventions?
   A. Benefit finding and finding meaning
   B. Play therapy and role reactioning
   C. Cognitive behavioral therapy
   D. A and C only
   E. A, B, and C

5. Family caregivers of patients with cancer are typically spouses, parents, and adult children. The informal caregiver may experience psychosocial burdens. Which of the following factors contributes most significantly to caregiver burden?
   A. Older age of the caregiver
   B. Lack of social networks
   C. Lack of time due to work
   D. Higher education

CHAPTER 33

Sexual and Reproductive Issues

Anne Katz, PhD, RN, FAAN

Introduction

Many factors affect sexuality, including mood, relationship satisfaction, and a multitude of illness-related considerations. Cancer and its treatments have direct and indirect effects on all aspects of sexuality and sexual functioning. Sexual functioning after treatment also is influenced by the person's sexual functioning prior to diagnosis and treatment. Sexuality is affected by all treatment modalities, including surgery, radiation, chemotherapy, and endocrine therapies; however, at this time, very little is known about the impact of molecular-targeted therapies.

Fertility in reproductive-age patients also is affected by all treatment modalities. Discussion about fertility preservation often is neglected in the face of the urgency, often on the patient's part, to start treatment. Assisted reproductive technologies are rapidly advancing, and it is difficult for oncology care providers to stay current with the latest changes in this area. Thus, patients may not be given the most accurate information or any information at all.

This chapter will address the sexual challenges faced by cancer survivors and their partners, as well as discuss the potential for loss of fertility and the current state of knowledge related to fertility loss and preservation for patients of reproductive age.

Sexuality and Sexual Health

The World Health Organization (2006) defined sexuality as

> a central aspect of being human throughout life and encompasses sex, gender identities and roles, sexual orientation, eroticism, pleasure, intimacy and reproduction. Sexuality is experienced and expressed in thoughts, fantasies, desires, beliefs, attitudes, values, behaviours, practices, roles and relationships. While sexuality can include all of these dimensions, not all of them are always experienced or expressed. Sexuality is influenced by the interaction of biological, psychological, social, economic, political, cultural, ethical, legal, historical, religious and spiritual factors. (p. 5)

A less formal approach comes from Weiss (1992), who described sexuality as a connection between the heart and the gut, a means of joining pleasurable physical sensations with the spirit. Sexuality often is euphemistically referred to as "intimacy," which by definition means something of a personal or private nature, closeness, or familiarity ("Intimacy," n.d.). Briefly, sexuality encompasses sexual preferences (whom a person loves and is sexual with) and sexual functioning (the behaviors a person engages in that are dependent on anatomy, physiology, and endocrine functioning), alone or with a partner.

The sexual response cycle is a way of conceptualizing how individuals function sexually. Masters and Johnson described the first model of the sexual response cycle in their 1966 publication. They suggested that men and women both experience four distinct stages in a linear fashion: excitement, plateau, orgasm, and resolution. These stages are purely physical and represent processes involving the nervous, muscular, and circulatory systems without any emotional or psychological components. Kaplan (1979) introduced a psychological component in her three-stage model comprising desire, excitement, and orgasm. This model is not intended to be linear, and the stages are seen as distinct and able to occur in any order; however, it has been widely interpreted as occurring in sequential stages, with desire as the first and necessary stage. Basson (2005) has developed a more recent model for women. This model recognizes the social and relationship context of female sexual functioning and focuses on reactive rather than spontaneous desire. This is of particular relevance for women who believe that sexual desire has to precede sexual touch or activity; recognizing that desire may result *from* sexual touch (reactive desire) may encourage sexual activity, rather than the woman refusing the advances of a sexual partner because she is not feeling spontaneous desire. Sociocultural factors also play a role, as these form the basis for attitudes and beliefs about sexuality that may profoundly influence how individuals view their sexuality.

It is estimated that 40%–100% of cancer survivors will experience treatment- and cancer-related sexual problems (Sadovsky et al., 2010). However, not all survivors will want to address these problems. Oncology nurses must recognize that sexuality is an important quality-of-life issue, and with many millions of cancer survivors affected, oncology care providers must pay attention to the needs and desires of patients.

Impact of Cancer on Sexuality

Healthy sexual functioning is dependent on functional anatomy of the sexual organs, nerves, and blood vessels, as well as emotional and cognitive health. Any treatment that affects these may have a negative impact on sexual functioning. Bober and Varela (2012) have proposed an integrative biopsychosocial model in which cancer-related sexual problems affect, and in turn are affected by, biologic, interpersonal, psychological, and sociocultural factors (see Figure 33-1).

All treatment modalities have the potential to affect sexuality and sexual functioning. Specific changes for different kinds of cancer will be described in greater detail in the next section of this chapter. Briefly, surgery affects sexual functioning when it involves removal of sexual organs (breasts, prostate, testes, uterus, vagina, vulva) but also by causing scarring that may be internal, leading to pain and alterations in nerves and blood vessels supplying the sexual organs. External scars may lead to alterations in body image, a significant issue for women with breast cancer, or may affect physical functioning by making sexual activity difficult because of pain or stiffness. Radiation therapies, including external beam, brachytherapy, and modern technologies such as CyberKnife®, cause global physical effects such as fatigue and local effects such as skin damage in the treated area. Radiation to the sexual organs can cause atrophy of tissues, for example, in the vagina, leading to pain with sexual intercourse, or genital shrinkage in the

Figure 33-1. Sexuality in Adult Cancer Survivors: Challenges and Interventions

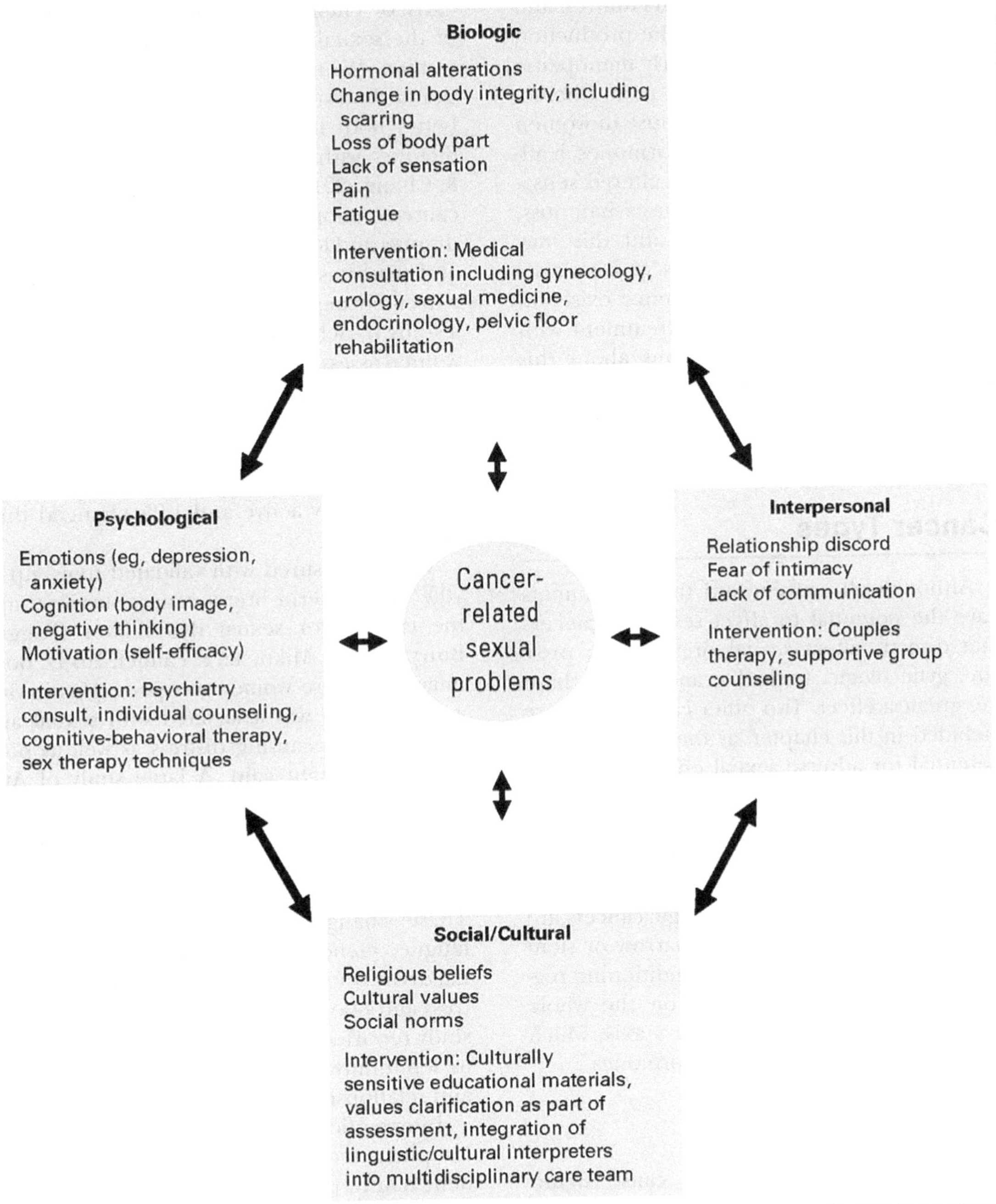

Note. From "Sexuality in Adult Cancer Survivors: Challenges and Intervention," by S.L. Bober and V.S. Varela, 2012, *Journal of Clinical Oncology, 30,* p. 3713. Copyright 2012 by American Society of Clinical Oncology. Reprinted with permission.

case of men. Radiation to the brain can interfere with hormonal functioning, causing problems with sexual development in children and adolescents. It also can affect the production of sex hormones, leading to early menopause for women and loss of libido for men. Chemotherapy can cause early menopause in women associated with the loss of sex hormones, leading to loss of desire, pain, and altered sensations. Chemotherapy often causes hair loss, including loss of pubic hair, and this may affect body image and feelings of attractiveness for both sexes. Little evidence exists on the sexual side effects during treatment with chemotherapy because questions about this aspect of life are not routinely asked in clinical trials and therefore are not reported as potential adverse effects.

Cancer Types

Although all cancers and their treatments have the potential to affect sexuality, cancers that directly affect sexual organs (i.e., prostate, gynecologic, testicular, and breast) have the greatest effect. Two other cancer types are included in this chapter, as they too have the potential for adverse sexual effects. The first, colorectal cancer, usually is treated with multimodality therapy, and surgery and radiation therapy can affect sexual organs because the colon and rectum are anatomically close to these organs. Second, hematologic cancers are sometimes treated with bone marrow or stem cell transplantation, and the conditioning regimens have significant effects on the whole body, including the hypopituitary axis, which governs the production of sex hormones.

Breast Cancer

Breast cancer is known to cause significant physical, emotional, and sexual side effects for survivors, and unfortunately, these effects persist for many years and cause distress. The effects on the body image of women combined with the exaggerated symptoms of early or chemical menopause lie at the root of the sexual problems experienced by these women. Women who have breast reconstruction or breast conserving surgery seem to have better body image than those who have mastectomy without reconstruction (Fang, Shu, & Chang, 2013). Adjuvant endocrine therapy causes menopausal symptoms such as vaginal dryness and loss of libido (Harrow et al., 2014) and aromatase inhibitors in particular have an extremely negative effect for many women. In a study by Schover and colleagues, 93% of the women assessed met the criteria for sexual dysfunction, and 75% of these women were distressed about this (Schover, Baum, Fuson, Brewster, & Melhem-Bertrandt, 2014). Of the women with sexual dysfunction, 24% stopped being sexually active and 13% changed therapy.

When measured with validated tools, up to 70% of long-term breast cancer survivors met the criteria for sexual dysfunction (Raggio, Butryn, Arigo, Mikorski, & Palmer, 2014). Body image for these women was poor, plus having a mastectomy was associated with sexual and body changes causing distress as well as post-treatment weight gain. A large study of Australian women revealed that frequency of sexual intercourse decreased following treatment. Sexual response and satisfaction were also negatively affected (Ussher, Perz, & Gilbert, 2012). These changes were associated with pain, fatigue, menopausal symptoms such as vaginal dryness and weight gain, and emotional distress and poor body image. The women in this study reported feeling unattractive and lacking in femininity, and this affected their partner and relationship.

Interventions for these women are largely nonpharmaceutical; the hormone-dependent nature of most breast cancers has led to extreme caution in the treatment of the vaginal dryness associated with menopause. A small feasibility study of a combination of pelvic floor muscle relaxation, vaginal moisturizer, and olive oil lubrication showed acceptability and effectiveness of these interventions (Juraskova et al., 2013). No U.S. Food and Drug Administration–approved medications exist for other sexual problems, such as low libido or lack of arousal. Local estrogen in pill, ring, or cream formulations is the only truly effective treatment for vaginal atrophy, but its use in women with breast cancer is highly controversial (Krychman & Millheiser, 2013).

Nonhormonal vaginal moisturizers such as Replens® or vitamin E oil can relieve minor dryness, and lubricants can be helpful for sexual activity. Caution should be used with products that claim to be warming or cooling. In addition, labels should be scrutinized for the presence of perfumes, dyes, and flavoring (Casey, Faubion, MacLaughlin, Long, & Pruthi, 2014).

Psychosocial interventions for women and their partner comprising skills-based training in communication, problem solving, education, and sex therapy have been found to be helpful (Taylor, Harley, Ziegler, Brown, & Velikova, 2011). A small feasibility study of a couple's intervention focused on communication, creation of intimacy, management of sexual problems, and dyadic coping found that a face-to-face or telephone-based program was acceptable to the couples; however, efficacy was not tested (Decker, Pais, Miller, Goulet, & Fife, 2012). In another study of a psychoeducational intervention, women who received the intervention who were the least satisfied with their sexual relationship improved the most (Rowland et al., 2009).

Colorectal Cancer

Treatment for colorectal cancer has many of the same side effects as treatment for prostate and gynecologic cancer. The colon, rectum, and anus are close to the sexual and reproductive organs; therefore, damage from surgery and radiation often results in sexual problems. In a study of men and women with rectal cancer who had surgical resection with or without preoperative radiation therapy, sexual problems were identified in 76.4% of men, erectile dysfunction in 79.8%, and ejaculatory problems in 72.2% (Lange et al., 2009). Women in the study experienced sexual problems (61.5%), including vaginal dryness (56.6%) and pain with intercourse (dyspareunia, 59.1%). The presence of a stoma was associated with these problems. Rectal cancer survivors also are known to experience urinary and fecal incontinence as long-term effects (Panjari et al., 2012). Chemotherapy may cause nerve damage affecting erections and ejaculation in men and often causes early menopause in women, resulting in vaginal dryness and other menopausal symptoms (Breukink & Donovan, 2013).

It is important to note the effects of a stoma on body image. In one study, researchers found body image to be strongly associated with poor sexual functioning (Philip et al., 2013). People with stomas often are worried about the ostomy bag leaking or coming off during sexual activity, and they may be concerned that their sexual partner finds the stoma distasteful. The ostomy may serve as a constant reminder of the cancer and treatment trajectory, which often is traumatic and invasive for patients.

For those who engage in anal intercourse, cancer of the anus or rectum may cause significant issues, including the inability to engage in this sexual activity if the rectum is closed off. Tissue friability or scar tissue causing rectal pain and bleeding may pose problems. This can be devastating to survivors who previously enjoyed anal intercourse and may leave them with significant emotional problems.

Gynecologic Cancer

Cancer of the vulva, uterus, or cervix may create sexual problems for women even before treatment, such as bleeding or pain. Treatment usually is multimodal and involves surgery, radiation therapy, and, for some, chemotherapy. In a study of 55 women with all types of gynecologic cancer, 55.6% reported alterations in their sexual functioning, including changes to body image (45%), vaginal dryness (25%), pain during intercourse (20%), and fear of physical harm from sex (20%) (Pilger et al., 2012). Qualitative studies suggest that the experience of women after treatment is more emotionally harmful than the previous statistics suggest. In a study of women with ovarian cancer, women reported that the treatment made them feel as if they were no longer whole. Physical as well as hormonal changes contributed to the intensity of the experience of these changes, regardless of the woman's age (Wilmoth, Hatmaker-Flanigan, LaLoggia, & Nixon, 2011). Women in another study spoke poignantly about how sex, once a source of pleasure, was now a source of pain. They felt unable to express their love for their partner in a physical way and had difficulty coming to terms with the sexual and relationship changes after treatment (Sekse, Gjengedal, & Råheim, 2013). This study was conducted with women who were five years after treatment. Women with vulvar cancer described their experience as one of "aloneness"; they felt separated from their partners because of the loss of sexual function and sexual pleasure after treatment (Jefferies & Clifford, 2011). Women with cervical cancer reported that sexual difficulties affected their quality of life, with reductions seen in overall sexual function, quality and quantity of sexual life, and relationship satisfaction at 12 months after treatment (Juraskova et al., 2012).

Surgery affecting the pelvis, particularly the cervix and vagina, can lead to shortening and narrowing of the vagina, causing pain with penetration. Women who are treated with radiation may experience vaginal atrophy, stenosis, and even fistula formation (Viswanathan et al., 2014). Women often are advised to use vaginal dilators to mitigate these adverse effects of treatment (Cullen et al., 2013). However, their use is not without consequences to women, as some may see the dilator as embarrassing and akin to a sex toy that is not acceptable, or as an aversive treatment that reminds them of the invasiveness of their original treatment for cancer (Cullen et al., 2012). The invasiveness of treatment has far-reaching effects for women who may dissociate from their bodies as sexual entities in the face of cancer and treatment and instead see their genitalia as diseased and the focus of scrutiny by healthcare providers, as well as a source of recurrence of the cancer (White, Faithfull, & Allan, 2013).

Some women may not prioritize a return to sexual activity as they recover, preferring to be grateful that they are alive and expressing willingness to live with diminished sexuality as a cost of survival (White et al., 2013). And yet in other studies, women with gynecologic cancer wanted information and assistance with sexual challenges (Hill et al., 2011). Gerestein et al. (2011) found that 37%–46.5% of the women in their study were interested in receiving help for sexual problems. However, these needs may not be met routinely; in this study, only 7% had sought help. In another study, although 51% of women wanted information or help, only 35% had initiated a discussion about their problems with a healthcare provider (Vermeer et al., 2015a). The same authors surveyed gynecologic and radiation oncologists as well as oncology nurses (Vermeer et al., 2015b) and found that most of the oncology care providers reported having at least one discussion with female patients about sexuality. They mostly reassured patients that sexual changes were normal after treatment, with only half of the healthcare providers offering practical suggestions. The patients were rarely referred for specialized sexuality help. McCallum, Lefebvre, Jolicoeur, Maheu, and Lebel (2012) found that gynecologic cancer survivors wanted specific information about changes to their anatomy as well as being offered a screening questionnaire to elicit problems, and they also wanted healthcare providers to be open to talking about sexual problems after treatment.

Beyond the use of vaginal dilators to maintain patency of the vagina, other treatments may mitigate the adverse effects experienced by women with gynecologic cancer. Vulvar, vaginal, and cervical cancers and some endometrial and ovarian cancers are not considered hormone dependent, and estrogen therapy can be prescribed to alleviate menopausal symptoms. Estrogen therapy is not recommended for endometrial stromal sarcomas or granulosa cell cancer of the ovary (Guidozzi, 2013). A professionally moderated online support group provided over 12 weeks showed general satisfaction from participants, with a small reduction in sexual distress (Classen et al., 2013). Mindfulness-based cognitive behavioral therapy sessions led to improvements in sexual response, including arousal, and a trend toward reducing sexual distress (Brotto et al., 2012).

Hematologic Cancer

Hematologic cancer presents global health challenges for many patients, including adolescents and young adults who often require urgent treatment. Bone marrow or stem cell transplant recipients face an arduous multimodality treatment journey with many side effects, including distress, depression, fatigue, and relationship problems (Majhail et al., 2012). Graft-versus-host disease may have skin and mucous membrane manifestations, making the survivor feel unattractive and also affecting sexual function for women who have a gynecologic presentation of this side effect. Majhail et al. (2012) recommended routine assessment of survivors and prompt and aggressive treatment of graft-versus-host disease.

In a recent study of men and women older than 50 years with diffuse large B-cell lymphoma, chronic lymphocytic leukemia, or acute myeloid leukemia, men experienced erectile difficulties as well as low desire and decreased sexual activity. Women in the study reported that sexual activity was not important to them, and the researchers concluded that the rigors of treatment may overshadow interest in sexuality (Olsson, Sandin-Bojö, Bjuresäter, & Larsson, 2015). Survivors of Hodgkin lymphoma also commonly report sexual problems, with low desire and decreased sexual activity being the most common challenges (Recklitis, Varela, Ng, Mauch, & Bober, 2010). In a study of 36 women of reproductive age with Hodgkin lymphoma, 31% of participants met the criteria for sexual dysfunction, with loss of libido being most commonly reported (Eeltink et al., 2013).

The International Myeloma Foundation Nurse Leadership Board suggested that the multiple medications used in myeloma treatment have global sexual side effects (Richards, Bertolotti, Doss, McCullagh, & International Myeloma Foundation Nurse Leadership Board, 2011). These medications include antidepressants, antihypertensives, antipsychotics, antiseizure medications, chemotherapies such as alkylating agents, immunomodulatory agents, interferon, proteasome inhibitors, and steroids.

Prostate Cancer

The cavernous nerves responsible for erections run alongside the prostate gland. Treatment of prostate cancer with radical prostatectomy or radiation therapy adversely affects these nerves, resulting in diminished erectile capacity. In the case of surgery, an immediate loss of erections occurs, with the potential for some improvement over time. Erectile difficulties occur in 14%–90% of men following surgery for prostate cancer (Salonia et al., 2012). Younger age and prior good erectile functioning are predictors of recovery, but one study showed that at two to four years after surgery, 58.5% of men saw no improvement and just 10.4% of men saw moderate improvement (Sivarajan, Prabhu, Taksler, Laze, & Lepor, 2014). Similarly, erectile dysfunction persisted at two years for 57% of men who were treated with external beam radiation and 31% of men treated with brachytherapy (Sanda et al., 2008). Androgen deprivation therapy is used in conjunction with external beam radiation to treat men with high-grade prostate cancer and men with metastatic disease (Pagliarulo et al., 2012). This treatment has profound effects on libido and erectile functioning, as well as body image (Walker, Tran, Wassersug, Thomas, & Robinson, 2013).

Other adverse effects of surgery that affect sexuality in men include delayed or absent orgasm, pain with orgasm, loss of urine during arousal or orgasm, penile shrinkage, and loss of sensation in the penis (Frey, Sønksen, Jakobsen, & Fode, 2014). Men experience loss of masculine identity as a result of the adverse sexual effects of both surgery and radiation, and this is distressing to them (Zaider, Manne, Nelson, Mulhall, & Kissane, 2012). Poor body image is associated with decreased quality of life (Harrington & Badger, 2009).

Adverse sexual effects have an impact on men's partners/spouses as well. In a study of 88 patient–partner pairs, treatment of prostate cancer was reported to have a negative impact on the couple's sexual relationship by 71% of partners at 12 months, particularly if the man had surgery (Ramsey et al., 2013). Female partners report distress related to the amount of distress or sexual bother the man experiences (Chambers et al., 2013). When sexual difficulties occur, the couple often does not communicate openly or effectively about these changes (Wootten et al., 2014), despite evidence that talking about their difficulties may alleviate the negative impact of sexual changes on the relationship (Badr & Taylor, 2009).

Treatment of prostate cancer poses unique challenges for gay men, including the loss of ejaculate, which plays an important role in the sexual experience for some gay men (Hartman et al., 2014). In this study, some gay couples found that opening their relationship to other partners helped mitigate the pressure to perform that was felt by the man with cancer and allowed for novelty in the relationship. However, gay men who are the insertive partners in penetrative sex may struggle with less rigid erections after treatment, even with the use of erectile aids (Hart et al., 2014). Referrals to sex therapists with experience working with this population are essential.

First-line therapy for erectile difficulties after treatment for prostate cancer involves taking oral medications (phosphodiesterase type 5 [known as PDE5] inhibitors such as sildenafil, tadalafil, and vardenafil). The evidence suggests that the use of these medications declines with time, implicating that either the cost is a barrier or perhaps they do not work (Plym et al., 2014). Second-line therapies include more invasive measures, such as vacuum devices, intracorporeal injections, and intraurethral suppositories (Chung & Brock, 2013). Penile implants may be considered for men who are not able to use other erectile aids successfully (Mirza, Griebling, & Kazer, 2011). A Cochrane review (Parahoo et al., 2013) concluded that psychosocial interventions (psychoeducation, counseling, cognitive behavioral therapy, relaxation, art or music therapy) may have short-term benefits on some aspects of well-being but showed no benefit on distress or depression.

Testicular Cancer

Testicular cancer incidence peaks in the adolescent and young adult years, a time at which sexual identity is being formed. It is also seen in men up to age 49 years, when they are usually otherwise healthy and sexually active. The multimodality treatment regimen for this cancer (orchiectomy, radiation therapy, and chemotherapy) has both short- and long-term effects on sexuality.

In a study of 161 men treated with orchiectomy and radiation, up to six months after the end of treatment, 61% of participants reported body image changes. These changes were associated with decreased sexual interest, erectile problems, and decreased sexual pleasure (Wortel, Alemayehu, & Incrocci, 2015). Another study reported that in 539 men who have orchiectomy alone, some also experienced sexual problems, including decreased libido (34.5%) and erectile dysfunction (31.5%), with 24.4% of the total sample able to achieve an erection but not able to maintain it during intercourse (Pühse et al., 2012). Ejaculatory problems were experienced by 84.9% of the participants, and 95.4% reported reduced global sexual satisfaction.

Researchers support the association between body image and sexuality (Rossen, Pedersen, Zachariae, & von der Maase, 2012), especially in the domain of erectile functioning. In a review of the factors affecting sexuality in testicular cancer survivors and their partners, Jankowska (2012) supported the role of psychological factors such as body image in the development of sexual dysfunction. This review concluded that men with partners experience less distress, and younger age appears to be protective as well. However, young age produces unique psychosocial challenges: testicular cancer survivors aged 18–34 years reported feeling different from others and feeling like damaged goods (Carpentier, Fortenberry, Ott, Brames, & Einhorn, 2011).

Special Populations

Young adults with cancer may be profoundly affected by cancer treatment. The sentinel developmental milestones of this phase of life (between the ages of 15 and 39 years) include developing a sexual identity, becoming sexually active, establishing romantic relationships, and becoming a parent (Morgan, Davies, Palmer, & Plaster, 2010). As described earlier in this chapter, all cancer treatments have the potential to affect sexuality and sexual functioning. Treatment during this developmental phase causes a biologic disruption, and most young adults have little life experience to draw on in coming to terms with the changes (Bakewell & Volker, 2005). Absences from school, college, or the workplace interrupt the normal socialization processes that are important in identity formation, and young adults with cancer may fall behind their peers in the social tasks related to peer identity, dating and flirting, and establishment of more committed relationships.

A study of young adult survivors revealed critical challenges after cancer, including loss of the ability to enjoy "normal" sexual activity due to early menopause and its symptoms, scars, and weight loss. Participants reported altered sexual responses to stimuli and loss of desire in response to these changes (Robinson, Miedema, & Easley, 2014).

Disclosing a history of cancer is not easy, and the experiences of young women with breast cancer highlight the vulnerability of trying to start a new relationship when lacking confidence in one's body and subjective attractiveness (Kurowecki & Fergus, 2014). Many of the women in this study felt that they were "damaged goods" and dating after cancer first required self-acceptance before they were willing to make themselves vulnerable with a potential new partner. Telling a prospective partner and closely watching the reaction was seen as a way of testing potential partners before any physical contact occurred. Disclosure was of particular importance to single women. These women are often fearful of the response of a new partner, especially if a previous partner had rejected them and their altered body (Holmberg, Scott, Alexy, & Fife, 2001).

Survivors of childhood cancer are at particular risk for physical, cognitive, and emotional late effects of treatment (Jacobs & Pucci, 2013). These effects are dependent on age at diagnosis and treatment, the type of treatment, and social history. Surgery or radiation affecting the reproductive organs may result in early menopause. Radiation to the brain may result in altered sexual development, as well as short stature, which may affect self-image in later years. Scars, amputations, and missing organs (for example, a testicle) may negatively influence body image and, as a result, social and romantic relationships.

Assessing Sexual Health

Communication about sexuality and sexual problems during and after treatment does not occur as often as it needs to. Multiple studies show that assessment of sexual functioning is not common, despite National Comprehensive Cancer Network® (NCCN®) guidelines recommending assessment at regular intervals (NCCN, 2017b). Patients want their oncology care providers to talk about sexuality, but this does not occur frequently or with any kind of regularity. Sporn et al. (2015) reported that of the 66 cancer survivors in their study, 96.9% stated that their oncologist rarely or never discussed this with them, and 94% said that their oncologist was unlikely to initiate the conversation. Provision of information about sexuality may also be dependent on sex. In Flynn et al.'s (2012) study, men were more likely than women to receive information from oncologists. In this study, 79% of men with prostate cancer were given information, compared to only 29% of women with breast cancer. Participants in this study said they were unprepared for the physical changes that affected sexual functioning. In a Swedish study, 48% of 104 women with a variety of cancers had not received information about changes to sexuality, and in particular, they wanted to know whether sexual activity should be avoided (Rasmusson, Plantin, & Elmerstig, 2013). Not knowing this may lead to avoiding sexual activity when it is permitted or being sexually active when it is prohibited or when barrier methods are needed. If the woman does not know about this, she may put her sexual partner or herself at risk for adverse events. Patients who experience sexual problems have a greater need for information (Hautamäki-Lamminen, Lipiäinen, Beaver, Lehto, & Kellokumpu-Lehtinen, 2013), but unless they raise this as a problem, they are unlikely to receive information or help.

Barriers to Sexual Health Assessment

Some patients do not broach the topic with their healthcare providers because they think that if it was important, the healthcare provider would have asked about it (Hordern & Street, 2007). Participants in this study also said that they felt as though they should just be grateful to be alive, and this left them angry when their needs and distress about sexual changes were not recognized.

Healthcare providers tend to take a biomedical approach to assessing sexual functioning in patients, while their patients want a more reflective approach that includes choice of treatment based on potential sexual side effects and an open and honest approach to the patient's needs (Hordern & Street, 2007). This incongruence serves to create distance between the patient and the healthcare provider and is unlikely to result in constructive interactions about a sensitive topic. In an analysis of the discourse about sexuality with oncologists and oncology nurses, Ussher et al. (2013) reported a similar biomedical approach with a focus on sexual pain, loss of libido, and changes to the body. Recognition was given to these problems in cancer of sexual or reproductive organs, neglecting other kinds of cancer that may have similar effects. However, in this study, oncology care providers situated sexuality in the domain of psychosocial support, in which discussions with patients can occur in the clinic with the aim of reducing distress, dispelling myths, and negotiating a different way of being sexual.

Ussher et al. (2013) also identified a number of common barriers cited by oncology care providers to discussions about sexuality. These include the sensitivity and private nature of the topic, lack of knowledge, lack of confidence and personal discomfort, a belief that this is the responsibility of another healthcare provider, lack of time in busy clinics, lack of privacy in the clinical setting, and patient attributes (e.g., age, sex, sexual orientation, relationship status, cultural background, type of cancer), as well as the sex of the healthcare provider vis-à-vis the sex of the patient. Of note in this study is the fear that the patient may negatively respond to introduction of the topic. Participants also mentioned that it is more difficult to talk about sexuality if the patient's partner was present. The perceived lack of services or other professionals to refer to was also cited as a reason to not talk about sexuality with patients. The authors of this study noted that almost all of these barriers are seen as outside of the control of the healthcare provider, thus abrogating personal responsibility for initiating meaningful discussions with patients as a part of routine care.

In a review of the attitudes and knowledge of nurses in providing sexual health care to people with cancer, Kotronoulas, Papadopoulou, and Patiraki (2009) suggested that while nurses recognize this as an important part of nursing care, they lack knowledge and communication skills and do not respond to patient concerns. Many of the same barriers are cited: assumptions about patients, lack of knowledge, discomfort, and work environment barriers. In another study, oncology nurses regarded their patients' need for sexuality information as being low but felt that they should talk about it with patients; however, they cited similar barriers (knowledge, skill, environment) to having the discussion (Olsson, Berglund, Larsson, & Athlin, 2012). In a study of Oncology Nursing Society members, Julien, Thom, and Kline (2010) found that age, years of experience, practice setting, and oncology nursing certification all influenced attitudes to sexuality discussion with patients. Nurses who were younger, had fewer years of experience, worked in inpatient units, and who were not certified identified more barriers to discussing this topic with patients. Nurses with oncology certification and those working in ambulatory settings identified fewer barriers. The largest barrier identified in this study was the belief that patients do not expect to discuss sexuality with nurses. In addition, nurses who thought the subject was too personal to discuss were more likely to think that this was the physician's responsibility. For oncology nurses caring for men with testicular cancer, although they recognized the importance of sexual issues in this population, few told their patients they were willing to discuss their sexual concerns (Moore, Higgins, & Sharek, 2013).

The Oncology Nursing Society recognizes the role of nurses in managing late and long-term effects of cancer treatment, including those on sexuality and sexual functioning, in the report *Red Flags in Caring for Cancer Survivors* (Baney et al., 2014). Addressing these issues with patients is an important part of the nursing role and one that nurses should perform. If the nurse finds the topic uncomfortable, there are ways to address this, including desensitization to increase level of comfort, assessing personal attitudes to sexuality, and gaining knowledge so that evidence-based information can be provided to patients (Shell, 2007). Shell suggested exposure to anxiety-producing material in a safe environment, which can be achieved by collaboration with a trusted colleague or attendance at a sexuality reassessment seminar. The American Association of Sexuality Educators, Counselors and Therapists (www.aasect.org) has information about these sessions. Nurses can assess their personal attitudes toward sexuality by listing personal values about sexual behavior, how these values may affect patient care, and recognition of what would be unacceptable to them and how they would handle a situation in which a patient presents with a problem in one of these areas. Finally, nurses should educate themselves about sexuality and cancer. Many options exist for this, including self-study (see the bibliography at the end of this chapter), courses through the Oncology Nursing Society (www.ons.org/education/courses-activities), conferences, and articles in nursing and health sciences journals.

Sexuality Assessment Models

A number of models exist to help nurses start the conversation about sexuality and address sexual concerns or questions raised by patients at any time in the cancer trajectory. For example, a biomedical approach is suggested in the NCCN (2017b) guidelines by using the Brief

Sexual Symptom Checklist for Women and the Sexual Health Inventory for Men. These contain closed-ended questions on satisfaction with sexual function (yes/no), identification of problem areas and of which problem is most bothersome, and whether the person wants to talk about it with their doctor (yes/no). However, these checklists are not cancer specific and are not recommended for use by oncology nurses due to the closed-ended questions and absence of psychosocial factors. Rather, the following models—BETTER, PLISSIT, and the 5 A's—are better suited for use by oncology nurses.

BETTER Model

The BETTER Model (Mick, Hughes, & Cohen, 2003) was created by oncology nurses and comprises 6 steps:

- B: Bring up the topic.
- E: Explain sexuality as a part of quality of life.
- T: Tell the patient about appropriate resources.
- T: Assess the timing of the discussion/intervention.
- E: Educate about side effects.
- R: Record the conversation in the medical record.

The following example shows how this model could be used with a young adult with lymphoma:

- Bring up the topic: "Many young adults with cancer have concerns about how their treatment will affect their sexuality or romantic relationship."
- Explain sexuality as a part of quality of life: "As a young adult, dating, relationships, and sex are some of the important tasks you have to accomplish. We recognize this, and that is why we talk to all young adults about this."
- Tell the patient about appropriate resources: "Online resources are available that you may find helpful. One of them is Stupid Cancer. They have an informative and user-friendly website, as well as conferences, retreats, and web-based groups and education."
- Assess the timing of the discussion/intervention: "If you don't want to talk about this now, we can plan to meet again to see how we can best support you and help you to find the resources that will be useful to you."
- Educate about side effects of treatment: "While not everyone gets all the side effects from treatment, you need to know what to look out for. Some men find that their interest in sex decreases after a stem cell transplant. If this happens to you, please let us know so that we can do something about this."
- Record the conversation in the medical record: "Sexual side effects of stem cell transplant were discussed with the patient. He is aware of the resources available."

PLISSIT Model

The PLISSIT Model (Annon, 1974) contains four levels of increasing complexity:

- P: permission
- LI: limited information
- SS: specific suggestions
- IT: intensive therapy

The following is an example of how this model could be used with a young adult with breast cancer:

- Permission: "Women with breast cancer often have questions or concerns about the impact of the cancer and treatment on body image and sexuality. I am here to answer your questions, now or in the future."
- Limited information: "Your breasts will feel numb for some time after the surgery. As the nerves that have been cut start to grow, you may feel tingling and other sensations. This does NOT mean the cancer is back."
- Specific suggestions: "It is not unusual to experience vaginal and vulvar dryness after chemotherapy; this can make sexual touch and penetration painful. I have a list of recommended lubricants that you may find helpful, as well as a list of stores where you can purchase them."
- Intensive therapy: "I think that you may benefit from seeing a sexuality counselor after hearing what is going on in your relationship. She will likely suggest that your partner come to your first session. I will send a referral to

her, and you can expect a call within the next 48 hours to set up an appointment."

The PLISSIT Model has been modified, referred to as the Ex-PLISSIT Model, to include explicit permission-giving at the core of each stage, review of all interactions, and reflection on the part of the practitioner (Taylor & Davis, 2007).

5 A's Framework

Finally, the 5 A's framework used in tobacco cessation counseling has been suggested as a way of assessing sexual health and sexual concerns in cancer survivors (Bober, Carter, & Falk, 2013). This model proposes the following actions: ask, assess, advise, assist, and arrange.

Examples of statements illustrating the 5 A's framework are the following:

- Ask: "What changes have you noticed to your sexual health/sexuality after treatment?"
- Assess: "Can you tell me more about the pain you are having with intercourse? Where exactly is the pain located, and what have you tried to do to help yourself with this?
- Advise: "What you are experiencing is quite common, and we can help you with finding a solution to these problems."
- Assist: "I have a handout about lubricants you can use, and we also have some books in the patient library that you may find helpful."
- Arrange: "I would like to see you again at your next visit to the oncologist. At that time, we can talk about how things have improved (or not) and plan for referrals as needed."

Given the evidence about the lack of attention paid to this aspect of quality of life, it is vital that nurses take a leadership role in assessing patients' sexual health, identify any problems associated with treatment, and offer assistance to help them resolve their issues. It is incumbent on nurses to know and understand the sexual side effects of cancer treatment for the specific populations they care for and to be able to normalize the situation for patients, which often will alleviate a great deal of anxiety for patients. In addition, nurses need to know where they can refer their patients for further help and do this in a timely manner; this begins with patient assessment.

Fertility

All cancer treatments have the potential to negatively affect fertility. Alkylating agents in particular have a negative effect for both men and women. When cyclophosphamide is coupled with total body irradiation in preparation for stem cell transplant, the risk to fertility is very high. In men, radiation to the testes affects sperm production. Radiation to the uterus may not affect a woman's ability to conceive but rather her ability to carry a fetus to term because the uterus may not be able grow with the pregnancy. Surgery to the reproductive organs has obvious consequences.

The American Society of Clinical Oncology guideline on fertility preservation (Loren et al., 2013) stated that all oncology care providers must discuss fertility preservation with patients of reproductive age and also with the parents and guardians of children and adolescents when a risk to fertility is present with the selected treatment modality. This guideline is echoed by NCCN (2017a).

Fertility Preservation

While many chemotherapy protocols do not allow for substitution of less damaging agents, radiation damage can be minimized by shielding the reproductive organs (Wallace, 2011). Some surgical approaches may help mitigate the damage to reproductive organs, for example, trachelectomy or conization for the treatment of cervical cancer, hormone therapy alone for endometrial cancer, or preservation of the contralateral ovary where possible in ovarian cancer (Kesic, 2008).

Fertility preservation includes sperm banking for postpubertal boys and men. This is a noninvasive and simple procedure; however, it must be done before treatment starts. Ideally, three semen samples should be collected with 48 hours between ejaculations, but even one specimen may be sufficient with modern in vitro fertilization techniques (Kelvin, 2015). For men who are unable to masturbate or are unwilling for religious or cultural reasons, electroejaculation may be necessary; this is done under general anesthesia. Testicular extraction of sperm or testicular tissue banking are two other alternatives, although the latter is regarded as experimental at this time (Johnson & Kroon, 2013). Spermatogenesis may return in men 12 months after treatment. Sperm production may be sufficient to allow for sperm banking at that time (Katz, Kolon, Feldman, & Mulhall, 2013).

Fertility preservation for women is more complex and requires a delay of treatment to allow for hyperstimulation of the ovaries and oocyte extraction for either in vitro embryo creation (the most well-established preservation technique) or oocyte cryopreservation. Women with hormone-dependent cancers are precluded from the high doses of hormones needed for hyperstimulation, and those who need to be treated urgently will not be able to take the necessary delay of treatment. Embryo cryopreservation requires the presence of a partner to donate sperm or the use of donor sperm. Ovarian suppression and ovarian tissue cryopreservation are two experimental techniques (Johnson & Kroon, 2013).

Significant psychosocial issues exist related to the potential threat to fertility and to the process of fertility preservation. For both men and women, the prospect of not being able to have biological offspring may be devastating (Levine, Kelvin, Quinn, & Gracia, 2015). Although some treatment regimens are known to cause post-treatment infertility, uncertainty remains with others, and factors such as age and comorbidities also may play a role. Discussing these complexities in the context of a new life-threatening cancer diagnosis can be difficult for oncology care providers and very challenging for patients and/or their parents to understand. The costs for fertility preservation are significant, and the subsequent costs for in vitro fertilization even more so; many insurance companies do not cover these costs. Financial programs can provide partial assistance, but great variation exists across jurisdictions (Levine et al., 2015).

Assessment and Guidelines

Despite clear guidelines on the need to discuss fertility preservation with patients of reproductive age (Loren et al., 2013), this is not always done consistently or effectively. When fertility is not discussed with patients, it may be seen as something not important to the oncology care provider and so is not asked about by patients, even if they are aware of the risks of treatment to fertility. Barriers to provision of this information include lack of knowledge, lack of time, discomfort with the topic, thinking the patient has a poor prognosis, and thinking the topic is not important to the patient (Duffy & Allen, 2009). In a review of the literature related to provider and patient factors concerning fertility information, Goossens et al. (2014) reported that 66%–100% of patients want information but a maximum of 85% received information.

The following websites have information that may be helpful to oncology care providers and patients:

- American Society for Reproductive Medicine: www.asrm.org
- Livestrong Fertility: www.livestrong.org/we-can-help/livestrong-fertility
- MyOncofertility: www.myoncofertility.org
- Oncofertility Consortium: www.oncofertility.northwestern.edu
- Oncology Nursing Society: www.ons.org, which offers an online course on sexual dysfunction and fertility impairment (www.ons.org/content/sexual-dysfunction-and-fertility-impairment), as well as courses specific to cancers affecting sexuality
- Save My Fertility: www.savemyfertility.org

Key Points

- Treatment for cancer may result in global sexual problems for survivors of all ages.
- Sexual changes are possible even with cancer of nonsexual organs.
- Sexual problems affect quality of life and cause distress in patients and partners.
- Nurses must be able to include a sexual health assessment as part of ongoing care of patients.
- Multiple models are available to assist nurses in a consistent approach to sexual health assessment.
- Fertility preservation must be discussed with all patients of childbearing age, as well as with parents of children whose future fertility is likely to be affected by treatment.
- Lack of information about potential for impact on fertility results in distress for survivors after treatment is over.

Conclusion

Sexuality is an important aspect of quality of life and is affected by all treatments for cancer. It remains a sensitive topic for both healthcare providers and patients, but as with all side effects of treatment, it is important for oncology care providers to ask about this and offer assistance. Fertility is another sensitive topic for patients of reproductive age, and it is imperative that healthcare providers address this issue with appropriate patients. This chapter has provided an overview of the sexual side effects for the most common cancers and effects on fertility, as well as suggestions to help oncology care providers start the conversation.

The author would like to acknowledge Judith A. Shell, PhD, LMFT, RN, for her contribution to this chapter that remains unchanged from the first edition of this book.

Bibliography

Katz, A. (2007). *Breaking the silence on cancer and sexuality: A handbook for healthcare providers.* Pittsburgh, PA: Oncology Nursing Society.

Katz, A. (2009). *Woman cancer sex.* Pittsburgh, PA: Hygeia Media.

Katz, A. (2010). *Man cancer sex.* Pittsburgh, PA: Hygeia Media.

Katz, A. (2011). *After you ring the bell . . . 10 challenges for the cancer survivor.* Pittsburgh, PA: Hygeia Media.

Katz, A. (2011). *Surviving after cancer: Living the new normal.* New York, NY: Rowman & Littlefield.

Katz, A. (2012). *Prostate cancer and the man you love: Supporting and caring for your partner.* New York, NY: Rowman & Littlefield.

Katz, A. (2014). *This should not be happening: Young adults with cancer.* Pittsburgh, PA: Hygeia Media.

Katz, A. (2015). *Meeting the need for psychosocial care in young adults with cancer.* Pittsburgh, PA: Oncology Nursing Society.

References

Annon, J. (1974). *The behavioral treatment of sexual problems: Brief therapy.* Honolulu, HI: Enabling Systems.

Badr, H., & Taylor, C.L. (2009). Sexual dysfunction and spousal communication in couples coping with prostate cancer. *Psycho-Oncology, 18,* 735–746. doi:10.1002/pon.1449

Bakewell, R.T., & Volker, D.L. (2005). Sexual dysfunction related to the treatment of young women with breast cancer. *Clinical Journal of Oncology Nursing, 9,* 697–702. doi:10.1188/05.CJON.697-702

Baney, T., Belansky, H., Gutaj, D., Hellman-Wylie, C., Mackey, H., Shriner, M., & Vendlinski, S. (2014). *Red flags in caring for cancer survivors.* Retrieved from https://www.ons.org/sites/default/files/media/Red%20Flags%20for%20Cancer%20Survivors.pdf

Basson, R. (2005). Women's sexual dysfunction: Revised and expanded definitions. *Canadian Medical Association Journal, 172,* 1327–1333. doi:10.1503/cmaj.1020174

Bober, S.L., Carter, J., & Falk, S. (2013). Addressing female sexual function after cancer by internists and primary care providers. *Journal of Sexual Medicine, 10*(Suppl. 1), 112–119. doi:10.1111/jsm.12027

Bober, S.L., & Varela, V.S. (2012). Sexuality in adult cancer survivors: Challenges and intervention. *Journal of Clinical Oncology, 30,* 3712–3719. doi:10.1200/JCO.2012.41.7915

Breukink, S.O., & Donovan, K.A. (2013). Physical and psychological effects of treatment on sexual functioning in colorectal cancer survivors. *Journal of Sexual Medicine, 10*(Suppl. 1), 74–83. doi:10.1111/jsm.12037

Brotto, L., Erskine, Y., Carey, M., Ehlen, T., Finlayson, S., Heywood, M., ... Miller, D. (2012). A brief mindfulness-based cognitive behavioral intervention improves sexual functioning versus wait-list control in women treated for gynecologic cancer. *Gynecologic Oncology, 125,* 320–325. doi:10.1016/j.ygyno.2012.01.035

Carpentier, M.Y., Fortenberry, J.D., Ott, M.A., Brames, M.J., & Einhorn, L.H. (2011). Perceptions of masculinity and self-image in adolescent and young adult testicular cancer survivors: Implications for romantic and sexual relationships. *Psycho-Oncology, 20,* 738–745. doi:10.1002/pon.1772

Casey, P.M., Faubion, S.S., MacLaughlin, K.L., Long, M.E., & Pruthi, S. (2014). Caring for the breast cancer survivor's health and well-being. *World Journal of Clinical Oncology, 5,* 693–704. doi:10.5306/wjco.v5.i4.693

Chambers, S.K., Schover, L., Nielsen, L., Halford, K., Clutton, S., Gardiner, R.A., ... Occhipinti, S. (2013). Couple distress after localised prostate cancer. *Supportive Care in Cancer, 21,* 2967–2976. doi:10.1007/s00520-013-1868-6

Chung, E., & Brock, G. (2013). Sexual rehabilitation and cancer survivorship: A state of art review of current literature and management strategies in male sexual dysfunction among prostate cancer survivors. *Journal of Sexual Medicine, 10*(Suppl. 1), 102–111. doi:10.1111/j.1743-6109.2012.03005.x

Classen, C.C., Chivers, M.L., Urowitz, S., Barbera, L., Wiljer, D., O'Rinn, S., & Ferguson, S.E. (2013). Psychosexual distress in women with gynecologic cancer: A feasibility study of an online support group. *Psycho-Oncology, 22,* 930–935. doi:10.1002/pon.3058

Cullen, K., Fergus, K., DasGupta, T., Fitch, M., Doyle, C., & Adams, L. (2012). From "sex toy" to intrusive imposition: A qualitative examination of women's experiences with vaginal dilator use following treatment for gynecological cancer. *Journal of Sexual Medicine, 9,* 1162–1173. doi:10.1111/j.1743-6109.2011.02639.x

Cullen, K., Fergus, K., DasGupta, T., Kong, I., Fitch, M., Doyle, C., & Adams, L. (2013). Toward clinical care guidelines for supporting rehabilitative vaginal dilator use with women recovering from cervical cancer. *Supportive Care in Cancer, 21,* 1911–1917. doi:10.1007/s00520-013-1726-6

Decker, C.L., Pais, S., Miller, K.D., Goulet, R., & Fife, B.L. (2012). A brief intervention to minimize psychosexual morbidity in dyads coping with breast cancer. *Oncology Nursing Forum, 39,* 176–185. doi:10.1188/12.ONF.176-185

Duffy, C., & Allen, S. (2009). Medical and psychosocial aspects of fertility after cancer. *Cancer Journal, 15,* 27–33. doi:10.1097/PPO.0b013e3181976602

Eeltink, C.M., Incrocci, L., Witte, B.I., Meurs, S., Visser, O., Huijgens, P., & Verdonck-de Leeuw, I.M. (2013). Fertility and sexual function in female Hodgkin lymphoma survivors of reproductive age. *Journal of Clinical Nursing, 22,* 3513–3521. doi:10.1111/jocn.12354

Fang, S., Shu, B., & Chang, Y. (2013). The effect of breast reconstruction surgery on body image among women after mastectomy: A meta-analysis. *Breast Cancer Research and Treatment, 137,* 13–21. doi:10.1007/s10549-012-2349-1

Flynn, K., Reese, J., Jeffery, D., Abernethy, A., Lin, L., Shelby, R., ... Weinfurt, K.P. (2012). Patient experiences with communication about sex during and after treatment for cancer. *Psycho-Oncology, 21,* 594–601. doi:10.1002/pon.1947

Frey, A., Sonksen, J., Jakobsen, H., & Fode, M. (2014). Prevalence and predicting factors for commonly neglected sexual side effects to radical prostatectomies: Results from a cross-sectional questionnaire-based study. *Journal of Sexual Medicine, 11,* 2318–2326. doi:10.1111/jsm.12624

Gerestein, C.G., Eijkemans, M.J., Bakker, J., Elgersma, O.E., van der Burg, M.E., Kooi, G.S., & Burger, C.W. (2011). Nomogram for suboptimal cytoreduction at primary surgery for advanced stage ovarian cancer. *Anticancer Research, 31,* 4043–4049. Retrieved from http://ar.iiarjournals.org/content/31/11/4043.long

Goossens, J., Delbaere, I., Van Lancker, A., Beeckman, D., Verhaeghe, S., & Van Hecke, A. (2014). Cancer patients' and professional caregivers' needs, preferences and factors associated with receiving and providing fertility-related information: A mixed-methods systematic review. *International Journal of Nursing Studies, 51,* 300–319. doi:10.1016/j.ijnurstu.2013.06.015

Guidozzi, F. (2013). Estrogen therapy in gynecological cancer survivors. *Climacteric, 16,* 611–617. doi:10.3109/13697137.2013.806471

Harrington, J.M., & Badger, T.A. (2009). Body image and quality of life in men with prostate cancer. *Cancer Nursing, 32*(2), E1–E7. doi:10.1097/NCC.0b013e3181982d18

Harrow, A., Dryden, R., McCowan, C., Radley, A., Parsons, M., Thompson, A.M., & Wells, M. (2014). A hard pill to swallow: A qualitative study of women's experiences of adjuvant endocrine therapy for breast cancer. *BMJ Open, 4,* e005285. doi:10.1136/bmjopen-2014-005285

Hart, T.L., Coon, D.W., Kowalkowski, M.A., Zhang, K., Hersom, J.I., Goltz, H.H., ... Latini, D.M. (2014). Changes in sexual roles and quality of life for gay men after prostate cancer: Challenges for sexual health providers. *Journal of Sexual Medicine, 11,* 2308–2317. doi:10.1111/jsm.12598

Hartman, M.-E., Irvine, J., Currie, K.L., Ritvo, P., Trachtenberg, L., Louis, A., ... Matthew, A.G. (2014). Exploring gay couples' experience with sexual dysfunction after radical prostatectomy: A qualitative study. *Journal of Sex and Marital Therapy, 40,* 233–253. doi:10.1080/0092623X.2012.726697

Hautamäki-Lamminen, K., Lipiäinen, L., Beaver, K., Lehto, J., & Kellokumpu-Lehtinen, P.L. (2013). Identifying cancer patients with greater need for information about sexual issues. *European Journal of Oncology Nursing, 17,* 9–15. doi:10.1016/j.ejon.2012.03.002

Hill, E., Sandbo, S., Abramsohn, E., Makelarski, J., Wroblewski, K., Wenrich, E., ... Lindau, S. (2011). Assessing gynecologic and breast cancer survivors' sexual health care needs. *Cancer, 117,* 2643–2651. doi:10.1002/cncr.25832

Holmberg, S.K., Scott, L.L., Alexy, W., & Fife, B.L. (2001). Relationship issues of women with breast cancer. *Cancer Nursing, 24,* 53–60. doi:10.1097/00002820-200102000-00009

Hordern, A.J., & Street, A.F. (2007). Constructions of sexuality and intimacy after cancer: Patient and health professional perspectives. *Social Science and Medicine, 64,* 1704–1718. doi:10.1016/j.socscimed.2006.12.012

Intimacy. (n.d.). In *Merriam-Webster's online dictionary* (11th ed.). Retrieved from http://www.merriam-webster.com/dictionary/intimacy

Jacobs, L.A., & Pucci, D.A. (2013). Adult survivors of childhood cancer: The medical and psychosocial late effects of cancer treatment and the impact on sexual and reproductive health. *Journal of Sexual Medicine, 10*(Suppl. 1), 120–126. doi:10.1111/jsm.12050

Jankowska, M. (2012). Sexual functioning of testicular cancer survivors and their partners—A review of literature. *Reports of Practical Oncology and Radiotherapy, 17,* 54–62. doi:10.1016/j.rpor.2011.11.001

Jefferies, H., & Clifford, C. (2011). Aloneness: The lived experience of women with cancer of the vulva. *European Journal of Cancer Care, 20,* 738–746. doi:10.1111/j.1365-2354.2011.01246.x

Johnson, R., & Kroon, L. (2013). Optimizing fertility preservation practices for adolescent and young adult cancer patients. *Journal of the National Comprehensive Cancer Network, 11,* 71–77.

Julien, J.O., Thom, B., & Kline, N.E. (2010). Identification of barriers to sexual health assessment in oncology nursing practice [Online exclusive]. *Oncology Nursing Forum, 37,* E186–E190. doi:10.1188/10.ONF.E186-E190

Juraskova, I., Bonner, C., Bell, M.L., Sharpe, L., Robertson, R., & Butow, P. (2012). Quantity vs. quality: An exploration of the predictors of posttreatment sexual adjustment for women affected by early stage cervical and endometrial cancer. *Journal of Sexual Medicine, 9,* 2952–2960. doi:10.1111/j.1743-6109.2012.02860.x

Juraskova, I., Jarvis, S., Mok, K., Peate, M., Meiser, B., Cheah, B.C., ... Friedlander, M. (2013). The acceptability, feasibility, and efficacy (phase I/II study) of the OVERcome (Olive Oil, Vaginal Exercise, and MoisturizeR) intervention to improve dyspareunia and alleviate sexual problems in women with breast cancer. *Journal of Sexual Medicine, 10,* 2549–2558. doi:10.1111/jsm.12156

Kaplan, H.S. (1979). *Disorders of sexual desire and other new concepts and techniques in sex therapy.* New York, NY: Simon & Schuster.

Katz, D.J., Kolon, T.F., Feldman, D.R., & Mulhall, J.P. (2013). Fertility preservation strategies for male patients with cancer. *Nature Reviews Urology, 10,* 463–472. doi:10.1038/nrurol.2013.145

Kelvin, J.F. (2015). Sperm banking: Fertility preservation for male patients with cancer. *Clinical Journal of Oncology Nursing, 19,* 108–110. doi:10.1188/15.CJON.108-110

Kesic, V. (2008). Fertility after the treatment of gynecologic tumors. In A. Surbone, F. Peccatori, & N. Pavlidis (Eds.), *Recent results in cancer research: Vol. 178. Cancer and pregnancy* (pp. 79–95). doi:10.1007/978-3-540-71274-9_9

Kotronoulas, G., Papadopoulou, C., & Patiraki, E. (2009). Nurses' knowledge, attitudes, and practices regarding provision of sexual health care in patients with cancer: A critical review of the evidence. *Supportive Care in Cancer, 17,* 479–501. doi:10.1007/s00520-008-0563-5

Krychman, M., & Millheiser, L.S. (2013). Sexual health issues in women with cancer. *Journal of Sexual Medicine, 10*(Suppl. 1), 5–15. doi:10.1111/jsm.12034

Kurowecki, D., & Fergus, K.D. (2014). Wearing my heart on my chest: Dating, new relationships, and the reconfiguration of self-esteem after breast cancer. *Psycho-Oncology, 23,* 52–64. doi:10.1002/pon.3370

Lange, M.M., Marijnen, C.A.M., Maas, C.P., Putter, H., Rutten, H.J., Stiggelbout, A.M., ... van de Velde, C.J.H. (2009). Risk factors for sexual dysfunction after rectal cancer treatment. *European Journal of Cancer, 45,* 1578–1588. doi:10.1016/j.ejca.2008.12.014

Levine, J.M., Kelvin, J.F., Quinn, G.P., & Gracia, C.R. (2015). Infertility in reproductive-age female cancer survivors. *Cancer, 121,* 1532–1539. doi:10.1002/cncr.29181

Loren, A.W., Mangu, P.B., Beck, L.N., Brennan, L., Magdalinski, A.J., Partridge, A.H., ... Oktay, K. (2013). Fertility preservation for patients with cancer: American Society of Clinical Oncology clinical practice guideline update. *Journal of Clinical Oncology, 31,* 2500–2510. doi:10.1200/JCO.2013.49.2678

Majhail, N.S., Brazauskas, R., Hassebroek, A., Bredeson, C.N., Hahn, T., Hale, G.A., … Hayes-Lattin, B.M. (2012). Outcomes of allogeneic hematopoietic cell transplantation for adolescent and young adults compared with children and older adults with acute myeloid leukemia. *Biology of Blood and Marrow Transplantation, 18,* 861–873. doi:10.1016/j.bbmt.2011.10.031

Masters, W.H., & Johnson, V.E. (1966). *Human sexual response.* Boston, MA: Little, Brown.

McCallum, M., Lefebvre, M., Jolicoeur, L., Maheu, C., & Lebel, S. (2012). Sexual health and gynecological cancer: Conceptualizing patient needs and overcoming barriers to seeking and accessing services. *Journal of Psychosomatic Obstetrics and Gynecology, 33,* 135–142. doi:10.3109/0167482X.2012.709291

Mick, J., Hughes, M., & Cohen, M. (2003). Sexuality and cancer: How oncology nurses can address it BETTER. *Oncology Nursing Forum, 30,* 152–153.

Mirza, M., Griebling, T.L., & Kazer, M.W. (2011). Erectile dysfunction and urinary incontinence after prostate cancer treatment. *Seminars in Oncology Nursing, 27,* 278–289. doi:10.1016/j.soncn.2011.07.006

Moore, A., Higgins, A., & Sharek, D. (2013). Barriers and facilitators for oncology nurses discussing sexual issues with men diagnosed with testicular cancer. *European Journal of Oncology Nursing, 17,* 416–422. doi:10.1016/j.ejon.2012.11.008

Morgan, S., Davies, S., Palmer, S., & Plaster, M. (2010). Sex, drugs, and rock 'n' roll: Caring for adolescents and young adults with cancer. *Journal of Clinical Oncology, 28,* 4825–4830. doi:10.1200/JCO.2009.22.5474

National Comprehensive Cancer Network. (2017a). *NCCN Clinical Practice Guidelines in Oncology (NCCN Guidelines®): Adolescent and young adult (AYA) oncology* [v.2.2017]. Retrieved from http://www.nccn.org/professionals/physician_gls/pdf/aya.pdf

National Comprehensive Cancer Network. (2017b). *NCCN Clinical Practice Guidelines in Oncology (NCCN Guidelines®): Survivorship* [v.1.2017]. Retrieved from https://www.nccn.org/professionals/physician_gls/pdf/survivorship.pdf

Olsson, C., Berglund, A.L., Larsson, M., & Athlin, E. (2012). Patient's sexuality—A neglected area of cancer nursing? *European Journal of Oncology Nursing, 16,* 426–431. doi:10.1016/j.ejon.2011.10.003

Olsson, C., Sandin-Bojö, A.K., Bjuresäter, K., & Larsson, M. (2015). Patients treated for hematologic malignancies: Affected sexuality and health-related quality of life. *Cancer Nursing, 38,* 99–110. doi:10.1097/NCC.0000000000000141

Pagliarulo, V., Bracarda, S., Eisenberger, M.A., Mottet, N., Schröder, F.H., Sternberg, C.N., … Studer, U.E. (2012). Contemporary role of androgen deprivation therapy for prostate cancer. *European Urology, 61,* 11–25. doi:10.1016/j.eururo.2011.08.026

Panjari, M., Bell, R., Burney, S., Bell, S., McMurrick, P., & Davis, S. (2012). Sexual function, incontinence, and wellbeing in women after rectal cancer—A review of the evidence. *Journal of Sexual Medicine, 9,* 2749–2758. doi:10.1111/j.1743-6109.2012.02894.x

Parahoo, K., McDonough, S., McCaughan, E., Noyes, J., Semple, C., Halstead, E.J., … Dahm, P. (2013). Psychosocial interventions for men with prostate cancer. *Cochrane Database of Systematic Reviews, 2013*(12). doi:10.1002/14651858.CD008529.pub3

Philip, E.J., Nelson, C., Temple, L., Carter, J., Schover, L., Jennings, S., … DuHamel, K. (2013). Psychological correlates of sexual dysfunction in female rectal and anal cancer survivors: Analysis of baseline intervention data. *Journal of Sexual Medicine, 10,* 2539–2548. doi:10.1111/jsm.12152

Pilger, A., Richter, R., Fotopoulou, C., Beteta, C., Klapp, C., & Sehouli, J. (2012). Quality of life and sexuality of patients after treatment for gynaecological malignancies: Results of a prospective study in 55 patients. *Anticancer Research, 32,* 5045–5049. Retrieved from http://ar.iiarjournals.org/content/32/11/5045.long

Plym, A., Folkvaljon, Y., Garmo, H., Holmberg, L., Johansson, E., Fransson, P., … Lambe, M. (2014). Drug prescription for erectile dysfunction before and after diagnosis of localized prostate cancer. *Journal of Sexual Medicine, 11,* 2100–2108. doi:10.1111/jsm.12586

Pühse, G., Wachsmuth, J.U., Kemper, S., Husstedt, I.W., Evers, S., & Kliesch, S. (2012). Chronic pain has a negative impact on sexuality in testis cancer survivors. *Journal of Andrology, 33,* 886–893. doi:10.2164/jandrol.110.012500

Raggio, G.A., Butryn, M.L., Arigo, D., Mikorski, R., & Palmer, S.C. (2014). Prevalence and correlates of sexual morbidity in long-term breast cancer survivors. *Psychology and Health, 29,* 632–650. doi:10.1080/08870446.2013.879136

Ramsey, S.D., Zeliadt, S.B., Blough, D.K., Moinpour, C.M., Hall, I.J., Smith, J.L., … Penson, D.F. (2013). Impact of prostate cancer on sexual relationships: A longitudinal perspective on intimate partners' experiences. *Journal of Sexual Medicine, 10,* 3135–3143. doi:10.1111/jsm.12295

Rasmusson, E.M., Plantin, L., & Elmerstig, E. (2013). Did they think I would understand all that on my own? A questionnaire study about sexuality with Swedish cancer patients. *European Journal of Cancer Care, 22,* 361–369. doi:10.1111/ecc.12039

Recklitis, C.J., Varela, V.S., Ng, A., Mauch, P., & Bober, S. (2010). Sexual functioning in long-term survivors of Hodgkin's lymphoma. *Psycho-Oncology, 19,* 1229–1233. doi:10.1002/pon.1679

Richards, T.A., Bertolotti, P.A., Doss, D., McCullagh, E.J., & International Myeloma Foundation Nurse Leadership Board. (2011). Sexual dysfunction in multiple myeloma: Survivorship care plan of the International Myeloma Foundation Nurse Leadership Board. *Clinical Journal of Oncology Nursing, 15*(Suppl. 1), 53–65. doi:10.1188/11.CJON.S1.53-65

Robinson, L., Miedema, B., & Easley, J. (2014). Young adult cancer survivors and the challenges of intimacy. *Journal of Psychosocial Oncology, 32,* 447–462. doi:10.1080/07347332.2014.917138

Rossen, P., Pedersen, A.F., Zachariae, R., & von der Maase, H. (2012). Sexuality and body image in long-term survivors of testicular cancer. *European Journal of Cancer, 48,* 571–578. doi:10.1016/j.ejca.2011.11.029

Rowland, J.H., Meyerowitz, B.E., Crespi, C.M., Leedham, B., Desmond, K., Belin, T.R., & Ganz, P.A. (2009). Addressing intimacy and partner communication after breast cancer: A randomized controlled group intervention. *Breast Cancer Research and Treatment, 118,* 99–111. doi:10.1007/s10549-009-0398-x

Sadovsky, R., Basson, R., Krychman, M., Morales, A.M., Schover, L., Wang, R., & Incrocci, L. (2010). Cancer and sexual problems. *Journal of Sexual Medicine, 7,* 349–373. doi:10.1111/j.1743-6109.2009.01620.x

Salonia, A., Burnett, A.L., Graefen, M., Hatzimouratidis, K., Montorsi, F., Mulhall, J.P., & Stief, C. (2012). Prevention and management of postprostatectomy sexual dysfunctions part 1: Choosing the right patient at the right time for the right surgery. *European Urology, 62,* 261–272. doi:10.1016/j.eururo.2012.04.046

Sanda, M.G., Dunn, R.L., Michalski, J., Sandler, H.M., Northouse, L., Hembroff, L., … Wei, J.T. (2008). Quality of life and satisfaction with outcome among prostate-cancer survivors. *New England Journal of Medicine, 358,* 1250–1261. doi:10.1056/NEJMoa074311

Schover, L.R., Baum, G.P., Fuson, L.A., Brewster, A., & Melhem-Bertrandt, A. (2014). Sexual problems during the first 2 years of adjuvant treatment with aromatase inhibitors. *Journal of Sexual Medicine, 11,* 3102–3111. doi:10.1111/jsm.12684

Sekse, R.J.T., Gjengedal, E., & Råheim, M. (2013). Living in a changed female body after gynecological cancer. *Health Care for Women International, 34,* 14–33. doi:10.1080/07399332.2011.645965

Shell, J. (2007). Including sexuality in your practice. *Nursing Clinics of North America, 42,* 685–696. doi:10.1016/j.cnur.2007.08.007

Sivarajan, G., Prabhu, V., Taksler, G.B., Laze, J., & Lepor, H. (2014). Ten-year outcomes of sexual function after radical prostatectomy: Results of a prospective longitudinal study. *European Urology, 65,* 58–65. doi:10.1016/j.eururo.2013.08.019

Sporn, N.J., Smith, K.B., Pirl, W.F., Lennes, I.T., Hyland, K.A., & Park, E.R. (2015). Sexual health communication between cancer survivors and providers: How frequently does it occur and which providers are preferred? *Psycho-Oncology, 24,* 1167–1173. doi:10.1002/pon.3736

Taylor, B., & Davis, S. (2007). The extended PLISSIT model for addressing the sexual wellbeing of individuals with an acquired disability or chronic illness. *Sexuality and Disability, 25,* 135–139. doi:10.1007/s11195-007-9044-x

Taylor, S., Harley, C., Ziegler, L., Brown, J., & Velikova, G. (2011). Interventions for sexual problems following treatment for breast cancer: A systematic review. *Breast Cancer Research and Treatment, 130,* 711–724. doi:10.1007/s10549-011-1722-9

Ussher, J.M., Perz, J., & Gilbert, E. (2012). Changes to sexual well-being and intimacy after breast cancer. *Cancer Nursing, 35,* 456–465. doi:10.1097/NCC.0b013e3182395401

Ussher, J.M., Perz, J., Gilbert, E., Wong, W.K.T., Mason, C., Hobbs, K., & Kirsten, L. (2013). Talking about sex after cancer: A discourse analytic study of health care professional accounts of sexual communication with patients. *Psychology and Health, 28,* 1370–1390. doi:10.1080/08870446.2013.811242

Vermeer, W., Bakker, R., Kenter, G., de Kroon, C., Stiggelbout, A., & ter Kuile, M. (2015a). Sexual issues among cervical cancer survivors: How can we help women seek help? *Psycho-Oncology, 24,* 458–464. doi:10.1002/pon.3663

Vermeer, W.M., Bakker, R.M., Stiggelbout, A.M., Creutzberg, C.L., Kenter, G.G., & ter Kuile, M.M. (2015b). Psychosexual support for gynecological cancer survivors: Professionals' current practices and need for assistance. *Supportive Care in Cancer, 23,* 831–839. doi:10.1007/s00520-014-2433-7

Viswanathan, A., Lee, L., Eswara, J., Horowitz, N., Konstantiopoulous, P., Mirabeau-Beale, K., … Wo, J. (2014). Complications of pelvic radiation in patients treated for gynecologic malignancies. *Cancer, 120,* 3870–3783. doi:10.1002/cncr.28849

Walker, J., Tran, S., Wassersug, R., Thomas, B., & Robinson, J. (2013). Patients and partners lack knowledge of androgen deprivation therapy side effects. *Urologic Oncology, 31,* 1098–1105. doi:10.1016/j.urolonc.2011.12.015

Wallace, W.H.B. (2011). Oncofertility and preservation of reproductive capacity in children and young adults. *Cancer, 117*(Suppl. 10), 2301–2310. doi:10.1002/cncr.26045

Weiss, K.E. (1992). *Women's experience of sex and sexuality.* Center City, MN: Hazelden.

White, I.D., Faithfull, S., & Allan, H. (2013). The re-construction of women's sexual lives after pelvic radiotherapy: A critique of social constructionist and biomedical perspectives on the study of female sexuality after cancer treatment. *Social Science and Medicine, 76,* 188–196. doi:10.1016/j.socscimed.2012.10.025

Wilmoth, M.C., Hatmaker-Flanigan, E., LaLoggia, V., & Nixon, T. (2011). Ovarian cancer survivors: Qualitative analysis of the symptom of sexuality. *Oncology Nursing Forum, 38,* 699–708. doi:10.1188/11.ONF.699-708

Wootten, A.C., Abbott, J.M., Osborne, D., Austin, D.W., Klein, B., Costello, A.J., & Murphy, D.G. (2014). The impact of prostate cancer on partners: A qualitative exploration. *Psycho-Oncology, 23,* 1252–1258. doi:10.1002/pon.3552

World Health Organization. (2006). *Defining sexual health: Report of a technical consultation on sexual health, 28–31 January 2002, Geneva.* Geneva, Switzerland: Author.

Wortel, R.C., Alemayehu, W.G., & Incrocci, L. (2015). Orchiectomy and radiotherapy for stage I–II testicular seminoma: A prospective evaluation of short-term effects on body image and sexual function. *Journal of Sexual Medicine, 12,* 210–218. doi:10.1111/jsm.12739

Zaider, T., Manne, S., Nelson, C., Mulhall, J., & Kissane, D. (2012). Loss of masculine identity, marital affection, and sexual bother in men with localized prostate cancer. *Journal of Sexual Medicine, 9,* 2724–2732. doi:10.1111/j.1743-6109.2012.02897.x

Chapter 33 Study Questions

1. A 54-year-old man treated with multimodality treatment for colorectal cancer mentions briefly that "things have shrunk 'down there'" since his surgery and radiation therapy. How should the nurse respond?
   A. "This is nothing to worry about. Just be glad you're alive."
   B. "I will refer you to a urologist to talk about this."
   C. "This happens quite commonly and is related to the radiation to the pelvis. You may find that once you regain your ability to have erections that your penis will return to its normal size. If that doesn't happen, please talk to me again and I will see what else can be done."
   D. "I'm not sure why this has happened. What do you want to do about this?"

2. A 55-year-old woman with estrogen receptor/progesterone receptor–positive breast cancer tells you that her primary care provider has prescribed oral hormone therapy for vaginal pain during penetration. She is not sure that she should be taking this. What would you advise her?
   A. "If this has been prescribed, then it is fine to take it."
   B. "Systemic hormone therapy is not advisable for women with hormone receptor–positive breast cancer. Nonpharmaceutical alternatives should be tried first."
   C. "Nothing can be done about this, but nonpenetrative activities should be considered."
   D. "Have you talked about this to your gynecologist?"

3. What strategies might be used when planning treatment for an adolescent with cancer affecting pelvic organs?
   A. Shielding of the ovaries, uterus, or testicles during radiation therapy when possible, which may mitigate the effects of radiation on these organs and protect future fertility
   B. Less-invasive surgery when possible
   C. Fertility preservation counseling and referral to a reproductive endocrinologist or fertility clinic before treatment starts, if possible
   D. All of the above

4. What is the responsibility of the nurse when a patient is diagnosed with cancer and is scheduled to start treatment that may affect his or her sexual health?
   A. Only answer patient questions if and when they arise.
   B. Describe the possible sexual side effects in detail.
   C. This is not a nursing responsibility.
   D. Refer the patient to a sexuality counselor or therapist.

5. A 27-year-old woman was treated for acute myeloid leukemia three years ago. She asks the nurse if it is possible that she is pregnant, as she has not had a period yet. What is the correct response to this question?
   A. "There is no way you could be pregnant. Your treatment will have made you sterile."
   B. "Have you taken a pregnancy test?"
   C. "When was your last period, and have your periods been normal since your treatment?"
   D. "Let me make an appointment for you with the gynecologist."

CHAPTER

34 Caring for the Cancer Survivor

Christy R. Smith, MSN, ACNP-BC, Julia J. Yates, MSN, RN, OCN®, and Nancy Rankin Ewing, DNP, APRN, ACNS-BC

Introduction

Who Is a Cancer Survivor?

In 1986, the National Coalition for Cancer Survivorship (www.canceradvocacy.org) defined cancer survivors as individuals with cancer from the time of diagnosis and for the balance of life (Ganz, 2011). In practical terms, the post-treatment phase of the cancer experience is targeted, with survivorship care beginning as treatment ends and follow-up care begins (Ganz, 2011).

Mullen (1985) and Miller (2009) have described the seasons of survivorship as progressing through a series of phases: acute, consisting of initial diagnosis and treatment; transitional, immediately following completion of initial treatment; extended, which includes a watchful waiting; and permanent survivorship, which occurs when patients are considered cancer free but suffer from late or long-term effects of treatment. Together these phases provide a framework that can be used to organize a comprehensive program of survivorship care that includes care coordination and prevention, identification, and management of acute, long-term, chronic, and late effects of treatment, including psychosocial consequences and surveillance for recurrence, as part of comprehensive follow-up care (Grant, Economou, & Ferrell, 2010).

Knowledgeable nurses are essential to meet the challenge of managing millions of cancer survivors who are currently living with an active disease or previously treated malignancies. The purpose of this chapter is to present the common medical, psychosocial, and quality-of-life issues faced by cancer survivors; highlight current models of care for providing long-term follow-up; discuss implementation of survivorship care plans (SCPs), and provide additional resources for providers and survivors.

Survivorship Care Plans

In 1971, approximately three million cancer survivors were living in the United States (Horner et al., 2009). In 2014, the number of adult cancer survivors in the United States reached nearly 14.5 million and is predicted to keep rising (American Cancer Society, 2016a), to an estimated 18 million by 2020 (Mariotto, Yabroff, Shao, Feuer, & Brown, 2011). Survivorship rates have risen so sharply in great part because of advances in early detection, diagnosis, treatment, and care (Ness et al., 2013).

Survival rates for children diagnosed with invasive childhood cancers show a five-year relative survival rate in the mid-1970s of 58%, increased to 83% in the period of 2005–2011 (Hurria et al., 2015). As of 2011, at least 388,501 of the cancer survivors in the United States had their first diagnosis before the age of 21 (National Cancer Institute [NCI], 2016). While the number of survivors continues to rise, care continues to be poorly coordinated and patient needs remain inadequately addressed (Stricker & O'Brien, 2014).

As one solution to this growing problem, the Institute of Medicine (IOM, now the Health and Medicine Division of the National Academies of Sciences, Engineering, and Medicine) in 2006 recommended the delivery of an SCP to each patient completing active treatment (Hewitt, Greenfield, & Stovall, 2006). The American College of Surgeons Commission on Cancer subsequently published its Program Standard 3.3, requiring accredited programs to implement treatment summaries and SCPs by 2015 to help improve communication, quality, and coordination of care for cancer survivors (Stricker & O'Brien, 2014). The goal of an SCP is to guide the content and coordination of care following acute treatment, facilitate care transitions, and foster greater self-management of health by cancer survivors (Stricker & O'Brien, 2014). Many templates for SCPs have been developed (see Table 34-1).

Survivorship Care Plan Format, Content, and Management

In a landmark report (Hewitt et al., 2006), IOM defined survivorship care as the phase of care following completion of primary treatment and recommended that it address four essential components: prevention of recurrent and new cancers and other late effects; surveillance for cancer spread, recurrence, and secondary cancers and assessment of medical and psychosocial late effects; intervention for consequences of cancer and its treatment; and coordination between primary and specialty care.

According to the IOM report (Hewitt et al., 2006), broadly speaking, SCPs should provide the following: a summary of an individual's cancer diagnosis and treatment information (the treatment summary); an overview of both physical and psychosocial effects of diagnosis and treatment; a detailed follow-up plan that outlines surveillance for recurrence and potential late effects, as well as recommendations for health-promotion strategies; and referrals and resources for physical, psychosocial, and practical needs.

Early and Late Effects

The role of the oncology nurse has traditionally been to coordinate care during treatment. That role needs to expand to include a focus beyond treatment to the continued needs of cancer survivors. Each type of cancer and its treatments are associated with certain long-term risks. The following sections of this chapter provide various resources to guide surveillance and management (see Table 34-2).

In a recent study to determine oncologists' and primary care physicians' (PCPs') awareness of late and long-term effects of chemotherapy (Nekhlyudov, Aziz, Lerro, & Virgo, 2013), the researchers found that although more than half of PCPs were aware of cardiac dysfunction as a late effect of doxorubicin, awareness of other late effects was limited. Because PCPs may not be directly exposed to chemotherapy-related late effects, oncologists must communicate this information to PCPs as patients transition to primary care settings. Education for all providers caring for the growing population of cancer survivors is needed.

Osteoporosis

Definition

The National Institutes of Health Consensus Development Panel on Osteoporosis Prevention, Diagnosis, and Therapy (2001)

Table 34-1. Survivorship Care Plan (SCP) Templates

Tool	Overview	Content	Format
American Society of Clinical Oncology Cancer Treatment Plan and Summary: www.cancer.net/survivorship/follow-care-after-cancer-treatment/asco-cancer-treatment-and-survivorship-care-plans	Intended to be a record of the patient's cancer treatment, as well as a brief outline of recommended follow-up care. Templates are available for breast, colorectal, lung, and lymphoma diagnoses. A generic form is also available.	Components include stage and pathologic details of the cancer; dose of chemotherapy, specific drugs used, number of cycles completed, and surgeries performed; additional treatments, including radiation, targeted therapies, and hormone therapy; recommended follow-up care, including a schedule of office visits and surveillance testing, with space to indicate the provider responsible for performing each aspect of follow-up care.	Forms that can be downloaded from the American Society of Clinical Oncology website and filled out by a member of the oncology care team
Journey Forward: www.journeyforward.org	Created through the collaborative efforts of Anthem Inc., Cancer Support Community, Genentech, National Coalition for Cancer Survivorship, Oncology Nursing Society, and UCLA Cancer Survivorship Center. SCPs can be downloaded from the Internet to the user's desktop.	SCPs in Journey Forward are based on the American Society of Clinical Oncology's Cancer Treatment Plan and Summary templates and surveillance guidelines. These include detailed summaries of cancer treatments, as well as follow-up care plans that incorporate education regarding late effects, recommendations for cancer surveillance and other healthcare issues, and links to relevant resources for cancer survivors.	Free online program
Oncolife Survivorship Care Plan: www.oncolink.org/oncolife	Product of a collaborative agreement between the University of Pennsylvania Abramson Cancer Center, OncoLink, and Livestrong. The care plan was developed to allow patients to create an SCP by inputting information regarding their cancer diagnosis, treatment, and current symptoms.	Output from the tool has extensive information about survivorship issues that the patient is at risk for or currently experiencing. Recommendations generated are based on available guidelines, such as those provided by the Health and Medicine Division of National Academies of Sciences, Engineering, and Medicine (formerly the Institute of Medicine), National Cancer Institute, and American Society of Clinical Oncology.	Electronic document that can be printed or converted to a PDF
Prescription for Living (see Haylock et al., 2007)	Paper care plan template developed by oncology nurses	Template presents cancer diagnosis, treatment details, and follow-up care plan in a checklist format that allows providers to individualize recommendations for follow-up care and surveillance testing, preventive behaviors, and education regarding potential late effects.	Available online

defined osteoporosis as "a skeletal disorder characterized by compromised bone strength predisposing a person to an increased risk of fracture" (p. 786). This definition continues to be supported by Lorentzon and Cummings (2015). The skeletal fractures in osteoporosis, called *fragility fractures*, occur with "minor or inapparent trauma, particularly in the tho-

Table 34-2. Cancer-Specific Geriatric Assessment and Nursing Implications

Domain	Recommended Tools	Tool Administrator	Nursing Implication
Cognition	Blessed Orientation-Memory-Concentration	Healthcare professional	Baseline deficit necessary to anticipate treatment tolerance
Comorbidities	Physical Health Section (subscale of OARS)	Healthcare professional	Rise in comorbidities related to rise in side effects
Functional status	Activities of daily living (MOS physical health subscale) Instrumental Activities of Daily Living (subscale of OARS)	Self-administered Self-reported or physician-rated	Identifies need for support in the home
	Karnofsky Self-Reported Performance Rating Scale Karnofsky Physician-Rated Performance Rating Scale	Self-administered Physician-rated	Karnofsky has significant relation to survival and global indicator of functional status
	Timed Up and Go	Healthcare professional	Timed Up and Go has shown gait speed as an important predictor of disability.
	Number of falls in prior six months	Self-reported or documented medical record review	Number of falls indicative of rise in risk of injury related to mobility, gait, and balance
Nutritional status	Percent of unintentional weight loss in prior six months Body mass index	Self-reported and healthcare professional Healthcare professional	Weight loss is associated with lower chemotherapy response and lower performance status.
Psychological status	Hospital Anxiety and Depression Scale	Self-reported	Depression related to potential for decreased self-care and loss of independence
Social support and social functioning	MOS Social Activity Limitations Measure and MOS Social Support Survey: Emotional and information and tangible subscales Seeman and Berkman Social Ties	Self-reported and healthcare professional Self-reported	Relates to loss of independence and identified need for care support resources post-treatment; identify family and community resources

MOS—Medical Outcomes Study; OARS—Older Americans Resources and Services

Note. From "Integrating a Cancer-Specific Geriatric Assessment Into Survivorship Care," by D. Economou, A. Hurria, and M. Grant, 2012, *Clinical Journal of Oncology Nursing, 16,* p. E79. Copyright 2012 by Oncology Nursing Society. Reprinted with permission.

racic and lumbar spine, wrist, and hip" (Bolster, 2015).

Quality-of-life data show a more severe impact in those with hip or multiple vertebral fractures than distal radial or single vertebral fractures (Lips & van Schoor, 2005). Quality of life improves with time after fracture, yet is never completely restored. Studies show that the burden of disease with osteoporosis is comparable to that of other chronic diseases (Lips & van Schoor, 2005).

Causes in Cancer Survivors

Cancer survivors are at risk for developing osteoporosis due to chemotherapy, steroid medication, or hormone therapies. Gynecologic oncology surgery requiring removal of the ovaries (bilateral oophorectomy) can lead to premature menopause and osteoporosis. Oral antiestrogen therapy, such as aromatase inhibitors, generally reserved for postmenopausal women, also can cause osteoporosis. Androgen deprivation therapy for prostate cancer increases the risk of osteoporosis in men (Miller et al., 2016).

Recommendations for Better Health

Prevention of osteoporosis due to cancer-related therapies is aimed at avoiding fractures and preserving bone mass. This involves risk factor modification; exercises to maximize bone and muscle strength, improve balance, and minimize the risk of falls; drug therapy to preserve bone mass or stimulate new bone formation; and calcium and vitamin D supplementation (1,000 mg/day for food and supplements for those aged 50 years and younger without risk, and 1,200 mg/day for those older than 50 years) (American Society of Clinical Oncology [ASCO], 2014). Patients can lower their risk of osteoporosis by avoiding tobacco products, eating foods rich in calcium and vitamin D, and engaging in regular physical activity (ASCO, 2014; Economou, Hurria, & Grant, 2012).

Cardiovascular Disease

Definition

Cardiovascular disease (CVD) includes diseases that involve the heart and blood vessels, especially in and around the heart and brain. These diseases cause diminished blood supply to organs and are associated with atherosclerosis and clots.

Causes in Cancer Survivors

Of the nearly 14.5 million cancer survivors in the United States today, many are more likely to die of CVD than their cancer. In fact, with the exception of people who smoke, risk factors for CVD are higher in cancer survivors than in the general adult population (Kaplan, 2013).

Cardiac toxicity is an important consideration for patients undergoing left-sided breast radiation, particularly with the increasing use of potentially cardiotoxic systemic therapeutic agents, including anthracyclines and targeted therapy such as trastuzumab. Motion management techniques such as deep inspiration breath hold can be effective in reducing radiation dose to the heart to decrease the risk of cardiac toxicity (Kron & Chua, 2014). People aged 65 or older and those who received higher doses of chemotherapy have a higher risk of developing side effects, which may include cardiomyopathy, heart failure, myocardial ischemia, and dysrhythmias (ASCO, 2014; Bovelli, Platanoitis, & Roila, 2010). Chest irradiation for Hodgkin lymphoma increases the risk of cardiac dysfunction, as well as breast cancer among women (Miller et al., 2016). Anthracyclines and HER2-targeted drugs can lead to cardiomyopathy and congestive heart failure (Miller et al., 2016).

CVD may compromise cancer survivors' long-term health and well-being, yet healthcare providers may overlook risk factors during survivorship care. Although CVD risk factors are common among cancers survivors, nearly one-third of survivors do not report having health-promotion discussions with their medical teams (Weaver et al., 2013). Survivors should be educated to be aware of their cardiovascular risk factors and initiate discussions with their medical teams about health promotion topics, if appropriate (Weaver et al., 2013). Careful monitoring of cardiovascular risk factors and serum glucose is recommended in men who have received androgen deprivation therapy for prostate cancer (Levine et al., 2010).

Recommendations for Better Health

Adherence to a Mediterranean diet, which typically includes legumes, cereals, fruits and nuts, vegetables, extra virgin olive oil, red wine in moderate quantities, and low amounts of red meat, poultry, and dairy products, is consistently linked to reductions in the risk of CVD. It has also been associated with significant reductions in the risk of overall (10%), colorectal (14%), and prostate (4%) cancer (Harvie, Howell, & Evans, 2015).

Other suggestions for better health include exercise during and after completion of treatment. The American Cancer Society (2014) includes suggestions for exercise while emphasizing the need for survivors to personally monitor the effects on their body and keep their caregiver team informed about the status of their exercise results.

Lymphedema

Definition

Lymphedema is the swelling of a limb and can be primary (due to lymphatic hypoplasia) or secondary (due to obstruction or disruption of the lymphatic vessels) (Douketis, 2015). Signs and symptoms are a brawny, nonpitting edema of one or more extremities. Diagnosis is made by clinical examination. The most common causes of secondary lymphedema are tumor obstruction, surgery, radiation therapy, and trauma (Douketis, 2015).

Causes in Cancer Survivors

Accumulation of lymphatic fluid in the upper extremities can be an effect of breast cancer surgery and radiation therapy, occurring in approximately 20% of women who undergo axillary lymph node dissection and 6% of women who undergo sentinel lymph node biopsy (DiSipio, Rye, Newman, & Hayes, 2013). Pelvic lymphadenectomy can cause development of lower extremity lymphedema, particularly in patients who also receive radiation therapy (Miller et al., 2016). Additional causes include obstruction of the lymphatic vasculature by tumors, clots, or scarring of the lymphatic ducts.

Recommendations for Better Health

Although the risk of upper extremity lymphedema has decreased with innovations in surgical management of breast cancer and lymph node removal, it is still important for lymphedema to be diagnosed as early as possible to optimize treatment and slow progression. Specially trained professionals and certified physical therapists are available to evaluate and manage this long-term effect with a gentle massage (manual lymphatic drainage) and other low-impact exercises based on assessment of the status of lymphedema.

Although not supported by research evidence, a personalized compression garment may be ordered and can be used for prevention of further lymphedema. These garments are fitted so that there is more pressure at the level of the fingertips than above the elbow. The use of these "sleeves" is especially helpful at high altitudes, such as when patients are flying. Edema occurs during air travel because the cabin pressure is lower than the pressure within the tissue, allowing the lymphatic fluid to move into the spaces between cells. These garments are expensive, need to be replaced every six months, and may not be effective once the fluid accumulation has reached a certain point (NCI, 2015).

Complex decongestive therapy consists of manual lymphedema drainage therapy, low-stretch bandaging, exercises, and skin care. Suggested by consensus panels, complex decongestive therapy is recommended as primary treatment and effective therapy for lymphedema unresponsive to standard elastic compression therapy. Intermittent external pneumatic compression is added when lymphedema persists after multiple treatment strategies have been ineffective (NCI, 2015).

Rehabilitation

The World Health Organization (n.d.) defines rehabilitation as "a process aimed at enabling [people with disabilities] to reach and maintain their optimal physical, sensory, intellectual, psychological, and social functional levels" and attain independence and self-determination. A goal is to maintain or improve quality of life for those with physical illnesses or conditions.

For many people, the transition to survivorship serves as strong motivation to make positive changes in lifestyle and health-related behaviors. Cultivating healthy habits is especially important for cancer survivors. As mentioned previously, survivors are often at higher risk for developing additional health problems as a result of their cancer treatment (e.g., CVD, bone disease). Healthy behaviors can help survivors regain or build strength, reduce the severity of side effects, reduce the risk of developing secondary cancers or other health issues, and enjoy life more (ASCO, 2014). Survivors as a group are excellent candidates for lifestyle and health behavior changes, as exercise and weight loss alone can improve their stamina, strength, mood, and quality of life (Kaplan, 2013).

Preliminary evidence exists in a number of areas that may be improved by rehabilitation interventions, such as pain, sexual functioning, cognitive functioning, and return to work, but further research is needed. A notable exception to limitations in the literature is that of rehabilitation interventions for breast cancer. Physiotherapy researchers in this area have performed extensive research and the result is a comprehensive rehabilitation guideline for prevention and intervention for mobility, pain, swelling, and function (Egan et al., 2013).

Health Maintenance

Overall, a typical person's cancer risk can be reduced with healthy choices such as avoiding tobacco, limiting alcohol use, protecting skin from the sun and avoiding indoor tanning beds, eating a diet rich in fruits and vegetables, maintaining a healthy weight, and increasing physical activity. Nearly one in five cancers diagnosed today occurs in an individual with a previous diagnosis of cancer, and these "second cancers" are a leading cause of morbidity and mortality among cancer survivors. Although long-term cancer survivors require similar preventive care and health maintenance as adults without cancer, they receive less counseling on diet, exercise, and smoking cessation than patients without cancer (Wilbur, 2015).

Smoking Cessation

Lung cancer survivors, particularly those who continue to smoke, are at an increased risk for additional smoking-related diseases, including second cancers, especially in the lung, head and neck, and urinary tract. Survivors may feel stigmatized because of the social perception that lung cancer is a self-inflicted disease, which can be particularly difficult for lung cancer survivors who never smoked (Chambers et al., 2012).

In 2013, ASCO issued an update to its policy statement on tobacco cessation to include that every individual should be queried about smoking status, with appropriate interventions and referrals to smoking cessation programs (Hanna, Mulshine, Wollins, Tyne, & Dresler, 2013). The update noted that 81%–84% of medical records documented a smoking/tobacco cessation discussion in the years 2009–2014. Although guideline adherence for smoking prevention or cessation is consistently greater than 80% (Mayer, Shapiro, Jacobson, & McCabe, 2015), the American Cancer Society (2016a) ranked smoking and tobacco-related diseases as the most preventable cause of death worldwide, and lung cancer was the leading cause of cancer death in the United States for both men and women.

Exercise

In a literature review and epidemiologic examination conducted on the link between physical activity and health outcomes among cancer survivors, Loprinzi and Lee (2014) found that cancer survivors are relatively inactive. Promotion of physical activity can be included within the SCP, as exercise has been shown to reduce the risk of recurrence and cancer-related mortality. Other benefits include reduced pain and other side effects of treatment, as well as improvements in physical and mental health (Loprinzi & Lee, 2014).

The Physical Exercise During Adjuvant Chemotherapy Effectiveness Study (PACES) was a multicenter randomized controlled trial of 230 patients with two intervention groups and a "usual care" control group. The intervention groups were randomly assigned to home-based, low-intensity, self-managed physical activity or moderate- to high-intensity combined resistance and aerobic exercise supervised by physical therapists. Both were encouraged to be physically active five days each week for 30 minutes per session. The control group did not involve suggestions for routine exercise. All groups started with the first cycle of chemotherapy and ended three weeks after the last cycle. The results of this trial revealed that moderate- to high-intensity exercise during chemotherapy has a beneficial effect on cardiorespiratory fitness, muscle strength, fatigue, and chemotherapy completion rates. For patients unable or unwilling to pursue a supervised, moderate- to high-intensity exercise program, the home-based, low-intensity physical activity represents a viable option (van Waart et al., 2015).

Nurses should take an active role in promoting strength exercise among cancer survivors using the Theory of Planned Behavior (TPB), particularly among survivors at higher risk of not performing strength exercise. TPB is generally assessed using Likert-type scale scoring from 1 (negative) to 7 (positive) that quantifies a person's attitude, subjective norm, perceived behavioral control, intention, and plan to engage in a behavior (Forbes, Blanchard, Mummery, & Courneya, 2015).

Research shows that any interventions that strengthen intentions to engage in strength exercise will be effective. Such interventions can focus on educating cancer survivors about the benefits of strength exercise and how to make strength exercise enjoyable, obtain social support for strength exercise, and overcome common barriers (Forbes et al., 2015).

Stress Management

A diagnosis of cancer, followed by treatment, recovery, and survivorship, can result in myriad stress-related symptoms. Cancer-related stress is defined as "a difficult, multifactorial experience that may interfere with the ability to cope effectively with cancer and its treatment" (American Cancer Society, 2016b, p. 3). Some consequences of acute stress are digestive symptoms, headaches, sleeplessness, anger, and irritability. Chronic stress can lead to immune-system depression, which results in more frequent viral infections and a decrease in the effectiveness of vaccines; hypertension; heart disease; diabetes; depression; and other illnesses (National Institute of Mental Health, n.d.).

Learning how to manage stress is extremely important for survivors' recovery. Big steps in reducing stress can be made through small lifestyle changes, such as learning to say "no" to tasks that require more time and energy than survivors can afford to expend. Nurses may advise patients to do their most important tasks first and get help with potentially challenging issues, such as finances. Other ways to manage stress include exercise, social activities, support groups, acupuncture, yoga, massage, and relaxation techniques, such as deep breathing (ASCO, 2014).

Recurrence

Fear of cancer recurrence or cancer progression is one of the most frequent distressing psychological symptoms in patients with cancer. Fear of recurrence describes an emotional response to the real threat of a life-threatening illness. Elevated levels of fear of recurrence can become dysfunctional, causing considerable disruption in social functioning, and affect well-being and quality of life (Mehnert, Koch, Sundermann, & Dinkel, 2013).

The probability of developing recurrence is multicausal and therefore depends on different determinants. The type of primary cancer itself and the cancer site have a major influence on the risk of recurrence.

Nurses can offer support to patients through referrals to psychosocial counselors, support groups, or face-to-face interactions with patients about their fears. Sometimes a discussion about signs and symptoms of recurrence provides patients with a sense of control instead of just "waiting" for the next surveillance to find out if they are still "cancer free."

Second Primary Neoplasms

The population of adult cancer survivors is growing; thus, the long-term effects of cancer treatment, including secondary cancer development, have become an increasingly important concern in the field of oncology (Lisik-Habib et al., 2015). In several cohorts, risk ratios were six times higher as compared with the general population: the cumulative incidence was 3%–4% after 20 years (Inskip & Curtis, 2007; Meadows et al., 2009). Risk factors include history of radiation therapy (usually 10 years after treatment), history of chemotherapy (usually 3–5 years after treatment), and individual factors (e.g., gender, younger age at diagnosis, type of first cancer, genetic predisposition) (Blatt, Olshan, Gula, Dickman, & Zaranek, 1992; Inskip & Curtis, 2007; MacArthur et al., 2007; Meadows et al., 2009; Neglia et al., 2001; Vasudevan et al., 2010).

The risk of second primary neoplasms (SPNs) after survival of primary cancers diagnosed and treated in adulthood is modest across cancers. A study in Finland from 1953 to 1991 with a cohort of 470,000 patients with cancer demonstrated no increased risk of developing an SPN compared to a matched healthy population (Sankila, Pukkala, & Teppo, 1995). In a separate study conducted on a U.S. cohort of 250,000 adult survivors, the risk of developing a second cancer was increased 1.3-fold compared to the general population (Curtis, Boice, Kleinerman, Flannery, & Fraumeni, 1985). The risk of SPN may be slightly higher for specific types of cancer, such as breast and prostate (Ng & Travis, 2008).

The risk of developing an SPN varies by patient factors, primary cancer type, primary cancer treatments, environmental exposures, and lifestyle factors (Travis et al., 2006). Patients with Hodgkin lymphoma are at risk for breast cancer, soft tissue sarcomas, thyroid cancer, secondary leukemia, and non-Hodgkin lymphoma (Bhatia et al., 2003). A study from the Late Effects Study Group followed more than 1,300 patients with Hodgkin lymphoma for a median length of follow-up of 17 years (Bhatia et al., 2003). The survivors had an 18.5-fold increased risk of developing an SPN compared with the general population (standardized incidence ratio of 18.5, 95% confidence interval [CI] [15.6, 21.7]).

The cumulative probability of developing a second cancer was 10.6% at 20 years from diagnosis, increasing to 26.3% at 30 years.

Survivors of acute lymphoblastic leukemia are at risk for central nervous system (CNS) tumors secondary to cranial irradiation, acute myeloid leukemia, and thyroid cancer (Bhatia et al., 2002). In a study of 8,831 patients with acute lymphoblastic leukemia enrolled on therapeutic protocols from 1983 to 1995, the cumulative incidence of any SPN was 1.18% at 10 years (95% CI [0.8%, 1.5%]), representing a 7.2-fold increased risk compared with the general population (Bhatia et al., 2002).

Surveillance

Early Detection

Current guidelines focus on cancer screening beginning in early adulthood for survivors who are at known risk (Oeffinger, 2003). Such early prevention strategies and surveillance are important in minimizing the mortality and morbidity associated with development of SPNs.

Breast Cancer Screening

The leading cause of premature death in women in the United States is breast cancer. Reduced morbidity and mortality is related to early detection. The American Cancer Society updated its screening guidelines for breast cancer in women at average risk in 2015 based on a synthesis of the most current evidence. These recommendations included the following:

- Yearly screening mammogram beginning at age 45 with the option to transition to biennial screening at age 55 or continue annual screening
- Opportunity to begin annual screening as early as age 40 if desired
- Continuation of screening mammography while overall health is good and life expectancy is at least 10 years
- No regular clinical breast examination or breast self-examination for screening at any age

Men and women with a previous history of breast cancer will follow the screening recommendations of their oncologist. Survivors with an identified *BRCA* mutation are at high risk to develop a breast cancer in the contralateral breast and should follow the National Comprehensive Cancer Network® (2016) guidelines for *BRCA*-related cancer syndrome (or specific suggestions of their oncologist), as follows:

- Females
  - Age 25–29: Perform annual breast magnetic resonance imaging (MRI) if a cancer diagnosis before age 30 is present.
  - Age 30–75: Perform annual mammogram and breast MRI.
  - Age older than 75 years: Determine management on an individual basis.
  - For women with a *BRCA* mutation who were treated for breast cancer: Continue annual mammographic screening and MRI of the remaining breast tissue.
- Males
  - Starting at age 35: Provide patient with breast self-examination training and education.
  - Starting at age 35: Perform clinical breast examination every 12 months.
  - Starting at age 40: Recommend prostate cancer screening for *BRCA2* carriers.

For women with a *PTEN* mutation, annual mammograms and MRI should begin at age 30–35 or 5–10 years prior to the earliest age of familial onset of breast cancer, whichever occurs first. For women who are older than age 75, individualized guidance should be considered. If a woman has undergone surgery for breast cancer, the annual screening mammogram and breast MRI should continue (National Comprehensive Cancer Network, 2016).

Colonoscopy

Colorectal cancer ranks in the top 3 of the 10 most common cancer sites for both male and female survivors. However, only 59% of survivors aged 50 years and older received colorectal cancer screening according to guidelines in 2010 (DeSantis et al., 2014). Regular screening and removal of precancerous polyps, beginning at age 50, is the key to preventing colorectal cancer. The U.S. Preventive Services Task Force recommends screening for colorectal cancer using high-sensitivity fecal occult blood testing, sigmoidoscopy, or colonoscopy beginning at age 50 and continuing until age 75 (Centers for Disease Control and Prevention, 2016). When colorectal cancers are detected at a localized stage, the five-year survival rate is 90%, compared to 71% for localized spread and 13% for distant metastasis (American Cancer Society, 2016a).

Lung Cancer Screening

In January 2013, the American Cancer Society issued guidelines for the early detection of lung cancer, which endorsed a process of shared decision making between clinicians who have access to high-volume, high-quality lung cancer screening programs and current or former (quit within the previous 15 years) adult smokers with at least a 30-pack-year history of smoking who are aged 55–74 years and in good health (Wender et al., 2013). Shared decision making should include a discussion of the benefits, uncertainties, and harms associated with lung cancer screening.

Survivors will thrive more efficiently if their healthcare provider not only provides the medical surveillance they need, but also screens and monitors them for psychosocial sequelae; provides education to improve their health-related knowledge deficits surrounding late effects and general health issues, insurance concerns, and vocational choices; and promotes socialization and autonomy in medical decision making (Freyer & Kibrick-Lazear, 2006).

Geriatric Survivors

Cancer survivorship care for the growing older adult population (Hurria et al., 2015) involves combining the expected late and long-term effects of cancer and cancer treatment with information about expected changes in health status that occur with aging. Individuals at a specific chronologic age vary in functionality, cognition, and the ability to handle stress (Walston et al., 2006). Assessing older adult cancer survivors beyond chronologic age to include changes in functional status is an essential process to help nurses anticipate cancer treatment impact and aid in planning individualized survivorship care (Economou et al., 2012). For cancer-specific geriatric assessment and nursing implications, see Table 34-2.

Because most older adult patients with cancer are treated by a number of clinicians in different specialties, PCPs must act as the gatekeepers (Routt, 2013). In general, advanced age is associated with inadequate cancer diagnosis and treatment and can translate into shorter survival time (Wedding, Röhrig, Klippstein, Pientka, & Höffken, 2007). Older adults with cancer have unique needs in all aspects of their survivorship. Although it is safe for older adults to receive treatment for cancer, proper assessment and careful consideration of all options is paramount. The ultimate goal of treatment is the preservation of physical and psychosocial function. It is vital that geriatric cancer survivors be continually assessed for the presence of geriatric syndromes, as these syndromes can limit treatment and quality of life. Geriatric syndromes are most likely to be identified and treated by PCPs (Routt, 2013).

As the aging population continues to grow, the quality of geriatric cancer survivorship will depend on accurate assessment of risk factors influencing prognosis. Functionality should be preserved at all costs by utilizing interventions that promote independence in activities of daily living. Clinicians have the responsibility of ongoing assessment of geriatric cancer survivors across the survivorship continuum. A collaborative approach to treatment, incorporating the entire oncology team and the PCP, provides the best outcomes for quality patient care (Routt, 2013). A geriatric assessment provides information beyond the standard history and physical assessment and identifies patients who are at increased risk for chemotherapy toxicity (Hurria et al., 2011). Incorporating this information in the older adult patient's SCP will allow for a truly individualized plan. Nurses will have the information needed to coordinate resources and support systems for appropriate and effective follow-up care of the older adult cancer survivor. Nurses can play an essential role in establishing a baseline screening for the unique needs of older adult patients with cancer, which will assist providers with direct treatment and survivorship follow-up services (Economou et al., 2012).

Children and Adolescent Survivors

The Children's Oncology Group (n.d.), an NCI-supported clinical trials group that cares for more than 90% of U.S. children and adolescents diagnosed with cancer, has developed long-term follow-up guidelines for the screening and management of late effects in survivors of childhood cancer (see www.survivorship-guidelines.org). It is important that survivors of pediatric cancers are monitored for long-term and late effects (Miller et al., 2016). Some effects are specific to children and adolescents, whereas others are consistent with long-term effects seen in adults.

Recurrence

Recurrent disease is the leading cause of death for adult survivors of childhood cancer (Mertens et al., 2001). Mortality rates from recurrence vary based on primary tumor type, with the highest rates being in survivors originally diagnosed with CNS tumors, leukemia, and bone tumors (Mertens et al., 2001). The lowest rate of mortality from recurrence is in patients with kidney tumors or Wilms tumor. A recent Childhood Cancer Survivor Study (CCSS) report focusing on non-Hodgkin lymphoma survivors found that chest irradiation as treatment for the cancer conferred additional risk of morality (Bluhm et al., 2008). Assessment for recurrence with a focus on early diagnosis and intervention may help to lower these mortality rates.

Second Primary Neoplasms

In contrast to adults with cancer, childhood cancer survivors in the CCSS cohort had a 6.4-fold increased risk of developing an SPN, with an estimated cumulative probability of 3.2% at 20 years after primary cancer diagnosis (Neglia et al., 2001). Screening and evaluation for SPNs in the at-risk population is essential because the associated mortality and morbidity is high.

Bone tumors, breast cancer, and thyroid cancer are among the most common SPNs in childhood cancer survivors and often are associated with specific treatments. For example, radiation therapy confers a 2.7-fold increased risk of developing a bone tumor with a dose response risk, and mantle radiation is associated with an increased risk of breast cancer. Similarly, exposure to alkylating chemotherapy agents is an independent risk factor for the development of bone tumors. In the CCSS, breast cancer was the most frequent SPN (Neglia et al., 2001). The majority of these tumors occurred in patients with Hodgkin lymphoma, who have a 16.2-fold increased risk of developing a second primary breast cancer when compared to the general population. The median time to development was 15.7 years. Women who were treated at a younger age initially were at higher risk compared to survivors diagnosed and treated later (Neglia et al., 2001).

The development of thyroid cancer also is associated with exposure to radiation, as shown in a cohort of 9,170 survivors, who had a 53-fold (95% CI [34, 80]) increased risk of thyroid cancer. As with bone and breast cancers, the risk for developing thyroid cancer increases with the radiation dose and with a younger age at the time of treatment (Tucker et al., 1991).

Transition of Care: Pediatric to Adult Transition

Transition of care has been defined as "purposeful, planned movement of adolescents and young adults with chronic physical and medical conditions from child-centered to adult-oriented healthcare systems" (p. 570) and ensures that their care will remain both medically and developmentally appropriate (Blum et al., 1993). It should begin in early adolescence with conversations directed to the individual to educate the young adolescent about his or her medical condition and to teach advocacy skills (Rosen, 1993). According to Suh et al. (2014), the correct timing of transition to survivorship care and correct survivorship team or provider and model of care often are difficult for both patients and providers to identify. In addition, providers who assume care of survivors often lack the knowledge needed to care for cancer survivors and ensure appropriate screening and follow-up.

Some have argued that an ideal survivorship clinic in a cancer center is one where a dedicated team of experts provide continuity of care from active treatment to follow-up and then provide a transition from pediatrics to adult medicine and from the cancer center to the community (Friedman, Freyer, & Levitt, 2006). The ease and effectiveness of transitioning survivors from pediatric- to adult-focused long-term follow-up care can depend on whether the pediatric cancer center is affiliated with an adult medical center or has a collegial relationship with an adult-focused physician group to work together to meet the needs of their survivor patients. All adult survivors, as with the general adult population, are recommended to develop a relationship with a PCP (e.g., internists; family medicine specialists; medicine-pediatric specialists; mid-level providers, including advanced practice nurses and physician assistants) as they reach young adulthood for general health issues.

Characteristics of adolescents and young adults, their parents, and providers play a critical role in successful transition. The CCSS identified predictors of lack of follow-up care in survivors, including older age, longer time from diagnosis, male sex, lack of health insurance, and lack of concern for future health (Lee, Santacroce, & Sadler, 2007). Survivors with physical symptoms, such as pain or increased anxiety, have been shown to have higher rates of follow-up care (Nathan et al., 2009). Granek et al. (2012) found that psychosocial variables, such as identification with being a survivor and fear and anxiety, could act as both a motivator for and a hindrance to successful transition.

Survivors' Concerns

Current literature documents that cancer survivors deal with myriad acute, chronic, and late effects of cancer and treatment. They face a host of physical, psychological, emotional, social, spiritual, and economic effects (Ness et al., 2013). Nurses should take a proactive role in assessing the needs of all cancer survivors, regardless of cancer type and time since diagnosis (Ness et al., 2013).

Barriers to Survivorship Care

Barriers to the provision of SCPs are numerous and include patient, provider, and system variables. Patient barriers include lack of awareness, and provider and system barriers include limited financial, time, and human resources.

Barriers appear particularly difficult to overcome in community settings, given limited resources and the demand for high practice volume (Grant et al., 2010; Irwin, Klemp, Glennon, & Frazier, 2011). Time often is quoted as the largest barrier to SCP delivery (Dulko et al., 2013; Salz, Oeffinger, McCabe, Layne, & Bach, 2012). The preparation of detailed treatment summaries and individualized follow-up care plans often is a time-consuming process, taking an average of 60–90 minutes per patient (Stricker et al., 2011). Beginning the preparation of SCPs at the time of diagnosis and prospectively capturing disease and treatment data over time is another strategy (Stricker & O'Brien, 2014). Harnessing the ability of electronic health record (EHR) systems and other health information technology solutions is one oft-quoted strategy for improving the efficiency of preparing SCPs (Houlihan, 2009; Jacobs et al., 2009). However, EHRs may fail to provide efficient solutions. Although some have begun to create SCP templates, limited diagnosis and treatment information can be pulled into EHR SCP templates, with a failure to provide automated customization of follow-up care plans. Reviewing the SCP with survivors presents a resource burden, often taking up to an hour per patient and typically performed by highly skilled providers (Salz et al., 2012; Stricker et al., 2011). There are growing efforts in attempts to interface survivorship templates with cancer registry records to improve accuracy and efficiency in SCP delivery. For example, the Centers for Disease Control and Prevention National Program of Cancer Registries (2015) is developing the Web Plus Survivorship Module, which will enable integration of cancer registry data and survivorship templates and information.

Other barriers to SCP delivery include patient factors such as the desire to stay with a specific oncology provider rather than receive SCPs within a survivorship clinic. Integrated models of survivorship care address this concern (Landier, 2009; McCabe & Jacobs, 2008).

The shortage of research to guide evidence-based guidelines for survivorship care is a major barrier to providing specific care recommendations within SCPs (McCabe et al., 2013); however, a variety of consensus-based guidelines (National Comprehensive Cancer Network) and guidance statements (ASCO, American Cancer Society) are becoming available to guide care while the evidence base grows (Cowens-Alvarado et al., 2013; McCabe et al., 2013).

The Institute of Medicine's report, *From Cancer Patient to Cancer Survivor: Lost in Transition* (Hewitt et al., 2006), described gaps in the cancer care system that undermined patients' transition from treatment to survivorship. Eight years later, the report *Delivering High-Quality Cancer Care: Charting a New Course for a System in Crisis* highlighted that with an additional four million survivors, the cancer system was then "in crisis" with a lack of patient-centered, accessible, evidence-based, or well-coordinated care (Levit, Balogh, Nass, & Ganz, 2013). Elements for inclusion in the SCP are (a) diagnosis and staging details, including biomarkers and specific tissue information, (b) recommended follow-up and surveillance, (c) education regarding short- and long-term side effects and symptoms of recurrence; and (d) a plan for addressing psychosocial needs. However, creating SCPs remains difficult and time consuming for nurses and often is inefficient and nonbillable. Although designed to be used for billing for the care of survivors, the process continues to be impossible or at least difficult to accomplish, even for institutions with EHRs (Darud, 2014).

Financial Concerns

Employment

Every survivor's work situation is different. Many people with cancer who took time off for treatment return to work afterward or may have worked throughout treatment, whereas others may not be able to return to work because of long-term side effects. Decisions about work will likely depend on patients' financial resources, health insurance, the type of work they do, and the nature of their recovery.

Survivors may stop working or work fewer hours during their treatment and recovery. They should be advised to discuss their plans with their doctor to set realistic expectations. The next step would be to contact their employer's human resources department for guidance regarding medical leave or short- and long-term disability options. Reasonable accommodations, such as telecommuting, reassignment, job sharing, and modified hours, are all permitted through the Americans With Disabilities Act (ADA) (see www.ada.gov). Although employers should not request medical records, they may request documentation verifying limitations, such as fatigue, pain, and cognitive difficulties, which qualify a patient for accommodations.

As evidenced by the results of the PACES trial, patients who participated in a physical exercise or activity program were more likely to have returned to work at six-month follow-up that those in the control group. This not only has financial implications, but also carries meaning in terms of quality of life and a sense of return to normalcy (van Waart et al., 2015).

Insurance

As in cancer treatment, racial/ethnic and socioeconomic disparities also exist in cancer survivorship care. Lack of access to survivor care services is a major barrier to the health and well-being of cancer survivors who lack health insurance or who experience exclusions or restrictions on their policies. The Patient Protection and Affordable Care Act, passed in 2010, addressed many of these issues. Components of the act that benefit cancer survivors include elimination of annual and lifetime benefit caps; elimination of copayments for select preventive services (e.g., mammogram, colonoscopy); elimination of preexisting condition clauses for new insurance plans; focus on delivery of high-quality coordinated care through accountable care organizations, community health teams, and medical homes; inclusion of screening and follow-up services as part of the essential health benefits package; and limitations placed on allowable amounts of out-of-pocket spending (McCabe et al., 2013).

Discrimination

Although many survivors can be as productive as they were before treatment, some find they are treated differently or unfairly. For example, some employers and colleagues may assume that a person's productivity will decrease or that performance will fall below the company's expectations. Other types of discrimination may include receiving a demotion for no clear reason, having an earned job promotion withheld, being overlooked for consideration in a new position, and finding a lack of flexibility in response to requests for time off for medical appointments (ASCO, 2014).

Whereas loss of occupational identity can be a source of significant anxiety and depression, remaining in or returning to the workplace allows many patients to maintain a sense of normalcy or control. The experience of discrimination can become a focus for strong feelings about fairness. Clinicians need to address work-related distress directly and appreciate the larger significance these themes may have in their patients' coping (Peteet, 2000).

It is important for survivors to understand that laws and regulations exist that prohibit discrimination, such as the ADA. To aid patients in transitioning back to work and avoiding discrimination, the healthcare team may suggest that they focus on catching up on new projects or developments that occurred in their absence; refreshing job skills, if necessary, by reviewing past work assignments or attending classes or workshops; seeking counseling from a professional about the transition back to work; or getting advice and tips from other cancer survivors through a support group. Healthcare providers also may need to write a letter confirming patients' ability to return to work.

Long-Term Follow-Up

Where should survivorship care take place and who is responsible? According to Ganz (2014), survivors must be engaged in their follow-up care for the remainder of their lives. They need to be concerned about recurrence, late effects of treatment, and second cancers, while often experiencing lingering physical and emotional effects of their prior treatments (Rowland, Hewitt, & Ganz, 2006; Yabroff, Lawrence,

Clauser, Davis, & Brown, 2004). These patient-survivors often find themselves educating their non-oncology clinicians about their cancer treatments and follow-up needs. It would be much more valuable for patient-survivors to have their primary treating oncologist act as a partner in this process, so that they are not solely responsible for designing and communicating a post-treatment plan (Ganz, 2014). Currently, survivorship care is delivered in a variety of settings, each with its own advantages and disadvantages (see Table 34-3). Most cancer survivors seek health care from PCPs who are unfamiliar with their unique healthcare needs. Regardless of where survivors are seeking care, it is critical that the healthcare team have some familiarity with the unique needs of this vulnerable population to ensure quality care (Hewitt et al., 2006; Oeffinger & Robison, 2007). Nurses must increase their knowledge base regarding optimal surveillance and follow-up strategies, as well as monitor for and intervene in the late effects of cancer treatment (Ganz, 2014). For resources for survivors and providers, see Figure 34-1.

Table 34-3. Models of Providing Long-Term Follow-Up Care

Model	Structure	Advantages	Disadvantages
Cancer center based (primary oncologist as lead)	Long-term follow-up occurs as continuation of one's therapy experience with the treating oncologist in oncology clinic.	Comfortable for the survivor and family who have developed relationship with treating oncologist Continuity of care Oncologists do not feel as though they have to "give up" their patients to another provider.	Provider attention may be distracted by acuity of on-therapy patients. Illness-focused, not wellness-focused Potential lack of provider interest/knowledge of late effects Relapse-focused follow-up rather than risk-adapted screening and health maintenance focus Research is difficult to coordinate.
Cancer center based (specialized long-term follow-up clinic)	Long-term follow-up is handled by a designated late-effects team in a separate clinic within or outside of the oncology clinic setting.	Providers with expertise in late effects Emphasis on improving survivor knowledge of cancer treatment and risk Provision of comprehensive risk-based screening and care Continued connection with treating physician and clinic setting; "comfort zone" for survivor Focus on modifiable risk factors and health education Opportunity to train healthcare professionals Structure for research Access to established network of subspecialists with commitment to survivor care	Cancer center has negative connotations for survivors, who want to "move on." For survivors of childhood cancer, as survivors get older, they may not feel comfortable in pediatric setting. May not be geographically convenient May discourage survivors' use of primary care Prevents survivors from negotiating their own health care in the community Requires multiple hospital resources For childhood cancer survivors, pediatric team lacks familiarity with issues that arise as survivors become adults.

(Continued on next page)

Table 34-3. Models of Providing Long-Term Follow-Up Care *(Continued)*

Model	Structure	Advantages	Disadvantages
Community based	Long-term follow-up is handled by the pediatrician, family practice physician, internist, or advanced practice nurse within the community.	Promotion of independence and reintegration of survivor into primary care Focus on wellness Convenience for survivor	Limited exposure to survivors in their practice on day-to-day basis Lack of provider training in late effects Limited knowledge of risk-based screening, particularly for those with more significant exposures Requires survivors to know their risk and advocate for their needs Lack of time to devote to complex physical and psychosocial needs of survivors Limited knowledge of cancer-related health education Lack of subspecialist resources with survivorship expertise Difficult to coordinate research
Combined approach/ consultative	Follow-up initially takes place in a cancer center–based program but then transitions to community-based primary care physician with ongoing interaction with cancer center as needed or at request of primary care physician.	Best of both worlds for survivors Allows for partnership between oncologist and primary care Cancer center always available as resource Access to cancer center network of subspecialists Encourages local providers to have knowledge of late effects Encourages primary care provider utilization of published screening guidelines for survivors	May be difficult for survivors to trust primary care provider Initial transition may be difficult for survivors. May not be well suited for survivors with more complex follow-up requirements Potential loss of patients for research initiatives Primary care providers are not experts on cancer late effects or issues.

Conclusion

This chapter outlined some of the most common medical and psychological late effects associated with treatments for cancer. It is important to recognize that those treatments resulted in more people surviving cancer than ever before. However, information on the long-term effects of treatments provided over the past several decades is being integrated into modified treatment protocols. The coming decade brings opportunity to make further advances in treatments that will minimize the unintended harm and improve the quality of long-term survivorship. It has provided information on the new recommendations regarding use of SCPs and available SCP templates, as well as resources for survivors and providers.

The authors would like to acknowledge Lisa K. Sharp, PhD, Karen E. Kinahan, MS, RN, PCNS-BC, and Aarati Didwania, MD, MS, FACP, for their contributions to this chapter that remain unchanged from the first edition of this book.

Figure 34-1. Survivorship Resources

For Survivors

- Cancer*Care*, www.cancercare.org: This site provides information for both survivors and providers regarding support groups, education, and information on financial support.
- Cancer.Net, www.cancer.net/survivorship: Cancer.Net's Survivorship section provides helpful information for cancer survivors and their friends and families on topics, including long-term side effects of treatment, dealing with recurrence, and life after cancer, as well as additional resources. It also offers a downloadable booklet in Spanish.
- Cancer Support Community, www.cancersupportcommunity.org: The site's mission is to ensure that all people affected by cancer are empowered by knowledge, strengthened by action, and sustained by community.
- Cancer Survivors Network, http://csn.cancer.org: The purpose of the Cancer Survivors Network is peer support. This site is noncommercial and provides a private, secure way for cancer survivors to find and communicate with others who share their interests and experiences.
- Centers for Disease Control and Prevention, www.cdc.gov/cancer/survivorship: The Cancer Survivorship section provides comprehensive cancer survivorship information for patients and caregivers.
- National Cancer Institute, www.cancer.gov/about-cancer/coping/survivorship: This page offers information pertaining to all areas of the survivor's life, including follow-up medical care, physical changes, family issues, and the new normal.
- National Children's Cancer Society, https://thenccs.org: This website is designed to provide information pertaining to all areas of the survivor's life. The Late Effects After Treatment Tool allows users to build an assessment of late effects specific to their diagnosis and treatment.
- National Coalition for Cancer Survivorship, www.canceradvocacy.org: This site provides survivorship education for patients, healthcare professionals, and caregivers, including the Cancer Survival Toolbox®.
- Stupid Cancer, http://stupidcancer.org: This 501(c)(3) nonprofit organization is the largest charity that comprehensively addresses young adult cancer through advocacy, research, support, outreach, awareness, mobile health, and social media.

For Providers

- American Society of Clinical Oncology, www.asco.org/practice-guidelines/cancer-care-initiatives/prevention-survivorship/survivorship/survivorship-compendium: The Survivorship Care Compendium has been developed as a repository of tools and resources to enable oncology providers to implement or improve survivorship care within their practices.
- Cancer*Care*, www.cancercare.org: This site provides information for both survivors and providers regarding support groups, education, and information on financial support.
- Children's Oncology Group, www.survivorshipguidelines.org: This site provides recommendations for screening and management of late effects that may result from pediatric cancer treatment and was developed as a resource for clinicians.
- CureSearch, www.curesearch.org: CureSearch for Children's Cancer's mission is to end children's cancer by driving targeted and innovative research with measurable results in an accelerated time frame.
- National Coalition for Cancer Survivorship, www.canceradvocacy.org: This site provides survivorship education for patients, healthcare professionals, and caregivers, including the Cancer Survival Toolbox.

References

American Cancer Society. (2014). Physical activity and the cancer patient. Retrieved from http://www.cancer.org/treatment/survivorshipduringandaftertreatment/stayingactive/physical-activity-and-the-cancer-patient

American Cancer Society. (2015, October 20). American Cancer Society recommendations for early breast cancer detection in women without breast symptoms. Retrieved from http://www.cancer.org/cancer/breastcancer/moreinformation/breastcancerearlydetection/breast-cancer-early-detection-acs-recs

American Cancer Society. (2016a). *Cancer facts and figures 2016*. Atlanta, GA: Author.

American Cancer Society. (2016b). *Cancer treatment and survivorship facts and figures 2016–2017*. Atlanta, GA: Author.

American Society of Clinical Oncology. (2014). *ASCO Answers: Cancer survivorship*. Retrieved from http://www.cancer.net/sites/cancer.net/files/cancer_survivorship.pdf

Key Points

- Survivorship care is a group effort and is the responsibility of the primary oncologist, the PCP, the oncology nurse, and the patient.
- Cancer survivors are at an increased risk for second primary cancers, making health maintenance and screening a necessity.
- Cancer survivors are at risk for late effects of cancer therapy and must be educated on the importance of knowing what treatment they have received and what screening is recommended.
- Survivorship care can take place in a variety of settings. It is important to determine the best setting for each patient individually.
- In 2006, IOM recommended the delivery of an SCP to each patient completing active treatment (Hewitt et al., 2006). Subsequently, the American College of Surgeons Commission on Cancer published its Program Standard 3.3, requiring accredited programs to implement treatment summaries and SCPs.
- Barriers to the provision of SCPs are numerous and include patient, provider, and system variables. Patient barriers include lack of awareness, and provider and system barriers include limited financial, time, and human resources.
- Mortality rates from recurrence vary based on primary tumor type, with the highest rates being in survivors originally diagnosed with CNS tumors, leukemia, and bone tumors.
- Cancer survivors who received chemotherapy, steroid medications, or hormone therapy may develop osteoporosis or experience joint pain. Patients can lower their risk of osteoporosis by avoiding tobacco products, eating foods rich in calcium and vitamin D, and engaging in regular physical activity.
- IOM defined survivorship care as the phase of care following completion of primary treatment and recommended that it address four essential components: prevention of recurrent and new cancers and other late effects; surveillance for cancer spread, recurrence, and secondary cancers and assessment of medical and psychosocial late effects; intervention for consequences of cancer and its treatment; and coordination between primary and specialty care.
- Reasonable accommodations, such as telecommuting, reassignment, job sharing, and modified hours, are all permitted through the ADA and can enable patients with cancer to maintain their employment during or after treatment.

Bhatia, S.S., Sather, H.N., Pabustan, O.B., Trigg, M.E., Gaynon, P.S., & Robison, L.L. (2002). Low incidence of second neoplasms among children diagnosed with acute lymphoblastic leukemia after 1983. *Blood, 99,* 4257–4264. doi:10.1182/blood.V99.12.4257

Bhatia, S.S., Yasui, Y., Robison, L.L., Birch, J.M., Bogue, M.K., Diller, L., … Meadows, A.T. (2003). High risk of subsequent neoplasms continues with extended follow-up of childhood Hodgkin's disease: Report from the Late Effects Study Group. *Journal of Clinical Oncology, 21,* 4386–4394. doi:10.1200/JCO.2003.11.059

Blatt, J., Olshan, A., Gula, M.J., Dickman, P.S., & Zaranek, B. (1992). Second malignancies in very-long-term survivors of childhood cancer. *American Journal of Medicine, 93,* 57–60. doi:10.1016/0002-9343(92)90680-A

Bluhm, E.C., Ronckers, C., Hayashi, R.J., Neglia, J.P., Mertens, A.C., Stovall, M., … Inskip, P.D. (2008). Cause-specific mortality and second cancer incidence after non-Hodgkin lymphoma: A report from the Childhood Cancer Survivor Study. *Blood, 111,* 4014–4021. doi:10.1182/blood-2007-08-106021

Blum, R.G., Garell, D., Hodgman, C.H., Jorissen, T.W., Okinow, N.A., Orr, D.P., & Slap, G.B. (1993). Transition from child-centered to adult health-care systems for adolescents with chronic conditions: A position paper of the Society for Adolescent Medicine. *Journal of Adolescent Health, 14,* 570–576. doi:10.1016/1054-139X(93)90143-D

Bolster, M.B. (2015, October). Osteoporosis. In *Merck manual professional version.* Retrieved from http://www.merckmanuals.com/professional/musculoskeletal-and-connective-tissue-disorders/osteoporosis/osteoporosis

Bovelli, D., Plataniotis, G., & Roila, F. (2010). Cardiotoxicity of chemotherapeutic agents and radiotherapy-related heart disease: ESMO clinical practice guidelines. *Annals of Oncology, 21*(Suppl. 5), v277–v282. doi:10.1093/annonc/mdq200

Centers for Disease Control and Prevention. (2015). Web Plus. Retrieved from https://www.cdc.gov/cancer/npcr/tools/registryplus/wp_survmodule.htm

Centers for Disease Control and Prevention. (2016). Colorectal (colon) cancer: What should I know about screening? Retrieved from http://www.cdc.gov/cancer/colorectal/basic_info/screening/index.htm

Chambers, S.K., Dunn, J., Occhipinti, S., Hughes, S., Baade, P., Sinclair, S., ... O'Connell, D.L. (2012). A systematic review of the impact of stigma and nihilism on lung cancer outcomes. *BMC Cancer, 12,* 184. doi:10.1186/1471-2407-12-184

Children's Oncology Group. (n.d.). About us. Retrieved from https://www.childrensoncologygroup.org/index.php/aboutus

Cowens-Alvarado, R., Sharpe, K., Pratt-Chapman, M., Willis, A., Gansler, T., Ganz, P.A., ... Stein, K. (2013). Advancing survivorship care through the National Cancer Survivorship Resource Center: Developing American Cancer Society guidelines for primary care providers. *CA: A Cancer Journal for Clinicians, 63,* 147–150. doi:10.3322/caac.21183

Curtis, R.E., Boice, J.D., Jr., Kleinerman, R.A., Flannery, J.T., & Fraumeni, J.F., Jr. (1985). Summary: Multiple primary cancers in Connecticut, 1935–82. *National Cancer Institute Monograph, 68,* 219–242.

Darud, M. (2014). Navigation and survivorship: Rationalizing your program costs. *Oncology Nurse Advisor.* Retrieved from http://www.oncologynurseadvisor.com/oncology-nursing/navigation-and-survivorship-rationalizing-your-program-costs/article/385395

DeSantis, C.E., Lin, C.C., Mariotto, A., Siegel, R.L., Stein, K.D., Kramer, J.L., ... Jemal, A. (2014). Cancer treatment and survivorship statistics, 2014. *CA: A Cancer Journal for Clinicians, 64,* 252–271. doi:10.3322/caac.21235

DiSipio, T., Rye, S., Newman, B., & Hayes, S. (2013). Incidence of unilateral arm lymphoedema after breast cancer: A systematic review and meta-analysis. *Lancet Oncology, 14,* 500–515. doi:10.1016/S1470-2045(13)70076-7

Douketis, J.D. (2015, October). Lymphedema. In *Merck manual professional version.* Retrieved from http://www.merckmanuals.com/professional/cardiovascular-disorders/lymphatic-disorders/lymphedema

Dulko, D., Pace, C.M., Dittus, K.L., Sprague, B.L., Pollack, L.A., Hawkins, N.A., & Geller, B.M. (2013). Barriers and facilitators to implementing cancer survivorship care plans. *Oncology Nursing Forum, 40,* 575–580. doi:10.1188/13.ONF.575-580

Economou, D., Hurria, A., & Grant, M. (2012). Integrating a cancer-specific geriatric assessment into survivorship care [Online exclusive]. *Clinical Journal of Oncology Nursing, 16,* E78–E85. doi:10.1188/12.CJON.E78-E83

Egan, M.Y., McEwen, S., Sikora, L., Chasen, M., Fitch, M., & Eldred, S. (2013). Rehabilitation following cancer treatment. *Disability and Rehabilitation, 35,* 2245–2258. doi:10.3109/09638288.2013.774441

Forbes, C.C., Blanchard, C.M., Mummery, W.K., & Courneya, K.S. (2015). Prevalence and correlates of strength exercise among breast, prostate, and colorectal cancer survivors. *Oncology Nursing Forum, 42,* 118–127. doi:10.1188/15.ONF.42-02AP

Freyer, D.R., & Kibrick-Lazear, R. (2006). In sickness and in health: Transition of cancer-related care for older adolescents and young adults. *Cancer, 107*(Suppl. 7), 1702–1709. doi:10.1002/cncr.22109

Friedman, D.L., Freyer, D.R., & Levitt, G.A. (2006). Models of care for survivors of childhood cancer. *Pediatric Blood and Cancer, 46,* 159–168. doi:10.1002/pbc.20611

Ganz, P.A. (2011). Q&A: The 'three Ps' of cancer survivorship care. *BMC Medicine, 9,* 14. doi:10.1186/1741-7015-9-14

Ganz, P.A. (2014). Cancer survivors: A look backward and forward. *Journal of Oncology Practice, 10,* 289–293. doi:10.1200/JOP.2014.001552

Granek, L., Nathan, P.C., Rosenberg-Yunger, Z.R., D'Agostino, N., Amin, L., Barr, R.D., ... Klassen, A.F. (2012). Psychological factors impacting transition from paediatric to adult care by childhood cancer survivors. *Journal of Cancer Survivorship, 6,* 260–269. doi:10.1007/s11764-012-0223-0

Grant, M., Economou, D., & Ferrell, B.R. (2010). Oncology nurse participation in survivorship care. *Clinical Journal of Oncology Nursing, 14,* 709–715. doi:10.1188/10.CJON.709-715

Hanna, N., Mulshine, J., Wollins, D.S., Tyne, C., & Dresler, C. (2013). Tobacco cessation and control a decade later: American Society of Clinical Oncology policy statement update. *Journal of Clinical Oncology, 31,* 3147–3157. doi:10.1200/JCO.2013.48.8932

Harvie, M., Howell, A., & Evans, D.G. (2015). Can diet and lifestyle prevent breast cancer: What is the evidence? *American Society of Clinical Oncology Educational Book, 2015,* e66–e73. doi:10.14694/EdBook_AM.2015.35.e66

Haylock, P.J., Mitchell, S.A., Cox, T., Temple, S.V., & Curtiss, C.P. (2007). The cancer survivor's prescription for living. *American Journal of Nursing, 107*(4), 58–70. doi:10.1097/01.NAJ.0000271186.82445.b6

Hewitt, M., Greenfield, S., & Stovall, E. (Eds.). (2006). *From cancer patient to cancer survivor: Lost in transition.* Washington, DC: National Academies Press.

Horner, M.J., Ries, L.A.G., Krapcho, M., Neyman, N., Aminou, R., Howlader, N., ... Edwards, B.K. (Eds.). (2009). *SEER cancer statistics review, 1975–2006.* Retrieved from http://seer.cancer.gov/csr/1975_2006

Houlihan, N.G. (2009). Transitioning to cancer survivorship: Plans of care. *Oncology, 23*(Suppl. 8), 42–48.

Hurria, A., Levit, L.A., Dale, W., Mohile, S.G., Muss, H.B., Fehrenbacher, L., ... Cohen, H.J. (2015). Improving the evidence base for treating older adults with cancer: American Society of Clinical Oncology statement. *Journal of Clinical Oncology, 33,* 3826–3833. doi:10.1200/JCO.2015.63.0319

Hurria, A., Togawa, K., Mohile, S.G., Owusu, C., Klepin, H.D., Gross, C.P., ... Tew, W.P. (2011). Predicting chemotherapy toxicity in older adults with cancer: A prospective multicenter study. *Journal of Clinical Oncology, 29,* 3457–3465. doi:10.1200/JCO.2011.34.7625

Inskip, P.D., & Curtis, R.E. (2007). New malignancies following childhood cancer in the United States, 1973–2002. *International Journal of Cancer, 121,* 2233–2240. doi:10.1002/ijc.22827

Irwin, M., Klemp, J.R., Glennon, C., & Frazier, L.M. (2011). Oncology nurses' perspectives on the state of cancer survivorship care: Current practice and barriers to implementation [Online exclusive]. *Oncology Nursing Forum, 38,* E11–E19. doi:10.1188/11.ONF.E11-E19

Jacobs, L.A., Palmer, S.C., Schwartz, L.A., DeMichele, A., Mao, J.J., Carver, J., ... Meadows, A.T. (2009). Adult cancer survivorship: Evolution, research, and planning care. *CA: A Cancer Journal for Clinicians, 59,* 391–410. doi:10.3322/caac.20040

Kaplan, B.W. (2013). A survivorship dilemma: The impact of cancer treatment on cardiovascular risk factors. *Oncology Nurse Advisor, 4*(3), 53–54.

Kron, T., & Chua, B. (2014). Radiotherapy for breast cancer: How can it benefit from advancing technology? *European Medical Journal Oncology, 2,* 83–90.

Landier, W. (2009). Survivorship care: Essential components and models of delivery. *Oncology, 23*(Suppl. 4, Nurse ed.), 46–53.

Lee, Y.-L., Santacroce, S.J., & Sadler, L. (2007). Predictors of healthy behaviour in long-term survivors of childhood cancer. *Journal of Clinical Nursing, 16,* 285–295. doi:10.1111/j.1365-2702.2007.01966.x

Levine, G., D'Amico, A.V., Berger, P., Clark, P.E., Eckel, R.H., Keating, N.L., ... American Urological Association. (2010). Androgen-deprivation therapy in prostate cancer and cardiovascular risk. *CA: A Cancer Journal for Clinicians, 60,* 194–201. doi:10.3322/caac.20061

Levit, L.A., Balogh, E.P., Nass, S.J., & Ganz, P.A. (Eds.). (2013). *Delivering high-quality cancer care: Charting a new course for a system in crisis.* Washington, DC: National Academies Press.

Lips, P., & van Schoor, N.M. (2005). Quality of life in patients with osteoporosis. *Osteoporosis International, 16,* 447–455. doi:10.1007/s00198-004-1762-7

Lisik-Habib, M., Czernek, U., Dębska-Szmich, S., Krakowska, M., Kubicka-Wołkowska, J., & Potemski, P. (2015). Secondary cancer in a survivor of Hodgkin's lymphoma: A case report and review of the literature. *Oncology Letters, 9,* 964–966. doi:10.3842/01.2014.2799

Loprinzi, P.D., & Lee, H. (2014). Rationale for promoting physical activity among cancer survivors: Literature review and epidemiologic examination. *Oncology Nursing Forum, 41,* 117–125. doi:10.1188/14.ONF.117-125

Lorentzon, M., & Cummings, S.R. (2015). Osteoporosis: The evolution of a diagnosis. *Journal of Internal Medicine, 277,* 650–661. doi:10.1111/joim.12369

MacArthur, A.C., Spinelli, J.J., Rogers, P.C., Goddard, K.J., Phillips, N., & McBride, M.L. (2007). Risk of a second malignant neoplasm among 5-year survivors of cancer in childhood and adolescence in British Columbia, Canada. *Pediatric Blood and Cancer, 48,* 453–459. doi:10.1002/pbc.20921

Mariotto, A.B., Yabroff, K.R., Shao, Y., Feuer, E.J., & Brown, M.L. (2011). Projections of the cost of cancer care in the United States: 2010–2020. *Journal of the National Cancer Institute, 103,* 117–128. doi:10.1093/jnci/djq495

Mayer, D.K., Shapiro, C.L., Jacobson, P., & McCabe, M.S. (2015). Assuring quality cancer survivorship care: We've only just begun. *American Society of Clinical Oncology Educational Book, 2015,* e583–e591. doi:10.14694/edbook_am.2015.35.e583

McCabe, M.S., Bhatia, S., Oeffinger, K.C., Reaman, G.H., Tyne, C., Wollins, D.S., & Hudson, M.M. (2013). American Society of Clinical Oncology statement: Achieving high-quality cancer survivorship care. *Journal of Clinical Oncology, 31,* 631–640. doi:10.1200/jco.2012.46.6854

McCabe, M.S., & Jacobs, L. (2008). Survivorship care: Models and programs. *Seminars in Oncology Nursing, 24,* 202–207. doi:10.1016/j.soncn.2008.05.008

Meadows, A.T., Friedman, D.L., Neglia, J.P., Mertens, A.C., Donaldson, S.S., Stovall, M., ... Inskip, P.D. (2009). Second neoplasms in survivors of childhood cancer: Findings from the Childhood Cancer Survivor Study cohort. *Journal of Clinical Oncology, 27,* 2356–2362. doi:10.1200/JCO.2008.21.1920

Mehnert, A., Koch, U., Sundermann, C., & Dinkel, A. (2013). Predictors of fear of recurrence in patients one year after cancer rehabilitation: A prospective study. *Acta Oncologica, 52,* 1102–1109. doi:10.3109/0284186X.2013.765063

Mertens, A.C., Yasui, Y., Neglia, J.P., Potter, J.D., Nesbit, M.E., Jr., Ruccione, K., ... Robison, L.L. (2001). Late mortality experience in five-year survivors of childhood and adolescent cancer: The Childhood Cancer Survivor Study. *Journal of Clinical Oncology, 19,* 3163–3172.

Miller, K.D. (2009, Summer). Revisiting the seasons of survival: Applying new wisdom to the phases of survivorship. *Cure.* Retrieved from http://www.curetoday.com/publications/cure/2009/summer2009/revisiting-the-seasons-of-survival

Miller, K.D., Siegel, R.L., Lin, C.C., Mariotto, A.B., Kramer, J.L., Rowland, J.H., ... Jemal, A. (2016). Cancer treatment and survivorship statistics, 2016. *CA: A Cancer Journal for Clinicians, 66,* 271–289. doi:10.3322/caac.21349

Mullen, F. (1985). Seasons of survival: Reflections of a physician with cancer. *New England Journal of Medicine, 313,* 270–273. doi:10.1056/NEJM198507253130421

Nathan, P.C., Ford, J.S., Henderson, T.O., Hudson, M.M., Emmons, K.M., Casillas, J.N., ... Oeffinger, K.C. (2009). Health behaviors, medical care, and interventions to promote healthy living in the Childhood Cancer Survivor Study cohort. *Journal of Clinical Oncology, 27,* 2363–2373. doi:10.1200/JCO.2008.21.1441

National Cancer Institute. (2015). Lymphedema (PDQ®) [Health professional version]. Retrieved from http://www.cancer.gov/about-cancer/treatment/side-effects/lymphedema/lymphedema-hp-pdq

National Cancer Institute. (2016). Childhood Cancer Survivor Study: An overview. Retrieved from https://www.cancer.gov/types/childhood-cancers/ccss

National Comprehensive Cancer Network. (2016). *NCCN Clinical Practice Guidelines in Oncology (NCCN Guidelines®): Genetic/familial high-risk assessment: Breast and ovarian* [v.2.2017]. Retrieved from http://www.nccn.org/professionals/physician_gls/pdf/genetics_screening.pdf

National Institute of Mental Health. (n.d.). 5 things you should know about stress. Retrieved from http://www.nimh.nih.gov/health/publications/stress/index.shtml

National Institutes of Health Consensus Development Panel on Osteoporosis Prevention, Diagnosis, and Therapy. (2001). Osteoporosis prevention, diagnosis, and therapy. *JAMA, 285,* 785–795. doi:10.1001/jama.285.6.785

Neglia, J.P., Friedman, D.L., Yasui, Y., Mertens, A.C., Hammond, S., Stovall, M., ... Robison, L.L. (2001). Second malignant neoplasms in five-year survivors of childhood cancer: Childhood Cancer Survivor Study. *Journal of the National Cancer Institute, 93,* 618–629.

Nekhlyudov, L., Aziz, N.M., Lerro, C., & Virgo, K.S. (2013). Oncologists' and primary care physicians' awareness of late and long-term effects of chemotherapy: Implications for care of the growing population of survivors. *Journal of Oncology Practice, 10,* E29–E36. doi:10.1200/JOP.2013.001121

Ness, S., Kokal, J., Fee-Schroeder, K., Novotny, P., Satele, D., & Barton, D. (2013). Concerns across the survivorship trajectory: Results from a survey of cancer survivors. *Oncology Nursing Forum, 40,* 35–42. doi:10.1188/13.ONF.35-42

Ng, A.K., & Travis, L.B. (2008). Second primary cancers: An overview. *Hematology/Oncology Clinics of North America, 22,* 271–289. doi:10.1016/j.hoc.2008.01.007

Oeffinger, K.C. (2003). Longitudinal risk-based health care for adult survivors of childhood cancer. *Current Problems in Cancer, 27,* 143–167. doi:10.1016/S0147-0272(03)00031-X

Oeffinger, K.C., & Robison, L.L. (2007). Childhood cancer survivors, late effects, and a new model for understanding survivorship [Editorial]. *JAMA, 297,* 2762–2764. doi:10.1001/jama.297.24.2762

Peteet, J.R. (2000). Cancer and the meaning of work. *General Hospital Psychiatry, 22,* 200–205. doi:10.1016/S0163-8343(00)00076-1

Rosen, D.S. (1993). Transition to adult health care for adolescents and young adults with cancer. *Cancer, 71*(Suppl. 10), 3411–3414. doi:10.1002/1097-0142(19930515)71:10+<3411::AID-CNCR2820711746>3.0.CO;2-E

Routt, M. (2013). Improving geriatric cancer survivorship. *Clinical Advisor, 16*(8), 48–64.

Rowland, J.H., Hewitt, M., & Ganz, P.A. (2006). Cancer survivorship: A new challenge in delivering quality cancer care. *Journal of Clinical Oncology, 24,* 5101–5104. doi:10.1200/JCO.2006.09.2700

Salz, T., Oeffinger, K.C., McCabe, M.S., Layne, T.M., & Bach, P.B. (2012). Survivorship care plans in research and practice. *CA: A Cancer Journal for Clinicians, 62,* 101–117. doi:10.3322/caac.20142

Sankila, R.P., Pukkala, E., & Teppo, L. (1995). Risk of subsequent malignant neoplasms among 470,000 cancer patients in Finland, 1953–1991. *International Journal of Cancer, 60,* 464–470. doi:10.1002/ijc.2910600407

Stricker, C.T., Jacobs, L.A., Risendal, B., Jones, A., Panzer, S., Ganz, P.A., ... Palmer, S.C. (2011). Survivorship care planning after the Institute of Medicine recommendations: How are we faring? *Journal of Cancer Survivorship, 5,* 358–370. doi:10.1007/s11764-011-0196-4

Stricker, C.T., & O'Brien, M. (2014). Implementing the Commission on Cancer standards for survivorship care plans. *Clinical Journal of Oncology Nursing, 18*(Suppl. 1), 15–22. doi:10.1188/14.CJON.S1.15-22

Suh, E., Daugherty, C.K., Wroblewski, K., Lee, H., Kigin, M.L., Rasinski, K.A., ... Henderson, T.O. (2014). General internists' preferences and knowledge about the care of adult survivors of childhood cancer: A cross-sectional survey. *Annals of Internal Medicine, 160,* 11–17. doi:10.7326/M13-1941

Travis, L.B., Rabkin, C.S., Brown, L.M., Allan, J.M., Alter, B.P., Ambrosone, C.B., ... Greene, M.H. (2006). Cancer survivorship—Genetic susceptibility and second primary cancers: Research strategies and recommendations. *Journal of the National Cancer Institute, 98,* 15–25. doi:10.1093/jnci/djj001

Tucker, M.A., Jones, P.H., Boice, J.D., Jr., Robison, L.L., Stone, B.J., Stovall, M., ... Fraumeni, J.F., Jr. (1991). Therapeutic radiation at a young age is linked to secondary thyroid cancer. *Cancer Research, 51,* 2885–2888. Retrieved from http://cancerres.aacrjournals.org/content/51/11/2885.long

van Waart, H., Stuiver, M.M., van Hartenm, W.H., Geleijn, E., Kieffer, J.M., Buffart, L.M., ... Aaronson, N.K. (2015). Effect of low-intensity physical activity and moderate- to high-intensity physical exercise during adjuvant chemotherapy on physical fitness, fatigue, and chemotherapy completion rates: Result of the PACES randomized clinical trial. *Journal of Clinical Oncology, 33,* 1918–1927. doi:10.1200/JCO.2014.59.1081

Vasudevan, V., Cheung, M.C., Yang, R., Zhuge, Y., Fischer, A.C., Koniaris, L.G., & Sola, J.E. (2010). Pediatric solid tumors and second malignancies: Characteristics and survival outcomes. *Journal of Surgical Research, 160,* 184–189. doi:10.1016/j.jss.2009.05.030

Walston, J., Hadley, E.C., Ferrucci, L., Guralnik, J.M., Newman, A.B., Studenski, S.A., ... Fried, L.P. (2006). Research agenda for frailty in older adults: Toward a better understanding of physiology and etiology: Summary from the American Geriatrics Society/National Institute on Aging Research Conference on Frailty in Older Adults. *Journal of the American Geriatrics Society, 54,* 991–1001. doi:10.1111/j.1532-5415.2006.00745.x

Weaver, K.E., Foraker, R.E., Alfano, C.M., Rowland, J.H., Arora, N.K., Bellizzi, K.M., ... Aziz, N.M. (2013). Cardiovascular risk factors among long-term survivors of breast, prostate, colorectal, and gynecologic cancers: A gap in survivorship care? *Journal of Cancer Survivorship, 7,* 253–261. doi:10.1007/s11764-013-0267-9

Wedding, U., Röhrig, B., Klippstein, A., Pientka, L., & Höffken, K. (2007). Age, severe comorbidity and functional impairment independently contribute to poor survival in cancer patients. *Journal of Cancer Research and Clinical Oncology, 133,* 945–950. doi:10.1007/s00432-007-0233-x

Wender, R., Fontham, E.T.H., Barrera, E., Jr., Colditz, G.A., Church, T.R., Ettinger, D.S., ... Smith, R.A. (2013). American Cancer Society lung cancer screening guidelines. *CA: A Cancer Journal for Clinicians, 63,* 106–117. doi:10.3322/caac.21172

Wilbur, J. (2015). Surveillance of the adult cancer survivor. *American Family Physician, 91,* 29–36. Retrieved from http://www.aafp.org/afp/2015/0101/p29.html

World Health Organization. (n.d.). Rehabilitation. Retrieved from http://www.who.int/topics/rehabilitation/en

Yabroff, K.R., Lawrence, W.F., Clauser, S., Davis, W.W., & Brown, M.L. (2004). Burden of illness in cancer survivors: Findings from a population-based national sample. *Journal of the National Cancer Institute, 96,* 1322–1330. doi:10.1093/jnci/djh255

Chapter 34 Study Questions

1. Many cancer survivors are at high risk for osteoporosis. All of the following are ways they can decrease their risk EXCEPT:
   A. Quitting smoking.
   B. Following a vegetarian diet.
   C. Exercising regularly.
   D. Following a diet high in calcium and vitamin D.

2. Through the Americans With Disabilities Act, survivors can expect all of the following reasonable accommodations EXCEPT:
   A. Transportation.
   B. Reassignment.
   C. Telecommuting.
   D. Job sharing and modified hours.

3. Which of the following is the definition of a cancer survivor?
   A. A person with no evidence of disease after five years
   B. Anyone diagnosed with cancer
   C. Someone who has undergone curative surgery
   D. Someone who has completed chemotherapy and/or radiation

4. Which of the following are considered essential components of survivorship care?
   A. Prevention of recurrent and new cancers and other late effects
   B. Surveillance for cancer spread, recurrence, and secondary cancers and assessment of medical and psychosocial late effects
   C. Intervention for consequences of cancer and its treatment
   D. Coordination between primary and specialty care
   E. All of the above

5. Who is responsible for survivorship care?
   A. Oncologist
   B. Primary care provider
   C. Patient
   D. Oncology nurse
   E. All of the above

Answer Key

Chapter 1

1. **C.** Nonsense mutations cause the premature stoppage of the translational machinery. This often results in a shortened and aberrant or nonfunctional protein.
2. **D.** *BAX* is a proapoptotic gene. A protein that upregulates this gene would result in increased apoptosis and antitumor activity.
3. **D.** Inflammation can aid in malignant transformation by providing the tumor microenvironment with growth factors, antiapoptotic factors, proangiogenic factors, and enzymes that alter the extracellular matrix and promote invasion and metastasis.
4. **B.** Cancer cells have a shift in their metabolism from oxidative phosphorylation to glycolysis as a result of increased metabolic needs. The increased metabolism seen in cancer cells causes them to be brighter on positron-emission tomography scans than normal cells, thereby aiding in identification.
5. **A.** Loss of heterozygosity means there was a mutation of the allele on the second chromosome, causing the chromosome to lose heterozygous status (loss of only one allele). Now, both alleles have been mutated, causing loss of heterozygosity.

Chapter 2

1. **A.** Metastasis occurs when the original tumor cells spread to a new location. The diagnosis would remain the original cancer type, identifying the location of the metastasis.
2. **A.** Pathologic examination of tissue samples by a pathologist is required to identify the correct type of cancer. Laboratory and radiologic information helps to understand the extent and behavior of cancer cells.
3. **B.** The correct answer is lung cancer. Multiple myeloma and non-Hodgkin lymphoma are hematologic disorders and staged using other systems. Ovarian cancer is usually staged using the International Federation of Gynecology and Obstetrics, or FIGO, system.
4. **B.** Grade 1 tumors are considered well differentiated and retain many of the behaviors and functions of the normal cells in the tissue of origin. Grade 3 or 4 tumors are more abnormal.
5. **D.** Performance status is considered when making decisions on the best treatment approach, as patients with a better performance status usually are more likely to tolerate aggressive treatment.

Chapter 3

1. **C.** Absolute risk is a measure of the occurrence of cancer, either incidence (new cases) or mortality (deaths), in the general population. It is helpful when a patient needs to understand what the chances are for all people in a population of developing or dying of a particular disease. The term relative risk refers to a comparison of the incidence or

deaths among those with a particular risk factor compared to those without the risk factor. Attributable risk is the amount of disease within a population that could be prevented by the alteration of a risk factor. Incidence is the number of new cancer cases in a year.

2. **A.** Primary prevention is any measure to avoid carcinogen exposure, improve health practices, and, in some cases, use chemoprevention agents or prophylactic surgery. Secondary prevention is the identification of individuals at risk for developing malignancy and the implementation of appropriate screening recommendations; it often is used interchangeably with early detection and cancer screening. Tertiary prevention is any measure aimed at individuals with a history of malignancy, including monitoring for and preventing recurrence and screening for second primary cancers.
3. **C.** Tertiary prevention is any measure aimed at individuals with a history of malignancy, including monitoring for and preventing recurrence and screening for second primary cancers.
4. **H.** Risk factor assessment suggests the chance of developing cancer; it does not determine if or when a person will develop cancer. Screening and prevention measures recommended for the general public might be modified based on a risk factor assessment if a person appears to be at higher risk for developing a malignancy. Assessment of family history is part of the risk assessment. When risk appears to be higher in a family, the family should be referred for genetic testing.
5. **B.** Secondary prevention is the identification of individuals at risk for developing malignancy and the implementation of appropriate screening recommendations; it often is used interchangeably with early detection and cancer screening.

Chapter 4

1. **C.** Bilateral breast cancer is a classic sign of hereditary breast and ovarian cancer. Answer A is incorrect because it is typically associated with early age at onset, especially before age 50. HER2-positive breast cancer is not necessarily associated with hereditary breast cancer, but it is an important prognostic marker that guides treatment; triple-negative (negative for estrogen receptors, progesterone receptors, and HER2) breast cancer is associated with some hereditary breast and ovarian cancer syndromes. Having one family member with breast cancer does not necessarily increase risk. Having multiple family members with breast cancer, especially across two or more generations, is suggestive of hereditary risk.
2. **D.** The patient has the same risk as the general population for developing colon cancer. He may have additional medical or lifestyle factors that increase his risk for developing the disease. This is a true negative, informative result.
3. **B.** Genetic testing is best managed by a genetic healthcare professional, such as a genetic counselor, an advanced practice nurse credentialed in genetics, or a medical geneticist. Individuals undergoing genetic testing should have counseling with a genetics healthcare professional, even though genetic tests typically are ordered as blood or saliva tests. The genetics healthcare professional typically evaluates the pedigree to determine if risk is high enough to offer testing and assists with preauthorizations when needed. Genetic testing is not a routine blood test.
4. **B.** The clinical implications of a genetic test can be challenging to interpret. Without the benefit of a genetics healthcare professional, it may be difficult or impossible for a consumer without clinical knowledge to correctly interpret results and select appropriate recommendations for prevention and early detection. When testing is done outside of formal counseling with a qualified professional, there may not be a plan to inform other members about the potential risk; family members cannot learn the results of genetic testing unless another family member tells them. Although genetic testing is expensive, if this is disclosed

to the patient during pretest counseling, it is not a risk. Genetic testing for cancer usually is predictive; seldom do patients know when they will be diagnosed with the cancer.

5. **B.** Individuals must understand the potential risks, limitations, and benefits to determine if genetic testing is appropriate in their own situation. Confirmation of the family history and estimation of the chance of carrying the mutation are critical components of determining if genetic testing is appropriate and typically are discussed with the patient, but it is not critical to the informed consent process. Informed consent does not depend on the patient's personal health status. Ideally, cancer genetic testing is initiated in a person who has the malignancy because there is the best chance that a mutation will be detected.

Chapter 5

1. **A.** The primary purpose of risk assessment is to determine appropriate recommendations for primary cancer prevention and cancer screening. People with an elevated risk for developing colon cancer might benefit from more frequent colonoscopys or want to consider chemoprevention with aspirin or a nonsteroidal anti-inflammatory drug based on their risk profile.
2. **D.** Breast MRI is a consideration in women with a lifetime risk of breast cancer of at least 20%. Because the patient's calculated lifetime risk is 32%, this is an appropriate consideration. The American Cancer Society recommends an annual mammography for all women starting at age 40. Women with a 20% or higher risk can add a breast MRI six months after the mammogram. This way, imaging is performed every six months in a high-risk woman.
3. **B.** Currently, lung cancer screening is reserved for those at increased risk. The only accepted strategy that has been demonstrated to result in the early detection of lung cancer is annual low-dose computed tomography. The American Cancer Society and other organizations state that clinicians should discuss this screening option for current and former smokers (those who have quit within the previous 15 years) who are 55–74 years old, in good health, and with at least a 30-pack-year smoking history.
4. **D.** Older age, light or fair complexion, and working outdoors are risk factors for developing skin cancer.
5. **C.** Several human papillomaviruses are directly linked to the development of cervical cancer. A history of multiple sexual partners, sexually transmitted infection, human papillomavirus infection, and early first coitus are major risk factors. Obesity is associated with an increased risk for developing endometrial cancer. Hereditary breast cancer syndromes can be associated with an increased risk for developing ovarian cancer. A pelvic examination is important for screening for endometrial cancer and possibly ovarian cancer. The Pap test and human papillomavirus testing are the best means to screen for cervical cancer.

Chapter 6

1. **D.** *UGT1A1* gene encodes for the phase II drug-metabolizing enzyme, UDP-glycosyltransferase 1A1, which inactivates irinotecan in the patients with cancer.
2. **D.** Missense is a variant change in which a substitution of one nucleotide for another is translated to an amino acid change in the protein sequence.
3. **C.** Nurses will play a key role in educating patients about pharmacogenomic information and how genetic polymorphisms influence drug treatment.
4. **A.** Breast cancer resistant protein is one of the main transporters that has been identified in chemotherapy drug resistance, especially for drugs such as methotrexate, gefitinib, and the irinotecan metabolite.
5. **B.** The use of 5-fluorouracil is dependent on the activity of the dihydropyrimidine dehydrogenase in the patient. If patients have

decreased or no functional activity of this drug-metabolizing enzyme, they could potentially die or suffer from toxicity because they are not able to inactivate and remove the chemotherapy agent from their body.

Chapter 7

1. **E.** The oncology cancer team is multidisciplinary and often includes all of the specialists listed.
2. **D.** Prophylactic surgery of the medulla would result in death.
3. **A.** All of the answers except "A" are correct. While prognosis may be addressed prior to surgery, the expectation of long-term survival is not.
4. **D.** A colonoscopy is a surgical technique used for colorectal cancer screening.
5. **B.** This is a known statistic for ductal carcinoma in situ–associated breast cancer.

Chapter 8

1. **A.** During radiation therapy, the skin may become irritated, decreasing the sensation of hot or cold to the area. Hot water may increase skin irritation, so the use of only lukewarm water for washing the treated area is recommended. Patients' skin may be extra sensitive to sunlight. If possible, patients should cover the treated skin with dark-colored or UV-protective clothing before going outside. They also should use sunscreen with SPF 30 or higher and reapply often. Patients should continue to give their skin extra protection from sunlight even after radiation therapy ends.
2. **D.** When providing education to patients, it is necessary to include that safety precautions must be maintained for at least a year after completion of therapy.
3. **B.** Principles of radiation protection follow the DTS system: distance (D), time (T), and shielding (S). Distance—at least three feet should be maintained when a nurse is not performing any nursing procedures. Time—limit contact to five minutes each time. Shielding—use a lead shield during contact with client.
4. **D.** Patients have varying degrees of side effects, especially skin reactions. These include itching, erythema, dryness, wet desquamation, rash, loss of hair at the site of radiation, radiation-induced necrosis, and general discomfort. Suppuration would be possible when a microbe is introduced from the environment.
5. **B.** The best treatment for dry desquamation is to cleanse the area with warm water and mild soap, and apply a thin coating of unscented, lanolin-free cream, such as Aquaphor®, Lubriderm®, or Cetaphil®, to the irradiated area to increase moisturization and decrease potential for wet desquamation.

Chapter 9

1. **C.** Personal protective equipment should be worn during drug preparation, administration, and disposal and when handling excreta while the patient is on chemotherapy precautions.
2. **A.** Antimetabolites such as folate antagonists (e.g., methotrexate), purine antagonists (e.g., 6-mercaptopurine), and pyrimidine antagonists (e.g., 5-fluorouracil) are included in the cell cycle–specific category of chemotherapy.
3. **C.** Petechiae are associated with bleeding. The other noted side effects are common but do not require immediate notification of a care provider.
4. **D.** Chemotherapy can cause a wide variety of acute toxicities. All of the toxicities noted in this question are included.
5. **B.** Oral hazardous drugs should not be crushed, mixed, or manipulated outside of a biologic safety cabinet and therefore must not be crushed or mixed in food in the patient's room.

Chapter 10

1. **C.** These medications should not be given in conjunction with everolimus: CYP3A4

inducers (i.e., carbamazepine, dexamethasone, phenobarbital, phenytoin, rifabutin, rifampin), as well as CYP3A4 inhibitors (i.e., amprenavir, aprepitant, atazanavir, clarithromycin, delavirdine, diltiazem, erythromycin, fluconazole, fosamprenavir, grapefruit juice, indinavir, itraconazole, ketoconazole, nefazodone, nelfinavir, ritonavir, saquinavir, telithromycin, verapamil, voriconazole).
2. **A.** Common adverse reactions of sorafenib include reversible skin rashes, hand-foot skin reaction, and diarrhea (40%, 30%, and 43%, respectively).
3. **C.** More than 60% of left ventricular ejection fraction abnormalities occur within the first nine weeks of lapatinib therapy.
4. **B.** CD20 is expressed on most malignant B cells, with nearly 90% of B-cell lymphomas expressing the CD20 antigen. B-cell acute lymphoblastic leukemia is CD20-positive in about 50% of cases.
5. **D.** If the name of the antibody ends in -momab, it is murine; -ximab is chimeric; -zumab is humanized; and -umab indicates a fully human antibody.

Chapter 11

1. **A.** Yes, anastrozole is the appropriate therapy for a postmenopausal patient because it blocks the synthesis of estrogen by inhibiting the enzyme aromatase.
2. **D.** Common side effects that she could experience include hot flashes, fatigue, headaches, mood swings, edema, weight gain, and osteoporosis.
3. **B.** No, it is not the appropriate therapy. The patient has lumbar spine metastatic disease. He should be started on an antiandrogen such as flutamide for at least one week prior to decrease circulating testosterone to avoid tumor flare.
4. **B.** The goal is either to reduce a specific hormone level in the body or reduce the cancer cells' ability to respond to the hormone, thus shrinking or preventing growth of the tumor cells.
5. **D.** Tamoxifen is more effective than raloxifene in preventing breast cancer, reducing incidence by almost 50% versus 38%, respectively.

Chapter 12

1. **C.** Many patients with cancer receive therapy that may affect their comfort and quality of life. Supportive care studies are clinical trials that monitor the quality of life of patients.
2. **B.** The goal of phase II clinical trials is to determine if the treatment has any beneficial effect in newly diagnosed patients with the same type of cancer. The number of participants enrolled in a phase II study is usually 80–300 patients.
3. **D.** Monitoring of patients includes a table that records all tests, office visits, etc., that are required at specific time points.
4. **A.** Following World War II, leading Nazi doctors performed experiments on people in concentration camps. The international military tribunal at Nuremberg opened criminal proceedings against those doctors. One of the main principles of the Nuremberg Code is the requirement of consent.
5. **C.** The Protecting Human Research Participants online tutorial covers all areas of human research protections. It includes review of historical studies, such as the Tuskegee syphilis study, informed consent, and all other vital aspects of human research protection. The International Council for Harmonisation of Technical Requirements for Pharmaceuticals for Human Use Good Clinical Practice is an international ethical and scientific quality standard for designing, conducting, recording, and reporting trials that involve the participation of human subjects.

Chapter 13

1. **A.** This is stated on the FDA MedWatch website.
2. **A.** This is the definition of integrative medicine.

3. **B.** Testimonial evidence and clinical trials now exist for many CAM therapies. Qualitative research also exists for some CAM therapies.
4. **B.** Nurses spend the most time with patients and families.
5. **C.** This answer is the most correct; something that is within the scope of nursing practice in one state may be outside the scope in another.

Chapter 14

1. **D.** Dry eyes is a manifestation of chronic graft-versus-host disease.
2. **A.** Engraftment is the process in which the donor stem cells make their way to the recipient bone marrow and begin producing healthy blood cells. It is indicated by the recovery of neutrophil counts to 500/mm^3. Hematopoiesis is blood cell growth, division, and differentiation. Myeloablation is the use of very high doses of chemotherapy to ablate the recipient's bone marrow to the point that without stem cell transplant, the marrow would not recover on its own.
3. **B.** Alcohol-based mouth rinse should be avoided in patients during conditioning and in the pre-engraftment phase, as it can lead to mucosal injury and pain.
4. **D.** Full siblings have a 25% chance of having an identical HLA haplotype.
5. **B.** Calcineurin inhibitors such as cyclosporine and tacrolimus are used in allogeneic transplant recipients as a form of immunosuppression to prevent and treat GVHD. Alkylating agents and antimetabolites are types of chemotherapy, and beta-blockers are antihypertensives.

Chapter 15

1. **B.** Although not life threatening, alopecia can have a great impact on a patient's emotional well-being. Providing a referral to Look Good Feel Better is an important resource, but it should not be a substitute for an honest discussion about her feelings and her body image.
2. **A.** Scalp cooling, although slow to gain popularity in the United States, can be an effective alternative treatment to prevent chemotherapy-induced hair loss.
3. **C.** Hair loss generally begins about two weeks after receiving treatment.
4. **A.** Irreversible alopecia has been reported after high-dose chemotherapy and hematopoietic stem cell transplantation, especially related to conditioning regimens containing busulfan and cyclophosphamide.
5. **D.** Doses greater than 40 Gy usually cause permanent damage to the hair follicles in the treated field. Doses of 30–35 Gy may cause temporary hair loss, and doses of 20–25 Gy may cause some hair shedding.

Chapter 16

1. **D.** Type II cardiotoxicity is associated with reversible cardiomyocyte dysfunction. Unlike type I cardiotoxicity, which is thought to be related to the cumulative dose, type II cardiotoxicity is not dose related. With cardiac damage due to type I toxicity, structural changes to the myocardium characterized by vacuoles, myofibrillar disarray, and necrosis may be seen; however, these are not apparent on microscopy with type II cardiotoxicity. Lastly, with type II cardiotoxicity, left ventricular dysfunction/heart failure typically recovers after treatment discontinuation of the anticancer therapy agent and initiation of HF therapy.
2. **B.** Doxorubicin is associated with only heart failure. Sorafenib is the correct answer because it has been implicated in causing all four cardiotoxicities. Nilotinib may cause hypertension, myocardial infarction, and QT prolongation; however, it is not known to cause heart failure. Lastly, ponatinib may cause hypertension, myocardial infarction, and heart failure; however, it is not known to cause QT prolongation.
3. **D.** Troponin I levels are used in the diagnosis of acute coronary syndromes. Troponin I is a cardiac biomarker that rises when the

heart muscle is damaged and begins to elevate 3–12 hours after the onset of an infarct and peaks in 12–24 hours. It remains elevated for 7–14 days, so it can be helpful in the diagnosis if the patient complains of angina symptoms that occurred several days prior. CK-MM is found in the skeletal muscle and the heart, whereas CK-BB is found mostly in the brain. BNP is a biomarker secreted from the ventricles in response to changes in pressure that occur when heart failure develops and worsens. The level of BNP corresponds to volume status. The BNP level in the blood increases when heart failure symptoms worsen and decreases when the heart failure condition is stable.

4. **C.** Endomyocardial biopsy is considered the gold standard for diagnosing anthracycline-induced cardiomyopathy because only the biopsy can show typical pathophysiologic changes caused by anthracycline cardiotoxicity (i.e., sarcoplasmic reticulum dilation, vacuole formation, myofibrillar disarray and necrosis). However, it is an invasive procedure; therefore, assessment of left ventricular ejection fraction by echocardiography and multigated acquisition scan have been commonly used in clinical practice for evaluation and monitoring of chemotherapy-induced cardiotoxicity.
5. **E.** Angiotensin-converting enzyme inhibitors, angiotensin receptor blockers, and beta-blockers are recommended medications for heart failure. Nondihydropyridine calcium channel blockers are generally contraindicated in heart failure because of their negative inotropic effects, as well as undesirable stimulation of the sympathetic nervous system and renin–angiotensin system.

Chapter 17

1. **D.** Although other nutritional deficiencies (e.g., thiamine, vitamin E) can influence cognitive function, vitamin C deficiency is not one of them. Diabetes mellitus can influence the brain via direct or indirect mechanisms as well as behavioral responses (as do other endocrine or metabolic disorders such as liver disease and thyroid dysfunction). For example, diabetes is associated with several macrovascular (e.g., artery disease, stroke) complications that can affect cognition. Psychiatric illnesses are known to affect cognitive function, as well as several medications used to treat those diagnosed with psychiatric disease. Drug or alcohol abuse can impair thinking and various cognitive domains.
2. **A.** Ginkgo biloba was found in two studies to have no effect on cognitive function and therefore was established as effectiveness unlikely. Vitamin E was found in one study to improve cognitive function. However, in another study, the use of vitamin E with donepezil showed no effect. Therefore, effectiveness has not been established as of yet. Methylphenidate studies have had mixed results, with some finding improvement in various cognitive domains and others finding no treatment effect. Therefore, similar to vitamin E, effectiveness has not been established. Erythropoietin studies have been poorly designed and have produced mixed results. Of concern, a warning by the U.S. Food and Drug Administration regarding an increased risk of severe cardiovascular and thrombovascular events and potential to increase tumor progression dictates that it is not recommended for practice.
3. **D.** Genetic mutations may play a role in patient susceptibility to cognitive changes but are not directly related to neuropsychological test performance. Stress and depression are known to reduce test performance. Anxiety may improve or diminish performance, depending on the level of anxiety. Lower levels may heighten performance, but increased anxiety will result in poorer neuropsychological test outcomes.
4. **B.** The temporal lobe, including the hippocampus and amygdala, is crucial for the laying down, strengthening, and storage (or consolidation) of memories. The frontal

lobe has a role for some aspects of memory but is more known for its role in psychomotor function, language, and executive functioning. The parietal lobe is associated with motor function, spatial attention, and visuospatial skills. The occipital lobe has primary responsibility for visual processing of color, motion, and shape.

5. **C.** Executive functioning involves the ability to initiate and generate hypotheses, plan, and make decisions. Attention is the ability to triage relevant inputs, thoughts, or actions while ignoring those that distract or are irrelevant. Information processing is the ability to rapidly and efficiently process simple and complex information. Memory is the ability to acquire, store, and recall learned information.

Chapter 18

1. **D.** Although ice packs have been found to be of use in some patients receiving liposomal doxorubicin, immersion of feet and hands in hot water is not recommended. Avoidance of pressure activities is recommended. Topical steroids have been recommended for some patients to reduce inflammation.
2. **D.** The incidence of nail toxicities in patients receiving taxanes is 0%–44% in widely published series. The appearance of white lines or grooves in the nails is cosmetically uncomfortable but not painful and is merely an interruption of nail bed growth. Paronychia refers to inflammation and infection of the nail bed; bloody collections are referred to as subungual hemorrhages.
3. **E.** All of the above can be seen in patients receiving EGFR inhibitor agents.
4. **D.** A proactive approach is now considered the best strategy, although no gold standard for treatment currently exists. Lotions without perfumes are appropriate, as perfume can be drying, and a maximal SPF product is critical to reduce symptoms.
5. **F.** All of the listed strategies are appropriate precautions nurses should take to manage extravasation. The best strategy is to avoid extravasation; prompt recognition and early intervention are important to reduce potential tissue damage.

Chapter 19

1. **B.** The exact cause is unknown, but CRF, unlike other types of fatigue, is not associated with exertion and can occur across the cancer trajectory.
2. **C.** Many definitions of CRF are found in the literature, and discrepancies have been noted partially because of a lack of consensus related to measurement of CRF. Generally, it is defined as a subjective and multidimensional symptom that includes physical, emotional, and cognitive components. Although many definitions state that CRF impairs functioning, patients have reported the experience of CRF while maintaining functional status.
3. **B.** Across populations of patients with different types of cancer and cancer treatment modalities, CRF has been demonstrated to exist in a symptom cluster consisting of fatigue, sleep disturbance, pain, and depression.
4. **C.** CRF is one of five common signs and symptoms that cancer survivors have indicated may continue even after cancer treatment is completed and into long-term survivorship.
5. **D.** Asking for help with important instrumental activities of daily living, such as shopping, transportation, house cleaning, food preparation, etc., contributes to two goals: conservation of energy for tasks that the patient values and allowing others the opportunity to give the gift of help during the cancer journey. The other three optional answers are incorrect (i.e., less energy is used in wearing shoes that slip on versus those with laces).

Chapter 20

1. **C.** Sialagogues increase flow of saliva and require residual salivary function. The use

of three-dimensional conformal radiation therapy can potentially deliver a lower dose of radiation to the parotid glands, decreasing the potential severity of xerostomia, not brachytherapy. Glycerin swabs and lidocaine mouthwash are not indicated for prevention of xerostomia.

2. **D.** Infection is a complication of mucositis. Prevention is the most effective way to avoid infection. Candida and herpes simplex virus are the two most common infections in patients with mucositis. They can occur independent of each other.
3. **A.** Endoscopy can provide a direct visualization of the causes, particularly intrinsic causes, for dysphagia. Biopsy can be done during endoscopy. A computed tomography scan and positron-emission tomography–computed tomography scan may identify extrinsic causes for dysphagia. Colonoscopy is a direct visualization of the colon and does not evaluate the esophagus.
4. **A.** Complications of diarrhea include the loss of fluid and electrolytes, with persistent or severe diarrhea resulting in life-threatening dehydration, renal insufficiency, and electrolyte imbalances that can lead to cardiovascular collapse.
5. **B.** The combination of a 5-HT_3 RA, dexamethasone, and an NK_1 RA has been demonstrated to be the most effective combination for prophylaxis of chemotherapy-induced nausea and vomiting for highly emetogenic regimens. This combination is endorsed by numerous national guidelines, including those published by the American Society of Clinical Oncology, the Multinational Association of Supportive Care in Cancer, and the National Comprehensive Cancer Network.

Chapter 21

1. **B.** The term genitourinary cancer is commonly used to describe cancers of the bladder, kidney (renal), penis, testicle, and prostate.
2. **D.** All of the choices are used. The American Urological Association Symptom Index (or symptom score, referred to as the AUASS) has seven items that measure symptoms in men on a six-point scale. The International Continence Society Short-Form Male Questionnaire, known as the ICSmaleSF, has two subscales, the ICSmaleIS (stress and urge incontinence) and the ICSmaleVS (voiding problems). The International Consultation on Incontinence Questionnaire Short Form (ICIQ-SF), which has three scored items assessing the frequency, severity, and perceived impact of incontinence and an unscored self-diagnostic item, can be used in both men and women.
3. **C.** The incidence of urinary incontinence after radical prostatectomy has been reported as high as 90%. More than 30% of patients continued to leak 12 months after prostatectomy, and 15% had leakage after 5 years.
4. **B.** PFME strengthens pelvic sphincter muscles and may improve urethral sphincter closure during periods of increased intravesical pressure. Increased strength of the external sphincter muscles is expected to increase urethral resistance to mitigate both stress and urge incontinence.
5. **A.** A range of conditions can aggravate urinary incontinence symptoms, including inadequate fluid intake, which can induce urinary tract infection; caffeine or alcohol intake, which stimulates bladder contraction; constipation or obesity, which adds pressure on the bladder; and certain medications or diseases (e.g., diabetes).

Chapter 22

1. **D.** All of the answers listed are common dose-limiting effects. The neutrophils, platelets, and red blood cells are all affected by systemic anticancer treatments.
2. **A.** Neutrophils' main function is phagocytosis. They are the body's first line of defense against microbial invasion. Their life span

is six to eight hours once they have been released from the bone marrow to the circulation.

3. **D.** All of these answers need to be addressed for the most successful patient outcome.
4. **B.** All of these chemotherapy agents can reduce the platelets, but gemcitabine has the greatest potential.
5. **D.** All of these interventions have been shown to combat fatigue during and after chemotherapy.

Chapter 23

1. **A.** Malignant biliary obstruction often is caused by tumor in the biliary tree or extrinsic compression by pancreatic cancer, cholangiocarcinoma, metastatic disease, or lymphadenopathy in the portal or distal biliary area. Elevated liver enzymes often indicate damage to the hepatocytes. Chemotherapy often has to be dose adjusted because of biliary obstruction but is not the cause.
2. **D.** Ascites is the excessive accumulation of extracellular fluid in the peritoneal cavity. The classic signs and symptoms include weight gain, abdominal distention, and early satiety due to the fluid accumulation.
3. **C.** The classic triad of symptoms for sinusoidal obstruction syndrome includes weight gain, tender hepatomegaly, and hyperbilirubinemia. The diagnosis often is a clinical diagnosis.
4. **B.** Hepatic artery chemoembolization is an alternative treatment for malignancies such as hepatocellular cancer and metastatic disease of the liver. It is used to suppress intrahepatic tumor growth, palliate symptoms, and improve survival. Postembolization syndrome symptoms often are self-limiting, and management includes symptom control.
5. **C.** This defines radioembolization. In chemoembolization, chemotherapy is delivered through the hepatic artery directly into the liver. Radiofrequency ablation is the use of high-frequency alternating current to a tumor that causes coagulative necrosis. Radiation uses external stereotactic or proton therapy to target the tumor.

Chapter 24

1. **C.** Four categories of HSRs exist: (a) immediate IgE mediated (type I), (b) antibody mediated (type II), (c) immune complex mediated (type III), and (d) delayed or cell mediated (type IV). As drug exposure increases cumulatively, the number of reactions to the agent can increase; therefore, answer A is true. Drug actions can produce immediate reactions, and those reactions usually are mediated by IgE. IgE is responsible for the degranulation of mast cells and basophils, which progresses to histamine and cytokine release, causing activation of complement.
2. **A.** Although any drug has the potential to cause an HSR, reactions are more frequently seen in patients receiving platinum agents versus methotrexate, 5-fluorouracil, and vincristine. Platinum agents often produce reactions later in the treatment cycle, and in particular, carboplatin reactions increase after several doses, leading to problems if patients require retreatment with the drug.
3. **E.** All of the symptoms listed may be experienced by the patient who is having an HSR.
4. **B.** Although it is not completely known how biphasic reactions may occur, it is thought that inadequate initial treatment of the original reaction is the culprit, allowing a resurgence of initial symptoms. Premedications can help to reduce HSRs, and certainly specific agents carry higher risk of reaction. Normal saline does not factor into biphasic reactions.
5. **E.** Dexamethasone, diphenhydramine, and H_2 antagonists are all strategies used to reduce the incidence of HSR. The use of opioids is certainly recommended in pain management but does not carry a significant role in the reduction of HSRs.

Chapter 25

1. **C.** Patients who are neutropenic have an inadequate number of functioning neutrophils to be able to mount a corrective response to infection. It is widely accepted that more than 50% of patients with febrile neutropenia or bacteremia will develop sepsis. Severe sepsis occurs in 20%–30% of these patients, while septic shock is seen in 5%–10% of patients (Ahn et al., 2013; Legrand et al., 2012).
2. **A.** When tumor cells are broken down, intracellular materials are released into the extracellular areas. These materials include potassium, phosphorus, and uric acid. The kidneys usually are able to compensate for the release of these agents, but with the rapid degradation of cells, the kidneys can become overwhelmed and unable to handle removing these electrolytes. When this happens, hyperkalemia with ensuing hypocalcemia, hyperuricemia, and hyperphosphatemia occurs.
3. **A.** The symptoms of hypercalcemia can develop slowly and may be unrelated to the actual calcium level. No absolute calcium level exists at which all patients become symptomatic; rather, the rate of rise appears more significant. Patients tolerate fairly high calcium levels if the increase is gradual (Behl et al., 2010). Older patients often experience more symptoms than younger patients.
4. **D.** Back pain for a prolonged period of time is the first symptom in 90%–98% of patients with metastatic spinal cord compression (Bowers, 2015). A hallmark sign is that the pain intensifies when raising legs in a supine position and often is rated at a high number. The next most common symptom is limb weakness to the point where the patient is unable to ambulate unassisted.
5. **D.** Symptoms of cardiac tamponade are dependent on the fluid volume and rate of accumulation. Most frequently, patients complain of exertional dyspnea, tachycardia, and chest discomfort as excess pressure from the accumulating fluids results in increased intrapericardial pressure.
6. **B.** Almost 75% of all cancer-related superior vena cava syndrome diagnoses are attributed to bronchogenic cancer, most frequently small cell lung cancer (Rice et al., 2006).

Chapter 26

1. **D.** Nociceptive (which may be characterized as visceral or somatic) and neuropathic pain are the main classifications of pain.
2. **A.** Renal function should be monitored because nonsteroidal anti-inflammatory drugs may rarely cause renal toxicities.
3. **C.** Meperidine is not recommended for the management of cancer pain because of its conversion to normeperidine, which can cause neurotoxicity.
4. **A.** Sedation is a common side effect of opioids that typically is transient.
5. **B.** Hypnosis is a type of integrative approach. All of the other options are examples of interventional strategies.

Chapter 27

1. **D.** A history of cumulative doses of specific chemotherapy agents (i.e., cisplatin, vincristine, and taxanes) is associated with peripheral neuropathy.
2. **A.** Patients at risk for developing peripheral neuropathy include patients older than 60 years of age.
3. **C.** Sensory peripheral neuropathies are commonly distinctive and distally progressive and usually manifest as sensory-type symmetrically distributed symptoms, such as tingling, numbness, burning, or increased sensitivity in a stocking-glove distribution.
4. **A.** Oncology nurses need to carefully assess and monitor for chemotherapy-induced peripheral neuropathy, educate patients, and notify physicians if peripheral neuropathy exists prior to initiation of a neurotoxic drug.
5. **A.** Only duloxetine and gabapentin have research evidence demonstrating effective-

ness in peripheral neuropathy. Pregabalin is effective in peripheral neuropathy associated with diabetes mellitus type 2.

Chapter 28

1. **C.** People older than 60 years of age are more likely to have chemotherapy-induced pulmonary toxicity.
2. **B.** Development of radiation-induced pulmonary toxicity can occur 6–12 weeks after ending treatment but can range from 1–6 months. Answer A is associated with cytokine release after targeted therapy. High-grade fever is always a symptom of an infection, and an asymptomatic dry cough is associated with targeted therapy treatment.
3. A = 1, 2, & 3; B = 1 only; C = 1 only.

Chapter 29

1. **C.** Young-old adults have most often entered retirement and a transitional status. They may review the past successes and failures of their life as they adjust to new roles, but for many, this is a time of welcome relief from the day-to-day stress of the work environment and satisfaction with their accomplishments. A cancer illness during the young-old developmental phase may have less psychological impact related to feelings of accomplishment for the completion of life tasks and less disruption of schedules.
2. **A.** Younger survivors were at greater risk for mood disturbance and reported higher levels of anxiety and depression than an age-matched comparison group related to the disruption in lifestyle and inability to complete age-related tasks. They often miss experiences common in this age group, such as dating, leaving home, and establishing independence (D'Agostino et al., 2011). Identity development is a key component of health development in the young adult. To minimize the disruption caused by cancer, it is important for young adults to stay connected with their peers.
3. **A and D.** Research has shown that some young survivors found that the cancer experience strengthened relationships, making the family closer as a result. Concerns about infertility and childbearing were a concern and seldom discussed prior to treatment. Fear of being left alone is expressed in caregivers of the young-old group. Physical decline is a concern for the old-old group.
4. **D.** As people age, they begin to experience declines in physical abilities and in managing complex medical regimens. Any impairment in physical, sensory, and cognitive function can have a serious effect on managing daily routines. Furthermore, age-related frailty, functional impairment, and social losses can stress older adults and make their tolerance to cancer therapy most difficult.
5. **C.** Middle adulthood is characterized by achievement of personal goals. A cancer illness can force early retirement and create a financial strain. Further loss of dignity related to the number of symptoms they are experiencing can bring about feelings of helplessness and depression. Ability to form close relationships, achieve career goals, and maintain independence are developmental goals of young adulthood. During the old-old developmental phase, cancer may have fewer psychosocial effects, as individuals are less concerned about recurrence and expect some health problems as a result of aging. Changes in socialization as a result of treatment can lead to loneliness in young-old individuals with cancer. Furthermore, treatment may make it difficult to fulfill dreams related to retirement.

Chapter 30

1. **D.** POLST is a legal order, protected by state statute, and must be honored in all care settings, including the home, and by emergency medical responders. The POLST form specifies the treatments to be withheld, such as resuscitation, as well as the treatments to

be provided, for example, tube feedings. It ensures the patient's end-of-life care wishes are honored.

2. **B.** Nurses must be sensitive to cultural and family norms. In situations like this, nurses should never lie to a patient; however, a team meeting with the family to discuss how best to disclose difficult information is helpful. The patient has a right to know the diagnosis, and the team and family can come up with the best way to discuss this with the patient.
3. **A.** Therapeutic misconception is when the patient believes that the protocol will be altered to benefit the patient's specific needs. The patient also may have an unrealistic belief that despite being told that it is unlikely the research will benefit the patient, and may even be harmful, as in phase I trials, the patient has hope that the research will be beneficial.
4. **C.** Rubin (1998) viewed futility as a negotiated reality where the patient, family, and the healthcare team engage in conversation to determine each other's goals and how to reach them. Treatment options and rationale are reviewed and a plan of care is developed.
5. **D.** When a patient's pain and suffering cannot be relieved by scrupulous pain and symptom management, it is permissible to provide nonopioid sedation, even to the point of unconsciousness, until the patient dies from disease progression. However, the use of palliative sedation for existential suffering, such as death anxiety or depression, is controversial and not supported by physician and nurse organizations for hospice and palliative care.

Chapter 31

1. **D.** Saunders proposed that "pain should be understood as having physical, psychological, social, emotional, and spiritual components" (Mehta & Chan, p. 27).
2. **B.** The simultaneous care model is recommended in current practice, that is, provision of PC concurrently with life-sustaining treatment. PC should be initiated at the time of a serious, life-limiting diagnosis.
3. **B.** The family meeting serves to establish the preferences and wishes of individuals in relation to their diagnosis and prognosis and to clarify goals in light of information provided. Ideally, the patient will be a full participant in these discussions. If the individual is unable to participate, then a surrogate decision maker acts in the patient's stead. In advanced illness, it may be problematic for the surrogate to determine preferences if prior conversations did not occur when the patient was lucid. This highlights the need to begin conversations at the time of diagnosis, or at least early after diagnosis. A series of meetings may better serve the patient and family, but depending on the state of illness and the setting, this may not be feasible.
4. **C.** The 3 C's of palliative care are communication, collaboration, and continuity.
5. **C.** Longer survival was accomplished even when compared to those who received aggressive treatment up to the end of life (Temel et al., 2010).

Chapter 32

1. **B.** The patient's fears are not based on fact or reasoned judgment. The patient has an excellent chance to fully recover and lead a normal life without sequelae. The extreme response to limited risk implies that an underlying psychological problem may exist that has been exacerbated by the diagnosis, and the patient is not able to comprehend or believe the likelihood of a favorable outcome.
2. **A.** According to the research conducted by Wedding et al. (2007), female patients, patients with solid tumors, and those with functional limitations had significantly higher scores for somatic and affective depressive symptoms on the Beck Depression Inventory. These data alert oncology nurses to the possible risk factors for depression, namely

female sex, tumor type, and functional status. Young age was not a factor.

3. **D.** Children with cancer experience all of these factors as distressing. Most aspects of cancer care are unknown to children, and these new experiences are frightening and can be painful. Even a young child will fear death. These stressors will be especially pronounced if the child has had negative, frightening exposures in the past.
4. **D.** One of the most significant acts of supportive care for patients and families is to help them clarify "meaning" in the context of cancer. Dignity therapy redirects the patient's thoughts to the individual's self-worth, self-respect, and desired esteem. Cognitive behavioral therapy targets problem areas and creates effective problem-solving techniques. Finding benefit and meaning helps patients to offset the negative effects. The therapist and client work collaboratively on problem identification, treatment planning, and outcome evaluation.
5. **B.** Among family caregivers, the highest burden was reported among those with more limited social networks, those with more restriction in their daily activities, and those who were younger.

Chapter 33

1. **C.** What he is describing is most likely genital shrinkage as a result of radiation to the pelvis. Reassurance that this is a common side effect and that regular genital massage may be helpful would be appropriate. It also is more likely that the penis appears to have shrunk when it is flaccid and that if he is able to have erections, his penis may appear more normal in size. Some men find that the regular use of a penile vacuum pump also helps, although men do not use this consistently over time.
2. **B.** Systemic hormone therapy is not approved for women with hormone-dependent breast cancer. A more appropriate treatment regimen would be to start with vaginal/vulvar moisturizers for daily comfort and lubricants for penetration during sexual activity. A consultation to a pelvic floor physiotherapist would also be appropriate. Additionally, sexuality counseling/therapy might be useful to educate this woman about alternatives to penetrative intercourse. Finally, local estrogen therapy might be useful if the other nonpharmaceutical interventions do not help.
3. **D.** All attempts should be made to preserve fertility where possible. At the very least, a referral to a fertility specialist should be made to enable the patient to hear about possible strategies for fertility preservation before or after treatment to reduce regret later.
4. **B.** It is incumbent on nurses to know and understand the sexual side effects of cancer treatment for the specific populations they care for and to be able to normalize the situation for patients, which often will alleviate a great deal of their anxiety. In addition, nurses need to know where they can refer patients for further help and do this in a timely manner; this begins with patient assessment.
5. **C.** The return of menses after treatment may be an indication that her ovaries are functioning. However, she needs to see a fertility specialist to assess whether she is indeed pregnant or amenorrheic and infertile.

Chapter 34

1. **B.** Survivors can lower their risk of osteoporosis by avoiding tobacco products, eating foods rich in calcium and vitamin D, and engaging in regular physical activity. Although some vegetables contain minerals or vitamins B and K, calcium and vitamin D are not common.
2. **A.** Reasonable accommodations, such as telecommuting, reassignment, job sharing, and modified hours, are all permitted through the Americans With Disabilities Act, but transportation is not among these.
3. **B.** In 1986, the National Coalition for Cancer Survivorship defined cancer survivors as individuals with cancer from the time of diagnosis and for the balance of life.

4. **E.** The Institute of Medicine defined survivorship care as the phase of care following completion of primary treatment, and recommended that it address four essential components: prevention of recurrent and new cancers and other late effects; surveillance for cancer spread, recurrence, and secondary cancers and assessment of medical and psychosocial late effects; intervention for consequences of cancer and its treatment; and coordination between primary and specialty care.
5. **E.** Survivorship care is a group effort and is the responsibility of the primary oncologist, the primary care provider, the oncology nurse, and the patient.

Index

The letter f *after a page number indicates that relevant content appears in a figure; the letter* t, *in a table.*

B

C

D

E

H

I

J

K

L

M

P

T

U

V

W

X

Y

Z